Rapid Review in Cardiology

Rapid Review in Cardiology

(For DM/DNB Cardiology, FNB Interventional Cardiology, Pediatric Cardiology, and MD/DNB Medicine Students)

Editors

Parin Chandrakant Sangoi
MBBS MD (General Medicine) DNB (Cardiology) FNB-PD (Interventional Cardiology)
Consultant Cardiologist
Wockhardt Hospitals
Mumbai, Maharashtra, India
International Associate
Society for Cardiovascular Angiography and Interventions (SCAI), USA

Ronak Vijaykumar Ruparelia
MBBS DNB Medicine DNB Cardiology
Interventional Cardiologist
Bankers Group of Hospitals
Vadodara, Gujarat, India

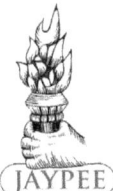

JAYPEE BROTHERS MEDICAL PUBLISHERS
The Health Sciences Publisher
New Delhi | London

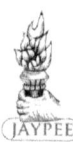

Jaypee Brothers Medical Publishers (P) Ltd

Headquarters
Jaypee Brothers Medical Publishers (P) Ltd
EMCA House, 23/23-B
Ansari Road, Daryaganj
New Delhi 110 002, India
Landline: +91-11-23272143, +91-11-23272703
+91-11-23282021, +91-11-23245672
Email: jaypee@jaypeebrothers.com

Corporate Office
Jaypee Brothers Medical Publishers (P) Ltd
4838/24, Ansari Road, Daryaganj
New Delhi 110 002, India
Phone: +91-11-43574357
Fax: +91-11-43574314
Email: jaypee@jaypeebrothers.com

Overseas Office
JP Medical Ltd
83 Victoria Street, London
SW1H 0HW (UK)
Phone: +44 20 3170 8910
Email: info@jpmedpub.com

EU GPSR Authorised Representative
Logos Europe, 9 rue Nicolas Poussin
17000, La Rochelle, France
Phone: +33 (0) 6 67 93 73 78
E-mail: Contact@logoseurope.eu

Website: www.jaypeebrothers.com
Website: www.jaypeedigital.com

© 2024, Jaypee Brothers Medical Publishers

The views and opinions expressed in this book are solely those of the original contributor(s)/author(s) and do not necessarily represent those of editor(s) or publisher of the book.

All rights reserved. No part of this publication may be reproduced, stored or transmitted in any form or by any means, electronic, mechanical, photocopying, recording or otherwise, without the prior permission in writing of the publishers.

All brand names and product names used in this book are trade names, service marks, trademarks or registered trademarks of their respective owners. The publisher is not associated with any product or vendor mentioned in this book.

Medical knowledge and practice change constantly. This book is designed to provide accurate, authoritative information about the subject matter in question. However, readers are advised to check the most current information available on procedures included and check information from the manufacturer of each product to be administered, to verify the recommended dose, formula, method and duration of administration, adverse effects and contraindications. It is the responsibility of the practitioner to take all appropriate safety precautions. Neither the publisher nor the author(s)/editor(s) assume any liability for any injury and/or damage to persons or property arising from or related to use of material in this book.

This book is sold on the understanding that the publisher is not engaged in providing professional medical services. If such advice or services are required, the services of a competent medical professional should be sought.

Every effort has been made where necessary to contact holders of copyright to obtain permission to reproduce copyright material. If any have been inadvertently overlooked, the publisher will be pleased to make the necessary arrangements at the first opportunity.

Inquiries for bulk sales may be soliticed at: jaypee@jaypeebrothers.com

Rapid Review in Cardiology

First Edition: **2024**

ISBN: 978-93-5696-155-5

Dedicated to
Our parents, teachers, and students.

Preface

It gives us immense pleasure to bring to you the first edition of *Rapid Review in Cardiology*. Cardiology is a vast branch, with lots of matter to be read from various sources. During our time while preparing for our DNB Cardiology and FNB Interventional Cardiology, we felt the dearth of having notes compiled from standard textbooks. During exam preparation and one day prior to the exams, it became very difficult to go back to all the various sources from where we had read previously and thus arose the need to compile and consolidate all the important matters into one place. That is when we started preparing these notes from various available literature. It has been compiled in such a manner that all the important points from a particular chapter can be rifled through quickly. It will be particularly useful for students appearing for DM/DNB Cardiology and FNB Interventional Cardiology. It will also be useful for those appearing for their DM/DNB and FNB entrance examinations. It might also prove useful for MD/DNB students with particular interest in cardiology where they can go through certain important topics.

It has been compiled in such a manner that it can be used both for theory and practical examinations and can prove to be your best companion for your previous day revisions.

We hope that this book proves as useful for you as it proved for us, and you enjoy reading it as much as we enjoyed compiling it.

Parin Chandrakant Sangoi
Ronak Vijaykumar Ruparelia

Acknowledgments

We are thankful to Shri Jitendar P Vij (Group Chairman), Mr Ankit Vij (Managing Director), Mr MS Mani (Group President), Ms Chetna Malhotra (Senior Director—Professional Publishing, Marketing and Business Development), Ms Pooja Bhandari (Director-Production), and Ms Manpreet Kaur (Development Editor) of M/s Jaypee Brothers Medical Publishers (P) Ltd, New Delhi, India, for being a source of help, encouragement, guidance, and coordination.

Contents

SECTION 1   DISEASE OF THE AORTA   1–13
1.1 Aortic Aneurysm..1
1.2 Aortic Dissection..7

SECTION 2   ARRHYTHMIAS   14–95
2.1 Cardiac Arrest and Sudden Cardiac Death...14
2.2 Syncope and Hypotension 23
2.3 Torsades..28
2.4 Various Ventricular Tachycardias 29
2.5 Ventricular Premature Contraction and Ventricular Tachycardia...31
2.6 Ventricular Tachycardia Storm 33
2.7 AVNRT, AVRT, Mahaim, PJRT 34
2.8 Genesis of Cardiac Arrhythmias (Anatomy of Card. System)..38
2.9 Bradyarrhythmia..40
2.10 Brugada Syndrome 42
2.11 Catecholaminergic Polymorphic Ventricular Tachycardia...44
2.12 Diagnosis of Cardiac Arrhythmias...45
2.13 Therapy for Cardiac Arrhythmias...50
2.14 Long QT and Short QT Syndromes 59
2.15 Premature Atrial Contractions and Atrial Flutter 62
2.16 Epicardial Ventricular Tachycardia 64
2.17 Therapy of Cardiac Arrhythmia 65
2.18 Mechanism of Arrhythmogenesis 71
2.19 Pacemaker and ICD 76
2.20 Atrial Fibrillation 84
2.21 Action Potential and Cardinal Ion Channels..89

SECTION 3   ATHEROSCLEROSIS   96–115
3.1 Complication of Atherosclerosis..96
3.2 Special Cases of Atherosclerosis 98
3.3 Novel Risk Markers..99
3.4 Vascular Biology and Atherosclerosis 103
3.5 Risk Markers and Primary Prevention of Cardiovascular Diseases 108

SECTION 4   CARDIOMYOPATHY   116–146
4.1 Arrhythmogenic Cardiomyopathy...116
4.2 Dilated Cardiomyopathy 119
4.3 Hypertrophic Cardiomyopathy..122
4.4 Left Ventricular Noncompaction 128
4.5 Myocarditis...129
4.6 Other Cardiomyopathies..134
4.7 Peripartum Cardiomyopathy 137
4.8 Restrictive Cardiomyopathy, Amyloidosis, and Sarcoidosis 139
4.9 Tachycardia-induced Cardiomyopathy 144
4.10 Takotsubo Cardiomyopathy: Stress Cardiomyopathy 145

SECTION 5   CONGENITAL HEART DISEASES   147–243

- 5.1 Truncus Arteriosus 147
- 5.2 Aortic Arch Anomalies and Vascular Ring 150
- 5.3 Anomalous Systemic Venous Connection 153
- 5.4 Complete AVSD 154
- 5.5 Coarctation of Aorta 159
- 5.6 Aortic Pulmonary Window 164
- 5.7 Conotruncal Anomalies 166
- 5.8 Congenital Coro Art Anomalies 168
- 5.9 Cong. Corrected TGA 173
- 5.10 Congenital AS 176
- 5.11 DORV 181
- 5.12 Duct Dependent Circulation 185
- 5.13 Ebstein's Anomaly 187
- 5.14 Eisenmenger Syndrome 191
- 5.15 Fontan Surgery 194
- 5.16 Hypoplastic Left Heart Syndrome 199
- 5.17 Fetal ECHO 202
- 5.18 Operability Assessment in LT ≥ RT shunt 204
- 5.19 Persistent LSVC 205
- 5.20 Interrupted Ao Arch 207
- 5.21 PA with Intact Vent Septum 209
- 5.22 Pulm Atresia with VSD 213
- 5.23 Congenital Pulm AV Fistula 217
- 5.24 Aneurysm of Sinus of Valsalva 219
- 5.25 Single Ventricle 222
- 5.26 Total Anomalous PV Connection 225
- 5.27 Tetralogy of Fallot 229
- 5.28 Cyanotic Congenital Heart Disease 234
- 5.29 TGA 239
- 5.30 Segmental Approach 242

SECTION 6   ENDOCRINE SYSTEM   244–252

- 6.1 Adrenal and CV disease 244
- 6.2 Amiodarone and Thyroid function 246
- 6.3 Endocrine Disorder and CV Disease 247
- 6.4 Parathyroid Disease 249
- 6.5 Pheochromocytoma 252

SECTION 7   HEART FAILURE   253–319

- 7.1 Left Vent Remodeling 253
- 7.2 Mechanical Circulation Support 258
- 7.3 Potential New Therapies for HF 264
- 7.4 Pathogenesis of Heart Failure 266
- 7.5 Sarcolemma Control of Calcium and Sodium 270
- 7.6 Heart Failure 272
- 7.7 Surgical Management of HF 274
- 7.8 Cardiopulmonary Exercise Test 276
- 7.9 Care of Patient with End Stage Heart Diseases 277
- 7.10 Contractile Cell and Protein 279
- 7.11 Device for Monitoring and Managing HF 282
- 7.12 Myocardial O_2 Uptake 284
- 7.13 Frank Starling Relationship 285

7.14	Cardiovascular Regeneration and Gene Therapy	287
7.15	HFrEF Management	290
7.16	HFpEF	298
7.17	Role of Ca^{++} in Cardiac Cont. Relax Cycle	304
7.18	Adrenergic Signaling System	306
7.19	Acute Heart Failure	308
7.20	Cardiac Transplant	314
7.21	Devices for Monitoring HF	318
7.22	Biomarkers and Natriuretic Peptides	319

SECTION 8 HEMOSTATIC SYSTEM   320–336

8.1	Antiplatelet Drugs	320
8.2	Hemostasis/Thrombosis/Fibrinolysis	328
8.3	Hypercoagulable States	332
8.4	NOACs	334

SECTION 9 HYPERTENSION   337–361

9.1	Practical Clinical Approach to Evaluation and Management of Ambulatory Hypertensive Patients	337
9.2	BP in Acute CVA	339
9.3	Approach to Patient with Chest Pain	340
9.4	Central Ao Pr	341
9.5	Device Based Treatment for HTN	342
9.6	Diagnosis and Initial Evaluation	343
9.7	HTN in Pregnancy	345
9.8	Systemic HTN: Management	346
9.9	Hypertension: Mechanism and Diagnosis	350
9.10	Management of HTN and Sprint Trial	354
9.11	Pathogenesis of Hypertensive Heart Disease	355
9.12	HTN and Erectile Dysfunction	356
9.13	Secondary HTN	359

SECTION 10 INFECTIVE ENDOCARDITIS   362–374

10.1	Cardiovascular Implantable Device INF	362
10.2	Infective Endocarditis Prophylaxis	364
10.3	Infective Endocarditis	365

SECTION 11 INTERVENTIONS   375–438

11.1	Carotid Artery Stenting	375
11.2	Coronary Perforation	378
11.3	CTO Intervention	379
11.4	Drug-Eluting Balloons	380
11.5	Dedicated Bifurcation Stent	381
11.6	Deferred Stenting	383
11.7	Distal Protection Devices	384
11.8	Endomyocardial Biopsy	385
11.9	FFR	386
11.10	Fick's Principle	391
11.11	Hybrid Revascularization	395
11.12	IABP	396
11.13	In-Stent Restenosis	398
11.14	Intravascular Ultrasound	401
11.15	LA Appendage and Closure	404
11.16	Leadless Pacemaker	406

11.17 MitraClip and Percutaneous Mitral Valve 408
11.18 Optical Coherence Tomography 412
11.19 Other Modalities of Intravascular 415
11.20 Radiation Hazards 416
11.21 Renal Stenting and Denervation 418
11.22 Rotational Atherectomy 421
11.23 Stent Thrombosis 423
11.24 Subcutaneous Implantable Cardioverter-Defibrillator 424
11.25 Transcatheter Aortic Valve implantation 426
11.26 TIMI-MBG-NO flow 431
11.27 Valve Area Calculation 433
11.28 Measurement of Vascular Resistance 436
11.29 Wearable Implantable Cardioverter-Defibrillator 437

SECTION 12 ISCHEMIC HEART DISEASES 439–496

12.1 STEMI: Pathology, Pathophysiology, and Clinical Features 439
12.2 Approach to Patients with Chest Pain 441
12.3 Cardiogenic Shock 442
12.4 Coronary Blood Flow and Management Ischemia 444
12.5 Coronary Collateral Circulation 447
12.6 Coronary Flow Reserve 448
12.7 Heart Muscle and Causes of Myocardial Injury 451
12.8 LVF in STEMI 453
12.9 Determinants of Coronary Vascular Resistance 455
12.10 Metabolic Management in CAD 456
12.11 Metabolic and Functional Consequences of Ischemia 458
12.12 Physiological Assessment of Coro Art Stenosis 460
12.13 NSTE-ACS 461
12.14 Causes of MI without Coronary Atherosclerosis 468
12.15 Coronary Vasospasm 469
12.16 Pathophysiology of STEMI 470
12.17 Prinzmetal Angina 473
12.18 Reperfusion Injury 474
12.19 STEMI: Management 475
12.20 Risk Stratification Post-STEMI 482
12.21 Stable Ischemic Heart Disease 483
12.22 Regulation of Coronary Microcirculation 493
12.23 Stunned Myocardium 495

SECTION 13 LIPID DISORDERS 497–518

13.1 Pharmacological Management 497
13.2 Nutrition and CV Metabolic Disease 501
13.3 Statin Intolerance 502
13.4 Secondary Causes of Hyperlipidemia 504
13.5 2013 ACC/AHA Guidelines (Management and Lipids) 505
13.6 Lipoprotein Disorders 506
13.7 Non-HDL Cholesterol 510
13.8 LA(A) and SGLT2 511
13.9 Emerging Therapies for Dyslipidemia Treatment 513
13.10 Lipoprotein Disorders and CV Disease 515
13.11 HOPE 3 Trial: Implication in India 518

SECTION 14 — MISCELLANEOUS — 519–553

- 14.1 CV Manifestation of Autonomic Disorders 519
- 14.2 Cocaine and Heart 525
- 14.3 Cardiorenal syndrome 527
- 14.4 Renal disease and CV Illness: Contrast Induced Nephropathy 530
- 14.5 Rheumatic Factor 533
- 14.6 Cardiovascular Abnormalities in HIV 539
- 14.7 Noncardiac Surgery in Cardiac Patients 541
- 14.8 Vascular Heart Disease 544
- 14.9 Ethanol and Heart 545
- 14.10 Traumatic Heart Disease 547
- 14.11 Rheumatic Disease and CV System 548
- 14.12 Vitamin D and Heart Disease 550
- 14.13 Ventriculoarterial Impedance (ZVA) 551
- 14.14 Exercise Cardiology 552

SECTION 15 — PERICARDIAL DISEASES — 554–570

- 15.1 Acute Pericarditis 554
- 15.2 Constrictive Pericarditis 557
- 15.3 Constrictive versus Restrictive 560
- 15.4 Pericardial Effusion and Tamponade 561
- 15.5 Pericardial Diseases 565
- 15.6 Relapsing and Recurrent Pericarditis 567
- 15.7 Specific Causes of Pericardial Disease 568

SECTION 16 — PERIPHERAL ARTERY DISEASE — 571–578

- 16.1 Acute Limb Ischemia 571
- 16.2 Peripheral Art Disease 573
- 16.3 Thromboangiitis Obliterans 578

SECTION 17 — PULMONARY DISEASES — 579–595

- 17.1 Sleep Apnea and Heart Disease 579
- 17.2 Pulmonary Embolism and Deep Vein Thrombosis 583
- 17.3 Pulmonary Hypertension 589

SECTION 18 — PREGNANCY AND HEART — 596–600

- 18.1 Pregnancy and Heart Disease 596

SECTION 19 — CLINICAL EXAMINATION — 601–608

- 19.1 Dynamic Auscultation 601
- 19.2 Hangout Interval 604
- 19.3 Second Heart Sound 605
- 19.4 History Taking and Physical Examination 608

SECTION 20 — ECG AND STRESS TEST — 609–615

- 20.1 Electrocardiography 609
- 20.2 Exercise testing 611

SECTION 21 — ECHO — 616–628

- 21.1 Intracardiac Flow Vortex Imaging 616
- 21.2 Speckle Tracking 618

21.3	3D-ECHO	621
21.4	Dobutamine Stress ECHO	623
21.5	TEE	625
21.6	ICE	626
21.7	Tissue Doppler Imaging	627

SECTION 22 NUCLEAR IMAGING 629–642

22.1	Radionucleotide Ventriculography	629
22.2	Viability, Hibernation and Stunning	630
22.3	Nuclear Cardiology	634
22.4	Use of Nuclear Imaging	637

SECTION 23 CARDIAC CT MRI AND PLAQUE RUPTURE 643–652

23.1	Plaque Rupture and Vulnerable Plaque	643
23.2	Cardiac Computed Tomography	645
23.3	Cardiovascular MRI	648

SECTION 24 TRIALS 653–687

24.1	Amulet Study	653
24.2	Best (2015)	654
24.3	Cantos Trial	655
24.4	AIDA	656
24.5	Castle AF	657
24.6	CAPTAF	658
24.7	Camera-MRI Trial	659
24.8	Viva Trial	660
24.9	Compass Trial	661
24.10	Clarify Study	662
24.11	Culprit Shock—2017	663
24.12	Champion Phoenix—2013	664
24.13	Courage Trial	665
24.14	Cross Boss First Trial	666
24.15	Decision-CTO	667
24.16	Favor 2 Studies	668
24.17	Fame 1, 2 and 3 Trial	669
24.18	Forma Trial	672
24.19	Fourier	673
24.20	HOPE 3 Trial: Implication in India	674
24.21	Ilumien 3 Trial: Optimize PCI	675
24.22	Impact AF	677
24.23	Fourier Trial	678
24.24	Symplicity HTN-3 Trial	679
24.25	Partner 1 and 2 SURTAVI	680
24.26	Sentinel Trial	683
24.27	Prevail Trial	684
24.28	Orbita Trial	685
24.29	Noble Trial	686
24.30	Vampire 3 Trial	687

SECTION 25 RCT versus REGISTRIES 688

Index 689

SECTION 1

Disease of the Aorta

1.1 AORTIC ANEURYSM

Q.1 Evaluation of abdominal aortic aneurysm (Abd Ao Ane or AAA), factors in the pathogenesis of Abd Ao aneurysm, endovasc therapy of Abd. Ao. Aneurysm (3+3+4)
(June 17)

Q.2 Discuss approach, evaluation and MLG dilatation of Asc. Ao (Dec 13)

Q.3 AAA: Pathogenesis, C/F, diagnostic imaging and mn. (Dec 12)

Q.4 Current concepts in mn of TAO Aney and dissection of AO (Dec 11)

Q.5 Nonsurgical treatment of Abd Ao Aney (Dec 10)

AORTIC ANEURYSM

Defn: Pathological segment of aortic dilatation that has propensity to expand and rupture.

What Dilatation to Call Aneurysmal?

Increase in diameter of at least 50% greater than expected for the same aortic segment in unaffected individuals of same age and sex.

In general cut off points:
- 4 cm for Thoracic Ao
- 3 cm for Abd. Ao

TYPES

Furiform	Saccular
More common	Less common
Symmetrical dilated with involvement of entire ao. circumference	Localized dilation involving only a portion of Aortic wall circ.
	Appears as focal outpouching

THORACIC AORTIC ANEURYSM

- Supracoronary Aneurysm—(MC)
- Annulo-Aortic Aneurysm—Marfanoid
- Tubular diffuse enlargement

Sites

- TAA much less common than AAA
- AO root on Asc Ao – 60%
- Descending Ao – 35%
- Aortic Arch – <10%

Etiology

- Genetic mutations
  - *Marfan syndrome:* Mutation of gene that encodes fibrillin 1
    → Deficiency of fibrillin 1 → excessive signaling by TGF B → Disruption of architecture of elastic fibers
  - EDS mutation of Type III procollagen
  - *Loeys-Dietz syndrome:* Mutation in gene that encodes for TGF B
    Receptor 1 and 2 → Disruption of the architecture of elastic fibers.
  - Familial thoracic Ao aneurysm syndrome
  - Turner syndrome
  - Osteogenesis imperfecta
  - Noonan syndrome
  - Alport syndrome
  - Bicuspid Ao valve
  - Cong heart disease (TOF, CDA, Supravalve As)
- Cystic medial necrosis
  - In Asc Ao and sinus of valsalva
  - Fusiform aneurysm

- Degen of collagen and elastic fibers.
- Medial cells replaced by multiple clefts of mucoid material.
- Seen in MFS, LDS, EDS, familial TAA, HTN, BAV.
- Degenerative/Atherosclerotic
  - In most Abdominal and Des. Thoracic Ao
  - Inflammation, proteolysis, biomechanical wall stress.
  - *Mediated by:* Degradation of elastin and collagen by B and T Lymphocyte, macrophages, inflammatory cytokines, MMP.
  - *Histopathological:* Destruction of elastin and collagen
    - Decreased vasc. smooth muscles
    - Ingrowth of new blood vessels
    - Inflammation
  - *Risk factor:* Aging, male sex, smoking, hypercholesterolemia, +ve F/H.
- *Infections:*
  - Syphilitic uncommon
    - 90% in Asc Ao or Arch
    - Peri and meso-aortitis causing damage to elastic fibers
    - Thickening and weakness of Ao wall
  - TB: Thoracic Ao
    - Direct extension of inf or bact seeding
    - Granulomatous destruction of medial layer
  - *Mycotic:* Rare variety
    Visually saccular type
    Due to Staphylococcal
    - Streptococcal
    - Salmonella
    - Aspergillus
  - HIV
  - Neisseria/candida
- Inflammatory/vasculitis
  - Takayasu's Arteritis/Giant cell arteritis 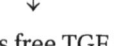 Ao arch and OTA
  - Spondyloarthropathies (AS, RA, psoriatic arthritis, relapsing polychondritis, reactive arthritis) → Asc Ao
  - *Other:* Behcet's syndrome, Cogan's synd, Idiopathic arthritis)
  - Kawasaki disease, SLE, Idiopathic Ao. sarcoidosis
- *Trauma:*
  - DTA just beyond ligamentum arteriosum is prone for trauma
  - After penetrating or non penetrating chest trauma.

Risk Factor
- Age
- Family history
- Smoking
- HTN
- COPD
- CAD

Pathogenesis
- Cystic medial degeneration
  (Degen and fragmentation of elastic fibers, loss of smooth muscles, increased deposition of collagen and replacement with interstitial "cysts" of mucoid appearance basophilic staining ECM)

  ↓

  Progressive weakness of Ao wall

  ↓

  Dilatation and aneurysm formation
  - CMD associated with many genetic disorder
  - Aging is associated with some degree of CMD which is accelerated by HTN.
- Marfan and Ao. Aneurysm
  - Mutated FBN, gene → Abnormal fibrillin-1
  - Fibrillin-1
    - Directs elastogenesis
    - Provide structural support to tissue
    - Interact with latent TGF B binding protein and control activation and signaling of TGF B

  Abnormal fibrillin-1 in MFS

  ↓

  Excess free TGF B

  ↓

  Stimulates both canonic and non-canonic pathway

  ↓

  Ao. dilatation via TGF B dependent ERK 1/2 cascade

  - Ao dilatation most pronounced in sinus of valsalva
  - Role of ARBs
    - Angiotensin is imp in TGF B signaling
    - ARB reduces SMAD and ERK activation both more effectively
    - Reduce Ao-growth.

C/F

- Most → Asymptomatic (incidentally discovered)
- Symptoms usually related to Ao mass effect, Prog AR, HF from Root dilatation, Syst Emboli from mural thrombus or atheroembolism mass effect
  - SVC or innominate vein → Congestion of head, neck and upper extremity
  - Trachea, Bronchus, Esophagus → Dyspnea, bronchospasm, cough, hemoptysis, dysphagia, chest pain
  - Direct mass effect
    - Persistent chest or back pain
    - sov = Sinus of valsalva
      - Cerebral ischemia ─┐
      - Arm ischemia
      - Spinal cord ischemia
      - Myocardial infarction ├─ Complications
      - Free rupture
      - Intestinal ischemia
      - Renal ischemia
      - Leg ischemia ──────┘

Complications

- Rupture and dissection
  - Sudden severe chest or back pain
  - Into pleural cavity (usually if) → Hypo t^n
  - Into the Esophagus → Hematemesis
  - Into bronchus/trachea → Hemoptysis
- Ac Ao, expansion, contained rupture and pseudoneurysm → severe chest/back pain
- Infected TAA → more common for fistulas.

Clinical Features

- *CXR:* Cordoned mediastinum, prominent to knob or displaced trachea
  Not useful for
  - Smaller aneurysm
  - Aneu. involving sov or Aoc root
  - Ao. tortuosity or unfolding in older adults mimics or masks TAA
- *TTE:* Excellent modality
  Can be used to visualize TAA involving sov and prox asc. Ao, Ao arch and prox desc. Ao
- *CECT and MRI:* Preferal over Aortography to define both Ao and branch vessel anatomy
  ECMO measures internal diameter, while CT and MRI measures external dia → 0.2-0.4 cm larger than internal diameter

Natural History

- Relatively indolent
- Growth rate = 0.1-0.2 cm/y
- Larger aneurysm grow faster
- Marked individual variability
- Desc. Ao aneurysm grow faster than Asc. Ao.
- MFS have faster growth rate
- BAV have faster growth rate

Rupture

<5 cm → 2% per year ─┐   <1/2 pt with
5-5 → 3% per year   │   rupture arrives
>6 → 7% per year   │   at hospital alive
MFS → 3.7% per year   │   Mortality
MFS(F) → 2-9% per year┘   @24 h >75%

Risk factor for rupture   *Aortic risk calculator*

Old age ─┐   Uses Ht, wt, Aortic size
Female sex │   Ao size index
COPD   │   → 2.75 cm/m^2 → 4% per year
HTN   │   → 2.75-4 cm/m^2 → 8%
Cigarette smoking │   → >4-25 → 20-25%
Rapid aneurysm growth
Pain
+ve family history ─┘

When to Operate

In general

- Asc Ao dia → 5.5 cm
- MFS, BAV, and familial TAA → 5 cm
- Adults with LDS → 4.2 cm
- Turner synd → 3.5 cm
- Descending Ao → 5.5 cm
- Thoracic abdominal → 6 cm

Surveillance

- Initial discovery of Aneurysm ──→ Repeat imaging at 6 mth to document stability
- Degen aneurysm
  3.5-4.5 cm → Annual imaging
  4.5-5.5 cm → Biannual imaging
- MFS, BAV, familial TAA
  3.5-4.5 cm → Annual
  4.5-5 → Biannual
- CDS
  <4 cm → At least annual
  >4 cm → Biannual

Management

- Medical management
  - Pharmacological:
    - Treating HTN (ARB preferred)
    - Chol lowring for pt with atherosclerotic TAA
    - BB for MFS
  - Nonpharmacological:
    - Smoking cessation
    - Awareness of condition and risk for dissection/rupture
    - Avoid strenuous physical activity especially weight lifting
    - Preg. Association with increased risk of dissection (especially MFS)
    - Ao imaging for first degree relatives
    (if first degree found to have TAA→screening of 2nd degree relatives)
- Surgical management
  - Ascending thoracic Ao aneurysm:
    1. Resection and grafting of Asc Ao with/without Concomitant AVR
       - Generally resected and replaced with prosthetic graft
         - Dacron tube with prosthetic aortic valve sewn into one end (composite aortic repair or modified Bentall procedure) is method of choice.
         - Valve and graft sewn directly into aortic annulus and coro arteries are reimplanted into Dacron graft
         - Risk of death /stroke - 1 to 5%
    2. Valve sparing root replacement
       - When AR is zi tp dilatation of sinotubular junction or aortic annulus.
       - David procedure – Reimplanting native valve within dacron Grafts
       - Yacoub procedure: Remodeling aortic root

       *Reimplantation preferable to remodeling
    3. Ross procedure
    4. Cryopreserved aortic allografts (cadaveric ao root and asc Ao.) less preferable due to its high rate of late ao. calcification.
  - Arch aneurysm
    - More difficult to treat
    - All branches need to be reimplanted
    1. *Proximal hemiarch resection:* Arch vessels are left intact with des. aorta as a root and remaining arch is replaced
    2. *Extended arch resection:* Removing entire arch tissue and using branched graft to replace the arch and great vessels (or) reimplanting an island of arch tissue that includes the origin of great vessels.
  - Arch aneurysm extending to descending Aorta
    1. *Frozen elephant trunk:* Covered endovascular stent graft attached to vascular graft.
       - Fixation of stent graft in descending Ao and vasc-graft reconstruct aortic arch
  - Descending thoracic aneurysm:
    - Resection and grafting with polyester graft
  - Thoraco-abdominal
    - *Crawford type I:* Repair extend from prox des. Ao above T6 vertebra to above renal artery.
    - *Crawford type II:* Starts from prox des. Ao above T6 vertebra to below renal artery.
    - *Crawford type III:* From distal des. Ao below T6 to below diaphragm
    - *Crawford type IV:* Extends from diaphragm and involve most of Abd. Aorta
- *Endovascular repair:*

Req-
- Suitable Aortic Anatomy
- 20-25 mm prox and distal landing zone
- Adequate area of Ao to accommodate endograft
- Adequate vascular access

Example:
- Gore TAG thoracic endoprosthesis
- Talent thoracic stent graft system
- Zenith Tx2 TAA thoracic endovascular graft

Compli:
- Mortality – 2%
- Stroke—2–4%
- Paraparesis—4.5–7%

In 50% of TEVAR, stent graft intentionally covers left subclavian - require grafting of LSCA to left carotid.

ABDOMINAL AORTIC ANEURYSM

- Most common form of aortic aneurysm
- Def. increase in size of des. Ao to >3 cm
- 3–9% of men older than 50 yrs
- >50% are in infrarenal aorta
- M:f = 5:1

Risk Factors

- Strong association with age and smoking (5 fold increase in risk in smokers)
- *Other risk factors:* Emphysema, HTN and hyper-lipidemia

Pathogenesis

- Chronic aortic wall inflammation (mediated by IL-1B, IL-6, and INF treatment)
- Increased local expression of MMP
- Degradation of structural connective tissue protein
  ↓
  Mechanical failure of medial elastin and adventitial collagen
  ↓
  Aneurysmal dilatation and rupture

C/F

- Mostly asymptomatic
- Abd palpation may reveal or pulsatile epigastric or periumbilical mass
- Symptoms due to:
  - Distal thromboembolism
  - Rapid expansion
  - Rupture
- Association with femoral
- Art Aneurysm in 85%
- Popliteal art aneurysm in 60%
- Aneurysmal pain is usually due to rupture (medical emergency)

Rupture:

- Into peritoneum
  - Acute stage, severe Abd. Pain, hypotension
- Into retroperitoneum
  - Contained periaortic hematoma
  - Severe abd. or back pain radiating to flank or groin
  - 30-50% die before hospitalization
  - 30-40% die after reaching hospital before start of treatment
  - Operative mortality—40-50%

Diagnosis

- *USG Abd.:*
  - High accuracy
  - Sens and spec 100%
  - Preferred over CT as screening test
  - Useful for follow up of AAA upto 4.5 cm.
- *CT Abd.:*
  - Extremely Accurate
  - CT Angio more accurate than USG
  - Esp. useful in demonstrating the extent of aneurysmal Disease.
  - 3D reconstruction is preferred
- *MRI:* Also has high accuracy

Screening

- Society for vasc surgical treatment – recommendations
- 1 time screening in all men >65 yrs or as early as 55 yrs in men and women with family history.
- Screening → 50% reductuion in rupture and 50% reduction in mortality

Natural History

- Gradual expansion over a period of years and eventual rupture
- Avg rate of expansion = 0.2-0.3 cm/yr
- Predictors of rupture
  - Size (most imp.)
  - Wall thickness
  - Peak wall stress
  - Intraluminal thrombus thickness
- Risk of rupture
  - 3-4 cm → 5%
  - 4-5.5 cm → 10-20%
  - 5.5-6 cm → 30-40%   } 5 yr risk of rupture
  - >7 cm → >80%

Surveillance

- Small AAA can be observed safely
- AAA repair recommended for asymptomatic pt with atleast 5-5.5 cm size
- Symptomatic aneurysm and rapid growth (>1 cm/yr) req repair
  - 2.5-3 cm → screen every 5 yrs
  - 3-3.5 cm → screen every 3 yrs
  - 3.5-4.5 cm → screen every year
  - 4.5-5.5 cm → screen every 6 months

Management

- Medical
  - Nonpharmacological
    - Smoking cessation
    - Small AAA - encourage to exercise regularly
  - Pharmacological
    - Statin
    - Appropraite measures of HTN, DM, dyslipidemia
  - Experimental
    - No benefit with BB
    - Doxycycline has suppressed AAA in animal model due to its action as MMP inhibition
    - ACEI/ARB being studied
- Surgical management
  - Depends on life expectancy and estimated risk of rupture (vs) estimated risk association with AAA

- Factors associated with operative morbidity and mortality
  - CAD
  - CKD
  - CDPD
  - DM

Tech: (OSR)
- Transperitoneal or retroperitoneal exposure
- Tube graft or bifurcation graft is directly sutured
- Aneurysm sac is sewn together to prevent
- Contact between prosthetic graft and GI tract
- Mortality 4–5%
- Annual follow up with CT @ 5 yr

- Endovascular Repair:
  - Req. adequate nonaneurysmal prox and distal site
  - Suprarenal or infrarenal fixation is possible
  - Risk of mortality is less
  - Low periop mortality 1–2%
  - Low complication 10–15%

DREAM AND EVAR -1 study
- EVAR was associated with greater number of late complications and reinterventions
- Initial reduction of mortality with EVAR was no longer available within 1–2 yrs
- *OVER:* EVAR demonstrated improved survival in pt younger than 70, but not in older pt.

Endoleaks: Persistent blood flow in aneurysmal sac outside endograft—seen in almost 25% of patients

Types:
  I. Attachment site
     Ia. Prox end of stent graft
     Ib. Distal end of stent graft
     Ic. Iliac occluder
  II. Branch leaks without attachment site leak
     IIa. Simple: One patent branch
     IIb. Complex: 2 or more patent branch
  III. Stent graft defect
     IIIa: Junctional leak or modular disconnect
     IIIb: Fabric holes
  IV. Stentgraft fabric porosity < body after placement

Endotertion: AAA enlargement associated with increase intra sac Pr. after EVAR but without an endoleak visualized on CTA.

Type II most common result from retrograde filling of aneurysm sac by lumbar or inf. mesenteric arteries.
Persistent type I/Type II endo leaks may req. OSR

Follow up CECT @ 1 mth, 6 mth and 1 yr after implantation.

1.2 AORTIC DISSECTION

INTRODUCTION
- Incidence ~2-3.5 /100,000 person years
  - M:F = 2:1
  - High mortality 1% per hour death rate in first several hours before surgical treatment.
  - Association Ao dissection more common in 50-60 yr
  - Dissociation Ao dissection more common in >60-70 yrs

HYPOTHESIS
- Primary tear in aortic intima with blood from ao. lumen penetrating into diseased media and leading to dissection
- Primary rupture of vasa vasorum leading to triage in aortic wall

With subsequent intimal disruption creating internal tear and ao dissection
↓
Arterial pressure and shear forces may lead to further tears in intimal flap and produce exit sites or additional entry sites
↓
Distension of false lumen with blood compresses true lumen and lead to malperfusion syndrome

CLASSIFICATION
Two main classification system
- Debakey classification:
  - *Type I:* Originate in asc. Ao and extends at least to ao arch and often to des ao.
  - *Type II:* Originate in the asc Ao and confined to this segment
  - *Type III:* Originate in des Ao, usually just distal to left subclavian and extend distally
    III a: above diaphragm
    III b: below diaphragm
- Stanford classification:
  Type A: Dissection involving the asc (with or without extension to des. Ao)
  Type B: Dissection not involving Asc. Ao
  - Most Asc Ao dissection begins just distal to Ao valve
  - Most des. Ao dissection begins just distal to LSCA
    65%   Asc Ao
    30%   Des. Ao
    <10%   Aortic Arch
    1%   Abd Ao
  - Acute <2 weeks
    Chronic >2 weeks
    Subacute between 2-6 weeks

CAUSES AND PATHOGENESIS
- Hypertension
- Genetically triggered thoracic Ao disease
  - Marfan
  - BAV
  - LDS
  - Familial thoracic aortic aneurysm
  - Vascular EDS
  - Aneurysm -osteoarthritis syndrome (sm AD 3)
  - TGF B2 mutations
- Congenital disease/syndrome
  - Coarctation of Ao
  - Turner synd
  - TOF
- Atherosclerosis
  - Penetrating atherosclerotic ulcer
- Trauma (blunt/iatrogenic)
  - Catheter/guidewire
  - IABP
  - Aortic/vascular surgical treatment
  - Motor vehicle accident
  - CABG
  - TEVAR
- Cocaine/methamphetamine use
- Inflammatory/infection disease
  - GCA/TA
  - Behcet disease
  - Aortitis
  - Syphilis
- Pregnancy (T. underlying aortopathy)
- Weightlifting (T. underlying aortopathy)

PATHOPHYSIOLOGY

Main — Disruption of normal architecture and integrity of aortic wall plus marked increase In ao wall shear stress

- HTN → Changes in wall structure: Intimal thickening calcification

  And adventitial fibrosis
  ↓
  Affect elastic property
  ↓
  Increased stiffness
  ↓
  Predispose to dissection

- Cystic medial degen (from TAA)
  - MFS account for 5% of all dissection especially in young adults
  - Young pt with Ao. dissection → MFS, EDS, VEDS, LDS
  - Familial TAA, BAV, Aneurysm osteoarthritis syndrome, TGFBZ mutation, TS, cocaine use, COA
- Marfan (fibrillin gene mutation) (From TAA)

CLINICAL MANIFESTATION
- Pain-MC
  - Severe, sudden onset, max intensity, occurring at inception → Accompanied by sense of doom
  - Sharp, severe, stabbing (More common) / tearing, ripping pain (Less common)
  - Chest burning, pressure or pleuritic pain
  - Migratory pain in approx. 17% → tends to follow path of dissection, through aorta
  - Pain in neck, jaw, throat, and head → involvement of Asc. Ao
  - Pain in back, abdomen or LL → involvement of Des. Ao
- Symptoms related to complication of dissection
  - CVS
    - Cardiac arrest
    - Syncope
    - AR
    - Coro ischemia
    - MI (IWMI-RCA)
    - Cardiac temponade
    - Pericarditis
  - Pulmonary
    - Pleural effusion (1+ sided)
    - Hemothorax
    - Hemoptysis
  - Renal
    - ARI
    - Renovase HTN
    - Renal ischemia/infarction
  - Neurologic
    - Stroke/TIA
    - Paraparesis/paraplegia
    - Encephalopathy
    - Coma
    - Spinal cord synd
    - Ischemic neuropathy
  - GI
    - Mesenteric ischemia/infarction pancreatitis
    - Hiage
  - Peripheral vasc-UL/LL ischemia
  - Systemic fever

(Complications)

- *Painless dissection:* In 6% and especially in pt with DM, prev Ao Aneurysm and prior cardiac surgical treatment

O/E
- Virtually unremarkable
- AR/HF/stroke/abnormal peri pulses
- Most pt with type B dissection are hypertensive
- Many with type A dissection are normotensive or hypotensive on initial evaluation
- Hypotension
  - AR
  - Temponade
  - HF

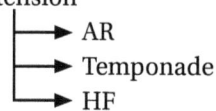

- Mch of AR in type A →
  - Incomplete coaptation of Ao. leaflets due to dilated aortic root and annulus
  - Aortic leaflet prolapse caused by dissection flap Propagating into aortic leaflet or commissure
  - Extensive or circumferential dehiscing intimal flap Prolapsing into LVOT during diastole and interfere with valve coaptation
  - Preexisting AR relayed to underlying root aneurysm or BAV
- *Comprehensive symptom:* Hoarseness, upper airway obstruction, dysphagia, svc syndrome pulsatile neck or abd mass, hematemesis, hemoptysis, ischemic pancreatitis, unexplained fever

LABORATORY FINDINGS
- *(CXR):*
  - May be normal
  - Nonspecific findings
  - May give clue to dissection
  - Abnormal aortic contour or widening of aortic silhouette or normal findings
  - Calcium sign separation of intimal calcification from outer soft tissue by >0.5–1 cm
  - Pl. effusion
- *ECG:*
  - Nonspecific
  - IWMI
- *Biomarker*:
  - D-dimer >1600 ng/mL with in first 5 h have high likelihood
  - D-dimer <500 in first 24 hrs → negative predictive valve of 5%

DIAGNOSTIC TECHNIQUES
- Imp to identify:
  - Type and location

- Entry site
- Extent
- Exit/reentry site
- Patency of false lumen
- Involvement of branch vessels
- Severity of AR
- Hemopericardium
- Coro. art. involvement
- Malperfusion
- Rupture
- CT:
  - MC used
  - 2 distinct lumina with intimal flap
  - 3D reconstruction
  - Sensitivity and specificity (95-100%)
  - Identify presence of thrombus, detecting Hemopericardium, periaortic hematoma, Ao. rupture, branch vessel involvement and blood supply from true and false lumina
  - Limitation:
    - Inability to evaluate coro. Art and Ao valve reliably
    - Motion artifact from cardiac movement
    - Streak artifact from device
    - Nephropathy (CIN)
- MRI:
  - Highly accurate
  - Similar to or higher than CT
  - Limitation:
    - CI with certain devices
    - Time consuming
    - Limited availability on emergency
- ECHO:
  - Presence of underlying intimal flap within the aortic lumen that separates true or false channel
  - Dissection flap has movt irrespective of surrounding str. and is contained within Aortic lumen.
  - Color flow Doppler → differential flow in lumina
    (TTE): Sens (77-88%) spec (93-96%)
    - Less sensitive for distal Ao dissection
    (TEE): Sens (98%) spe (95%)
    Limit
    - Linear reverb artifact common in dilated Asc Ao → can be mistaken as dissection
    - May not visualize distal Asc Ao and prox Ao arch.
  - Adv.
    - Can detect thoracic des. Ao dissection
    - Can detect AR with 100% sensitivity
    - May define mechanism of AR
    - Visualize prox coro art
- (Aortography)
  - Rarely used for initial diagnosis of aortic disease Sens (90%) spec (94%)
- *(CAG):* Routine CAG not recommended for type A dissection before surgical treatment.

EVALUATION ALGORITHM

Step 1: Identify pt at risk for AoD:
Consider AoD in pt presenting with
- Chest, back or abd pain
- Syncope
- Symptoms of perfusion deficit
(CNS, mesenteric, myocardial, limb ischemia)

Step 2: Bedside risk assessment:

High-risk condition	High-risk feature	High-risk exam feature
• Marfan syndrome • FIHIO aortic disease Know Ao. valve Disease (BAV) • Recent to Manipulation • Known TAA	• Chest/back/abd pain • Abrupt onset • Severe • Ripping/tearing	• Elo perfusion deficit (pulse, deficit, SBP diff, FND) • murmur of AI • hypotension/shock

Determine risk by calculating number of categories in which any title risk factor of +n+

Step 3: Risk Based diagnostic evaluation:

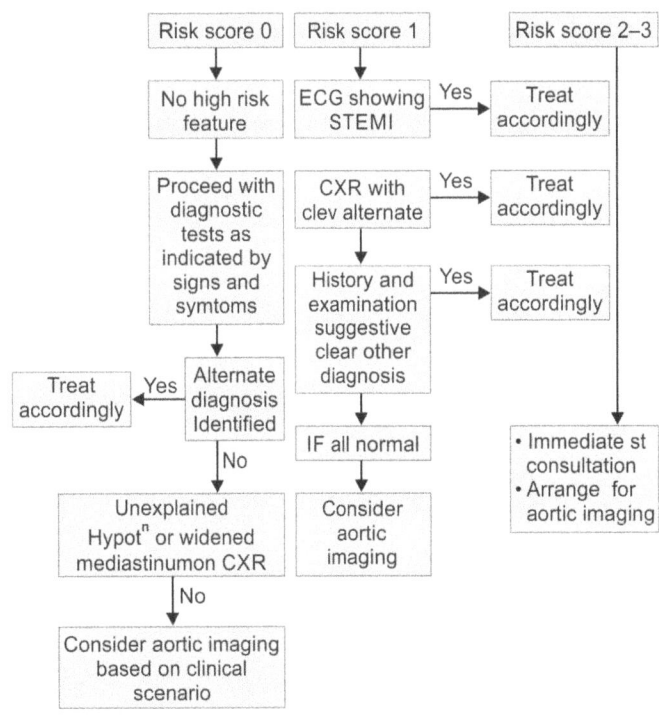

Step 4: AOD +n+ → Yes → Proceed to management pathway
→ No → if high suspicion → 2nd Ao imaging

Disease of the Aorta

Management Algorithm

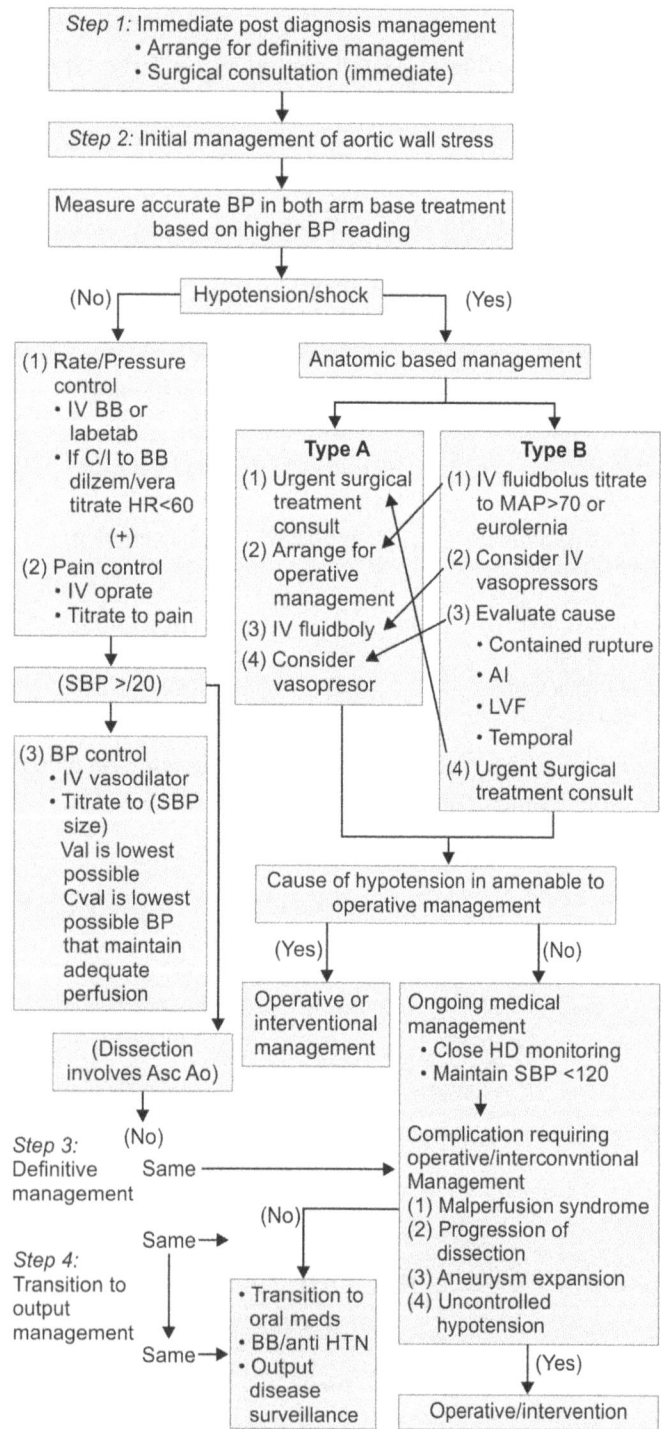

MANAGEMENT

Imp:
- Stabilize pt
- Control pain
- Lower BP
- Reduce rate of rise in dp/dt (force) of uv contraction-BB

Risk of Mortality with Type-A Dissection
- First 24 hr → 15-30%
- Between 24-48 hr → 10-20%
- Between 5-30 d → 1% per day

Beta-blocker
- Administer even if pt does not have HTN
- Target HR 60/MIN
- Esmolol bolus 500 mg/kg → infn 50-200 mg/kg/min
- Labetalol bolus 20 mg over 2 min → 40-80 mg every 15 mins → infusion 2-10 mg/min (max 300 mg)
- Propranolol/metroprolol
- BB CI → vera/diltiazem
- Na+ Nitropruside: Rapid reduction of BP
  - But may increase dp/dt
  - Must be used with BB
- IV ACE -Enalaprilat/
- IV NTG

*Refractory HTN in AOD
- Underlying severe HTN
- Uncontrolled pain
- Acute cocaine use
- Renal Art involvement → renovasc HTN

Tamponade
Pericardiocentesis:
- Recurrence bleeding and acute HD collapse
- In stable pt with type A dissection risk of pericardiocentesis outweigh its benefits

DEFINITIVE TREATMENT: DIAGNOSIS

IRAD study:
- 26% mortality in surgical treatment yr
- 58% in medical management group
  Indication for surgical treatment/endovasc/medical management
- Surgical treatment
  - Acute Type A dissection
  - Retrograde dissection into Asc Ao
- Endovascular/surgical
  - Ao type B dissection complicated by
  - Visceral ischemia
  - Limb ischemia
  - Rupture/impending rupture
  - Aneurysmal dilatation
  - Refractory pain
- Medical management
  - Uncomplicated Type B dissection
  - Uncomplicated isolated arch dissection

Mortality rate in Type B dissection = 1-6%

SURGICAL TREATMENT

Type A Dissection (Options)

- Supracommisural replacement of Asc Ao.
- Hemiarch replacement
- Total arch replacement
- Trifurcated graft
- Frozen elephant trunk
- Modified bentall (composite valve and root replace)

Basic: Excise the prox entry tear

Aims
- Prevent pericardial rupture
- Prevent or treat coro artial dissection
- Correct AR
- Restore flow into true lumen
- Correct malperfusion
- If possible obliterate false channel distally

Type B Dissection

Surgical treatment/endovascular device

Endovascular
- Aortic fenestration technique with or without additional aortic branch stenting
- Balloon fenestration of intimal flap allows blood flow from false to true lumen (when dead end false lumen dynamically compress true lumen)
- Percutaneous stenting of affected arterial branch in which dissection process has compromised flow.
  - STABLE trial: 2/3rd of pt treated with endovasc stenting have persistent of perfused false lumen, which can require reintervention and surgical conversion
  If malperfusion of SB persists branch vessel stenting or the technique of provisional extension to induce complete attachment (PETTICOAT) in which entry point is sealed with endograft and remaining thoracic aorta and potentially the abdominal aorta are stented open.

  IRAD: OSR mortality 33% ⎤
          TEVAR mortality 11% ⎦ Type B dissection

Uncomplicated Type B
- *INSTEAD:* TEVAR had no advantage over medical management regarding survival, Ao rupture or need for reintervention @ 2yr
- *But:* TEVAR had significantly higher rate for Ao Remodeling – False lumen thrombosis and true lumen expansion

LONG-TERM FOLLOW-UP

- Survival:
  - 90% @ 1 yr ⎤
  - 75% @ 5 yr ⎬ Poor surgical treatment
  - 54% @ 10 yr ⎦
- Long term management:
  - Anti-hypertensive therapy (BB/CCB)
  - Screening 1st degree relative for Ao. Asc.
  - Serial imaging of aorta over time
  - Lifestyle modification and education
  - Smoking cessation
- CT/MRI @ 1 to 3, 6, 12, 18 and 24 months
- Partially thrombosed false lumen have high mortality compared to completely patent or completely thrombosed lumen.

ACUTE AORTIC SYNDROMES

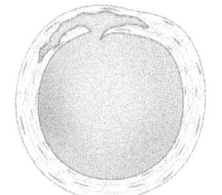
Ao dissection

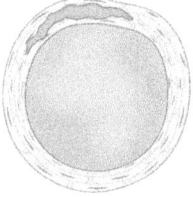
Intramural hematoma

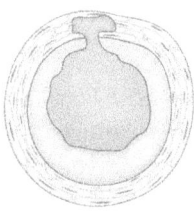
Pentrating athrosclerotic ulcer

AORTIC INTRAMURAL HEMATOMA (Q. DEC 14)

5-10% of pt with Ac Ao. syndrome

Definition

Hematoma develop within medial layer of aortic flap without any evidence of initial flap or false lumen. This non-communicating dissections are called IMH.

Causes

- One degree rupture of vasa vasorum and subsequent mural hemorrhage
- Nonvisualized small intimal defect

Incidence

- IRAD study—6%
- Asians—25%
- Compared to AOD, IMH more commonly involve elderly and more common in Asc Ao.

Classification

Type A ⎤ According to classification scheme used for
Type B ⎦ AoD

C/F

- Risk factor and clinical features similar to AoD
- Chest pain/back pain—predominating feature
- Freq. coexistence of pleural and pericardial effusion due to proximity of IMH to adventity
- Higher risk of Ao rupture
- Asc Ao IMH—can lead to AR, hemopericardium or rupture

Investigation

- *TEE:*
  - Focal crescentic or circumferential aortic wall thickness
  - Eccentric Ao lumen
  - Displaced intimal calcification
  - Areas of echolucency within aortic wall
  - No elo intimal flap
- *CT:* Area of high attenuation in wall of aorta
- *CECT:* Area of low attenuation
- *MRI:* Focal thickening
  - Phased contrast cine and gradient echocardio demonstrating no flow in aortic wall
- Aortogram-less sensitive

D/D

- Aneurys with mural thrombus
  - IMH has smooth lumen and curvilinear walls
  - Thickening beneath intima → IMH; thickening on luminal side → mural thrombus
- Severe Ao atherosclerosis (Diffuse Irregularity)
- AoD with thrombosis of false lumen

Fate of IMH

- Progression to acute AoD
- Complete resolution of hematoma
- Persistence without progression
- Prog Ao dilatation and aneurysm formation

Risks

- *Type A:* High risk (mortality >30% with medical management)
- *Type B:* Low risk (10-15% mortality)

Management

- *Type A:* Surgical treatment
- *Type B:*
  - Medical management
  - Surgical treatment (progression, impending rupture, rupture)
- Complete resolution of type B IMH = 50%
- Predictor of resolution
  - Young age
  - Small ao dia (<4-4.5 cm)
  - Hematoma Thickness <1 cm
  - Post op use of BB
- Endovasc repair pomble

PENETRATING ATHEROSCLEROTIC ULCER

Definition

Atherosclerotic lesion penetrate through interval elastic lamina into the media

- Often associated with variable degree of IMH
- Single or multiple
- May lead to pseudoaneurysm formation
- 2-7% of all aortic syndrome
- Common in elderly with coro atherosclerotic risk factor
- Or coexisting vasc disease
- May have concomitant dilatation Ao elsewhere
- In: CT, MRI, TEE.
  - CT—Focal ao ulceration, association IMH and calcified displaced intimal
  - Typically crater like outpouching with irregular edges occur in setting of heavy atherosclerosis
- Uncertain NA+ history with variability in life value
- PAV may stabilize or lead to complication (IMH, Distal embolization, Ao rupture, pseudoaneurysm, AoD, saccular or furiform aneurysm)
- In general, pt with ascending PAV → surgical treatment Stable type B PAV → Medical management
- Endovasc repair is possible

AORTOARTERITIS (BACT INF. OF AO)

- Infected aortic aneurysm
  - Rare but
  - Lethal
  - <1% of all aneurysm

Route of Spread

- Contiguous spread from adjacent str (Mediastinitis, abscess, infected LN, emphysema, paravertebral Abscess)
- Septic emboli from endocarditis
- Hematogenous septic
- IV drug abuse
  - Most commonly involve diseased aorta (Aneurysmal, atherosclerotic, traumatized)

ODP
- Insidious onset and
- Fulminant course (freq rupture >50%)
- High mortality rate (>25-50%)

C/F
Classical triad: fever
- Abd./back/chest pain ⎤ Most pt do not have
- Reliatile tendor mass ⎦ classical triad

Febrile
- Leukocytosis
- Increased ESR
- +VE Bd. culture
- Organism established only at time of operative repair → (in some cases)
- Underlying DM/chronic disease/immunocomprostatic or chronic

Steroid therapy
- (Most common):
  - Infrarenal aorta
  - Paravisceral and juxtarenal ao involved rarely
  - Infected TAA are rare
- (Most common):
  - Microorganisms
  - *Staphylococcus aureus*
  - Salmonella
  - Amvi and fuyd can occur

(Ix)-CT/MRI aortography
- Saccular aneurysms are common
- *CT:* Disruption of calcification, irregular way thickening, perioaortic mass, rim enhancement, periaortic standing
- Most des ao aneu are atherosclerotic
  - Lack of catt suggest
  - Infected aneurysm

Complication
- Aneurysm or pseudo aneurysm
- Prosperity to rupture (expand rapidly)
- Salmonella - propensity to expand
- Mortality (only medical management → 50%

Treatment
- Surgical treatment
- Excision of infected aortic tissue
- Debridement of infected tissue
- Antibiotics
- Arterial reconstruction

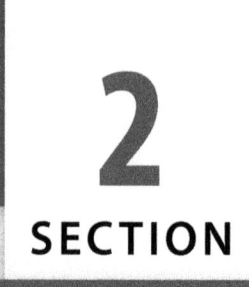

Arrhythmias

2.1 CARDIAC ARREST AND SUDDEN CARDIAC DEATH

DEFINITION

SCD is natural death from any cardiac cause heralded by abrupt loss of consciousness within 1 hour of the onset of acute change in cardiovascular states:
- Preexisting heart disease may or may not have been known
- Time and mode of death unknown

- Natural, rapid, and unexpected

Four temporal elements:
1. Prodromes
2. Onset
3. Cardiac arrest
4. Biological death

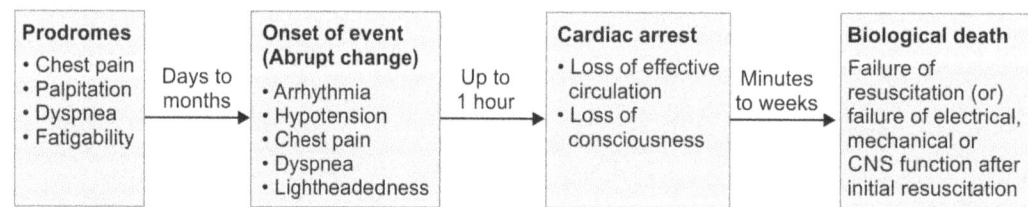

- Unwitnessed death continues to use definition of SCD for a person known to be alive and functioning normally 24 hours before
- *Various terminologies*
- *SCD:* Sudden *irreversible* cessation of all biological function
- *Cardiac arrest:* Abrupt cessation of cardiac mechanical function which may be reversible with prompt intervention
- *CV collapse:* Sudden loss of effective blood flow because of cardiac and/or peripheral vascular factor that may reverse spontaneously [(e.g., neurocardiogenic/vasovagal syncope/or require intervention (e.g., cardiac arrest)]

RISK FACTORS

Environmental
- Both excessive heat and excessive cold has been linked to SCD
- Transient ambient air pollution has been linked to increased incidence of vent arrhythmia

Age/Sex and Hereditary
Age:
- Bimodal peak
  - Within first year of life (including sudden infant death syndrome)
  - Between 45 and 75 years

- Adult > 35 years → Incidence of SCD is 1/1,000 person/year
- Incidence increases with advancing age

Sex: M > F (during young adult and middle age)
- Female enjoys protection from coronary atherosclerosis (Before menopause)
- Female with postmenopausal status → similar risk as male

Hereditary
- Familial pattern of SCD
- Due to genetic variation
- *Four categories:*
  1. *Genetically based 1° arrhythmic disorder*
     - Cong. LQTS, SQTS
     - Brugada syndrome
     - CPVT, VF
  2. *Inherited structural disorder with risk for SCD*
     - HCM
     - ARVD
  3. *Genetic predisposition to induced arrhythmias*
     - Drug-induced acquired LQTS
     - Electrolyte and metabolic arrhythmogenic effect
  4. *Genetic modulation of complex acquired disease*
     - CAD and ACS
     - CHF
     - DCMP

General Profile of Risk Factors

Risk factors for coronary atherogenesis, For example, age, DM, SBD, HR, ECG abnormality, vital capacity, relative weight-obesity, cigarette consumption, serum cholesterol level:
- HIO DM and LQT on ECG are potential markers of interest
- HTN is clearly established risk factor
- No relationship established between cholesterol conc and SCD
- TVCD association with disproportionate number of SCD
- WEF is a marker of SCD (<30% → single most powerful predictors)
- High resting HR; small increase in HR during 1st min pf recovery predict high risk of SCD

Micro T wave alternance Indices of QT duration and dispersion Genetic Profile	Also predictive

Functional Capacity

SCD does not found to vary with function classification.

Lifestyle and Psychosocial
- Cigarette smoking → 2-3 risk fold of SCD
- Obesity
- Significant correlation between lower level of physical activity and SCD
- Association between acute physical exertion and myocardial infarction
- Moderate consumption of alcohol is associated with lower risk of SCD

Electrocardiographic Markers
- PVC/Short runs of NSCT → Benign prognosis in absence of str heart disease
- Exception, polymorphic form of NSVT that occur in pt without str heart disease but can have molecular, functional, drug related or electrolyte related
- Exercise induced VPC and NSVT indicates some level of risk for SCD
- PVC in survivor of MI (esp. freq. PVC) and having complex forms such as repetitive PVC s predict increased risk for SCD (VPL >10/her as threshold for risk)
- Arrhythmias in recovery phase is more predictive than arrhythmia during exercise
- CAST trial (Cardiac Arrhythmia Suppression Trial)
  - *Hypothesis:* Suppression of VPC with antiarrhythmics alter risk factor for SCD after MI
  - Surprising result
    - Death rate in randomized placebo gr. was lower than expected
    - Death rate among pt in encainide and flecainide arm exceeded control group by > 3-fold

Emerging Risk Factors
- Microvolt T wave alternans
- Contrast-enhanced MRI of port infarct border
- QT variability
- HR variability
- MIBG imaging
- Genetic risk profile
- Clustering (familial) of SCD as an expression of CAD

CAUSES OF SUDDEN CARDIAC DEATH

Coronary Art Disease
- 80% of SCD
  - Atherosclerotic CAD
  - Nonatherosclerotic
    - Congenital coronary artery anomalies
    - Coronary arteries

- Coronary artery embolism
- Mechanical obstruction (dissection in Marfan, dissection in preg, prolapsed of aortic valve myxomatous polyp into coro. artia)
- Function coro art obstruction (spasm/bridge)

Ventricular Hypertrophy and Hypertrophic Cardiomyopathy

- WH association with CAD
- Hypertensive heart disease
- HCM v to VHD
- HCM obstructive/nonobstructive
- 1° or 2° PH

All association with increased SCD

- Clinical markers for SCD in HCM
  - Young age
  - Strong FIH
  - Magnitude of LV mass
  - Vent arrhythmia
  - Worsening symptoms
  - NSVT on Holter
  - Inducibility of potent lethal arrhythmias
  - Fall in BP during exercise
  - High resting gradient

Chronic Congestive Heart Failure

- Ischemic cardiomyopathy
- Idiopathic DCMP, acquired
- Hereditary DCMP
- Alcoholic cardiomyopathy
- Hypertensive cardiomyopathy
- Peripartum cardiomyopathy

Acute and Subacute Heart Failure

- Massive AMI
- Fulminant myocarditis
- Acute alcoholic cardiac dysfunction
- Takotsubo
- Ball value embolism in AS
- Mechanical disruption of cardiac str
- Acute PE
- Absolute risk of SCD increases with deteriorating LV function
- Worsening function class → worsen mortality
- Unexplained syncope → High risk
- *HFPEF:* Risk of SCD is similar to HEREF

Inflammatory, infiltrative, degenerative, and neoplastic

- Viral myocarditis
- Myocarditis associated with vasculitis/giant cell arteritis
- Sarcoid/amyloidosis
- Hemochromatosis
- ARVD
- Neuromuscular disease
- Intramural tumors
- Intracavitory tumors
- Sarcoid—67% death due to SCD
- Amyloidosis—30% death due to SCD

Valvular Heart Disease

- AS/AR
- MS
- MVP
- Endocarditis
- Prosthetic valve dysfunction
- High rate of SCD with stenotic lessons
- Chronic AR and acute MR cylo has risk for SCD

Congenital Heart Disease

Most common:
- Cong. AS
- AASD with Eisenmenger
- Late after surgical treatment repair of ToF

Electrophysiological

- Abnormality of conduction system
  - Lenegre disease – 1° degeneration
  - Lev disease – 2° degeneration to fibrom
  - And calcification of cardiac skeleton
  - Postviral conducting system fibroma
  - WPW
- Abnormality of repolarization
  - LQTS, SQTS
  - Acquired long QT (drugs, electrolyte, etc.)
  - Brugada
  - Early repolarization
- VF of unknown or uncertain case
  - Idiopathic VF
  - Short coupled TDP
  - Sleep death in SE Asians
  - IVCD in CAD → Risk for SCD
  - AMI and RBBB (or) bifascicular block → SCD
  - Congenital AV block or interventricular block
  - Sodium channel gene mutation

- *Kearns Sayre syndrome:*
  - Ext ophthalmoplegia; retinal pigmentation, Prog
  - Conduction system disease
  - Association with mitochondrial DNA
  - High grade AV block and pacemaker dependence
- High-risk features of LQTS
  - Female sex
  - Greater degree of QT prolongation
  - QT alternans
  - Unexplained syncope
  - F/H/O premature SCD
  - Documented Tdp or Prev VF
- High-risk feature in Brugada
  - Persistent Type 1 ECG pattern
  - Syncope
  - Life-threatening arrhythmias
  - Strong F/H/O SCD
  - QRS fragmentation
  - Effective vent refractory period <200 milliseconds

Electrical Instability Related to Neurohumoral and CNS Influence
- CPVT
- Other catecholamine-dependent arrhythmias
- CNS related (psychic stress, auditory related, voodoo death, and disease of cardiac nerves)

Sudden Infant Death Syndrome
- Immature respiratory control function
- LQTS
- Cong. heart disease
- Myocarditis

Sudden death in children:
- (35-40%) → Eisenmenger, AS, HCM.PA/PS
- (25%)—After corrective surgical treatment
  - Myocarditis
  - LQTS

Miscellaneous
- Sudden death during extreme physical activity
- *Commotio cordis:* Blunt chest trauma
- *Mechanical interference with venous return*
  - Acute tamponade
  - Massive PE
  - AC intracardiac thrombosis
- Dissecting aneurysm of AO
- Toxic and metabolic disturbance
  - Electrolyte disturbance
  - Metabolic
  - Proarrhythmic effect of antiarrhythmic dry

- *Mimics of SCD*
  - Cafe coronary
  - Acute alcoholic states (holiday heart)
  - Acute asthmatic attacks
  - Air or amniotic fluid embolism

PATHOLOGY AND PATHOPHYSIOLOGY
Coronary atherosclerosis is major risk factor.

Pathology of SCD Caused by CAD
Coronary Arteries
- Plaque fissuring
  - Plaque erosion or rupture — Major mechanics of onset of cardiac arrest
  - Platelet aggregation
  - Thrombosis
- Less commonly nonatherosclerosis pathology
  - Coronary art spasm
  - Deep myocardial bridges with patchy fibrous
  - Coronary vasculitis

Myocardium
- Healed MI—common finding in SCD (40-70%)
- Large or small (<1 cm^2) scar

Vent Hypertrophy
- Independent risk for mortality
- Can also coexist and interact with acute/chronic ischemia
- Heart weight is higher pt than SCD
- Hypertrophy associated mortality is also independent of LV function and the extent of CAD

Conducting System
- Fibrosis (Lev and Lenegre)
- Ischemic damage
- Focal disease (sarcoid, Whipple, and RA)

Mechanism and pathophysiology:

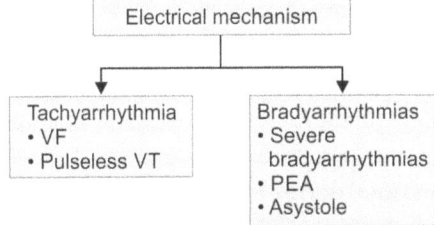

- Occurrence of potentially lethal tachyarrhythmias or severe bradyarrhythmias or asystole is end of a cascade of pathophysiologic abnormality that results from complex intervention between coro-vasc events, myocardial injury, variation in autonomic tone and electrolyte state.

Pathophysiologic Mechanisms of Tachyarrhythmias

- *Coronary artery str and function*
  - Simple increase in myocardial on demand in presence of fixed supply → exercise-induced arrhythmias and SCD during intense physical activity
  - Acute ischemia → Arrhythmia and SCD
  - Coronary spasm due to endothelial dysfunction double hazard of transient ischemia and reperfusion
  - Platelet aggregation and thrombosis also play a role
- *Effect of acute ischemia:*

Acute ischemia
↓
Arrhythmias directly related to ischemic injury (initial 10 mins)
↓
Either reperfusion or evaluation of different injury (20–30 mins) pattern in epicardial and endocardial muscle

  - Propensity of vent arrhythmias are max in first 30 minutes
  - After that it reduces
  - Reappear after several hours

At myocyte level:

- Alteration in cell membrane physiology ⎤
- Efflux of K^+, influx of Ca^{++} ⎬ Ischemia
- Reduction of transmembrane resting potential and enhanced automaticity ⎦

Followed by reperfusion changes:

- Continued influx of Ca^{++} → electrical instability ⎤
- Altered response to α and β-stimulation ⎬ Reperf.
- After depolarization ⎦
- Other possible mechanism:
  - Superoxide radicles
  - Differential response of endocardial and epicardial muscle activation time ← refractory period
- ATP-dependent K^+ current (which is inactive during normal condition)
  - Activated during ischemia
  - Strong efflux of K^+ ions from myocyte
  - Markedly shortening of repol
  - Leads to slow conduction and ultimately to inexcitability
  - More marked in epicardium than in endocardium
  - Prominent dispersion of repol across myocardium ◀

- Ischemia alter distribution of connexin 43 (Gap junction protein between myocyte)
Uncoupling of myocyte
Altered pattern of excitation and conduction velocity
Arrhythmogenic
- Tissue heated after MR is more susceptible to electrical destabilization
- Role of metabolic changes and neurohumoral changes
  - Increase in interstitial K^+ levels
  - Decrease in tissue ph <6.0
  - Change in adrenoceptor activity
  - Alteration in autonomic nerve traffic

Create and maintain electrical instability
So

Triggering event:
- Electrophysiological
- Ischemia
- Metabolic   + Susceptible myocardium
- Hemodynamic

↓
Initiation of potentially lethal arrhythmias

Bradyarrhythmia and Asystolic Arrest

- Asystolic arrest MC in terminal events
- PEA: Two forms
  - *Primary:*
    - No obvious mechanical factor
    - Occurs as an end stage event
    - Can occur in acute ischemia
    - More common after prolonged resuscitation
  - *Secondary* due to:
    - Abrupt cessation of cardiac venous return (e.g., massive PE, cardiac tamponade)
    - Acute malfunction of prosthetic valve
    - Exsanguinated

CLINICAL FEATURES OF PATIENT WITH CARDIAC ARREST

Prodromal Symptoms

- Chest pain
- Dyspnea
- Weakness/fatigue
- Syncope
- Nonspecific complain
- Symptoms that occur within last hours or minutes before cardiac arrest are more specific and that includes symptoms of arrhythmias and ischemia and HF
  ↓ Days to months

Onset of Terminal Event

- Period of 1 hour or less between acute change in cardiac status and cardiac arrest
- Increasing HR and advancing grades of vent ectopy is common antecedent of VF (due to alteration in autonomic system tone)

C/F

Arrhythmias:
- Chest pain
- Dyspnea
- Hypotension/shock

Cardiac Arrest

- Abrupt loss of consciousness caused by lack of adequate cerebral
- Blood flow as a result of cardiac pump
- Leads to death in absence of successful intervention

Mechanical VF (MC)

- Asystole/PEA (2nd)
- Pulseless VT (3rd)
- Mechanical factors
  - Rupture of vent
  - Cardiac tamponade
  - Acute mechanical obstruction to flow
  - Acute disruption of major vessel
- Only 14% pt receiving CPR were discharged from hospital alive and 20% of these died within next 6 months
- Prog better for VF/VT

Predictors of Mortality after CPR

Before arrest	During arrest
• Hypotension • Pneumonia • Renal failure • Cancer • Homebound • Lifestyle	• Arrest duration >15 minutes • Intubation • Hypotension • Pneumonia *After resuscitation* • Coma • Need for pressors • Arrest duration >15 minutes

Progression to Biologic Death

Progression from arrest to biologic death depends on:
- Mechanism of arrest
- Nature of underlying disease
- Delay between onset and resuscitation

- Onset of irreversible brain damage begins within 4-6 mins after loss of cerebral circulation
  ↓
- Biological death quickly follows
- Young pt with less severe cardiac disease and absence of coexistent multisystem disease have a higher probability of a favorable outcome after such delays
- PEA—asystole have poor prognosis because they usually have advanced heart disease
- Sometimes pt with VT have marginally sufficient cerebral blood flow
  - If not treated promptly
  - Progress to VF/PEA/asystole

SURVIVORS OF CARDIAC ARREST

Hospital Course

- Cardiac arrest during phase of MI
  - *Primary:* Electrical event not associated with HD dysfunction
  - *Secondary:* Electrical events linked to HD dysfunction
- Survivor of cardiac arrest may not have repetitive vent arrhythmias during initial 24-48 hours
  - Variable response to antiarrhythmics
  - Overall rate of recurrent to cardiac arrest = 10-30
  - Mortality rate in pt with recurrent arrest ≅ 50%
- Most common cause of death
  - Noncardiac events related to CNS injury
  - Anoxic encephalopathy
  - Sepsis
- Approximately 40% of those who arrive at hospital in coma never awaken and die at median survival of 3-5 days
  - 2/3rd of those who regain consciousness have no gross deficit
  - Additional 20% have persistent cognitive deficit
- Cardiac causes of delayed death
  - HD deterioration
  - Arrhythmic

Clinical profile of SCD survivor:
- Most common cause is CAD—80%
  - Cardiomyopathy 10-15% ⎤
  - Structural heart disease ⎥
  - Functional abnormality ⎬ Rest
  - Environmental cause ⎥
  - LQTS, CPVT, ARVD, ERS ⎥
  - Spasm, BS ⎦

- *LV function:*
  - Abnormality in most of survivor
  - Wide variation
  - Severe dysfunction
  - Stunning—improve in 24–48 hours
  - Cardiac arrest and nonlife threatening arrhythmias both are associated with transient elevation of troponin level
  - Failure to beginning of improvement in LVEF in first 48 hours → poor short-term prognosis
  - Reduced EF → poor long-term prognosis
- CAG:
  - Acute coro lesions often +n+
  - Mod-sense stenosis of LMCA is as common as in gen population
- *Exercise test:* No longer used commonly
- ECG:
  - New Q wave in association with ST segment elevation
  - Repolarization abnormality (ST depression flat T wave prolonged QT)
- *Blood biochem:*
  - Lower serum K^+ level
  - Low ionized calcium level with total Ca^{++}
  - Higher resting lactate levels

Long-term prognosis:
- 2 years mortality = 15–25%
- Outcome improved by –ICD
  - β-blockers
  - Antiischemic procedures
  - HF treatment
- Risk of recurrent cardiac event are highest during first 6 months

MANAGEMENT OF CARDIAC ARREST

- *Principles:*
  - Maintain cont. artificial cardiopulmonary support until return of sport circ
  - Restore rose as quickly as possible
- *J elements:*
  - Initial assessment and summoning emergency response team
  - BrS
  - Early defibrillation by first responder
  - ACLS
  - Postcardiac arrest care
  - Long-term management
- Clinical findings associated with poor neurological outcomes
  - Absence of pupillary reflex to light 72 hours post-arrest
  - Presence of status myoclonus (not myoclonic jerks) during first 72 hours
  - Presence of marked reduction of gray-white ratio on brain CT obtained within 2 grs after arrest
  - Extensive restriction of diffusion on MRI brain at 2–6 days after arrest
  - Persistence absence of sea reactivity to external stimuli at 72 hours postarrest
  - Persistent burst suppression or intractable status epilepticus on ECG after rewarming

Postcardiac Arrest Care

- Four elements
  1. Brain injury
  2. Myocardial dysfunction
  3. Systemic ischemia/reperfusion responses
  4. Control of persistent precipitating factor
- Four categories
  1. Management of 1° cardiac arrest in AMI
  2. 2° cardiac arrest in AMI
  3. CA association with noncardiac disease, drug affect or electrolyte disturbances
  4. Survival after out of hospital CA
- 1° CA in AMF:
  - Almost always reverted successfully in properly
  - Antiarrhythmic discontinues after 24 hours if no arrhythmics
  - Bradyarrhythmias in IWMI respond to atropine/pacing
  - Bradyarrhythmias in large AWMI → poor prognosis
- 2° CA in AMF:
  - Due to H.D or mechanical causes
  - Incidence of PEA-1 asystole higher in 2° CA
- CA due to noncardiac cause
  - Those with life limiting disease, e.g., malignant neoplasm, sepsis, organ failure, end stage pulmonary disease, advanced CNS disease
  - Those with acute toxic or proarrhythmic state that are potentially reversible
- CA core in pt with survival of out of hospital SCD
  - Stabilize cardiac electrical system
  - Supporting HD
  - Supportive care for reversal of organ damage
  - Amiodarone to prevent recurrent arrhythmias
  - Anoxic encephalopathy is strong predictor of in hospital cleats

Long-term management of survivor
- Goal of work up
  - Identify specific causative and triggering factors

- Clarify function states
- Establish long-term therapeutic strategies
■ Role of therapeutic Hypothermia

PREVENTION OF CARDIAC DEATH AND SUDDEN CARDIAC DEATH

Prevention divided in five subgroups
1. Secondary prevention of recurrent events in survivor of SCD (Trials: AHD, CIDS, CASH)
2. Primary prevention in pt at high risk because of advanced heart disease with low EF and EF and other markers risk
3. Primary prevention in pt with less advanced common or uncommon Str heart disease
4. Primary prevention in pt structurally normal heart, subtle or minor Str abnormality
5. Primary prevention in gen population

Four antiarrhythmic strategies:
1. Antiarrhythmic drugs
2. ICD
3. Catheter ablation
4. Antiarrhythmic surgical treatment

Methods to Estimate Risk

■ *General medical and CV risk measures*
- Coro atherosclerosis and associated myoischemia
- MRI defined scar pattern
- LV dysfunction and vent volume and HF
- HTN/DM/CRF/dyslipidemia
- Cig smoking

Other measures being evaluated
■ Noninvasive measure of autonomic function
■ QT interval stability
■ Genetic influences on risk for SCD

Role of Holter/loop recorder:
■ For profiling risk for dev. of life-threatening arrhythmias
■ Esp in pt with HCM, DCMP, HF, post MI

Role of programmed electrical stimulation
■ Less used now
■ For pt with symptomatic arrhythmia or those considered to be at potentially high risk PES is used
■ Inducibility of sustained, HD unstable arrhythmias, initiated with appropriate protocols is considered positive and predictive

Strategy to reduce risk:
■ *Antiarrhythmic drug:*
- Memb active antiarrhythmic drugs
- *CAST trial:* Showed that certain class I antiarrhythmics are neutral or harmful
- BB and amiodarone might have some benefits
■ *Catheter ablation*
- With rare exceptions catheter-based techniques not used for treatment of high risk vent arrhythmias or for definitive treatment
■ ICD: Preferred for 2° and 1° prevention
■ *Surgical strategies*

Specific groups:
■ *2° prev in survivor of SCD*
Antiarrhythmic esp Amiodarone
Trials
- AVID −27% relative risk reduction with ICD as compared to Amiodarone
- CIDS
- CASH
 also showed benefit of ICD

ICD has emerged as preferred strategy regardless of EF for survivors without identifiable and correctable transient cause of CA

■ *1° prev in pt with advanced disease of heart*
- *CAST:* Lack of efficacy and adv-event with class I antiarrhythmias
- *Amiodarone:* EMIAT and CAMIAT
Both trials showed antiarrhythmic benefit
No total mortality benefits
Concomitant use of BB conferred mortality benefits
- *Amio versus ICD:* (MADIT)
  ♦ EF <35%, NSVT on Holter, inducible VT that was not suppressible by procainamide 54% reduction in total mortality with ICD
  ♦ *CABG* Patch trial → No benefit of ICD on mortality
  ♦ *MUSTT*—pt who received ICDs because they fail to respond during
  drug treatment accounted for all benefits
  ♦ *MADIT II:* ICD provided mortality benefits
  ♦ *DINAMIT*→No survival benefit attributed to early implantation of ICD
- *Revascularization +BB+DAPT +statin*
  ♦ Reduce risk of arrhythmia and SCD
- *Define:* Pt with nonischemic cardiomyopathy, accompanied by HIO
HF, EF<35% or NSVT/PVC benefit from prophylactic ICD.
- *SCD HEFT:* In contrast to definite, pt with class II symptoms achieved greater survival benefit as compared to class III amiodarone provided no additional benefit

- *1° prev in pt with less advanced CV disease*
- *1° prev in pt with str. normal heart*
- *1° prev in gen POP*
  - Family screening
  - Athlete screening

INDICATIONS FOR IMPLANTABLE CARDIOVERTER-DEFIBRILLATORS

HCM:
- *Secondary protection:*
  - Previous SCA, pulseless VT = class I
    ↓
    Unexplained syncope = class IIa
- *Primary protection:* LV wall thickness >30; High = class IIa LVOT gradient, NSVT, F/H, Bluntreal BP response to ex

ARVD:
- 2° prev SCA, sustained VT –Class I
  ↓
  Unexpected syncope = Class IIa
  1° prev: Induced VT, ambient = Class IIa
      NSVT, ext disease

Secondary prev in:
- LQTS
- SQT
- Brugada
- CPVT/F

with prev SCA → class I

1° prev in:
- *LQT:* VT or syncope while on BB,   Class IIa
  QTc >500, F/H of phenol SCD
- *Brugada:* Symptomatic VT,   Class IIa
  unexplained syncope, F/H of SCD
- *CPVT/F:* Syncope or VT while on BB   Class IIa
- *1° prev in:* Familial SQT = class IIb/III

2.2 SYNCOPE AND HYPOTENSION

DEFINITION

Syncope for transient loss of consciousness caused by transient global cerebral hypoperf, and characterized by rapid onset, short duration, and spontaneous recovery.

- LOC develop due to decrease blood supply to reticular activity system in brainstem
- LOC within approximately 10 seconds of cessation off blood flow to brain
- Immediate recovery with appropriate behavior and orientation
- Bimodal peak: (1st) 10–20 years
  (2nd) 60–80 years

CLASSIFICATION

Causes of Real or Apparent Transient LOC

- Syncope
- Neurologic or cerebrovascular disease
  - Epilepsy
  - Vertebrobasilar TIA
- Metabolic syndrome and coma
  - Hyperventilation with hypocapnia
  - Hypoglycemia
  - Hypoxemia
  - Intoxication with drugs or alcohol
  - Coma
- Psychological syncope
  - Anxiety, panic disorder
  - Somatization disorder

Causes of Syncope

- Vascular cause—most common approximately 1/3rd of all
  - *Anatomic* (rare)
    - Vascular steal syndrome (subclavian steal)
  - *Orthostatic*
    - Autonomic insufficiency
    - Idiopathic
    - Volume depletion
    - Drugs and alcohol induced
  - *Reflex mediated*
    - Carotid sinus hypersensitivity
    - Neurally-mediated (common faint, vasodepressor, neurocardiogenic, and vasovagal)
    - Glossopharyngeal syncope
    - Situational (cough, defecation, laugh, sneeze swallow
- Cardiac

Anatomic	Arrhythmic
• Obstructive valves	• Bradyarrhythmias
• HCM	• Tachyarrhythmias
• AOD syndromes	• BS, ARVD, LQTS
• Myxoma	• Drug-induced
• Pericardial tamponade	• ICD/ PPI malfunction
• MI	
• PE	
• PHTN	

- Syncope of unknown origin

Approach to Evaluation of LOC

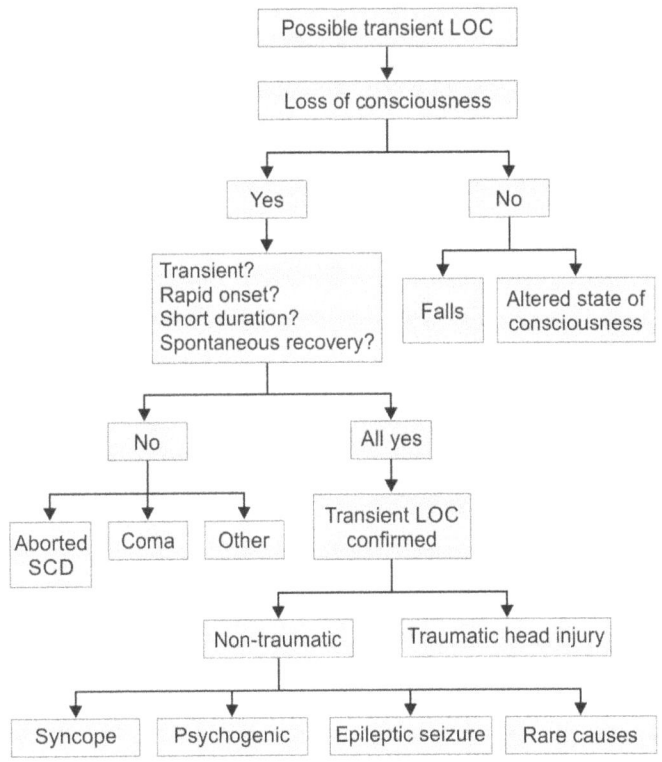

- *Most common:* Neurally mediated syncope and reflex-mediated syncope
- *2nd most common:* Cardiac tachy and bradyarrhythmias

ORTHOSTATIC HYPOTENSION

Definition

20 mm Hg draws in SBP or 10 mm Hg in DBP within 3 minutes of standing.

- *Initial OH:* <40 mm Hg decrease in BP immediately on standing with rapid return to normal in <30 seconds
- *Delayed prig OH:* Slow prog decrease in SBP on standing

Arrhythmias

C/F
- Can be asymptomatic
- Can have symptoms of orthostatic
  - Syncope
  - Lightheadedness/presyncope
  - Tremulousness
  - Weakness
  - Fatigue
  - Palpitation
  - Diaphoresis
  - Blurred vision

Mech

Standing displaces 500–800 mL blood to abdomen and LL
↓
Sudden decrease in venous return
↓
Decreased cardiac output
↓
Stimulate aortic carotid and cardiopulmonary baroreceptors
↓
Reflex increases in symp activity
↓
HR, cardiac contractility and PVR increases to maintain SPB on standing (abnormality in any of these steps leads to OH)

Causes

Drugs
Most common:
- Diuretic
- α-blockers, labetalol, and terazosin
- Adrenergic neuron blocking drugs-avanithidine
- ACE I
- Antidepressant MAO inhibitors
- Alcohol
- Ganglion blocking drugs—hexamethonium
- Tranquilizers—barbiturates
- Vasodilators
- Centrally acting hypertensive drugs

Primary Disorder of Autonomic Failure
- Pure autonomic failure (Bradbury-Eggleston syndrome)
- MSA (Shy-Drager syndrome)
- Parkinson's disease with autonomic failure

Secondary Neurogenic
- Aging
- *Autonomic disease:* GBS, MCTD, RA, SLE
- Carcinomatous autonomic neuropathy
- Central brain lesion multiple sclerosis
- Dopamine-β-hydroxylase deficiency
- *General medical disorder:* DM, amyloid, alcoholic, renal
- *Infection of nervous system:* HIV, Chagas, and syphilis
- *Metabolic:* Vitamin B_{12} deficiency, porphyria, tangier

DIAGNOSIS OF SYNCOPE

History and Examination
- Determine whether patient actually had syncope?
  - Complete LOC?
  - Transient flow with rapid onset and short duration?
  - Spontaneous recovery?
  - No sequelae?
  - Loss of postural tone?
  ↓
  If answer to anyone is "no"
  ↓
  Consider other cause of LOC
- *To determine cause and other parameters*
  - H/O cardiac disease
  - F/H/O: Cardiac disease/syncope/SCD
  - Identify mechanism of probable syncope
  - Quantify number and chronicity of prev syncope and presyncopal episode
  - Identify precipitating condition of any
  - Quantity type and duration of prodrome and recovery symptoms
  - History from witness

Neurally-mediated	Arrhythmia	Seizure	Psychogenic
1. Clinical setting			
F>M	M>F	Any sex	F>M
Young age (<55 years)	Old age (>54)	Younger	Young (<40)
More episodes (>2)	Few episodes (<2)	Any setting	Often many
Standing warm room	during excretion/ supine		episode in a day no identifiable
Emotional upset	Family H/O SCD		trigger

Contd...

Contd...

Neurally-mediated	Arrhythmia	Seizure	Psychogenic
2. Premonitory symptom			
Longer duration (>5 s) Palpitation, blur vision, nausea Warmth Lightheadedness Diaphoresis	Shorter duration <6 sec palpitation	Sudden onset Brief aura	Usually absent
3. During event			
Pallor, diaphoresis Dilated pupil, slow pulse, low BP, incontinence may occur, brief clone movt may occur	Blue, not pale incontinence Brief clonic movt	Blue face frothing, tonic clonic movt, incontinence	Normal color Not diaphoretic Eyes closed Normal pulse/BP No incontinence Prolonged duration Common
4. Residual symptoms			
Common, prolonged Fatigue (>90%)	Uncommom	Common disonented Headache	Uncommon
Oriented	Oriented	Slow recovery	Oriented

- *Petit mal seizure:* Lack of responsiveness in absence of loss of postural tone
- *Examination*
    - Whether structural heart disease is present?
    - Defining patients level of hydration
    - Detecting level of neurological abnormality suggestive of dysautonomia
    - CVA
    - BP and HR in supine and standing
- *Carotid sinus massage*
    Caution: Elderly patient
    Presence of carotid bruit
    HIO TIA/CVA
    Procedure: CSM done on one side and then another
    5-10 seconds each side
    Supine and upright poster
    Normal response: Transient decrease in HR (sinus rate)
    Prolongation of AV condition or both

Carotid sinus hypersensitivity:
Defined as sinus pause > 35 seconds in duration
and/or fall in SBP of ≥50 mm Hg
↓
Cardioinhibitory (asystole) or vasodepressor
(fall in SBP) or mixed
↓
Diagnosis of carrot sinus hypersensitivity

Above character + Reproduction of patient's symptoms
Treatment: PPI for recurrent falls/syncope
Class I indication
- Blood tests
    - Not recommended routinely
- Tilt table test
    - Performed for 30-45 minutes following 20 minutes horizontal free tilt stabilization
    - Done at angle between 60 and 80° (70° common)
    - Positive response → susceptibility to neurally mediated syncope
    - Sensitivity increased by: Prolonged tilt
        Steeper tilt angle
        Provocative agents
        (Isoproterenol/NTG)

Isoproterenol: Infusion
- Incrementally from 1-3 mg/min to increase HR 25% greater from baseline
- *NTG*: 300-400 MG NTG spray after 20 mins of unmedicated tilt when provocative agents used → specifically decreases dramatically
- Tilt test not recommended in patients whom can be established from initial history and examination
- Induction of reflex hypotension bradycardia without reproduction of symptoms
    - Indicative of neurally mediated syncope but is a less specific response

- In patients with known CV disease other causes of CV syncope must be excluded before till test
- Tilt test also indicated in patients with determined case for syncope (e.g., asystole) but presence of neurally mediated syncope would influence treatment
- Also helpful in patients with psychogenic Case (LOC within normal BB response)
- ECMO
  - Only in patients with suspected str heart disease
  - Severe AS, tamponade, Aod, HCM, congenital abnormality
- Stress test
  - Reserved for patients in whom syncope or presyncope occur during or immediately after exertion in association with chest pain in patient with high risk of CAD
    - Syncope during exercise → Cardiac case
    - Syncope after exercise → neurally mediated
- ECG
  - Diagnostic in 5-10% patients
  - LQTS, WPW, BS, AMI, AV block, T inversion (ARVD)
  - Most patients with syncope have apparently normal ECG

Signal averaged ECG
- Noninitiative technique
- Detect 100 amplitude signals in terminal portion of QRS complex (late potential)
  ↓
  Substrate for vent arrhythmias
  Useful especially in case of ARVD
- Holter
  - Low yield
  - Absence of arrhythmia and symptoms during Holter does not rule out arrhythmia
- Event recorder/ Loop recorder
  - Indicated in early phase of evaluation of patients with syncope of uncertain origin
  - Also indicated in high risk patients in whom comprehensive evaluation did not demonstrate cause of syncope
  - Implantable record for patient with very infrequent episode
  - *Current guideline:* When mech of syncope is uncertain after full evaluation → implantable event recorder is indicated in patient with ECG feature suggestive of arrhythmia
- *EP testing:* Establish assessment of SSS, CSH, heart block, SVT and VT

Indications
- In patient with IHD when initial evaluation suggest arrhythmic case and there is no established induction for ICD (I)
- In patient with BBB when noninvasive test do not establish diagnosis (II)
- In patient with syncope preceded by sudden and brief palpitation
- In patient with syncope and BS, ARVD or HCM (IIb)
- In patient with high risk occupation

Not recommended in patient with normal findings on ECG no palpitation, no heart disease, clinical history do not suggestive of arrhythmic cause.

Diagnostic criteria on EPS
- Sinus brady and prolonged CSNRT (>525 msec)
- BBB and either of base line HV interval ≥100 msec or second or third degree His Purkinje block during incremental atrial pacing which pharmacological challenges — Class I
- Indication of MMVT inpatients with prev MI
- Induction of SVT the reproduction and symptoms
- HV interval between 70 and 100 (IIa)
- Induction of PMVT /VI In patients with BB, VD are patients resuscitated from arrest (IIB)
- Induction of poly VT/VF in patients with ischemic make disease should not be considered a diagnostic finding (III)
- Test screen for cases neurologic cases:
  - CT scan
  - ECG
  - Carotid duplex scan

MANAGEMENT OF PATIENT WITH SYNCOPE

Three goals:
1. Prolong survival
2. Prevent traumatic injury
3. Prevent recurrence of syncope

Indication for hospitalization:
1. *Severe str heart disease*
   - Low EF, prev MI, HF
2. Clinical or ECG features
   - Syncope during exertion while supine
   - Palpitation at time of syncope
   - F/H/O SCD

- NSVT
- Bifascicular block/QRS >120
- Severe sinus Brady
- Pre-excitation
- Brugada pattern
- ARVD
- ECG s/o HCM
- Suspected PE

3. *Comorbid condition*
   - Severe anemia
   - Significant electrolyte abnormality

Treatment is individualized
For example, WPW—ablation
- VT-ICD
- CHB -PPI
- CHB WITH IWMI → revasc

Factors to be considered before making any recommendations
- Potential for reassurance
- Presence of dissection of warning symptoms
- Syncope while seated or only standing
- How often and in what capacity patient drives
- Applicable state or national laws
  Usually driving is prohibited for several months ←

I. *Neurally mediated syncope*
   1. Reassurance and education
   2. Isometric physical counter pressure maneuvers with prodrome (lying or sitting)
      - Leg crossing hand grip with arm tensing
   3. Precipitating factor avoidance example: dehydration, prolonged standing, alcohol, diuretics, vasodilators
   4. Volume expansion by salt supplement
   5. Injection of 500 mL water acutely improve Roth static tolerance
II. 6. Tht training
   7. Head up tilt sleeping greater than 10 degree
   8. Moderate aerobic and isometric exercise
   9. Standing training leaning against the wall with heel 20 inches from the wall for prog or longer period for 2–3 months (5 min BD initially → 40 min BD)
   10. Pharmacological maneuvers
       - BB
       - Fludrocortisone   For patient refractory to
       - Midodrine   conservative treatment
       - SSRI
   11. Pacing in patient with dominant cardioinhibitory carotid sinus hypersensitivity
       - Patient with frequent recurrent reflex syncope, age 40 documented cardioinhibitory response
       - After alternative treatment has failed

Pacing algorithms: 1. Rate drop hysteresis
2. Closed loop stimulation
Rate adaptive pacing that responds to myocardial contraction dynamics by measuring variation in RV intracardiac impedance

- Trigger of situation including syncope must be avoided
- Hypotensive drug discontinued or modified
- BB not indicated until necessary
- Pacing not indicated in absence of cardioinhibitory reflex

2.3 TORSADES

TORSADES DE POINTER

- Refers to VT char. by QRS complexes of changing amplitude that appear to twist around the isoelectric line and occur at a rate of 200-250/min
- Originally described in setting of bradycardia
- It connotes a syndrome rather than ECG finding
  └─ Char by prolonged QT int >500 milliseconds
      → + Prolonged vent repol.
- Abnormal repol need not be present in all beats, but it may be apparent only on the beat before the onset of TDS.
- (Long Short RR cycle) commonly precede onset of TDP from acquired course
- Relatively late PVC can discharge during termination of long T wave and precipitate successive burst of VT
  ECG: Peaks of QRS complexes appear successively on one side and then on other side of isoelectric baseline
- TDP can terminate with progressive prolongation of CL and larger and more distinctly formed QRS complex
  ↓
  Culminate into - Return to SR
                  - Period of vent standstill
                  - New attachment of Tdp/VF (short coupled variant)
                  - Less common form
                  - Malignant and high mortality
                  - Arrhythmia begin with close coupled PVC
                  - Does not involve preceding pause or brady

Note: VT similar in morphology to Tdp and occurs in patient without QT prolongation, whether spontaneous or electrically induced, should generally be classified as PMVT (not as TDP).

EP Features

- EP mechanism not completely understand
- *Data suggest:* EAD are responsible for its initiation
- Perpetration (continuation) can be caused by triggered activity, re-entry resulting from dispersion of ↓ repolarization (produced by EAD) or abnormal automaticity
  Transmural re-entry is most likely mechanical as suggested by data

C/F Predisposing Factors

- Severe brady (most common)
- Hypokalemia
- QT prolonging drugs

C/F depends whether cong/Acq. LQT caused Tdp
Symptoms of VT—Palpitation → Syncope → Death

Treatment:

- H.D unstable → Defibrillation
- IV MgSo$_4$ initial drug of choice
- Temp vent or atrial pacing
  └─ Isoproterenol can be used to increase rate until pacing can be done (cautiously because it may exacerbate arrhythmia)
- Avoid class IA, IC, and III drugs → further prolong QT and worsen arrhythmia
- Lidocaine, mexiletine, or phenoline can be tried
- TDP from long IQTS
  ↓
  BB+ pacing of ICD

DRUG-INDUCED TORSADES

- Incidence 1-8%
  - *I_{KR} channel blocker and repolarization reserve*
    └─ Majority of such drugs → I_{KR} channel blocker S/E
    └─ Also known as HERG channel blocker
- *QT prolonging drug produced LQT_2 type phenotype*
  └─ Reduce repolarization efficiency and lengthen AP
  - *Repolarization reserve:*
    Cardiac repolarization relies on interaction of several ion channels
    ↓
    All channels provide some level of redundancy in protecting against extreme prolongation by QT liability drugs
    ↓
    Known as repolarization reserve
    Repolarization reserve in drug-induced Tdp due to anomalies in repolarization machinery
    ↓
    Loss of repolarizing current I_{KS} and I_{KR}
  - *Genetic:*
    Polymorphism of KCNH$_2$ encoding I_{KR} potassium channel
    ↓
    Loss of function mutation
    ↓
    Somewhat weaker than classic autosomal dominant mutation of LQTS
    ↓
    Multiple hypothesis of reduced repolarization reserve

2.4 VARIOUS VENTRICULAR TACHYCARDIAS

J WAVE SYNDROME

- Junction of QRS complex and ST segment
- Also referred as Osborn wave
- J wave syndrome is part of spectrum of early repolarization syndrome
- Can lead to PMVT/VF
- J wave syndrome defers from Brugada and SQT by magnitude and lead location and has an ECG pattern of early repolarization.
  J point elevation in inf or lat precordial leads

Other causes: Ischemia
              Hypothermia

- Linked to abnormality in I_{TO} current
- J point elevation >0.2 mv associated with SQT or distinct J wave should raise suspicion, especially when they appear in Inf. Leads (II, III, and AVF)

IDIOPATHIC VENTRICULAR TACHYCARDIA

- Defined as MMVT in patient without any str heart disease or CAD
  - Outflow tract VT
  - Annular tachycardia
  - Fascicular VT

Outflow Tract Ventricular Tachycardia

- *(1) Paroxysmal VT* and *(2) Repetitive MMVT*
- Originate from RVOT or LVOT
- Rarely VT originate from proximal PA
- *RVOT:* LBBB contour in V_1 and inferior axis
- *LVOT:* Presence of S wave in lead I and early R wave transition (V_1 to V_2)
- Vagal maneuver, including Adenosine can terminate VT
- Exercise, stress, isoproterenol infusion and rapid atrial stimulation initiate or perpetuate VT.
- *Paroxysmal form:* Induced by ex or stress
- *Repetitive form:* Occurs at rest
- BB or verapamil can also help
- Very small number of patients, tachycardia seems to arise in inflow tract or apex of RV
- *Prognosis:* Good
- *Treatment OC:* RFA → Drugs

Annular Ventricular Tachycardia

- VT arising from mitral or tricuspid annulus
- 4–7% of cases of idiopathic VT
- Mostly *repetitive MMVT*

- (Mitral annular) RBBB pattern (transition in V_1 or V_3) S wave in V_6 and monophasic R QRS in lead V_2 through V_6
- (Tricuspid annular) foci generally in septal region typical findings on ECG IS LBBB pattern (QS in lead V_1) and early transition in precordial leads (V_3) and narrower QRS
- *Prognosis:* Good
- *Treatment OC:* Ablation → Drugs

Fascicular Ventricular Tachycardia

- Most often arise in left postseptal
- Frequently preceded by fascicular potential
- Most commonly arise from left port fascicle
- LPFVT, RBBB + LAD (like typical LAPB)
- *LAFVT:* Like typical LPFB
- Re-entry circuit
- Shows phenomena of entrainment
- Verapamil/Diltiazem sensitive
- Adenosine rarely terminates this VT.
- *Paroxysmal and sustained*
- Can be initiated by rapid atrial or vent pacing and sometimes by exercise or isoproterenol
- Prognosis good
- RF ablation

IDIOPATHIC VF

- 1–8% of out of hospital VF
- Structurally normal heart
- Overlap with SQTS and J wave syndrome
- Treatment ICD
  Ablation of short coupled PVC that initiates VF

BIDIRECTIONAL VENTRICULAR TACHYCARDIAS

- Uncommon type of VT
  - *ECG:*
    - QRS of RBBB pattern
    - Polarity in frontal plane alternating from -60 to -90 ↔ +120 - +130
    - Regular rhythm
    - Rate 140–200 BPM
- *Mech and site:*
  - Controversial
  - Most evidence supports ventricular origin
- *Cause:* Digoxin toxicity (especially in elderly or severe moyamoya disease)
         Otherwise → CPVT
                PROG-POOR

BUNDLE BRANCH REENTRANT

- ECG depends on circuit established by BB or fascicle (MC)
  1. Retrograde over LBB and anterograde
     ↓
     QRS complex like LBBB
     Axis +30°
  2. Conduction in opposite direction
     ↓
     RBBB contour
  3. Re-entry can also occur over Ant-Post fascicle

EP:
- HV interval of BB re-entrant complex equals or exceeds HV interval of spontaneous normally conducted QRS
- Usually seen in patient with STR heart disease, e.g., DCMP

BRADYARRHYTHMIA

HYPERSENSITIVE CAROTID SINUS

ECG:
- Vent A systole often caused by cessation of atrial activity as a result of sinus arrest or SA exit block
- AV block noted less frequently because SA nodal dysfunction precludes its occurrence
- AV junction or vent escape generally do not occur or are present at very slow rates → suggesting that heightened vagal tone and sympathetic withdrawal can suppress subsidiary pacemaker located on vent as well

2.5 VENTRICULAR PREMATURE CONTRACTION AND VENTRICULAR TACHYCARDIA

PREMATURE VENTRICULAR COMPLEXES

- Frequent PVC can lead to LV dysfunction over time
- PVC burden >24% over 24 hours Holter
- Very wide QRS PVC
- PVC of epicardial origin

↓

Favors development of PVC included cardiomyopathy

↓

Ablation of PVC may be required

VT

- >30 seconds → sustained
- <30 seconds and stops spont → nonsustained

SVT	VT
Slowing or termination by vagal or adenosine onset with premat P P and QRS rhythm linked to suggest that vent activation depends on atrial discharge AV block, rsr1 IV v1 Long movement cycle sequence	Fusion beat/capture beat AV dissociation P and QRS rate and rhythm Linked to suggest that atrial activation depends on vent discharge, e.g., 2:1 v4 block LAD, QRsd >140 specific QRS counter

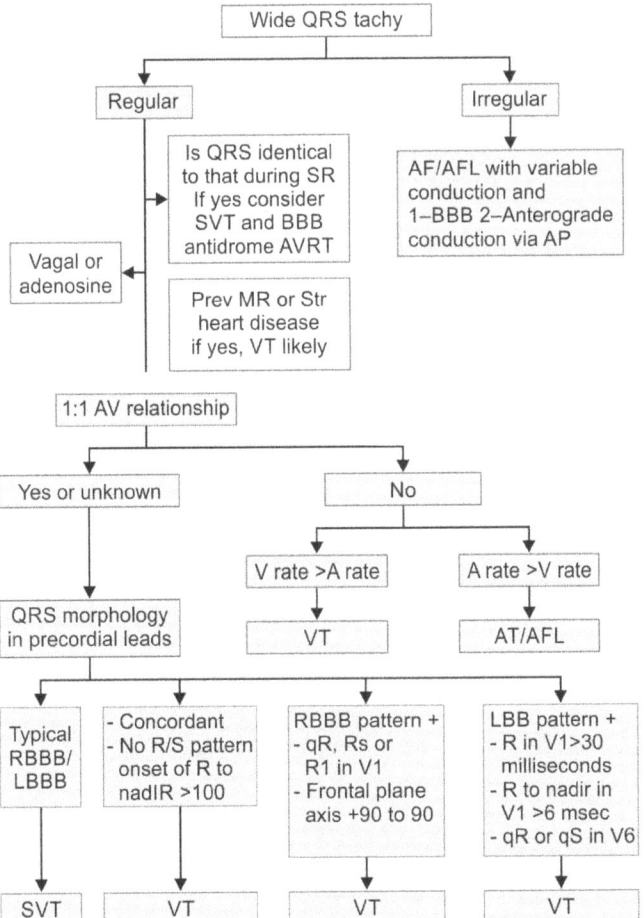

VARIOUS ALGORITHMS

Kindwall

- R > 30 msec in v1 or v2 → VT
- >60 milliseconds to S wave in v1 or v2 → VT
- Any Q in v6 → VT
- Notched downstroke S wave in V1 or v2 → VT

Wellers

- AV dissociation → VT
- QRS >140 → VT
- LAD >-30° → VT
- If RBBB, monophasic or biphasic QRS in v1 → SVT R to S ratio <1 in V6 to VT
- If LBBB S in v1, v2 → VT

Brugada

- Absence of RS complex in all precordial leads→VT
- Longest interval >100 milliseconds in any precordial → VT
- AV dissociation VT
- If RBBB, monophasic R or qR in V1→VT
  - R > R1→VT
  - Rs in V6→VT
- If LBBB, initial R >40 milliseconds >VT
  - Slurred or notched s in v1 or v2→VT
  - Beginning of Q or QS in V6→VT

Miller

- Initial R wave in aVR→VT
- aVR with notch on descending limb of negative onset and predominantly negative QRS VT
- In aVR mv of initial 40 milliseconds/terminal 40 sec (v1/v6 ← 1) → VT

VT LOCALIZATION

VT origin/exit site can be determined

- VT from LV free wall → RBBB
- VT from RV or septum → LBBB
- Apical VT → Negative precordial lead, concordance Basal site → Positive concordance
- VT from posterior (inf) LV or RV → predom -ve QRS in leads I, III aVF
- OT VT +ve QRS in leads II, *III* aVF
- Intrinsicoid deflection exceeding >55% of QRS is likely to be epicardial

- Inducibility of VT on ERS
- Reduced LV function
- Spont VT
- Late potential on SA-ECG
- QT dispersion
- T wave alternans
- Prolonged QRSD
- HR turbulence
- Decreased HRV
- Decreased baroreceptor sensitivity

} Risk factors for SCD

Drugs for VT
- Procainamide
- Amiodarone
- Lidocaine

Treatment of VT

NSVT
- Asymptomatic, low risk population (preserved WEF)
  - No treatment required
- Symptomatic
  - BB
    Class I C/amio/sotalol for BB refractory patient (Class I C should be avoided in patient with str heart disease and CAO → Increased mortality) (due to their proarrhythmic effects)

VT with Decreased EI
- For 2° prev in patient with str heart disease/IHD
  1. Class I antiarrhythmics → worse outcome
  2. Empiric amiodarone
  3. ICD better than amiodarone in EFC <35%

VT with Normal EF (in Patient with CAD)
- Empiric amiodarone
- Holter guided sotalol
- Ablation
- Other drugs—procainamide, mexiletine, and flecainide
- ICD → need antiarrhythmic to decrease shock frequency

CPVT
- Uncommon
- Occurs in absence of overt str heart disease
- Mutation in RYR2 or calsequestrin
- Syncope or aborted SCD
- During exercise typical response include initial S. Tach and vent extrasystole followed by MMVT or bidirectional VT
  - Eventually PMVT if ex continued
  - Treatment BB and ICD/Flecainide (inhibit R1R2 receptor)

2.6 VENTRICULAR TACHYCARDIA STORM

DEFINITION

Life threatening syndrome that involves recurrent episodes of vent arrhythmias.

Defined as 3 or more sustained VT/VF or appropriate ICD shocks during 24 hours period.

Sustained VT/VF that resumes immediately after efficacious therapy (≥1 sinus cycle and within 5 minutes) by defibrillation is regarded as severe form of electrical storm.

- Electrical storm is deemed to be resolved if the patient is free from VT for at least 2 weeks
- Most patients with electrical storm have severe underlying Str heart disease
- Less frequency reported in patient with normal heart (Brugada, LQTS, etc.)

INCIDENCE

- AVID trial (ICD for 2° prev) = 20%
- MADIT II (Primary prev) = 4%

TRIGGER AND RISK FACTORS

- Underlying Str heart disease
- Drug toxicity
- Electrolyte disturbance (Hypokalemia and Hypo MG^{++})
- New or worsened HF
- AMI
- Hyperthyroidism
- Infection/Fever
- Prolonged QT (congenital/acquired)
- Psychological stress
- Severely compromised LV function
- Advanced age
- Male sex
- NYHA III/IV HF

Trial of

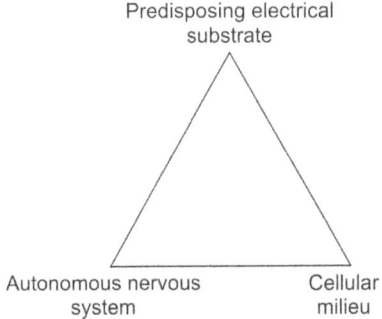

CLINICAL FEATURES

Depends on
- VR
- Underlying heart disease
- LV dysfunction
- Presence/absence of ICD
  Patient with ICD
  - Multiple ICD shocks + or - ATP
  - Patient with vent arrhythmia slower than detection setting may present with symptoms similar to patient without ICD

  Patient without ICD
  - Palpitations/syncope/presyncope
  - Cardiac arrest
  - Dyspnea

Type of Arrhythmia

(Most common)→ 1. MMVT—80–97%
2. 1° VF—1–21%
3. Mixed VT/VF—3–14%
4. PMVT—2–8%

EVALUATION AND MANAGEMENT

- Resuscitation of patient
- Routine blood tests including cardiac biomarkers and electrolytes
- 12-lead ECG
- ECMO
- Interrogation of ICD
- EDS (if required)
  Overdrive pacing

Treatment

- ICD
  - Amio/B.B
  - Lidocaine/procainamide (class IA)
  - Adrenergic blockade:
    - Catecholamine (may be arrhythmogenic)
    - Propranolol/esmolol
    - Left stellate ganglion blockade
- *Anesthetic*: Propafenone and benzodiazepines
- RF oblation
- IABP/ECMO/transplant

VT Storm in Patient with ICD

- Check ICD for malfunction
- Search for underlying triggers
- Sotalol, amiodarone, BB

SUMMARY

- Clue about trigger can be obtained from morphology of arrhythmia and ECG
- After acute management, treat underlying cause

2.7 AVNRT, AVRT, MAHAIM, PJRT

ATRIOVENTRICULAR REENTRANT TACHYCARDIA

- QRS complex of supra-vent origin
- Sudden onset and termination
- Rate—150-250 BPM
- Rhythm regular
- P buried in QRS Pseudo-s or Pseudo-r1
- AVNRT begins after a *PAC that conducts with prolonged PR* variation in cycle length esp at the onset of tachy or just before its termination is usually caused by variation in anterograde AV node conduction time.
- Very rarely VPC can also initiate AVNRI
- Most cases P wave buried beneath QRS 30% cases it is just after QRS
- Short RP tachy RP inr <50% of RR int
    Typical = Anterograde slow and retrograde fast
  (5-10%) Atypical = Anterograde fast and retrograde slow
    Slow-slow AVNRT= 2 slow pathways or
    Anterograde intermediate and retrograde slow
  - *Typical AVNRT*: AV/VA ratio < 0.75
  - *Atypical AVNRI*: Long VA and short AV interval
  - *Slow-slow*: p wave in midway in cardiac cycle
- Spont. AV block can occur = esp. at onset of arrhythmia
  - *Site:* AV node distal to reentry circuit, between AV node and bundle of His, within bundle of His or distal to His (*MC*) and rarely in between re-entry circuit and atrium
- Retrograde atrial activation is concentrate
       ↓

Means, during retrograde conduction over fast pathway is recorded first in His bundle electrogram → followed by electrogram recorded from as of CS and then spreading to depolarize rest of RA and LA.

C/F: Late 20's or Teens

- No str heart disease
  Symptom = Palpitation
               Anxiety   / Syncope
               Angina   Shock
               HF

Syncope can be due to:
- Rapid VR → decreased CO → decreased cerebral circ
- Asystole post SVT because of depressed sinus nodal automaticity

Management

- Rest, reassurance
- Vagal maneuver
  - CSM
  - Valsalva
  - Müller maneuver
  - Gagging
  - Exposure of face to ice cold water
- Adenosine 6-12 mg ⎤ Depress cond
- Verapamil/Dilzem   ⎬ in anterograde conducting
- BB   ⎦ slow pathway
- Class IA and IC → depress cond in retrograde fast pathway Not neg. usually
  DC shock C.I in pt with Dig toxicity → Can lead to post shock vent arrhythmias
- Rarely DC shock: sync
                   10-50 J
- Competitive atrial or vent pacing
- Cath ablation >95% success

Long-term

- Infrequent SVT   ⎤
- Short interval   ⎥
- Well tolerate   ⎬ No prophylactic treatment
- Early terminated by pt ⎥
- No HD compromise   ⎦
- Longer and more freq ⎤
- HD instability   ⎬ Cath ablation
- Syncope/near syncope ⎦

ACCESSORY PATHWAYS

Drugs that slow cond and increases RP in pathways and AV node
- AP → class IA
- AV node → Class II
            Class IV
            Adenosine
            Digitalis
- Both → Class IC
         Class III (Amiodarone)

Anterograde conducting path + symptoms of Tachy → CPW synd

Only retrograde cond → No preexcitaton → concealed path
- Reentry over concealed pathway:
  - Only retrograde conduction
  - ECG feature of WPW are absent
  - Orthodromic AVRT

ECG:
- Normal QRS complex

- P. retrograde after QRS completion in ST/T
- Sometimes P wave not clearly visible and seen as depression of ST segment
  ↓
  So ST depression during Tachy, mostly its AVRT
  Contour of retrograde P is different
  Because it's from abnormal direction
  ↓
  Atria activated *eccentrically*
  ↓
  Sequence other than usual retrograde activation sequence
- Concealed path is mostly on left side
  - LA activated first on retrograde conduction
  - Retrograde P neg in lead I

| AVRT does not change with function BBB | If function BBB occur in vent involving the AD VA interval and CL changes lengthening of tachy cycle by >30 ms during II function BBB is diagnostic of a free wall AP (if lengthening can be shown by prolongation of VA interval and not HV interval) |

Septal AP (Concealed)

- Retrograde atrial activation is *concentric*
- VA interval or CL increases by 25 milliseconds or less by function BBB.
- Vagal maneuver can terminate this tachy
  ↓
  Tachy ends in P wave (Lat retrograde P fails to conduct to ventricle)

Diagnosis of Concealed AP

EPS:
- PVC activates atria before retrograde depol of His bundle.
- Vent can be stimulated prematurely during tachy at a time when His bundle is refractory and impulse still conducts to the atrium
- Eccentric atrial stimulation (retrograde)
- His bundle refractory VPC can terminate tachycardia → suggesting AVRT

C/F

- Concealed pathway present in 30% of pt with apparent SVT
- Most of pathway between LV and LA or in posteroseptal
- Rate slightly more than AVNRT (≥200 BPM)
- Syncope (sum mech as AVNRT)
- S1 constant
- JVP can be elevated

Management: Similar to AVNRT

PREEXCITATION SYNDROME

- (Occurs when atrial impulse activates the entire ventricle or some part of it)
  Or
  (Ventricular impulse activates the entire atrium or some part of it)
  Earlier than would be expected if the impulse travelled only by way of normal specialized conduction system
- *Three basic features:*
  1. PR<120
  2. QRS>120 and slurred slowly rising onset of QRS in some leads (delta wave) and usually normal terminal QRS
  3. Two degree ST-T changes in opposite direction of delta wave and major QRS deflection

LOCALIZATION OF PATHWAY

See Flowchart below

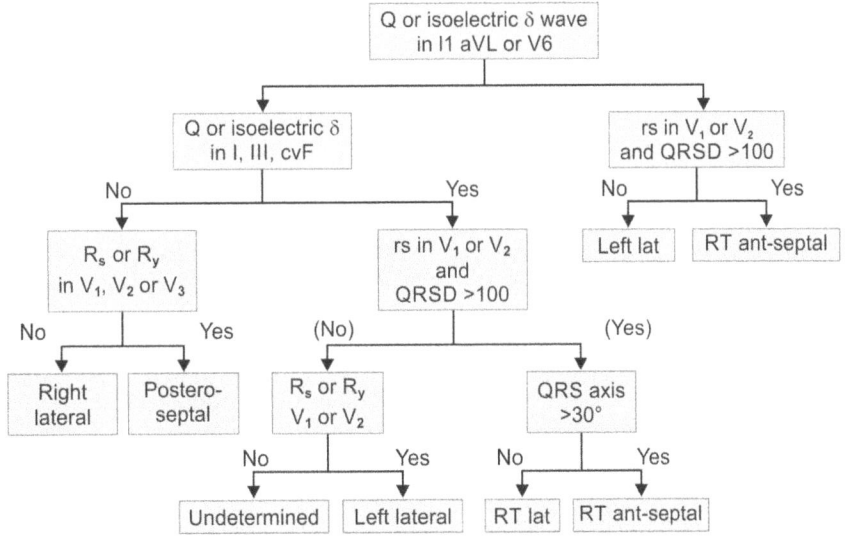

Tachy: Sudden onset and termination
- Normal QRS—orthodromic
- Wide QRS—antidromic
- Rate = 150–200
- Rhythm = regular
  Variants:
  - Atrio-Hisian pathway → short PR; Normal QRS: (James fiber) Lown-Ganong-Levine syndrome (LGL)
  - Atriofascicular ⎤ Mahaim
  - Nodofascicular ⎦ fibers
  - Nodoventricular
  - Fasciculoventricular
- In Mahaim fibers, progressive increases in AV interval is noted in response to atrial override pacing (in other AP, preexcitation occur with short AV interval)
  - Mahaim fibers generally insert onto rt bundle branch
  - Generally have LBBB
  - Apical end lies close to tricuspid annulus and conducts slowly (like AV node property)
  - Distal portion of fibers insert into distal rt bundle branch
  - Or apical region of PV
  - No retrograde conduction (only antidromic AVRT)
  - Preexcited tachy has LBBB pattern, long AV interval and short VA interval
  - RBBB can be proarrhythmic by increasing length of tachy circuit and tachy becomes incessant
    - *EP feature of preexcitation*:

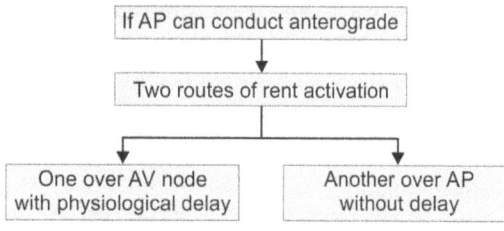

   - QRS develop due to fusion of depol of ventricle over both the pathways
   - δ represent activation of ventricle over AP
   - IV AV node delay occurs because of rapid atrial pacing or PAC → more of rent activated over AP and QRS become more anomalies during sinus rhythm HV interval is short or even vent gets activated before His bundle due to conduction over AP
         ↓
So short HV or Neg HV occurs in either cond over AD or *VT*
- Usually AP conducts fast
But ERP of AP is more esp. during long cycle length (SR)

PAC can occur early when AP is in refractor period
         ↓
PAC conducts over AV node
         ↓
HV and QRS can be normal
         ↓
Such an event can initiate MC type of reciprocating tachy
(Orthodromic AVRT)
- Less commonly AVRT is antidromic
- Rarely multiple pathway
- Very rarely tachy caused by anterograde conduction over 1AP and retrograde conduction over another AP

PJRT
- Long RP Tachy
- Usually a *posteroseptal* AP
- Most often RV
- Conducts slowly because of long and tortuous route
- Orthodromic tachy
- ECG usually normal during NSR

Location of AP in preexcitation:
- Mapping technique provides accurate assessment of position of AP which can be anywhere in AV groove except in intervent trigone between MV and AoV annuli.
- Retrograde cord. Over septal AP vs AVNRT can be differentiated by His-refractory VPC
- *Other forms of Tachy in WPW:*
  1. Other Tachy with bystander AP. For example, AVNRT or AT
  2. AF/AFL (AP is not requisite part of tachy mechanic)
  3. Pre-excited AF
  (*Note:* Interruption of AP and elimination of AVRT usually prevent recurrence of AF) in pre-excited AF at very rapid rate ERP of AD can be shorten significantly and permit extremely rapid VR and can lead to VE.
- An impulse bypassing AP and failing over vulnerable period of T wave can also precipitate VF

Wide QRS Tachy in AP
- AT/AF/AFL conducting over AP
- Antidromic tachy
- Orthodromic tachy with BBB (function or preexisting)
- Tachy using nodofascicular or nodofascicular fibers
- VT

C/F: Incidence 15/1000

- Left free wall path—(MC) followed by posteroseptal, rt free wall and anteroseptal
- All age group (Prev. decreased with age)
- M > F
- Most adult with preexcitation have normal heart
- *CHD: Ebstein*, MVP, cardiomyopathies
  ↓
  Often multiple
  Rt sided pathways
  (Postseptum, post-iot freeway)
- Incidence of reciprocating tachy increases with age
- Prog usually good
- SCD 0.1%

Risk stratification
- Stress test
- EP study (Procainamide)
- Pt with multiple pathways → family screening is advisable

Treatment asymptomatic patient
- Intermittent preexcitation—do not require further evaluation or treatment observe
- Persistent preexcitation—(no arrhythmias)
  - Stress test to determine whether abrupt loss of preexcitation occurs
  - EP if no loss of preexcitation on TMT
- Symptomatic tachyarrhythmias → treatment

- *Two therapeutic options*
  1. Pharmacotherapy
  2. Cath ablation
- Drugs chosen to stop conduction over AV node or AP or both
- CCB, BB, adenosine → prolongs conduction over AV node
- Digitalis can shorten ERP of AP → Better to avoid in possibility of AF with AP
- Class IA drugs prolong RP in AD ⎤
- Class IC and Amio and sotalol ⎥ Can be used in
  prolong RP in both   ⎦ preexcited AF
  - For acute episode:
    - Vagal maneuver
    - Adenosine
    - Verapamil/Dilzem
  - For acute preexcited AF
    - DC cardioversion
    - Procainamide
  - Prevention/long-term
    - Cathartic ablation—Preferred
    - Drug treatment is option
      - Difficult to determine which drug will be most effective
      - Flecainide and propranolol can be effective by decreasing conduction capability in both anterograde and retrograde limb
      - Amio and sotalol can increase ERP in both AV and AP → effective

2.8 GENESIS OF CARDIAC ARRHYTHMIAS (ANATOMY OF CARD. SYSTEM)

SA NODE
- Spindle shaped
- Closely packed cells
- 10–20 mm long
- 2–3 mm wide and thick
- Tends to narrow caudally towards FVC
- Lies <1 mm from epicardial surface at junction of SVC and RA (in right atrial sulcus terminalis)
- *Blood supply:* SA nodal Br from RCA (55–60% times)
  Or LCX (40–45% times)
- *Cellular str:*
  1. Spindle and spider-shaped cells
  2. Rod-shaped cell with striation
  3. Small round cell corresponding to endothelial cells
- Electrophysiological property of pacemaker cells

Function
Two theories:
1. Hyperpolarization activated cyclic nucleotide gated (HCN) ion channels are main regulator of HR
2. Intracellular Ca^{++} oscillations affects Ca^{++} sensitive ion channels and ion transporter in outer memb → diastolic depolarization → trigger propagating SA node AD.
- Mech of entrainment that enable synchronized electrical activity of multiple individual SA nodal cells to give rise to discharge of SA node has been uncertain
- Functioning of SA node as a pacemaker require delicate balance of intercellular electrical coupling.
- Connexin 40 and 45 expressed in central part of SA node. Major part of crista terminalis SA node border exhibits a sharp demarcation boundary of connexin 43 expressing SA nodal cells

↓

Disparate connexin create specific types of hybrid channels that ensures the maintenance of SA nodal pacemaker activity

↓

Electrical impulse originates in central part

↓

Spreads bidirectionally (1–14 con/sec) within tiny node

With failure to conduct laterally to crista terminalis and IAs

↓

After a delay of 50 milliseconds within SA node impulse reaches atrial myocardium via 2 main (superior and inferior) pathways

Innervation
- Densely innervated by postganglionic adrenergic and cholinergic nerve terminates.
- ACh, acetylcholinesterase and choline acetyltransferase (enzyme necessary for synthesis of acetylcholine) have been found in high core in SA node
- β_1, β_2 and muscarinic receptors present on SA node

Symp stimulation	Parasymp stimulation
↓	↓
B1	ACh
↓	↓
GTP	M2
↓	↓
GS	• Neg chronotropy
↓	• Increased infranodal conduction time
Positive chronotropy	• Increased refractoriness in center of SA node

AV NODE
- Normal AV junction area composed of
  - Transitional tissue
  - Inferior nodal extension
  - Compact portion
  - Penetrating bundle
  - HS bundle
  - Atrial and vent muscle
  - Central fibrous body
  - Tendon of Todaro
  - Valves
- Tract of nodal tissue divided into two major components
  1. Inferior nodal extension
     - Located between CS and TV
     - End of inf extension covered by transitional tissue
     - Myocyte in inf ext do not exhibit connexin 43 (while myocyte in transition zone exhibit connexin 43)
     - Inf nodal extension is cont with penetrating bundle
  2. Penetrating bundle
     - Continues from mf nodal extension
     - Penetrates fibrous tissue separating atria and ventricles
     - Emerge in ventricle as bundle of His
- Compact portion of AV node:
  - Superficial str lying just beneath the RA endocardium art to ostium of CS and directly above insertion of septal leaflet of TV

- It is at apex of triangle is formed by tricuspid annulus and tendon of Todaro
- Triangle of Koch:
  Superiorly: Tendon of Todaro
  Inferiorly: Attachment of septal leaflet of TV ;
  Fibrous commissure of the flap guarding openings of IVC and CS
  Bore: Mouth of CS
- *Blood supply:*
  - 85–90% branch from RCA
    - Originate at crux
  - 10–15% from LCX
- *Function:* Main function is to delay transmission of atrial impulse to ventricles.
- *EP:*

  Electrical impulse from SA node
  ↓
  Atrial tissue
  ↓
  Enters AV node at 2 points

  1. At the end of inferior nodal extension (most likely corresponds to fast pathway)
  2. Toward beginning of inferior nodal extension (slow pathway)

  [*Note:* AP can't enter nodal tissue at any other point because the nodal and atrial tissue are isolated from each other by a vein]
  ↓
  AP entering nodal tract via transitional zone also propagates into compact node and then reaches His bundle and propagates down to bundle branches

HIS BUNDLE

- Continuation of penetrating bundle on vent side
- *Blood supply:* Branches from LAD and PDA
  Supply upper muscular FVS
  ↓
  Makes this site more impervious to ischemia (unless ischemia is extensive)

BUNDLE BRANCHES

- Begins at margin (upper) of muscular IVS immediately beneath membranous septum

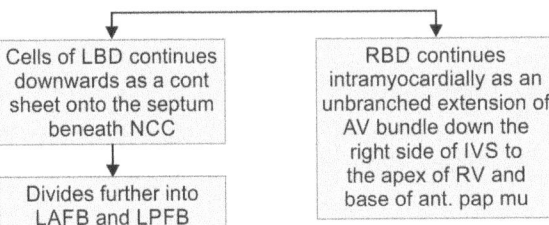

TERMINAL PURKINJE FIBERS

- Connects with ends of BB to form interweaving network on endocardial surface
- Less concentrated at base of ventricle and at papillary muscle tip.
- Penetrates only inner 1/3rd of endocardium
- More resistant to ischemia than ordinary fibers
- Are capable of contraction also
- *Main function:* Conduction of impulses
- AP propagates within Purkinje fibers from base to apex before activation of surrounding myocardium occurs
- Purkinje myocyte lacks transverse tubules
  - Fat conduction
- Propagation of AP within His-Purkinje system and working myocardium is mediated by connexins (vent myocyte 43 His Purkinje system-40 and 45)
- Innervations of AV node, His bundle and vent myo
- AV node and His bundle—rich supply of cholinergic and adrenergic fibers (density exceeds that found in vent myocardium)
  - *Sidedness:* Autonomic neural input to heart exhibit some sidedness
  - Rt sided sympathetic and vagus nerves affects SA node more
  - Left sympathetic nerve affects AV node more
    ↓
  - Stimulation of rt stellate ganglion → Tachycardia with less effect on AV nodal conduction
  - Stimulation of lt stellate ganglion generally produce a shift in sinus pacemaker to an ectopic site constantly shorter AV nodal conduction time e refractoriness
  - Stimulation of rt vagus primarily slows SA nodal discharge
  - *Stimulation of left vagus prolongs AV nodal conduction time and refractoriness*
- Neither sympathetic nor vagal stimulation affects conduction in His bundle
  - Neg dromotropic effect of vagal stimulation mediated via activation of I_{kAch} which result in hyperpolarization of nodal cells
  - Positive dromotropic effect of symp. Stimulation is due to increased cytoplasmic Camp and ensuring activation of L-type Ca^{++} channel

ARRHYTHMIAS AND ANS

Damage to nerves extrinsic to heart (stellate ganglion) and intrinsic cardiac nerves from disease that may affect primarily nerves (such as viral inf) or from disease that secondarily cause cardiac damage may produce cardiomyopathy

- Numerous studies have suggested primary role of altered cardiac sympathetic innervations in arrhythmogenesis
- In pt with HF→SNS is upregulated→leads to adv myocardial effect including arrhythmia

2.9 BRADYARRHYTHMIA

HYPERSENSITIVE CAROTID SINUS

ECG:
- Vent asystole often caused by cessation of atrial activity as a result of sinus arrest or SA exit block
- AV block noted less frequently because SA model dysfunction precludes its occurrence
- AV junction or vent escape generally do not occur +n1-ot very slow rates → suggesting that heightened vagal tone and sympathetic withdrawal can suppress subsidiary pacemaker located in vent as well

C/F—2 types:
1. *Cardioinhibitory:* Vent asystole exceeding 3 seconds.
2. *Vasodepressor:* Fall in SBP ≥ 50 mm Hg without associating cardiac slowing (or) decreasing in SBP > 30 mm Hg when pt's symptoms reproduced in elderly asymptomatic pt/pt with syncope CSM producing above finding may not be related as a cause of syncope always

↓

Direct pr on carotid sinus as a result of head turning, neck tension and tight collars can also be source of syncope by reducing blood flow to cerebral arteries
- Hypersensitive carotid sinus synd is mostly associated with CAD
- Mech of HCS syndrome is unknown

Management
- Atropine can abolish cardioinhibitory response
  - Most symptomatic pt req. PPI (some form of vent pacing) with or without atrial pacing is required
  - Atropine/PPI do not abolish vasodepressor reflex
  - In mixed form vasodepressor can continue to be a cause of syncope even after PPI
  - Elastic support hose and sodium retaining drugs may be helpful
- Asymptomatic pt → no treatment required

SICK SINUS SYNDROME
- Term applied to no. of sinus node abnormalities comprising
  1. Persistent spont sinus brady not caused by drugs and inappropriate for physical circumstances
  2. Sinus current or exit block
  3. Combination of SA and AV conduction disturbances
  4. Tachy-brady syndrome
- *Categorized as:*
  1. Intrinsic SA node disease unrelated to autonomic abnormalities or
  2. Combination of intrinsic and autonomic abnormalities
- *Causes:*
  - Children:
    - Long or acquired heart disease esp. after corrective surgical treatment can also occur in STR. Normal heart
- *Course:* Unpredictable because it is influenced by underlying heart disease
- *Anatomic basis:*
  1. Total or subtotal destruction of sinus node
  2. Areas of nodal-atrial discontinuity
  3. Inflammatory or degenerative changes in nerves or ganglia surrounding node
  4. Pathological changes in atria
  5. Occlusion of SA node atria
- Patho:
  - Fibrosis and fatty infiltration
  - Sclerodegen process involving SA and AV node
- Management
  - Asymptomatic → Observe
  - Symptomatic → PPI

AV BLOCK—SALIENT FEATURES
- Normal retrograde conduction can occur even in presence of advanced anterograde AV block
- High grade AV block ≥ 2 blocked consecutive impulses

First Block
- Sometimes PR can exceed PI interval

↓

Phenomenon known as skipped P waves
- Acceleration of atrial rate or enhancement of vagal tone by CSM can cause 1st degree AV block to progress to type 1 2 degree AV block

Second Degree Block
- During Wenckebach, increases in PR interval is greatest in 2nd beat of Wenckebach group and absolute increase in condition time decrease progressively over subsequent beats
- Classic Wenckebach group beats
  1. Interval between successive beats progressively decreases, although conduction time increases

2. Duration of pause produced by nonconducted impulse is less than twice the interval preceding the blocked impulse
3. The cycle that follows the nonconducted beats is longer than the cycle preceding the blocked impulse
   ↓
   The characteristics found in < 50% patients with type 1
   2 degree AV block

Type I AV block
- Benign ⎤
- Usually associated with IWMI ⎥ Almost drugs at AV node level
- Transient ⎥ Uncommonly type I infrahisian
- Do not request TPM ⎦

Type II AV block
- Associated with Stokes – Adams syndrome
- May progress to CHB ⎤
- Malignant ⎥ Localized to system His-Purkinje
- Associated with AWMI ⎥
- Requires TPM/PPM ⎥
- High mortality ⎦

Differentiation of type I from type II
1. 2:1 AV block can be type I or II
   - QRS normal → Type I
   - QRS with BBB morphology → Type II
2. AV block can occur simultaneously at 2 levels
3. If atrial rate varies it can alter conduction time and cause type I AV block to stimulate Type II block and vice-versa
4. Abrupt alteration in autonomic tone can cause block of 1 or more p waves without altering PR interval → Produce type II block clinically bust of vagal tone usually lengthens PP interval as well as produce AV block
5. CSM improves AV conduction ⎤
   Atropine worsens AV conduction ⎥ in patients with His-Purkinje block
   Exercise/Isoproterenol worsen AV conduction ⎦
   Opposite occurs in patients with nodal block
6. 1° AV block and Type I/2° AV block can occur in normal healthy children and trained athletes

Third Degree AV Block
- Atrial pacemaker can be sinus/ectopic or can result from AV junction region
- Vent focus is usually located just below region of block (can be above or below His bundle bifurcation)
- Acquired CHB rate = 40 BPM with congenital CHB → it can be higher
- CHB site of block can be at AV node (congenital) within bundle of His, or distal to it in Purkinje system (acquired)

Paroxysmal AV Block
- Hyper-responsiveness of AV node to vagal tone
- Surgery
- Electrolyte disturbance
- Myoendocarditis
- Tumors
- Chagas disease
- Calcific AS
- Myxedema
- Polymyositis
- Infiltrative process (amyloid, sarcoid)
- Tachy dependent AV block → Rapid rate can sometimes followed by block (due to phase 3 block) incomplete recovery.
- Pause dependent AV block → AV block after a pause or brady (due to phase 4 block)

Autonomic Modulation for Arrhythmias
1. *AF:*
   - BB
   - Ablation of ganglionated plexi
   - Symp. denervation
   - Renal denervation
2. *Acquired VT:*
   - BB
   - Partial and transient HCT Cardiac symp. denervation (Ropivacaine injection)
   - Renal denervation
   - Vagal stimulation (INNOVATE- HF and NECTAR- HF) Trials
   - Spiral cord stimulation (DEFEAT-HF)—ongoing

2.10 BRUGADA SYNDROME

CLINICAL MANIFESTATION

- Heritable arrhythmia syndrome
- Cored-type ST seg elevation (≥ 2 mm) followed by negative T wave in right precordial lead V_1–V_3 (referred as type-1 Brugada)
- Increased risk of SCD from PMVT.
- *C/F:* Lifelong asymptomatic to SCD during 1st year of life
- Involves young males
- Average age of 40 years
- SCD typically occurs during sleep

GENETICS

AD (~50%)
- 50% are sporadic
- Loss of function mutation in SCN5A (Brs Type-1) 20–30%
- Mutation can be
  1. Nonsense
  2. Missense
  3. Frame shift
  4. Splice site
  5. In frame deletion / insertion

  SCN5A mutation → Brs (Depends on other env. Or genetic modifying factors)

  ↓

  WTS.3
- 13 other Brs susceptibility gene has been identified decrease in inward Na^+ or Ca^{++} current or increase in outward K^+ current
- Mutation in interacting prot can also cause Brs for example, glycerol-3-phosphate dehydrogenase 1-like prot (GPDIL) → mutation → reduce overall Na^+ current → Brs

GENOTYPE-PHENOTYPE CORRELATE

- Not analyzed to the extent of LQTS
- SCN5A mutation associated with higher incidence of conduction abnormality in Brs patient
  Long PQ interval may be indicative of SCN5A mediated ⎤
  Short QT interval may be indicative of LTCC mediated Brs pathology ⎦ Brs1
- Genetic testing for Brs is limited due to relative absence of therapeutic contri. From knowledge of genotype

EARLY REPOLARIZATION SYNDROME

- Char. by ECG finding of elevation (≥ 1 mm) of QRS-ST junction (so called J point) manifested as either QRS slurring (at transition of QRS to ST segment) or notching (positive deflection inscribed on terminal S wave), ST segment elevation with upper concavity and prominent T waves in 2 or more contiguous leads
- Prev 1–13%
- J point elevation in IL lead was significantly over expressed and greater in magnitude in patient who experienced cardiac arrest 2° idiopathic VF
- M > F
- Syncope or CA in sleep
- Increase in risk for both cardiac death and arrhythmias
- Risk further elevated with increasing elevation pH J point (≥ 2 mm)
- ER pattern localized to only lateral leads did not show significant association with increase in risk for arrhythmic death

Genetics

- CACNA1C-12_p → voltage gated L-type Ca^{++} channel
- CACNA2D1-7_q → voltage gated L-type Ca^{++} channel δ subunit
- CACNB2-10_p → voltage gates L-type Ca^{++} channel B_2 δ subunit
- KCNJ8-12_p → inward rectifier K^+ channel KIR 6.1

SICK SINUS SYNDROME

- ANK-B-4q—Ankyrin-B
- HCN4-15q—Hyperpolarization activated cyclic nucleotide gated channel 4
- SCN5A-3p

BRUGADA SYNDROME

- Distinct form of idiopathic VF
- Patients have RBBB and ST elevation in Ant precordial leads
- Without any C/O Str heart disease
  Type 1: Coved ST segment
  Type 2: Saddle shaped
  Type 3: Saddle shaped
- ECG finding can be transient and subtle changes on ECG similar to these findings can be found in patient without Brugada

- Brs suspected in patient with type I ECG pattern m >1 right precordial lead (V_1 to V_2) if there is [1]Document VF, [2]Poly VT, [3]F/H/O SCD, [4]Brs pattern in other family members or [5]syncope
- Type 2 and 3 finding an ECG is not diagnostic of Brs
- If type 2 and 3 changes to Type 1 ECG with challenge with procainamide

↓

Consider Brs if above clinical criteria (AY.1)
Note: Quinidine has been shown to normalize ECG in patient with Brs B_1 blocking I_{TO}

Genetics

↓

SCN5A mutation and Ca^{++} channel mutation

↓

Heterogeneous loss of dome of AP in PV epicardium

↓

Propagation of dome from site where it is maintained to site where it is lost (Phase 2 re-entry)

↓

Vent arrhythmia

High-risk Group

- Spontaneous ECG pattern of Type 1 Brs
- HIO syncope
- Vent refractoriness < 200 msec
- QRS fragmentation

Treatment

1. ICD
2. Quinidine
3. Ablation

Characteristics of Br pattern:

	Type 1	Type 2	Type 3
J wave amplitude	≥2 mm	≥2 mm	≥2 mm
J wave	Negative	positive/biphasic	positive
ST.T configuration	cored	saddle back	saddle back
ST segment terminal portion	Gradually descending	Elevated ≥1 mm	Elevated ≥1 mm

2.11 CATECHOLAMINERGIC POLYMORPHIC VENTRICULAR TACHYCARDIA

INTRODUCTION
- Heritable arrhythmia syndrome
- Manifested as ex-induced syncope or SCD
- Predominantly in young pt (infancy to 40 years)
- Closely mimic phenotype of LQT1
- More fatal than LQT1
- Swimming is also potential trigger

ELECTROCARDIOGRAPHY
- Complete normal resting ECG
  - May show bradycardia and mild U wave
  - Postexercise (catecholamine stress)
  - Shows vent ectopy/(bidirectional VT)
    ↓
  (Pathognomic) of CPVT

DIAGNOSIS
Ex induced syncope and QTC ≤ 460 milliseconds should prompt suspicion of CPVT (rather than so called concealed LQT or normal QT interval LQT1)

Ex induced bigeminy are more common than bidirectional VT associated with structurally normal heart

PROGNOSIS
Highly lethal
- Mortality rate 30–50% by age 35 years
- Positive F/H/O SCD in young in >33% pts

GENETICS
60%-   CPVT1-RYR_2-1_q-Ryanodine receptor-2
(AD)   CPVT2-CASQ-1_p-Calsequestrin 2
         CPVT3-KCNT-2-17_q-I_{K1} K^+ channel
AR   CALM-1-14_q-calmodulin-1
Form   TRDN-6_q—triadin

Components of Ca^{++} induced Ca^{++} release from SR serves as basis for pathogenesis of CPVT
- (AD) inheritance
- CPVT-1 (RYR_2 mutation) is most common

Gain of function mutation
↓
Leaky calcium release channels
↓
Excessive release of Ca^{++} esp during sympathetic stimulation
↓
Calcium overload
↓
Delayed after depolarization
↓
Vent arrhythmias

Surgical treatment cardiac symp denervation was shown to be effective in CPVT.

CATECHOLAMINERGIC POLYMORPHIC VENTRICULAR TACHYCARDIA
- Uncommon
- Occurs in absence of overt str heart disease
- Mutation in RYR_2 or calsequestrin
- Syncope or aborted SCD
- During exercise typical response include initial S.TACH and vent extrasystole followed by MMVT or bidirectional VT
  - Eventually PMVT if ex. continued
  - Treatment BB and ICD/flecainide (inhibit RYR_2 receptor)

2.12 DIAGNOSIS OF CARDIAC ARRHYTHMIAS

HISTORY

- *Palpitation:*
  - Syncope
  - Presyncope
  - Dyspnea
- *Mode of onset*
  - Provide clues about type of arrhythmias

Example:
- Palpitation caused in setting of exercise Fright or anger are often caused by catecholamine sensitive automatic or triggered tachycardia
- Palpitation at rest → vagal inhibition such as AF
- Syncope in tightly fitting collar showing the neck for turning head → carotid sinus hypersensitivity
- *Mode of termination:* Terminated by Valsalva or vagal maneuver or breath-holding → Arrhythmia involves AV node as part of tachy circuit
- Freq and severity of symptoms
- Characteristics of palpitation
  - Rapid/ slow
  - Regular/irregular
- Drug and dietary history
  - Nasal decongestant can cause tachycardia
  - BB eye drops may cause bradycardia
- Presence of systemic illness
  - OPD, thyrotoxicosis pericarditis CHF
- F/H LQTS, AF, HCM, muscular myotonic dystrophy

PHYSICAL EXAMINATION

- *HR and BP:* HD stable or not
- JVP and waveforms
  - Cannon a wave in CHB
- Maneuvers
  - Valsalva
  - Carotid sinus massage
  - vagal stimulation
- Focal AT and VT occasionally terminates in response to vagal stimulation
- S Tachy close slightly but returns to its original rate soon
- VR during AF slows transiently
- Terminates AVRT/AVNRT
- Blocks VA conduction—establish diagnosis of VT by demonstrating AV dissociation

ECG

- Primary tool
- Determine tachy or bradyarrhythmias

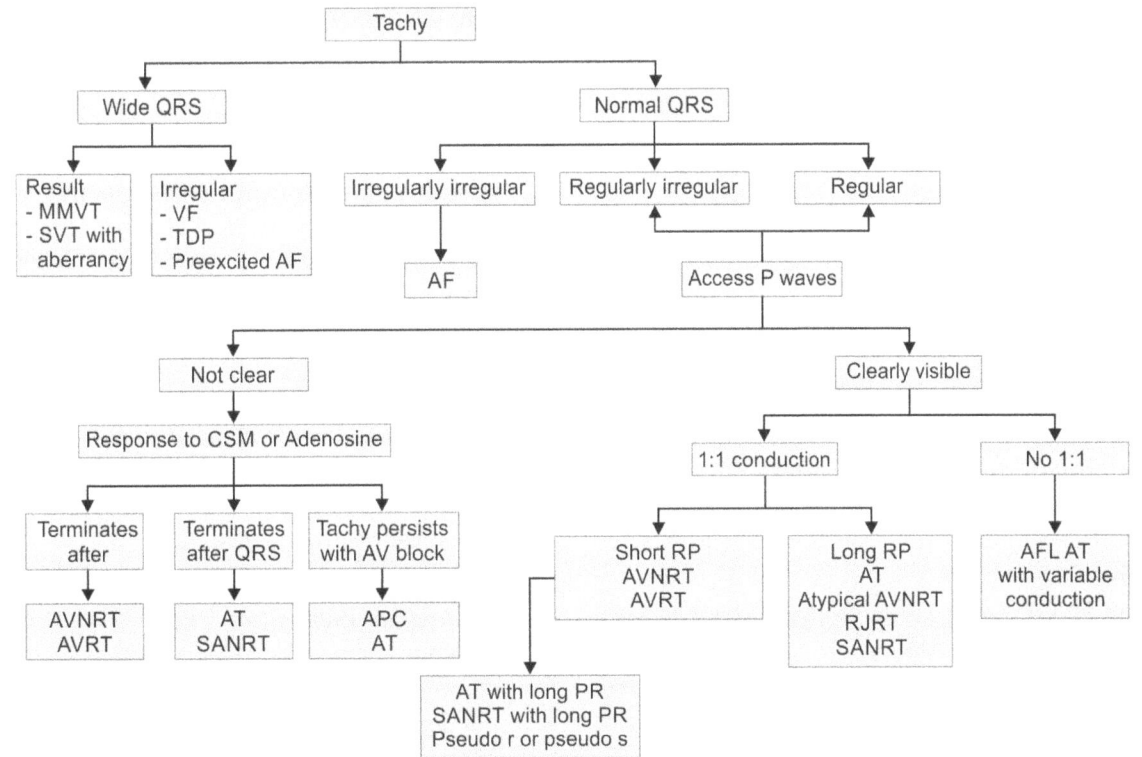

Wide QRS Tachy

Favors SVT with aberrancy	Favors VT
• Initiation with premature P	• Initiation with premature QRS
• Tachy complex identical to those in resting rhythm	• Tachy beats identical to PVCs during SR
• Long short sequence preceding changes in RR interval	• Short long sequence preceding changes in PP interval
• QRS contour consistent with aberrant conduction	• QRS inconsistent with aberrant conduction
• Slowing or termination with vagal	• AV dissociation or non 1:1 relation
• Onset with QRS to peak <50 ms	• Onset with QRS to peak >50 ms
• QRS d ≤ 0.14 ms	• QRSd >140 ms
	• LAD (−90–180°)
	• Concordant R wave pattern
	• Contract BBB (for resting rhythm)
	• Initial R, q or r >40 ms Or notched Q in a awR
	• Absence of rs complex in Or precordial ed

- Special Tech
  - Lewis led to demonstrate hidden P
  - Esophageal electrode
  - Intra-atrial ECG
  - Ladder diagram derived from ECG
    - Used to depict the depolarization and conduction schematically
    - Straight or slightly slanting line drawn on framework

EXERCISE TESTING

- Can induce various types of SVT and VT
- VPC develop in 1/3rd of normal person in response to exercise testing
- 3-6 beats of VT can also occur in normal person
  - Does not predict presence of IHO of or structural heart disease or predicts increased CV mortality or morbidity
- Persistent elevation of HR postexercise is associated with worse CV prognosis
- Frequent DVC (>7/min) or complex ectopy e is associated with worse prognosis
- Prolonged amputate retesting is more sensitive than exercise test stress testing is frequently useful in patients with LQTS and CPVT

IN HOSPITAL ECG RECORDING

Holter Monitoring

- Recording for 24-48 hours
- Symptomatic events and important findings (asymptomatic)
- Frequent PVC >1 5% of total had been shown as marker of cardiomyopathy and HF
- Frequent and complex PVC post MI or associated with two to five fold increase risk of cardiac or SCD in patient forth MI
- CAST showed that suppression of such PVC with flecainide and encainide was associated with increased mortality

Event Recorder

- Device are about the size of a page
- Kept by patients for 30 days
- Monitoring can be made during symptomatic period and transmitted to receiving station over a standard telephone line at patients convenience
- 30-60 seconds recording can be saved when event button pressed by a person
- Only one channel is recorded usually

Drawback

If syncope occurs without warning and patient is unable to stress response button—device can't provide data about the event with some system device continuous to begin automatic recording with change in the rate outside preset parameters some system automatically notify central system about extreme Tachy/brady.

Implantable Loop Recorder

- For patient with very in frequent symptoms
- Device is inserted under skin at about second rib of left front aspect of chest and is activated by passing a special magnet over device
- Record up to 42 minutes (1 to 7 episodes)
- Single channel recorded
- Up to 20 minutes of free activation ECG can be saved
- Saved data can be downloaded to a programming unit for analysis
- Device can save patient activated episode as well as automatically activated recording

Various parameters of interest:
- *Heart rate variability:*
  - Used to evaluate vagal and sympathetic influence on SA node and to identify patients at risk of CV Events or death
  - Freq domain and time domain analysis

- RR variability predicts all case mortality, LVEF nonsustained VT inpatient post MI
- Reduce RR variability → marker of increased risk
- Indicates loss of physiologic periodic SA node fluctuations
- *HR turbulence:*
  - Index of change in sinus discharge rate after a PVC that is followed by compensatory pause
  - *Normal:* SR initially accelerates and then slows
    ↓
  - This is absent or blunted in patient with various heart disease
  - HR turbulence is a measure of reflex vagal control of the heart whereas HR variability is measure of overall vagal tone
  - Abnormal HR turbulence → Predictor of mortality
- *QT dispersion:*
  - Difference between longest and shortest QT on 12-lead ECG can be adjusted for HR and number of leads sampled
  - Abnormal high QT dispersion → high mortality

SIGNAL AVERAGED ECG AND LATE POTENTIAL

- Signal averaging method to improve signal to noise ratio
- Require appropriate filtering and other method of noise reduction can detect cardiac signal of few microvolt in amplitude and reduced noise amplitude such as muscle potential
- Very low amplitude electrical potential generated by the sinus node AV not His bundle and BB can be detected
- In patients with prev MI → Conclusion is slowed → damaged areas are activated later → this led potential can be recorded by SA ECG criteria for late potentials
  - Filtered QRSd >114–120 ms
  - <20 mV of root mean square signals amplitude in last 40 msec of filtered QRS
  - Terminal filter QRS remaining below 40 mv for >3.9 ms
- Late potential can be detected as early as 3 hours after onset of coronary occlusion; increase in prevalence in patient week after MI and disappeared in same after 1 year
- Late potential also reported in patient with VT not related to ischemia (example DCMP)
- Late potential—Sensitive but not specific
    ↓
    Limited prognostic use
- In patient with suspected ARVD and IWMI
    ↓
- Absence of late potential suggest very low arrhythmia risk overall use is limited at present
5. *T wave alteration*
   - Beat to beat alteration in amplitude and morphology of ST segment and T wave
   - Found in condition following dev of VT such as ischemia LQTS
   - *Electrophysio basis*: Alteration of repolarization of vent myocyte (beat to beat repol changes in mid myocardial cells)
   - *Method*: Testing required to exercise for atrial pacing (HR >120 bpm)
   - Positive T wave alterations → worse arrhythmic prognosis
   - Negative test → strongly predict freedom from VT and VF in all groups low risk of life-threatening arrhythmia

BARORECEPTOR REFLEX TESTING

- Increase in sinus cycle length per mm Hg increase in SBP is measure of sensitivity of baroreceptor reflex
- Decreased baroreceptor sensitivity → identify patient susceptible to VT/VF

BODY SURFACE MAPPING

- Used to define complete picture of effects of current from heart to body surface
- Used clinically to:
  - Localize and size area of MI
  - Localize ectopic foci
  - Localize AP
  - SVT with arbitrary vs VT
  - Recognize patient at risk of arrhythmia
- Technique is cumbersome and analysis is complex

TILT TABLE TEST

(Read from chapter of syncope)

ESOPHAGEAL ECG

- Record atrial potentials
- Occasionally pacing can also be done
- When recorded simultaneously with surface ECG St can be used to differentiate SVT with arbitrary from VT

INVASIVE EP STUDY

Tech: Introducing multipolar electrodes in venous or arterial system position them at various intracardiac site records or stimulate cardiac electrical activity.

False negative = not finding a particular electrical abnormality known to be present
False positive = induction of nonclinical arrhythmia

Sinus Node: Dysfunction

- EPS considered inpatient with symptoms attributable to bradycardia or asystole
- Demonstration of slow sinus rate sinus exit block or sinus pauses related to symptoms suggests a casual relationship and do not require EP testing
- Carotid sinus hypersensitivity also do not repair EP study

Parameters to be Checked

- *SNRT:* Sinus node recovery time
- *SACT:* Sinoatrial conduction time

SNRT: Interval between last paced high RA response and first (spontaneous) sinus high RA response after termination of pacing spontaneous SR influences SNRT

So value is corrected by subtracting spontaneous sinus node cycle length (before pacing) from SNRT corrected SNRT <5-25 ms

SA nodal dysfunction:
- CSNRT increases
- Secondary pauses after first return sinus cycle

SACT:
- Estimated by simple pacing technique based on the assumptions that
  1. Conduction time into and out of SA node is equal
  2. No depression of SA nodal automaticity
  3. Pacemaker site it doesn't shift after premat stimulation

  Normal result doesn't exclude sinus node disease
  - SNRT and SACT can also be calculated directly with special recording techniques
  - Sensitivity of SNRT and SACT is 50%
  - Also measure AV nodal parameters in patient with SA node dysfunction

AV Node Dysfunction

- AH interval (measure of AV nodal conduction time)—60-125 ms
- HV interval (measure of infranodal conduction)—35-55 ms

Indications

- Symptomatic patients in whom His Purkinje block suspected but not established
- Patients with AV block treated with pacemaker but continue to be symptomatic

Tachycardia

EPS can be used to:
- Diagnose arrhythmia
- Determine and deliver therapy
- Establish anatomic site involved
- Identify patients at high risk of serious arrhythmia
- To gain insight into mech of arrhythmia

SVT → HV interval equals or exceeds that recording during NSR.

VT → HV interval shorter than normal his deflection can't be recorded clearly because of superimposition of large ventricular electrogram consistently short HV interval occasion (only two):
1. During retrograde activation of HS bundle from activation originating in ventricle (example PVC vent pasting VT)
2. During AV conduction over AP (preexcitation)

VT → atrial pacing at higher rate than VT can demonstrate wide QRS Tachy by producing fusion and capture beats and normalization of HV interval.

Only VT that exhibit HV interval equal to or slightly exceeding normal sinus HV interval is bundle branch reentry.

Indications for EDS

- Patient with symptomatic recurrent or dry resistant SVT Or VT
- In patient with tachyarrhythmias occurring too in frequently
- To diff SVT with aberrancy from VT
- Whenever nonpharmacological treatment example electric device catheter ablation for surgical treatment is contemplated
- Patient surviving an episode of cardiac arrest occurring >48 hours after AMI
- For assessment of risk of sustained VT in patient with prev MI EF < 40% and NSVT on ECG

Unexplained Syncope

- 3 common causes: SA node dysfunction, AV block and tachyarrhythmias
- EPS helps when it can induce arrhythmia that can replicate patient symptoms or is associated with significant hypotension
- When tachyarrhythmias have been thoroughly sought and excluded and clinical suspicion for AV block is high → PPI may be justified
- In patient with nondiagnostic EPS Injection of adenosine, triphosphate (diff from adenosine) distinguishes patient who may benefit from permanent pacing from those who may not benefit

Palpitation

EPS indicated in patients with palpitation who have had a pulse documented by medical personnel to be inappropriately rapid or slow.

Complications of EPS

- Small risk
- Myocardial perforation with tamponade
- Pseudoaneurysm at arterial site
- System thromboembolic complication (AF ablation)
- Valve damage
- Phrenic nerve injury

Direct Cardiac Mapping

- Recording potentials directly from heart
- Potentials are specially depicted as a function of time in integrated manner
- Location of recording electrode epicardial/intramural/endocardial
- Recording mode unipolar/bipolar
- Method of display isopotential, isochronal, unipolar, bipolar, voltage maps

Conditions amenable for diagnosis
- AP in WPW
- Pathway of AVNRT
- AV-node His bundle ablation
- Focal AT
- AF
- Mapping information required in this way can be displayed on the screen to show relative activation time in color coded sequence
- Dozens or even hundreds of site can be sampled quickly
- Some mapping system can acquire data from several thousand points simultaneously
- Current mapping system have the ability to both integrate previous imaging studies (CT/MRI) into the procedure for additional anatomic reference and derived anatomic information by having a catheter throughout a cardiac chamber

2.13 THERAPY FOR CARDIAC ARRHYTHMIAS

VAUGHAN WILLIAMS CLASSIFICATION

Class I: Predominantly Block Fast Na⁺ Channels

They can also block K⁺ channels.

Class IA:
- Reduce Vmax [rate of rise in AP upstroke (phase 0)]
- Prolongs APD
- Kinetics of onset and offset in blocking Na⁺ channel is intermediate rapidly (<5 seconds)
- Quinidine, procainamide, and disopyramide

Class IB:
- Does not reduce Vmax
- Shorten APd
- Kinetics of onset and offset in blocking Na⁺ channel is rapid (<500 sec)
- Mexiletine, Phenytoin, Lidocaine

Class Ie:
- Reduce Vmax
- Slow conduction velocity
- Prolong refractoriness minimally
- Slow onset and offset (10–20 seconds)
- Flecainide and propafenone

Class IIa:
- Block beta adrenergic receptors
- Propranolol, metoprolol, nadolol, nebivolol, carvedilol

Class III:
- Predominantly blocks K⁺ channel prolong repolarization
- Sotalol, amiodarone, dronedarone, ibutilide

Class IV:
- Predominantly blocks slow Ca⁺⁺ channel
- Verapamil, diltiazem, nifedipine
  Classification based on modification of vulnerable parameter

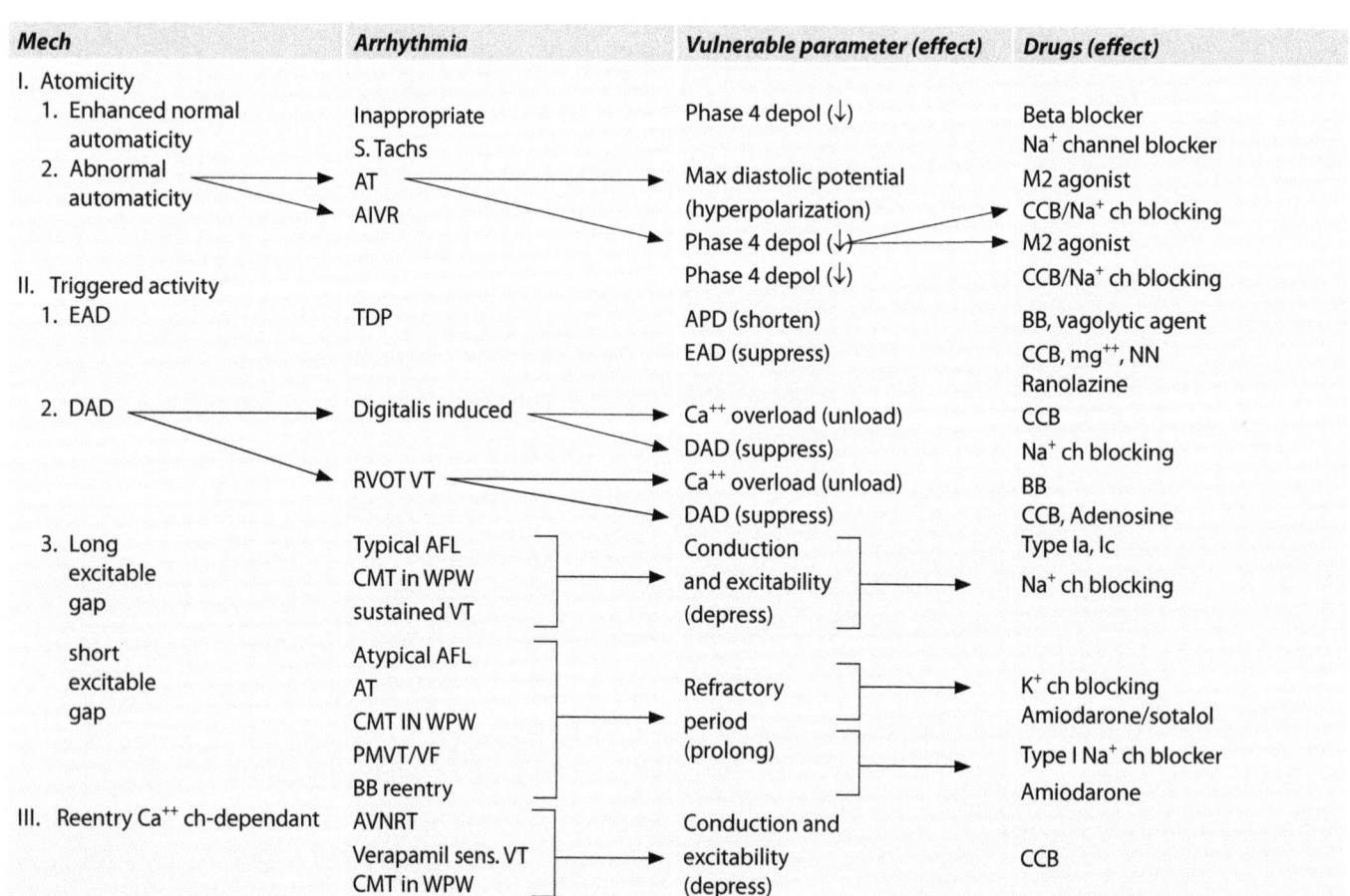

Antiarrhythmic (In General)

- **Use dependence:**
  - Some drugs exert greater inhibitory affects on the upstroke of AP at more rapid rates of stimulation and after longer period of stimulation → k/as use dependence
  - Use dependence means the depression of Vmax is greater after the channel has been "used" (i.e., AP depol rather than after a rest period)
  - Class IB agents exhibit fast onset and offset and have use dependent block of fast channels
  - Class IC drugs (slow kinetics) and class IA drugs (Intermediate Kinetics)
    ↓

  With increased time spent in diastole (slower rate) a greater portion of receptors become drug free and drug exert less effect

- **Reverse use dependence:**
  - Some drugs exert greater effect at slower rate → known as reverse use dependence
  - True for drugs that lengthen depol
  - QT interval becomes prolonged at lower HR than higher
    ↓

  Effect is not what ideal antiarrhythmic agent would do. Ideally it should prolong QT at higher HR to terminate and prevent arrhythmia.

- **MOA:**
  - Antiarrhythmics can slow spont discharge frequency of automatic pacemaker cell by depressing slope of diastolic depolarization → shifting threshold voltage towards zero or hyperpolarizing memb potential
  - Most antiarrhythmic drugs depress automatic firing rate of ectopic size while minimally affecting discharge rate of normal SA node
    - CCB and BB and amiodarone also depress spont. Discharge of sinus node
    - Disopyramide and quinidine (vagolytic effect) → increases sinus discharge rate
  - Antiarrhythmics also prevent/stop re-entry, e.g.,
    1. Improving conduction can eliminate unidirectional block so that reentry cannot begin
    2. Improving conduction facilitates conduction in reentrant loop so that returning wave front reenters too quickly → encounter cells that are still refractory → circuit breaks
    3. Drugs that decreases conduction can transform unidirectional block into bidirectional block and terminate re-entry

- **Proarrhythmia:**
  - Can be manifested as
    - Increase in freq. of preexisting arrhythmia
    - Sustaining of prev nonsustained arrhythmia
    - Development of new arrhythmia
  - Electrophysiologic Mech
    - Prolongation of repolarization
    - Increase in transmural dispersion of repolarization
    - Development of EAD → Tdp
    - Alteration in reentrant pathway
  - *Incidence:* 5-10 % pt receiving antiarrhythmic agents
    - HF increases risk ⎤
    - Reduced LVEF   ⎥ Increased
    - Treatment with digitalis and diuretics ⎬ risk of drug induced VF
    - Longer pretreatment QT ⎦
    - Profile
      1. Incessant VT ⎤ Within several days of
         Long QT synd ⎬ beginning treatment
         Tdp   ⎦ or changing dosage
      2. Late proarrhythmic effects may be related to drug induced exacerbation of the regional myocardial conduction delay caused by ischemia and due to heterogeneous conduction that can provoke reentry

Class IA Agents

- **Quinidine**
  - Blocks – Rapid inward Na+ channel
    - Ikr
    - Ito
  - To a lesser extent ⎱ Slow inward Ca^{++} channel
    - Iks
    - ATP sensitive K$^+$ channel
  - EP action:
    - Little effect on automaticity of SA node
    - Suppress automaticity in normal Purkinje fibers
    - In pt with SSS → pt can depress sinus node automaticity
    - Produces EAO → responsible for Tdp
    - Can reflexely increase SA nodal discharge rate and improve AV node conduction
    - Reverse use dependence (increases repol at slow HR) because of Na$^+$ channel
    - Also use dependence block because of block of Na$^+$ channel
    - Also blocks Ito → responsible for suppressing vent arrhythmia in Brugada

- HD effect: Vasodilatation by blocking α receptor significant hypotension
- Pharmac IV (Avoid Ion dose)
  - 80% P.P. Bound
  - Both liver and kidney remove quinidine
  - Elimination t1/2 = 5-8 hours
- Indi:
  - Previously used to treat premolar supravent and vent complexes
  - ↓
  - Because of its s/e and potential for causing TDP
  - ↓
  - Use had been restricted to
  1. Treat 1 degree VF
  2. Vent arrhythmias in pt with pros
  3. Sqt related arrhythmias
- S/E:
  - (MC) GI induced N/V/D, abd pain, anorexia
  - *CNS:* Tinnitus, hearing loss, visual disturbances, confusion, delirium and psychosis
  - Allergic reaction
  - CVS:
    - Slow cardiac conduction
    - Prolonged QPSD/sinus external/AV conduction
    - Prolong QT significantly
    - Syncope

- *Procainamide:*
  - *EP Action:*
    - Resembles Quinidine
    - Predominantly block inactivated state of INa
    - Prolongs ERP more than it prolongs APD prevent reentry
    - Does not affect normal 8A node automaticity
    - NADA, metabolic of Procainamide acts as class III action (Ikr blocker) and prolongs APD
  - *Dose:* Oral/IM: 25-50 mg over 1 min → repeat every 5 minutes until arrhythmia controlled, hypotension ensues or QPsd increases >50%
  - Indi:
    - Supravent and arrhythmia
    - Conversion of recent onset AF to NSR
    - Prior treatment with BB/CCD is recommended to prevent acceleration of VR
      - Can block conduction in AP of WPW
      - Can block His-Purkinje conduction → used during EP to stress His Purkinje system to check for need for PPI
      - More effective than lidocaine in terminating sustained VT.

- Diagnostic use:
  1. In pt with BrS suspected with normal resting ECG → Drug infusion results in characteristic Brugada syn.
  2. In pt with WPW drug causes sudden loss of preexcitation → suggest AP with long ERP → Low risk pt
- S/E:
  - aI S/E are less frequent
  - Rash, myalgia, digital vasculitis and Raynaud
  - Fever, agranulocytosis
  - CNS S/E less frequent
  - Various conduction disturbance
  - NAPA can cause prolonged QT and Tdp
  - Arthralgia, rash, pleuropericarditis, hepatomegaly and hemorrhagic pericardial effusion described in SLE like syndrome related to procainamide (slow acetylator group)
- Disopyramide
- Ajmaline

Class IB Agents

- Lidocaine
  - EP action:
    - Blocks Ina
    - Rapid onset and offset kinetics
    - Does depress abnormal automaticity and EAD/DAD in Purkinje fibers
    - Faster rate of stimulation ⎤
    - Reduced PH   ⎥ Changes that can
    - Increased extracellular K⁺ conc ⎥ result from ischemia
    - Decreased memb potential   ⎦
    - Increased ability of lidocaine to block Na⁺ channels
    - Convert unidirectional block to bidirectional block → inhibit development of UF
    - Lidocaine has little effect on atrial fiber and does not affect conduction AP.
  - Pharmac: Only parenterally
    - Hepatic metabolism
    - Elimination $t_{1/2}$ = ⎤ 1-2 hours
      ⎦ >10 hours in HF
    - Maintenance dose decreases to 1/3rd in pt with decreased EF.
  - *Dose:*
    - *Bolus:* 1-2 mg/kg body weight at a rate of 20-50 mg/min
    - *2nd stg:* Half dose 20-40 minutes later

- If required 2 more boluses can be given 5 minutes apart
  Maintenance: 1-4 mg/min
  Reduce dose in pt with HF and cardiogenic shock
- Indi:
  - Efficacy against vent arrhythmia
  - Rarely effective for SVT/MMVT
- S/E:
  - Dizziness, paresthesia, confusion, delirium, stupor, coma, seizure SA node depolarization and His Purkinje Block

■ *Mexiletine:* Local anesthetic congener of ledexaine with anticonvulsant properties
- *EP action:*
  - Similar to lidocaine
  - Shorten APD and ERP of Purkinje fibers
  - Depress Vmax of phase 0 (Ina blocking)
  - Does not affect SA nodal automaticity in normal portion in pt with SA nodal disease → Severe sinus brady and abnormal SNRT
  - Does not affect AV nodal conduction
  - Does not affect atrial AP
  - Does not affect QT
- HD effect
  No major HD effect
- *Dose:*
  - 200 mg every 8 hourly when rapid arrhythmia control is not essential
  - Can be increased or decreased by 50-100 mg every 2-3 d
  - Max 1200 mg/d
- *Indi:*
  - Acute and chronic VT
  - But not SVT
  - LQT3
  - Very useful in child with CHD and vent arrhythmia
- *S/E:*
  - Tremor, dysarthria, dizziness, paresthesia, diplopia, nystagmus, confusion, coma
  - Hypotension, Brady and exacerbation of arrhythmias

■ *Phenytoin:*
- *EP action:*
  - Abolish abnormal automaticity caused by digital induced DAD in Purkinje fibers
  - Suppress certain digitalis induced arrhythmias
  - Some of effect may be neurally mediated because it can modulate with time and vagnus efferent activity
- *Dose:*
  - 100 mg IV over 5 minutes until arrhythmia is controlled, 1 g has been given or adv effect develop
  - JVP line to avoid phlebitis
  - Oral:
    - 1000 mg loading on D1
    - 500 mg on D2 and D3
    - 300-400 mg there after
- *Indi:*
  - To treat atrial and vent arr. caused by digitalis
  - Less effective for vent arr. caused by ischemia or nondigitalis drugs

Class IE Agents

■ *Flecainide:*
- *EP action:*
  - Blocks rapid Na^+ channel → decreased Vmax
  - Slow onset-offset kinetics → marked drug effect occur at physiological HR
  - Sinus node function remains unchanged in normal person.
  - Conduction time in atria, ventricles, AV node and His-Purkinje system prolonged
  - Shorten diversion of AP in Purkinje fiber but prolongs it in vent muscle
  - In high dose also inhibit slow Ca^{++} channels
  - Minimal increase in QT interval
  - Anterograde and retrograde refractoriness in AP can increase significantly
  - Flecainide can facilitate or inhibit reentry and transform AF to APC
- *HD effect:*
  - Depress cardiac performance esp in pt with compromised vent syst function
  - Should be used cautiously/Avoid in pt with mod-severe IV dysfunction
- Pharmac elimination $t_{1/2}$ = 20 hours
- *Dose:*
  - Starting dose 100 mg every 12 hours
  - Increase in increments of 50 mg BD every 3-4 d
  - Max 400 mg/d
- *Indication:*
  - Life-threatening VT
  - SVT (AT, AFL)
  - Paroxysmal AF
  - CPVT
  - Effective in totally suppression VPC/NSVT
    (*Flecainide produces use dependent prolongation of VT cycle length ≥ improve H.D. tolerance)
    (*Imp to slow VR before flecainide in AF to avoid 1:1 AV conduction of slowed APC)

- Fetal arrhythmias and arrhythmias in children
- Diagnostic for Brugada synd
- S/E:
  - Proarrhythmic effect
  - Marked slowing of conduction
  - Negative inotropic effect
  - pt with SA node dysfunction develops sinus arrest
- Propafenone:
  - EP action:
    - Blocks fast Na^+ current in use dependent manner in Purkinje fibers and to a lesser degree in vent muscle
    - Use dependent action ≥ ability to terminate AF
    - Decreased excitability (AH, HV, QRS interval increases)
    - Suppress automaticity and triggered activity
    - Weak blocker of I_{Kr} and beta receptors
    - QT increases because of increase in QPSD
    - Effect greater on ischemia than in normal tissue
  - *HD effect:* Negative inotropic action
  - Worsening symptoms in pt with LV dysfunction
  - *Dose:*
    - 150–300 mg 8 hourly
    - Max 1200 mg/d
    - $t_{1/2}$ = 5–8 hours
  - Indi:
    - Paroxysmal SVT
    - AF
    - Life-threatening VT/VF
    - Suppress spont PVC and NSVT
    - Acetic termination of AF (600 mg single oral dose)
  - S/E:
    - Proarrhythmic response (less than flecainide)
    - Dizziness, disturbance in taste, blurred vision
    - GI S/E

Class II Agents

Beta Blockers

- Metoprolol, Propranolol, carvedilol, atenolol, esmolol
  - Decreases overall mortality and SCD post MI
  - Nadolol particularly effective for pt with LQTS
  - Low dose → selectively block β_1
  - High dose → Blocks both β_1 and β_2
  - Some BB has intrinsic sympathomimetic activity (As effective as BB without ISA)
  - EP Action:
    1. Competitively inhibit catecholamine binding to β-receptor
    2. Direct memb stabilizing action occurs at core 10 times than the dose need to block β-receptor ≥ Insignificant antiarrhythmic role
    3. Also block ICaL stimulated by β agonists
    4. Propranolol can flows normal automaticity in SA node and Purkinge fibers
  - Conc. That causes BB but no memb stabilizing effect
    ↓
    Do not alter
    1. Resting memb potential
    2. Max diastolic potential
    3. Vmax
    4. Repol
    5. Refractoriness
  - Conc exceeding 3 mg/mL (due to depression of Ina)
    - Depress Vmax, AP amplitude, memb responsiveness, conduction in atrial, vent and Purkinje fibers
    - Do not alter RMP
    - Slows sinus discharge rate sever brady occ. Results if the heart is dependent on symp. Tone or if SA node is dysfunctional
    - PR interval increases
    - AV nodal conduction time increases
    - AV node ERP and functional RP T
    - Refractoriness and conduction in His Purkinje system remains unchanged even at high dose
    - Do not affect conduction in vent ≥ No effect on QT or QPSd
  - Indication:
    - *IV:* 0.25–0.5 mg (increasing to 1.0 mg if req) every 5 minutes effect or side effect develops
    - Arrhythmia association with thyrotoxicosis or pheochroma
    - Arrhythmia related to catecholamines surge, e.g., those initiated by cocaine, exercise, emotion, etc.
    - Rate control in AF
    - Inappropriate sinus Tach, AT   can slow or
      AVRNI, AVRT   terminate
    - LQTS
    - CPVT
    - Can be effective for digitalis induced arrhythmias such as AT, DVCs, VT, nonparoxysmal AVJET.

Class III Agents

Amiodarone

- EP action:
  - (Chronic) Prolongs APD and refractoriness of all cardiac fibers without affecting RMP.
    (Acute) Amio and its metabolite (desethylamiodarone) prolong APD of vent muscle but shorten APD of Purkinje

- Decreases Vmax by use-dependent block of inactivated Na⁺ channel
- Decreases SA nodal discharge rate and prolong AV conduction time
- *Use dependence action:* Blocks conduction at fast rate more than at slow rate.
- Time dependent effect on refractoriness.
- Desethylamiodarone has relatively greater effect on fast channel tissue → contribute significantly to antiarrhythmic action if this metabolic not generated rapidly delay in antiarrhythmic activity
- Other action:
  - Noncompetitive antagonist α and β receptor
  - Blocks conversion of T4 to T3
  - Slows tiny rate by 20-30y.
  - Prolong QT interval
  - Changing contour of T wave
  - Produce U wave
  - ERP of all cardiac muscle increases ⎫
  - HV interval increases, QPSD increases ⎬ Less with oral disease
  - AV nodal conduction time CPR increases ⎭
  - Additionally
    Blocks Ina (Class I action)
    Antiadrenergic (Class II action)
    Blocks ICaL (Class IV action)
  - Amiodarone action approximates those of ideal antiarrhythmic
- Use dependent Na⁺ channel blockade with fast diastolic recovery from block and use dependent prolongation of APD
- *HD effect:* Peripheral and coro vasodilators
  IV—decreases HR, SVR, Lr contractility and LV dp/dt
  Oral—no not depress contractility.
- Pharmac:
  - Peak conc 3-7 hours after oral dose
  - Hepatic extraction
  - Extensive hepatic metabolism
  - Accumulate in liver, lung, fat, blue skin
  - Renal extraction is negligible
  - Not palpable
  - (IV) → onset of action within 1.2 hours
    (oral) → onset of action in 2-3 days (often 1-3 weeks)
  - Elimination t1/2—multiphasic
    - Initial 50% reduction in 3-10 d
    - Terminal half-life—26-107 d (53 days)
    - To achieve steady state conc. Without loading dose takes about 265 days

- *Dose:*
  i. 800-1200 mg/d for 1-3 weeks
     - 400 mg/d for next several weeks
     - 300 mg/d maintenance after 2-3 months
  ii. IV:
     - 15 mg/min for 10 minutes
     - 1 mg/min for 6 hours
     - 0.5 mg/min for 18 hours
  Supplement infusion of 150 mg over 10 minutes can be used for breakthrough VT/VF can be continue up to 2-3 weeks
  Caution: pt with decreased VVEF
- Indi:
  - SVT and VT termination and prevention
  - Useful in improving survival in pt with HCM, asymptomatic vent arr post MI, vent arr during or after resuscitation
  - Superior to class I and sotalol in maintains, SR in pt with AF.
  - Fewer shocks of FCD if concomitant Amio
- S/E:
  - 75% of pt
  - Most are reversible
    - Pulm toxicity more severe
      - Unclear mech
      - May be hypersensitivity reaction
      - Amiodarone must be discontinued
      - Uncommon at maintain dose ≤ 300 mg/d
    - Asymptomatic elevation in live enzyme uncommonly—cirrhosis
    - Neurologic dysfunction
    - Photosensitive
    - Bluish skin discoloration
    - GI disturbance
    - Hypo/Hyperthyroidism
    - Corneal micro deposits—in almost 100% pt receiving drug >6 months optic neuritis and atrophy with visual loss
    - CVS:
      - Symptomatic Brady
      - Worsening of VT
      - Hypotension
      - Depress W

Dronedarone

- EP action:
  - More potent blocker of rapid Na⁺ current than amio
  - Effect on atrial Ach-activated K⁺ channel and antiadrenergic effects are significantly more potent than amio
  - Rest same as amio

- *HD:* Little effect on cardiac performance except in pt with compromised IV
- Pharmac:
  - Elimination $t_{1/2}$ = 13–19 hours
  - 85% during excreted unchanged in feces and remaining in urine
- *Dose:* 400 mg into 12 hourly with food
  No v form available
- Indi:
  - To facilitate cardioversion of AF/AFL ⎤
  - To maintain SR in AF ⎦ Slightly less effective

  ANDROMEDA / DALLAS ⎤ greater mortality, stroke, systemic embolism or MI in dronedarone compared to placebo
- S/E:
  - Predictable increase in S. creat
    High mortality in class III and IV NYMA group
    QT prolonged
    Rarely proarrhythmic
    Rash, photosensitivity, nausea, diarrhea, dyspepsia, headache, asthenia
    No hepatotoxicity
    Low thyroid and lung toxicity
  - C.I in Preg and lactation

Sotalol

Nonspecific BB without ISA

- *EP action:*
  - Beta blocking
  - Prolong repol
  - No α-blocking or Na⁺ blocking property
  - Prolong atrial and vent repol time by reducing I_{Kr} ≥ prolongs plateau of AP
  - Reverse use dependent—APP prolongation is greater at slower rates
  - RMP, AP amplitude and Vmax—Not significantly altered
  - Prolongs atrial and vent refractoriness
    AH, HV and QT interval increases sinus cycle length increases
- HD effect:
  - BB → Neg inotropic effect (predominantly)
  - It can also increase strength of contraction by increasing repol time (which occurs maximally at slow HR precipitate overt HF use cautiously in pt with borderline W function
- Dose:
  - Oral—80-160 mg 12 hourly
  - Monitor ECG for QT and arrhythmia
  - $-t_{1/2}$ = 10–15 hours
- Indi:
  - Vent arrhythmia ⎤ More effective than Approved → conventional atrium and
  - AF ⎦ Equally effective as amiodarone
  - SVT, AFL, AT, AVNRT, AVRT
- S/E:
  - Proarrhythmia—most serious S/E
  - Tdp
  - New or worsened vent arr
  - SWORD Trial:
    - This proarrhythmic effect was the cause of excess mortality in pt given dI-sotalol (enantiomers without BB activity)

Ibutilide: Class III Antiarrhythmic

- Approved by USFDA in 1999
- Classified as "Pure" class III antiarrhythimic
  ↓
  - Pure APD prolonging drug
  - No neg inotropic effect
- EP action:

  K⁺ channel blocker
  ↓
  Prolong repol by activation of a slow, inward current
  ↓
  Prolongs APD

  - Blocks also inward Na⁺ current
  - No effect on QRS or AV conduction
  - Dose related prolongation of QT int
  - Prolongs APD, ERP in both atria and vent
- HD:
  - No significant effect on HD
  - No decrease in CD
  - No effect on MPAP
  - No effect on PeWP
- Pharmac
  - Route i.v (High 1st pass metabolism → so no oral)
  - Onset of action: After 90 minutes of start of infusion
  - PP binding: 40%
  - Metabolism: Hepatic via oxidation
  - Excretion: Via urine (+2%)
  - Elimination $t_{1/2}$ = Avg 6 hours

- Dose and admin
  ≥ 60 kg → 1 mg bolus over 10 minutes
  <60 kg → 0.01 mg/kg over 10 minutes
  ↓
  If no termination of arrhythmia
  ↓
  Second bolus can be given
- Postcardiac surgical treatment dose:
  - ≥ 60 kg → 0.5 mg over 10 minutes
  - <60 kg → 0.005 mg/kg over 10 minutes
  - Can repeat after 10 minutes

Caution:
1. More than 2 infusions not recommended
2. More rapid infusion not recommended
3. Not recommended in pt with
   - QTc>400 ms
   - Polymorphic VT/Tdp
   - Uncorrected hypokalemia
   - Hypomagnesemia
   - Bradycardia
4. Monitor for at least 4 hours or until QTC returns to normal
- Indi:
  1. Recent onset AF/AFL
  2. Persistent AF/AFL
     - As standard treatment
     - Pt already on amiodarone
     - To facilitate electrocardioversion (increased success rate; decreased energy required)
     - Facilitate cardioversion by overdrive pacing
  3. Post op AF/AFL
  4. Preexcited AF
  5. AF/AFL during EP study
- C.I:
  1. Hypersensitivity reaction
  2. Proarrhythmic if given with drug prolonging QT interval
  3. Not to give with class Ia/III agent prolong refractoriness
- S/E:
  1. Vent. Extrasystole
  2. NSVT—sustained PMVT
  3. Tdp (at prolongation)
  4. Hypotension/Bradycardia
  5. Nausea/vomiting/Headache
- How to reduce Tdp
  1. Pretreatment with class Ic dugs
  2. Combine with esmolol or $MgSO_4$
- ACE/AHA 2014
  Class I:
  For AF/AFL

For pre excitation synd in WPW
Class IIb: DOA cardiac surgical treatment AF

Dofetilide

- Approved for acute conversion of AF → NSR as well for ch
  Suppression of recurrent AF
- EP Action:
  - Block I_{Kr} (more prominent in atria than in vent)
  - Prolong refractoriness without slowing conclusion
  - Prolong QTc
- *HD effect:* No significant effect
- *Dose:* Oral only
  0.125-0.5 mg BD
  In hospital setting only (Prolong QT)
- *S/E:* QT prolong

Class IV Agents

Verapamil/Diltiazem

- EP action
  - Blocks I_{CaL} in all cardiac fibers
  - Reduce plateau height of AP
  - Slightly shorten AP (muscle)
  - Slightly prolong AP (Purkinje)
  - No effect on Vmax, RMP
  - Depress slope of diastolic depol in SA node cells
    Vmax of phase 0 and max least potential and prolongs Cond. Time and refractory period of AV node
  - Use dependence
  - Voltage dependence
  - Prolongs cond time through AV node
    - Increased AH interval and lengthen AV nodal anterograde and retrograde refractor period
    - No effect on HV or QPSd
  - Sinus rate does not change significantly (because of reflex increase in sinus rate due to peripheral hypotension)
  - Can dangerously increase VR in preexcited AF reflex symp stimulation
- HD effect:
  - Coronary and perivasodilatation
  - Neg inotropic action (masked by reflex symp activation)
  - Direct myocardial depressant (high dose)
  - BB + verapamil → marked myodepression
  - All HD action occur within 3-5 minutes
  - SVR and MAP decreases
  - LV dp/dt decreases
  - LV EDP increases

- *Dose:*
  1. For Ac termination of SVT or rapid rate control in AF
     - 10 mg over 1-2 minutes
     - 2nd injection 30 minutes later
     - Cont inf 0.005 mg/kg/min
     } Vesa
  2. *Oral:* 240-480 mg/day in divided doses } Vesa
  3. Dilzem IV 0.25/kg over 2 minutes 2nd dose in 15 minutes
- *Indi:* AVNRT/AVRT—after vagal and adenosine
  - As effective as adenosine
  - Rate control in AF
  - Possibly convert small no. to surgical treatment
  - Can terminate some AT
  - Fascicular VT
  - Left septal VT
  - RVOT VT

Others

Adenosine

- Endogenous nucleotide
- Present throughout body
- EP action:
  1. Adenosine
     ↓
     A1 receptor on extracellular surface of cardiac cells
     ↓
     Activates I_KAch, I_KAdo
     ↓
     Increased K⁺ conductance

     - Shortens APD
     - Hyperpolarize memb potential
     - Decreases atrial contractility
  2. Effect mediated through Gi and Go
     ↓
     Antagonize adenylyl cyclase
     ↓
     Decreasing CAMP
     ↓
     Decreasing I_{CaL} and If in pacemaker cells
     ↓
     Decreasing Vmax
     Decreasing sinus node rate
     Transient increasing A-H interval
  - His Purkinje conduction is not affected
  - Does not affect conduction in AP
  - Myo mediate phenomena and preconditioning
- *Pharmac:* → t1/2 = 1-6 seconds
  - Methylxanthine are competitive antagonist
  - Theophylline at therapeutic core totally block exogenous effect
- Dose:
  - *Peds:* 0.1-0.3 mg/kg
  - *IV:* 6 mg → 6 mg → 12 mg (92% success)
  - *CVP:* 3 mg
- Indi:
  - Doc for SVT (AVRT/AVNRT)
  - Can terminate ATs or SNRT
  - Can be useful as diagnostic test in APC
  - Also terminate a group of VT that depends on adrenergic drive
  - RVOT VT

Ranolazine

- Approved by FDA for chronic arginines
- Decreased incidence of AF, SVT and VT
- EP action:
  - Blocks I_{Kr} as well as late ING current
  - P, PR and QPS unaffected
  - QT mildly prolonged
- *H.D:* No significant H.D effect
- *Dose:* 500 BD-1000 BD

Ivabradine

2.14 LONG QT AND SHORT QT SYNDROMES

GENETICS OF CARDIAC ARRHYTHMIAS

LONG QT SYNDROME

- Majority → Autosomal dominant pattern (Romano ward)
- Rarely → Autosomal recessive Jervell and Lange-Nielsen
  - 10 LQTS susceptibility gene
  - Hundreds of mutation
    - Gain-of-function or loss-of-function mutations
  - Nucleotide substitution/Insulation/deletion
    - Missense mutation
    - Nonsense mutation
    - Frameshift mutation
    - Splice site mutation
- *Major LQTS genes* (75 %)
  - *LQT1:* KCNQ1 (35%)-11_p-I_{Ks} K^+ channel α-subunit
  - *LQT2:* KCNH1 (30%)-7_q-I_{Kr} K^+ channel α-subunit
  - *LQT3:* SCN5A (10%)-3_p-cardiac Na^+ channel α-subunit
- *Minor LQTS genes*
  - *CACNA 1C:* (3-5%)-12_p-voltage gated L type Ca^{++} channel
  - *KCNE1:* 21_q-K^+ channel β-subunit
  - *KCNE2:* 21_q-K^+ channel β-subunit
  - *KCNJ5:* 11_q-Kir 3.4 subunit of I_{KAch} ch   ⎫
  - *SCN4B:* 11_q-Na^+ channel subunit   ⎬ 5%
  - *AKAP9:* 7_q-Yotiao
  - *CAV3:* 3_p-caveolin 3
  - *SNTA-1:* 20_q-syntrophin α -1   ⎭

Anderson Trial (former LQT 7)

KCNJ2- 17_q-I_{K1} potassium channel.

Timothy synd (former LQTS)

CACNA1C-12_p-voltage gated L type Ca^{++} ch.

Ankyrin B Syndrome (former LQT4)

- LQTS   KCNQ1   Loss of function mutation
         KCNH2
         SCN5A   Gain of function mutation

Genotypes phenotype correlation:
- *Genetics and risk assessment*
  - C loop missense mutation (6 fold than '3')   ⎫
    - Highest risk of exercise and arousal triggered events (increasing rate of sleep/rest-related event)   ⎬ LQT1
  - Transmembrane spanning domain missense mutation (2 fold increased risk than '3')
  - N and C terminal mutations   ⎭

- Pure region mutation—highest risk
- Frameshift nonsense mutation in any region—intermediate
- Missense mutation in C terminus—lowest risk
    ↓
  - Poor region mutations have greater risk for arousal triggered events   ⎫ LQT2
  - Nonpoor loop region have seven fold increased risk for or exercise triggered events ⎭
- *Triggering events*
- Genotype phenotype correlation suggests gene specific triggers
  - KCNQ1 (LQT1)—Swimming and excision induced
  - KCNH1 (LQT2)—Auditory stimuli and postpartum events
  - SCNJA (LQT-3)—During sleep or rest
- *ECG pattern*
  - LQT1—Broad base T wave
  - LQT2—Low amplitude notched/bifid T wave
  - LQT3—Long isoelectric segment followed by narrow base T wave
"Exceptions do exist"
"MC clinical mimicker of an LQT3 appearing ECG is seen in patient with LQT 1
- *Response to pharmacotherapy*
  - Genetic bases also affect response to treatment
  - BB—Extremely protective in LQT1
    ↓
    Moderately protective in LQT2 band 3
  - Mexiletine, flecainide, and ranolazine → represent gene-specific treatment for LQT3
- *Others*:
  - Incomplete penetrance   ⎫ Hallmark of LQTS
  - Variable expressively   ⎭
  - Various mutation produce subclinical phenotype with asymptomatic course
  - While some zero type produce overt diseases representing mark QT prolongation and pre-syncopal episode
- *Besides cardiac ion channel:* Single nucleotide polymorphism (SNP) of nonion channel also modified disease severity
    ↓
  e.g., Gene encoding for NoS-1 adaptor protein:
  α-2 adrenergic receptor
  β-1 adrenergic receptor
- Strong disease modifying effect of 3 and translated region 3 untranslated region (3 UTR)-KCN Q1 allele specific halotype

↓
If normal KCNQ1 gene allele expression is suppressed
↓
More KCNQ1 mutant α subunit translated and assembled
↓
More severe manifestation of disease

Anderson Tawit Former LQT 7

- Sporadic or AD
- Multisystem disorder
- *C/F:* Trial of
  1. Periodic paralysis (mean age of onset J years)
  2. Dysmorphic features
  3. Vent arrhythmias (mean age 13 years)
- *ECG:* Prolonged QU interval
  Prominent U wave
  Vent ectopy/bigemine/poly VT/Bidirectional VT
  SCD extremely rare

Timothy Syndrome

- Extremely rare (<30 cases worldwide)
- Multisystem disorder
- *Cardiac:* Fetal brady, extreme prolongation of QT, macroscopic T wave alternans, 2:1 AV block at birth
- *Extracardiac:* Syndactyly, dysmorphic, facial feature, abnormal dentition, immune deficiency, severe hypokalemia, developmental delta (autism)
  Most die before reaching puberty

SHORT QT SYNDROME

- QT ≤ 320 milliseconds
- Associated with paroxysmal AF, syncope and increased risk of SCD cardiac arrest (most common) symptom and frequency (1st) manifestation of syndrome
- 25% had syncope
- 30% had F/H/O SCD
- 33% had AF
- Most frequency syncope during rest or sleep
- SCD observed during infancy also

Genetics (AD inheritance)

- *SQT1:* KCNH2-7_q-I_{Kr} K$^+$ channel β-subunit
- *SQT2:* KCNQ1-11_p-I_{Ks} K$^+$ channel β-subunit
- *SQT3:* KCNJ2-17_q-I_{K1} K$^+$ channel
- *SQT4:* CACNA1C-12_p-voltage gated L type Ca^{++} ch
- *SQT5:* CACNB2-10_p-voltage gated L type Ca^{++} ch (β-subunit)
- *SQT6:* CACNA2D1-7_q-voltage gated L type Ca^{++} ch (β-subunit)
- SQTS
  - KCNQ1 and KCNH2 gain of function mutation
  - KCNT2 gain of function mutation

Genotype-Phenotype

- <60 cases have been described
- Typical ECG pattern
- QT int <320 milliseconds (QTc ≤ 340)
- Tall peaked T wave in precordial leads
- No or short ST segment

Gene specific pattern:

- SQT1: T waves tend to be symmetrical
- SQT2: Asymmetric T: Inverted T possible
- SQT3: Asymmetric T
- SQT4: Asymmetric T
- SQT5: Brs like ST elevation in rt precordial leads
  SQT1 (KCN H2) mutation has shorter QT interval and greater response to hydroquinidine therapy then patient with non KCNH-2 mediated SQTS

DRUG-INDUCED TORSADES

Incidence 1–8%

- I_{Kr} channel blocker and repolarization reserve
  - Majority of such drugs ≥ I_{Kr} channel blocker S/E
  - Also known as HERG channel blocker QT prolonging drug produce LQT2 type phenotype
  - Reduce repolarization efficiency and lengthen AP

SHORT QT SYNDROME

- Increased risk of SCD
- Idiopathic VF
- Also prone to develop AF
- Gain of function mutation in genes sine as long QT loss of function mutation
- QTC ≤ 350 milliseconds at rate lower than 100 BPM

- Conventional formulas to correct QT may not apply to SQT because QT does not change usually with HR
- *Risk markers*:

  F/H/O SCD
  Palpitation / In absence of this SQT on ECG is
  AF / not a marker of increased SCD
  Syncope / RISK

(ECG)—patient often have persistently SQT intervals, short or absent ST segments and tall and narrow T wave in precordial lead.

Other causes:
- Hyperkalemia
- Hypercalcemia
- Hyperthermia
- Acidosis
- Digitalis

Treatment:
- ICD should be considered
- Antiarrhythmic drugs that increases refractoriness
- Quinidine shown to be effective in patient with KCNH2 gene mutation

2.15 PREMATURE ATRIAL CONTRACTIONS AND ATRIAL FLUTTER

SPECIFIC ARRHYTHMIA

Inappropriate Sinus Tachy

Definition

- SR >100 at rest with average 24 hours HR >90 in absence of 1° cause and associated with distressing syndrome of palpitation.
- Accelerated phase 4 diastolic depol. of sinus nodal cells is responsible for Sinus Tachy
- S. Tach can be cause of inappropriate shock in patient with ICD
- *Syndrome of Inappropriate Sinus Tachy*
  - In otherwise healthy person
  - Due to increased automaticity of SA node or automatic atrial focus near SA node
  - Due to defect in either sympathetic or vagal nerve control of SA automaticity
- *Treatment: BB/CCB.*
  - Sinus node RF/SX ablation
  - Ivabradine

PAC

- Most common cause of irregular pulse and palpitation
- Premat P wave with PR >120 msec
- Morphology of P wave differ from sinus P wave
- Can be blocked or conducted
  1. *Noncompensatory pause:* Interval between 2 P wave that comprises APC is < twice the PP interval of sinus rhythm (because PAC has reset sinus node
  2.
     - Less commonly PAC encounters sinus node refractory → sinus node not reset by PAC → basic sinus rhythm is not altered.
     - Interval between 2 P wave comprising PAC is twice the normal PP interval ≥ *Compensatory* pause
  3. Rarely *interpolated PAC* can occur.

PAC can conduct down with:
  1. Normal morphology of QRS
  2. RBBB (due to increased ERP of right bundle branch in setting of bradycardia (long cycle length) (Because RBBB has longer refractory period at long cycle length)
  3. LBBB at shorter cycle length the RP of LBB exceeds that of RBB

C/F PAC Occur in Various Situation

- Infection
- Inflammation
- Ischemia
- Medication
- Tension
- Tobacco/Alcohol/Caffeine
- Aging (without any cause)

Prognosis PAC'S have Benign Prognosis

- Treatment
  - Do not require treatment generally
  - BB/CCB can be used

Atrial Tachy

- Can be Automatic/Triggered/Re-entrant
- Adrenergic stimulation can initiate automatic and triggered atrial tachy
- Burst pacing may initiate triggered and microreentrant atrial tachy

Atrial Flutter

- Prototype macroreentrant atrial arrhythmia
- Typical AFL is re-entrant rhythm in RA
- Circuit bounded anteriorly by tricuspid annulus and post by crista terminalis and Eustachian valve
- *Typical:* Counter clockwise
- *Atypical:* Clockwise

Various Types of AFL

1. Typical counter clockwise—Tricuspid Annulus dependent on cavotricuspid isthmus
2. Atypical counter clockwise—Tricuspid annulus dependent on cavotricuspid isthmus
3. Lower loop re-entry—Cavotricuspid isthmus
4. Upper loop re-entry—SVC and upper crista terminalis
5. RA free wall-around area of scar in lat or POA RA wall
6. Septal AFL—Atrial septum typically postsurgical treatment
7. Mitral annular flutter—Around mitral annulus
8. Post AF ablation/maze flutter-variable circuit

ECG: Atrial Rate 250–350 BPM

- *Rhythm:* Regular/Irregular
- Can be slow if patient on arrhythmic
- Saw tooth waves on ECG
  - *Typical:* Positive in V_1, increases in II, IIIavF, and V_6
  - *Atypical:* Positive in II, IIIavF and V_6, negative in V_1
- Lack of isoelectric interval between flutter wave conduction 1:1, 2:1, 3:1, 4:1 or variable

C/F

- Occur due to atrial dilatation 2° to aging, HTN, HF, PE, MV/TV disease or idiopathic
- Thyrotoxicosis, alcohol or pericarditis can cause AFL
- Can follow surgical treatment repair of CHD
- S_1 normal intensity
- S_2 normal split

Management

- H.D unstable → cardioversion (sync) 50J
- Ibutilide → success 60-90%
- Procainamide ⎤ less effective
- Amiodarone   ⎦ than ibutilide
- Rapid atrial pacing with catheter in esophagus or RA
- Ablation—preferred choice (90% success)
- Indi for anticoag are similar to AF
- Rate control in AFL is much more difficult
  - Than in AF (rhythm control preferred)
  - Verapamil 2.5-10 mg IV
  - Dilzem 0.25 mg/kg IV
- Adenosine can be used for diagnostic purpose
- Esmolol (9 mm $t_{½}$) can be used to slow VR
- Digoxin (if CCB + BB is inadequate)
- If AFL persist/returns → class I_{A1}/I_C/III drugs can be tried
- Treatment of underlying disease (example thyrotoxicosis)

Caution:

- Class I drug should not be used until VR is controlled with BB/CCB. Because class I drugs slow AFL rate and facilitate AV conduction → can lead to 1:1 response to flutter.

2.16 EPICARDIAL VENTRICULAR TACHYCARDIA

INTRODUCTION
Categorized as idiopathic VT as well as associated with various CV diseases.

INCIDENCE
- Exact prevalence not known
- Some studies—10–20% of all

COMMONLY ASSOCIATED WITH
- Dilated nonischemic cardiomyopathy
- Arrhythmogenic RV cardiomyopathy
- Chagas disease

ECG PARAMETERS
- Broad QRS tachycardia with AV dissociation
- Pseudo-delta wave
  - Slow rate of rise in QRS voltage
  - Pseudo delta >34 ms ⎤ favors
  - Intrinsicoid deflection >85 ms ⎦ epicardilal VT
- Maximum deflection index (MDI) >0.55
  - Calculated by divided the earliest time to maximum deflection in any precordial lead by total QRS duration
  - Highest sensitivity (100%) and specificity (98%)
- Shorter Rs complex duration >121 ms
- QRS duration more in epicardial VT
- Q waves in I present ⎤ epicardial VT
  Q waves in I II-avF absent ⎦
- avR/avL amplitude ratio higher in epicardial VT

DIAGNOSIS
Which criteria to apply and when?

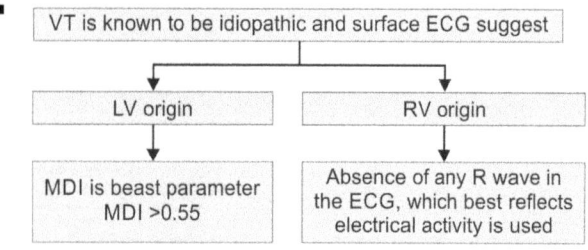

- *Nonischemic cardiography*

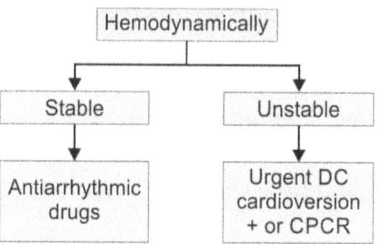

- Patient with history of IHD
  Q wave criteria should not be used
- Electrophysiological study with BD mapping is investigation of choice for differentiating endocardial-ubendocardial VT from epicardial VT

TREATMENT (SAME AS ENDOCARDIAL VT)

```
           Hemodynamically
           /            \
       Stable          Unstable
         |                |
   Antiarrhythmic     Urgent DC
       drugs         cardioversion
                      + or CPCR
```

RF ABLATION
Simultaneous epicardial and endocardial mapping (because both VTs can coexist together in patients with organic heart disease).

Method
- Conscious sedation or GA
- Continuous hemodynamic monitoring

Approaches
- Pericardial approach pericardial fluid input and output should be matched to avoid cardiac tamponade
- Coronary sinus approach
  RF ablation via coronary sinus
  CAG is must for pericardial approach to check for proximity of RF catheter with coronaries → prevent inadvertent injury to coronaries

PROTOCOL
Mid diastolic potential recorded from VT site entrainment may be carried out to confirm their participation in mechanism underlying VT.

COMPLICATIONS
- RV puncture
- Hemopericardium
- Tamponade
- Pericardial effusion
- MI/coronary thrombosis
- Coronary stenosis
- Pericarditis
- Pulmonary embolism
- Phrenic nerve injury

2.17 THERAPY OF CARDIAC ARRHYTHMIA

DC CARDIOVERSION

Two types:
1. Synchronized
2. Unsynchronized (Defibrillation)
   - Obvious advantage over pharmacy cardioversion
   - Restore surgical treatment immediately and safely

Mechanism

- Most effective in tachy of reentrant mech CAFL, AF, AVRT, AVNRT, array with WPW, most form of VT and VF)
  - Mech by which it terminates VF is uncertain
  - Electrical shock:
    - Depolarize all excitable myocardium
    - Prolonging refractoriness
      ↓
    Interrupt reentrant circuit
      ↓
    Establish electrical homogeneity
    Which terminates re-entry
- Arrhythmias of automaticity
  E.g., AT, parasystole, JT, AIVR
    ↓
  Not terminated with shock
    ↓
  It may restart soon after cardioversion
  It may get exaggerated due to release of endogenous catecholamines by shock
- Not established whether cardioversion can terminate tachy caused by enhanced automaticity or triggered activity

Technique: Monophasic vs Biphasic

- Synchronized
  - Timed to QRS complex
  - Lower energy
  - Avoids vulnerable period of T wave

To improve success rate
1. Admin maintenance antiarrhythmic drugs 1-2 days before planned cardioversion
   - Can revert some pt to SR
   - Help prevent recurrence of AF
2. Statin/AECI/ARB also prevent recurrence of fibrillation
3. Ibutilide admin
   - Paddle or Pads
   - 12-13 cm patches

Position

- Standard apico anterior or (anteroposterior) ← More effective by placing more of atrial way in shock vector
- Do not apply pad over subcut device or dermal patch

Dose

SVT: 25-50 J
AF:
- 100 J monophasic
- 50 J biphasic

Can accelerate the dose if unsuccessful

Patient Prep

- Short acting barbiturates (methohexital); sedative (propofol) or amnesic (midazolam)
- 100% or 5-15 mm before shock
    ↓
  Success rate: 90-95% pt with AF
    ↓
  In 5% of pt (unsuccessful)
1. If AF restarts early → does not responds to higher dose because AF has been terminated but restarted soon
2. If AF not terminated (esp in obese pt and/or COPD) → escalate dose or can try internal cardioversion with special catheter
3. Defibrillation: For VF and pulseless VT
4. Internal cardioversion
   - With specialized catheters
   - Placed in CS or lateral part of RA
   - So that vector is across atrial mess
   - 2-15 J

Indications

- Arrhythmias (Tachy) with HD instability
  1. Hypotension
  2. Mental state change
  3. Angina
  4. HF
  5. Shock
- Preexcited AF responds well to cardioversion

Favorable Candidate for DC Cardioversion of AF

1. Symptomatic AF <12 hours duration
2. Pt cont to have AF after precipitating cause has been removed (example after treatment of thyrotoxicosis)
3. Rapid VR that is difficult to slow
4. Symptoms of decreasing CO attributable to loss of atrial contraction

Unfavorable Candidate (AF)

1. Dig toxicity
2. No symptoms and well controlled VR
3. Sinus node dysfunction and various supravent tachy or bradyarrhythmias—tachy brady synd
4. Little or no sympt improvement with restoration of SR who promptly revert to AF
5. Large LA and long standing AF
6. AF that reverts spont to SR
7. No mechanical atrial systole after establishment of electrical atrial activity
8. Cardiac surgical treatment planned in near future
9. Antiarrhythmic drug intolerance
   Pt with high chance of recurrence
   1. COPD
   2. CHI
   3. MV disease (esp. MR)
   4. Enlarged LA (>45 mm)
   5. AF > 1 year

Compli

Rarely pt develop hypotension, decreases CO. or CHF post.

Cardioversion: May be due to embolism, myocardial depression from anesthesia/shock itself, hypoxia, lack of restoration mechanical LA contr, postshock arrhythmia:
- Can produce VF (esp. unsync)
- Rarely asystole

POSTSHOCK

- Observe till conscious
- If ibutilide used → 8 hours
- Anticacy into 4 weeks

ABLATION FOR ARRHYTHMIAS

- Purpose of ablation = Destroy myocardial tissue by delivery of energy
  - Electrical energy
  - Cryo energy
- For tachy with focal pathology (e.g., Automaticity, triggered activity or Microre-entry circuit ≥ Target for ablation is narrow portion of myocardium between inexcitable area (e.g., Scar)
- Types of energy used
  1. RF energy
  2. Cryothermal catheter ablation
  3. Laser and microwave energy

RF energy → causes resistive heating of tissue (transducer electrical energy into thermal energy → when tissue temp exceeds 50 °C

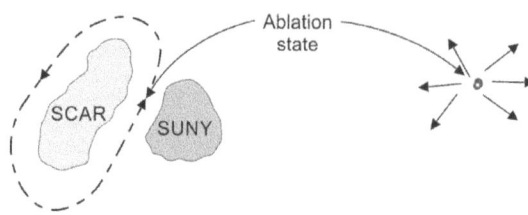

- Irreversible damage
  Note: RF induced heating of tissue that has inherent automaticity (e.g., His bundle, foci of automatic tachycardia) results in initial acceleration followed by termination
- RF delivery to reentrant arrhythmia typically causes slowing and followed by termination

Cryothermal Ablation

- In some cases RF ablation is ineffective
- Amount of damage required is more
- Standard cath can deliver 55°–70°C
- Tip temp of >90°C are associated with coagulation of blood element on electrode
  ↓

Cooled tip ablation has been used to good advantage in cases with failed std. ablation (cooling of catheter tip by cont irrigation of fluid keep heat under control and allow great delivery of power)

Cryoablation catheter causes tissue damage of freezing cellular structure

- Cooling of tip achieved by nitrous oxide
- Temp as low as -80°C
- Cooling to 0° causes reversible damage → can be used as diagnostic

Purpose:
- Catheter cooled further to damage tissue irreversibly
- Also be used for PV isolation by balloon inflated with 80°C No.
- Cryoablation causes less endocardial damage than RF energy

ABLATION OF AP

RF ablation is treatment of choice for AVRT and AFL.

Location of Pathway

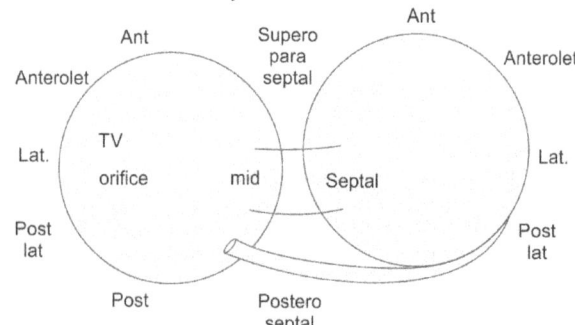

- Superoseptal pathway near His bundle
- Midseptal near AV node
- Rt and lt posteroseptal pathways are near CS.

Ablation Site

- Found by direct recording of AP
- Vent insertion site can be identified by finding site of earliest onset of vent electrocardiogram in relation to onset of δ wave
- Major vent potential sync with onset of the δ wave can be a target site in left-sided preexcitation whereas, in right-sided path vent potential earlier to δ wave is site of ablation.
- Atrial insertion site of manifest or concealed pathway (δ wave present or about respectively) can be found by locating the site showing earliest atrial alteration during retrograde conduction.
- Left-sided AP typically crosses MV annulus obliquely earliest site of retrograde activation of atria and anterograde activation of ventricle are not directly across AV groove
- Successful ablation site
  - Exhibit stable fluoroscopic and electrical characteristic
  - During SR, local vent activation at successful ablation site precedes onset of delta wave on the ECG by 10–35 ms during orthodromic AVRT the interval between onset of vent activation and local atrial activation is usually 70–90 msec.
- Retrograde transaortic and trans-septal route used with equal success

Cryoablation useful in pt with septal AP.
↓
Test done with reversible cooling injury

If AV cond hampers quickly rewarm catheter case irreversible prevent permanent damage to AV node

If AV cond preserved and conduction through AP fails Deeper cooling plane achieved for injury to AP
Atriofascicular pathway = Decremented conduction

Indications

1. Symptomatic AVRT with
   - Drug resistance
   - Drug intolerance
   - Do not desire long-term drug treatment
2. AF/AT with AP and rapid VR
   - Drug-resistant/intolerant
   - Do not desire long-term drug treatment
3. AVRT/AF with rapid VR identified during EDS of other arrhythmias
4. Asymptomatic pt with preexcitation whose livelihood, profession, important activity in insurability or public safety affected by tachyarrhythmias
5. AF and controlled VR over AP
6. F/H/O SCD

Results

- Success rate >95%
- Slightly less for RV force well pathways in which stable cath position is problematic
- Recurrence rate—2%
- Complication 1–2% (Bleeding, vasc. damage, myocardial perf with tamponade, valve damage, stroke, MI)
- *Heart block:* <3% of septal pathway

ABLATION FOR AVNRT

i. Fast pathway ablation:
   - Rarely performed because its association prolonged PR interval, higher recurrence rate (10–15%) and higher risk for complete AV block (2–5%)
   - May be preferred in pt with markedly prolonged PR interval at rest and no evidence of anterograde fast pathway conduction in such situation slow path ablation causes complete AV block

ii. Slow pathway ablation:
   - Located by mapping along posteromedial tricuspid annulus close to CS os.
   - Multicomponent atrioventricular electrocardiogram obtained
   - Single RF application usually eliminate slow pathway
   - Accelerated junction rhythm usually occurs when RF energy is applied at site → followed by successful elimination of SVT
   - Success rate = 100%   Recurrence = 5%
     <10% chance of CHB   Re-ablation always successful
   - Cryoablation can also be used successfully
     - Slightly higher recurrence rate
   - Slow path ablation—increased anterograde AV block cycle length and AV node ERP without change in AH intamol
   - Surest end point for successful ablation is elimination of sustained AVNRT with and without an infusion of isoproterenol
- Pts in whom slow path cond. Is completely eliminated, almost never have recurrent SVT
  - Slow path ablation is preferred
  - Safe and effective

Indications

1. Recurrent sympt AVNRT
   - Drug-resistant/intolerant
   - Pt do not desire to take drug for long
2. Sustained AVNRT found during ERS of another arrhythmia
3. Dual AV node physiology with atrial ECMO but without AVNRT in pt clinically suspected of AVNRT.
   - Result
     - Success 98%
     - Recurrence <2%
     - Heart block ≤1%

ABLATION OF SA NODAL ARRHYTHMIAS

- Can be identified anatomically and electrophysiologically
- Ablative lesions usually placed between SVC and crista terminates at site of early atrial activation

Indi:
1. Sinus node reentrant tachy
2. Inappropriate sinus Tachy—Failed medical management

ABLATION OF AT

Can be focal tachy/re-entry

| Can occur irrespective of str. heart disease | Occur in structurally damaged heart/postsurgical treatment |

i. Focal AT:
   - Activation mapping used to determine site of AT
   - Practically nonincludible during EPS
   - 10% pt can have multiple foci
   - Tends to cluster near PV and mouth or LAA and along crista terminals in RA
   - Care must be taken to prevent damage to phrenic nerve
ii. Reentrant AT:
   - Ablative strategy is to identify regions with mid-diastolic atrial activation during tachy
   - Technique analogous to AFL ablation
   - 80–90% success but 20% recurrence

ABLATION OF AFL

Reentrant circuit:
- Retrograde activation of RA
- LA passively activated
- Caudocranial activation along RA septum and craniocaudal activation is across isthmus

- Typical site for ablation is across isthmus of atrial tissue (cavotricuspid isthmus) between IVC orifice and tricuspid annulus ⎫
- Success oblation can be accomplished at the point where flutter wavefront (1) enters in cavotricuspid isthmus in lower inf-lat RA; (2) Exit from this zone or (3) in between ⎬ Cavotricuspid isthmus dependent flutter ⎭
- In other rapid atrial arrhythmias there may be different circuit in RA/LA → more difficult to ablate

Indications

1. Recurrent AFL
   - Drug resistant/intolerant
   - Pt do not wish to take drugs
2. Pt with AF and concomitant AFL

Results

- 90% success
- Recurrence <5%

ABLATION AND MODIFICATION OF CONDUCTION FOR ATRIAL TACHYARRHYTHMIAS

- In some pt with atrial tachyarrhythmias with rapid VR in spite optimal medical management; less amenable to ablation, RF ≥ His can help
- Catheter placed across TV and positioned to record a small His bundle electrogram associated with large atrial electrogram.
- RF energy applied until complete AV block is achieved and cont for additional 30–60 seconds.

Indi

1. Symptomatic atrial arrhythmias with inadequate ventricular rates and failed OMT/ablation
2. Similar pt when drugs are not tolerant or pt does not wish to take drugs
3. Pt with symptomatic nonparoxysmal junction tachy that is drug-resistant/intolerant
4. Patients resuscitated from SCD related to AF/AFL with rapid VR in absence of AP
5. Pt with dual chamber pacemaker and PMT that cannot be treated effectively by drugs

Result

- Success in almost all
- Recurrent conduction <5%

RF ABLATION FOR VT

- Slightly lower success rate than AVRT/AVNRT ablation (may be because this is last resort in pt with drug-resistant VT and extensive str heart disease + more difficult mapping in ventricles)
- VT must be
  1. Reproducible
  2. With uniform QRS morphology
  3. Sustained and HD stable so that pt can tolerate VT long enough during procedure to undergo extensive necessary to localize site of ablation
  4. Target of ablation must be fairly circumscribed and preferably endocardial.
- Very rapid VT, PMVT and infrequent /NS VT are less well suitable to this ablative treatment.

Location: VT divided into:
1. Idiopathic VT—Pt with str normal heart
2. VT in various disease setting—without CAD
3. VT in pt with CAD and prev MI
   1. Idiopathic VT
      - RV origin: Usually PVOT (LBBB + Inf. Axis)
      ↓
      LV origin: Usually LV septal (RBBB + Sup Axis)
      Uncommon: LVOT; sinuses of Valsalva
   2. VT in abnormal heart without CAD can be due to
      → Intramyocardial re-entry
         Or focal process
      → Bundle branch re-entry
      → (e.g., in pt with DCMP) sarcoid; HCM, Chagas)
      - Epicardial foci commonest in this group
      - In pt with BB re-entry, ablation of rt bundle branch can eliminate tachy
   3. Scar based VT:
      - Finding of potential region of diastolic activation
Used as a critical part of reentrant
Circuit is desirable
↓
Ablation at this site eliminates VT.

Techniques

1. Activation mapping ⎤ In pt with
2. Pace mapping   ⎦ idiopathic VT
- Timing of endocardial electrogram sampled by mapping cath is compared with onset of surface QRS
- Site which are activated 20–40 ms before QRS on surface are near origin of VT
- Ablation at a site at which unipolar ECG shows QS complex → greater yield than rs potential

- Pace making (low sensitivity than activation mapping) involve stimulation of various vent site produce QRS contour similar to that of spont VT
- Presystolic Purkinje potential or very low mid diastolic potential can be observed
↓
Ablation of this site terminates VT
- Such localization in pt with ischemic (Port MI VT) is more difficult
- In scar VT
- Region of diastolic activation can be used to determine part of reentrant circuit
- Entrainment can be used to test whether a site is a part of reentrant circuit or a bystander
↓
Entrainment → pacing for several seconds during a tachy-cardia
At a rate slightly faster than VT → After pacing stopped original VT resumes → Timing of last paced beat to first complex determine how close the pacing site to a part of VT circuit
↓
Pacing within critical produces QRS complex exactly similar to VT

3. Substrate mapping
   - When activation or pace making is unsuccessfully because of HD
     Instability on induction of arrhythmia
   - Substrate mapping, in which area of low electrical voltage or with
     Delayed potential are recorded during SR
   - Good result in many cases

Note: In pt with idiopathic VT usually only single VT is present in pt with ischemic VT many VT are present and ablation of VT is only palliative and does not preclude antiarrhythmic therapy.

Limitation

Many cases with PMVT/VF are not amenable to treatment because of HD instability and beat-to-beat change in activation sequence.

Indi

1. Symptomatic sustained MMVT
   - Drug-resistant/intolerant
2. Pt with str heart disease BB reentrant VT sustained MMVT receiving multiple ICD shock
3. Occasionally NSVT or very frequent PVCs

Results

- Success approximately 85% (Idiopathic VT) 70% (postinfarction VT)

Mapping Technologies

a. Magnet based mapping
   CARTO
b. Impedance-based mapping
   Ensite velocity syst (St. Jude)
c. Ultrasound-based mapping
   RPM (Real time position management) (Boston)
d. Hybrid magneto-impedance based
   CARTO 3: Rhythmia system
   (Biosense) (Boston)
e. *Newer:*
   - Novel noninvasive EP mapping
   - Topera 3D mapping

NEW TECHNOLOGY

1. *Multielectrode mapping system:*
   - Mapping of multiple sites simultaneously and incorporate sophisticated computer algorithm for analysis and display
2. *Epicardial cath mapping:*
   - Often required in pt with cardiomyopathy
   - Long spinal anesthesia needle introduced from subxiphoid under fluoroscopy

   ↓

   Entry into periocardium is confirmed by injection of small amount of contrast

   ↓

   Guidewire introduced and needle exchanged with sheath

   ↓

   Usual mapping technique that can be adopted

   ↓

   CAG is must to avoid delivery of RF energy near coro artery
3. *Chemical ablation:*
   - With alcohol or phenol
   - To create AV block

2.18 MECHANISM OF ARRHYTHMOGENESIS

DISORDER OF IMPULSE FORMATION

A1. *Automaticity*
- Normal automaticity (normal in vivo or in retro SA nodal, AV noda and Purkinje cells)
  - S. Tachy or brady inappropriate for clinical situation possible vent parasystole
- Abnormality (depolarization-induced automaticity in Purkinje myocyte)
  - Possibly AIVR after MI

A2. Triggered activity
- EADs drugs like sotalol, N-acetyl procainamide terfenadine, barium, and low K^+)
  - Acquire LQTS and association vent arrhythmias
- DADs (Gain-of-function mutations in gene encoding RYR2)
  - CPVT

DISORDER OF IMPULSE CONDUCTION

B1. *Block*
1. Bidirectional or unidirectional without re-entry (SA nodal, AV, bundle branch, and Purkinje muscle) SA/AV/BB block
2. Unidirectional block with free entry (AV node, Purkinje muscle junction, infarcted myocardium) AVNRT BB re-entry VT caused by BB re-entry reciprocal tachy in WPW

B2. *Reflection* (Purkinje fibers with area of in excitability)
- Unknown clinical example

COMBINED DISORDERS

C1. *Interactions between automatic foci* (depolarizing or hyperpolarizing subthreshold stimuli speed or slow the automatic discharge rate)
- Modulated parasystole

C2. *Interaction between automatic foci and conduction* (deceleration dependent block overdrive separation of conduction entrance and exit block)
- Experimental

ABNORMAL AUTOMATICITY

- Can arise from cells that have reduced maximum diastolic potential often at membrane potentials positive to -50 mv
- Automaticity at membrane potential more negative than -70 mv may be caused by I_f
- Automaticity rate speeds up with progressive depolarization
- Abnormal automaticity in Purkinje cell can also originate secondary to spontaneous submembrane Ca^{++} sensitive membrane conductance

NORMAL AUTOMATICITY

2 modes:
1. HCN channels activated by hyperpol → increasing their probability of being open → conduct both Na^+ and K^+; but at negative membrane potential attacks as Na^+ inward current—together with inflow of Ca^+ channel inward current through Na^+-Ca^{++} exchanger and decaying out word K^+ currents depolarize cell membrane of pacemaker cell → generate AP
2. *Ca^{++} clock:* Periodic increase in $[Ca^{++}]$: → serves as internal generator → signal transform in membrane voltage via modulation of Ca^{++} sensitive ion channels and transporters in outer membrane

Periodic SR Ca^{++} release events rhythmically activate NCX invert current exponential increase in membrane potential that promotes activation of surface membrane l type Ca^{++} channel to initiate AP

Once AP is generated 2 highly interacting concurrent series of events proceed during a normal SA node cell cycle
1. Depolarization-induced activation of delayed rectifier K^+ current (I_K)
2. AP induced Ca^{++} release from SR

- Rhythm resulting from abnormal automaticity are
  - Slow atrial
  - Junction — escape rhythm
  - Ventricular
  - Certain AT (those produced by digitalis those coming from PV ostia)
  - Accelerated junction rhythm
  - Inherent rhythm
  - Parasystole

TRIGGERED ACTIVITY

After depolarization: Depolarizing oscillators in membrane voltage induced by one or more preceding APs—so triggered activity is a pacemaker activity that result as a consequence of a preceding impulse or series of impulse:
- It's not automaticity
- These depolarization of occur before or after full repolarization

EAD: when they arise from reduced level of membrane potential during phase 2 (type 1) and phase 3 (type 2) of AP

DAD: When they occur after completion of repol (Phase 4)

DAD

- Results from activation of Ca^{++} of sensitive inward current elicited by spontaneous increase in intracellular force Ca^{++} iron concentration
  Rapid mobilization of Ca^{++} from SR into systole is mediated by synchronous opening of ryanodine sensitive Ca^{++} release channels

RYR: Encoded by RYR2 gene	
During systole	*During diastole*
Small influx Ca^{++} through L type Cav channels	RyR2 channel closes
Trigger massive release of Ca^{++} from SR via synch. opening of RYR2 channels	Ca^{++} recycled into SR via Ca^{++} pumps
Caused Ca^{++} induced Ca^{++} release	Refilling SR Ca^{++} stores for next release cycle

Mutation in R1R2 gene
Mutation in CASQ2 (calsequestrin gene) ⎤ increased sensitivity of RyR2
↓
Both
Linked with
CPVT

Channel to luminal Ca^{++} activation on adrenergic stimulation
↓
Enhance spont. Diastolic Ca^{++} release from SR
↓
Delayed after Depolarization

Ip3 Receptor

- Another Ca^{++} release channel
- Activated by second messenger IP3 and Ca^{++}
- Predominant subtype in atrial myosite
- Located near RYR channel of SR
- Contribute to alter excitation contraction coupling and arrhythmogenesis
- IP3 dependent Ca^{++} signaling has been implicated in arrhythmia attributable to ischemia and reperf injury, inflammation process and cardiac failure

Events Leading to DAD (Mech.)

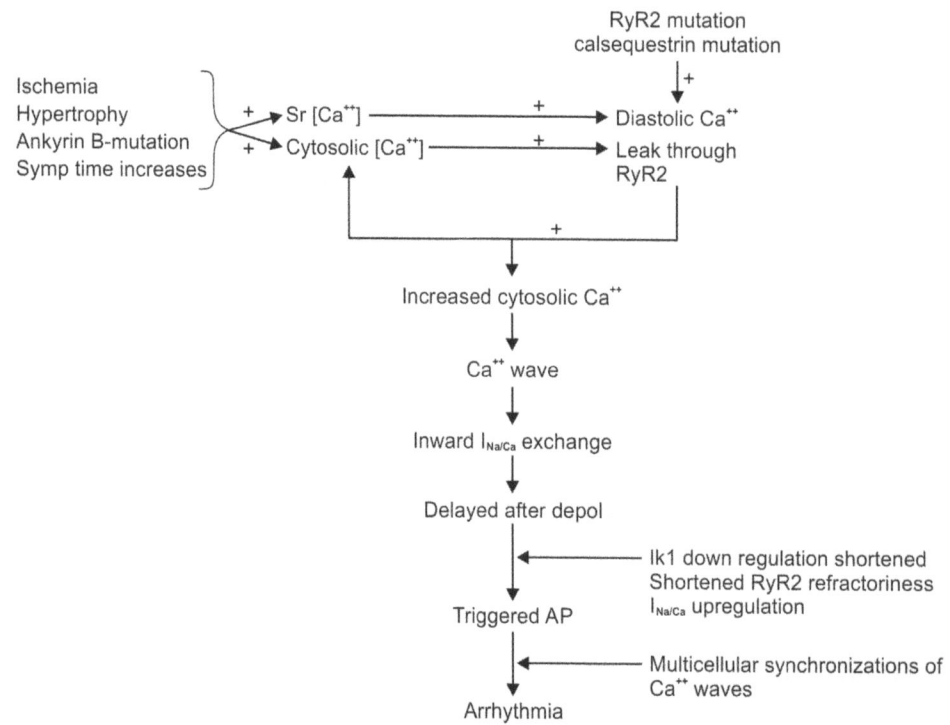

DAD most likely to play a role in arrhythmogenesis in failing heart because of
- Up regulation of $I_{Na/Ca}$
- Down regulation of inward rectifier K^+ current (I_{K1})
  ↓
  Facilitates DAD

Clinical Implication

1. Short coupling interval and overdrive pacing increasing the amplitude and shorten the cycle length of DAD after cessation of pacing rather than suppressing DAD
   ↓
   Tachyarrhythmias caused by DAD are not suppressed by overdrive pacing in fact it may be precipitated by rapid rates either spontaneously or during pacing
2. Single premat stimulus can initiate and terminate triggered activity
   ↓
   Important to differentiate from re-entry
   ↓
   Response to overdrive pacing helps in differentiation

EAD

Responsible for lengthened repolarization time and ventricular tachyarrhythmias seen in several clinical situations suggest LQTS.

Mech

Increased intracellular Ca^{++} release from SR coupled with dispersion of repolarization plays important role in LQTS in association arrhythmias

Lengthening of AP
↓
Increased influx of Ca^{++} true L type Ca^{++} channel
↓
Excessive accumulation of Ca^{++} in SR
↓
Spontaneous release from SR
↓
Elevation of intracellular free Ca^{++}
↓
Can depolarize cardiomyocyte membrane by
1. electrogenic Na^+/Ca^{++} exchange current
2. activation of Ca^{++} of dependent chloride current
   ↓
   Evoke EAD
2. Marked transmural dispersion of repolarization
   ↓
   Create a vulnerable window for development of re entry

3. Sympathetic stimulation (especially left) can also increase EAD amplitude to provoke vent arrhythmias

Clinical Implication

EAD associated with:
1. LQTS association vent arrhythmias
2. Acquired LQTS and TDP
3. Parasystole

DISORDERED IMPULSE CONDUCTION

Brad arr: When propagating impulse is blocked and followed by a systole or slow escape rhythm.

Tachy arr: When delay and block produce reentrant excitation
1. *Deceleration dependent block*
   - Bradycardia-dependent block
   - Diastolic depolarization is suggested as a cause
2. *Tachycardia dependent block*
   - Impulse block that rapid rate
   - Caused by incomplete time or voltage-dependent recovery of excitability
3. *Decremental conduction*
   - Property of fiber changes along its length such that AP loses its efficacy as a stimulus to exile the fibers ahead of its stimulating efficacy of propagating AI diminishes progressively
4. *Re-entry*: Group of fiber not activated during initial cave of depolarization recovers excitability in time to be discharge before impulse dies out
   ↓
   Serves as a link to reexcite site areas that were just discharged.
5. *Entrainment*
   - Entraining tachy (i.e., increasing rate of tachy by pacing) with resumption of intrinsic rate of tachy when pacing is stopped → Establish presence of re-entry
   - Criteria of entrainment can be used to prove reentrant mechanism of clinical test and form the basis for localizing the pathway
6. *Anatomic re-entry*
   AVNRT: For re-entry of this type, the time for conduction within the depressed but unlocked area (slow pathway) and excitation of distal segment it must exceed the refractory period of initially blood pathway (fast pathway) and tissue prox to site a block
   ↓
   Means cont. re-entry require that anatomical length of the circuit travel to be equal or exceed reentrant wavelength
   ↓

- Anatomical length of circuit is fixed
- Conditions that depress conduction velocity promote development of re-entry whereas feeding conduction velocity and prolonging refractoriness hinder re-entry

↓

Re-entry frequently exhibit excitable gap time interval between end of refractoriness from one cycle and beginning of depolarization in next
During excitable gap tissue in circuit is excitable
Excitable gap occurs because wavelength of reentrant circuit is < length of path way

↓

Electrical stimulation during this period can invade reentrant circuit and terminate tachy/reset its timing

7. *Functional re-entry*
   - Occurs in contagious fiber that exhibit functionally different EP properties
   - Caused by difference in transmembrane AP
   For example, Purkinje, myocyte, transition

Tachycardia caused by re entry
1. Atrial flutter
   - Macro reentrant circuit
   - Typical = counterclockwise in cardiocranial direction in interatrial septum and craniocaudal direction in RA free wall
   - Area of slow conduction presents in postero K^+ posteromedial inf area in RA

   ↓

   Area of successful ablation
2. *AF:* Micro reentrant circuit
3. *Sinus re-entry:* Reentrant circuit can be entirely within SA node or involve both SA node and atrium
4. Atrial re-entry
5. AVNRT
   - Slow-fast type counterclockwise reentrant circuit
   - Fast-slow type clockwise reentrant circuit
   - Slow-slow type anterograde conduction over intermediate pathway and retrograde conduction or slow pathway
   Clinical implication:
   - Slow pathway involved in all types
   - Ablation of slow pathway is responsible for termination of all AVNRTs
   - Triangle of Koch's involved in all AVNRT
6. Pre-excitation syndrome (WPW)
   - Orthodromic Tachy
   - Antidromic Tachy
   - In some patient with antidromic tachy, 2 AP can form a circuit

In some patient AP may be capable of only retrograde conduction (concealed)
LaL. (James fibers)—Connects atrium to distal portion of AV node and His bundle

7. *VT caused by re-entry*
   - Re-entry in vent muscle with or without contribution from specialized tissue
   - Responsible for many VT in patient with IHD
   - Can be microentry (around scar)
   - Surviving myocardial tissue separated by connective tissue provide route of activation traversing infarcted areas → establish reentrant pathways
   - BB re-entry can also cause VT
   - Functional block at and re-entry at Purkinje vent myocyte interface is also described
   - Collagen matrix formed by fibrosis after MI → establishes the basis for slowed conduction, fragmented electrocardiogenesis and cont electrical activity → leads to re-entry

   During ischemia:
   - Elevated $[K]_o$ ⎤ create depressed AP
   - Reduced PH ⎦ in ischemic cells

   ↓

   Retard conduction

   ↓

   Leads to re-entry

8. *Brugada syndrome*
   - Phase and re-entry implicated in genesis of VT-VF in patient with inherited BrS
   - Alteration in sodium current

   ↓

   Loss of AP dome during plateau phase (phase 2)
   In PV epicardium

   ↓

   Marked dispersion of repol and refractoriness

   ↓

   Potential for phase 2 re-entry

9. *CPVT*
   - Stress induced PMVT in str normal heart
   - Increased leakage of Ca^{++} from SR
   - Carvedilol and flecainide → can suppress CPVT via direct inhibition of R1R receptor mediated Ca^{++} release

10. *APVC/D*
11. *VF*

Classic theory: VF maintained solely by re-entry
New theories: Restitution kinetics

Wavefront	⎤ suggested as
Wave break	replacement for
Focal discharge	classic re-entry
Rotor	⎦ theory

Cardiac Fibrillation

- Hallmark is *wave break*
  ↓
  Caused by conduction block
  ↓
  His localized block
  ↓
  2 hypothesis ←—— Wave break
  Splitting of mother wave into 2 daughter wavelets

Mother rotor hypothesis
VF maintained
By single
Stationary
Intramural
Stable
Reentrant
Circuit
↓
Fastest acting
Rotor rather than
Wave break is the
Engine driving
Fibrillation

Wandering wavelet hypothesis
dynamic wave breaks
plays a fundamental role in inhibition maintenance of VF
↓
VF maintained by wavelets with constantly changing reentrant circuit

VT Caused by Nonreentrant Mech

- Catecholamine dependent
- Can be terminated in Valsalva, adenosine and verapamil
- Generally located in RVOT
- May be caused by triggered activity, possibly DADs
- LV fascicular tachy can be suppressed by verapamil (but not adenosine)
  ↓
  Some of these may be caused by triggered activity and not by re-entry

2.19 PACEMAKER AND ICD

CARDIAC ELECTRICAL STIMULATION

Local and Global Effect

Local

- *Pacing* require local stimulus sufficient enough to depolarize myocardium during diastole and initiate a wave-front of depol
- Electrode with small surface area 1-6 m
- Field strength 1v/cm
- Stimulus needs to capture fully excitable myocardium and propagate to myocardium which is also fully excitable

ATP: Must interact with specific reentrant circuit during tachycardia that is removed from the pacing side

- ATP stimulus must capture local myocardium in relative refractory period—propagate to reentrant circuit through relative refractory myocardium → enter reentrant circuit during excitable gap and causes bidirectional block
- So stimulus strength required is high

Global

- Termination of VF or AF shock require global field effects
- Electrode require larger surface area
  - Transvenous 400-800 mm^2
  - Subcut/epicardial 35-70 cm^2
  - Transthoracic patch 75-100 cm^2 strength 3-4 v/cm (biphasic) 5-6 v/cm (monophasic)

DFT: Minimum shock strength that results in defibrillation during testing

Programming — Strength duration and polarity of pacing
Defibrillation pulses

- Duration of pacing and defibrillation pulses are optimized to achieve desired physiological result with minimum energy consumption
- Voltage output set at 1.5-2 times threshold
- Pulse duration 0.4-0.5 milliseconds
- Pacing chronaxie 1.5-2 times
- Shock strength of ICD programmed near ICD's max output of 750-800 V or 30-40 J with pulse duration of 3.5-6 milliseconds for first phase of biphasic

Binary search protocol for ICD

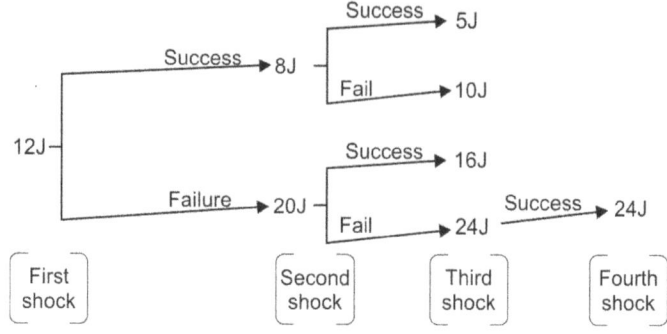

Metabolic effect and threshold

- Hypokalemia → Raises pacing and ICD threshold
  ↘ Alter sensing by conduction delay
- Marked acidosis/Alkalosis—reuse pacing threshold (but not ICD)
- Profound hypothyroid—reuse pacing threshold (but not ICD)

HD RELATED TO PACING

A. *Chronotropic response*
   - Ability of HR to increase during accession
B. *AV synchrony*
   - Coordination of atrial and ventricular electrical activation and mechanical contraction is called AV synchrony
   - AV synchrony increases CO by 25-35%
   - Patient with impaired systolic and/or diastolic function are most dependent on atrial transport

     PPI: Retrograde VA conduction
     ↓
     VA synchrony
     ↓
     Most of atrial contraction while AV valve is closed
     ↓

     A cause of pacemaker syndrome in single chamber pacing (In dual chamber pacing with retrograde conduction and loss of atrial pacing/unreliable sensing can also lead to pacemaker syndrome)
   - Patients with long PR on pacing (depending on PR length)
     ↓
     Mechanical dyssynchrony despite electrical synchrony

1. *If PR extremely long:* Atrial cont occurs during prev vent systole acts like VA condition
2. *If PR slightly short:* Atrial cont in early diastolic filling period → Possibility of diastolic MR during later part of diastole
3. *If PR interval too short* → Contribution of atrial cont is insufficient because MV closes before completion of atrial systole.

C. *RV pacing*

RV pacing
↓
Intraventricular dyssynchrony
↓
Impair vent function
↓
Incidence of HF and AF

INDICATION AND DEVICE SELECTION

A. *Pacemaker*
 1. Relive or prevent symptomatic Brady
 2. Relief of symptoms confirm to be due to bradycardia
 3. Asymptomatic Brady
 4. Symptoms thought to be due in Brady although Brady not documented but other causes excluded and symptoms are severe
 5. To prevent symptomatic Brady in asymptomatic patient if the risk for rapid progression to severe symptoms is high

B. *ICD*
 - Prevention of SCD from VT/VF (either 2°/1° prev)
 - MADIT II and SCD HEFT demonstrated absolute mortality reduction of 5–7% over a period of 2–4 years in high risk patient

C. *Single vs dual chamber ICD*
 - No recommendations

Advantages: Dual-chamber ICD provides
1. Diagnostics for AF
2. Discriminators of SCT and VT
3. Dual chamber pacing
4. Higher diagnostic accuracy

Disadvantages of dual chamber ICD
1. Higher cost
2. Atrial lead complication
3. Decreased longevity

Meta-analysis: Dual chamber ICD
1. Modest benefit of SVT vs VT discriminators function in 2° prevention patients in whom MMVT occurs at rate that overlaps VR in SVT or S.Tachy
2. No benefit in 1 degree prevention
3. Unlikely to benefit 2° patient whose only arrhythmia is VF

HARDWARE

A. *Pacing and defibrillation leads:*
 - Screw-in or tine leads
 - Inner and outer coil
 - Ring electrode
 - Active HP electrode (screw-in) for positive tip electrode (tine)
 - *Unipolar pacing lead* → only 1 electrode is used for both sensing and pacing
   - Other electrode is in pacemaker generator
   - At high output can lead to pectoral muscle stimulation
   - Much more likely to have over sensing

- *Bipolar pacing leads*
  - 2 electrodes between which sensing and pacing occurs over sensing less common

- *Defibrillation lead*
  - 1 or 2 sensing and pacing electrode +1 or 2 defibrillation coil
  - If two electrode (a tip and ring electrode)—'true' bipolar sensing and pacing occur
  - If only tip electrode—"Integrated" bipolar sensing and pacing occur between electrode and distal coil
    2 coils: 1 in SVC
    └→ 2 in RV
    If any need to remove lead, SVC with fibrosis creates problem

For PCD left pectoral implants preferred because the defibrillation vector to the can includes more of LV

B. *Generator*
 10–15 cm³ for (PPI): Lithium iodine batteries
 30–35 cm³ for (ICD): Lithium silver vanadium oxide
 ↓ Or Lithium manganese dioxide
 Need high voltage for long time to deliver shock and ATP.

PACING MODES

APEC/BPEG coding
 NAPSE = North American Society of Pacing and Electrophysiology
 BPEG = British Pacing and Electrophysiology Group
- 1st letter = chamber paced
- 2nd letter = chamber sensed
- 3rd letter = function (I = inhibition, T = triggered, D = dual tracking of atrial activity and inhibited in vent)
- 4th letter = R for rate adaptive

1. *VVI:* Indicated for patient with permanent AF
2. *AAI:* Appropriate for SA node dysfunction and interact AV conduction
3. *DDD:* Preferred
   - Maintain AV synchrony
   - Has upper rate limit

BLANKING AND REFRACTORY PERIOD

- After each sensed event sensing every FIDE is turned off for a short period (20–250 milliseconds) to prevent multiple sensed events single cardiac depol—this period is known as blanking period
- Following each blanking period there is refractory period during which events may be sensed or tachyarrhythmia detection algorithm but do not alter pacemaker timing cycle.
- Blanking period and refractory period in ventricle after atrial sensed or paced event and in atrium after vent sensed or paced events are called cross chamber blanking and refractory period.

↓

It reduces over sensing of casing artifact after a paced event in opposite chamber

PVARP: Postventricular atrial refractory period
- In DDD mode
- Starts with any ventricular event and defines with period on atrial channel during which a spontaneous atrial event is not tracked
- Especially important in patient with retrograde conduction
- If PVARP too short → PVC may be conducted retrogradely sensed on atrial channel and tracked-resulting in a second (paced) vent beat that can conduct retrogradely → This repetitive sequence leads to PMT
- PVARP has important implication regarding upper rate behavior

↓

Sinus rate higher than upper paced rate
↓
Vent rate can't exceed upper programmed rate
↓
Activates algorithm for extending AV delay
↓
Eventual P wave will occur progressively earlier after each successive vent patch beat
↓
Until a P wave falls in PVARP and not tracked
↓
Pseudo AV Wenckebach
↓
If sinus rate increases even further
↓
Every alternate P falls into PVARP
↓
2:1 atrial tracking

TARP: Programmed AV delay + PVARP

Imp to keep TARP below max sinus rate during exercise
↓
Otherwise 2:1 tracking occurs
↓
Decreased vent rate
↓
Exercise intolerance

Rate adaptive pacing:
- Adjust pacing rate to metabolic demand of body
- Sensor located in generator or lead monitor
- Commonly used sensors
  1. Body motion (accelerometer)
  2. Respiration (minute ventilation)
  3. Cardiac motion (endocardial acceleration)

Algorithm to avoid unnecessary RV pacing → AAI pacing
↓
VVI pacing with back up 40 rate
(AAIR = DDDR mode switch)
1. AAIR pacing with backup went packing
   - Switch to DDDR when AV block detected
   - Switch back to AAAIR to when AV conduction improves
2. Prolong AV interval to allow intrinsic AV conduction
   - If intrinsic AV conduction detected → AV delay remains extended
   - IV intrinsic AV conduction not detected in a specified delay period → vent pasting resumes
3. Positive search hysteresis periodic extension of AV delay to detect intrinsic AV conduction

DETECTION OF VT/VF IN ICD

Rate, Duration and Detection Zone

- Primary criteria used for VT/VF detection are rate and duration
- ICD has three vent detection zones that permits programming of zone-specific therapy and SVT-VT Discriminations
- 2 zones are sufficient in many patients VT zone and VF zone

For secondary prev:
- VT detection rates should be programmed at least 20 beats/min slower than any documented VT
- B zone programming indicated in many such patients to permit different ATP for two distinct rates of VT

Typical values for this zone are:
- 300–500 milliseconds for slower VT
- 300–350 milliseconds for faster VT
- 240–300 milliseconds for VF

For primary prev
- Programming higher rate cut often safe and reduce in appropriate therapy
- Typically set at 180–200 *BPM*
- In VF zone ATP is programmed during or before charging for shock

Duration: It is the time or number of intervals required to satisfy the rate criterion longer durations permit unnecessary therapy for VT/VF that could have terminated spontaneously if therapy has been delayed

SVT-VT discriminators:
Various algorithms
1. Single chamber discriminators:
   - Sudden onset
   - Vent rate stability (regularity)
   - Morphology of vent EGM
   - Uses of a difference in cycle and that is greater than programmed percentage or a diff in value can cause under detection of VT that begins slower than VT rate criterion
   - To discriminate irregular conduction during AF from regular rate during MMVT
   - Detects VT based on change the morphology of dRs in vent EGM
2. Dual chamber discriminators:
   1. Comparison of atrial and vent rate
   2. AV relationship
   3. Absolute atrial rate during AF
      ↓
   - If vent rate > atrial rate ≥ VT
   - If vent rate = atrial rate
   - Additional single or dual chamber discriminator must be used to discriminate 1:1 AV conduction of SVT from 1:1 VA conduction of VT
     - If atrial rate > vent rate
   - Additional criteria must be used to discriminate rapidly conducted atrial arrhythmia from VT to VI

ELECTRICAL THERAPY FOR VT/VF

Once VT/VF detected → ICD can deliver up to 6 therapies consists of ATD/high voltage shock
↓
After each therapy ICD monitor for
1. Resumption of NSR
2. Persistence of some VT/VF
3. Change in VT/VF
   ↓
If VT/VF persists
Therapy can escalate from low voltage ATP to progressively high voltage shock therapy can be individualized on zone detection in primary and secondary prevention

A. Antitachycardia pacing consists of 3–10 beat train of pulses at a cycle length shorter than VT cycle length first pulse set to percentage of preceding VT cycle length (Typically 85–90% for faster VT and 75–85% for slower VT) can be delivered in bust or ramp mode

Burst mode: Pulses within a train have a fixed cycle length
- CL can be decreased 10–30 milliseconds between successive trains if first train does not terminate VT

Ramp mode: Sequential pulse within each train are delivered at a progressively shorter CL until a minimum value is reached
- For ATP to be successful at least one pulse must enter reentrant VT circuit in excitable gap period and terminate VT
  ATP is 1° treatment for MMVT
  ATP rarely effective for PMVT or VF

Success: ATP terminates approximately
- 50% of FVT
- 50% of slow VT

Usually 1–2 ATP sequence (trains) programmed for FVT
          2–4 VT ATP sequence (trains) programmed for slow VT

B. Cardioversion and shock
Imp: MMVT can be Orphan terminated with low-energy cardioversion (≤ 5 J)
↓
Problem with this
↓
If VT not terminated and shock falls into vulnerable period
↓
Cycle length changes
↓
Rate of VT accelerates

Another problem
- Changing period
- Imp during VF
- Higher joules require longer changing period → Harmful during VF

Note: Amount of shock does not determine shock pain strategies
1. Patient-specific
   - 1st shock value is programmed to a patient-specific value (weakest shock strength that can achieve defibrillation)
2. Maximum shock
   - 30–40 J
   - 98% of all spontaneous VT/VF is terminated by first 2 shocks
   - In some cases VT does not appear to terminate despite multiple shocks and low DFT possibly because shock reinduces VT

C. Shock reduction
   1. Nondevice-related interventions
      - Treat metabolic abnormality
      - Treat ischemia and HF
      - Use of BB/antiarrhythmics
      - Catheter ablation
   2. Programming principle
      - Not treating self-terminating VT
        SVT
        Slow VT (in 1degree prev)
      - Minimizing shock energy delivered
      - Minimizing shock delivery due to sensing problem
      - Use of ATP as initial therapy
      - Programming high energy shock for arrhythmias that require multiple shocks

TROUBLESHOOTING PPI

- History
- ECG
- CXR
- Stored device data (programming lead impedance and trends, stored EGM during packet manipulation and arm movt)

i. *Failure to capture*
   Causes
   - Pacing output below threshold
   - Changes at electrode myocardial interface (fibrosis)
   - Lead displacement
   - Lead insulation failure or conductor fracture
   - Connection problem between header and lead
   - Functional failure to capture (under testing for async pacing)

   Defined as pacing stimulus without subsequent cardiac depolarization

ii. *Failure to pace:* (Most common)—over sensing of physiological or nonphysiological signals → can be corrected why magnet or programming to asynchronous mode
   - Failure in pulse generator ⎤ Not corrected by magnet or
   - Lead conductor failure/ ⎬ or programming in
     fracture ⎦ asynchronous mode
   - Connection problem between (header) and (lead) header-failure to insert lead fully into connection block failure to tighten the screw
   - Signals are in indistinguishable from lead
   - But impedance trend may vary
   - Crosstalk (atrial impulse sensed by rent lead)
     Can be avoided by went blanking period
     Cross talk increasing in setting of
   1. High atrial output
   2. Vent sensing parameter program to very sensitive value
   3. Short duration of went blanking

iii. *Pacing at a rate not consistent with prog rate*
   1. Shorter than expected escape interval
      → Indicates undersensing
   2. Longer than expected escape interval
      → Indicates over sensing
   3. Battery depletion

iv. *Unanticipated rapid pacing*
   1. Pacemaker mediated tachy
   2. Inappropriate ventricular tracking of rapids sensed atrial rate
   3. Electromagnetic interference
   4. Myopotential
   5. Sensor driven PMT (unrelated to patient activity)
      Sensor increases pacing rate unrelated patient activity
      E.g. Vibration in helicopter sensed by accelerometer volume sensor responding to asthma attack

v. *Other problems*
   1. Pacemaker syndrome
   2. Extracardiac pacing from stimulation of pocket
   3. Phrenic nerve diaphragm for intercostal muscle stimulation
   4. Brady PPI can be proarrhythmic, e.g., if normal function results in pores causing short long short sequence in vent
      - Can lead to pause dependent VT/VF
   5. It very rarely rapid pacing during threshold testing can cause VT

vi. *Misinterpretation of PPI function*
   - Fusion and pseudofusion beats
   - *Fusion* depolarization partially by intrinsic activation and partially by PPI
   - *Pseudofusion* PPI simulation does not alter QRS morphology on surface ECG

This occurs after normal depolarization of when it has already started and it is not allowed by PPI stimulus

TROUBLESHOOTING ICD

- Determination of reason for shock
- Failure to deliver treatment
  1. Troubleshooting shocks
     Three step approach
     1. Determine whether shock was delivered in response to over sensing or to a tachycardia
     2. Determine whether tachy was VT/VF or SVT
     3. Determine whether VT might have terminated with ATP or spontaneously

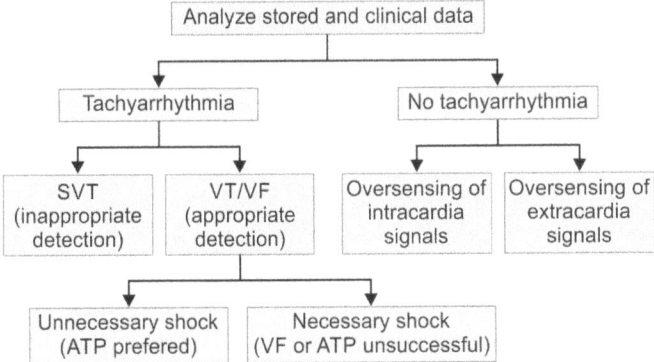

  2. Over sensing
     - When nonarrhythmic physiologic or nonphysiologic signal are oversensed
       a. Nonphysiologic signal
          Usually extracardiac
       b. Physiologic signal
          Usually intracardiac or extracardiac
          P.R or T wave
          Myopotential
     P wave over sensing and r wave double counting are manifested as alternating cycle length of sensed RR interval and alternating morphologies
     ↓
     Can occur if the distal coil is too close to TV
     R wave double counting occurs if duration of sensing EGM exceeds the vent blanking period
     T wave over sensing may occur in setting of normal or low amplitude R waves
     When extracardiac signals are over sense isoelectric baseline is replaced by high frequency "noise" signals over sensing can lead to
     - Failure to pace
     - Failure to deliver necessary shock
     - Deliver unnecessary shock → can induce VF

  3. *VT vs SVT:* Inappropriate detection of SVT as VT of can be minimized by programming VT and VF detection rate and duration, optimal programming of VT SVT discriminators, appropriate use of BB and antiarrhythmic drugs for SVT and catheter ablation of SVT
  4. *NSVT:* Shock can be prevented by increasing duration of detection
  5. *Unnecessary shop for MMVT*
     - Can be minimized by programming ATP
  6. *Approach to patient experiencing ICD shock*
     - ICD interrogated within 24–48 hours
     1. Inappropriate repetitive shock due to over sensing or miss discrimination between SVT and VT
        - VT/VF detection can be described by programmer or magnet
     2. Repetitive shock for VT can be due to VT storm or by multiple unsuccessful shocks for single episode (VT storm caused by acute ischemia, exacerbation of HF, metabolic abnormalities hypokalemia and proarrhythmic drug effect or noncompliance reversal of precipitating case BB antiarrhythmic drug (sotalol)/ amiodarone) catheter ablation ⎤ VT Storm
  7. Unsuccessful shock
     - Failure of 2 Max output shocks to convert VI

  Reason
  - True failure of reversion
  - ICD fails to recognize NSR pot conversion of VT/VF and restart of VT/VF in a short period
  - Postshock SVT in VT/VF rate zone

  Causes
  A. Misclassified therapy
     - VT/VF recurs before device can determine that it has terminated
     - Failure to terminate sinus Tachy
     - Postshock SVT as missed determined as VT
  B. *Patient-related factors*
     - Metabolic (hypokalemia)
     - Ischemia
     - Prog of HF
     - Some antiarrhythmic drugs example amiodarone
     - Pleural or pericardial eff
  C. *Device system related*
     - Insufficient programmed shock strength
     - Battery depletion
     - Failure of generator component/lead
     - Incorrect device lead connection
     - Load dislodgement
     - Delayed detection resulting in prolonged episode that increases shock strength required

COMPLICATIONS

May be related to:
1. Vascular access
2. Lead placement
3. Pocket integrity
4. Hemodynamics
5. Infection

Incidence: 4–5% of device (new) implantation
2–3% of generator charge

A. Venous access-related compli
   1. Injury to lung → Pneumothorax/hemothorax
      Vasculature
      Nerve
      Other str
   2. Placement of lead into LA or LV via PFO
   3. Placement of lead into LV via inadvertent subclavian artery puncture and retrograde passage of lead into LV

Pneumo: Most common with subclavian approach almost 0% extrathoracic axillary vein puncture and cephalic vein cutdown

B. Lead placement related
   1. Lead dislodgement most common require lead revision micro dislodgement increases pacing threshold but may not require lead revision
   2. Cardiac perforation-hemopericardium/tamponade
   3. Extracardiac stimulation phrenic nerve intercostal left hemidiaphragm
      • RA pacing along free wall can cause right phrenic nerve stimulation
   4. *Tip extrasystole:* Lead placement can cause extrasystole beat because of mechanical effect of tip of the lead against myocardium → usually resolved within 24 hours
   5. TR rarely with RV lead
   6. Chest pain due to pericardial irritation or pericarditis
   7. Thrombosis of axillary Or subclavian vein SVC thrombosis rare but most serious
   8. Loose screw or inadequate connection of lead terminal pin to header may result in over sensing of nonphysiologic stimuli

C. *Device-related infection*
   1. Erosion
   2. Pocket infection
   3. Bacteremia
   4. Endocarditis

Early infusion usually by *Staph aureus*/strepto late inf by intra op containment or by hematogenous infections.

FOLLOW-UP

A. Remote monitoring
   • Via analoge telephonic system
   • Determine status capture sensing
   • Can be schedule transmission
     ↘ Patients initiated transmission about event
     ↙ Automatic and schedule transmission based on pre-specified alerts

It permits:
   • Identification of increased frequency of NSV
   • Asymptomatic sust VT terminated by ATP
   • Early asis of device cyst problem
   • Premat batt depletion
   • High voltage circuit failure (lead problems)

■ *Monitoring of comorbid condition:* AF and HF
   • AF can be reliably monitored by device with atrial lead
   • AF is most common reason for remote monitoring alerts in ICD patients
   • Device collected data
     HR
     HR variability
     Activity level estimation   ⎤
     intrathoracic impedance   ⎥ Provide insight
     (Indirect measure of log water)   ⎥ into diagnosis
     endocardial acceleration   ⎥ and prog of HF
     (Indirect measure of contractility) ⎦

B. Psychological factors
   • More with ICD than PPI
   • ICD shocks associated with reduced qdl

C. *Lifestyle issue*
   1. *Driving and flying*
      ICD for one degree prev—no restriction
      ICD for 2 degree prev—soft driving for 6 months post-implant stop trying for 6 months after each shock
   2. *Sports*
      • Swimming is associated with risk of drowning even if VT/VF treated promptly
      • Most expert's advice for ICD patient against swimming
      • Also depends on baseline disease (HCM, ARVD, LQTS, CPVT)
   3. *Drug interaction*
      • Antiarrhythmics in patient with BPI to prevent AF
      • *IMP:* Whenever antiarrhythmic prescribed

        Important to slow the detection rate of VT/VF

4. *Electromagnetic interference*
   PPI—switch to asynchronous mode
   ICD—stops functioning VT/VF detection
   ↳ Does not alter pacing function
5. *Nonmedical source of interference*
   - Cell phone: Not to carry in pocket hold on c/l ear
6. *MRI*
   Relatively CI if MRI compatible device-reprogramming PPI two asynchronous and disabling ICD VT/VF Detection during scanning and close monitoring limit specific absorption rate of tissue during imaging to <2 W/kg MRI not advisable in 4–8 weeks of implantation
   ↳ patient with abandoned leads
7. *Surgical cautery*
   - Over sensing with unipolar cautery
   - For ICD oversensing is more with integrated bipolar (rather than with true bipolar) leads

2.20 ATRIAL FIBRILLATION

ELECTROCARDIOGRAPHY FEATURES

- Supravent arrhythmias
- Low amplitude baseline oscillation (fibrillatay or f waves)
- Irregularly regular
- 300–600 bpm (f waves)
- Vent rate = 100–160 BPM
- With pre-excited AF vent rate can be 250/min

CLASSIFICATION

- *Paroxysmal:* AF terminates within 7 d
- *Persistent:* AF present cont. for >7 d
- *Permanent*: AF present for 1 year or more where rhythm control is no longer planned or has failed
- *Long-term*: AF + n + for >1 yr
  Confounding faction: Antiarrhythmic drugs and cardioversion can switch AF from one class to another and interfere with its classification

LONE AF

- AF that occurs in pt <60 years
- No or minimal str heart disease
- No associated HTN
- Lower risk of thromboembolic complications
- Rhythm control is safer option

ROLE OF ANS

Paroxysmal AF subdivided into:

- *Vagotonic AF (25%)* occurs in condition with high vagal tone (e.g., during sleep or during rest esp. at late evening)
  Drugs with vagotonic action aggravate it (Digitalis)
  Drugs with vagolytic (disopyramide) can terminate it
- *Adrenergic AF* (10–15%)
  - Initiated alluring heighten eel adrenergic tone, for example, during exercise
  - BB provides rate control as well as prevents initiation of such AF
- Most pt have mixed form

EPIDERMIC

- MC arrhythmia treated in clinical practice
- MC arrhythmia for which pt are hospitalized
- 33% arrhythmia-related hospitalizations are due to AF
- 5 fold increased risk of stroke

RISK FACTORS

- Advanced Age
- Obesity
- OSA
- HTN
- HF
- AoV and MV disease
- LAE on ECMO

MECH

2EP mechanism:

1. *Drivers*: Automatic, triggered or microreentrant
   Foci → fire at rapid rate
2. *Multiple reentrant circuits:* Perpetuating AF by producing daughter wavelets
   - PV astia are MC trigger drive
   - In persistent AF, change in atrial substrate (including interstitial fibrosis) contributes to slow, discontinuous and anisotropic conduction
     - So persistent AF rarely respond to only PV isolation

CAUSES

- VHD
- IHD
- Str heart disease (LVH with HTN)
- CM pathy (HCM, DCM)
- Restrictive CMpathies
- CP and cardiac tumors—less commonly
- Obesity → Atrial dilatation and increased syst inflam^n
- OSA → Hypoxia, dysautonomia → AF
- Severe PH association with AF
- Alcohol birge
- Immediate post op period of CABG/Open heart surgical treatment
- Hyperthyroidism

MANAGEMENT

A. *Acute management*

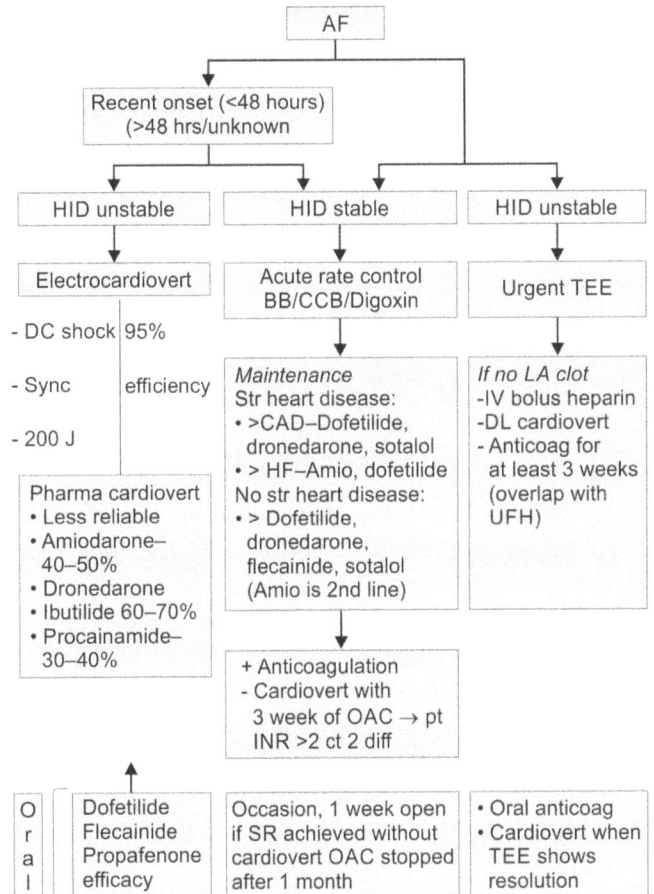

- *Adv of early cardioversion*
  1. Rapid relief of symptoms
  2. Avoid need for TEE
  3. Avoid need for therapeutic anticoagulation (which is required for 3-4 weeks before delayed cardioversion)
  4. Lower risk for early recurrence of AF
- *Reason to defer early cardioversion*
  1. Unavailability of TEE (in pt with AF >48 hrs)
  2. LAA thrombus
  3. Suspicion (Based on prev history) then AF will convert spontaneously within few days
  4. Correctable case (hyperthyroidism)
- *Types of failure of cardioversion*
  i. Complete failure to restore SR
     ♦ Increases shock strength
     ♦ Ibutilide infusion prior to shock
  ii. Immediate recurrence within few seconds
     ♦ 25% for episode <24 hrs
     ♦ 10% for episode >24 hrs
  • Increasing shock strength is of no. value

Long-term Management

Two alternative strategies:
1. Rate control
2. Rhythm control
   - *Largest AFFIRM Trial:* No diff between 2 strategies in terms of mortality stroke risk and QDL but incidence of rate control is significantly lower in rate control arm repeated hospitalization also less in rate control arm.
   - Choosing strategy depends on various factors

Favors rate control	Favors rhythm control
• Recurrent, long standing AF	• Newly discovered AF
• Persistent AF	• Paroxysmal AF
• Age >75 years	• Age <75 years
• Minimal or asymptomatic AF	• Highly symptomatic AF
• Ext. str heart disease esp. with cardiac chamber enlarge	• Lack of ext. str heart disease esp. chamber enlargement
• Multiple poorly treated comorbidities	• Comorbidities absent or well treated
• Prev failure of antiarrhythmic drugs and/or abortion	• No known prev. failure of antiarrhythmic drugs
• Informed pt preference	• Informed pt pref

- Cardioversion gives advantage of avoiding long-term antiarrhythmic drugs and adverse reaction related.
  - Esp in part in whom AF episodes are brief and separated at least by 6 months.

A. *Rate control*
   - Strict rate control (Resting HR <80 and rate during moderate ex <110)
   - Lenient rate control (Resting rate <110) small studies shows no diff between these 2 strategies strict rate control is still an appropriate goal for relief of symptoms, improvement in F^n capacity and avoidance of tachy induced CM-Pathy ideal VR during AF is
     ♦ 60-75/min during rest
     ♦ 90-115/min during mild to mod exercise
     ♦ 120-160/min during strenuous exercise
     Agents BB, CCB, *Digitalis*, amiodarone

B. *Rhythm control*
   - Class I A—Quinidine, procainamide, disopyramide
   - Class I C—Flecainide, propafenone
   - Class II—Sotalol, amiodarone, ibutilide, dofetilide
   - Class I A and III can prolong QT interval → TDP
   - Class I C can increase QPSd and precipitate MMVT
- Choice of antiarrhythmic depend on pt's comorbid condition
  1. Lone AF or minimal str, heart disease → flecainide, propafenone, sotalol, dronedarone are first line, amio considered if these drugs fails

2. Pt with substantial LVH → Amio is DUC
3. Pt with CAD - Class I drugs harmful
   - Dofetilide and sotalol 1st line Rp
   - Amiodarone 2nd line Rp
4. HF → only 2 drugs known to have neutral effect on mortality are Amio and Dofe

PALLAS trial

Dronedarone increases risk of HF, stroke and CV death in
1. 65 years or older with permanent AF and either CAD, prev stroke or sympt HF
2. 75 years or older with HTN and DM

C. *Rhythm control other than antiarrhythmics*
   - ACEI
   - ARB
   - Statin

ORAL ANTICOAGULANTS

Risk Stratification

- Strongest predictor of risk = TIA/HIV stroke/MS
- Other = DM
          HTN
          HF
          Age >70 years
  Simple risk score
- CHA2DS2 VASc score: (Better than CHADS score)

C—CHF	-1
H—HTN	-1
A—Age ≥ 75	-2
D—DM	-1
S—Stroke/TIA/Thromboembolism	-2
V—Vascular disease	-1
A—Age 65-74	-1
S—Sex (Female)	-1
	Total 9

Point	Risk of stroke	
0	0	← (*)
1	1.3%	←(*)
2	2.2%	←(*)
3	3.2%	
4	4%	
5		
6		
7		
8		
9	15.2%	(*)

HAS-BLED Score

H—HTN	-1
A—Abnormal renal or liver F^n (1 point each)	-1 or 2
S—Stroke	-1
B—Bleeding	-1
L—While INR	-1
E—Elderly (>65 years)	-1
D—Drugs or alcohol (1 pt each)	-1 or 2

Score	Bleeding risk per 100 pt year
0	1.13 ← (*)
1	1.02
2	1.88
3	3.74
4	8.70
5	12.5
6-9	Insufficient data ← (*)

- Net clinical benefit of warf defined as no. of stroke while not taking warf mMG no. of ICH episodes while taking warf.
- With CHA_2DS_2-vasc ≥1 → Benefit of giving warf exceeds risk of bleeding compli.
- HAS-BLED developed for pt on WARF (Except for labile IMR, it is likely that components of HAS-BLED also applies to pt on NOACS)

But predictive value of HAS-BLED for pt on NOACS is not yet defined.

1. Warf:
   - INR between 2 and 3 provides best balance between stroke prevention and hemorrhagic risk
   - Even a small decrease in INR from 2.0→1.7 doubles risk.
   - Annual risk of major hemorrhagic complication with warf is in range of 1-2%
   - C.F: Uncontrolled HTN. HIV bleeding
2. Aspirin + Warf
   - Increased risk of major bleeding
   - But does not decrease risk of thromboembolism
3. Dabigatran: (150 BD)
   - Oral DTI
   - Rely study—Noninferiority trial
   - Lower risk of stroke with syst embolism than warf and similar rate of major hemorrhage
4. *Rivaroxaban*: (20 OD)
   - Rocket—AF
5. *Apixaban* (5 mg BD)
   - ARISTOTAL

6. *LMWH* rarely used on routine basis
- *How to switch*
  (Read from articles)

NONPHARMACOLOGICAL MEASURES TO AVOID THROMBOEMBOLISM

LAA closure/surgical treatment excision
- 90% of thrombi form in LAA
- PROTECT AF = Device closure of LAA is noninferior to warf

Nonpharmacological Management of AF

A. Pacing to prevent AF:
  1. DDD pacing with RV pacing + RA pacing decreases AF incidence. Studies suggest that higher incidence of AF during vent pacing maybe at least partially due to proarrhythmic effect of vent pacing
  2. Dual site RA pacing or pacing of IAs near Bachmann bundle prevents AF
  3. Pacing algorithm to prevent AF
     - Burst of rapid atrial pacing at onset of AF (But rarely useful)
     ↓
     Because of insufficient evidence to support its use, atrial pacing is not indicated for prevention of AF in pt without brady
B. Catheter ablation:
  - Arrhythmia substrate of AP is not well understood
  - Its widespread
  - Variable between patients
  - May be progressive

  } AP ablation is not so much successful It recurs 2-3 years after initial successful ablation

- *Pt selection*:
  - Pt on at least 1 rhythm control drug (because of efficacy of ablation is lower for persistent AF than for paroxysmal AF)
  - Ideal candidate lone AF or minimal str heart disease
  - C.I in:
    1. pt with LAA thrombus
    2. Who can't tolerate anticoagulation for at least 6-8 weeks?
       Post ablation
  - Inappropriate in pt with CHA_2DS_2-vasc score >1 and asymptomatic whose only motivation to undergo the procedure is to eliminate the need for anticoag.
- Cath ablation can be appropriate in
  1. Age <35 with symptomatic AF
  2. 8A node dysfunction in whom antiarrhythmic therapy is likely to create a need for PPI
  3. Pt who express aversion to drugs
- Strategies
  1. PV isolation by
     - Ostial ablation
     - Wide area ablation 1-2 cm away from ostia
     - Wide area ablation has better result
     - PV isolation is often sufficient to eliminate paroxysmal AF but is usually insufficient for persistent AF.
  2. Linear AF across LA roof, mitral isthmus or cavotricuspid isthmus
  3. Ablation of CFAE in LA1 CS or RA
  4. Ablation of ganglionated plexus
  5. Various combinations

  } Can be tried in persistent AF

  - *Postablation*
    - Recurrence is common in 1st 3 months due to inflammatory response
    - Even in pt with sympt AF, postablation recurrence are asymptomatic
    ↓
    So accurate efficacy of ablation require monitoring for 7 days and preferably for 1 month (even for asympt episodes)
  - Compli
    - Cardiac tamponade
    - PV stenosis
    - Cerebral thromboembolism
    - Atrioesophageal fistula
    - Silent cerebral ischemic lesson
C. Cryoablation
  - Balloon designed to fit PV ostium and create circumferential ablation via cryo energy (liquid No@-80°C)
  - 1 year freedom from AF -75%
  - Less likely to cause PV stenosis
D. AV node ablation
  - Improves LVEF in pt with tachycardiomyopathy
  - All pt will require PPI
E. Surgical treatment:
  1. Cut and seal maze procedure developed by Cox
     - Includes 12 atrial incision to bolate PV
  2. Pulm vein isolation
  3. LAA excision
     - Good option for pt who are undergoing cardiac

POST-OP AF
- 25-40% pt
- 2 fold increase in risk of post of stroke
- Deals on 2nd DOD
- Pathogenesis—multifunctional
  - Adrenergic activation
  - Inflammation
  - Atrial ischemia
  - Electrolyte disturbance (hypomagnesemia)
  - Genetic factors
- Risk factors
  - Age >70
  - HIO prev AF
  - Male sex
  - LV dysfunction
  - LA enlargement
  - COPD
  - DM
  - Obesity

Treatment:

BB   /   sotalol   /   Amiodarone
↓   ↓   ↓
30%   50-65%   50-65%

Increased risk of post op AF

- RA or BiA temporary pacing electrodes reported to decrease risk for post op AF by 40%
  - Atorvastatin
  - Hydrocortisone   } Also decreases risk
  - Colchicine
  - Omega 3 PUFA

2.21 ACTION POTENTIAL AND CARDINAL ION CHANNELS

ACTION POTENTIAL

Definition

AP is short-lasting event, in which the electrical membrane potential of a cell rapidly rises & falls, following a consistent trajectory.

- Mediated by transient change in ion channel conductance major ion channels involved are
  1. Na^+ channels: I_{Na}
  2. Ca^{++} channels: I_{CaL} and I_{CaT}
  3. K^+ channels: I_{to}, I_{Kur}, I_{Kr}, I_{Ks}, I_{K1}
  4. I_F (only in pacemaker cells)
  5. N_{Cx} Na^+-Ca^{++} exchanger

Phase

0. *Rapid depolarization*
   Mainly due to opening of I_{Na} channel
1. *Rapid repolarization*
   Due to $I_{to, f}$ and $I_{to, s}$
2. *Pleathe phase*
   Due to I_{CaL} and I_{CaT} channel
3. *Final repolarization*
   Due to inward rectifier K^+ current
   Via I_{KUR}, IKR, IKS and I_{K1}
4. *Resting potential* maintained at -90 mv with help of I_{k1} I_{kAch} N_{Cx}.

AP in Various Parts of Heart

AP differ in pacemaker cells as compared to AP in working myocardium in to following terms

- RMP is -50 to-65 mv (Phase 4)
- Slow depolarization to merge in phase 0
- Rate of depolarization in phase 0 is much slower (θ = 0.1–0.2 m/s) (in myocardium θ = 1 m/s)

AP Also Varies from Endocardium to Epicardium

Epicardium: Shortest AP and prominent phase 1
Mid-myocardium: Longest AP
- AP duration of ventricular muscle represents QT interval on ECG
- QT interval,
  Early childhood—Male = Female
  At puberty—Male < Female

Epicardium has shortest AP because I_{t0} is maximum here → which leads to notch in AP at end of phase 0.

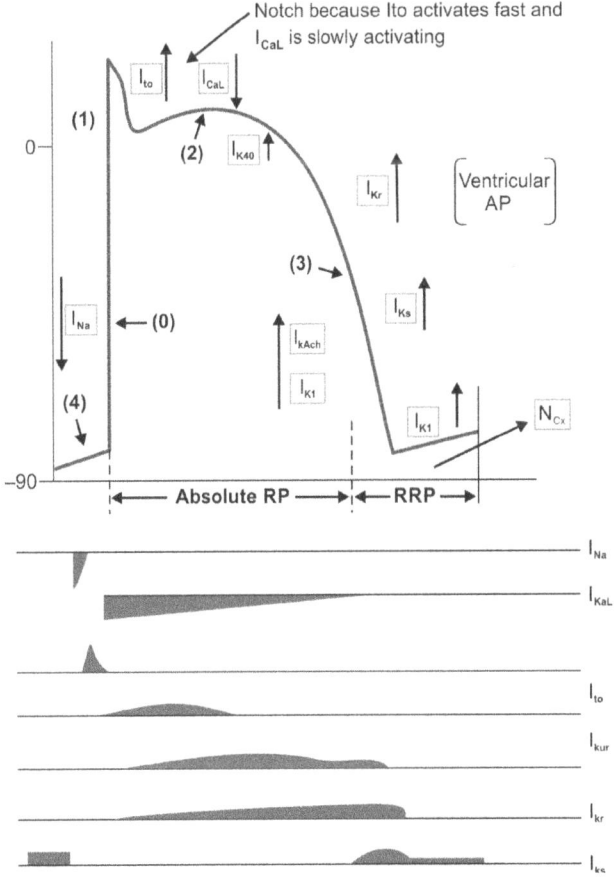

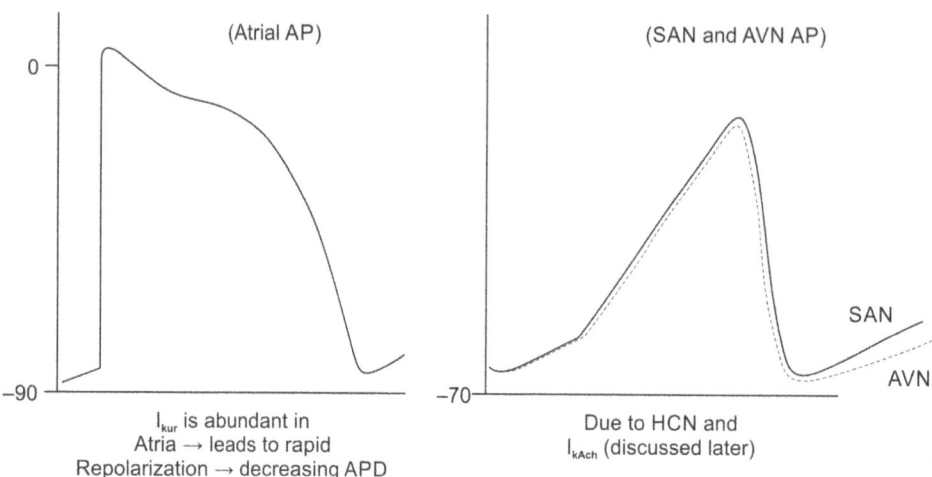

I_{kur} is abundant in Atria → leads to rapid Repolarization → decreasing APD

Due to HCN and I_{kAch} (discussed later)

Q: Physiology of Ion channels (Dec 14)

ION Channels

During AP permeability of ion channel changes and ion moves passively down its electro-chemical gradient.

$$\Delta V = \Delta V_m - V_x$$

ΔV = electro-chemical gradient
V_m = membrane potential
V_x = reversal potential of Ion x.

2 fundamental properties of ion channel
(1) Permeability and (2) Gating.

Permeability

- Ion channel are not simple fluid-filled pores
- Provide multiple binding sites
- Binding is saturable
- Ohm's law: $I = \Delta V_g$

  I = current
  ΔV = Driving force of ion mort.
  G = channel conductance

- In other words, flow of current across myocardium via Ion channels ohmically.
- But cardiac ion channels are nonohmical means, they have non-linear current voltage relationship (This property termed as rectification)
- *Mech,* e.g., in Mg^{++}, induce strong inward rectification current of K^+ channels

Gating 3 Mechanism

1. *Voltage Gated*
   - Commonest
   - Majority of ion channel opens in response to depolarization
   - I_f channels open in response to hyperpolarization

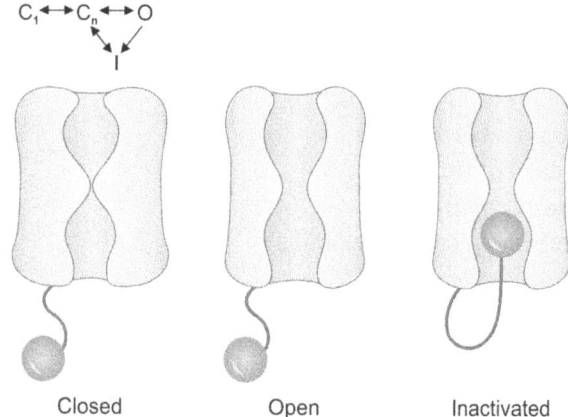

C_1 = Initial closed state
C_N = Closed state before O
O = Open state
I = Inactivated state

- Inactivation is basis of refractoriness
- Na^+ and Ca^{++} channels enter inactivated state during maintained depolarization and must undergo hyperpolarization to become active again.

2. *Ligand-gated*
   - Second major mechanism
     2.1 *Ach activated K^+ channel:*

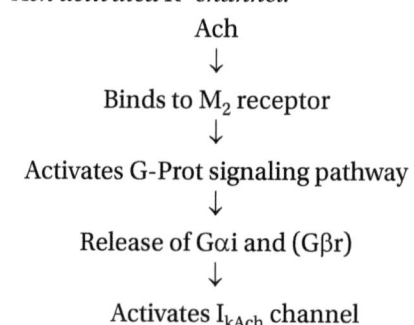

2.2 *ADP activated K⁺ channel:*
   Activated during ischemia
      (ADP|ATP ratio increases)
         ↓
   Abbreviate action potential
         ↓
   Less force generation (cardio protective)
         ↓
   Ischemia Preconditioning

3. *Mechano-sensitive channels:*
   - Stretch mediated
   - For example:
   - Acute cardiac dilatation induced arrhythmia
   - *Commotio cordis:* Blunt chest wall impact at appropriate timing may precipitate VPC or VF.

Structure

- α-subunit:
  - Central portion
  - Makes pores for ion passage
  - Highly selective for one ion
- β-subunit:
  - Regulate surface expression
  - And opening and inactivation
  - Kinetics

Channel	α subunit	β subunit
I_{Na}	$Na_v1.5$	$Na_v\beta$
I_{Ca}	$Ca_v1.2$	$Ca_vB2|\alpha2|\delta$
I_{to}	$K_v4.3$	$KCh|P_2$
I_{Kur}	$K_v1.5$	
I_{Ks}	$K_v7.1$	KCNE1
I_{Kr}	$K_v11.1$	KCNE2
I_{K1}	$K_{ir}2.x$	

Current	α subunit	β subunit	gene (α)	gene (β)
I_{Na}	$Na_v1.5$	B_1	SCN51	SCN1B
		B_2		SCN2B
		B_3		SCN3B
		B_4		SCN4B
I_{tof}	$K_v4.3$	$M1RP_1$	$KCND_3$	KCNE2

Contd...

		$M1RP_2$		KCNE3
		KCHIPs		multiple
I_{tos}	$K_v1.4$	K_vB1-4	KCNA4	KCNB1-4
I_{CaL}	$Ca_v1.2$	Ca_vB2	CACNAIC	CACNB2
		$Ca_v\alpha_2\delta_1$		CACNA2D1
I_{CaT}	$Ca_v3.1$		CACNAIG	
	$Ca_v3.2$		CACNAIH	
I_{Kur}	$K_v1.5$	$K_v\beta_{1-2}$	KCNA5	KCNAB1-2
I_{Kr}	$K_v11.1$	M_1RP_1	KCNH2	KCNE2
I_{Ks}	$K_v7.1$	MmK	KCNQ1	KCNE1
I_{K1}	$K_{ir}2.1$		KCNT2	
I_f	HCN1-4		HCN1-4	

*ION Channels

Pacemaker cells

1. I_f *(funny channel)*
   - *Activated by:* Hyperpolarization (≤55 mv)
   - *Mech:* Cyclic nucleotide –gated
   - HCN = Hyperpolarization-activated
   - Cyclic nucleotide gated
   - 4 members:
     • HCN1-4
     • Most abundant = HCN4
     • Permeable to both Na⁺ and Ca⁺⁺
     • *β-subunit:* KCNE-2
         Increases surface expression

2. K_{Ach}
   - Mech G-protein coupled inward rectifier (GIRK)
   - Arch/Adenosine/ATP

   ↓

   Activates G-Protein signaling pathway (M2 receptor)
         ↓
   Gα and Gβr
         ↓
   Activates GIRK
         ↓
   Slows the depolarization (phase 0)
         ↓
   Negative chronotropic action
         ↓

Arrhythmias

HCN and I_{Kach} relationship
- As pacemaker cells enter phase 0 of depolarization → HCN (I_f) enters inactive state and primarily transmit Na^+
- At the same time, I_{KAch} is activated and leads to outward K^+ current

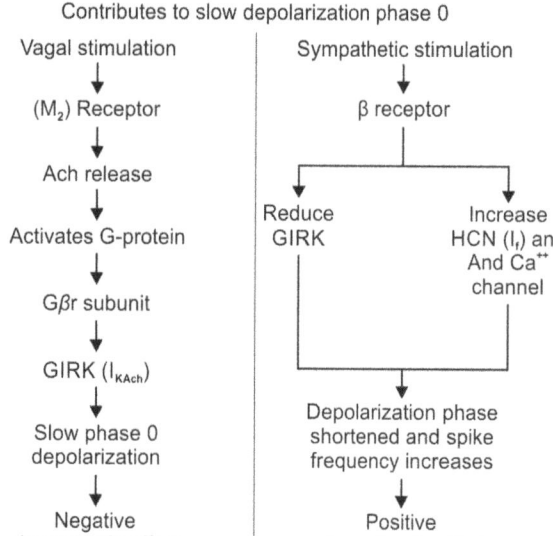

ALL CARDIAC CELLS

Sodium Channel

- Only in non-nodal tissue
- Primary determinant of depolarization
- Very fast activation and deactivation
- –85 to +25 mv within 10th of msec.
- α subunit = $Na_v1.5$
- Subunit - $Na_v\beta$

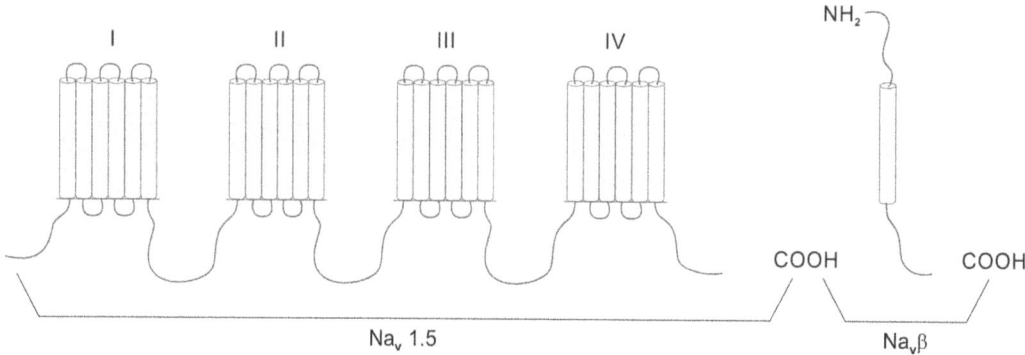

$Na_v1.5$:
- 220 kilo Dalton
- 4 homologous domains
- each have 6 transmemb protein

$Na_v\beta$:
- One transmembrane spanning β subunit
- *Genes involved*
  - $Na_v1.5$ encoded by SCN5A
  - β-subunit ($Na_v\beta_1-\beta_4$) encoded by SCN1-4B.
- *Mutation*
  - SCN5A → long QT syndrome (type 3)
  - SCN1B → Brugada syndrome/AF
  - SCN2B → AF
  - SCN3B → Brugada syndrome/AF
  - SCN4B → Long QT synd/sudden Infant Death Syndrome

Phosphorylation of $Na_v1.5$:
- Phosphorylation mediates ion channel.

Glycerol-3-phosphate dehydrogenase 1-like (GPDIL)
↓
Activates PKC (Protein kinase C)
↓
Phosphorylation of serine residue of $Na_v1.5$
↓
Reduce current activation
↓
Mutation in GPDIL → Brugada syndrome
Sudden infant Death Syndrome

- *Clinical Implication*
1. Mexiletine and flecainide decreases late component of sodium current and restores Qt interval
↓
Used to treat LQTS-3

2. Brugada syndrome due to synthesis of non-functional protein (failure of protein to be targeted to cell membrane) ↓accelerated inactivation of channel
3. Primary cardiac conduction defect (PCCD) sinus node Dysfunction, Atrial stand still, Av block and infra-Hisian block.
4. Overlap syndrome of LQTS, Brugada, and PCCD.
5. Dilated cardiomyopathy (mechanism not well understood)

Calcium Channel

- 2 types (L-type and T-type)
- Voltage gated
- *T-type channel:* expressed during development but drastically reduce during development.
- In adult heart t-type channel seen in SA nodal cells

Site	L-type	T-type
Site	Everywhere	SA nodal/Purkinje cell
Activation	low-threshold	High threshold
Inactivation		
↳Voltage Dependent	Slow	Fast
Ca^{++} Dependent	Yes	No

- α-subunit: $Ca_v1.2$
- Structure–similar to Na^+ channel
- β-subunit-total 4 types (like Na^+ channel)
- α-subunit encoded by CACNA1C
- β-subunit encoded by CACNB1-4
- 2 accessory subunits $α_2$ and δ

Unique Features

1. Sympathetic stimulation → β receptor → cAMP release → Increases amplitude of Ca^{++} current → positive chronotropic and inotropic effect
2. Ryanodine receptor, located on sarcoplasmic reticula → activated by Ca^{++} influx → major contributor in contractile machinery.
3. Calmodulin dependent protein kinase II
 ↓
 Phosphorylate I_{CaL} channel
 ↓
 Regulates Ca^{++} influx
 ↓
4. Calcium released from sarcoplasmic reticula (v/a RYR2 receptor)
 ↓
 Binds to calmodulin
 ↓

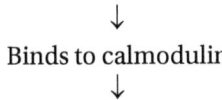

5. | Low memb potential (depolarized) | Normal Resting potential |
|---|---|
| ↓ | ↓ |
| Recovery of I_{Ca} is slow | Recovery from inactivated state is fast |
| ↓ | ↓ |
| I_{Ca} declines in Response to repetitive stimuli | I_{Ca} progressively increase during repetitive stimuli |
| ↓ | ↓ |
| Negative staircase of contractility | Positive staircase of contractility |

Inactivates I_{CaT} channel

Clinical Implication

1. *Timothy syndrome:* Multisystem disease with LQTS, cognitive abnormality, immune deficiency, hypoglycemia, syndactyly (mutation of $Ca_v1.2$)
2. Sudden death syndrome: Brugada + short QT syndrome (loss of Function of I_{CaL})
3. *Rule of class IV antiarrhythmics (CCB)*

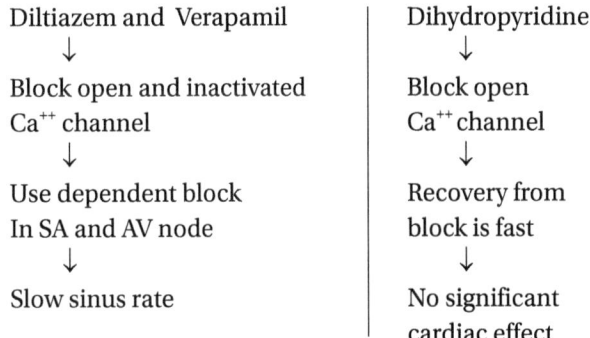

Diltiazem and Verapamil	Dihydropyridine
↓	↓
Block open and inactivated Ca^{++} channel	Block open Ca^{++} channel
↓	↓
Use dependent block In SA and AV node	Recovery from block is fast
↓	↓
Slow sinus rate	No significant cardiac effect

4. *EAD generation*
 If there is prolonged depolarization
 ↓
 Reuptake of Ca^{++} by sarcoplasmic reticula
 ↓
 Release of I_{CaT} from Ca^{++} dependent inactivation
 ↓
 Enable 2 degree depolarization
 ↓
 Early after depolarization
 ↓
 Polymorphic VT in LQTS

*Potassium Channel

- Many subtypes
- I_{to} important in atria and in subepicardial vent myocytes
- I_{Kur} predominantly in atria

Transient Outward (I_{to})

- 2 components
    1. Ca^{++} dependent chlorine channel
    2. Ca^{++} independent potassium channel
- Subdivided into
    1. $I_{to, f}$: rapidly activating and inactivating
    2. $I_{to, s}$: slow recovery kinetics
- α-subunit – $K_v4.3$
- β-subunit – $KchiP_2$ (K_v channel interacting Prot2)
  – KCNE-β subunit (total-5)
- Mutation in KCNE 3 and 5 → Brugada and VF

Clinical:
1. Brugada syndrome
2. In MI, I_{to} is down regulated by increased activity of calcineurin
3. Sustain Tachy in HF reduce I_{to} by similar mechanism

Delayed Rectifier (I_{Kr})

- Present in atria, nodal tissue, Purkinje cells and ventricles
- α subunit $K_v11.1$/β subunit KCNE-2 also termed as "ether —a-go-Go related gene 1 (ERG 1)
- Fast activation followed by slow deactivation conducts minor potassium current during early depolarization

And pleathe phase
↓
When membrane potential moves slightly towards repolarization (due to L-type Ca^{++} channel inactivation and I_{Ks} activation
↓
ERG1 channel released from inactivation
↓
Slowly progress to closed state (deactivation)
↓
Large K^+ current conducted through I_{Kr}

Low external K^+ → reduce activity
High external K^+ → increase activity

Clinical
1. Loss of F^n mutation of ERG1 → LQTS 2
2. Gain of F^n mutation → SQTS

Slowly Delayed Rectifier (IKs)

- α-subunit-$k_v7.1$
- β-subunit – KCNE1
- gene KCNQ-1
- Slowly activating and deactivating
- "I_{Ks} is the only potassium current which is upregulated with increased beating frequency"

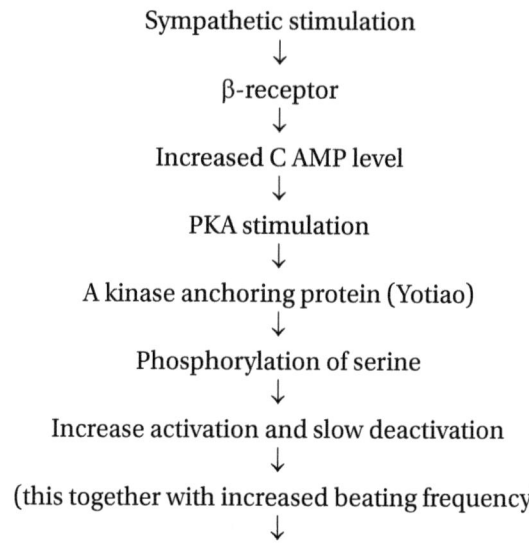

Sympathetic stimulation
↓
β-receptor
↓
Increased C AMP level
↓
PKA stimulation
↓
A kinase anchoring protein (Yotiao)
↓
Phosphorylation of serine
↓
Increase activation and slow deactivation
↓
(this together with increased beating frequency)
↓
Essential for AP shortening at higher heart rate

Clinical significance
1. Ischemia → increased extracellular Hyperosmolality → activates KCNQ1
2. I_{Ks} loss of p^n → LQTS1 (most common type)
↓
Mutant I_{Ks} does not increase sufficiently during β adrenergic stimulation
↓
Arrhythmia during exercise and emotional stress
3. Loss of F^n mutation in both alleles of KCNQ-1
   - Jervell and Lange—Nielsen syndrome

Inward rectifier (IK1)/(IKir)
- Four pair forming subunit
- Each subunit has 2 transmembrane Protein
- Responsible for terminating AP
- α-subunit: Kir2.1
- gene KCNJ2

Clinical significance
1. Loss of F^n mutation:
   - Andersen–Tawil syndrome
   - Skeletal development abnormality
   - Periodic paralysis
   - NSVT
   - Mild QT prolongation (LQTS 7)

Arrhythmias

1. *Long QT syndrome*
   LQT1-KCNQ1-I_{Ks}-α subunit-loss of f^n
   LQT2-KCNH2-I_{Kr}-α subunit-loss of f^n
   LQT3-SCN5A-I_{Na}-α-subunit-Gain of F^n
   LQT4-ANK2-Ankyrin-B
   LQT5-KCNE1-I_{Ks}-α-subunit
   LQT6-KCNE2- I_{Kr}-α-subunit

LQT7-KCNJ2- $I_{K1}\alpha$ subunit
LQT8-CACNA1E-Ca^{++} channel

2. *Short QT syndrome*
S4T1-KCNH$_2$-I_{Kr}
S4T2-KCNQ$_1$-I_{Ks} → gain of F^n
S4T3-KCNJ$_2$-I_{K1}

3. *Brugada syndrome*
BrS1-SCN5A –I_{Na}-Loss of f^n
BrS2-GPDIL-G3PD1- Altered f^n
BrS3-CACNA1c-ICa^{++}- Loss of f^n
BrS4-CACNB2b-ICa^{++}- Loss of f^n
BrS other –Ankyrin-B- Altered f^n

4. *CPVT (catecholaminergic Polymorphic VT)*
RVR2-ryrodin receptor- Gain of f^n
CASQ-calsequestrin-Gain of f^n

Intercalated discs
- Family of ion channel prot that contain gap J^n channels
- 3 types of specialized junction makes up each intercalated disc
  - Macula adherence or desmosome and fascia adherence
  - Form areas of strong adhesion between cells
- Nexus or gap J^n is the region in intercalated disc adhere Cells are in f^n contact with each other
  - Gap J^n provides biochemical and low resistance Electrical coupling between adjacent cells
  - Gap J^n allow movt of ion and small molecules (C Amp, C GMP, IP3)
  - Cardiac conduction is discontinuous due to Discontinuity created by gap J^n
  - Gap J^n also provides biochemical coupling, which Permits cell to cell movt of ATP, C AMP, Ip3 coordinated response of myocardium to physical Stimuli
  - Altered distribution and F^n of cardiac gap J^n are association with increased susceptibility to arrhythmias
- Defect in cell-cell adhesion prevent normal localization of connection in gap J^n → contribute to SCP from tachy arrhythmias
- For example: Carvajal synd-mutation in desmoplakin
Naxos disease
ARVD

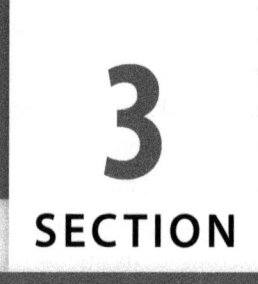

SECTION 3

Atherosclerosis

3.1 COMPLICATION OF ATHEROSCLEROSIS

ARTERIAL STENOSIS AND CLINICAL IMPLICATION

After the plaque burden exceeds the capacity of artery to remodel outward
↓
Encroachment on arterial lumen begins
↓
Eventually it impedes blood flow
↓
Lesion of >60% stenosis causes limitation of flow under increased demand
↓
Produce chronic stable angina pectoris or intermittent claudication
↓
Can progress to critical stenosis
↓
Myocardial infarction

- Even small atheromatous lesion can lead to MI when they rupture – form thrombus and occludes artery

THROMBOSIS AND COMPLICATIONS

Modes of plaque disruption
(2/3rd) (1) Fracture of plaque's fibrous cap (Plaque rupture)
(1/3rd) (2) Superficial erosion
    More common in females

Plaque Rupture

Due to imbalance between
- Forces that impinge on plaque's cap
- Mechanical strength of CAP

Factors Responsible

- Factors that decrease collagen synthesis
    T-cell derived cytokine INFY
    ↓
    Decreased collagen content of plaque cap
    ↓
    Prone to rupture
- Increased catabolism of ESM macromolecules that forms the fibrous cap of plaque
    - MMP enzymes
    - Elastolytic cathepsin
    ↓
    Breakdown collagen and elastin
    ↓
    Thinning of fibrous cap
    ↓
    Prone to rupture
- *Relative lack of SMC*
    Inflammatory mediators   T-cell
        ↓   ↓
    Induce programmed cell death of SMC
    ↓
    Weakening of plaque cap
    ↓
    Prone to rupture
- Prominent accumulation of macrophage with large lipid pool
    Large lipid pool   Activated macrophage
        ↓   ↓
    Increased biomechanical force   Cytokines and matrix degrading enzymes
        ↓   ↓
    On shoulder region of plaque   Degradation of collagen and SMC
        ↓   ↓
    Fracture of plaque   Plaque prone for rupture

Superficial Erosion

More likely to cause MI in women and in patients with hypertriglyceridemia and DM
- Underlying molecular mechanism is obscure

Possible mechanisms:
- Apoptosis of EGs → desquamation of EGs in areas of superficial erosion
- MMPs (such as certain gelatinases) degrade nonfibrillar collagen (Type-4) in BM
  - Tethering of EG to subjacent basal lamina → promote their desquamation

Mural platelet thrombi can complicate plaque erosion without causing arterial occlusion → Most plaque erosion do not give rise to clinically evident coronary events

↓

Repetitive cycles of plaque disruption, mural thrombosis in sites and healing contributes to lesion evolution and plaque growth

↓

This nonocclusive thrombi precedes the fatal event more frequently

Healing
- By PDGF and TGF-B released from platelet granules at the site of thrombosis

↓

Stimulate migration of SMC and increase collagen synthesis
(and)
- Thrombin generated at site of mural thrombi

↓

Stimulate SMC proliferation

This burnt-out fibrous and calcific atheroma represents late stage of plaque that previously uses lipid rich with characteristic association with plaque rupture but has become fibrous and hypocellular because of wound healing response.

PLAQUE SUSCEPTIBILITY TO RUPTURE AND INFLAMMATION IN ATHEROGENESIS

"Vulnerable Plaque"

CAG, OCT, IVUS, MRI, and CT all have shed light on morphology of plaques that causes Acs

Inflammatory markers (e.g., CRP) also increased in patients with MI)

Imaging + Inflammatory markers suggest widespread, diffuse and systemic nature of instability of atheromas in individual with or at risk of ACS.

THROMBOSIS DEPENDS ON

- *Solid state of plaque:* That may rupture or erode to trigger, thrombosis
- *Fluid state of blood:* That determine consequences of a given plaque disruption
  i. Amt of tissue factor in lipid core of a plaque
     - Control degree of clot formation
  ii. Level of fibrinogen in fluid determine whether plaque rupture leads to occlusive thrombus or mural thrombi
  iii. Elevated level of inhibitor of fibrinolysis (e.g., PAI)
     - Impede the ability of endogenous thrombolytic enzyme to limit thrombus growth

- Inflammation limits both thrombotic vs fibrinolytic
- Balance in both solid state and fluid state
- PAI-1 and fibrinogen both are acute phase reactants
- As well as inflammation mediator CD40 ligand induces tissue factor expression

3.2 SPECIAL CASES OF ATHEROSCLEROSIS

RESTENOSIS AFTER PCI

After Balloon Angioplasty

- SML prolifiration in intimal thickening (relatively less important)
- *Negative remodeling:* Due to advential inflammation caused by balloon-scar formation-wound contraction by healing process – arterial constriction-narrowing of lumen.

After Stent

Depends on intimal thickening rather than negativity remodeling stents prevent constriction from adventitia.

ACCELERATED ATHEROSCLEROSIS AFTER TRANSPLANT

- Limitation to long term survival
- Difficult to diagnose
  - No angina (denervated heart)
  - Diffuse and concentric disease/difficult to diagnose by CAG
- Selective environment of AN-grafted vessel with sparing of host's native arteries suggest-accelerated arteriopathy does not necessarily resulted from immunosuppressive therapy or other systemic factors in transplantation recipient
- Immunologic difference between host and recipient vessel might contribute to pathogenesis of disease
- Homozygous familial hypercholesterolemia—can detect fatal ath in 1st decade of life due to elevation in LDL
- EC in engrafted coronaries express MHC antigen-activate T cell-secrete INF—increasing adhesion molecule-increases leukocyte accumulate-enhance plaque formation (diffuse)

So graft arteriosclerosis represents extreme case of immunologically derived arterial hyperplasia

ANEURYSMAL DISEASE

- Dorsal surface of infrarenal aorta is prone to develop fatty streaks
- Because of absence of vasa vasorum the relative lack of blood supply to tunica media in this portion of abdominal aorta can explain susceptibility of these portions to develop aneurysm
- Additionally lumbar lordosis may alter the hemodynamics of blood flow-flow disturbance may promote lesion formation

Atherosclerosis	*Aneurysm*
Expansion of intimal lesion produces stenotic lesion	Transmural destruction of arterial structure
Tunica media underlying the lesion is thinned but with well preserved structure	

INFECTION AND ATHEROSCLEROSIS

- Infection may cause atherosclerosis
- Certain bacteria (e.g., *Chlamydia pneumonia*) and certain virus (e.g., *Cytomegalovirus*) has been shown to be responsible in seroepidemiological studies
- Multiple clinical trials have not shown benefit of antibiotic therapy in 2° prevention of atherosclerosis events

Confounding Factors

C. Pneumoniae: High incidence of bronchitis in smoker occurs due to *C pneumonia*

This *C pneumonia* infection is merely a marker for tobacco use, which is in turn a risk factor for ath events

Theories: Infection may potentiate the action of conventional risk factor, e.g., hypercholesterolemia

1. Cells within the plaque itself may harbor the infection (macrophage in plaque harboring infection with a pneumoniae)
   This can activate and accelerate inflammatory pathway
2. Specific microbial product (e.g., lipopolysaccharide or HSP) may act locally at level of arterial wall to potentiate atherosclerosis)
3. Minor breach in intestinal epithelium—breach by endotoxin—vascular reactivity and inflammation in adipose tissue – Insulin resistance and other factors of metabolic syndrome – CV death
4. Extravascular lesion also potentiate ath lesions, e.g., circulating endotoxin or cytokines produced in response to remote infection can act locally at level of artery wall to promote activation of vascular cells and lenocytes in preexisting lesion
5. Acute phase reactants also affect vascular inflammation and leucocyte activation
6. Acute infection can produce H.D alteration that can provoke coronary events (e.g., Tachycardia and hypotension)

3.3 NOVEL RISK MARKERS

INTRODUCTION
Basic requirement for risk marker
- There should be standardized and reproductive assay method
- Series of prospective study should have demonstrated predictive risk status of positive marker
- There should be evidence that novel marker adds to risk stratification by lipids
- It should add to global risk prediction score
- It should have proven intervention to reduce risk

hs-CRP
- Inflammation characterize all phases of atherosclerosis (including plaque formation, rupture and thrombus formation, occlusion, infarction)
- Various inflammatory markers associated
  ↓
  Most studied and most easily applied is acute phase reactant-CRP

CRP
- 5(23 k-Da) subunits
- Circulating member of penetration family
- Function in human innate immune response
- Primary derived from lives
- Cells in coro circulation can also elaborate CRP
- Whether CRP simply marks the risk or has direct role in atherothrombotic risk is controversial
- CRP measured with high sensitive (hs-CRP) independently predict risk of MI, stroke, PAD, SCD, among apparent healthy person (even when LDL cholesterol level are low)
  Patients with high hs-CRP but low LDL → higher risk ⎤
  Patients with low hs-CRP but high LDL → lower than above subgroup ⎦ Absolute risk

AHA Guidelines Cut-off
- Low risk ≤1 mg/L
  Intermediate = 1–3 mg/L
  High risk ≥3 mg/L
- Screening of hs-CRP should be done as a part of global risk and not as a replacement for LDL and HDL cholesterol
  - Greatest used in patients with intermediate risk (anticipated risk between 5 to 20%)

- hs-CRP evaluation recommended by CSS 2009 guidelines and 2011 guidelines from National Leopard Association USA
- hs-CRP >8 mg/dL ≥ represents acute phase response caused by underlying inflammatory disease are intercurrent infection
  ↓
  Repeat testing in 2 to 3 weeks
- hs-CRP: Minimal circadian Variation
  Do not depend on prandial state
- hs-CRP Incorporated into Reynolds risk score
- hs-CRP >3 → Predict recurrent coronary events
  Thrombotic complications after angioplasty
  Poor outcome in sitting of UF
  Vascular complication after CABG

AMT-additionally High hs-CRP Acute MI Suggest Enhanced
Inflammatory response at the time of hospital admission (even without troponin elevation) can determine subsequent M. rupture
↓
Patient with high hs-CRP likely to be benefited more with aggressive (early) intervention

Synd X
hs-CRP level also increased in syndrome X suggesting role of inflammation in coronary micro vascular function

AMI
hs-CRP elevation are more common in patients with frankly ruptured plate than those with plaque erosion

Prognosis
In patient with CRF and dialysis ⎤ High CRP
allograft vasculopathy ⎦ suggest pov short term prognosis

*hs-CRP also predict onset of T2 DM
*hs-CRP also adds prognostic info at all level of Met synd

Intervention
- Diet ⎤
- Exercise ⎬ First line intervention
- Smoking cessation ⎦
- *Use of statin therapy:* To reduce vascular risk among patients with elevated hs-CRP (even with low LDL)

JUPITER Trial

Healthy male and female with high hs-CRP (>2 mg/L) with low LDL (<130 mg/dL)

↓

Use of rosuvastatin resulted in 44% reduction in 1° endpoint of all vascular event 54% reduction in MI; 4% reduction in stroke; 46% reduction in arterial revasc; 20% reduction in all-cause mortality

↓

All subgroup significantly benefited with statin therapy "Low risk" group (women, nonsmoker, those without ms, those with Framingham score <10%)

- Jupiter trial also demonstrated significant reduction of hs-CRP and LDL level by rosuvastatin

PROVE IT-TIMI 22

Acs created with statin, achieving hs-CRP <2 mg/L conferred long term event free survival as achieving LDL cholesterol <70 mg/d. Those who net both this goal → greater benefit

Drawbacks

- With chronic inflammatory disease such as RA, IBD, psoriasis—Have elevated hs-CRP and on average are somewhat at higher vascular risk
- Low grade infection (gingivitis) are those with chronic carriers of *chlamydia pneumoniae, H. pylori*, herpes simplex, cytomegalovirus, also may have high CRP level and height and risk of CV disorder due to chronic inflammatory response.

OTHER BIOMARKERS OF INFLAMMATION

- Cytokines such as IL-1 and IL-6
- Soluble intercellular adhesion molecule (SICAM-1)
- p selectin
- CD 40 ligand
- Marker of leukocyte activation (myeloperoxidase)
- Preg. associated plasma protein A (PLAP-A)
- IL-1 receptor family member (ST-2)

↓

- Some have analytic limitation
- Some have too short half life
- Some have limited ability to predict risk
- No large scale trials
- Soluble CD40 provide insight into efficacy of specific antithrombotic agents
- Myeloperoxidase provide prognostic information in case of acute ischemia
- ST2 is novel association in HF and ischemia

8. Fibrinogen
   - Positive association with age, obesity, smoking, DM and LDL cholesterol level and negative association with HDL cholesterol level, alcohol use, physical activity, and exercise level
   - Fibrinogen was among the front "novel" risk factor evaluated
   - Linear association was seen between usual fibrinogen level and the risk of CAD and stroke
   - hs-CRP and fibrinogen showed addictive ability to predict risk
   - Fibrinogen has highest predictive usefulness in patients with other concomitant elevation of Lp(a) or homocysteine

Anti-inflammatory Modulators

- Broad based
  Aspirin, statin, colchicine, methotrexate
- Anti-pro-inflammatory cytokines
  IL-1: canakinumab, anakinra
  IL-6: tocilizumab
  INF: infliximab, etanercept, adalimumab, golimumab, certolizumab
- Delivery of anti-inflammatory cytokines (TGF-β, IL-10, IL-19)
- Treg cell induction
- In vivo transfection
- Lp-PLA2
  - Only other marker available commercially
  - Positive relation between Lp-PLA2 and vascular risk
  - LP-PLA2 bound to apo B100 (So its level closely related to LDL cholesterol)
  - 2 large scale clinical trial
    Lp-PLA2, no longer predicted residual risk after aggressive LDL cholesterol reduction with statin

Interventions

4 clinical trials → Disappointing result
- Bezafibrate → No reduction in risk
- Hormone replacement therapy → lower fibrinogen but not improve clinical outcome

Therapies under evaluation
- Darapladib (inhibitor of Lp PLA2)
- Canakinumab (monoclonal ab against IL-1β)
- Generic anti-inflammatory agent low dose methotrexate (already in use for methotrexate)

LIPOPROTEIN (A)

- Consist of LDL particle with its apo B100 component link bi disulfide bridge to apolipoprotein(a)
- Lp(a) level varies inversely with apo(a) isoform
- >25 forms available
  1. Homology between lp(a) and plasminogen → raised possibility that it Lp may inhibit endogenous fibrinolysis by completing with plasminogen binding site
  2. Lp(a) binds and inactivate tissue factor pathway inhibitor and augment expression of plasminogen activator inhibitor for the linking Lp and thrombosis
  3. Lp(a) also colocalizes with ath lesion and may have local action through oxidized phospholipids pathway

Lp(a):
- Prognostic information to overall risk in 1 prevention remains uncertain
- In most studies lp(a) has proven to be e credit to for person already known to have high risk because of elevated LDL levels
- Predicts risk non-linearly
- At present laboratories lp(a) in a manner independent of apo(a) isoform size

Interventions
1. High dose niacin
2. LDL chol reduction markedly reduce hazard associated with Lp(a)
3. New agents: PCSK9 inhibitors
   Anacetrapib
   Mipomersen

HOMOCYSTEINE

In patient with inherited defect of methionine metabolism severe hypercholesterolemia can develop
↓
Elevated risk of premature atherosclerosis as well as venous thromboembolism.

Mechanism

Endothelial dysfunction, accelerated oxidation of LDL cholesterol, impairment of flow mediated endothelial derived relaxing factor, platelet activation, and oxidative stress.

Cause

1. Mild-mod elevations (1.5 mmol/L) are more common in gen pop because of insufficient dietary intake of folic acid
2. Patients receiving folate antagonist-methotrexate, carbazine
3. Impaired homocysteine metabolism due to hypothyroidism or renal insufficiency
4. Mutation in MTHFR (methylenetetrahydrofolate reductase)-can elevate homocysteine level

Recent guidelines has not advocated its use

Intervention

Trials: None of trials has shown substance benefit
1. *VISP:* High dose and low dose regimes containing folate and pyridoxine → no diff between 2 regimes
2. *NORVIT:* In patient with acute MI: Harmful effect with combined vit B supplement
3. *HOPE2:* 5 years of therapy with folate, vit B6 and vit B12 resulted in no benefit

Subgroups who can't get benefited with treatment
1. Those taking traditional risk factors
2. With renal failure
3. With markedly premature atherosclerosis or family h/o, MI or stroke at young age

DIRECT PLAQUE IMAGING

1. Ultrasound measure of carotid—IMT
2. Coronary art calcium scoring (CAC)
   - Recent meta-analysis—IMT is of doubtful prognostic importance
   - MESA-CAC, ADI, hs-CRP and family history (not IMT) can independently predicts vascular event among persons at intermediate risk

Drawback:
1. However CAC has high false positive rate
2. Radiation exposure
3. CT detect place with least likely to rupture and does not detect noncalcified thin capped lesion
4. Absence of CAC does not preclude ath risk
   New-functional imaging
   Potential targets for function imaging
   - Measure of glucose uptake, specific adhesion molecule, biomarker of apoptosis and protein degradation (proteinases, MMPs, cathepsins)
   - MRI, PET and contrast enhanced ultrasound all are under evaluation
   - Function measure of vascular reactivity also decreases evaluation

Intervention

- No trials showed benefit of treatment based on imaging
- DIAD trial underscores the importance of performing such trials
- EISNAR trial did not show any beneficial effect as estimating CAC

GENETIC MARKERS

- 95 genetic loci association with normal lipid variation and extreme lipid phenotypes
- Most loci appears to act on process of atherosclerosis independent of traditional risk factors
- Magnitude of risk associated with any one genetic variant tends to be small
- Individual SNP (single nucleotide polymorphism) or multiple genetic panels to predict CV risk has proved to be disappointing
- Reynolds risk score which included F/H and traditional risk factors highlights the importance of F/H as a variable of shared genetic and environmental factors

Intervention

[Pharmogenetic study of inherited and acquired genetic variation in drug response that can affect both individual and selected population]

E.g., Statin induced myopathy
Clopidogrel resistance
Warfarin dosing

1. *SEARCH trial:* Common variant in (SLCOIBI) found strong association with increased risk of simvastatin induced myopathy
Encodes organic anionic transporting protein known to regulate hepatic uptake of statin
2. TIMI group found genetic variation in cytochrome p450 system responsible for clopidogrel resistance

Newer Biomarkers

1. Plaque instability markers
   - Preg associated plasma protein
   - Myeloperoxidase
   - MMPG, MMP-2, TIMP-1
   - Myeloid related Port 8/14
   - Interleukin 6 and 18
   - Soluble lectin like oxidized LDL
2. Inflammatory markers
   - hs-CRP
   - Homocysteine
   - Pentraxin -3
   - Serum Amyloid-A
   - Fibrinogen
   - Lipoprotein associated phospholipase A2
3. Endothelial markers
   - ET1/CT pro ET1
   - Mid regional pro adrenomedullin
4. Biomarkers of cardiac necrosis
   - Hs TnI assay
   - Heart FA binding prot
   - Ischemia modified albumin
5. Markers of biomechanical stress
   - BNP
   - Copeptin
   - Mid—regional pro-ANP
   - GDF-15 and ST 2
3. Several genetic polymorphisms has been found to be related with warfarin dosing

So to conclude: Family history can be considered important to know and predict CV disease related risk

ENVIRONMENTAL FACTORS

- Depression and mental stress
  Depression
  Chronic stress
  Anxiety   } Risk of CAD
  Chronic hostility and anger
  Social isolation
- Depression doubles the risk of CVD (INTERHEART)
- Effect of depression:
  - Effect on inflammation
  - Endothelial dysfunction
  - Increased platelet activity
  - Increase whole blood serotonin
  - Enhanced activity of HP-A axis
  - Alteration in cardiac autonomic tone
  - Adverse lifestyle factors (poor diet, smoking, lack of exercise, nonadherence to medication)
- Mental stress adrenergic stimulation—Increased myocardial oxygen requirement and aggravate myocardial ischemia; coronary vasc constrictions platelets and endothelial dysfunction; metabolic syndrome and induction of vent arrhythmias

3.4 VASCULAR BIOLOGY AND ATHEROSCLEROSIS

STRUCTURE OF NORMAL ARTERY

Cells of Normal Artery

1. Endothelial cells:
   - Directly in contact with blood
   - Maintain blood in liquid state

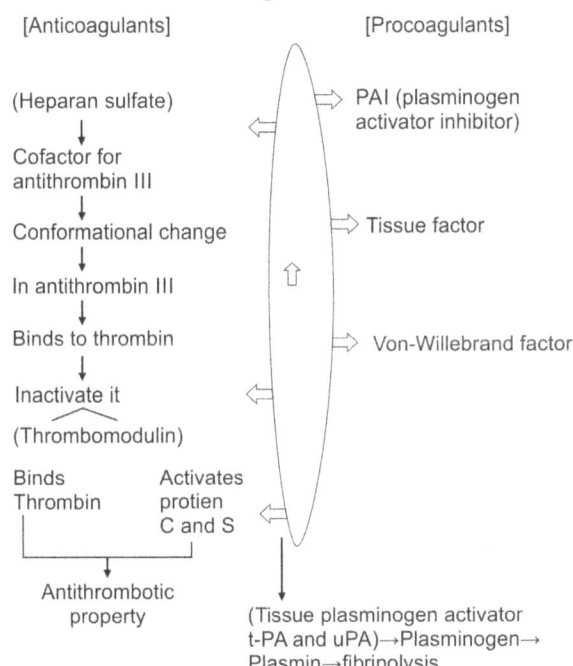

Embryology

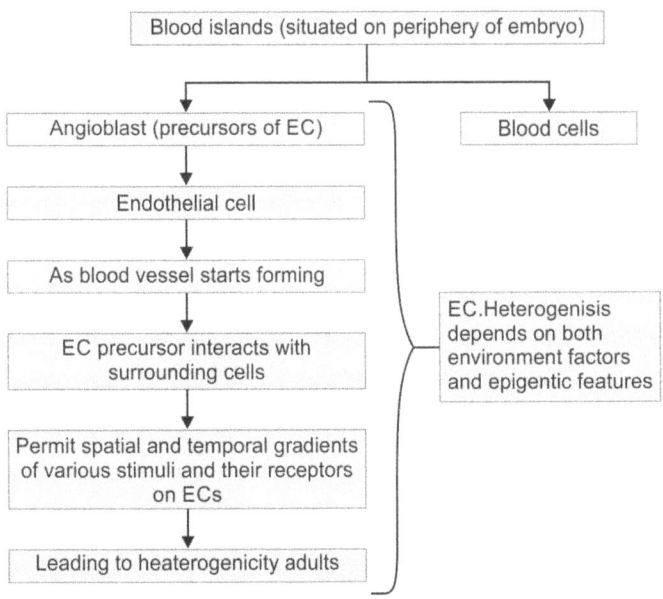

Postnatal Life

Cells that make various components of arterial wall originate

From bone marrow
↓
Peripheral blood contains endothelial precursor cells
↓
Helps repair areas of endothelial desquamation

2. *Arterial smooth muscle cells*
   - Second major cell type
   - Function
     1. Contract and relax → control blood flow through various arterial beds (especially muscular arterioles) → abnormal SMC contraction → vasospasm
     2. Synthesize bulk of complex ECM → plays key role in normal vascular homeostasis → formation and complication of atherosclerosis
     3. Migrate and proliferate → formation of intimal hyperplastic lesions (atherosclerosis and restenosis) (e.g., restenosis after PCI and anastomatic hyperplasia complicating vein grafts)
     4. Death of SMC → destabilization of atheromatous plaque ecstatic remodeling and ultimately aneurysm formation

Embryologically: Arise from many sources

- Neural crest
- 2nd heart field
- Somites
- Various stem cells
- Mesoangioblasts
- Proepicardium
- Splanchnic mesoderm
- Mesothelium

After ECS form tubes (rudimentary blood vessels)
↓
ES, recruit SMC and pericytes
↓

- Descending aorta and its branches from regional mesoderm
- Distal aorta and its branches from somites
- Arteries and carotids from neuroectoderm
- Asc aorta and carotids from proepicardial mesoderm
- Coronary artery from proepicardial mesoderm

Various SMC arise from

↓
Heterogenicity of SMC
↓
Decide about capacity of certain arteries or regions to develop atherosclerosis of heightened response to injury or its medial degeneration (e.g., marfan)

Small population of precursor cells may reside in tunica media of normal arteries → gives rise to SMC that accumulate in injured atherosclerotic arteries

Layers of normal arteries:
1. *Intima:* Innermost layer
   - Thin at birth (monolayer)
   - Resides on basement membrane containing non fibrillar collagen (such as Type IV)
   - With aging human arteries develop complex intima containing arterial SMC and fibrillan form of collagen type I and III. SMC produce ECM of arterial intima
   - Precursor of complex adult intima is diffuse intimal thickening (characterize most adult human arteries)
   - Some region develop thicker intima even in absence of atherosclerosis (e.g., Prox LAD)
   - Internal elastic memb bound turned intima abluminally and serve as border between intima and media
2. *Media:*
   Elast Art—Contains well developed concentric layer of SMCs interlaced with layers of elastin rich ECM.
   Modular Art.
   - SMCs embedded in surrounding matrix in more continuous than lamelle array
   - SMCs seldom proliferate
   - SMCs rate of division and cell death is low
     CSM—Neither accumulates nor atrophies matrix synthesis and dissolution balances each other
   - Tunica media bounded by EEL
3. *Adventitia:*
   Contains:
   1. Collagen fibrils (loose than intima)
   2. Vasa vasorum and nerve endings
   3. Fibroblast and mast cells
      (Evidences suggested role of mast cells in atherosclerosis but human importance is still speculative)

INITIATION OF ATHEROSCLEROSIS

A. *Extracellular Lipid accumulation*

   Diet rich in cholesterol and saturated fat
   ↓
   Small lipoprotein particles accumulate in Intima
   ↓
   Lp decorates the proteoglycan in intima and tends to coalesce into aggregate
   ↓
   [Lp + proteoglycan] retained by intima for prolonged time
   ↓
   Increase susceptibility of oxidative or other chemical modification
   ↓

B. *Leucocyte recruitment and retention*

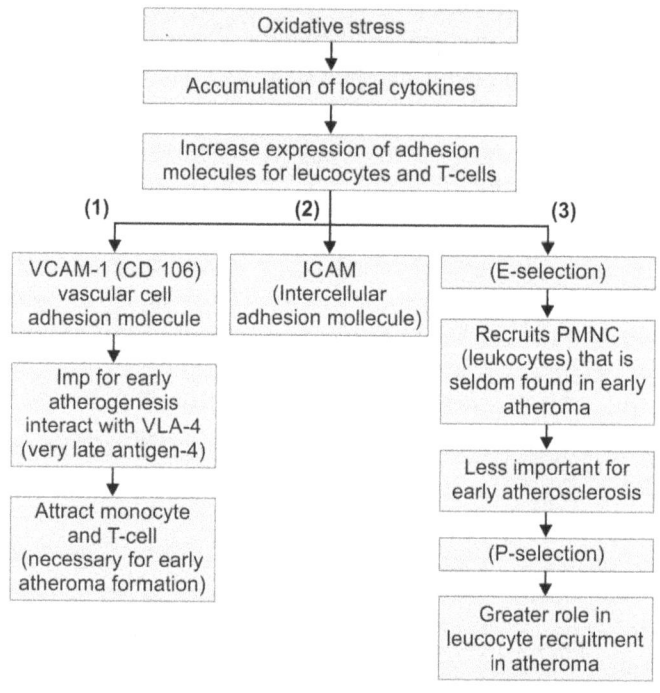

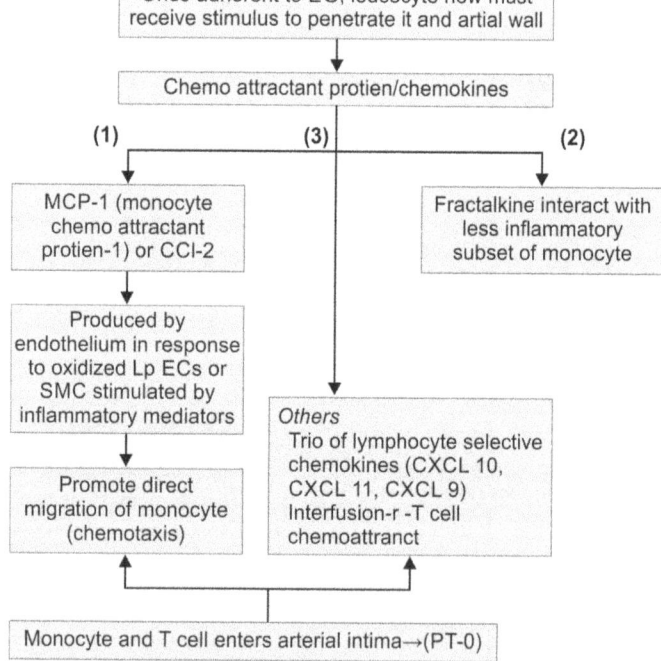

C. *Focality of lesion formation:*
   Why atheroma is focal?
1. *Multicenter origin hypothesis:*
   - Atheroma arise as benign leiomyomas of arterial wall

2. *Hydrodynamic basis hypothesis:*
   - Prediction of proximal portion of arteries after branch point or bifurcation at flow dividers
   - Arteries without many branches (e.g., IMA and radial tend not to develop atherosclerosis
- *Laminar flow:* Antiatherogenic
- Decreases sheer stress at branching → atherogenic

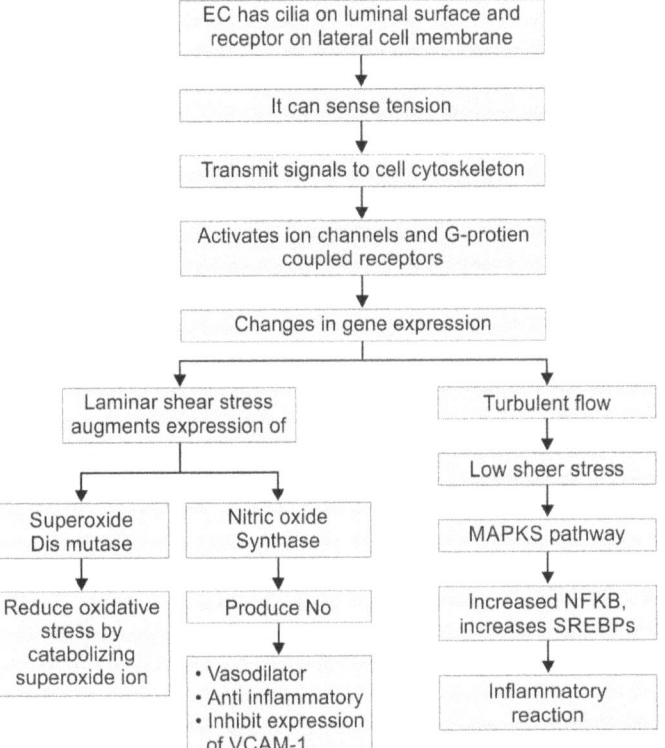

[Transcription factor KLF-2 –(Kruppel-like factors 2) Regulate anti-inflammatory activity of EC]
[KLF2 enhance no synthase expression and inhibit NFK-β function]

D. *Foam cell formation*

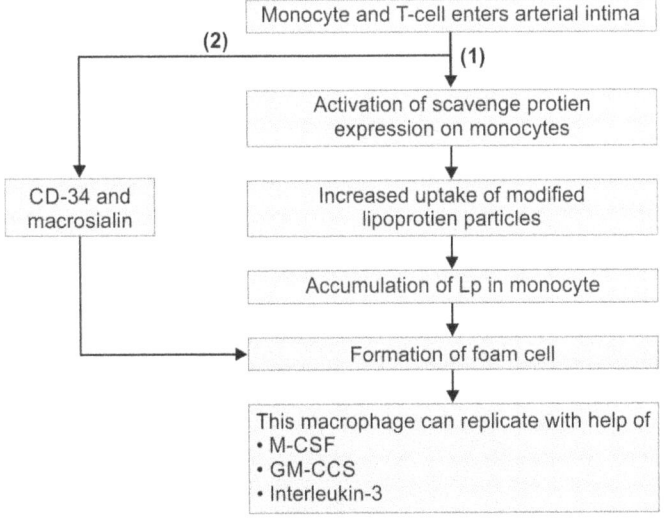

Fatty streak: Lesion consists primarily of lipid engorged macrophages. No thrombosis, No calcification
- Its precursor lesion of atheroma
- Can regress to some extent

E. *Fatty streak to atheroma*

$$\text{Foam cell}$$
$$\downarrow$$
Produce additional cytokines
- Hypochloric acid
- Superoxide anion (O_2)
- MMP

$$\downarrow$$
Stimulate migration of SMC
$$\downarrow$$
From media to intima
$$\downarrow$$
SMC can divide and elaborate ECM
$$\downarrow$$
ECM accumulate in growing atherosclerotic plaque
$$\downarrow$$
Fatty streak evolve into fibrofatty lesion
$$\downarrow$$
Ca^{++} accumulation can occur

Sometimes SMC death (apoptosis) leads to relatively acellular
Fibrous capsule surrounding lipid rich core that may also contain
Dying or dead cells and their debris

EVOLUTION OF ATHEROMA

A. Role of innate and adaptive immunity: Mechanism of inflammation:

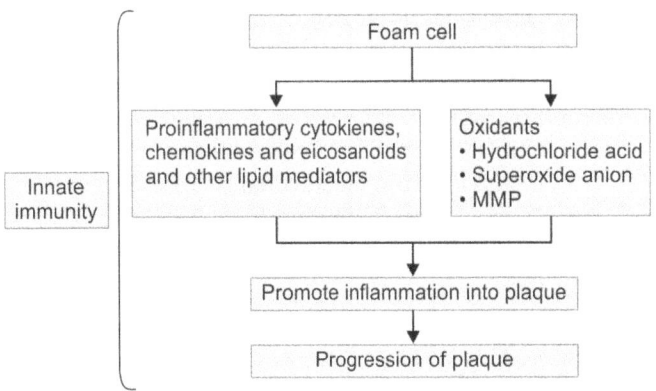

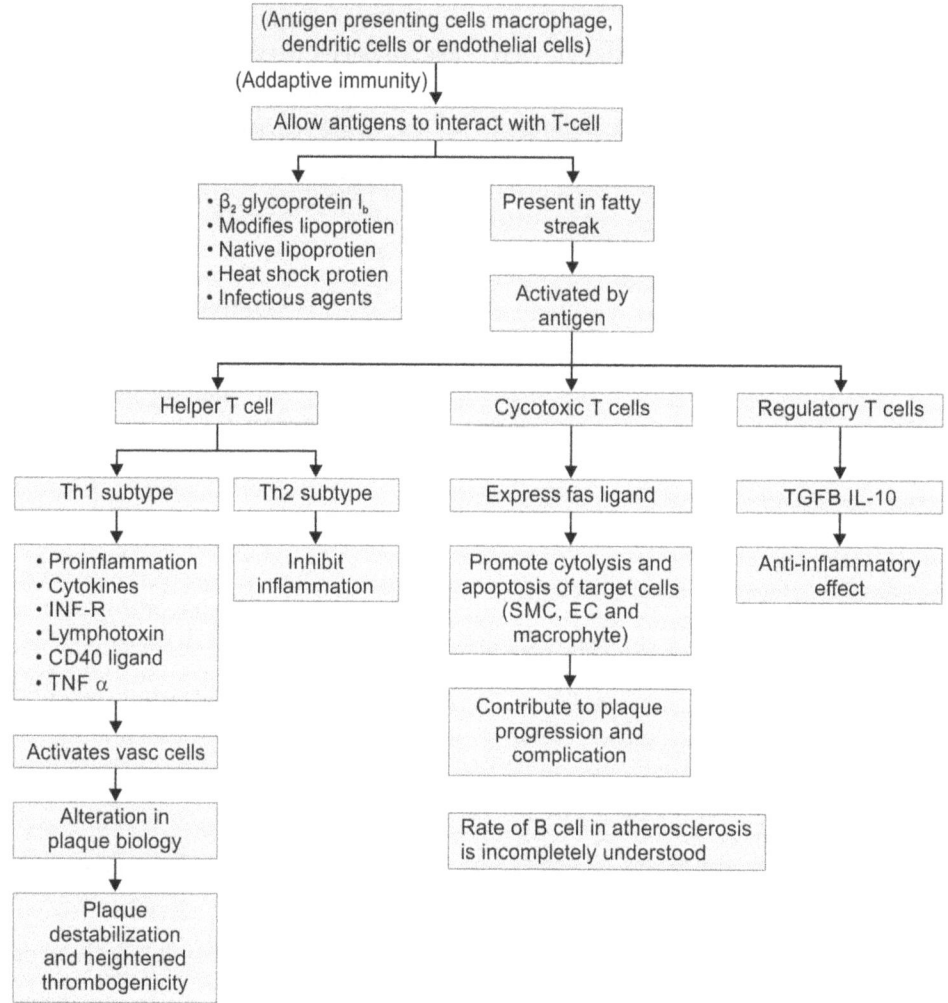

B. SMC migration and proliferation
- SMC in intima is less mature than that in arterial medial layer
- Intimal SMC has higher embryonic isoform of myosin
- So SMC in intima is of embryonic type and it can recapitulate
- It contain more ER and fewer contractile fibers

(How intimal SMC differ from medial SMC)

Burst of SMC replication may occur during life history of a given atheromatous lesion

Note: Accumulation of SMC and growth of intima may not occur in linear pattern

C. *Smooth muscle cell death during atherogenesis*
- Apoptosis/programmed cell death
  • Due to inflammatory cytokines or
  • Due to T-cell in atheroma
  (Fas ligand on T cell birds to Fas on SMC → SMC death)

So SMC accumulation in plaque depends on
1. SMC replication
2. SMC death

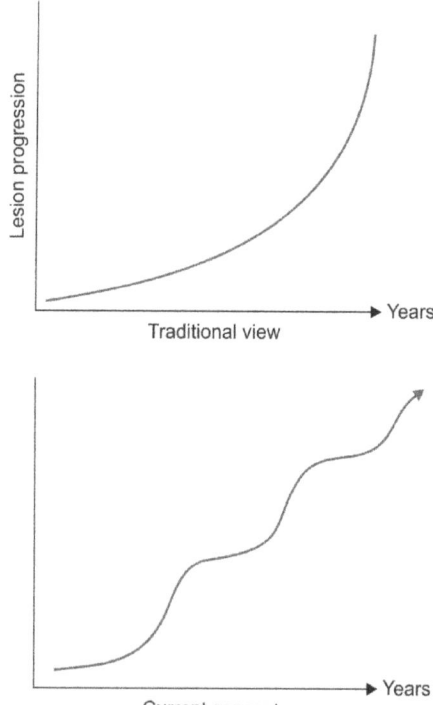

Arterial ECM:
- ECM makes up much of plaque
- ECM macromolecules that accumulates in atheroma
  1. Collagen (Type I and III)
  2. Proteoglycans (versican, biglycan, aggrecan, decorin)
  3. Elastin fibers
     - Stimuli for excessive ECM production by SMC: PDGF and TGF-β
     - MMP dissolution of ECM by MMP contributes to migration of SMC from media to intima
     ↓
  Leads to arterial remodeling
     ↓
  Initial plaque growth occur outwards in an abluminal fashion (increasing the caliber of entire artery) (positive remodeling)
     ↓
  Must involve tumor of ECM to accommodate circumferential growth of artery
     ↓
  Luminal stenosis tends to occur only after the plaque burden exceeds approx 40% of cross sectional area of artery

D. *Angiogenesis in plaque:*
   Ath. Pl. develop their own microcirculation as they grow because of endothelial migration and replication

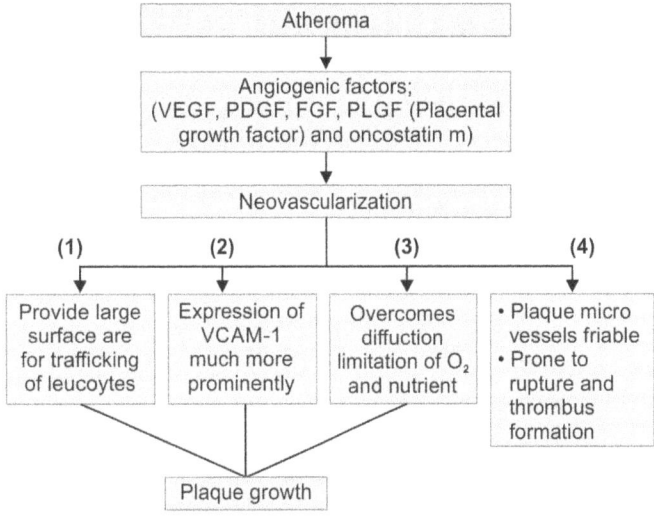

E. *Plaque mineralization:*

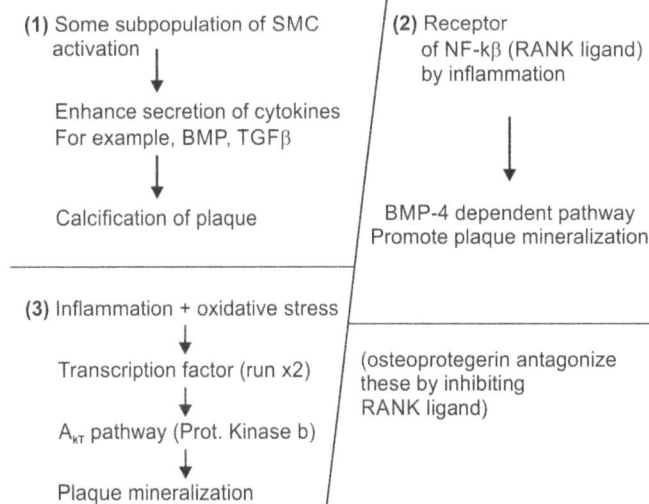

*Micro particles elaborated by macrophage provides nidus for plaque calcification (link between inflammatory cell and CV disease)

3.5 RISK MARKERS AND PRIMARY PREVENTION OF CARDIOVASCULAR DISEASES

INTRODUCTION

Core approach to 1° prevention (historically)
Global risk estimating algorithm
1. Framingham risk score
2. Reynolds risk score
3. European risk evaluation (SCORE)

Stratified patients into B group
- Low risk
- Intermediate risk
- High risk
- Lifestyle intervention for low and intermediate risk
- Pharmacological intervention for higher risk

Current concept
- 1° prevention strategy should be based on RCT and not on epidemiological data
- This scoring system themselves are not tested in a random manner.

CONTROVERSY WITH STATIN

Multiple RCTs do not support statin therapy
1. CORONA (Controlled rosuvastatin multinational trial in HF)
2. AURORA (A study to evaluate use of rosuvastatin in subjects on regular hemodialysis)
3. 4D (Gorman analysis and diabetes study)
4. GISSI-HF
↓
All enrolled high absolute risk patients who achieved large LD4 chol reduction with statin but none showed significant clinical benefit
5. JUPITER (Justification for use of statin in prevention: and international trial evaluating rosuvastatin)
6. AFCAPS/Tex CAPS (Air force/texas coro ath. prev prog)
7. MEGA (Management of elevated cholesterol in adult Japanese)
↓
32621 1° prevention patients
↓
Enrolled low risk patients (most of whom will not qualify for statin treatment due to current guidelines)
↓
- All 3 showed marked benefit with statin therapy
- Greatest relative risk reduction ever achieved with statin therapy
↓
Interference from above 7 trials

1. Not used statin in patients with
   - Heart failure (CORONA, GISSI-HF)
   - Renal failure (AURORA, 4G)
2. Used statin aggressively as 1 prevention in
   - In elevated LD2 cholesterol (MEGA)
   - Low HDL cholesterol (AFCAPS/Tex CAPS)
   - Elevated CRP (JUPITER)
↓
Cardiologist in US or Canada and Europe has suggested following five recommendations
1. Adjunct to diet, exercise and smoking cessation for 2° prevention in patients with prev. HIO MI, smoker clinically apparent ath.
   (Trials: 4S, HPS, CARPs, LIPID)
2. Can be considered as adjunct to diet exercise and smoking cessation in setting of 1° prevention for those age >50 years and with either diabetes (CAEDS)
   - Elevated LDL chol. (WOSCOPS) (MEGA)
   - Low HDL (AFCAPS)
   - High hs-CRP (JUPITER)
   Physician may limit statin prescription to above group who also has at least one additional risk factor (HTN/smoking)
3. Physician should maximize intensity of treatment and then focus on compliance and long-term adherence
   (Trials: PROVEIT, TNT)
   Dose should not be selected close to or at higher level the individual patient can tolerate without S/E
4. Non-statin lipid lowering agent for monotherapy or combination with statin should be limited during the wait for evidence that such an approach further reduces CV event rates in specific patient group.
   (Trial: AIM-HIGH, HPS2 THRIVE, ACCORD, FIELD)
5. Guidelines based on trial (what works) and trial entry criteria (in whom) is simply practical and consistent with evidence based principles.

CONVENTIONAL RISK FACTORS

Smoking
- Important risk factor
- Second hand smoke exposure too
- Smokes lose 1 decade of life expectancy compared to nonsmoker
- Increased risks are now equal for male and female
- Increased risk of CAD and stroke both
- Smoking → vasoconstriction → greater risk of developing PVD and Abd Ao. Aneurysm

- Second hand smoke → increased risk of heart disease by 25-30%
- Smoking—doubles risk of CAD
  - Increases CV disease related mortality by 50%
  - Increases sudden death
  - Increases Ao. aneurysm formation
  - Increases asymptomatic PVD
  - Increases ischemic stroke
  - Increases hemorrhagic stroke (IC and SAH)
  - Recurrent MI
- Risk increases with age and number of cigarettes smoked
- Passive smoking → Ham per endothelial dependent
  Vasodilatation + increases bronchial responsiveness + pulmonary dysfunction
- Smoking acts synergistically with OC pills
- Smoking especially hazardous for women with DM

Effects of Smoking

1. In favorable effects on BP and sympathetic tone
2. Decreases myo oxygen supply
3. Contribute to pathogenesis of atherosclerosis
4. Enhance oxidation of LDL
5. Impair endothelial dependent coro vasodilatation
6. Impair endothelial NO biosynthesis
   Smoker's Paradox: Smokers have better outcome after various reperfusion strategy. Reason is that smokers undergo procedure at younger age and have lower rate of comorbid illness at that age.
7. Adverse hemostatic and inflammatory effect
   - Increases CRP level
   - Increases ICAM-1, fibrinogen, homocysteine
8. Spontaneous platelet aggregation
9. Increases monocyte addition to endothelial cells
10. Adverse alteration in endothelium derived fibrinolytic and antithrombotic factors (e.g., T-PA and PAI)
11. Increases coronary spasm
12. Decreases threshold for vent arrhythmias
13. Insulin resistance

*Intervention for smoking cessation
Smokers who quit
1. Decreases risk of coronary event by 50% within 2 years (much house benefit even in first few months)
2. Risk approximates to nonsmoker within 3 to 5 years
3. Stroke risk decreases (approximate nonsmoker within 5-15 years)
   1. Advice and assistance by treating physician
   2. Counseling
   3. Behavioral therapy
4. Medications
   1. Nicotine patch, gum, lozenges
   2. Nicotine inhaler/spray

Even after smoking cigarette → risk of COPD, CA king, CA pancreas, CA stomach persists for decades

Hypertension

- Major risk factors for
  - CAD
  - HF
  - CVA
  - DAD
  - Renal failure
  - AF
  - Total mortality
  - Loss of cognitive function
  - Dementia
- Degree of BP lowering relates timely to risk reduction
- For 40-70 years age,
  - Each 20 mm Hg increases in SBP ⎤ Doubles risk of
    Or 10 mm Hg increases in DBP ⎦ CV disease
  - Prehypertension (SBP 120-139 and DBP 80-89)
    Doubles the risk of MI and stroke in women
  - Below 45 years M>F ⎤
    45-65 years M=F   ⎬ Prevalence
    >65 years F>M   ⎦
  - HTN increases with age in all race and ethnicity

Risk for developing HTN: Increasing age, ethnicity, family history, genetic factors, low education, low SE level greater weight, low physical activity, stress, tobacco use, sleep apnea, high Na^+ and low K^+ intake, increases dietary fats and excessive alcohol intake

- High risk group for developing HTN
- Obese, DM, metabolic syndrome, ckD
  - 69% patients with 1st heart attack ⎤
  - 77% patients with 1st stroke   ⎬ BP 140/90 or higher
  - 74% patients with CHF   ⎦
- Recent (within last 10 years) and remote BP also contributes importantly to risk
- HTN in young
  - Decreasing life expectancy
  - Decreasing life years free of CV disease
  - Increasing years lived with CV disease
- SBP, DBP/PP contributes equally
- PP (indicates vascular wall stiffness) also predicts first and recurrent MI
- Ambulatory BP provide strong prediction rather than office BP
- Nocturnal HTN: increases risk of CHF

Interventions to decrease BP:
1. Diet and lifestyle modification
2. Weight reduction
3. Limited alcohol intake
4. Smoking cessation
5. Salt restriction; adequate K^+ and Ca^{++} intake (DASH diet); reduce context of saturated fat; abundant fruits, vegetables and low fat dairy products
6. ACEI/ARBS/CCB/thiazide diuretics-1st line
7. Beta blocker -no 1st line treatment
   HYVET: HTN in very elderly trial
   - Diuretic and ACEI safe in >80 years age

ACCORD: Decreases SBP to 140 or 120 → a composite of rates of MI, nonfatal stroke and death from CV disease did not differ significantly
- Intensive therapy group experience fever stroke but heightened S/E
- *Conclude:* No additional benefit of BP of <130 in DM

SPRINT: Provided same information in nondiabetics patient
- *Sprint senior:* Age> 75 years; CKD
- *Sprint mind:* Cognitive function and memory

LDL Cholesterol

- Best established risk factor
- Mutation in LDL receptor that produce hypercholesterolemia on monogenic basis leads to accelerated atherosclerosis as early as first decade of life (homozygous)
- Heterogenous-10-15 years late
- PCSK of mutation results in lifelong LDL reduction and reduced risk of lifetime events
- Concept of threshold for cumulative Lifting LDL exposure
  1. Low threshold with homozygous LDL-R mutation
  2. Slightly low threshold and normal people for heterozygous LDL-R mutation
  3. Higher threshold for PCSKg mutation

Cholesterol level in youth → long-term risk of MI

Interventions
1. Diet and exercise
2. Statin in both 1° and 2° prevention
   - Every 1 mmol/L decreases in LDL ≥22% reduction in vascular events and 10% reduction in all cause mortality
   - Those with higher absolute risk attend greater absolute risk reduction with statin use
     S/E of statin myopathy/generally determined slight increase in risk of DM
- Not all agents that reduce cholesterol level will reduce vascular events → cause and is required in prescribing nonstatin drugs

HDL Cholesterol

Each increase in HDL C by 1 mg/dL → 2–3% decrease in CV disease
1. Process of 'reverse cholesterol transport may' contribute to protective role of HDL
2. HDL could ferry cholesterol from vessel wall, augmenting peripheral catabolism of cholesterol
3. Also carry antioxidant enzyme that reduces levels of oxidized phospholipids in ath lesion
4. Increased expression of APO-AI also reduce the risk of atherosclerosis development
5. IDL also may have anti-inflammatory properties
   (Ratio of total: HDL cholesterol is most potent liquid based predictor of CV risk)

Interventions
1. Large-scale trials failed to show so any benefit with any intervention for HDL increases
2. *AIM-HIGH trial:* Significant increase in HDL but no clinical benefit
   HPS2-THRIVE No CV benefit from Niacin
3. *ACCORD trial:* Fenofibrate decreases TG and increases HDL but no clinical benefit
4. *Illuminate:* CETP (cholesteryl ester transfer protein) inhibitor—Torcetrapib showed an increase in all-cause mortality
5. Dalcetrapib also failed to show reduction of CV events. Still all observational data continued to show HDL as a risk marker → search for agent to show clinical benefit is still on

Alternative lipid and lipoprotein measures:
1. Small dense LDL particles + association with high level of TG + low HDL → increases inflammation and considering increase CV risk
2. Large and less dense LDL particles appen less likely to be associated with acute vasc events
   - APO B (Major apolipoprotein of LDL) → predicts CV risk better than LDL cholesterol
   - Non-HDL (total chol-HDL chol) provide risk info as strong as APO B.
   - *Total chol:* HDL ratio: very strong predictor (Even superior to APO B: APO A ratio)
   - On-treatment LDL, non-HDL, apo B and a lipid ratio → suggests residual risk

- Measurement of core lipid composition and lipoprotein particle size provide better measurement for or risk prediction
  (Small LDL particles more atherogenic than large particles)
- HDL particle concentration (HDLP) (measured by NMR) also predict residual risk after statin therapy. (Better than HDL size and chemical HDL cholesterol)
- LDL particle concentration also predict better than standard LDL assay.

Most Recent Recommendations

- Caution when using any novel lipid measure among those at lower risk
- LDL-P and apo B levels are considered "reasonable" for use among patients with intermediate risk.

Triglyceride

Produced in:
1. Intestine dietary chylomicrons
2. Liver TG assembled from de novo synthesized fatty acids

Rate of TG is uncertain reason:
1. Inverse correlation of TG and HDL
2. Dietary production of TG interfere with risk prediction
   (Guidelines recommend fasting state TG level → evidences indicates that post prandial level is much more prognostic importance)
   - Interventions to reduce TG level
     1. Diet
     2. Exercise and weight reduction
     3. Omega 3 fatty acid
     4. Fibrates

Trial

1. Meta-analysis of Omega 3 fatty acids did not show clinical benefit
2. *ORIGIN:* Omega 3 fatty acid decreases TG level but no clinical benefit
3. FIELD and ACCORD failed to show so TG Lowering and clinical benefit with fibrate
4. Current guideline
   - Do not recommend pharmacological reduction of TG
   - Do not set target level TG

2° causes (should be exclude)
1. Excessive alcohol
2. Renal disease
3. Cushing syndrome
4. Hypothyroidism

Concomitant medications (e.g., estrogen, corticosteroids, cyclosporine and protease inhibitors)

Metabolic Syndrome: Insulin Resistance and DM

- Insulin resistance and DM are major risk factors
- DM = Smoking risk
- DM = Equivalent to risk of aging by 15 years elder
- DM—2-8 fold risk of future CV events
- 75% of all debts in DM patient are from CV events
- DM—increasing risk of ath. complications
- Insulin resistance also increases risk of CHF
- Risk of CV disease starts to increase long before onset of clinical DM

Metabolic Syndrome

1. Waist circumference >102 (male) and 88 (female)
2. Serum TG ≥15 mg/dL
3. HDL-C <40 mg/dL (male) and <50 mg/dL (female)
4. BP ≥130/85
5. Sr Glucose conc of ≥110 mg/dL

3/5 criteria → MS

MS is cluster of all above + hypofibrinolysis + Micro-albuminuria and predominance of Dense LDL

- Various definitions available—decreasing reliability of metabolic syndrome of risk predictor
- All definition include waist hip ratio but none includes visceral fat deposition measurement
- Recent definition of MS by NHLBI include pro-inflammatory state → hs-CRP may help stratifying further risk
  (hs-CRP >3 mg/L ≥ imp prognostic factor for CV risk at all levels of MS)
  (hs-CRP <1 mg/L ≥ substantially lower risk)
- Obesity per se itself does not increase CV risk
  - Person with predominant subcut fat has less CV risk
  - Person with centripetal Android or Apple pattern → higher CV risk
    ↓

So BMF itself does not predict CV risk as well as biomarkers

Conclude: Risk of CV events with MS is no longer greater than that for some of its parts

- Treatment of syndrome is not it different than treatment of its components
- Medical value of diagnosing MS is unclear

1° prev
Aspirin for prevention:
- Low dose aspirin
- Clearly shown benefit in meta-analysis
- Reduce mortality nonfatal CV events among those with previous MI, stroke, bypass surgery, angioplasty, peripheral vascular surgery and angina
  - Dose above 75 only showed benefit (nonsignificant benefits with dose <75)
  - Other antiplatelet did not offer superiority over aspirin
  - Absolute increase in GI and other extra cranial bleeding

2° prev
- In Primary prevention, Aspirin has less Clear benefit: risk ratio
- Primary prevention trial meta-analysis
- 12% reduction in serious vascular events
- 23% reduction in nonfatal MI
  - No significant effect on stroke/vasc mortality
  - 32% increase risk of hemorrhagic stroke
  - Significant increase in G and extra-cranial bleeding

- Aspirin reduce risk of coronary events in male but not in female
- Aspirin reduce risk of stroke events in female but not in male

Ongoing studies
1. ACCEPT-D (Aspirin and simvastatin combination for CV event prevention trial in diabetics)
2. ASCEND (a study of CV events in diabetics)
   ↓
   Will provide beneficiary effect/not about use of Aspirin in diabetics
- FDA has not approved aspirin in 1° prevention
- US preventative service task force (2009) recommends Aspirin in

  Men: 45 to 79 years if benefit of reduction of MI
  Female: 55 to 79 years if benefit of reduction of stroke

  European guidelines do not recommend Aspirin for 1° prevention
  European guidelines do not recommend Aspirin in Diabetics with low risk of vasc events

Polypill
- E.g., Aspirin + statin + AECI
- Cost effective in 2° prevention
- Controversial in 1° prevention

ENVIRONMENTAL FACTORS
Depression and Mental Stress

Depression
Chronic stress
Anxiety   } Risk of CAD
Chronic hostility and anger
Social isolation

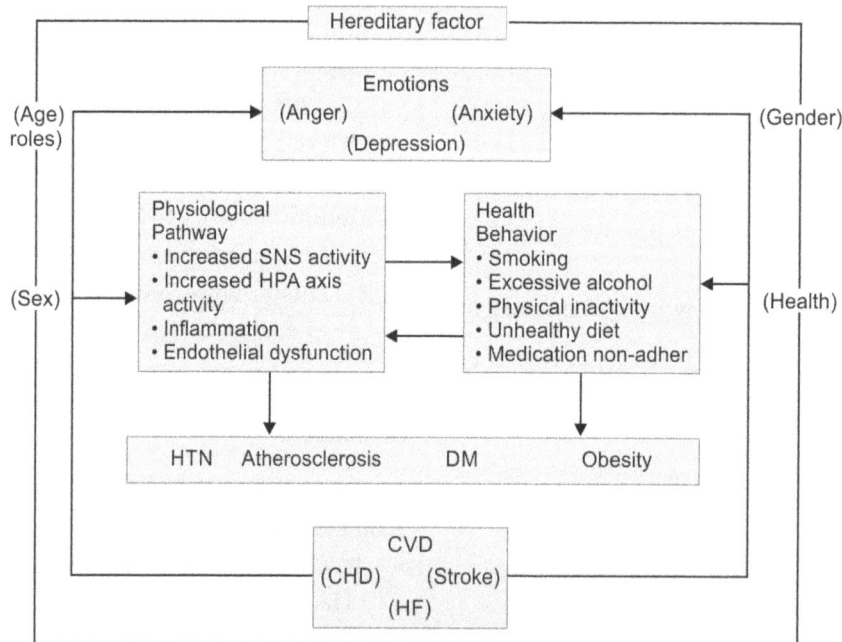

- Depression doubles the risk of CVD (INTERHEART)
  - Effect of depression:
    - Effect on inflammation
    - Endothelial dysfunction
    - Increased platelet activity
    - Increase whole blood serotonin
    - Enhanced activity of HP-A axis
    - Alteration in cardiac autonomic tone
    - Adverse lifestyle factors (poor diet, smoking lack of exercise nonadherence to medication
- Mental stress adrenergic stimulation—Increased myocardial oxygen requirement and aggravate myocardial ischemia; coronary Vasc Constrictions Platelets and endothelial dysfunction; metabolic syndrome and induction of vent arrhythmias
- Depression and mental stress also associated with
  - Increased prevalence of HTN
  - Smoking
  - Lack of physical activity
  Depression +DM ≥ great increase in risk
- Job strain
- Effort reward imbalance ⎤
- PTSD   ⎬ Double risk of MI
- Anger or anxiety   ⎦

Intervention
1. Cognitive behavior therapy
2. Antidepressant drugs
3. Physical activity

Trials
1. SADHART-CHF tested sertraline versus placebo in patients with chronic syst HF and major depression sertraline found to be safe but did not provide greater reduction than placebo in depression or improved CV status
2. ENRICH D cognitive behavior—drug therapy modestly improves depression and social isolation but did not improve CV risk rates
3. Heart and soul study D 50% increase in CV events in patients with depressive symptoms; physical inactivity (associated with depression) largely explain this association
4. UPBEAT: Both exercise and sertraline show trends towards improvement of CV biomarkers

Conclude
- RCT has not established weather screening for depression
- +SSRI treatment will improve survival benefit
- SSR1 provide significant benefit in depression symptoms but not in CV risk
- ACC/AHA because of high prevalence of depression any patient with CAD, all patients should be screened for depression

European: Prudent approach for clinically significant anxiety or depression treatment

Physical Activity
- Associated with reduced rate of CV mortality as well as cause mortality
- 2008: At least 150 minutes of moderate intensity physical activity/week (example: walking) for 75 minutes of vigorous activity per week (example: jogging) or combination of activities of both intensities
- "Some physical activity is better than none"
- Activity for both 1 and 2 prevention

Mechanism
1. Reduced myocardial oxygen demand and increased exercise capacity improving CV fitness
2. Lower systolic and diastolic pressure
3. Improve insulin sensitivity and glycemic control
   - Reduction in hBA1C along with reduced requirement for therapy
4. Improve dyslipidemia
5. Improve vascular inflammation
6. Lower CRP level, tissue type PA, fibrinogen, Von Willebrand factor, fibrin d dimer and plasma viscosity
7. Helps control body weight and lower levels of adiposity
   - Compared with in active people active people are at lower overall risk for CV disease

Obesity and Weight Loss
- Overweight and obesity are associated with increased all-cause mortality
- Obesity strongly predict CV disease and CAD as well as T2DM and other chronic conditions
- Obese children → grown to obese adults have increased risk of T2DM
- Obese children grand 2 nonobese adult it has very similar to adults who were never obese
- Obesity alone is associated with all-cause mortality regardless of level of physical activity
- Abdominal obesity   ⎤ Independently
- Increased waist hip ratio ⎦ predicts risk

Intervention

1. Dietary counseling
2. Behavior modification
3. Increase physical activity
4. Psychosocial support
5. Pharmacotherapy
6. Bariatric surgical treatment
   - Long term results, long-term risk and cost effectiveness needs the further evaluation
   - Modest weight loss of 5 to 10% it is associated with significant improvement in BP among person with and without HTN
   - No long-term studies available
     1. *LOOK-AHEAD study:* No reported reduction in (total mortality CV disease CHD) because of subjects inability to maintain long-term weight loss

Dietary Habits

Diet:
- Dietary factors influence multiple CV risk factors
  - Established risk factors BP lipoprotein glucose level and obesity
  - Novel risk factor inflammation
- Dietary patterns — Emphasize fruits vegetables other plant food such as beans whole grain fish limited occasional dairy products limiting red meat or processed Meat fewer refined Carbohydrate and processed food
  1. Healthy eating index
  2. Alternative healthy eating index
  3. Western versus prudent diet
  4. Mediterranean diet
  5. DASH type diet

Recommendations
- Food those are higher in dietary fiber, healthy fatty acid, vitamins, antioxidants, potassium, other minerals and phytochemicals
- Food that are lower in refined carbohydrates, sugar, salt, saturated fatty acid, dietary cholesterol and trans fat

DASH Diet

- Fruit and vegetables 4.5 cup/day
- Fish 3.5 O_2 serving or more per week preferable fish
- Fiber rich whole grain (1.5 gram fiber aur more per 10 gram of carbohydrate; three or more 102 equivalent servings per day)
- Sodium <1500 mg/d
- Sugar sweetened beverages: 450 kcal or less

ACC/AHA Recommendations

1. Choose whole grain, high fiber food
   Whole grain ≥3 02/d; Dietary fiber ≥2 gm/d
2. Consume a diet rich in vegetables and fruit
   Fruit including 100% juice ≥2 cups/day
   Vegetables including juice/sauce ≥25 cups/day
3. Consume fish, especially oily fish at least twice/week
   Fish and shellfish ≥7 02/week
4. Minimize intake of beverages and food with added sugar:
   <36 02/week (beverages)
   <125 g/week (sweets and Bakery dessert)
5. Balance calorie intake and physical activity to achieve or maintain healthy body weight
7. Limit intake of saturated fat to 7% of energy transferred to 1% of energy and chol 300 mg/d
8. Choose and prepare food with little or no salt

Moderate Alcohol Consumption

- Habitual heavy alcohol consumption increase total mortality, CV disease mortality, coronary heart disease and stroke
- Light to moderate alcohol consumption—associated inversely with risk of Mi, ischemic stroke, PVD, SCb, DM and death from all CV causes
  - Both 1° and 2° prevention
  - Both men and women
- Up to one drink per day for women and up to 2 drinks per day for men
- Correlated with decrease in CV risk by 20–40%
  Effects: increases HDL
  - Improve fibrinolytic capacity
  - Improve insulin resistance
  - Decrease platelet aggregation
  - Decreases inflammation

Red wine: Particular cardioprotective property because of its nonalcoholic component RESVERATROL and other components

Other Dietary Supplements

- Multi vitamins and minerals
- Large-scale RCT did not show any significant benefit
  1. Vitamin E-antioxidant
     Delay or prevent various steps in inflammation
     High-dose decreases CAD risk
     Trials for 1° prevention → no significant benefit
     Trials for 2° prevention → little benefit
  2. *Vitamin D:* Small RCTs have suggested role of vitamin D against CV disease

Mechanism: Inhibition of inflammation
Inhibition of vascular smc proliferation
Inhibition of vascular calcification
Volume homeostasis
Regulation of glucose metabolism
- RCT suggested u-shaped relation between vitamin D level and CV disease risk
    - Lowest risk at mod level
    - High risk at low and high level
3. Omega 3 fatty acids (eicosapentaenoic acid docosahexaenoic acid). Has shown considerable promise to reduce CV disease risk
    Mech: Hypertriglyceridemic effect
    Hypotensive effect
    Decreases platelet aggregation
    Decreases susceptibility of heart to vent arrhythmias
    - *Meta analysis:* Modest benefit only with Omega 3 fatty acid
    - AHA guidelines consider Omega 3 fatty acid consumption in form of fish oil or capsule form (e.g., EPA 1800 mg/d) in women with hypercholesterolemia and or hypertriglyceridemia for 1° and 2° prevention
    - No trials have suggested Omega 3 fatty acid as 1° prevention strategy
    - α linolenic acid: Found in Walnuts → whether this provide benefit as 1/2 prevention → will require more research ongoing trial-VITAL: (Vitamin D and Omega 3 trial)

Menopause and Postmenopausal Hormone Therapy

- Age specific CAD death rates in women lag approximately 10 years behind that in men
- By age of 60 years, CAD is leading cause of death among women
- Increased risk after menopause
    1. Adverse change in lipids and glucose metabolism → increased LDL c and decreases HDL C
    Increases glucose tolerance
    2. Change in hemostatic function
    3. Change in vascular function
    All due to hormonal shift towards androgen dominance as estradiol level fall

Estrogen's Cardioprotective Effect

1. Reduce LDL and increase HDL
2. Reduce Lp la
3. Decreasing plasminogen activator inhibitor I
4. Decreasing Insulin level
5. Inhibit LDL oxidation
6. Improves endothelial vas function
7. Complex effect on inflammation
    - Level of fibrinogen decreases
    - Level of hs-CRP increases

Intervention

- Observational study did show benefit of HRT
- RCT has not demonstrated any significant cardio protection with estrogen plus progesterone
- *NHLBI WHI-arm:* Recommend stopping off trial three years early due to increased overall risk benefit ratio of estrogen and progesterone therapy

Risk: Increase in CAD stroke venous thromboembolism, breast cancer exceeds the benefit of reduction of # and colon of CA

- NHBI-WHI Arm of oestrogen versus placebo also stopped early
    ↓
    Discrepancy in observations and RCT
- Women who start with HRT >10 YRS beyond menopause had increased risk for CAD, but this woman in in home heart disease was normalize within 10 years of menopause tend to have lower risk for heart disease

Trials

1. *ELITE* — No increase in CV risk during short term use of HRT
2. *KEEPS* — Neither hormone regimen significantly reduced or accelerated progression of atherosclerosis

Conclusion

- Current evidences support start of HRT near menopause to treat menopause related symptoms and to prevent osteoporosis
- HRT comes with low absolute CV risk in short term in women with 50 to 59 years of age
- Long term HRT or HRT initiation in elderly comes with high CV risk

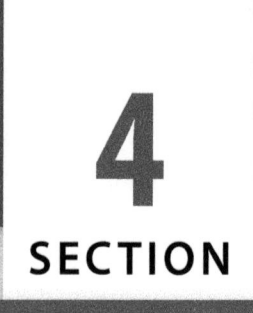

Cardiomyopathy

4.1 ARRHYTHMOGENIC CARDIOMYOPATHY

INTRODUCTION
- Genetically determined cardiomyopathy
- Char by fibro fatty replacement of myocardium
- Biventricular (BiV) involvement occurs as 50%
- Small proportion of cases involve LV only

PATHOPHYSIOLOGY
3 stages
- Subclinical (1) Early subclinical phase in which imaging studies are negative but SCD can occur
- Preclinical (2) Phase in which RV abnormality are obvious without clinical manifestation of RV dysfunction but with development of symptomatic ventricular arrhythmia
- Clinical (2) Progressive – fibro fatty replacement and infiltration of myocardium leading to severe RV dilatation and aneurysm formation and associated RV failure

Phase-4: LV (4) sometimes LV dilatation and failure may occur: Referred to as phase 4

Electrical Manifestation
- Early stage
  - Slow conduction and electrical uncoupling can lead to arrhythmia
- As fibro fatty infiltration progress
  - In homogenous activation and further delay in conduction

TRIANGLE OF DYSPLASIA
- Sub tricuspid area
- Apex
- RV out flow tract

Most common area of RV thinning, regional dilatation and aneurysm formation

ECG
- Typical ECG shows—T inverted in ant precordial leads
- Epsilon potential early during vent repolarization—represents late depolarization of area of RV
- Monomorphic VT – LBBB + LAD (superior axis)

WHY RV?
Hypothesis
- RV being thinner than LV is more susceptible to mechanical stretch, particularly during exercise mechanotransduction or conversion of mechanical stimuli to biochemical intracellular signals may further increase dysfunction at cellular level

GENETICS
- Alteration in genes encoding proteins that are key for cell-to-cell adhesion: E.g., genes encoding desmosomes
- Fibro fatty replacement occurs due to
  1. Aberrant cont. signaling of desmosomal proteins and
  2. Direct plakoglobin signaling which transform myocyte in to adipocytes with disease progression

Molecular Genetics
- Mutation in gene encoding
  1. Plakophilin
  2. Desmoglein-2
  3. Desmoplakin

  Account for most genetic causes

Clinical Genetics
- Autosomal recessive syndrome: (NAXOS disease)
  - (Discovered on Greek island of Naxos)
  - (ACM + Palmoplantar keratoderma + wooly hair)
  - (due to frameshift mutation of junctional plakoglobin)

- Autosomal recessive syndrome: Carvajal syndrome
  - Resembles Naxos disease
  - DCM + palmoplantar keratoderma + wooly hair No ACM
  - Frame shift mutation in desmoplakin
- Other mutation in desmoplakin
  - Only ACM or only skin/ hair manifestation

*Converted recommendation currently discourage use of genetic testing for ACM

DIAGNOSIS

- Diagnosing early cases presenting with aborted SCD is difficult
  - Role of CMRI
  - In ACM fatty infiltration + fibrous replacement both has to be present (only fatty infiltration can be a normal variant)
- Diagnosis depends on
  - Clinical + Electrocardiographic + genetic findings

↓

(I) Global and/or Regional Dysfunction and Structural Alteration

Major:

By 2D ECHO: Regional RV dyskinesia/akinesia/Aneurysm and one of the following:
- PLAX view of RVOT ≥ 32 mm (end diastole)
- PSAR view of RVOT ≥ 36 mm (end diastole)

By MRI: Regional RV dyskinesia/akinesia/dyssynchronous contraction and one of following:
- Ratio of RVEDV to BSA ≥ 110 ml/m² (M)
  Or   ≥ 100 ml/m² (F)
- RVEF ≤ 40%

By RV angio: Regional RV dyskinesia/akinesia/Aneurysm

Minor:

By ECHO: Regional RV dyskinesia/akinesia and one of following:
- PLAX RVOT 29-32
- PSAR RVOT 32-36
- FAC 33-40%

By MRI: Regional RV dyskinesia/alkinesia/dyssynchrony contraction and one of the following:
- Ratio of RVEDV to BSA 100-110 (M)/100-110(F)
- RVEF 40-50%

(II) Tissue Characterization of Wall

Major

Residual myocyte <60% by morphometric analysis with fibrous replacement of RV free wall myocardium in at least 1 sample with or without fatty infiltration on endomyocardial biopsy.

Minor

Residual myocyte 60-75%.

(III) Repolarization Abnormality

- *Major:* Inverted T in rt precordial leads (V1 9) or beyond in Individuals >14 years (in absence of RBBB)
- *Minor:* Inverted T in V1 and V2 or V4, V5 or V6 (in absence of RBBB)
- Inverted T wave in V1-V2, V3 and V4 in presence of RBBB

(IV) Depolarization/Conduction Abnormality

- *Major:* Epsilon wave (reproducible low amplitude signals between end of QRS to onset of T wave)-in rt precordial lead (V1-V3)
- *Minor:* Late potential by SA-ECG
  Filtered QRSd ≥ 114 msec
  RMS voltage of terminal 40 msec <20 uV
  Terminal activation duration of QRS ≥ 55 msec

↓

Definite Diagnosis = 2 major (or)
                     1 major + 2 minor (or)
                     4 minor
Borderline: 1 major + 1 minor (or)
            3 minor
Possible: 1 major (or)
          2 minor

Endocardial Biopsy: Septum is rarely involved, so septal biopsy lead to false negative diagnosis
- RV free wall biopsy carries significant risk esp if pathological thinning present
- In early stage, biopsy may be negative

D/D

- *In early stage:* Idiopathic and RVOT -VT
  - Morphology of VT differ
  - Precardial T inversion during NSR favors ACM
- Cardiac sarcoid
  - Indistinguishable

TREATMENT

- Suppression and prevention of vent arrhythmias and risk of SCD
  - Arrhythmics often successful
  - BB have not been shown to be of value
- ICD is recommended in patient with aborted SCD, syncope or decreased LV function
- Ablation (endocardial + epicardial) are most successful
- Use of ACEI and/or nitrate has been suggested but no clinical trials available

*MMVT of ACM is usually well tolerated

4.2 DILATED CARDIOMYOPATHY

Q.1 Discuss the management of DCMP.
Q.2 Discuss the newer trends in management of DCMP.
Q.3 What are the genetic causes of cardiomyopathy? Describe the gene mutation causing.

Hypertrophic, metabolic and dilated cardiomyopathy (June 14)

- DCM is characterized by dilated LV with systolic dysfunction that is not caused by ischemic or valvular heart disease

CLINICAL PRESENTATION

- Latent period of Asymptomatic LV systolic dysfunction
- Risk of arrhythmic and SCD may be seen during this period
- Angina may occur even in absence of epicardial coronary disease
  - Should raise possibly of CAD either coexistent or as a major causative factor
- H/O alcohol consumption
- F/H/O HF or SCD
- Combi of defines
  - Maternity inherited DM ⎤ mitochondrial
  - HF in relatively young ⎦ cardiomyopathy

ECG

- LVH
- Nonspecific ST-T changes
- Bundle branch block
- Pathological Q waves may be present
- Low voltage limn leads (in advanced cases with extensive fibrosis)

ECHO

- BiV dilatation (mild – severe)
- LV systolic dysfunction
- LV wall thickness – Normal but
- LV mass – invariable increase
- Global LV hypokinesia
- Septal dyskinesia in patient with LBBB (Disproportionate thinning of dyskinetic wall should rise possibly of CAD)
- MR and TR
- Mitral and tricuspid valve – structurally normal
  Restrictive diastolic function (most often seen in volume overloaded "decompensated" heart failure → improve with initiation of diuretic or vasodilator therapy)

CAG OR CCFA

Should be considered in all patients with risk factor or who are at an age where CAD is common

CMR

- Pattern of nontransmural delayed gadolinium enhancement in noncoronary distribution in dilated LV suggest nonischemic cause
- Able to evaluate extent of myocardial fibrosis in DCM and may provide info complimentary to that obtained with cardiac biopsy

CARDIAC BIOPSY

- Often unrewarding
- May provide unexpected diagnosis

GENETICS OF DCM

- 25–35% DCM are familial DCM
- Recent study demonstrated that genetic causes can be found be in at least 30% of cases (as high as 40–50% in some studies)

*Molecular Genetics

Genes causing DCM (classified by sub cellular location)

Sarcomere

- ACTC-1 – Cardiac actin
- MYH7 – β myosin heavy chain
- MYH6 – α myosin heavy chain
- MYBPC3 – Myosin binding protein C
- TNNT-2 – cardiac Troponin T
- TNNC-1 – Cardiac Troponin C
- TNNI-3 – Cardiac Troponin I
- TDM -1 – α tropomyosin
- TTN – Titin (25% of cases of DCM)

Cytoskeleton

- DMD – Dystrophin
- DES – Desmin
- LDB 3 – cipher
- SGCD – Delta – sarcoglycan
- PDLIM3-LIM domain prot-3
- VCL – metavinculin
- CRYAB – Alpha B crystallin

- ILK – Integrin linked kinase
- LAMA4 – Laminin a4

Z Disk
- TCAP – titin Cap
- CSRP3 – Muscle LIM protein
- ACTN2 – α actinin-2
- MYPN – myopalladin
- ANKRD1 – Ankyrin repeats domain protein
- NEBL – Nebulette
- NEXL – Nexilin
- MURC – Muscle restricted coil

Ion Channels
- ABCC
- SCN5A – sodium channel

Mitochondrial
TAZ/G4.5

Nuclear Envelope
- LMNA – laminin A/C
- TMPD – thymopoietin

Gamma – Secretase Activity
- PSEN-1   Presenilin-1
- PSEN-2   Presenilin-2

Sarcoplasmic Reticula
PCN – phospholamban

Transcription Factor
EYA-4

RNA Binding
RBM20 – RNA binding protein

Chaperone Heat Shock Protein
BAG-3
- Most of implicated genes encode sarcomere, z disk and cytoskeleton protein
  - 30 genes have been found to cause DCM
- This sub cellular location of gene causing DCM differentiate it from HCM and arrhythmogenic CM, which are caused by variants in gene

Encoding sarcomeric/desomosomal protein respectively
- DCM – sub cellular location of gene
- HCM – sarcomeric gene
- ACM – desmosomal genes

*Clinical Genetics
- No unique or distinguishing genotypic or phenotypic features have been associated with specific gene mutation
- Only general phenotype variation has been noted is "DCM with prominent conduction system disease" observed in all cases of laminin A/C DCM and in some cases of SCN5A and desmin DCM
- Most familial DCM are AD
- Offspring of mutation carrier having 50% chance of inheriting mutation
- AR pattern noted in consanguineous families
- X-linked DCM—Duchene muscular dystrophy
- Mitochondrial DCM also reported (esp. syndromic DCM)

Familial DCM:
- Age dependent penetrance (DCM causing allele will manifest evidence of DCM with increasing age)
  - Most occur in 4th–7th decade
  - Incomplete penetrance (Incomplete means an individual with disease causing allele may not manifest any aspect of the disease phenotype
- Variable expression-clinical feature and phenotype varies significantly
  - Both environmental + genetic factor
  - Intrinsic (hypertension) and extrinsic (toxin, virus, adverse or favorable drug exposure)

Second hit
From a second mutation in different disease gene
- *Allelic heterogeneity:* Mutation in one gene can give rise to different and distinct phenotypes seemingly unrelated to one another, e.g. LMNA (which encodes for laminin A/C)
  - Mutation causes DCM in which conduction system disease and arrhythmia occur before onset of DCM
  - Mutation also causes variety of syndromic diseases including striated muscle, adipose, nerve, and vascular tissue
  - Collectively known as laminopathies
    - skeletal myopathies (AD Emery-Dreifuss muscular dystrophy, limb girdle muscular dystrophy)
    - lipodystrophy syndrome
    - peripheral neuropathy
    - accelerated aging syndrome (Progeria)

*Disease Model

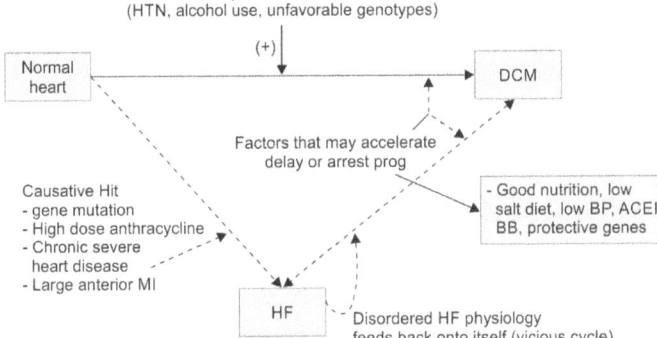

APPROACH TO CLINICAL GENETIC EVALUATION

- Comprehensive F/H of 3-4 generation for any evidence of type of cardiomyopathy, muscular dystrophy or syndromic disease
  - F/H might be negative as DCM has long talent asymptomatic period
- Clinical screening for all NT degree relatives (History, physical examination, ECG, ECMO)
- Referral for genetic evaluation
  - Identification of disease associated mutation can permit
    Molecular genetic testing of other preclinical but at risk family member and their risk stratification

- Those negative for familial DCM → low risk
- Those positive for familial DCM → enhanced screening,
- Early intervention with ACEI/BB
- Genetic counseling for all patient and family members
- Therapies based on phenotype
- ICD considered for primary prevention depending on genotype and phenotype data

THERAPY FOR PCM

- Similar to all type of systolic dysfunction
- Avoid excessive dietary salt
- ACEI/ARB/BB – mainstay of treatment
- Diuretic to reduce pulmonary edema and congestion
- Aldosterone antagonists in advanced cases
- Ivabradine
- Treatment of atrial arrhythmias
- ICD/CRT
- LVAD or cardiac transplant may be required

*Alcohol and Diabetic Cardiomyopathy

- Excessive alcohol intake → cardiotoxic
- Rarely occurs without a history of drinking at least 90 g of alcohol daily for at least 5 years (≅ min 8 standard drink daily)
- May be reversible if abstinence from alcohol. Progress if patient continues to drink heavy alcohol use → HTN → worsen DCM

4.3 HYPERTROPHIC CARDIOMYOPATHY

Q.1 Signs of HCM on examination. Natural history and management of non obst HCM (5+5) (June 17)
Q.2 Alcohol ablation vs surgical treatment myomectomy (June 16) (Dec 14)
Q.3 Genetics in etiopathogenesis and management of HCM (Dec 12)
Q.4 Pathology, genetic basis and phenotype variation in HCM (Dec 11)
Q.5 AV block in Alcohol ablation
Q.6 Genetics of HCM
Q.7 Assessment of High risk patient with HOCM (June 02)

- HCM is most common of genetic CV disease
- HCM is MC cause of SCD in young, including competitive athletes and responsible for HF related disability at virtually any age

DEFINITION

- HCM is characterized by thickened but non dilated LV in absence of other cardiac or systemic condition (e.g., AS, HTN, some expression of physiologic athlete's heart) capable of produce LVH.

Incidence: 1 in 500 patients approximately one-third have nonobstructive HCM

GENETICS

- Autosomal Dominant disease
- Equal find in men and women
- No relation between gender and SCD risk or overall HCM related mortality

Other Genetic and Non-genetic Causes

Inborn Error of Metabolism
- Glycogen storage disease: Pompe, Danon
- Carnitine disorder
- Lysosomal storage disease: Anderson–Fabry

Neuromuscular Disease
- Friedreich Ataxia
- FHLI (four and half L/M prot.)

Mitochondrial Disease
- MELAS and MERFF

Malformation Syndrome
- Noonan
- LEOPARD (lentigines, ECG abnormality, ocular hypertelorism, PS, Abnormal genitalia, Retarded growth, SNHL)

Amyloidosis
Drug induced:
- Tacrolimus, HCQ, steroid
- Autosomal dominant inheritance
- Every offspring of affected individual has 80% chance of developing disease
- Mutation in thick and thin contractile myofilament components of cardiac sarcomere or adjacent 2 disk
- 2 sarcomere gene those encoding

Most common
(1) B-myosin heavy chain (MYH7)
(2) Myosin binding protein C (MYBP C3)

Strong Evidence of Pathogenicity

- *Thick filament:*
  - B myosin heavy chain (MYC 7)
  - Regulatory myosin light chain (MYL 2)
  - Essential myosin light chain (MYL 3)
- *Thin filament:*
  - Cardiac Troponin T (TNNT2)
  - Cardiac Troponin I (TNNI3)
  - Cardiac Troponin C (TNNC1)
  - α Tropomyosin (TPM)
  - α cardiac actin (ACTC)
- *Intermediate filament:*
  - Cardiac myosin binding protein C (MYBPC3)
- *2 disks:*
  1. α Actinin-2
  2. Myozenin 2

Lesser Evidence

- Titin (TTN)
- α myosin heavy chain (MYH 6)
- Muscle Lim protein
- Vinculin
- Calsequestrin
  - (50%): No mutation
  - (15%): Myosin binding protein C
  - (15%): B-myosin heavy chain
  - (7%): Troponin T
  - (7%): α Tropomyosin
  - (5%): Others (Troponin I, α-Actin, α-Actinin 2, myosin light chain)
  - Predicting prognosis and risk of SCD in individual patients with HCM based on specific sarcomere mutation has proven to BE unreliable.

MORPHOLOGY AND ROLE OF CARDIAC IMAGING

HCM Phenotype/LV Hypertrophy

Can be detected by
1. 2D-ECMO
2. CMR

- CMR allow for quantification of fibrosis (late gadolinium Enhancement): allow risk stratification as well as identification of disease progression to end-stage phase
- CMR is complementary to ECMO
- Areas of segmental hypertrophy in anterolateral free wall or posterior portion of septum, or pathology in apical LV chamber such as hypertrophy and aneurysm are better identified by CMR.
- Diverse pattern of hypertrophy is char of HCM
- Absolute increase in wall thickness to 21-22 mm on avg
- One or more regions of LV chamber are hypertrophied with sharp transition in thickness between adjacent areas
- Hypertrophy frequently is extensive involving LV free wall and septum
- In minority wall thickening is limited to segmental areas (e.g., apical HCM)
- In 20%: LV mass may be normal
- Genetically affected family member; without LVH (gene-positive, phenotype Negative → incomplete penetrance) may show
- Ancillary signs of disease
  - Sub clinical diastolic dysfunction
  - Blood filled myocardial crypts
  - Mitral leaflet elongation
  - Collagen biomarker and myocardial scarring

} Spectrum of HCM

Mitral Valve Apparatus

- May be more than twice normal size as a consequence of Elongation of both leaflets, or segmental enlargement of only AML/mid scallop of PML.
- Congenital and anomalous antero lat papillary muscle insertion directly into AML without interposed chordate may occur

Histopathology

- Hypertrophied cardiac myocyte
- Bizarre shapes often maintain intercellular correction with adjacent cells.
- Areas of cell disarray evident in 95%

- Majority of patient with HCM exhibit intramural coronaries with marked thickening of vessel wall 2° to smooth muscle hyperplasia

In media

- This micro vascular small vessel disease probably is responsible for repeated bursts of silent myocardial ischemia leading to myocyte death and repair process leading to replacement fibrosis.
- Disorganized cellular architect, microvascular ischemia and replacement fibrosis hampers electrophysiological impulse transmission and increased dispersion of depol and repol.

PATHOPHYSIOLOGY

LVOT Obstruction

- 70% patient shows dynamic LVOT obstruction with gradient 30 mm Hg or more
- True Nonobstructive HCM-1/3rd of cases
- Long standing LVOT O: Prog HF symptom and CV death
- Weak correlation between LVOT O and SCD
- LVOT O: Increases interventricular pr: increases myocardial wall stress and O_2 demands
- LVOT O occurs due to SAM
- MR is 2° to SAM (Posteriorly directed jet)
- Occasionally mid-systolic gradient noted due to contact of septum with PAP muscle (anomalously positioned and may insert directly into AML)
- Sub aortic gradients in HCM are often dynamic

  | Heavy meal or Alcohol can also transiently increase sub ao. gradient |

  - Decreases by:
    1. Decreasing by myocardial contractility (e.g., BB)
    2. Increasing vent volume/Art pr (e.g., squatting, isometric hand grip, Phenylephrine)
  - Increases by:
    1. Decreasing vent vol./vent vol. (e.g., Valsalva, administration of NTG or amyl nitrate, blood loss, dehydration)
    2. LV contractility increasing (e.g., PVC, exercise, dobutamine, or isoproterenol)

Diastolic Dysfunction

- Impaired LV relaxation and filling is present in most patient with HCM
- DD is likely cause of limiting symptoms in patient with nonobstructive HCM
- It represents mech by which prog – HF occurs despite preserved LV function

- DD occurs due to
  - Hypertrophy ⎫
  - Replacement fibrosis ⎬ Decrease elastic property
  - Interstitial scarring ⎭
  - Disorganized cellular architecture
  - Abnormal energetic handling and diastolic Ca^{++} overload
- MC pattern noted in HCM is impaired relaxation characterized by prolonged rapid filling phase associated with decreased rate and volume of LV filling and compensatory increase in contribution of atrial systole to overall LV filling.
- Restrictive pattern have adverse prognosis

Microvascular Dysfunction

- Microvascular dysfunction → myocardial ischemia → adverse LV remodeling → affect clinical course (poor prognosis) and increased CV mortality
- Microvascular dysfunction occur both in Hypertrophied and non hypertrophied areas
- Marked reduction in coro reserve demonstrated early in clinical Course

CLINICAL FEATURE

*Symptoms

- Symptoms of HF develop at any age
- Exertional dyspnea/fatigue → functional limitation orthopnea/PND
- chest pain (typical/atypical) due to microvascular abnormality
- syncope/near syncope and light headedness due to obstruction or arrhythmias
- Nature and severity of symptoms may be similar in patient with or without OT obstruction

*Physical Examination

In patient with obstructive HCM
- Medium pitched systolic ejection murmur at lower left sternal border and apex
- Murmur varies with intensity of sub aortic gradient
- Increases with Valsalva, on standing, during or immediately after exercise
- Lack of radiation of murmur to neck
- HCM and loud murmur (>3/6) → likely to have LVOT gradient 30 ≅ mm Hg
- Bisferiens pulse
- Double/triple apical impulse

In Patient without OT Obstruction

- Subtle findings
- No or soft systolic murmur
- Forceful outward thrust at apex (systolic) may arouse suspicion.

ECG

- Abnormal in >90% patient
- Abnormal >75% Asymptomatic relatives
- Wide variety of pattern [none are unique to disease]
- Most common findings are
  - Increasing voltage consistent with LVH
  - ST-T changes (marked T wave inversion in lat precordial leads)
  - LA enlargement
  - Deep and narrow Q waves
  - Diminished R wave in lateral pre cordial leads
- ECG do not reliably distinguish between obstructive and nonobstructive HCM
- Normal ECG → Associated with less severe phenotype and favorable outcome

CLINICAL COURSE

Natural History

- Presents during all phase of life (infancy to adult to old age)
- Mortality 1% per year
- HCM compatible with normal life expectancy and good QOL with little or no disability; No major therapeutic interventions to achieve these outcomes subgroups with high risk are:
  - Sudden and unexpected death
  - Progressive heart failure with exertional dyspnea and functional limitation
  - Atrial fibrillation with embolic stroke and HF risk

Heart Failure

- Some degree of HF with exertional dyspnea-common
  - Severe functional limitation is uncommon
    - 10–15% of patients
  - Risk factors
    - LVOT obstruction
    - AF
    - Diastolic dysfunction
- 3% of patient developed advanced HF associated with systolic sysfunction (EF <50%)—due to microvascular disease related myocardial ischemia and scarring

- Risk factors
    1. F/H/O HCM with systolic dysfunction
    2. LV remodeling—wall thinning, chamber enlargement or Both
    3. Atrial fibrillation
- End stage HF with severe symptoms warrants cardiac transplant
- Survival after transplant is similar or more favorable than other diseases

Sudden Death

- MC in adolescent and young adults (<30-35 years)
- Less common in >60 years
  (Note: In elderly COD is non cardiac or other cardiac condition)
- HCM is most common CV cause of SCD in competitive athletes including high school, college and marathon participants
- Recommended to disqualify HCM athletes from intense competitive sport to reduce the risk
- Risk factors:
    - F/H/O SCD due to HCM
    - Unexplained syncope
    - Multiple/repetitive NSVT on Holter
    - Hypotensive/attenuated BP response to exercise
    - Massive LV hypertrophy (wall thickness ≥ 30 mm)
    - Extensive late gadolinium enhancement (>15% of LV)
    - End stage phase (LVEF ≤ 50%)
    - LV apical aneurysm/scarring
    - Young age
    - Cardiac arrest/sustained VT - aborted SCD
    - Sub stained LVOT gradient at rest ⎤
    - Multiple sarcomere mutation   ⎥ 2° prev
    - Modifiable risk factors - CAD,   ⎬ Potential
      competitive sports prognosis is   ⎥ arbitrators
      benign in patients with genotype   ⎥
      positive but phenotype negative for ⎥
      HCM   ⎦

ATHLETES

- Intensive and long term athletic training can
    - Increased LV diastolic cavity dimension ⎤
    - Increased wall thickness   ⎬ k/as Athlete's heart
    - Increased calculated mass   ⎦
- Absolute increase in LV wall thickness usually are modest and seen in some athletes only (e.g., rowing and cycling) - not seen in athlete with isometric exercise (e.g., weight lifting)

*Distinguish between HCM and athlete's heart.

	HCM	Athlete's heart
Focal pattern of LVH	+	+
LV cavity <45 mm	+	−
LV cavity >55 mm	−	+
LA enlargement	+	+
Bizarre ECG pattern	+	+
Abnormal LV filling pattern	+	+
F/H/O HCM	+	−
Decreasing wall thickness with		
Deconditioning	−	+
VO_2 increases >110%	−	+
Late gadolinium enhance	+	−
Pathologic sarcomere mutation	+	−

Screening for sport participation
- Complete personal and family history
- Detailed physical examination
- ECG for all participants
- ECHO for all - not recommended

FAMILY SCREENING

- *Age <12 years:*
    - Imaging optional unless:
        - Malignant F/H/O premature death from HCM
        - Competitive athlete in intense training
        - Onset of symptoms
        - Other clinical evidence s/o early LVH
- *Age 12-21 years*
    - Imaging every 12-18 months
- *Age >21 years*
    - Imaging at onset of symptoms or possibly at 5 year interval throughout mid life

MANAGEMENT

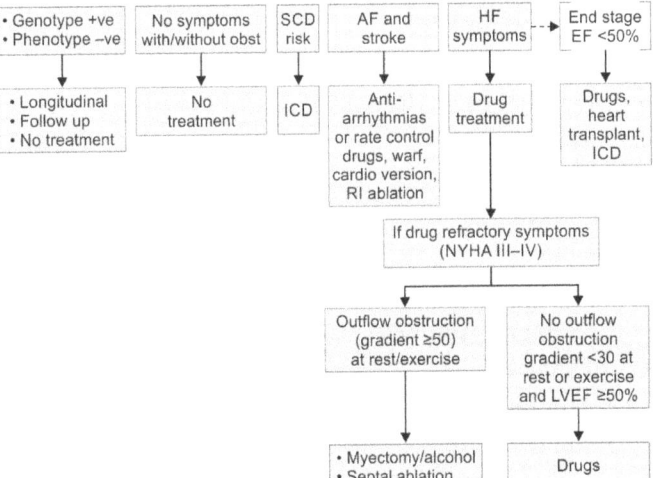

*Prevention of SCD

ICD
- Both for 2° prevention of SCD (11%/year)
  1° prevention of SCD (11%/year)
- More in young patient
- Elderly are at low risk of arrhythmic death in HCM → ICD is not recommended for 1° prevention

Pharmacological Treatment (Amiodarone)
- Obsolete strategy
- No proven efficacy for SCD prevention
- Can be used for supraventricular arrhythmias

*Medical Management of HF
HF occurs due to:
1. Diastolic dysfunction
2. Outflow obstruction
3. Micro vascular ischemia

- Beta blocker – Relieve symptoms of HF in obstructive and non-obstructive HCM by slowing HR and decreasing force of LV contraction
  ↓
  Augment vent filling and decreasing myo O_2 consumption
- Verapamil – Improve symptom and exercise capacity in patient with/without obstruction by controlling HR and beneficial effect in vent relaxation and filling.
- *Disopyramide:* In patient with obstructive HCM
- Diuretics should be avoided because dehydration worsens no added advantage of BB+CCG

  Treatment for end stage HF with systolic dysfunction is same as patient with HFREF

*Atrial Fibrillation
- MC arrhythmias in HCM
- 25% patient with HCM develop AF
- Risk factors
  - Increasing age
  - Magnitude of LA enlargement and dysfunction
- Problems
  - Embolic stroke (1%/year)
  - Prog HF symptoms
- *Treatment:*
  - Amiodarone – most effective
  - Beta-blocker
  - Verapamil
  - Anticoagulant
  - RFA

*Surgical Myectomy
- Prefaced primary management option for
  - Severe drug refractory NYHA III/IV HF
  - Obstruction to LVOT under basal condition or with exercise (gradient ≥ 50 mm Hg)
- Morrow procedure: Transaortic ventricular septal myectomy
- Resection of small portion of muscle (usually 3-10 g) from basal septum.
- Some surgeon perform aggressive myectomy with muscle resection extended more distally within the septum to base of pap muscle
- Operative mortality <1%
- 1° Cum: Reducing HF symptoms and improved QOL by relieving SAM and OT obstruction

Results: 95% patient undergoing myectomy experience permanent abolition of basal outflow gradient with/without compromising LV function.

- Long term relief of symptoms in 85%
- Extended survival as comparable to normal population
  - Not recommended for asymptomatic or mildly symptomatic patients.

*Alcohol Septal Ablation
- Alternative to myectomy
- Injection of 1-3 mL of 95% alcohol into major septal perforator artery
- To create necrosis and permanent transmural infarction localized to proximal IVS progressive thinning enlargement and decreasing LVOT gradient alos decreasing MR resolves HF symptoms
- Procedure complication and mortality are equal to or more than myectomy
- Gradient and symptom reduction are similar to myectomy
- Patients up to 65 years experience better symptom resolution with myectomy than alcohol ablation problems:
  - Multiple procedure required (10-20%) due to inadequate gradient symptom relief
  - CHB: Permanent pacing (10-20%)
  - Alcohol induced transmural scar: potentially unstable arrhythmogenic substrate + vent tachyarrhythmias (10%)

Current guideline – ASA is alternative strategy for patient with obstructive HCM who are not optimal candidate for myectomy (e.g., advanced age, significant comorbidities and increasing operative risk)

*Dual Chamber Pacing

Benefit is much less consistent than can be achieved by myectomy or ASA

*Other Management Issues

- No increasing risk during pregnancy
  - Maternal mortality confined to high risk gr
    - Severe HF
    - Vent arrhythmias
    - Marked LVOT O
  - Most women can undergo FTND
- Bacteria endocarditis – uncommon complication
  - Vegetation MC on AML or septal endocardium at site of MV contact.
  - Prophylaxis before dental procedure

*Follow-up

Regular follow up—12-18 months

4.4 LEFT VENTRICULAR NONCOMPACTION

INTRODUCTION

- Type of genetic cardiomyopathy
- Controversy: Cardiomyopathy (or) congenital development abnormality?
- AHA (2006) - LVNC is genetic CMPATHY
- ESC (2208) - LVNV cardiomyopathy or mainly a congenital or acquired morphological trait that is shared by many phenotypically distinct cardiomyopathies recent genotype - phenotype model support both entity
- AD>x linked | LVNC does not have its own genetic ontology but it overlaps DCM, HCM, ACM
- Familial & AR also noted (Mutation in mitochondrial, cytoskeletal, z - line and sarcomeric proteins)
- Point mutation in x linked a 4.5 α dystrobrevin (in pediatric pop) LVNC may be found in
  - Otherwise physiologically normal heart
  - No apparent W dysfunction
  - In associated with all types of cardiomyopathies
  - Some congenital heart disease

DIAGNOSTIC CRITERIA

Echocardiographic Criteria

- *California criteria*
  - X/Y ratio ≤ 0.5
  - This criteria evaluate trabeculae at the LV apex on PSAX and apical view and by using LV free wall thickness at end diastole
- *Zurich criteria*
  - Bilayered myocardium with thin c layer and much thicker NC layer with deep endomyocardial recess: NC/C>2

> **Embryology**
> - Gradual compaction of spongy meshwork of fibers and intertrabecular recess 5-8 weeks of embryonic life
> - Compaction progress from epicardium to endocardium; from base to apex and from septum to free wall so apex always involved

- Predominant location is mid lateral, mid interior and apex
- e/o intertrabecular recess filled with blood from LV cavity
- Imaging in SAX with measurement of NC/C ratio of end systole

- *Vienna criteria:*
  - 4 or more trabeculations protruding from LV wall, located apically to the pap muscle and visible in 1 imaging plane
  - Trabeculations with some echogenicity as myocardium and sync Movt with vent contraction
  - Perfusion of intertrabecular recess from LV cavity
  - Imaging in AP4C, modified views
- *Milwaukee criteria:*
  - Evaluation of trabeculation sizes (NC myocardium) in relaxation to c wall thickness in multiple windows and at diff ventricular levels throughout cardiac cycle
  - NC/C ratio >2

MRI Criteria

- Ratio between NC/C >2.3 at end diastole
- Trabeculated LV mass >20% of global LV mass at end diastole
  *LV size and function are not diagnostic criteria

GENETICS

- LVNC observed in all cardiomyopathy phenotypes
- In some cases WNC with LV systolic function, physiology and Chamber dimension → increased risk for later development of systolic dysfunction and risk of thromboembolism
- Mutation in some genes causing DCM /HCM has also been identified to cause LVNC

Approach: If LVNC found in concert with other cardiomyopathy, genetic testing should be as per primary cardiomyopathy

- If LVNC found in isolation, not clear at this time whether family based screening is warranted or not.

MANAGEMENT

- Not clear if any specific management for dilated LVNC
- LVNC + other cardiomyopathy: Treatment as per primary cardiomyopathy
- Stroke rate in LVNC is uncertain
  - No 1° prevention is required as such
  - 2° prevention strongly advised
- Arrhythmias also noted in LVNC for cases
  - 1° prevention not recommended

4.5 MYOCARDITIS

Q.1 List common causing acute myocarditis. What are the clinical syndrome of Ac myocarditis. Immunity in Ac myocarditis. Immunity in Ac myocarditis.
(3 + 5 + 2)
(June 17)

DEFINITION

Myocarditis refers to inflammation of heart muscle occurring as a consequences of exposure to either (1) discrete external antigen (such as virus, Bacteria, parasite, toxins or drugs) or (2) internal triggers (such as autoimmune activation against self Antigen)

Most common:
- Viral infection
- Most freq. = Parvovirus B19 and Human Herpes virus -6
Fortunately for most patients, clinical myocarditis is self-limited.

EPIDEMIO

- 3rd leading cause of SCD (1st is HCM and 2nd is CAD)
- 4–12% of SCD
- 10–50% of nonischemic cardiomyopathy cases with symptom duration less than 6 months are due to myocarditis
- 0.5–4% of HF cases are due to myocarditis
- Slight male predominance
- *Prevalence:* Myocarditis as a cause of empathy
High in 1st year of life: declines during late childhood and peaks in early 20s.

ETIOLOGICAL AGENTS

- *Initiating event:* Infection/toxin/drugs activate immune response

Virus

- Commonest cause of myocarditis
  - Parvovirus B19 ⎤ most common
  - Human herpes virus-6 ⎦ currently
  - Coxsackie virus B ⎦ Most common historically

Other

- Adenovirus
- Enterovirus
- HIV
- HCV
- Herpes simplex
- Influenza virus
- Yellow fever
- Epstein-Barr virus
- *Cytomegalovirus*
- Polio
- Rabies
- Rubella
- Varicella-zoster
- Dengue

Bacterial

- Virtually any bacterial agent can cause myocardial dysfunction
- It does not necessarily mean that bact has infected myocardium
- In case of sepsis or other severe bacterial infection: myocardial dysfunction attributed to activation of inflammatory mediators
  - *Corynebacterium diphtheriae*
    - Damage myocardium and conduction system due to exotoxin: Particular affinities for cardiac conduction system
  - MC cause of death in diphtheria
- Streptococcal infection
  - Rarely produce nonrheumatic myocarditis (distinct from rheumatic carditis)
  - Occur coincident with acute infection or in few days of pharyngitis
- Tuberculosis
  - Involvement of myocardium is rare
- Whipple disease
  - *Tropheryma whipplei* (gram negative bacilli)
  - PAS positive macrophage can be found in myocardium, pericardium, coronary arteries and heart values
- Lyme carditis
  - Char rash (erythema chronicum migrans) followed by acute neurological, joint or cardiac involvement
  - MC manifestation is transient AV block
- *Other:*
  - *Leptospira*
  - Syphilis (*Treponema pallidum*)
  - *Staphylococcus*
  - *Salmonella*
  - *Neisseria*
  - Cholera (*Vibrio cholerae*)
  - *Mycoplasma*
  - *Chlamydia*
  - Tetanus (*Clostridium tetani*)
  - Relapsing fever

Protozoa

- Chagas disease (*Trypanosoma cruzi*)
  - Major cause of nonischemic cardiomyopathy
  - *Host:* Armadillo or domestic cat
  - *Vector:* Reduviid bug
  - Parasite infection of heart activates immune system
    - Clinical presentation of myocarditis
  - Symptoms start 1-2 weeks after bite
  - Acute phase 4-8 weeks
    - CV abnormalities: nonspecific ECG changes, 1° AV block, cardiomegaly
  - Up to 90%: resolve spontaneously
  - 20-30% leads to chronic Chagas disease
    - CV abnormalities: Myocardial fibrosis, destruction of conduction tissue, vent dilatation, thinning of apex
    - H, arrhythmia, AV and double branch block, possible thromboembolism
  - *Treatment:* Antitrypanosomal treatment for all patients
- Leishmaniasis
- Malaria

Helminths

- Echinococcosis (Hydatid cyst)
  - Cardiac involvement <2%
  - Cyst usually invade IVS or LV free wall
  - Rupture into pericardium leads to acute pericarditis and into cavity leads to systemic or pulmonary emboli
  - Circulatory collapse due to anaphylactoid reaction
- Trichinosis - *Trichinella spiralis*
  - Cardiac involvement in 25% of patients
  - Cardiomyopathy and arrhythmias
  - MC electrocardiographic abnormalities are repolarization abnormally and VPC

Cardiotoxins

- Ethanol
- Anthracycline drugs
- Arsenic
- Carbon monoxide
- Heavy metals – copper, mercury, lead
- Lithium
- Radiation
- Excessive heat
- Insect bite
- Snake bite

Drugs

- Usually within 8 weeks of initiation of a new drug but can occur any time
  - Antiepileptics
- Antimicrobials
- Sulfa based drugs
- Allopurinol
- Dobutamine
  - Associated with eosinophilic myocarditis
  - Need to be stopped when eosinophilia appears or any decrease in LV function noted
- Cephalosporin
- Clozapine
- Tetanus toxoid

Miscellaneous

Kawasaki, Sarcoidosis, Wegener's

PATHOGENESIS

- Prototype: Coxsackie virus – induced myocarditis
- Basic steps
  - Viral infection and replication
  - Innate and acquired Immunity
  - Cardiac remodeling

*Viral Infection

Coxsackie virus
↓
Enters host through variety of locations CGI tract or respiratory system
↓
Initial replication in liver/spleen/pancreas
↓
Reaches heart via blood/lymphatics
↓
Birds to virus specific receptor
↓
(e.g., CAR for Coxsackie virus)
↓
Internalization of viral capsid protein and viral genome DAF-Decay Accelerating factor promote this)
↓
Activation of P50, Abl and Fyn kinase
↓
Entry of single strand RNA of virus into nucleus of cell and its translation
↓
Replication of virus genome
↓
Forms new virus with positive strand RNA and capsid
↓
Release from myocardial cells with cell lysis and disruption

- Generally, activation of innate and adaptive, antigen specific immune response greatly reduce replication of virus

*Role of Innate Immunity

- Effective during earlier stage of viral infection
- Antigen – independent mechanism
- Protect host from broad range of pathogens
- Initiated on 1st day of infection
  Inhibit viral infection and replication during first 4-5 days

E.g.: *Activation of Interferon signaling*
  - Type I Interferon signaling
    - Binds to IFN-receptor
  - Type II Interferon (INF r)
- *Toll-like receptor*
  - Earliest innate immune mechanism
  - Most common
  - Recognize pathogen-associated molecular pattern
    ↓
    Activates defense against pathogen (reacts more quickly as they do not have high specificity toward B or T cells) ↓
    Increased cytokine and interferon

*Role of Acquired Immunity

- Begins usually 4-5 days after infection
- Antigen specific response: directed to a single antigen
- Mediated by T and B cell
  - T cell attempt to limit infection by destroying host cells through cytokines or perforins death of host cell via Necrosis/Apoptosis can have detrimental effect on host cells appropriate regulation of T cell is needed to control infections and at same time avoid inappropriate destruction of host tissue such as myocardial cell
  - Activation of T cell also activates B cell
  Secretion of antigen specific antibodies against invading pathogen (cross reaction with host tissue is possible due to molecular mimicry by pathogen)

*Cardiac Remodeling

Virus can directly enter the endocardial cells and myocardial cells and subsequently lead to intracellular interaction direct cell death or hypertrophy DCM

CLINICAL SYNDROME

- Wide ranging array of clinical presentations
  - *Bimodal distribution*
    - Acute presentation common in young children and teenage
    - Chronic presentation with subtle and insidious presentation in older adult preparation: may lead to DCM and HF

↓
Difference in presentation is due to
  - Immune system response
  - In young population, exuberant response to initial exposure of provocative antigen
  - In older, greater degree of tolerance and show chr inflammatory response only to chronic presence of foreign antigen
- Presentation can also vary by cause:
  Parvovirus B19: freq. chest pain from endothelial dysfunction
  Giant cell myocarditis: Arrhythmia with heart block are more common
- May be asymptomatic ECG or ECMO abnormality
- Diagnosis of chest pain, cardiac dysfunction, arrhythmia, HF and/or HD collapse
  - Chest pain may be typical, atypical angina
  - May precipitate by Coro vasospasm
  - Can also occur from pericarditis
- *O/E:* Enlarged LN with hilar adenopathy on CXR: Suggest systemic sarcoidosis
  - Pruritic, maculopapular rash with increased eosinophil count suggest hypersensitivity reaction to drug or toxin
  - DCM complicated by vent arrhythmia or heart block: suggest giant cell myocardosis or cardiac sarcoidosis
- Pt who fail to recover from acute episode of myocarditis → Ongoing immune activation → chronic myocarditis → persistent LV dysfunction

Reason:
- Failure to clear virus
- Recognition of endogenous protein as foreign

DIAGNOSIS

*Classification

- *Possible subclinical acute myocarditis*
  - In context of possible myocardial injury without cardiovascular symptoms but with at least one of following:
    - Biomarker of cardiac injury increased
    - ECG finding s/o cardiac injury
    - Abnormality cardiac function on ECMO or CMR
- *Probable acute myocarditis*: In clinical context of possible myocardial injury with cardiovascular symptoms: Any one of above 3
- *Definite myocarditis:* Histologic or immunohistologic evidence of myocarditis.

Diagnostic Criteria (ESC)
- Myocarditis suspected when patients presents with following:
    - ≥1 clinical presentation (with or without ancillary findings)
    - ≥1 Diagnostic criteria from diff categories (in absence of)
        - CAG detectable CAD (≥50%)
        - Known pre-existing CV disease
        - Extra cardiac cause
- Suspicion is higher with higher number of fulfilled criterion
- If patient asymptomatic ≥2 criteria should be met

Presentation
- AC pericardial/pseudo – ischemic pain
- New onset (<3 months) or worsening of dysp at rest or exercise and/or fatigue, with/without left and/or rt heart failure
- Palpitation and/or unexplained arrhythmia sympt. And/or syncope, and/or aborted SCD
- Unexplained card shock

Diagnostic Criteria
- ECG/Holter/stress test
- Markers (Trop I/T)
- Function and str abnormality (ECMO/CMR)
- Tissue characterization by CMR

*Lab Testing
- Cardiac injury biomarkers to screen for myocarditis in patient with acute viral illness
    - Elevated cTn helps to confirm case of myocarditis
    - Fulminant myocarditis associated with higher level of cTn than acute myocarditis
    - High cTn level associated with low LVEF
- Other biomarkers
    - Sr. creatinine, Lactate, AST/SCOT — Associated with increase in hospital mortality in fulminant myocarditis in children
    - IL-10, Soluble Fas — Associated with high mortality
    - High NT proBNP: associated with Ac. DCM due to myocarditis
    - Nonspecific biomarker of inflammation (ESR, CRP, leukocyte count) have low specificity
    - Circulating viral antibody titer does not correlate with viral infection and are rarely of diagnostic use

*ECG
- No Pathognomonic finding
- Nonspecific repolarization changes and sinus tachy
- PR depression and diffuse ST elevation
- QRS >120 and abnormality Q wave: associated with greater mortality

*Cardiac Imaging
- ECMO:
    - No specific features
    - MC – Dilated, spherical vent with reduced syst function
    - Fulminant myocarditis present with small cavity and mild reversible vent hypertrophy due to inflammation
    - RV dysfunction – less common → if present—Poor progno
    - Segmental wall motion abnormality may be present
- CMR:
    - Can distinguish myocarditis
    - T1-weighted delay enhancement can quantitate region of damage and possibly predict risk of CV death and arrhythmia
    - Sensitivity and specificity are low (63 and 40%) after 14 days in suspected myocarditis
- PET: Remain useful to diagnose cardiac sarcoid

*Endomyocardial Biopsy
- Remain essential for diagnosis of specific myocarditis
- Highly useful in giant cell myocarditis fulminant lymphocytic myocarditis

*Dallas Criteria for Diagnosis (EMB)
- Definition – Idiopathic myocarditis – An inflammatory infiltrate of the myocardium with necrosis and/or degeneration of adjacent myocyte not typical of ischemic damage.
- Classification:
    - First biopsy:
        - Myocarditis with/without fibrosis
        - Borderline myocarditis
        - No myocarditis
    - Subsequent biopsy:
        - Ongoing myocarditis with/without fibrosis
        - Resolving myocarditis with/without fibrosis
        - Resolved myocarditis with/without fibrosis

MANAGEMENT

- First line therapy: Supportive case

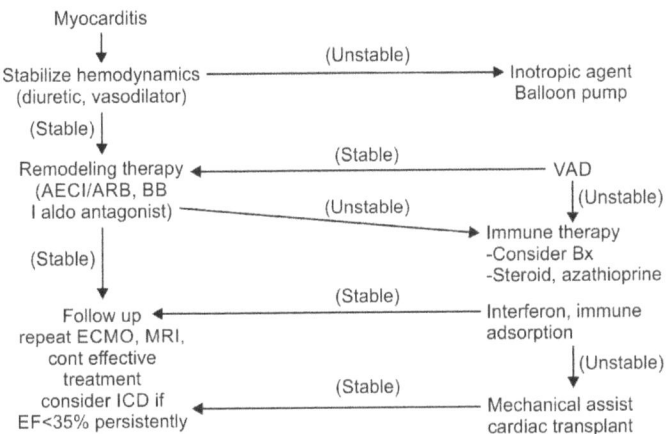

- Routine treatment with immunosuppressive drug is not recommended for adults
- Exceptions are
  - Giant cell myocarditis
  - Cardiac sarcoid
  - Eosinophilic myocarditis
  - Myocarditis associated with inflammatory connective tissue disease
- IVIG and immunosuppressive drugs are neutral to favorable in pediatric age group
- No trials for anti-viral drugs
- Arrhythmias managed conventionally indication of ICD are same as non-ischemic CMpathy

PROGNOSIS

- Poor prognosis in patient with myocarditis and poor W function
- RV dysfunction – poor outcome
- High DAD – poor outcome
- Presence of viral genome on EMB: Poor outcome
- Late gadolinium enhancement: High CV mortality

4.6 OTHER CARDIOMYOPATHIES

*FABRY DISEASE

- Lysosomal storage disease
- Accumulation of neutral glycosphingolipids
- Due to def of α galctosidase A (encoded by GLA)
- GLA situated on X chromosome

S/S

- Angiokeratoma, Acroparesthesia, Anhidrosis, ocular change and
- CVS, renal, CNS disease

Central Pathophysiology

- Small vessel disease, due to deposition of glycosphingolipid and consequent vascular insufficiency

C/F

- Angiokeratoma
- Acroparesthesia
- Anhidrosis
- Ocular change
- Systemic involvement
- Age of onset depend on degree of α-galactoridase A activity

*CVS Involvement

- 3rd or 4th decade
- LVH-MC finding
- LVH progress with age
- May precipitate angina due to small vessel involvement

ECG

- Short PR interval
- LVH
- Later on – heart block
- Nonspecific IVCD
- Bradycardia common

ECHO

- Mild to severe LVH
- Mild to significant diastolic dysfunction
  *Atypical cardiac variant: Unexplained LVH in 6th or 8th decade. Accompanied by cardiomyopathy, MR, mild proteinuria, little or no renal dysfunction

Diagnosis

- Showing reduced α-glactosidase A activity
- Molecular genetic testing showing mutation in GLA
- Endomyocardial biopsy

Management

Enzyme replacement

*GAUCHER AND GLYCOGEN STORAGE DISEASE

- AR
- Deficient B-glucocerebrosidase enzyme activity
- Mutation in GBA
- Cardiac involvement uncommon to rare

*HEMOCHROMATOSIS

- Iron overload
- Iron infiltrates major organs (liver, heart, thyroid, gonads, skin, and pancreatic islet cells)
- Lead to cirrhosis
  - Cardiomyopathy
  - Diabetes
  - Endocrine disease

Etio

- Hereditary (Primary) or
- Secondary (caused by increased absorption associated with thalassemia sickle cell disease or sideroblastic anemias or when related to excess blood transfusions for myelodysplasia or aplastic anemia
- Autosomal recessive
- Homozygous mutation in HFE gene

C/F

- Nonspecific
- Insidious onset

Cardiac

- Restrictive nondilated phenotype with advanced disease
- Progress to systolic dysfunction, mid to mod LV dilatation
- Consistent with DCM
- Eventually HF
  - Arrhythmias and conduction system disease
  - AV and bundle branch disease
  - Brady arrhythmias
  - Syncope and SCD

Investigation
- Cardiac MRI
- End myocardial biopsy
- Serum ferritin and % TS
- Genetic testing for HFE

Treatment
- Iron removal by phlebotomy in HFE – associated
- Hereditary hemochromatosis
  - Cardiac function improve in most as iron stores depleted

*CARCINOID HEART DISEASE
- Occur as a part of carcinoid syndrome
- Elevated circulating level of
  - 5 HT (serotonin)
  - 5 hydroxytryptophan
  - Histamine
  - Bradykinin
  - Tachykinin
  - Prostaglandin

  Due to rare metastatic neuro endocrine malignancy - carcinoid

C/F
Trial of:

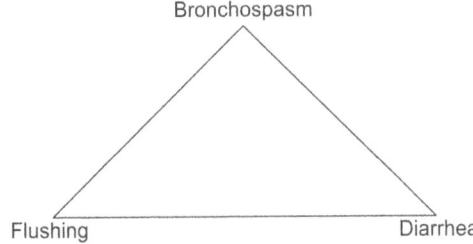

- In association with Hepatic mets: Produce 5HT carcinoid heart disease
- High level of 5HT in rt heart (via venous circulation) produce progressive fibrotic endocardial plaque
- Right sided valve thickening and retraction due to myofibroblast proliferation along with deposition of collagen, SMC and elastic tissue
- Tricuspid annular and subvalvular involvement and pulmonary root constriction
- Valvular dysfunction
- RV vol. and Pr overload with murmur of TR and PR/TS and PS
- Peripheral edema and ascites with low CO

Investigation
- Elevation of urinary 5HIAA – highly specific
- ECMO and CMR – thickened and immobile tricuspid and pulm valves with stenosis and regurgitant lesion

Prognosis
- Poor
- Carcinoid syndrome untreated – 3 - 4 years
- Cardiac involvement <1 year

Treatment
- Debulking hepatic mets by
  - Embolization
  - Partial hepatic resection
  - Octreotide
- Valve replacement can be done
  - Carries risk of development of acute carcinoid crisis char by profound hypotension, severe flush-bronchospasm and arrhythmias

*EOSINOPHILIC (LOEFFLER) ENDOCARDITIS
- Eosinophils invades and damage tissue in a variety of organs including endocardium and myocardium
- Causes of eosinophilia
  - Helminthic or parasitic infection
  - Malignancy: CA or eosinophilic leukemia
  - Allergy: E.g., drug reaction
  - Idiopathic hyper eosinophilia
- Hyper eosinophilia = chronic absolute eosinophilic count >1,500 cells/mL x at least 1 month or pathological e/o eosinophilic tissue invasion

3 stages:
1. *Acute phase:*
   - Few or no high symptoms
   - Eosinophils invade myocardium
   - Intense inflammation
   - Eventually myo necrosis
   - CMRI can detect it
   - Myocardial biomarkers elevated
2. *Second stage:*
   - Thrombus favoring apices covers affected endocardium
   - Chest pain/dyspnea
   - MR/TR
   - Cardiomegaly
   - HF
   - Embolism to brain and other organs
   - ECG: T inversion
3. *Third fibrotic stage:*
   - Diffuse scarring that result in endocardial fibrosis and RCM
   - Commonly involve MV and TV-Regurgitation

Treatment
- Treat underlying cause
- Corticosteroid
- Cytolytic therapies
- Fibrotic stage: Surgical treatment to release valve, repair or replacement

*ENDOMYOCARDIAL FIBROSIS
- Unusual disease
- Char by fibrosis of LV and RV apical endocardium causing RCM
- Found in tropical region of Africa, SE Asia
- M>F
- Family clustering
- Bimodal peak – onset in 1st decade and 2nd peak in 2nd-4th decade
- No consistent underlying cause
- Env exposure to cerium

C/F
- HF from rt/lt restrictive physiology
- DOE
- FND
- Edema
- Ascites
- Atrial enlargement

Management
Surgical resection of endocardial fibrosis with valve repair or replacement

*REVERSIBLE CARDIOMYOPATHY
Usually manifest as DCMP

Etiology
- Endocrine disorders (Hyperparathyroid, pheochromocytoma, thyrotoxic Cushing, 1° aderal insufficiency)
- Toxin and drugs (Adriamycin, Amphotericin B, anagrelide alcohol, cocaine use, and scorpion bite)
- Obesity
- End stage renal disease
- Cirrhosis
- Tachy induced
- Stress induced
- GBS, hypophosphatemia, SIRS, and Selenium def
- Tyrosinemia Type I

Obesity Induced CM-pathy (Mech)
- Increased blood volume and CO
- Increased preload and after load
- Compensating LV dilatation and eccentric hypertrophy
- LV syst and diastolic dysfunction
- OSA and PH
- Activation of RAAs
- Activation of SNS
- Fatty infiltration of myocardium

4.7 PERIPARTUM CARDIOMYOPATHY

DEFINITION
No universally accepted definition

ESC
"PPCM is idiopathic cardiomyopathy presenting with HF 2°
To LV systolic dysfunction toward end of pregnancy or in months following delivery when no other cause of HF is found.
LV may not be dilated but EF is nearly always <45%
- Life threatening disease
- In last months of preg or within 5 month postpartum

EPIDEMIOLOGY
1 in 2,500 to 1 in 4,000

ETIOLOGY
*Risk factors – Excessive prolactin production
- Old age
- Multipathy
- Black race
- Multiple fetal pregnancies (twin preg)
- Selenium deficiency
- Viral myocarditis
- Abnormal immune response
- Malnutrition
- Preeclampsia/history of HTN

*Genetic mutation reported in
- α and β myosin heavy chain
- Myosin binding protein C
- Cardiac Troponin T
- Presenilin-2
- SCN5A

PATHOPHYSIOLOGY
- Poorly understood
  - Inflammation may play a role
    - CRP, INF – r and IL-6 elevated
  - Autoimmune process ⎤
    - Apoptosis and   ⎬ Also may play a role
    - Endothelial dysfunction ⎦
  - Recent studies PPCM is vascular disease

(I) Placenta in late preg secrete and VEGF inhibitor (SFI+1)
↓
Excessive antiangiogenic signaling
↓
Cardiac angiogenic Imbalance

(II) Preeclampsia multiple gestation
↓
also have marked increase in SFI+1

- Unbalanced peripartum oxidative stress proteolytic cleavage of prolactin 16 kDa subform potent antiangiogenic, proapoptotic, and proinflammatory
- Bromocriptine found to be useful as preventive measure in animal studies
- Inhibition of prolactin increase in risk of thrombosis so bromocriptine given with heparin

C/F
- Symptoms and signs of HF
- Rapid progression
- Recovery is more likely to occur
- Mild cases in postpartum period is overlooked and never diagnosed
- Less likely to occur in women who enter 2nd preg with normal EF than in those with persistent reduction in EF

SELF-TEST FOR EARLY DIAGNOSIS
- Score each symptoms 0 = none
  1 = mild
  2 = mod-severe
- Orthopnea None = 0
  Need to elevate head = 1
  Need to elevate >45° = 2
- Dyspnea = climbing 8 or more steps = 7
  Walking on level = 2
- Unexplained cough = at night = 1
  Day and night = 2
- Swelling lower extremities below knee = 1
  Above and below = 2
- Excessive weight gain <2 pound/week = 0
  2-4 pound/week = 1
  >4 pound/week = 2
- Palpitation: when lying down at night = 1
  Day and night any portion = 2
  >4 = needs further evaluation; ≥ 5 = Always associated with syst dysfunction

MANAGEMENT
- Pentoxifylline (By its anti TNF α action) ⎤ Both shown to
- Bromocriptine   ⎦ be beneficial
  - Same as that of CHF
  - Na⁺ and fluid restriction
  - Hydralazine, BB, and digoxin–safe
  - Diuretics – use cautiously as it decreases placental flow
  - Avoid Aldosterone antagonist – it has antiandrogenic effect on fetus
  - Nitrate and inotropes may be required
  - Heparin in patient with EF < 35 (because intra cardiac Thrombus and embolisms are common)

- Early fetal delivery (if possible)
  - Preferably CS
- IABP/WAD/ECMO may be required
- Cardiac transplant in patient refractory to management

FOLLOW UP
- Normalization of LV function in 25-50%
  - More likely if EF >30%
  - Recur in 30% of cases

(most physician counsel against 2nd preg)

BIOMARKERS
- NT pro BNP = Not specific
- 16 kDa Prolactin = Astic accuracy needs to be evaluated
- Interferon r = Astic accuracy needs to be evaluated
- Asymmetric Dimethyl Arginine (ADMA) = Astic accuracy needs to be evaluated
- Cathepsin D = Astic accuracy needs to be evaluated
- Soluble fms like tyrosine kinase = Astic accuracy needs to be evaluated
- Motor RNA = Astic accuracy needs to be evaluated

4.8 RESTRICTIVE CARDIOMYOPATHY, AMYLOIDOSIS, AND SARCOIDOSIS

RESTRICTIVE AND INFILTRATIVE CARDIOMYOPATHY

RCM

- Heterogeneous group of disease characterized by nondilated LV, often with preserved EP
- Predominant manifestation is diastolic dysfunction
- Some infiltrative cardiomyopathies
  - Amyloidosis: Produce RCM
  - Sarcoidosis: Produce DCM

Approach to RCM

- Endomyocardial biopsy: RCM may be caused by infiltrative cardiac process without systemic involvement or with subclinical involvement of other organ
- Familial RCM is uncommon (c.f. DCM)
- Even though, detailed clinical history of 1st degree relatives and their screening is advised

Molecular and Clinical Genetics

- Clinical genetics is similar to PCM
  - Reduced Penetrance
  - Variable age at onset
- Genetic similarity with HCM suggest that in these cases the RCM Phenotype can be viewed as a minimally hypertrophic HCM with prominent restrictive physiology
- Overlap or crossover phenotype of RCM and HCM is also observed

C/F of Idiopathic RCM

- Rare
- From infancy to late adulthood (median age = 68 years)
- Poor prognosis in children
- Symptoms are nonspecific
- Presence of Heart failure
- Dyspnea in most of patients
- Edema in approx. 50%
- Palpitation, fatigue, orthopnea
- O/E: BiV failure; Jugular venous distention
  - Ascites and significant edema in advanced cases
  - AF – common
  - Murmur – Not a feature
  - S^3 in 25% of patients

Investigation

ECG
Usually normal

ECMO
- Biatrial enlargement + Nondilated ventricles + Typical normal LVEF and LV thickness
- Both RV and LV filling pr. Increased

Endomyocardial biopsy
Nonspecific findings such as myocyte hypertrophy, interstitial fibrosis and endocardial fibrosis

Progno
Survival is reduced 5 to 10 years survival rate -64 and 37% death due to cardiac causes SCD or 2 to HF

D/D
Infiltrative cardiomyopathy
(e.g., Amyloidosis
- Increased LV wall thickness
- Subtle abnormality in LVEF constrictive pericarditis)

Treatment
Limited to treatment of HF advanced cases-transplant

CARDIAC AMYLOIDOSIS

- Infiltrative cardiomyopathy
- Associated with toxic component
- "Amyloid" refers to proteinaceous material derived from misfolded products of a variety of precursor protein
- Amyloid deposit contain: Extracellular, nonbranching fibrils, amyloid P component, heparin and dermatan sulfate, glycosaminoglycans, apolipoprotein E, type IV collagen and laminin

Types

1. AL amyloidosis-abnormal light chain produced by plasma cells
2. Senile systemic amyloidosis-derived from wild type transthyretin (TTR)
3. Familial ATTR amyloidosis – mutant TTR
4. Localized atrial amyloid – mutant TTR
5. Secondary amyloidosis

Cardiomyopathy

Type	Age at onset	Main organs involved	Avg. untreated survival	Specific treatment
1. AL (1°)	50+	All except CNS heart in 50%	Non-cardiac – 2 years HF <9 month	Chemotherapy aimed at plasma cells
2. Familial ATTR	20–70	Peripheral and auto nomic neuropathy heart	7–10 years	Liver transplant investigational agent (tafamidis)
3. Senile syst amyloidosis	70+	Heart	5–7 years	Investigational agent (tafamidis) to prod. Of TTR
4. Isolated atrial amyloidosis	Unknown	Cardiac atria (in disease heart)	No effect on survival	None needed
5. 2° amyloidosis	Depends on underlying condition	Liver, kidney renal heart	10+ years	Treatment of underlying condition

AL Amyloidosis

- Abnormal light chain produced by plasma cells
- Closely correlate with multiple myeloma
- Involve all organs except CNS
- 50% has heart involvement
  - Clinically significant in 75%
- C/F:
  - Rapidly progressive HF
  - BiV failure
  - Rt sided signs predominant

Like RCM vessel and RV failure	- May have typical angina – due to amyloid deposit in small - Postural syncope due to autonomic dysfunction

- O/E:
  - NSR or AF (less common)
  - JVP markedly increased
  - Kussmaul sign
  - Heart sounds normal
  - Absence of S4 despite small stiff ventricle
    - Due to atrial systolic dysfunction 2° to atrial infiltrate
  - S3-indicates RV dysfunction
  - Pleural effusion – often present
  - Congested hepatopathy – common
  - Ascites – may be detected
- Noncardiac:
  - Periorbital purpura (pathognomonic)
  - Heavy proteinuria
  - Peripheral/Autonomic neuropathy
  - Macroglossia
  - Cachexia
- ECG:
  - Low voltage limb leads
  - Rightward axis
  - 1° AV block common
  - Q in V1-V3 frequently seen

- ECHO:
  - Normal to small LV cavity
  - Increasing LV and RV thickness ⎤
  - Increasing myocardial echogenicity ⎦ Common
  - Mild to mod MR
  - No AoV involvement
  - Elevated LV filling pr
  - Normal LVEF
  - Severely impaired longitudinal LV systolic function
- Speckle tracking:
  - Classical appearance of regional longitudinal
  - Dysfunction char by relative apical sparing and
  - Prolonged diastolic relaxation
- Occasionally ASH present
- Cardiac cath:
  - BLL elevated filling pr
  - Dip and plateau tracing (But unlike constrictive pericarditis, equalization of diastolic pr is uncommon)
  - Simultaneous recording of LV and RV pr during respiration demonstrate concordant changes in systolic pr in amyloidosis and other RCM [Discordant changes (inspirational increase in RV syst pr with simultaneous decrease in LV pr) in constrictive pericarditis]

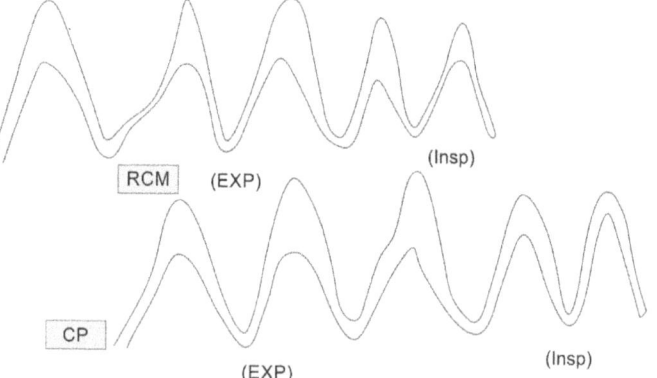

- CMR – Useful diagnostic tool
  - Classical feature
    - BiV thickening

- Normal cavity sizes
- IAS thickening
- Delayed gadolinium enhancement of sub endocardium - diffuse or patchy - and may involve atrium in many cases
- *PET with vasodilator stress:* may slow diffuse widespread stress induced subendocardial ischemia related to small vessel disease

Familial and Senile Systemic Amyloidosis
- A.D
- High penetrance
- Point mutation in TTR
- TTR sense or carrier of thyroid hormone Thyroxin (T4) and retinol binding protein (TTR = Transports Thyroxin and retinol)
- Involve cardiac + Peripheral + ANS
- 2 mutations common
    1. Val30Met
        - Neuropathy + cardiac involvement
        - Younger patient: SA nodal dysfunction
        - After middle age: Cardiomyopathy
    2. Val 122 Ile-Almost no neuropathy
        - Amyloid cardiomyopathy in 6th-7th decade

Senile syst Amyloidosis
- Wild type TTR
    - Even though "systemic"-Heart is almost always the only organ to be involved
    - 7th decade onward, Predom meds (20:1)
    - Prog BiV failure with No neuropathy

*In AL amyloidosis, toxic component from circulating free light chain may exist: survival poor

C/F:
In contrast ti AL amyloidosis
- *ECG:* Normal voltage
    - Nonspecific conduction disturbance
    - Nonspecific ST-T changes
    - LBBB more common(less with AL Amyloid)
    - High degree AV block may occur
    - Indolent course
    - Unrelated survival considerably longer

Investigation: Pyrophosphate screening is useful tool

Isolated Atrial Amyloidosis
- Cannot be diagnosed other than on a biopsy
- Increases prevalence of AF
- Not associated with vent amyloidosis

DIAGNOSIS
- Clinical features as mentioned above
- Serum and urine immunofixation reveals monoclonal gammopathy
- Serum free kappa and lambda light chains (increased in AL amyloidosis)
    - Patient with TTR Amyloidosis has normal serum
- Bone marrow Biopsy Plasma cell in AL Amyloid in range of 10-20% (>30% plasma cell: overlap synd)
- Biopsy for definitive diagnosis
    - Subcutaneous fat pad aspiration
    - Endomyocardial biopsy - always positive in cardiac amyloidosis
- Laser microdissection of amyloid deposit with subsequent proteomic analysis - Gold standard treatment differ as per type of amyloid deposit

MANAGEMENT
Aim:
- Treatment of heart failure
- Management of amyloidogenic protein
- *For HF*
    - Diuretics are mainstay
    - ACEI poorly tolerated - worsens hypotension
    - BB doesn't affect outcome
        - But can be used for AF
    - CCB contradicted - it worsens HF
    - Low dose dopamine may help
- *For amyloid:*
AL Amyloidosis:
- Chemotherapy for pharma cell dyscrasia
    - Autologous stem cell transplant
    - Bortezomib based regimen
    - Normalization of serum free light chain is associated with significant improvement in HF (mostly because of removal of cardio toxic effect of amyloid precursor)
Familial ATTR:
- Removal of source of amyloidogenic protein -i.e. liver transplant
Some patient continues to have progression of infiltrative cardiomyopathy even after many years due to wild type TTR combined liver heart transplant considered
Senile systemic ATTR:
- No role of liver transplant
- Heart transplant may be considered
- High degree AV block: BiV Pacing (only PV pacing will be determined in patient with small cavity)

*SARCOID CARDIOMYOPATHY

- Multisystem disorder of unknown cause
- Noncaseating granuloma
- Cardiac involvement: Vent dysfunction
  Heart block
  Vent arrhythmias
- MC phenotype—DCM with Aneurysm formation (occasionally)
- Isolated cardiac sarcoidosis is also noted
- Usually in association with pulmonary or systemic sarcoidosis

Pathology

- Hallmark = Noncaseating granuloma
- Granulomatous lesion associated with edema and inflammation, and widespread myocardial fibrosis in late disease: Sever systolic dysfunction
- Occasionally RV may be severely involve
  - Mimic ACM
  RV function can be impaired in patient with pulmonary sarcoidosis and PHTN

C/F

Cardiac

BiV failure

- DCM type
- MR – severe (due to pap mu. dysfunction)
- Prediction for conduction system
  - High grade AV block/CHB
- Atrial and vent arrhythmias
- SCD
- Rare: Acute sarcoid myocarditis
  - High grade AV block, malignant vent arrhythmias, HF

Noncardiac

- MC site = lung (50% had avert parenchymal disease Rest 50% - B/L hilar lymphadenopathy)
- Other: Hepatic → GI → ocular → Neurologic

Diagnosis

- Increased ESR (nonspecific)
- Increased immunoglobulin (nonspecific)
- Hypercalcemia due to activation of vitamin D by macrophages in sarcoid granuloma useful clue
- Elevation of serum ACE level – useful
- CMRI with gadolinium enhancement – sensitive test for detecting abnormality in cardiac sarcoid
- Gadolinium enhancement is nontransmural and involve basal and/or mid ventricular septum
- *FOG PET:* Complementary to MRI
  Reveals area of inflammation in active disease and permits
  Serial evaluation of response to therapy
- Tissue biopsy: positive cardiac biopsy showing noncaseating granuloma is diagnostic
- Patchy nature of granulomatous infiltration results in low yield of positive biopsy

Diagnosis Algorithm

(I) (1) Unexplained 2nd/3rd degree AV block in young patient (<55 yrs) and/or
(2) Sustained MMVT/DCM
↓
HRCT/CMR/PET
↓
(1) CT s/o plum sarcoidosis
(2) CMR/PET suggestive of cardiac sarcoid

- 1 or more of 2 → High probability of cardiac sarcoid → Biopsy (Extra cardiac if possible or guided EMB to confirm diagnosis)
  - (Positive) → Cardiac sarcoidosis diagnosed
  - (Negative) → Consider repeat biopsy in 4–6 months
- Neither of 2 → Low probability of cardiac sarcoid → Consider alternate diagnosis

(II) Biopsy proven extracardiac sarcoid
↓
12 lead ECG, Holter, 2-D ECMO
↓
1. Bundle branch block or abnormal Q waves on ECG
2. Sustained 2nd/3rd degree AV block
3. VT, freq PVC
4. RWMA, wall aneurysm or basal septum thinning
5. LVEF <50%

- One or more of 5 → CMR and/or PET → Suggestive of cardiac sarcoidosis
  - Yes → High probability of cardiac sarcoid
  - No → Low probability of sarcoid
- None of 5 → Low probability of sarcoid → Consider annual monitoring

Management:
- Standard HF therapy
- Steroid – especially early is disease when irreversible fibrosis has not developed prednisolone 1 mg/kg and 40 mg daily
- Infliximab – monoclonal antibody against TNF α for non – pulm sarcoidosis
- Pacemaker and/or ICD for arrhythmias
- Cardiac transplant

4.9 TACHYCARDIA-INDUCED CARDIOMYOPATHY

DIAGNOSIS OF EXCLUSION

Definition: Atrial and/or vent dysfunction 2° to rapid and/or dyssync/irregular myocardial contraction – Particularly or completely reversible after treatment of arrhythmia

- Tachycardia for prolonged period: systolic and diastolic dysfunction (even in absence of other cardiac diseases)
- Diagnosis should be considered in any patient with tachycardia and LV systolic dysfunction, who is not in sinus rhythm.
- Diagnosis can be ascertained only retrospectively when correction of arrhythmia improves ventricular function
- It can also superimpose on other cardiomyopathy e.g., DCM patient with atrial arrhythmia
  - Decompensated HF due to loss of atrial function as well as systolic dysfunction due to irregular vent contraction

CAUSES

(Purest form of tachy cardiomyopathy)
- Incessant or very freq. atrial tachy
- Permanent reciprocating junction tachy
- Very freq. PVCs (>20,000/24 hrs)
- Recurrent NSVT

All Tachy + Pacing abnormality

Duration of arrhythmia is more important than rate of tachycardia

NAT HISTORY

- Most patient with tachycardiomyopathy, improve within 3-6 months after correction of arrhythmia
- Some patient has late improvement up to 1 year
- Following restoration of NS, 2, subtle abnormality in LV function may remain (e.g., mild LV dilatation despite of normalization of LVEF)
- Tachy induced LV diastolic – dysfunction can also occur

Pathophysiology

- TIC is rate dependent: Those patient with higher tachy rate develops it early
- Time of onset also depends on existing str heart disease; type of arrhythmia, age, duration and other comorbidities
  Tachy → High VR → initiates cardiac dilatation → MR → increases filling
  PR → decreases contractility → HF
  Tachy → short diastolic phase → increases level of Ca^{++} within sarcoplasma → could not move to SR

Other

Oxidative stress, ACE gene polymorphism, depletion of myo energy store and ischemia ionic channel remodeling.

4.10 TAKOTSUBO CARDIOMYOPATHY: STRESS CARDIOMYOPATHY

INTRODUCTION
- Acute reversible
- First recognized in 1990

C/F
- Variable
- Acute onset regional LV dysfunction
- Associated with chest pain
- Sometimes HF
- ST-T changes that may mimic acute MI
- Common in postmenopausal women
- M = F
- Freq. have preceding emotional or physical event that is believed to act as **trigger**
- 1.2% patients have trop T positive

ECHO
- Prominent LV contractible abnormality
- Most commonly involve apex (LV apical ballooning)
- RWMA may be limited to mid-vent wall
- RWMA lack single coro. Art. Distribution
- CAG – No obstructive CAD
- Compensatory hyperdynamic contraction of basal LV + Apical LV dyskinesia
  ↓
- Acute LVOT obstruction by Ant motion of MV
  ↓
- Hypotension

PATHOPHYSIOLOGY (HYPOTHESIS)

Catecholamine surge
↓
Regional microvascular dysfunction in susceptible patient
↓
Cellular calcium overload

PROG
- Good long term prognosis
- In-hospital mortality 1.2% (due to irreversible cardiogenic shock, LV rupture or embolization)
- Rarely associated with arrhythmia
  - Tdp
  - QT prolongation
  - CHB
- Recurrence is uncommon (2–5%)

MANAGEMENT
- Self-limited disorder
- Rapid resolution of symptoms and LV dysfunction
- Avoid QT prolonging drugs
- Anticoagulants if thrombus
- Beta blockers may help to alleviate catecholaminergic effect

  Diff vent morphology in patient with stress cardiomyopathy

  1) Takotsubo type   2) Reverse Takotsubo

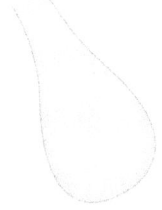
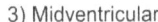
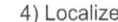

  3) Midventricular   4) Localized

Type	Morphology	Physiology	Pathology	Systemic condition or diseases clinical Associations	Non syndrome usually single gene	Syndromic
1. DCM	LV/RV dilatation with minimal or no wall thickening	Reduced contractility variable degree of diastolic dysfunction	Myocyte hypertrophy scattered fibrosis	HTN, alcohol use, thyrotoxicosis myxedema, persistent tachy toxin cg chemotherapeutics radiation, drug	Diverse gene ontology (>30 genes)	• Muscular dystrophies, Emery–Dreifuss limb girdle • Duchenne/Becker Kearns–Sayre barth syndrome
2. RCM disease	Normal chamber size, minimal wall thickening	Contractility normal with marked increase, in end-diastolic filling pr	Amyloid, iron, glycogen storage disease	EMF, amyloid, sarcoid scleroderma, Churg–Strauss cystinosis, lymphoma pseudoxanthoma Elasticum, hypereosinophilic	Sarcomeric gene mutation	Gaucher hemochromatosis fabry disease familial amyloidosis mucopolysaccharidosis
3. HCM	Normal or reduced interval chamber dimension septal thickening	Syst function increase to normal	Myocyte hypertrophy classically with disarray	Syndrome, carcino Severe HTN con confound diagnosis	Mutation of gene encoding sarcomeric proteins	Noonan synd Noonan/leopard/ Danon, Fabry, WPW Friedreich, ataxia, MERRI, MELAS
4. Arrhythmogenic CM	Scattered fibro fatty infiltration classically of RV RV ± LV dilatation	Vent arrhythmias	Islands of fatty replacement fibrosis	Palmoplantar keratoderma wooly hair in Naxos syndrome	Mutation of genes encoding protein of desmosomes	Naxos syndrome
5. LV NC	Ratio of non-compacted to compacted myocardium increased. Normal chamber dimensions varying to a DCM phenotype	Normal to reduce systolic function	Myocardium normal and ranging to findings consistent with other coexists CMpathy		Uncertain which genetic cause or developmental defect	
6. Infiltrative		Restrictive physiology	Amyloid, iron, glycogen storage disease		See RCM	See RCM
7. Inflammatory			Inflammatory infiltrate	Hypereosinophilic syndrome acute myocarditis		
8. Ischemic	Normal or dilated without hypertrophy	Reduced systolic function	Areas of infracted myocardium	Hypercholesterolemia, HTN, DM, cigarette smoking	Familial hyper-cholesterolemia other heritable lipid disorder	Familial hypercholesterolemia
9. Infectious						

SECTION 5

Congenital Heart Diseases

5.1 TRUNCUS ARTERIOSUS

DEFINITION
Single arterial trunk exiting from heart through common valve, giving origin to aorta (systemic circulation); pulmonary artery (PA) (pulmonary circulation) and coronary arteries

EMBRYOLOGY
(Conotruncal anomaly)
- Failure of absence of separation of conotruncal segment
- Failure of development of subpulmonary conus (van Praagh)
- Inadequate migration of neural crest cell

ETIOLOGY
Environmental Factors

Infant of diabetic mother embryonic exposure to retinoic acid:
- Deletion of 22q11
- CHARGE syndrome, DiGeorge syndrome,
- CATCH 22 (cardiac defect, abnormal facies, thymic hypoplasia, cleft palate, hypocalcemic)

EPIDEMIC
- 1.4–2.1% of all congenital heart defects (CHDs)
- 0.04–0.09 cases per 1,000 live birth

CLASSIFICATION
(Most common):
A. Collett and Edwards
   Type 1: Single pulmonary trunk arise from posterolateral aspect of common trunk
   Type 2: Left and right PA arise separately but closely from the posterior wall of trunk
   Type 3: Right, left or both PA arise independently from either side of truncus

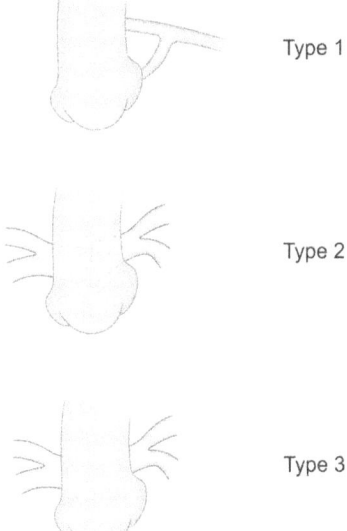

(Rarely only 1 PA arises from trunk and other pulmonary stenosis (PS) absent or may have been supplied by ductus. Absent PA is on same side of arch of aorta)

Type 4: No PA arise from the common trunk and lungs supplied by systemic to pulm collaterals aka pseudo truncus

[No longer considered as truncus PA with intact atrial septum (IAS)]

B. Van Praagh's classification
   A1-similar to Type 1
   A2-resembles type 2 and 3
   A3-one PA from truncus and other from patent ductus arteriosus (PDA)/collaterals
   A4-Truncus with Interrupted Aorta arch

C. Hemitruncus one PA arise from ascending Aorta and other comes off normally from main PA arising from right ventricular (RV) (modified Van Praagh classification included this in A3 type)
D. Physiological classification
   Gr-1: High pulmonary blood flow (PBF) with low pulmonary vascular resistance (PVR)
   Gr-2: Normal or slightly increases PBF, increasing PVR
   Gr-3: low PBF due to ostial narrowing or due to progressive pulmonary vascular disease
Latest
E. Russel et al. (to determine surgical outcome)
   2 groups:
   A. Aortic Dominant
   B. Pulmonary Dominant

ANATOMY

Truncal valve
- Truncal valve overrides large what is large Ventricular septal defect VSD with overriding aorta?
- VSD: committed to both vent
- 2–5 cusps (in 70% there are cusps)
- Thickened, dysplastic, polypoid, and unequal cusp
- Truncal valve insufficiency is common
- Truncal stenosis is less common

- Fibrous continuously between Truncal valve and mitral valve (MV)
- Hyperplasia of aortic arch with or without coarctation
- Interrupted Aorta Arch in 1/5th cases
- Right sided arch in 1/3rd
- Coronary anomalies frequent—Arise higher and post

HEMODYNAMICS

- Demands on PBF amount and truncal regurgitation
- Both ventricle pump blood in common trunk
- Systolic pressure in ventricles, Aorta and PA are same
- Soon after birth: PVR fall + Systemic Vascular Resistance (SVR) increases → increased PBF
  - Congestive Heart Failure (CHF) in first week of birth (cyanosis is negligible or mild)
  - *Truncal regurgitation:* Contributes to volume overload
  - *Interrupted Aorta Arch:* System circulation is duct dependent—PDA closure is life threatening
  - With PS—PBF decreases—cyanosis is deeper
  - *Over a time:* PVR decreases—Eisenmenger

CLINICAL FEATURE

- *Most of infants:* Present in early infancy with CHF due to increased PBF: Feeding difficulty; failure to thrive; excessive sweating; tachypnea; repeated respiratory infection, O/E -hyper dynamic precordium, cardiomegaly, hepatomegaly, minimal cyanosis. High volume pulse if truncal regurgitation is associated

  Auscult: S1 normal; S2 single and loud (due to dilatation of trunk), ejection click, ESM -Gr 3-4/6 over left third 4th LICS due to increased flow across truncal valve. Early diastolic murmur (high pitched) due to truncal regurgitation (ESM + EDM → to and fro murmur)
- Small number of infants, survive initial crisis phase develops pulmonary vascular disease become asymptomatic as PVR increases. Gradually becomes cyanotic (deeper) and symptoms of exertional dyspnea, easy fatigability and chest pain Eisenmenger syndrome.

ECG

Normal sinus rhythm (NSR), tall and peaked P [Right atrial enlargement (RAE)], Right axis deviation (RAD)
   Right ventricular hypertrophy (RVH) universally present
   In infant with large PBF—left ventricular volume overload (LVVO)—q waves in V5 and V6

Chest X-ray (CXR)

Varies with magnitude of PBF
Comma sign: High origin of dilated left PA (Described by Abraham)
- Right sided arch in 1/3rd
- Right arch + increasing PBF—strongly suspect Truncus arteriosus (TA)
- Pulmonary pruning with enlarged central PA—Pulmonary veno-occlusive disease (PVOD)

ECHO

- Visualization of only 1 outlet from vent
- Abnormal, thick, multicuspid truncal valve with regurgitation
- Large nonrestrictive VSD
- Main or branch PA from common trunk (short axis)
- Aortic arch abnormality
- Coronary anatomy
- Any associated lesions

Cath

Indications
- Doubt about anatomical issue by ECHO
- To delineate coronaries and PAs
- Doubt about operability, PVR calculation

NATURAL HISTORY

75% infants die within 1st month of life either due to CHF or bronchopneumonia.

MANAGEMENT

Medical Management

- Vigorous anti congestive measures with Angiotensin-converting enzyme (ACE) inhibitors
- Frequent associated with Digeorge syndrome
  - Sr Ca^{++} and Mg^{++} correction
  - Only irradiated blood used during surgical treatment (because of insufficient time for evaluation of immune status accurately)
  - Treatment and prophylaxis of pneumococcal and streptococcal infection (Thymus based immune deficiency)
  - Immunization with live vaccine should be avoided

Surgical

- *Palliative:* PA banding for increased PBF (was advocated in post) high mortality 30%
- *Definitive surgical treatment*
  - Within first week of life
  - When diagnosis is delayed, surgical treatment should be performed on urgent basis after 2-3 days of medical stabilization
- Various modification of Rastelli procedure
  - VSD closure in such a manner that left ventricle LV ejects into truncus
  - *For type 1:* Aortic homograft between right ventricle (RV) and PA
  - *For type 2&3:* Circumferential band of truncus which contains both PA is removed and connected to RV

  Aortic continuity with Dacron graft
- Repair of regurgitation truncal valve or truncal valve replacement

Postoperative

Follow-up every 4–12 month

- Check for truncal insufficiency
- Small RV-PA conduit need to be changed after 2-3 years of age
- Calcification of valve of conduit may develop
- Vent arrhythmia due to RV ventriculectomy
- Balloon dilatation/stenting of RV-PA conduit
- Nonsurgical percut PVR implantation
- Subacute Bacterial Endocarditis (SBE) prophylaxis throughout life
- No competitive sports

5.2 AORTIC ARCH ANOMALIES AND VASCULAR RING

VASCULAR RING

Broad term refers to several arterial anomalies having common feature of tracheal and/or esophageal compression by surrounding blood vessels part of which may or may not be patent (arteritic).

SIDEDNESS OF ARCH

- Determined by which bronchus it crosses
- Determined by CXR ⎤ Shows indentation on
  - Bronchogram   trachea/esophagus on
  - Esophagogram ⎦ Respective side
- ECHO ⎤
- CT   ⎥ Determined by branching pattern of
- MRI   ⎥ Brachiocephalic vessels
- CAG ⎦

CLASSIFICATION

A. Edward's Classification

- Double aortic arch
- Right aortic arch
- Left aortic arch
- Other rare anomalies

B. Anatomical Classification

- Abnormal branching
- Abnormal arch (rt, lt, double, cervical arch and supernumerary arch)
- Interrupted arch
- Anomalous origin of PA from Asc Ao

C. Clinical Classification

Vascular ring malformations divided into two groups: (1) complete and (2) incomplete
1. *Gr A* [complete]:
   - Produce clinical symptoms
   - E.g., Double Ao arch, rt Ao arch with lt ductus, anomalous innominate art and lt Ao arch with rt ductus
2. *Gr B* [incomplete]:
   - Do not produce symptoms
   - Anomalous rt subclavian from Ao, rt aortic arch with left des. Ao and lt Ao arch with rt des Ao.

C/F

- May remain asymptomatic
- Incidentally detected
- May produce
- *Mainly-respiratory distress:* Stridor, dyspnea, cough, occ wheezing, respi sound such as crowing/choking
  Brassy cough due to compressed recurrent laryngeal nerve by vascular ring
- Rarely diff in swallowing
- It is not possible to diagnose individual lesions independently only on clinical examination

INVESTIGATION

- ECHO cardiography (1st choice)
- Barium swallow (1st choice in post)
- Bronchoscopy gives useful info but it may be hazardous for children
- Aortography is mandatory
- MRI/CT gives better info than ECHO

A. Left Sided Arch

- Normal arch
- Formed due to regression of right dorsal root (between rt subclavian and desc Ao) and rt ductus arteriosus
- Curves over left main stem bronchus at level of T5 vertebrae
- Continue as desc Thoracic aorta, which remains over left side till it enters the diaphragm
- First branch is right brachiocephalic
- Ductus joins distal to LSCA
- Rt innominate and left carotid may arise from a common trunk (10%) known as Bitruncus
- Left vertebral artery may arise separately from arch prox to LSCA (10%)

Aberrant RSCA

- Most common Ao arch anomaly
- Occurs in 0-5% of general population
- Occurs in about 20% of cases of vasc ring
- RSCA arise independently from Ao and course behind esophagus
- 15% runs between eso and trachea
- Exceptionally it may run ant to trachea
- ARSCA may compress esophagus from post side, producing dysphagia (Dysphagia lusoria)

Majority: no compression

Asymptomatic Associated with:

- TOF
- VSD
- CoA
- Down syndrome

B. Rt Aortic Arch

Ao arch crosses over rt main stem bronchus and passes on rt side of trachea-occurs due to persistence of rt 4th bronchial arch and rt dorsal aortae

Associated with:
- TOF (13-34%)
- TA (30-40%)
- dTGA (8%)
- Tricuspid Atresia (7.7%)
- CTGA (10%)
- Pulm atresia with VSD (20%) [Not reported in PA with IVS]

Abnormal branching
- Mirror image branching
- Retro esophageal LSCA
- Retro esophageal diverticulum of Kommerell
- With aberrant innominate

B1. Associated with cyanotic CHD (98% cases)

Rt Aortic Arch with mirror image branching
- Due to regression of left dorsal aortic root between left ductus and descending Ao
- Ao arch crossed over right mainstem bronchus
- Upper part of desc Ao remains rt to midline, but after a short distance it deviates to left to enter normally placed left sided Diaphragmatic hiatus

  1st branch: Left innominate:
  - LSCA
  - LSR

  2nd branch: Rt common carotid (rec)

  3rd branch:
  - RSCA
  - Ductus usually on (lt) side Rt sided and BIC ductus also noted
  - Rarely ductus connects to LPA and upper descending aorta-forming vasc ring
- C/F: Asymptomatic (no vasc ring)
  Symptoms due to associated cardiac anomalies

B2. *Rt Ao arch with retro esophageal diverticulum of Kommerell*
- No innominate artery
- 1st branch is LCC
- 2nd branch is RCC
- 3rd branch is RSCA
- LSCA is a continuation from the large diverticulum from the arch behind esophagus
- Diverticulum is equal to diameter of desc Ao at its origin-that abruptly tapers to form LSCA
  This arrangement of vessels with left sided ductus produce complete vasc ring

C/F: Due to vasc ring (described above)

B3. *Rt Ao arch with retro esophageal LSCA*
- Sequence is similar to B2
- But prox part of LSCA is not longer in caliber as in diverticulum of Kommerell
- Presence of left sided ductus produce vasc ring
- When ductus on rt side-no vasc ring

B4. *Rt Ao arch with aberrant innominate art*
- 10% of patients
- Left innominate takes off too far to the left from rt Ao arch or posteriorly after RCC and RSCA-courses behind the esophagus
- Together with ductus or ligamentum arteriosus it completes vasc ring and produce compressive symptoms

C. Double Ao Arch
- MC vasc ring seen in 40% of cases
- Rt arch gives rise to RSCA and RCC
- Lt arch gives rise to LSCA and LCC
- Rt arch longer than lt arch
- Rt dominant pattern
- Double Ao arch is commonly an isolated anomaly
- Rarely associated with TOF, VSD, TGA, and PDA
- *Embryo:* Persistence of both dorsal aorta and both 4th aortic arch
- Left arch passes in front of trachea and crosses over left main stem bronchus
- Rt sided arch passes over rt main stem bronchus and proceeds behind trachea and esophagus to join desc Ao
- Almost always left sided ductus or ligamentum
- Both arches join to form des Ao
- Dominant arch is contralat to the side of desc Ao
- Rare anomaly
- 0.3-0.9% of all CHD
- C/F: Infant becomes very sick after birth (due to compression)
- Swallowing diff less severe
- No abnormality on clinical examination (Investigation) CXR, Barium swallow, ECHO, Aortogram

D. Cervical Ao Arch
- Ascending Ao ascends abnormally to neck and arch S found in cervical region between C3 and C8

Two types
1. *Common form:* Right ao arch and desc Ao crosses behind esophagus to opp side about T4 level and give rise to anomalous LSCA

   Rarely: Arch on lt side of trachea and crosses to rt behind esophagus where aberrant RSCA found

   If associated with contralateral ductus, forms complete vasc ring

2. *Other group:* Left aortic arch with normal branching
   ↓
   Does not produce vascular ring
   Long tortuous retro esophageal course of des Ao may compress esophagus.

E. Other Rare Anomaly

- Circumflex Ao arch
  - Left Ao arch with rt descending aorta
  - Right Ao arch with lt descending aorta
- Isolation of any branch of Asc aorta
  MC–is LSCA isolation–isolated branch does not take origin from Ao, instead remain cont with PDA
- Usually associated with cyanotic CHD-TOF

F. Anomalies of Pulm Art

Rare

F1. Aberrant LPA
- LPA arising from RPA
- Anomalous course over prox portion of rt main stem bronchus (behind trachea and in front of esophagus)
- Can compress both Trachea and Esophagus

Vascular sling: In contrast to aortic arch anomaly that surrounds the trachea and esophagus
- Known as vascular sling
- Trachea bifurcates at lower pace with wide angle, which is known as inverted T sign
→ Associated with PDA, VSD, AVCD

F2. Absence of one PA
- Usually associated with CHD (esp TOF)
- One PA is absent to contralateral side of aortic arch
  Distal PA is usually present—it is also known as occult PA
  Involved lung gets blood from cyst collaterals Bronchial arteries or PDA

F3. One PA arising from asc Ao
- Usually RPA arise from Asc Ao above sinus of valsalva
- Always associated with CHD.

5.3 ANOMALOUS SYSTEMIC VENOUS CONNECTION

EMBRYOLOGY

- Primitive veins
  B/L symmetrical
  1. Vitelline vein
  2. Umbilical vein
  3. C cardinal vein (anterior and post)
     - Ant cordial veins drain from upper part of body and UL
     - Post cardinal veins drain lower part of body
       ↓
       Interconnection occurs between these 2 veins with prominence of certain parts and regression of after
       ↓
     - Rt cardinal vein become more prominent and form
       1. SVC- extra cardiac (rt ant cardinal)
       2. Intracardiac SVC (rt common cardinal)
     - Posterior cardinal vein regress gradually (when subcardinal and supracardinal vein forms)
     - Left cardinal and Vitelline vein regress
     - Rt sinus horn incorporated into PA
     - Lt sinus horn separated from LA
       - Transverse portion of sinus venosus and proximal lt sinus horn becomes CS
- Distal left sinus horn and left common cardinal vein becomes ligamentous
  structure (ligament of Marshall)

  IVC develops from 5 diff embryonic venous channel
  1. Posterior cardinals
  2. Supra cardinals
  3. Sub cardinals
  4. Communication of rt sub cardinal with Hepatic vein
  5. From part of hepatic veins that develop from rt vitelline vein

CLASSIFICATION

A. Abnormality of SVC
- Persistent LSVC communicating to CS
- LSVC communicating to LA
- Absent normal RSVC with persistent LSVC

B. Anomalies of IVC
- IVC interruption with Azygous continuation
- IVC communicating to LA

C. Anomalies of CS
- Unroofed CS
- Atresia/hypoplasia of CS
- Stenosis of ostium of CS
- Diverticulum of CS

D. Anomalies of Ductus Venosus
- Anomalies of umbilical vein
- Persistent ductus venosus

E. Total Anomalous Syst Venous Communication

F. Anomalies of Valves of Sinus Venosus

5.4 COMPLETE AVSD

INTRODUCTION

Also known as AV canal defect
Endocardial cushion defect
Essence of group of hearts described as AVSD

- Presence of common AV junction with one fibrous ring at one horizontal plane (No separate TV and MV annuli)
  ↓
- Complete absence of AV valve
- Common AV ring has 5 leaflets

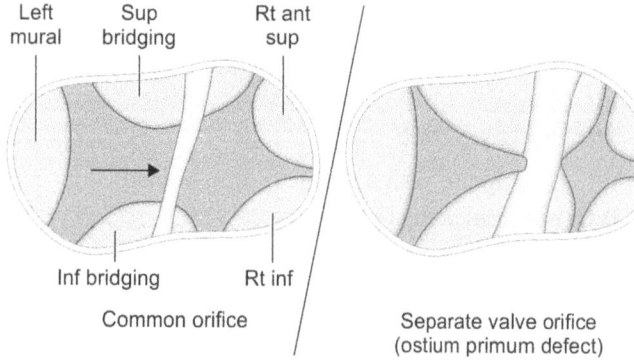

- This basic anomaly is uniform to all types of AVSD
  Complete AVSD—common AV orifice with a common fibrous ring and partially shared valve leaflets, large primum ASD and in general large VSD

INCIDENCE

- 0.19/1000 live births
- 2–9% of CHF
- 3/5th defects are only partial
- Associated AVSD with Down's syndrome
  - 33–50% of all AVSD has Downs
  - 1/3rd of down could have complete AVSD
  - Down uncommonly associated with partial AVSD
- 10% recurrence risk in offspring (double if mother has AVSD
- 10% occurrence in 1st degree relatives
- No sex prediction

EMBRYO

- No exact understanding
- Widely prevalent theory
  Lack of fusion of endocardial cushion as the prominent problem
  Normal at D-28: The common atrium is dorsal to vent
  ↓
  These 2 communicates with AV canal
  ↓
  35d: Two thickening on the dorsal and vent side of AV canal grow (endocardial cushion)
  ↓
  Divide AV canal in lt and rt
  ↓
  Mesenchyme around each proliferate to form valve leaflets (AVSD)

- Superior and inferior cushion do not close completely and so can't fuse with septum Primum—1 degree ASD
- Failure of fusion of endocardial cushion—abnormally low position of AV valve and high position of AoV—goose neck deformity
- Small portion of AV valve also arise from endocardial cushion—As cushions do not fuse, most patients has ant and post component to AML (cleft mitral value)

ANATOMY/PATHOLOGY

AV Junction

Common AV junction (Hallmark of ACSD)

- Normally AV septum formed partly by membranous tissue and partly by atrial tissue. This overlap in postero inf area is overlapped by extension of fibrofatty tissue and therefore is not truly septal (termed AV muscular sandwich)
- Absence of AV muscular sandwich along with AV fibrous septum is near universal phenomena

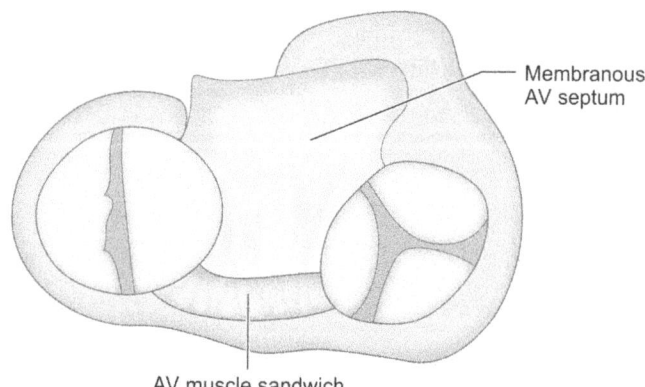

Position

In both partial and complex AVSD, AV valve lie in same plane with respect to base of vent septum

- Annulus of AV valve lies in one plane but in patient with complete AVSD annulus of AV valve is convex toward cardiac apex

Normal wedging of sub aortic area between 2 AV annuli does not occur-ant displacement of LVOT

AV Valve

- Common AV valve has 5 leaflets
- 2 exclusively in RV (Ant sup and inf)
  1 exclusively in LV (mural)
  2 bridging leaflet (sup and inf)
- Pap muscle also align differently
  - Left side has superior and inf pap muscle
  - Rt side has medial, anterior and inf pap muscle
- Cleft mitral valve is not defect in mitral valve but it's due to incomplete opposition of 2 bridging leaflet on septal side

↓

Leading to regurgitation into either atria
Dilated common AV ring can also lead to central jet of MR and appear as prolapsing anterior leaflet

IAS

Mostly 1 degree ASD
- Rarely additional 2 degree ASD
- Very rarely absent IAS

IVS

Manner of attachment of AV valve tissue determine presence or absence of VSD

- Inf bridging leaflet often fuse with vent crest
- Attachment of sup bridging leaflet determine size of VSD
- In heart with exclusive atrial shunting 2 bridging leaflets are joined by tough of tissue running along IVS crest
- If this fusion is incomplete—lead to single inlet type VSD. (Size depend on sup bridging leaflet attachment)

↓

Such defect termed as intermediate/transitional

↓

Transitional AVSD
- Type of partial AVSD
- Small inlet VSD (due to dense chordal attachment to septum)
- Large primum ASD
- 2 separate AV valve orifice

Intermediate AVSD
- Type of complete AVSD
- Large inlet VSD
- Large primum ASD
- 2 separate AV valve orifice
- Common AV ring

Outlet dimension of LV aspect of septum is appreciably longer than inlet: pathognomonic of AVSD

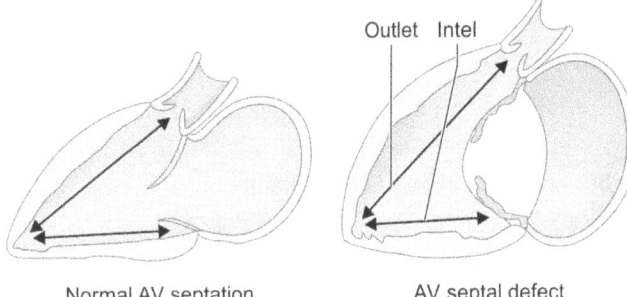

Normal AV septation | AV septal defect

- Additional perimemb or muscular VSD may coexist
- VSD in AVSD is typically inlet

Unbalanced AVSD

Condition in which one vent is hypoplastic and other receives most of AV valve

LVOT

Abnormal position (shifted Ao)
- Vulnerable to obstruction
- LVOT is elongated and narrow
- HD significant obst is uncommon

Conduction System

- Abnormal AV conduction
- AVSD—only inf limb of atrial septum comes in contact with vent septum at crux

↓

AV conduction axis and nodal axis displaced postero-inferiorly

↓

Elongated nonbranching bundle that runs either on the crest or to its left

↓

Bundle branches located more posteriorly

↓

LVOT (Ant) nowhere near conduction system (like in normal heart)

Associated Anomalies

- Double inlet ventricle or discordant AV connection
- DORV or discordant vent-arterial connection
  - Associated with situs ambiguous and asplenia/polysplenia syndrome
- PS or TOF
- LVOT obstruction; CoA; Ao arch interruption (50%)-LSVC to LA or unroofed CS with coronary sinus type ASD

CLASSIFICATION
A. Rastelli Classification

- Traditionally classified in 3 types
- Based on attachment of SBL to rt side in otherwise normal (S, D, S) heart in situs solitus
- *(50–70%)-Rastelli type A:* SBL is tightly tethered to crest of IVS. There is no VSD
- *(3%)-Rastelli type B:* SBL is not attached to IVS rather it is attached to an anomalous RV papillary muscle and is almost always associated with unbalanced AV canal with rt dominance
  - VSD extends up to aortic cusp
- *(30%)-Rastelli type-C:* Free floating SBL is attached to anterior papillary muscle

B. Complete-partial

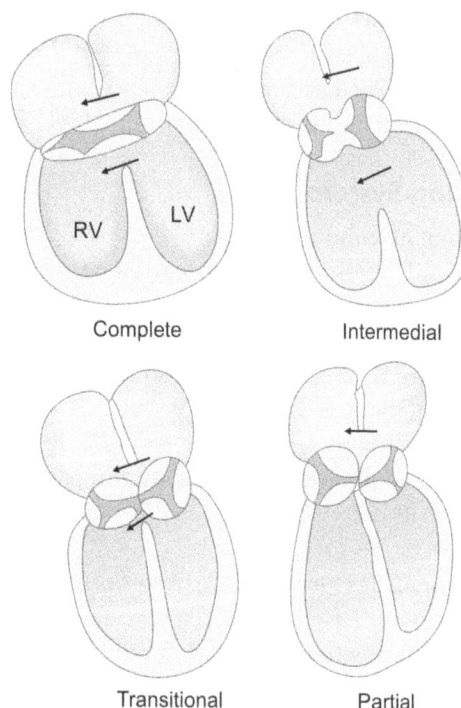

Complete   Intermedial

Transitional   Partial

ASSOCIATED ANOMALIES

- Partial AVSD
  - Most common 2 degree ASD and LSVC to CS
  - Less Freq PS, TS or atresia, cor triatriatum, CoA, PDA, memb VSD, PV anomalies, HLV

Complete AVSD:
- Type A is Freq in patient with Down syndrome
- Type C—TOF, DORV, TGA and heterotaxy syndrome

PHYSIOLOGY

- Intrauterine life
- SVC blood which is usually directed through the tricuspid valve, will shunt across the ASD to LV, decreasing the O_2 sat diff between Asc and dB Ao

↓

Concomitant increase in sat of blood ejected by RV

↓

Increasing DO_2 in blood flowing to pulm vessel and affect their development.

If a large VSD is present, shunting of additional PV blood across the defect into Ao could occur. This would further decrease PO_2 in Asc Ao and increase PO_2 of blood perfusing lung.

LV-RA shunt decreases LV stroke volume

(Post natal)
- Partial AVSD:
  - Interatrial shunt is large and left AV valve regurgitation is mild or absent HD identical to isolated 2 degree ASD
  - When important left AV valve regurgitation is present lt or rt shunt becomes larger and causes vol. overload of RV as well as LV and produce CHF in early life
- Complete AVSD
  - Large VSD
  - Systolic PAP are equal to Ao pr
  - Left AV valve regurgitation will increase LV VO
  - Increased PBF early in life with CHF and Freq. respi infection
  - This patient will develop irreversible PVD early in life (6–12 months) (even earlier in Downs)

C/F

(Partial):
- Patient with 1 degree ASD usually asymptomatic during childhood
- Dyspnea, easy fatigability, recurrent RTI and growth retardation (if associated with major MR or common atrium)

(Complete):
- Tachypnea and failure to thrive (increased PBF) early in life usually all patient have symptoms by 1 year of age

C/F depends on
- Size of VSD
- Severity of AV valve regurgitation

↓

Both leads to early onset of CHF or LRTI

EXAMINATION

- Usually undernourished and have signs of CHF
- Hyperactive precordium with systolic thrill at lower (lt) sternal border
- S1 is accentuated, S2 narrow split (PHTN), P2 increases intensity (S2 can be widely split—2 degree ASD)
- Gr 3-4/6 holosystolic murmur (AV valve regurgitation)
- Peripheral pulse: severe MR can give rise to so-called water hammer like pulse
- PVS3 and LVS3 may be heard
- Pulm ejection click (due to dilated PA)
- ESM in pulm area (due to increased flow)
- MDM over lower left precordium and apex (due to large diastolic flow across AV valve leaflets)

INVESTIGATION

CXR

Cardiomegaly
- Apex mostly RV type (may be LV type in some)
- RA is prominent chamber
  - LA also may be enlarged (in patient with VSD and significant shunt or because of left AV valve regurgitation)
- Lack of cardiomegaly does not exclude AVSD
- MPA prominent
- Signs of increased PBF
- Peripheral pruning if PVD present.

ECG

Classical ECG pattern
- Superior axis (LAD) with counter clock depolarization (initial lt to rt septal depolarization does not occur in usual way because of post displaced AV conduction axis)
- PR prolonged
- RAE/LAE
- RVVO-IRBB, rsR1 or dsR1
- LVVO if lt AV regurgitation (Peripheral smear) and (vsa)
- Asplenia may be suspected by appearance of Howell-Jolly bodies in RBC

ECHO

- Diagnostic
- Situs should be carefully examined
- Most AVSD has situs solitus
- If associated with situs ambiguous—search for complex association
- Associated with persistent LSVC + unroofed CS
- Pulm venous drainage should be confirmed to ascertain presence or absence of TAPVC
- RA/RV dilated in partial AVSD
- All in chamber enlarged in complete AVSD
- Morphology of common AV valve
- Absence of central hinge point (aortomitral tricuspid continuity) is lacking
- Large single AV orifice that is opening into ventricles and central coaptation in systolic reveals 1 degree ASD and VSD clearly
- 3rd leaflet in LA can be found if searched diligently

Color Doppler—ASD
- VSD
- Jet of left AV regurgitation (Seen kissing IVS (unlike Rheumatic MR Which is central))
- Additional control jet of left AV valve regurgitation can be seen too. (due to dilated annulus and cleft)
- Shunting from LV—RA and RV → LA (obligatory shunting)
- Associated 2° ASD can be seen
- Inlet VSD
- Chordal attachment, pap muscle arrangement and size of vent
- Typical AVSD has normally related great arteries

Cardiac Cath

- Indicated when there is concern regarding PVD or when multiple associated cardiac defect persists
- Classical goose neck deformity of LVOT and also presence of AV valve regurgitation
- Difficult to enter RV and PA—tendency for catheter to enter LA

D/D

- Gerbode defect
- Inlet type VSD with TV tissue allowing LV-RA shunt
- Isolated cleft in AML and straddling of AV valve
- TGA with VSD
- TAPVC

Compli

- Failure to thrive
- CHF
- Repeated respi infection
- Eisenmenger syndrome
- IE
- Rhythm problem

NATURAL HISTORY

- Severe CHF in early infancy (1st month of life)
- Significant PVD appear by 6 months

- Irreversible PVD (>90% of patients) by age 3–5 years
- 80% die by 2 year (if no surgical treatment)
- Severe pneumonia in early infancy leads to respi failure

MANAGEMENT

A. Medical

- Management of CHF
- Nutrition should be optimized

B. Surgical

- *Indi:* All patients will require surgical treatment
- *Timing:* 2-4 month of age usually
- Early surgical treatment repair for patient with Dacron syndrome because of their tendency to develop PVR early

Palliative Surgical Treatment

- PA banding
- 15% in-hospital mortality
- Not recommended unless other association abnormalities make complete repair high risk (e.g., unbalanced AVSD)

Corrective Surgical Treatment

- Closure of primum of ASD and VSD (inlet) and construction of 2 separate and competent AV valves
- Single patch or 2 patch
- Left AV valve is allowed to persist as 3 leaflet structure
- MVR in few patients
- Unbalanced AVSD -PA banding followed by fontan

Mortality

3–10%

Factors that increases surgical treatment risk

- Young age
- Severe AV valve regurgitation
- Hypoplasia of LV
- Increased and fixed PVR
- Severe pre op symptoms
- Associated complex lesions

COMPLICATION

- MR become persistent or worsens (10%)
- SA node dysfunction
- Post op arrhythmias (usually supravent)

Special Situation

- Unbalanced AVSD
  PA band—Fontan
  DKS surgical treatment: Fontan
- Downs and AVSD
  Pre op cardiac cath to evaluate PVR (even before 3 months) and decide timing accordingly
- *TOF+ AVSD* (+ severe cyanosis)
  - Syst to PA shunt in infancy
  - Complete repair at 2–4 year

Follow-up

- Every 6 months –1 year
- Diuretic, captopril, digoxin if residual HD abnormality present
- Some restriction of activity.

5.5 COARCTATION OF AORTA

DEFINITION
Obstruction in descending Ao, located in typically near aortic attachment of the ductus arteriosus or ligamentum arteriosum.

INCIDENCE
4th MC cong heart disease
- M:F = 3:1
- 0.2–0.6/1000 live births
- 7.% of CHF

Associated with Turner, Noonan, William-Beuren syndrome.

EMBRYO
- Abnormal dev of left 4th and 6th aortic arch
- 2 theories
  1. Ectopic ductal tissue theory (Skodiac theory)
  2. HD theory (Hemodynamic theory)

Ectopic ductal tissue theory (Rudolph)
Coarct develop as migration of smooth muscle cell into periductal aorta with subsequent constriction and narrowing.

HD THEORY
Most acceptable
- Hemodynamic disturbance lead to reduction of volume of blood flow through fetal Ao arch produce CoA

Because intracardiac lesions which reduce LV outflow such as VSD and LVOT obstruction are more commonly associated with coarctation.

CLASSIFICATION

Bonnet Classification
- *Infantile type:* Prox to aorta ductal junction with patent duct
- *Adult type:* Distal to insertion of arterial ligament, associated with collaterals

Lev Classification
- *Fetal coarct:* Elongated, narrow, and preductal
- *Adult coarct:* Localized and postductal

Recent Classification
MC- 1. Preductal
Rare- 2. Para ductal or juxtaductal
3. Postductal

Three types of constriction in main preductal lesion
1. Isthmal hypoplasia
2. Discrete ductal shelf with isthmal hypoplasia
3. Waist lesion with closed duct

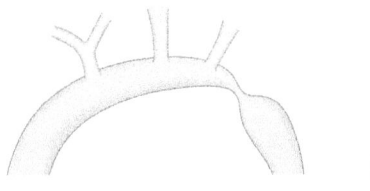
A-1 Waist lesion with closed duct

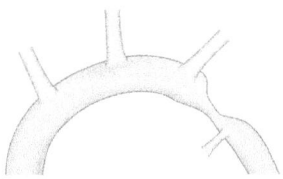
A-2 Discrete ductal shelf with isthmal hypoplasia

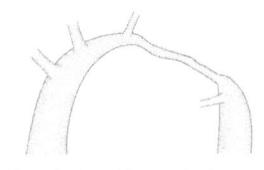
A-3 Isthmal hypoplasia

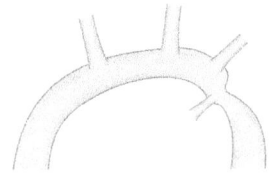
B Juxta ductal

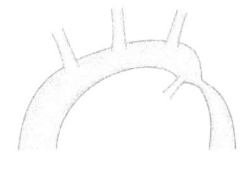
C Postductal

TYPES OF COARCTATION
- *Simple coarctation:* Without intracardiac lesion
- *Complex coarctation:* Associated with intracardiac lesion (VSD/PDA/MR)
- *Pseudocoarctation:* Kinking of aorta near the ligamentum arteriosum due to elongation and dilatation of distal Ao arch and prox des ao
  - No significant gradient
  - Benign
  - Rare
- Reverse coarct UL pulses not palpable but LL pulses are well palpable
  - One form of Takayasu arteritis where there is diffuse so involvement including renal art but Femoral art spared
- *Function coarctation:* Due to ext pr on Aorta either by mediastinal mass/tumor
- Multiple coarct
- *Residual coarct:* Presence of gradient across coarct segment after repair
- Recurrent coarct

- Abdominal coarct
  - Due to Takayasu arteritis
  - Or congenital due to hypoplasia of abd aortic intima.

ASSOCIATION

- *PDA and ASD/PFO: Part* of coarct
- *Acyanotic:* VSD, AS, cong MS and BAV BAV-MC
- *Cyanotic:* dTGA without TA, Taussig-Bing, AKCD, truncus, DORV, HLHS
- *Shine's complex:*
  - Multiple (lt) sided obstructive lesions including- coarctation of Aorta
  - Sub aortic stenosis
  - Congenital MS:
    - Supravalvular mitral ring
    - Parachute MV
- *Extracardiac association:*
  - Aneurysm of aortic root, circle of willis and intercostal arteries
  - Dissection of prox aorta
  - Retinal art anomaly
  - Subclavian steal syndrome

HEMODYNAMICS

- Fetal circ—not much affected
- After birth—foramen oracle closes and Ductus closes
  ↓
  Entire CO has to cross coarct seg
  ↓
  When there is significant obstruction LV has to work more to push blood to circulation to maintain CO
  ↓
  LV pr and Ao syst pr increases
- Pr gradient between Asc Ao and des ao
  <20 = mild
  69–70 = severe
- Pr gradient persists during both phase of cardiac cycle
- When CoA is severe-Infant develop severe CHF
- Additional lesion (large VSD, PDA, or MR)
  Increased LVEDV and EDP
  ↓
  Ppt CHF and lead to PHTN
- Postductal coarctation and hypoplasia of Ao arch
  ↓
  When associated with systemic RV pr
  ↓
  Leads to rt to lt shunt through PDA
  ↓
  Known as coarctation syndrome

PATHOLOGICAL CHANGES

Intimal and medial thickening with protruding ridges into aortic lumen
↓
Cystic medial necrosis in aorta close to coarctation site
↓
Infant who survive early crisis develop LVH and blood flow to LL increase by collateral
↓
HD changes are not significant in childhood and adolescent period
↓
Remain relatively asymptomatic

C/F

A. Neonate and Infant

- Tachypnea   esp during feeding and irritability
- Sweating   (due to CHF)
  ↓
  Most of these infant die due to shock, renal failure OV necrotizing enterocolitis
  ↓
  Those who survive early crisis, they become gradually asymptomatic and attend adulthood

Signs:
- Pulse in LL is diminished ⎫
- Once ductus close LL pulse absent ⎬ Hallmark of CoA
- Pr diff between UL and LL is significant when more than 20 mm Hg ⎭
- Tachypnea ⎫
- Mattled sun ⎬ All due to CHF
- Peripheral cyanosis ⎬ and low CO
- Hepatomegaly ⎭

Auscultation: RV impulse, gallop sound, short ESM over left sternal border and over back
- When CoA is severe -no murmur because CO is low

B. Children and Adults

- 2/3rd–free from symptoms
- Gen appearance may be Turner phenotype or athletic appearance with muscular nature of upper body and relative thinning of lower half

Upper limb HTN due to (theories)
- *Mechanical theory:* Persistence to circulation at the zone of CoA leads to disproportionate UL HTN
- *Neural theory:* Distensibility of pre coarct segment of aorta—elevated during pr in proximal ao during infancy

will reset baroreceptor to higher basal rate which leads to HTN
- *Renal theory:* Renal art originating from low pr post coarct aorta will lead to reduced RBF with activation of RAS system:
  - HTN may persist or appear later after a successful repair because change in vascular reactivity, arterial wall compliance and abnormal baroreceptor reflex persists even after surgery
  - Incidence of hypertensive retinopathy and papilledema is rare
  - Incidence of toxemia of preg is also rare
  - *Preg:*
    - Decreased risk of CHF
    - Increased risk of IE, ICH, and Ao rupture

OTHER SYMPTOMS

- Epistaxis, headache (due to HTN)
- Leg fatigue, intermittent claudication, add lower limb
- Hematemesis due to post coarct aneurysm rupture to esophagus (rare)
- Dysphagia (rare)
- ICH due to rupture of aneurysm of circle of Willis
- Dissection or rupture of prox Asc Ao
- Premature CAD
- Fainting and/or palpitation due to VT,

SIGNS

- Abnormal diff between UL and LL pulse (Hallmark) (Brachial-Femoral-Radial)

It's not delayed arrival of pulse, it's slow rate of rise with a delayed peak is the cause
- Dilated Asc Ao—pulsation occur rt 2nd and 3rd des
- Visible pulsation over suprasternal area with systolic thrill may occur
- Visible and palpable pulsation over infraclavicular on both side may be due to collaterals
- Diminished left brachial pulse—presubclavian coarct to
- Diminished rt brachial—aberrant origin of rt subclavian distal to coarct
- If femoral appears normal in setting of coarct—suspect 'pseudo coarct'
- Forceful carotid and suprasternal pulsations

Increasing with ex-imp feature of coarct
- O/E: Apical impulse normal—as age advance apical impulse is LV type and hearing
- Collateral pulsation in intercostal or interscapular
- S1 normal; S2 normal split

Ao ejection click-suspect BAV
ESM-at upper left sternal border radiating to interscapular
—flow across coarct
  At base due to associated BAV
  Collaterals may also produce ESM/cont murmur over chest ant, lat and post
  (Suzman's sign)

COLLATERALS IN CoA

Between pre- and postcoarct segment
- Superior intercostal arising from subclavian

Post-intercostal br of des thoracic Ao
- Intercostal arteries from int mammary

Intercostal arising from postcoarct segment of Ao
- Sup epigastric branch of int thoracic artery

Inf epigastric br of femoral art
- Axillary art system—desc so
- Ant spinal art—intercostal arteries

INVESTIGATION

ECG

Infants: Normal ECG (normal RV dominance pattern)
If findings of LVH with strain—suggests presence of associated As or endocardial fibroelastosis
Older children: Feature of LVH
- *LAD in CoA:* Indicate presence of associated AVCD, DORV or 1 degree myocardial disease
  Persistent RVH beyond infancy—suggests associated lesion such as VSD or ms producing PHTN

CXR

Asymptomatic infant and young children—normal

Infant with CHF: Mod cardiomegaly and pulm venous HTN
- *Later in course of disease:* Dilated LSCA and coarct segment with dilated descending aorta—classical radiological appearance of figure of three due to pre- and poststenotic dilatation
- Rib notching seen on inf border of post rib (common from 3rd to 8th) known as Dock's sign
- Rib notching can be B/L or UL

U/L rib notching needs to be differentiated from notching due to AT shunt.

Barium swallow shows E sign in LAD projection also known as reverse 3 sign.

Rib Notching not found in upper 3 and lower 3 ribs as they do not form collateral with internal mammary.

ECHO

Suprasternal long axis:
Delineates CoA as a localized narrowing of thoracic Ao beyond origin of LSCA, posterior shelf appear as a thin fibrous memb protruding from post aspect of Ao. Poststenotic dilatation. cw will detect high velocity—high velocity flow persists in diastole called diastolic tail depending on severity of coarct
- Assess mitral valve—LV function
- Size of transverse ao arch—often stenotic or hypoplastic

MRI and CT

Better than ECHO

Cardiac Cath

Mandatory before surgical intervention
- Defines anatomy (location and extent of collaterals and other intracardiac lesions + assess W function
Pressure gradient <20→ mild CoA
But; pr gr may be underestimated
In:
1. Left sided obstructive lesions
2. LV dysfunction
3. Presence of PDA

COMPLICATION

- CHF during infancy
- Rupture of diseased aorta
- Dissection of Ao
- IE or infective endocarditis
- Cerebral hemorrhage due to HTN causing rupture of circle of Willis or rupture of BCM aneurysm
- Premature CAD

DIAGNOSIS

Acyanotic infant with CHF- suspect CoA
UL-LL pulse diff-suspect CoA

PROGNO

- Long term Prognosis adversely affected by systemic HTN and premature CAD

- Mean age of death = 90 years (without surgery) 3/4th die by age 45 years
In infant: CHF—survival is poor
1 year survival is 16% only
COD: CHF (infants)
HTN causing ApD (adults)

MANAGEMENT

A. Asymptomatic CoA

Medical management: HTN or hypertensive crisis should be detected and treated. Arm and leg BP should be checked frequently
- *Intervention*:
  - Balloon angioplasty for CoA is controversial
- *Indications*:
  - Trans catheter systolic gradient >20 mm and suitable anatomy irrespective of age
  - Trans catheter gr <20 mm Hg with suitable anatomy in
    - Presence of significant collateral
    - Patient with univent heart
    - Patient with significant LV dysfunction
  - As a palliative procedure for
    - Patient with LV dysfunction
    - Severe MR
  - Balloon expandable stainless steel stent implanted concurrently with angioplasty
  For older patients (8-10 years of age)
    - Stent should be expanded to an adult size (min 20 mm in diameter)
    - Indicates similar to balloon angioplasty
    - In whom balloon failed—stenting
  - Absorbable metal stent is in experimental phase
- *Surgical:*
  - Indication
    - PG >20-30 mm Hg with reduction of aortic diameter by 50% at level of coarct
    - Significant narrowing of Ao with Doppler PG >20-30 mm Hg
    - Gradient developing with exercise is not a reliable marker (it may be due to peripheral amplification of syst pr in arm
  - *Preferred age*
  If done <1 year = low rate of HTN but high recurrence rate
  Some center prefer 2-3 years of age
  Others 4-5 years age
  - *Procedure:* Resection of coarct segment with end to end anastomosis—preferred

Other:
- Subclavian patch
- Patch aortoplasty

B. Symptomatic Patient

- *Medical management*
  - Anticongestive treatment
  - PGE 1 infusion to keep duct open before any surgery or intervention
- *Intervention*
  - Balloon coarctoplasty
    - High rate of recoarctation (>50%)
    - High complication rate
    - Some center use cutting balloon
  - Stenting
    - Cannot be expanded to adult size
    - Require surgical removal at a later date
- Surgery
  - Urgent if CHF develop
  - *Options*
    - Resection and end to end anastomosis
    - Subclavian flap aortoplasty
    - Patch aortoplasty

FOLLOW-UP

If done in infancy
- Reexamination over 6–12 months because re coarctation is possible
- Balloon coarctoplasty if re-CoA
- Surveillance and treatment for systemic HTN

If surgery not done
- Annual examination with attention to (1) BP difference, (2) status of associated abnormality, and (3) gradient across CoA

Possible late compli-aneurysm formation

MRI/CT performed every 2–5 years

5.6 AORTIC PULMONARY WINDOW

DEFINITION

Rare congenital cardiac malformation resulting from def in AP septum

- Large single defect present between Asc Ao and MPA just above SLV

INCIDENCE

- Not well established
- 0.1–0.2% of all CHD
- Male dominance
- No tendency to close spont

EMBRYOLOGY

- Non fusion of embryonic AP (spiral) septum or failure of embryonic AP septum
  Localized defect between 2 great arteries
  ↓
- Malalignment of AP septum and truncal septum

ANATOMY

- 5 mm–3 cm or greater
- Usually involves left side of Asc Ao and right wall of pulm trunk
- Inferior edge of defect 1–2 cm above coronary ostia
- Situated midway between AV and bifurcation of PA
- IVS intact in majority patients
- Nearly always single-large oval shaped

D/D

Truncus arteriosus: In AP window, both great arteries arise from separate infundibulum and outflow tract

ASSOCIATED ANOMALIES

- Isolated anomaly in 50%
- May be associated with PDA
  - Interrupted Ao arch (type A)
  - Anomalous RCA from PA
  - Severe CoA
  - Rt Ao arch
  - VSD
  - TOF
  - TGA
  - TA

CLASSIFICATION

Morris Classification

- *Type 1:* Proximal defect midway between SLV and bifurcation of pulm Art (70–98%)
- *Type 2:* Distal defect with I'll defined or absent posterior border and Anomalous origin of ROA from Aorta (13–25%)
- *Type 3:* Large defect—combination of 2 types
  Total absence of AP septum (5%)

Morphological Classification (Kutsche and VCM Merop)

- Circular and localized detect midway between SLV and bifurcation of PA
- Helical shaped in a similar position
- Large defect with no post or distal border

Modified Morris Classification

Type 4: Intermediate type (with adequate superior and inf rim)

HD

- Large (lt) to (rt) shunt
- PHTN related to size of defect, associated lesion and relative resistance between SVR and PVR
- Lt-rt shunt establish within few weeks of birth
  By end of infancy usually there is high pulm vasc persistence and infant develops Eisenmenger physiology

C/F

Similar to large VSD/PDA

- Symptomatic very easily
- CHF, dyspnea, diaphoresis, feeding difficulty band failure to thrive
- Cyanosis not usually present
- May be seen when associated with TGA, TOF or aorta atresia
- Those who survive to teenage—develop signs of Eisenmenger physiology
- Very few patients with small defect remains asymptomatic in childhood

SIGNS

Tachypnea/Tachycardia

- High volume pulse wide pulse pr
  Forceful apical impulse (due to LV vol overload) and left parasternal lift (RV pr overload)

Narrow split S2/single S2 with increased P2 component (suggesting PHTN)

- Pulm ejection click
- Harsh long syst murmur in upper left parasternal border
- Cont murmur is unusual but may be hard of defect is small
- If MDM heard over apex (increases flow across MV) PDA or VSD may be associated and clinical feature of AP window are masked
  Graham steel murmur (if severe PHTN)

INVESTIGATION

ECG

BiV vent hypertrophy

- LV forces predominate in patient with large PBF
- In patient with PHTN, RV forces predominate
- LVH (tall qR or qRs in 3, cvF and qR in V5-V6)
- RUH (rSr in V1 and V2)

CXR

No specific clues

- Cardiomegaly
- MPA prominent due to dilated pulm trunk

ECHO

High PSAX view—when scan angle is extended superiorly, communication between Ao and PA can be seen

- T artifact at edges of the defect helps to differentiate false dropout and true defect
- Both arterial valve seen arising from 2 diff OT
- Dilated LA and LV
- RVH
- Significantly enlarged PA
- Forward flow coming from rt border of PA differentiate this condition from PDA, where the flow in PA is retrograde along left border
- Significant aortic diastolic retrograde flow is found in both the prox aortic arch and the descending aorta—This is in contrast to PDA where there is no retrograde flow in prox arch
- Can also be detected by fetal ECHO

Cardiac Cath

- Often not indicated
- Certain associated defect such as Anomalies of origin of RPA from Ao may be detected better by Aortography
- Cath should be done in patient with PHTN to determine operability
  Cath findings: lt to rt shunt
  RV and PA pr systemic
  LAP and LVEDP increased
  Widened Ao PP
- PA/PV/LA/LV Ao sats are equal
  Cath cause is typical-when passed from IVC catheter enters RA-RV
  MPA-Asc Ao-diagnostic of AP window

D/D

- Large VSD
- PDA
- *Truncus arteriosus (type 1):* EDM of truncal regurgitation over left 2nd and 3rd ICS and presence of mild central cyanosis arouse suspicion of TA VSD is always associated in truncus and rt Ao arch is very common. In AP window both uncommon.

Compli

- CHF
- PHTN, Eisenmenger
- Infective endocarditis (rare)

Natural History

- Large AP window with CHF—poor survival
- 20-30% does in 1st year
- Minority survives up to childhood
- 50% die during neonatal period due to CHF

MANAGEMENT

- No specific medical management
- CHF and Freq chest inf treated with conventional anti failure treatment (digoxin and diuretics) and suitable antibiotics
- Transcatheter device closure (amplatzer duct occluder)- for small and intermediate type
- *Early surgical closure*—(with Dawon patch or pericardium or PA flap)
  - As soon as diagnosis is made patient referred
  - Anterior sandwich patch technique
  - Elective surgical repair before 3 months of age
  - Surgery on priority bases when coro or PA arising abnormally—from Ao

5.7 CONOTRUNCAL ANOMALIES

INTRODUCTION

Defined as malformations of the outflow tract of the heart, resulting from, abnormal alignment of embryonic structure named conotruncus.

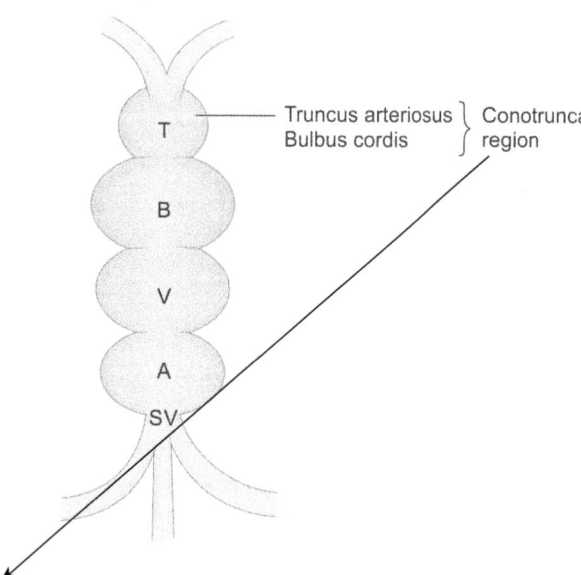

Conus: Segment between primitive vent and semi lunar valves which gives rise to sub arterial coni

Truncus: Segment between semi lunar valve and aortic sac which gives rise to great arteries

EMBRYOLOGY

A. Septation of Conus and Truncus

4 truncal and 2 conal cushion

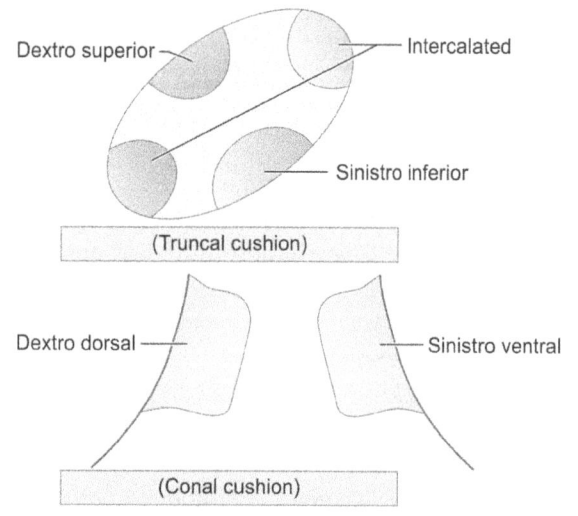

Intercalated cushion forms semilunar valve
Dextro-sinistro cushions of both conus and truncus fuses to form conotruncal septum

B. Septation of Conus and Truncus

In truncus arteriosus; cushions are not in straight line
- Lower part → Rt and lt ridges
- Middle part → Ant and port ridges
- Upper part → Rt and left ridges.

Develop during 5th week

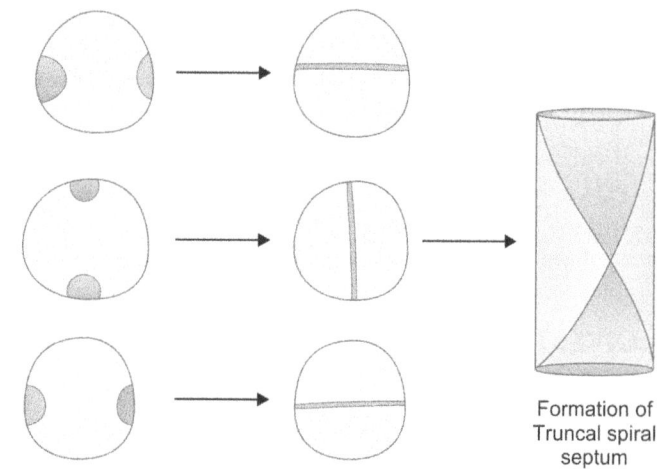

Formation of Truncal spiral septum

C. Rotation

Two rotations occurs:
- 1st at conoventricular junction—brings aorta in continuation with LV and PA with RV
- 2nd at conotruncal junction—brings normal position of aorta in relation to PA (Ao is to the left and post to PA)

D. Absorption

- In normal heart, sub aortic conus is absorbed completely
- Subpulmonic conus persists and grows—pushes pulm art more anterior and superior
  (Detection 22q11 aka CATCH -22)
  C-cardiac defect   C-cleft palate
  A-abnormal facies   H-hypocalcemia
  T-thymus aplasia

E. Formation of SLV

Form:
1. Intercalated cushions at vent level
2. Conotruncal cushions

Note: Conotruncus formed from 2nd heart field cells and neural crest
   Cell play important role in development of conotruncus
- *Genetics association*
  - Recombinant 8-TOF, DORV
  - Partial trisomy 8q-truncus arteriosus
  - Deletion 7q 11.2-TOF

- Trisomy 13-VSD, DORV, TOF
- Trisomy 18-VSD, DORV, TOF
- Trisomy 21-VSD
- Deletion 22q11 spectrum
  - *Digeorge:* Interrupted Ao Arch
  - *Velocardiofacial syndrome:* VSD, TOF, DORV
- *Autosomal dominant syndrome*
  - CHARGE-truncus, interrupted Ao arch
  - Alagille-TOF
  - Adams Oliver-TOF
  - Jones-Waldman-TOF
- Autosomal recessive
  - TAR (thrombocytopenia + absent radius) -TOF

CLINICAL SIGNIFICANCE

Conotruncal anomaly comprise of
1. Truncus arteriosus.
2. TOF.
3. DORV.
4. DOLV.
5. D-TGA

Spectrum
No conus decreased Ao-TOF
No conus decreased PA-TGA
DORV is in between

6. Conoventricular septal defect
7. Interrupted Ao arch (type B)

ASSESSMENT

- History of cyanotic spells
- Maternal history of rubella or on other infections, DM
- Maternal consumption of thalidomide, isotretinoin
- Familial history of conotruncal anomaly
- ECHO (investigation of choice)
- CXR (TOF: core en sabot and D-TGA: egg on string)
  Cardiac MRI
  Cardiac cath

MANAGEMENT

Corrective surgical treatment

5.8 CONGENITAL CORO ART ANOMALIES

EMBRYOLOGY

- Develop from primitive cardiac sinusoids during the process of myocardial compaction

  ↓

  Very small islands present over epicardial surface forms small vascular channels without any connection with vent cavity

  ↓

  Gradually a vascular channel is established between small epicardial capillaries and the outgrowth or buds from aortic sinus

  ↓

  Completed by 7th week of gestation

  ↓

  Blood starts flowing from aorta to epicardial coronary vessels

WHAT IS NORMAL CORONARY

- No of ostia—2 to 4
- Location—rt and lt ant sinuses
- Proximal orientation—40-90 degree off aortic wall
- Proximal common stem or trunk—only left
- Proximal course—direct from ostium to destination
- Mid cause—extramural
- Branches—adequate for dependent myocardium
- Termination—capillary beds

ANOMALIES

(Angelini classification)

A. Anomalies of Origin and Course

- Absent LM trunk
- Anomalous location within aortic root
  - High
  - Low
  - Commissural
- Anomalous location outside aortic sinus
  - Right posterior/non coronary sinus
  - From ascending aorta
  - From LV or RV
  - From pulm artery
    - ALCAPA
    - ARCAPA
    - AC x PA
  - From aortic arch
  - From innominate artery
  - From right carotid artery
  - From internal mammary artery
  - From sub clavian artery
  - From descending aorta
- Anomalous origin from opposite looking sinus
  - RCA arising from left anterior sinus with anomalous course
    - Post atrio ventricular groove or retro cardiac
    - Retro aortic
    - Between aorta and PA
    - Intraseptal
    - Postero-anterior interventricular groove
  - LAD arising from rt ant sinus with anomalous course
    - Between Ao and PA
    - Intraseptal
    - Ant to pulm outflow or pre cardiac
    - Postero-anterior interventricular groove
  - LCX arising from rt ant sinus with anomalous course
    - Retroaortic
    - Post atrioventricular groove
  - LCA arising from rt ant sinus with anomalous course
    - Between Ao and PA
    - Retro aortic
    - Post atrio ventricular groove or retro cardiac
    - Intraseptal
    - Ant to pulm outflow tract or pre cardiac
    - Postero-anterior interventricular groove
- Single coronary artery

B. Anomalies of Intrinsic Coro Art Anatomy

- Congenital ostial stenosis/Artesia
  - Coro ostial dimple
  - Coro ectasia or aneurysm
- Absent coro art
- Coro hypoplasia
- Intramural coro art (myocardial bridge)
- Subendo cardiac course
- Coro crossing
- Anomalies origin of post descending art from Ant descending or septal perforator
- Absent PDA (split RCA)
- Absent LAD variants
  - LAD + first large septal br
  - LAD, double
- Ectopic origin of 1st septal branch

C. Anomalies of Termination

- Inadequate arteriole/capillary ramifications
- Fistulas from RCA, LCA or infundibular art to—RV, LV, RA, LA, CS, SVC, PA, PV multiple

ALCAPA

Definition
Whole of the left main trunk arise anomalously from left posterior facing sinus
- It can also arise from MPA or rarely from RPA

Incidence
Rare
- 1 in 300,000 live births
- 0.5% of CHD
- Generally isolated anomaly
- Can be associated with PDA, VSD, TOF, COA
- M>F 3:1

Embryology
Several theories:
- Abrikossoff → (1) Abnormal septation of conotruncus into Ao and PA
- Hackensellner → (2) Persistence of pulm bud + involution of Aortic bud
- → (3) Persistence of PA–coro art analgen with involution of aortic-coro analgen

Anatomic Abnormality
Coronary

Arise from left:
- Posterior facing cusp/MPA
- Runs a normal course
- *Thinner than normal LCA:* Resembles a vein
- RCA arise normally; but it becomes dilated and gives collaterals to LCA

Ventricle

Blood supply to AL post of LV is diminished
- Vulnerable for ischemia
- Diffuse fibrosis in subendocardial layer
- 2° subendocardial fibroelastosis
- LV dilated/Aneurysmal

MV Incompetence
- Existence fibrosis/calcification in PAP muscle
- Endocardial fibroelastosis in mitral apparatus and LV

Hemodynamics
In Fetal Life

No abnormal HD changes occurs as LV gets adequate supply from PA

In Neonatal Period

Stage 1: LV myocardium gets adequate blood from PA till PVR is high: No ischemia

Stage 2: As neonatal PVR falls, flow through anomalous LCA decreases and infant develop myocardial ischemia/infarction

Stage 3: Later on, adequate collaterals develop

Stage 4: As time passes
- LCA behave as conduit between PCA and PA
- So coronary steal occurs
- Lt to rt shunt is established
- LV is not well perfused—ischemia, Infarction, LV dysfunction, CHF
- Increased volume load due to lt—rt shunt and MR combined with LV dysfunction causes increased LVEDP and increased LVEDV = passive pulm venous Congestion

CLINICAL FEATURE
Three categories

A. Infant
Born healthy:
- Asymptomatic for about 6-8 weeks
- Subsequently becomes critically ill dyspnea, tachypnea, chest pain (restlessness, irritability or Freq. Cry) during feeding
- Develops CHF
- 85% die within 1st year

B. Few Infants (10%)
- Improve dramatically without any efforts
- Leas almost asymptomatic life
- Have restricted physical activity
- Reason: not clear; may be due to adequate collaterals
- May present later on with angina/MR

C. Rarely (5%)
Asymptomatic from beginning:
- Grow Normally
- Possible cause: early dev. Of collaterals

When ALACAPA associated with VSD
- LV gets adequate blood (oxygenated) from RV
- ALCAPA is not manifested by itself
- VSD closure without ALACAPA surgical treatment will be catastrophic

O/E

- Tachycardia
- Increased JVP ⎤
- Cardiomegaly with LV apex ⎬ CHF
- Hepatomegaly ⎦
- S1 normal or decrease
- S2 normal or closely split
- P2 loud due to PHTN
- S3 often present (due to WF/MR)
- Short ESM or PSM (due to MR)

May have cont. Murmur over upper left sternal border due to CAVF (retrograde blood flow through intercoronary communication)

INVESTIGATION

ECG

Very typical

- In a click infant or toddler when ECG shows myocardial ischemia or infarct pattern (pathological Q and ST T changes)—suspect ALACAPA
- Abnormal Q (deep and narrow Q)
  ST deviation ≥2 mm.
  T inversion
  LVH is usual ⎬ Myo infarct

CXR

Cardiomegaly with LA-LV enlargement
- Pulm venous HTN/pulm edema
- Neither sensitive nor specific

ECHO

LV dilatation/hypertrophy
- Global or regional WMF
- Decreased LV function
- MR
- Aneurysm formation
- In some infant, bright endocardial ECHO is observed—Indicates endocardial fibroelastosis

Main diagnostic feature: Delineate origin of coronary arteries and especially show flow pattern (direction of flow) by color Doppler

Nuclear MPI

- Thallium 201-reduce tracer uptake in myocardium
- Sensitive but not specific

CT/MRI

Very accurate for demonstrating coro anatomy

Cardiac Cath

- Gold standard
- Mandatory before surgical treatment
- Clear delineation of coro art origin and its course is necessary

COMPLI

- Myocardial infarction
- MR
- CHF
- LV aneurysm
- LV fibroelastosis
- SCD

NATURAL HISTORY

- Majority (>85%) die during infancy (1st year) due to CHF (if not treated)
- 15% patients present beyond infancy
  - Life expectancy 30-40 years
  - Subsequently die of CHF or SCD

MANAGEMENT

A. Medical Management

Anti-failure treatment

B. Palliative Surgical Treatment

- In very sick infant
- Simple ligation of LCA close to its origin from PA (to prevent steal phenomena)
- To be followed later on by definitive surgical treatment

C. Definitive Surgical Treatment

- Preferred (of not critically ill)
- *Options*
  - Intrapulmonary tunnel surgical treatment (Takeuchi repair)
    - 5-6 mm AP window and orifice of LCA
    - High mortality (0-20%)
    - Late Compli supravalvular PA stenosis by tunnel (75%), baffle leak (52%)
  - LCA reimplantation from PA-AO
  - Tashiro repair: Narrow cuff of MPA, including orifice of LCA is transected—upper and lower edge of cuff are closed to form a new LM CA—Anastomosed to aorta
    Divided MPA is Anastomosed end to end
  - Sub clavian to LCA anastomosed—end to side
  - CABG

CORONARY ANEURYSM

Definition
Coronary dilatation that exceeds the diameter of normal adjacent segments or the diameter of patient's largest coronary vessel by 1.5 times

Etiology
- Congenital
- Atherosclerosis
- Kawasaki disease
- Marfan
- Ehler-Danlos
- Complication of PTCA
- Endarteritis
- Polyarthritis
- Scleroderma

Incidence
0.15-0.49% of patients undergoing CAG

Types
1: Diffuse in 2-3 vessels
2: Diffuse in 1 vessel + localized in other
3: Diffuse in 1 vessel
4: Localized in 1 vessel

Complication
- Thrombosis
- Embolization
- Rupture
- Vasospasm

Surgical Strategies
- Coro astula closure
- Coro art aneurysm resection
- Embolectomy

CONGENITAL CORO AV FISTULA

Definition

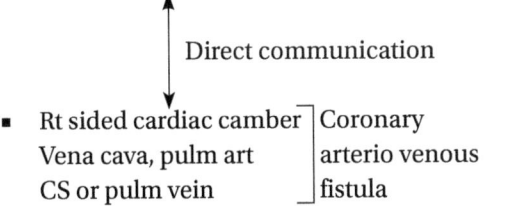

CORONARY AV FISTULA

Incidence
MC coro artery is RCA (50%) >LCA (35%)
MC site of fistula = RV (40%)>RA (25%)>PA>CS>LA>LV>SVC
- 0.2-0.4% of all CHD
- M=F

Embryology
- Persistence of portion of coronary sinusoid that connects primitive coro art-cardiac chambers (those entering RV)
- Coro art to LV fistula results from direct flow through well-developed intramyocardial well developed thebesian venous channels
- Coro art to PA fistula develop from persistent communication between primitive coro arteries and mediastinal plexus of vessels

Anatomical Abnormality
- Proximal part of coro art from which fistula originates becomes dilated and tortuous
- Distal to fistulous branch, the coronary artery remains normal
- Coro fistulas gradually increase in size
  ↓
  Behave like a shunt
  ↓
  Increased hemodynamic burden

Hemodynamics
Depends on three factors
1. Vol of blood that flows through fistula
2. Chamber or vessel that receive fistula
3. Myocardial ischemia that occurs due to steal phenomena

Normally 10% of aortic blood enters coronary
In setting of coro fistulas
↓
Longer vol enters coro bed
↓
Stolen from coronary by fistula if it is connected to low pr chamber
↓
Run off of coro blood into receiving chamber
↓
- Myocardial ischemia
- Left to rt shunt (fistula to RA, RV, PA, CS)
- Volume overload of distal chamber

C/F

- *<20 years:* Asymptomatic
- *>20 years:* Gradually becomes symptomatic
- Many times detected on routine examination as prominent cont murmur

Symptoms

Exertional dyspnea, fatigue, Anginal pain, palpitation

G/E

Physical app is normal
- Growth and dev normal
- Acyanotic
- Arterial pulse normal
- If fistula is large-high vol and collapsing pulse

CVE Examination

Normal precordial examination
- PV impulse may be felt when fistula drains to RA or RV
- S1 normal
- S2 normal split
- Rarely wide split if RV receive large blood
- Cont murmur (louder in diastole) is hallmark
   - *Fistula to RA:* Cont murmur is maximal at either the upper or lower rt sternal border and systolic competent is louder
   - *Fistula to RV:* Max murmur at mid lower left sternal border or subxiphoid. Intensity of murmur varies from cycle to cycle
   - *Fistula to RVOT:* Max murmur along upper to mid left sternal border

Investigation

ECG
- Usually normal
   - May be chamber enlargement
   - With coro steel-changes of ischemia

CXR
Not specific/sensitive
Depending on site, chamber enlargement can be seen

ECHO
- PSAX at base can show dilated proximal coronaries
- Fistula entry into chamber/PA can be ascertained by color flow

Cardiac Cath
- Gold standard
- Step up in O_2 sat may be noted in rt sided chamber in which fistula terminates
- Aortic root angio/selective CAG—can delineate fistulous track and it is opening

Compli
- CHF
- Rupture of fistula
- Arrhythmias
- SCD
- Infective endocarditis
- Embolism
- Myocardial Infarction

Nat History
- Survival into adult life is expected
- Life span is not normal
- Complication present in
  11% of patients <20 years
  31% of patients >20 years

Management
- No specific medical management
   - Anti failure medications
- Asymptomatic
   - Tiny fistula between coronary and pulmonary artery, detected incidentally, should be left alone and monitor for spontaneous closure or increase in size
   - Small fistula in asymptomatic patient may be monitored (Qp/Qs<1.3): give anticoag
- Surgery/Intervention
   - Moderate to large fistulas (even if asymptomatic)
   Possible modalities:
   - Percutaneous closure
      - Coils and vascular plugs
      - Amplatzer duct occluder
      - Fistula closed near entry into cardiac chamber to avoid compression to coro circulation
   - Surgical closure

KUGEL'S ARTERY
- Also known as Artesia anastomotica auricularis magna
- Passes from either the prox RCA or LCA down along the ant margin of atrial septum to anastomose with AV node branch of distal RCA

5.9 CONG. CORRECTED TGA

INTRODUCTION
- Anomaly where there is both atrioventricular and ventriculo arterial discordance (Double discordance)
- Also known as l-TGA

EPIDEMIO
- 1 in 13,000 live births
- 0.5% of all CHD

EMBRYOLOGY
- Exact morphological and biological factors unknown
    1. Embryonic heart tube bends to left known as l-ventricular loop
    ↓
    So morphologic PV comes to lie on left and posterior of morphologic LV
    ↓
    Developing LA communicates with morphologic RV and developing RA communicates with morphologic LV
    ↓
    (+)
    2. Straight course of conotruncal septum puts great vessel paired to each other (developmental defect in both infundibular and arterial segment of primitive heart tube)

PATHOPHYSIO
- Situs solitus in 95%
- Heart position — Levocardia
                  Mesocardia
                  Dextrocardia (20%)
- Aorta arise from RV and course is Any and left to PA
- Pulm trunk arises from LV
    - Mitral and pulm continuity maintained

But: Right AV valve (actual mitral valve now) is separated from aortic by muscular infundibulum of RV

CIRCULATION
- Oxygenated blood from pulm vein comes to LA—enters morphologic RV through left AV valve (anatomic TV)
- Aorta and systemic circulation
    Deoxygenated blood from vena cava enters RA—enters morphologic LV through rt AV valve (anatomic MV)—pulm circulation and lung

CORONARIES
Relatively thick walled morphologic PV
   β Exposed to systemic circulation and
   β Supplied by concordant RCA
   (Concordant supply)
   ↓
Myocardial perfusion abnormally and WMA are common in syst RV with decreased EF
   ↓
RV function deteriorates gradually by end of 2nd or 3rd grade

ASSOCIATED DEFECT
- VSD (60-70%)
- PS (30-40%)
- Dextrocardia
- Abnormality of left AV valve
- Conduction system (AV block)
- Rarely no associated lesion (1%)
- Ebstein anomaly of AV valve
    - Ant leaflet normal in size rather than long and sail like
    - Valve ring is not dilated
    - RV sinus not enlarged

OTHER
- PDA/ASD (20%)
- Supravalvular LA ring
- COA
- Left Juxtaposition of atrial appendages

CONDUCTION SYSTEM
- AV node and HiS bundle abnormally situated
- Normal AV node replaced by anomalous ant AV node
- Bundle of HiS descends on any aspect of IVS
- Fibrosis of bundle of his responsible for various degree of AV block
- CHB approx 2%/year
- WPW associated in some case of cTGA

C/F
- Asymptomatic (uncomplicated TGA)
- Associated lesion predicts C/F
- Signs of CHF ⎤
- Growth failure ⎬ Lt to rt shunt across VSD
- Ex intolerance ⎦
- In contrast to usual VSD, no sign of increased PBF Because of sub pulm LVOTO, which restrict PBF

- Mild to mod cyanosis and effort intolerance ⎤ May occur due to VSD with PS
  ↓
  - 30% cases in infancy
  - With advancing age, cyanosis present in more number of cases as subpulmonic LVOTO increases
  - In some adults cyanosis is due to development of Eisenmenger's reaction

O/E

Bradycardia is common (10–30%)
- JVP shows
  - Prom a wave (if associated with isolated PS)
  - Cannon a wave: CHB
- A2 may be palpable because of anteriorly placed Ao
- S1 variable due to CHB/prolonged PR interval
- Ejection sound present due to dilated ant placed aortic root
- Loud A2
- P2 soft (posteriorly placed PA)
- Holosystolic murmur of VSD
- Mid diastolic flow murmur across (L) AV valve
- Murmur of PS-3rd -4th LICS (due to subpulmonic LVOTO)
- (L) AV valve regurgitation murmur

INVESTIGATION

ECG

Usually NSR
- AV conduction defect
  - 75% = 2:1 block
  - 30%= CHB
  - (Degree of block varies from time to time—sometimes it's progressive)
- p wave
  - Normal in uncompromised c TGA
  - LAE if large VSD or (L) AV regurgitation
  - RAE if PS or PHTN
- q wave: Q in III, avF
  - Small Q in V1-V2 and absence of a in V5-V6 is characteristic of ccTGA

Because of ventricular inversion causes septal activation from rt to lt
- LAD: Cause not clear
  - Not due to LAFB
- Associated anomalies like
- Severe PS with IVS—qR in V1 and rs in V6
- Non-restrictive VSD with large lt to rt
  - Shunt—large biphasic RS complex in mid precordial leads

- *Other:* Preexcitation commonly seen AF due to atrial enlargement
- Chamber enlargement with (L) AV regurgitation
- Dextrocardia
- IDD variant

CXR

Normally, upper part of cardiac border formed by Asc Ao on the rt, Aortic knuckle and PA on left

In CTGA: Absence of normal PA segment and smooth convexity of left supracardiac border produced by displaced asc Ao
↓
- Very characteristic
- But present only in 50%
- MPA trunk is displaced posteriorly and to rt—so it remains behind cardiac silhouette
- RPA often prominent and elevated LPA is displaced downward
- If both branch of PA at same level-produce rt sided waterfall appearance
  Left cardiac border formed by RV-char 'hum-shaped' appearance

ECHO

- RA identified by insertion of IVC
  LA identified by PV insertion
- Vent identified by features given in table on next page
- PSAX—Both arteries appear as double circle—aorta anterior and left to PA
- Ao and PA identified by their branching pattern
- Can also diagnose associated abnormalities

		Morpho LV	*Morpho RV*
1.	AV valve	- More toward base - Bicommissural (MV) With fish mouth Appearance in diastole (PSAX)	- More toward apex - Tricommissural (TV)
2.	PAP muscle and chordae	- Paired pap muscle - Chordae tendinea that inserts only into vent free wall	- Multiple irregular pap muscle

		• Chordal attachment to IVS
3. Shape and trabeculation	Ovoid or ellipsoid with fine apical trabeculation	Crescent shape with coarse apical trabeculation
4. Av valve and great vessel	Fibrous continuity between AV valve and great art	Discontinuity between AV valve and great art

Cardiac Cath

- PA IRs post and to rt—venous catheter follow course close to spine
- With PS—gradient between morphologic LV and PA
- Frontal and lat ventriculogram with 30 degree RAO view profiles vent Septum, LVOT and MV inflow

MRI

One of best modality to syst RV function

NATURAL HISTORY

- Depends on severity of association malformation and function of morphologic RV
- Survival in uncomplicated cTGA is good but not normal
- Morphologic PV ultimately fails
- Mortality is high in infancy (if untreated)
- If infant survives
  ↓

Mortality is 1–2% per year
- With PS: Better prognosis (develop symptoms later)
- Syst AV valve regurgitation is strongly associated with RV dysfunction and CHF
- Present surgical treatment evaluation:
  Survival: 5 yr–92%
  10 yr–91%
  20 yr–75%
- *CHB:* 5–10% at birth
  Increases to 10–15% by adolescence and 30% by adult life

MANAGEMENT

A. Medical Management

- Treatment of CHF
- Treatment of arrhythmias
  • Antiarrhythmic

B. Surgical

- Palliative procedure
  • PA binding for uncontrollable CHF due to large VSD
  • BT shunt for patient with severe PS
- Corrective procedure
  Presence or absence of TR (systemic AV valve regurgitation) determines type of surgical treatment that can be performed
  • No TR—classic repair is done which leaves anatomic RV as systemic vent
  • TR or RV dysfunction—attempts made to make LV the syst vent
  • *Complex anatomy:* Fontan type surgical treatment
- Other surgical treatment
  • Valve replacement for significant TR
  • Pacemaker for CHB

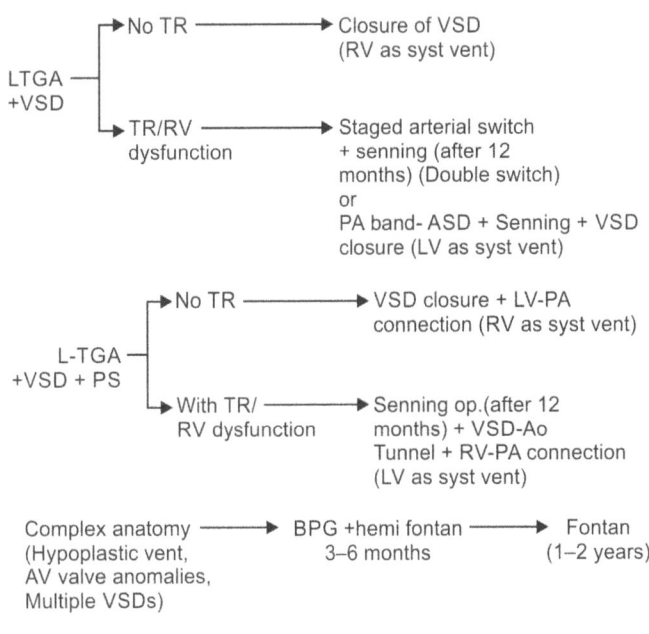

FOLLOW-UP

- Every 6-12 month for possible prog of AV conduction disturbance, arrhythmias, worsening TR
- Routine pacemaker care if pacemaker
- Varying degree of activity restriction based on HD abnormality

5.10 CONGENITAL AS

INTRODUCTION
- Valvular (75%)
- Subvalvular (23%)
- Supravalvular (2%)

VALVULAR AS
- 5% of all cong. Heart disease
- BAV in 1-2% of gen. Population
- MC cause of valvular As in pediatric age gr.
  BAV (75%)
- In pediatric age gr. As is mainly congenital (Because Rheumatic As takes time to develop)
- BAV: Male predominance
  4:1

Embryo
- Aortic valve develops from swelling appearing from (lt) side of conotruncus (Bulbar cushion) Hollows out to form Aortic cusps

Various Theories
1. Due to abnormal development of Bulbar cushion → AoV may be deformed with absent commissures
2. Some postulate that abnormal valve is due to fibroelastosis of Ao valve
3. Myxoid dysplasia of tricuspid or bicuspid AoV

Anatomy
MC tricuspid
2nd bicuspid → All BAV do not develop As (only 20-30%)
Unicuspid → No commissure; Always pathological
→ Severe As from intrauterine life
  (Rare) quadricuspid

BAV
- Unequal 2 leaflets
- False commissure seen in one of leaflet
- With time AoV thickened due to high turbulent flow
- AoV become rigid and fusion of dysplastic cusps with commissure →As
- Slow calcification ⎫
- Fibrotic changes   ⎬ May contribute to
- Myxomatous degen ⎬ Deformity and
- Lipid deposition   ⎬ Dysfunction
- Inflammatory changes ⎭
- All changes occur slowly
- Patient remains asymptomatic till late adulthood

Associated Lesions
- CoA
- VSD
- PDA
- Peripheral PA stenosis (Rubella syndrome)
- Turner syndrome
- Jacobsen syndrome
- Autosomal Dominant transmission of NOTCH-1 gene mutation

HD
- Normal Ao area = 2.6-3.7 cm^2/m^2
- HD significant As occurs when orifice size reduce to < ⅓ rd of its normal size
- When orifice size reduce to 50% → clinically systolic murmur audible

Classification
A. Acc to valve area (cm^2/m^2 of BSA)
   - Normal = >2.6 (2.6-3.7)
   - Mild As = 0.7-1.2
   - Mal As = 0.5-0.7
   - Severe As <0.5
B. Hemodynamic classification
   Acc to peak transvalvular gradient
   - Trivial As < 25 mm Hg
   - Mild As 25-50
   - Mod As 50-75
   - Severe As > 75

Forgotten HD Criteria
Severe As
1. LV ejection time index > 0.42 sec
2. Rate of rise of Max syst carotid arterial pulse <500 mm Hg/sec
3. Time from q wave on ECG to peak R > 0.19 sec

Pathophysiology
- As → increased work load to LV → LVH
- LV remodeling (myofibrillar hypertrophy) → Eccentric LVH
- LA has to contract forcefully → increased LA a wave
- LV systole and ejection phase are prolonged
  - AV closure is delayed
  - Paradoxical split in severe As

- Demand-supply mismatch
  ↓
  As reduce blood flow → Subendocardial ischemia /Infarction
  ↓
  LVH increases myo O₂ demand
- Tachycardia due to any cause decrease diastolic filling time and worsen ischemia

C/F

- Infantile type critical As (discussed separately)
- Mild mod As
  - Born with normal BCD
  - Milestones normal
  - Asymptomatic till adulthood
  - Fatigability and DOE
  - Systolic murmur (many times ignored as function murmur)
  - PULSE, BP, PP within normal limit
  - S1 normal, S2 normal split
  - Ejection click (also heard over apex)
    - Due to 1. Opening of thickened AoV
    - 2. Sudden distention of dilated Ao wall
    - No change with respiration
  - Low pitch ESM over So area-may transmit to carotids
3. Severe As
  - Usually symptomatic
  - Some patient-SCD
  - Symptoms become apparent in adulthood
    - Anginal pain
    - dyspnea.   On mild → rod execution
    - syncope
  - Dyspnea and fatigability → LV dysfunction
  - Low volume pulse
  - Low PP
  - Anacrotic pulse (slow rise)
  - *Coanda effect:* Pulse in rt arm and rt carotid is better felt compared to lt due to powerful jet that is directed straight into rt innominate artery
  - JVP prom a wave (d/t decreased compliance of PV because of gross WH)
  - Heaving apex
  - S2 normally split/single (F2 absent/Paradoxical split)
  - Severe As → Ao closure occur later than palm closure so during expiration splitting become apparent (not inspire) (Paradoxical split)
  - [Splitting heard in expiration on case of PS and ASD → falsely interpreted as Paradoxical split (Pseudo paradoxical split)]
  - EC may be absent (decreased S1–EC gap)
  - S4 (d/to distensibility of LV)
- ESM (3-4/6) conducted to carotid surgical treatment with EC and end before f2)
- Severe symptoms—larger and louder murmur
- Syst murmur faintly audible when decreased CO or CHF

Symptom/sign	Transvalv gradient
Easy fatigability	>25
Anginal pain	>50
Syncopal attack	>80
Syst thrill over Ao area	>50
Paradoxical split (child)	>00
(Adult)	> 75
S4	>50
Gr 2 murmur	<50 (mild)
Gr 5 murmur	>50

Investigation

ECG

Normal in mild case
- Normal in 50% mod As
- LVH main feature
- LAE
- LVH with strain (Gr>50)
- Upright T in lat leads → mild mod As
- LBBB pattern
- Prog changes in ECG current further study and indicate increasing severity of lesion

CXR

Not changed even in severe cases
- Cardiomegaly → CHF/AR
- Asc Ao prominent (post stenotic dilatation)

ECHO

Eccentric closure line ⎫
Cuspal separation   ⎬ M-node
Valve thickening and calcification ⎭

PLAX

Thickening of valve
Doming b.f leaflet
Assess Ao annulus
Supravalvular pulm
Sub Ao area

PSAX

No of leaflets
Valve area

- TEE more accurate
- Continuity equation
- Other way of measuring severity of stenosis
- Peak velocity (mild <3, mod 3-4.5, severe >4.5)
- Ao valve area <0-15 → severe As

Cardiac Cath

- In complicated cases when other cong anomalies are associated and in certain specific condition
- With presence of AR if Gr > 70 ⎤ -severe
- With CHF of AR if Gr > 30 ⎦ As

In infant balloon valvuloplasty is indicated when peak to peak syst gradient exceeds 69 mm Hg, valve area <0.5 cm²/m², ECG shows LVH with strain and mean systolic gr by echo >50 mm Hg

Compli
- CHF
- IE
- SCD

Progno
- Mild—normal life
- *Campbell:* Overall life expectancy decreases, they reach 40 years age (60% die)
  Avg longeving:
  - Angin—5 yr
  - Syncope—3 yr
  - CHF/dyspnea—1.5-2 yr

CRITICAL AS

In infant with peak systolic gr > 80 mm Hg ⎤
  Mean syst ge > 60 mm Hg. ⎬ Nadas Criteria
  Valve area < 0.5 cm²/m². ⎦

- Real emergency. ⎤
- May not have significant murmur ⎦ CF severe As
- Common case of intractable CHF in neonate and infant
- Can be diagnosed on iv echo
- During fetal life HD changes as aortic flow is maintained by ductus

Patho

Usually tricuspid valve
- Small LV cavity and associated with endocardial fibroelastosis
- May be associated with HLHS
- Persistence of ductus is essential to maintain life

C/F

- Florid CHF after some days to weeks of birth (depends on duct closure)
- Even on 1st day of life neonate may be very symptomatic
- ESM may not be audible

Investigation
- (ECG) RAD with RVH
- (CXR) cardiomegaly
- (2DECHO) very specific

D/D
- HLHS
- 1 degree fibroelastosis
- Large VSD /PDA
- CoA

Management

Asymptomatic mild-mod As → observe
                         IE prophylaxis
                         2 yearly ECG

ACC/AHA: peak gr → 70 (even if asymptomatic patient) → balloon valvuloplasty

- Severe/critical as with symptoms → BAV (neonate/infant with LVEDP >17 and AI annular dia 6-8 mm are suitable for BAV)

Surgical Treatment

If BAV fail   AR

SUPRAVALVULAR AORTIC STENOSIS
- Localized or diffuse narrowing of Asc Ao over sinus of valsalva, just above level of coro arteries
- Least common (2-4%) of all As
- Associated with abnormal calcium metabolism
        Infantile hypercalcemia (William-Beuren synd)
        Abnormal development of in folding of Ao wall

Types
- Hour glass type (MC)-localized narrowing
- Diffuse narrowing
- Diaphragmatic/membranous type

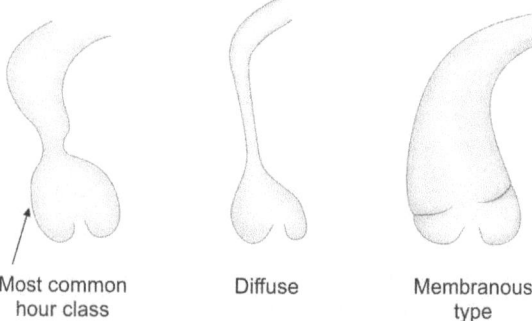

Most common hour class | Diffuse | Membranous type

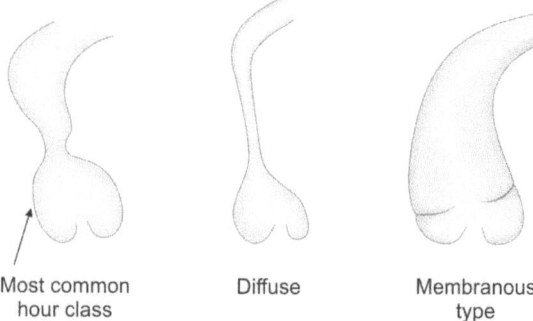

Pathology

- In diffuse type, diffuse narrowing involving entire length and circumference of Asc Ao
  - May be aortic valve thickening
  - Associated with cerebral art stenosis

  Coro art stenosis. ⎤
  Renal art stenosis   ⎬ Thickening
  Iliac and innominate stenosis ⎦

  Infancy: Williams/Rubella syndrome associated

  ↓

  Diffuse involvement of Aorta /PA

- Wall thickening ⎤
  SMC hypertrophy. ⎬ Diffuse
  Disorganization   ⎬ + arterial
  Increases collagen and ⎬ changes
  Luminal narrowing ⎦

  Histopathology findings of aorta are described as mosaic pattern by Edward

C/F

William syndrome

- Mental retardation, elfin facies
- Symptomatic due to absolute constipation or repeated vomiting (probably due to abnormal Ca^{++} metabolism)
- Adult patient often express ex. dyspnea and Anginal pain
- Coandă effect
- Systolic thrill over suprasternal notch and over carotids
- LV apex
- S1 normal; S2 normal by split with loud A2
- No EC
- ESM (2-3/6) over rt upper sternal border
- When ESM heard on both side of sternal border → consider branch PA stenosis

Investigation

ECG
WNL in majority
  Some cases LVH

CXR
Absence of post stenotic dilatation

ECHO
Diagnostic (PLAX and suprasternal)
  Pwd localize site of obstruction
- Peak instantaneous gradient >60 mm Hg
  Across obstruction → surgical treatment is advised

MRI/CT
Helpful in diagnosis

Cardiac Cath
- No pr gradient between LV and Asc Ao proximal to obstruction
- With further withdrawal of catheter, pr drop is noted

Natural Course

- Symptomatic for long period
- Gradual regression of this lesion occurs in due course of time
- When CHF/Angina appear → poor prognosis

Management

No specific medical management
- Dyspnea/angina/syncope, mean Gr >50 or peak gr >70 → surgical treatment
- Balloon dilatation and stenting is under trial

SUPRAVALVULAR AS

- Obstruction immediately within few millimeters below aortic valve
- Etiology not clear-contributed by both congenital and acquired factors
  - Obstruction by fibrous ring below the Ao valve is attributed congenital persistence of a part of bulbus cordis
  - Progressive nature of this lesion is attributable to acquired cause
- 20-25% of all As
- Male dominance (2:1)
- 5-10% among all CHD
- Forms a part of shone complex

Types

- Fixed type
  - Discrete fibrous membrane (most common) 80-85%
  - Fibromuscular ridge type obst
  - Fibromuscular tunnel type obst
- *Dynamic type:* HOCM/IHSS

Embryo

- Discrete subvalvular As due to incomplete evolution of bulbus cordis

  ↓

  Persistence of bulbus cordis

  ↓

  Sub aortic ridge

Muscular hypertrophy subvalvular As is due to localized hypertrophy of septal portion of LVOT (rarely seen in infant even if its congenital origin)

Patho

- Progressive lesion
- Observed from early childhood
- Membranous diaphragm mainly encircle LVOT
- Sometimes tissue derived from membranous septa, TV or MV causes subaortic stenosis
- Fibromuscular tunnel type causes diffuse obstruction below ao. Valve

↓

Result in high velocity jet producing constant trauma to valve

↓

Prog AR in 30-40%

C/F

- Usually asymptomatic
- Pulse and BP WNL
- Apical impulse normal
- Heart sounds normal
- No EC
- ESM over Erb's area/rt 2nd/3rd IC space
- Murmur not conducted to neck vessels

Investigation

- ECHO is method of choice
- TEE clearly delineates discrete ridge or membrane
- Peak syst gradient >40-50 → surgical treatment
  Cardiac cath—can be done

MANAGEMENT

- No specific medical management
- PG > 50 is indication for surgical treatment
- If associated with AR/VSD → surgical treatment
- Progression of gradient is more rapid than valvular As after surgical treatment
  - Valvular As- slowly progressive
    - Subvalvular As-progressive/very progressive
    - Supravalvular As-regressive/slowly progressive

CONGENITAL AR

Cause of Congenital AR

- Bicuspid aortic valve (most common)
- Cong aneurysm of sinus of valsalva
- Aortic root dilatation
- VSD causing AR (AV prolapse)
- Rarely quadricuspid AoV
- Sub aortic obst due to subvalvular discrete memb producing deformity of AoV → AR
- Supravalvular As may cause AR
- Coronary art to LV fistula
- Aorta—atrial tunnel

Main Causes of Severe AR

- Large LCA- LV fistula
- Aortico -LV tunnel
- Absente Al valve (non immune hydrops)
- Quadricuspid Ao valve

AORTIC-LV TUNNEL

(Aka Aortico-cameral tunnel)

- Abnormal tunnel communicating between aorta and LV cavity
- Endothelial small communication
- Begins above rt coronary sinus, course along post aspect of RV infundibulum to connect with LV

Types

- Aortic sinus of valsalva ⎤
- Coronary arteries   ⎥ Not involved
- Aortic valves   ⎦

Main diff between Aortico-cameral and coronary-cameral fistula → coronary fistula pusses through myocardium and drains into cardiac chamber

C/F

- Depends on size of the tunnel and degree of AR (not valvular AR)
- One of the causes of severe AR in infants
- AR → CHF, hyperdynamic precordium, LV impulse, loud A2; to and fro murmur over both sides of upper precordium
- ESM—due to large volume ejected through AV
- DM—due to flow through tunnel (loud and harsh)

Investigation

ECHO

Retrograde flow through tunnel in diastolic CT and MRI may help

Treatment

Treat CHF
   Surgical treatment for tunnel

5.11 DORV

DEFINITION
(By Kirklin and Barret-Bayes)
- Congenital cardiac anomaly in which both great arteries (AO and PA) arise wholly or in large part from RV.

HISTORY
- 1st described by John Abernathy (1793)
- Witham termed it to be DORV
- 1st repair Kirklin (1957)

CLASSIFICATIONS
- *Neufeld's:* Postulated that both are great arteries and arterial
  Trunks arise from RV
  - Absence of fibrous continuity between SLV and AV valves
  - VSD is only outlet from LV
  - Classify DORV based on (1) presence of PS
    And (2) position of VSD
- Lev and Anderson's conotruncal mal position:
  Postulated: One complete and at least half of the other
  Arterial trunk arise from RV ±mitral-AO continuity
  - Widely accepted
    a. DORV with sub aorta USD (commonest)
       (15%) 1. Without PS | Low PVR
       (40%) 2. With PS | High PVR
    b. DORV with sub pulmonic USD
       (20%) 1. Without PS (Taussig Bing) | Low PVR
             2. With Arch anomalies | High PVR
                and sub aortic stenosis
    c. (<10%) DORV with doubly committed VSD
    d. (10%) DORV with noncommitted VSD
    e. (rare) DORV with intact septum
- Van praagh's conal under development
  - *Type I:* Isolated conotruncal anomaly
  - *Type II:* Conotruncal anomaly with associated malformation of AV valves and ventricle
  - *Type III:* Heterotaxy/polysplenia, Asplenia, Atrial Isomerism

EPIDEMIO
- 0.03–0.2/1000 live births
- <10% of all cardiac defects
- No racial/sexual prediction

Embryo
Development of conal septum determine position of SLV to Ventricle
↓
More coral muscle beneath SLV → more it is pushed ant and Superior and it gets aligned with RVOT
↓
If sub aortic conus gets hypertrophied or fails to get absorbed
↓
Ao gets aligned to RV
↓
Gives rise to DORV

ANATOMY
- Almost always associated with visceral situs solitus
- Both great arteries arises predominantly from RV
- Well developed LV
- Four types of association of great arteries
  1. Aorta to right and posterior of PA (Normal arrangement)
  2. Side-by-side: Aorta to right of PA (Commonest)
  3. Aorta to right and anterior to PA (d- malposition)
  4. Aorta to left and anterior to PA (l- malposition)

Type of VSD
1. Sub aortic (50%)
2. Sub pulmonic (35%)
3. Doubly committed (10%)
4. Noncommitted (5%)

VSD to Arterial Relationship
Total 16 possible combinations
  Most common—sub aortic VSD with side by side great Arteries with Ao directly to the right of PA
- Sub aortic obstruction in 1/3rd
- Pulmonic stenosis: ½–2/3rd
  - Valvular/subvalvular
  - PV can be bicuspid
  - Rarely pulm atresia
- B/L infundibulum (double conus) ⎤
  >50% aortic override   ⎬ Clues to diagnose DORV
  Aortic mitral discontinuity   ⎦
- ASD in 25% (secundum type)

- MV abnormalities
  - Mitral atresia
  - Parachute MV
  - Supravalvular mitral ring
  - Straddling mitral valve

PHYSIOLOGY

Depends mainly on
- Position of VSD
- Great art relationship

Also depends on
- IPS
- Presence of pulm vasc. Obst. Disease
- Sub aortic stenosis
- Size of VSD

A. Sub Aortic VSD

- Most common type
- Aorta to rt and anterior of PA
- Ao conus, pulm conus and conus septum present
- VSD is posterior inf and closely related to Ao
  - A1. *Sub aortic VSD without PS*
    - With low PVR
      - Resembles non-restrictive perimerb VSD
      - LV blood preferentially enter Ao
      - RV blood exclusively enter PA
      - Aortic SPO_2 is virtually normal
    - With PVR
      - Resembles Eisenmerger synd
      - LV blood enters Ao
      - RV blood diverted into Ao
      - PBF decline and Aortic SPO_2 declines
  - A2. *Sub aortic VSD with PS*
    - Resemble TOF
    - RV and LV both empties to Ao due to PS
    - Ao SPO_2 falls

B. Subpulmonic VSD (Taussig–Bing)

- Pulm trunk markedly dilated
- VSD antero superior and adjacent to PA
  - LV blood enters PA
  - RV blood enters Ao
  - PA SPO_2 > Ao SPO_2

C. Doubly Committed VSD

- VSD closely related to both SLV
- VSD in superior position
- Aortic and pulm conus present

D. Non-committed VSD

- Significant amt of conus beneath each great vessels
- VSD opens primarily into body of RV

E. Unusual Form

E1. *Intact vent septum*
  - Varying degree of hypoplasia of LV
  - Anomalies of MV
  - LV → MV → ASD → great arteries

E2. *DORV + DRCV*

E3. *DORV + dextrocardia + atrio ventricular discordance*

DORV with sub aortic VSD (no PS)	DORV with sub aortic with PS	DORV with sub pulmonic VSD
Transient neonatal cyanosis mild/absent cyanosis in infant	Cyanosis can be present since birth	Cyanosis from birth (due to RV → Ao flow)
Rise in PVR → cyanosis reappear	Squatting episode	SPO_2 high (at cost of high PBF)
CHF (due to LVVO) → catabolic state	No CHF (PBF effectively regulated)	• VHF due to LVVO • Rise in PVR → CHF reduce but cyanosis worsen can show features of CoA
Art pulse – Brisk	Normal	
• JVP: Prom A and V wave 2° to CHF – High PVR → JVP normal	Normal	• Prom A and V wave 2° to CHF • High PVR → JVP normal
• RV and LV impulse + – Impulse of dilated PA + Palpable P2	RV impulse in 4th–5th LICS and subxiphoid	• RV and LV impulse + • Impulse of dilated PA+ Palpable P2
Thrill generated by VSD	Systolic thrill of VSD	Thrill due to VSD
PVR rise → LV impulse absent	LV impulse not palpable	PVR rise ≥ LV impulse absent
• Auscultation – Loud P2 (hypertensive and dilated pulm trunk)	P2 delayed	Loud P2 (hypertensive and dilated pulm trunk)
– Loud A2 (Anterior aorta) Inspiratory split +		– Inspiratory splitting preserved

Apical MDM (Rise in PVR)		Apical MDM
– Loud S2, pulm ejection sound, Graham steel murmur		
• Murmur of VSD since birth: (flow from LV->RV is obligatory	Murmur of VSD -at lower left sternal border	• Murmur of VSD – PSM of VSD as high as 2nd
And does not await neonatal (fall in PVR)	Duration varies inversely with severity of PS	LI cs (PVR rises):
• Intensity increases as PVR falls (Rise in PVR) • Murmur become soft • Never disappear		• S2 loud and single • VSD murmur decreases • MDM disappear • Pulm ejection sound • Graham–steel murmur

ECG

- PR interval prolonged (long course of common AV bundle)
- RAE and LAE
- RAD/LAD
  - LAD with counterclockwise loop in DORV + sub aortic VSD (no PS) + increasing PBF
  - When PVR rises → RAD
  - If PS present → RAD
- QRS duration normal (RV conduction defect can occur –RBBB)
- RVH (obligatory) Tall R in V1-V2 and deep S in V5-V6
- LVVO-large RS complex in midprecordial lead and tall R in left
  Precordial lead
  Taussig-Bing
  - Clockwise loop
  - RAD (not LAD)
  - RAE, RVH

CXR

- DORV with sub aortic VSD without PS
  - Resembles nonrestrictive perimemb VSD
  - Increased PBF (now PVR)
    ◆ Cardiomegaly (LA and LV enlargement)
    ◆ Palm trunk prominent
  - High PVR (Resembles Eisenmenger)
    ◆ Lung fields dynamic
    ◆ RV copes with systemic resistance without enlarging significantly
- DORV with sub aortic VSD with PS (TOF like)
  - Mild PS → pulm vascularity increased and LV dilated
  - PS severe → Pulm vasculartiy decreased, heart size normal
  - Pulm atresia → Asc. Ao is enlarged, MPA segment is Concave, apex is boot shaped
- Taussig – Bing (DORV with subpulmonic VSD)
  - Cardiomegaly (all 4 chamber enlarged)
  - Increased pulm vascularity
  - Egg-lying on side appearance (like TGA)
  - When PA and Ao side by side
    ◆ Dilated pulm trunk project to lt
  - When dilated PA is posterior
    ◆ PA is not border forming
    ◆ Resembles TGA (except presence of thymus)

ECHO

To define
1. Great artery relationship
2. Position of VSD
3. Outflow obstruction
4. AV valve abnormalities
5. Associated lesion
6. Coronary artery anatomy and abnormalities
   - PLAR and PSAR → degree of commitment to RV
   - Subcostal and APLC → separation between semilunar and AV Valve (ventricular infundibular fola)
A. DORV with sub aortic VSD
   - Ao entirely from RV
   - Pulm Trunk predominantly from RV
   - *PSAR:* Double circle (Ao to rt of PA)
   - B/L sub arterial conus
   - *Outlet septum:* Curves leftward towards ventricular Infundibular fold (sub aortic VSD)
   - Aorta mitral discontinuity
B. DORV with sub pulmonic VSD
   - Pulm trunk overrides sub pulmonic VSD
   - *PSAX:* Side by side (Ao on rt)
   - B/L sub arterial coni
   - Outlet septum: straight and parallel to trabecular Septum → sub pulm

Cardiac Cath

- When catheter easily enters to PA and Ao from LV
  - Subpulmonic VSD is strong possibility
- PA sats are > Ao sats (subpulmonic VSD)
- Char findings of DORV
  - Opacification of both Great Art from RV
  - Both SLV at same level
  - Malposed Ao in Lat view
  - Tounge like filling defect in frontal view
  - Aortic mitral discontinuity

NATURAL HISTORY

- Infant without PS
  - May develop severe CHF
  - Pulm vasc obstructive disease (if untreated)
  - Spont closure of VSD (rare) → fatal
- Infant with PS
  - Develop complication similar to cyanotic cong. Heart Disease (polycythemia, CVA)
- Taussig–Bing:
  - Severe pulm vasc obstructive disease develops early

MANAGEMENT

A. *Medical:* Treatment of CHF with diuretic
   ACE inhibitor
   Digoxin

B. Surgery
  - Palliative surgical treatment
    - PA binding – for increases PBF and CHF
      (Not recommended for sub aortic VSD or doubly Committed VSD)
    - *For Taussig-Bing:* Balloon atrial septostomy to receive LA
      Pressure → relieves pulm venous congestion and allow
      Better mixing of blood
    - *Syst to PA shunt:* For patient with PS and reduced PBF
  - Definitive surgical treatment
    (Timing)
    - *VSD type:* One stage complete repair as neonate or young
      Infant because of palm over circulation
    - *TOF type:* One stage within few months or 2 stages with
      Initial palliative shunt followed by complete repair >6 months of age
    - *Taussig Bing:* One stage complete repair as neonate before LV becomes unprepared
    - Noncommitted: Complete BiV repair deferred up to 6 months because of complexity

A. Sub aortic VSD (<5% mortality With treatment) → Interventricular tunnel between VSD and sub aortic outflow by Dacron patch ± RVOT reconstruction (req. if tunnel Obstructs RVOT)

B. Sub aortic VSD +PS(TOF type)
  - BT shunt
  - Tunnel VSD closure + Rastelli operation (to receive PS)
  - RVE procedure
  - Nikaidoh procedure

C. Taussig-Bing → ASD Enlargement
  - VSD-PA tunnel + Atrial switch op less desirable (high mortality)
  1. VSD-PA tunnel + senning
  2. VSD-AO tunnel ±RVOT Augmentation
  3. VSD-PA tunnel + Damus-Kaye-Stansel +RV-PA conduit

D. Multiple VSD or Remote VSD → PA banding ± → VSD-Ao tunnel (2-3 yr)

E. Hypoplastic LV or RV → BT shunt → BDG or hemifontan → Fontan

5.12 DUCT DEPENDENT CIRCULATION

- Duct dependent pulm circulation
  - Pulm Atresia—intact septum or VSD
  - Severe TOF
  - Neonatal Ebstein
  - Critical PS-Isolated or with complex CHD
  - Severe TR
- Duct dependent syst circulation
  - Hypoplastic left heart
  - Critical As
  - CoA
  - Interrupted Arch
  - Mitral atresia
- *Mixing:* TGA with IAS with IVS

PULM VS SYSTEMIC
C/F

- *Pulm*
  - Cyanosis predominant
  - Hypoxia dominating C/F
  - Relatively well (at least initially)
  - Present within 24–48 hrs of life
- *Systemic*
  - Poor perfusion
  - Decreased CO
  - Sick infants from birth
  - Present in first 24 hours of life

Suspect duct dependent syst circulation
- Anybody with shock or collapse after 24 hrs "duct dependent syst circulation"
- Poor perfusion, absent pulse, pallor, shock

Suspect duct dependent pulm circulation
- Cyanosis
- Differential cyanosis
- Respi symptoms but lungs clear
- No response to O_2 or worsening with O_2

HYPEROXIA TEST

100% O_2 for 10 mins (by blow mask or intubation)
↓
Measure rt arm PO_2 (not pulse ox)
  PO_2 >250 - unlikely to be cyanotic CHD
  PO_2 100–250 - possibly cyanotic CHD
  PO_2 <100 = cyanotic CHD

DIAGNOSIS OF DUCT DEPENDENT CIRCULATION

ECHO is gold standard
- Delineate the anatomy
- Assess the size of PDA, degree of constriction/restriction
- Assess PVR/SVR ratio on the flow pattern across the duct

MANAGEMENT
(A-B-C and drugs)
- Ensure airway
  - Optimize oxygen
  - *Ventilate:*
    - Off load work of breathing
    - Ensure good oxygenation
2. Maintain circulation
3. When doubt?
   - Blue Baby
   - Baby in shock
        ↓
   Start prostaglandin

PGE1
(1 mL ampoule = 500 µg/mL)
  Dilute 0.1 mL (50 µg) in 50 mL 5% D
  Remaining PGE1 stored in fridge 2–8 degree Celsius
  Each ml contain 1 µg of PGE1

  Start infusion of 0.1 µg/kg/min
  Infusion rate can be increased up to 0.4 µg/kg/min
  (Depending on clinical response—saturation, femoral pulse, VO)

  Once desired response obtained, maintain patency by cont infusion at 0.01–0.05 µg/kg/min

Monitoring PGE1

- Hypotension—cold extremities, delayed capillary refill >3 min, tachycardia low U.O
  Treatment IV fluid bolus 5–10 mL/kg NS
- *Apnea:* Often noted in initial hours
  Common in preterm
    <2 kg weight
  Treatment stimulation, hand banging
    Intubate and ventilate

- *Fever:* Often in first 24 hrs
  treatment
  - Tepid sponging
  - Make sure that insensible losses met adequately
- Fluid retention
- *Seizure:* Rare
  May need cessation of PGE1
- *Bradycardia:* Stop infusion of severe
- *Other:* Flushing, diarrhea, hypokalemia, sepsis, DIC
- *> 7 d use:* Long bone hyperostosis
  Gastric outlet obstruction

- Other option to maintain PDA patency
  - PDA balloon/stent
- Surgical treatment
  BT shunt
  Problems
  1. *Shunt blockage:* Acute thrombosis
  2. *Shunt overflow:* CHF, pleural eff
  3. Chylothorax
  4. Late-PA distortion or stenosis
  Surgical treatment for underlying heart disease

5.13 EBSTEIN'S ANOMALY

Q.1 Discuss in detail, the pathophysiology of Ebstein's anomaly of TV; it is diagnosis and management (June 2000).

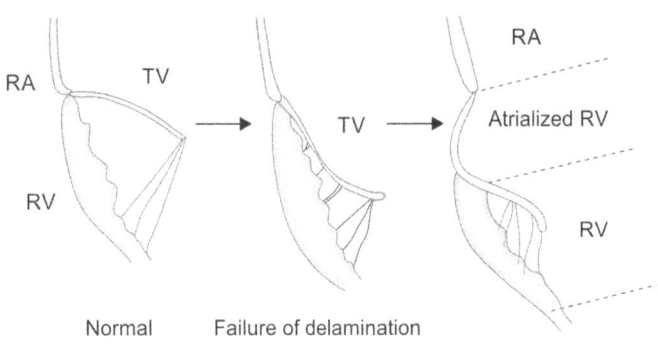

Normal   Failure of delamination

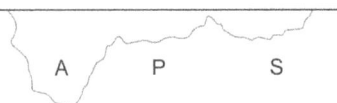

Septal leaflet—always affected
Posterior leaflet—nearly always
Anterior leaflet—seldom affected

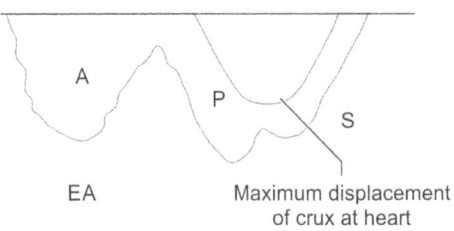

DEFINITION

Downward displacement of tricuspid valve into right ventricle due to abnormal attachment of posterior leaflet and septal leaflet to the ventricular wall
↓
Thereby creating 2 chambers inside the RV; the proximal atrialized RV and distal real functional ventricular chamber

HISTORY

- First described in 1886 (Wilhelm Ebstein)
- Term (EA) was coined by Alfred Arnstein
- 1st case clinically diagnosed (1949) Tournair

INCIDENCE

- 0.3–0.8% of all Congenital heart disease
- 1 in 20,000–50,000 live births
  Male=female

ETIOLOGY

Congenital disease of uncertain origin

ENVIRONMENTAL FACTORS

- Maternal ingestion of lithium in 1st trimester
- Maternal use of benzodiazepine, varnishing substance

EMBRYOLOGY

Main feature (failure of determination)

Normally: TV leaflet and tensile apparatus of AV valve formed by undermining of inlet portion of RV (delamination)
↓
Ebstein's anomaly: This process of delamination is impaired (esp. post and septal leaflet)
↓
Delamination fall short of reaching the level of AV junction
↓
Downward displacement of TV into RV
↓
Forms and character inside RA
↓
RA proper and atrialized RV

Anatomical Abnormality

TV

- Origin of TV from AV ring and its chordal attachments are malpositioned
- Leaflets are malformed, dysplastic, thickened
- Anterior leaflet is enlarged-Sail like
- Posterior and septal leaflets reduced in size

RA

- Dilated
- Circumference of true AV junction is enlarged

RV

- Smaller than normal
- Thinner wall with fewer muscles
- Infundibulum/RVOT is well developed
  Sometimes obstructed by Sail like anterior leaflet

ARV
- Thin walled
- Moves paradoxically during systole and atria
- Electrical potentials are ventricular, but pressure pulse is atrial

Associated Anomalies
- ASD or PFO (90%)
- VSD, AV canal defect
- Pulmonary stenosis/atresia (20-25%)
- WPW syndrome (esp. Type B)
- Down, Marfan, Noonan

Genetics
- NKx2.5 mutations
- MYHZ gene mutation

Classification

Carpenter Classification

Based on degree of atrialized RV and mobility of anterior leaflet

Type A = RV volume adequate
     B = large ARV; mobile ant leaflet
     C = Restricted movement of ant; leaflet; may cause infundibular obstruction
     D = near complete atrialization of RV

Pathophysiology
- Failure to delaminate
↓
Abnormal attachment of tricuspid valve as well as abnormal structure
↓
Incomplete closure of tricuspid valve
↓
 Severe TR -TR begets more TR
↓
Enlargement of RA
↓
Right to left shunt (via OS ASD /PFO)
↓
 Cyanosis -Mixing of blood in LA
↓
Increased LVVO and LVEDP + unoxygenated blood in LV
↓
Fibrosis; hypertrophy; dysplasia
↓
 LV dysfunction → Congestive heart failure

- Sail like anterior leaflet
↓
Can obstruct RVOT/infundibulum
↓
Decreased PBF
↓
Increased TR
- Atrialized RV
↓
Behave as a part of RV
↓
Behaves paradoxically during contraction of RA
↓
May bulge or form aneurysm
↓
Reduce RV filling
↓
- RV dysfunction
↓
Inadequate pumping portion (trabecular portion) of RV
↓
Thinning and loss of myocardial fibers
↓
RV systolic dysfunction
↓
Further hamper PBF
- Role of Arrhythmias
Right sided accessory pathways
↓
Tachyarrhythmias
↓
Shorten diastolic period and loss of atrial kick
↓
Contribute to right heart failure
- Neonates (at birth)
↓
High PVR
↓
RV is unable to propel blood   Functional
Into Pulmonary circuit   Pulm atresia
↓
Decreased PBF
↓
Increased rt to left shunt and cyanosis

Clinical feature
- Fetal life

Diagnosed incidentally by ECHO

- Neonatal life
  Mild case—asymptomatic
  Severe case—cyanosis/CHF/respi distress
  Tachycardia/tachypnea/feeding difficulty
  ↓
  Improves as PVR falls
  (Duct depend circulation may worsen when PDA closes)
- Children/adolescent
  Fatigue, exercise intolerance, exertional dyspnea, cyanosis, tricuspid regurgitation and/or right heart failure

Clinical Examination

- *Cyanosis:* Commonly present
  Plays hide and seek game
  Disappear when PVR falls
  Reappear in children/adolescent
  Mild cases may develop cyanosis in adult life
  Once infant develop deep cyanosis—worse prognosis
- Clubbing
- Precordium—usually silent
  "Although there is huge cardiomegaly, cardiac apex and its activity are weakly palpable
  - Absence of RV (left parasternal) activity
- JVP usually normal
  (No prominent V wave of TR because it is absorbed by compliant enlarged RA)
- Heart sounds
  Split S1 (wide) with loud T1
  Split S2 (wide)
  S3   triple/quadruple   } Plethora of sounds
  S4   Rhythm
  Sail like sound of ant tricuspid leaflet
- Murmurs
  - Systolic murmur of TR
  - Diastolic (flow) murmur across tricuspid valve
  - Opening snap of TV may be used

Complications

- CHF
- SCD
- Bact endocarditis
- Brain abscess
- Paradoxical emboli
- TIA
- Stroke

Twelve Lead ECG

- Himalayan P wave (enlarged RA)
- Atrial arrhythmias
- WPW Type B preexcitation.
- Splintered QRS
- Prolonged PR (d/t intra RA conduction time)
- RAD
- RBBB

CXR

- Cardiomegaly (round or box like contour)
- Small aortic root and MPA
- Decreased pulmonary vasculature
- Enlarged RA (fill retrosternal space, may overlap spine posteriorly)

ECHO

2D imaging and M-mode
- Enlarged PA
- Increased amplitude and velocity of ant tricuspid leaflet
- Paradoxical septal motion
- Delayed source of ATL (>50 ms)
  (Normally TV closes within 30–50 ms after MV)
  Downward displacement of septal leaflet

>8 mm/m²	-EA
>15 mm (below 14 years)	- EA
>20 mm (adults)	- EA

  Excessive elongation of ATL
  Leaflet tethering to underlying myocardium
  Enlarged TV annulus

Color and Doppler Imaging

- TR
- ASD/PFO
- Any associated shunts

High Risk Features

- Functional RV area <35%
  Calamager Index/Gose score
  (RA + aRV area/RV +LV+LA area)

Grade	Ratio	Mortality
1	<0.5	8%
2	0.5–1	9%
3-(acyanotic)	1–1.5	10% (neonate) and 45% later
3-(cyanotic)	1–1.5	100%
4	>1.5	100%

- Aneurysmal dilatation of RVOT (RVOT: Ao root>2:1) severe TR

Treatment

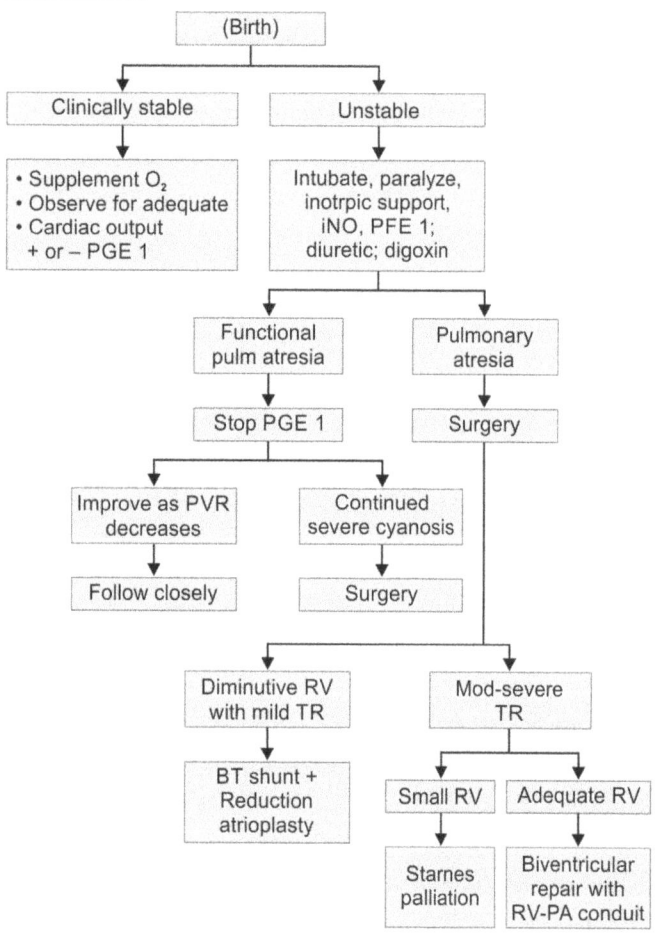

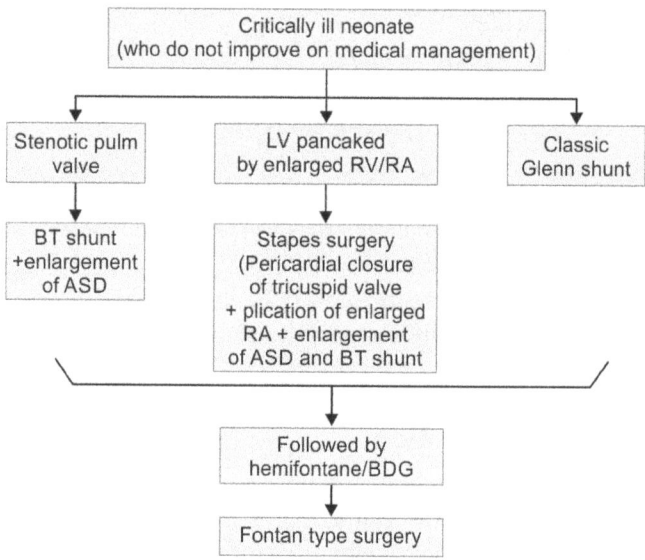

2. Definitive surgical treatment

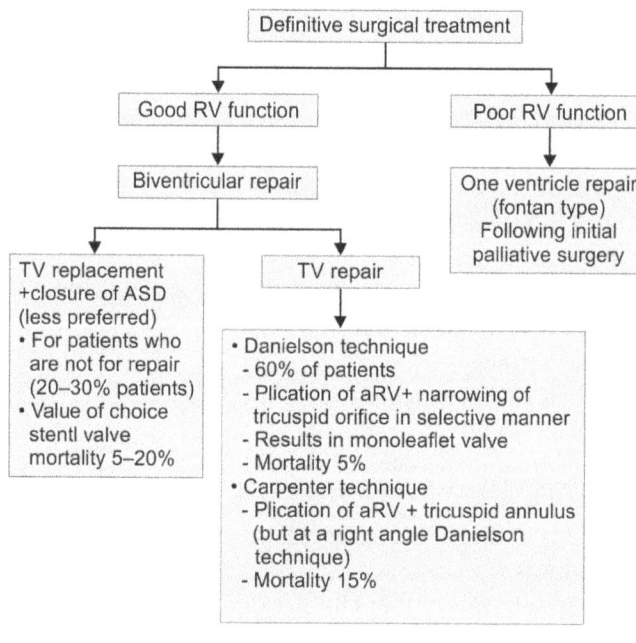

Indication for Surgery

- Critically ill neonate who show symptoms within first week of life
- Moderately severe or progressive cyanosis (<80%)
- Polycythemia (>16 g/dl)
- CHF
- RVOT obstruction by redundant TV
- Severe activity limitation (NYHA 3 or 4)
- History of paradoxical embolus
- Life threatening arrhythmias
  - Palliative surgery for

POST OP CASE

- Frequent follow-up: ECG for arrhythmias
- Freq 2D—ECHO to look for complications associated tricuspid valve interventions
- No participation in competitive sports

LEFT SIDED EBSTEIN'S

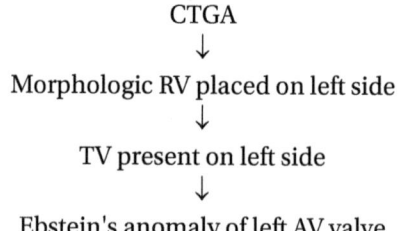

5.14 EISENMENGER SYNDROME

DEFINITION

- *Eisenmenger complex:* Clinical conditions having large VSD+ reversal of shunt known as Eisenmenger complex
- *Eisenmenger syndrome:* (Paul wood coined the term)
All cardiac defects, initially having large lt->rt shunt (irrespective of its sites) who subsequently develop PH and reversal of shunt
- *Eisenmenger reaction:* "Gradual process of development of pulm HTN and pulm vasc disease"

CAUSES

A. *Pretricuspid shunts:* ASD; PAPVC; TAPVC
   - Normal resolution of neonatal PAH occurs and then shunt is established—high compliant pulm are handles large left to right shunt for a long duration until PVD sets in
B. *Posttricuspid shunt:* (VSD; PDA; AP window)
   - Transmission of LB syst pr to pulm vasc prevents normal process of lowering of PVR after birth—Early PVD
C. OS 1° ASD associated with AVCD or Down
   - PVR develops very early in postnatal life
D. Surgically created shunts
   - BT shunt, Waterson's shunt
E. *Other cases:* TGA with VSD no RS; persistent truncus arteriosus, cc TGA with VSD and no PS; single vent without PS; DORV with large VSD without PS; common atrium; TA with nonrestrictive bVSD and No RS and Interrupted Ao Arch with PDA

INCIDENCE

Unoperated patient—AP window and truncus → 100% patients develop ES
- VSD and PDA → 50% patient develops ES
- Large ASD → only 10% patients develop ES
  Mean age:
  - PDA—19 years
  - VSD—22 years
  - ASD—35 years

CHANGES AFTER BIRTH

In fetus: Pulm circulation is hardly 5-10% of CO
   Systemic and pulm pr are same
   PVR is high (8-10 wu)
   ↓
After birth: PVR fails rapidly to 1-3 wu
   (by about 6-8 weeks of age)

- Rapid progression of medial muscle layer of large po Ulm arteries and arterioles
- Reasons for sudden decrease in PVC are
  - *Onset of breathing:* Expand lungs and pulm vessels
    - Distal vessel becomes straight (coiled in fetus) and expand
  - Blood flow through these arteries—they no more remains function less tubes—thick muscular arteries becomes thin and dilate
  - Increased O_2 content—vasodilatation—decreased PVR
  - Elasticity of pulm art—helps for more distensibility—reduces PVR
  - Many new small intra acinar art develops and participate in pulm circ
- Factors not allowing normal physiologic decrease in PVR
  - Failure of regression of thickened muscular arteries (present in fetus)
  - Decreased arterial O_2 content (shunt lesions)
  - Inappropriate vasoconstriction (abnormal contractile response of pulm vasculature to increased flow)

PATHOLOGY

- Constant high flow—shear stress—gradually progressive structural abnormality
  ↓
  - Damage to endothelial cells of initial layer
  - Rapid development of SMC in peripheral arteries leads to muscular hypertrophy of media
  ↓
Narrowing of lumen
(Esp. pulm arterioles with 30-100 um diameter and having single elastic lumina and endothelial lining)
  ↓
At some place, thrombosis and complete occlusion develops
  ↓
  PVOD

As shunt persists
Pathological changes progress from Gr1-Gr3
Heath Edwards classification and ultimately becomes irreversible
Health Edwards classification

Reversible
- Gr1—medical hypertrophy in small PA
- Gr2—cellular initial proliferation and hyperplasia
- Gr3—prog intimal fibrosis with lumen occlusion

Irr.
- Gr4—From early generalized dilatation of arterial lesions (muscular arteria) to advanced stage (Appearance of plexiform lesions)
- Gr5—Thinning and fibrosis of media (widespread) without angiomatoid formation
- Gr6—Necrotizing arteritis and fibrinoid necrosis

- Increasing PAP leads to bidirectional shunt and ultimately rt to lt shunt (PVR > 12 wu and PVR:SVR 1:1)
- Genetics also play role
  In some Eisenmenger reaction is rapid (hyper reactor)
  In some Eisenmenger reaction is slow (hypo reactor)
- *Role of matrix glycoprotein:* Tenascin, fibronectin, TGF-B, pro collagen, Ca^{++} binding prot, serotonin, transporter, SMC migration, angiogenesis, imbalance between thromboxane - endothelin-1 and no prostacyclin

HEMODYNAMICS

- PA pr = RV output (pulm flow)
- So PAP increases due to (1) increased RV flow (hyperkinetic) and (2) Increased PVR
  ↓
  Initially all PHTN are due to hyperkinetic type
  PHTN = when PA P > 30/18 (mean 22) at rest
  MPAP has to be > 25 for development of ES
  ↓
  Initially RV hypertrophies
  ↓
  So RA contracts more forcefully to fill RV
  ↓
  "a" wave of RA increases
  ↓
  As PAP rises progressively
  ↓
  RV dilates and subsequently fails
  ↓
  TR develops PS
  ↓
  Raised "V" above
  ↓
  Ultimately CO falls
  ↓
  Systemic hypotension
  (PH begets PM)

C/F

- Timing of development of symptoms depends on type of lesion
- Central cyanosis → indicated (1) reversal of shunt
- Dyspnea
  Fatigue; syncope   (2) due to decreased CO
  Decreased ex tolerance
  Symptoms of (3) hyper viscosity: myalgia, lassitude, headache, light headedness, visual disturbance, H/O bleeding tendency, Brain abscess
- Anginal pain: (4) (RV hypoxia)
- Repeated hemoptysis (due to (5) pulm infection 2 degree to thrombosis)
  (6) CHF
  (7) Paradoxical emboli /TIA
  (8) Prone to IE

PDA is well tolerated because head-neck and upper extremity gets saturated blood

Signs: Central cyanosis
- Differential cyanosis (PDA)
- Clubbing
- Low volume pulse (decreased CO) in late stage

Left parasternal heave, diffuse apical impulse (RV type impulse), palpable P2, Prominent "a" and "v" wave in JVP
- S1 normal
- S2 single (VSD + ES)
- Closely split (PDA+ES)
- Wide and fix split (ASD + ES)
- Loud pulm ejection click
- RVS4 in ASD + ES

In PDA diastolic component of murmur disappear early as PA rises—with suprasystemic PAP, systolic part of murmur also disappears

INVESTIGATION

Blood Tests

CBC (give info about hyperviscosity)

ECG

RAE, RVH, RAD
- qR and T inversion in V1 and no Q in V5-V6 → ASD
- Good LV force and q in V5-V6 - PDA/single vent/AVCD

CXR

Cardiac size normal or slightly increased (VSD/PDA)
- Huge cardiomegaly in (ASD)
- ES—centralization of pulm vasc
    Dilated MPA-RPA-LPA
    Peripheral pruning
- RT sided arch indicates VSD (never ASD/PDA)

CT/MRI

6 minutes walk test

ECHO

M-mode of pulm valve
- Characteristic absent "a" wave
  Reduced EF slope
  Mild systolic closure
  Other:
  • RVH, RAE, dilated PA
  • Calculate PAP

Cardiac Cath

- To study any possibility + closure
- To exclude intracardiac and extracardiac shunts
- Accurate measure of RV, RA, PA pr and LV filling pr
- To determine reversibility

Pulm vasc resistance index (PVRI) >= 8 => CI to repair ((in post-tricuspid shunts)

Fall of PVRI <10% or <8 U/m² = suitable for surgical treatment

COMPLI

Brain abscess
- IE
- Repeated hemoptysis
- Pulm infarct
- CVA
- Arrhythmia
- SCD
- CHF

PROGNO

Mean age of death = 33 year (VSD/PDA)
                    46 year (ASD)
Poor survival predicted by
- Repeated hemoptysis
- Arrhythmias
- CHF

Maternal mortality 27%

MANAGEMENT

No specific drugs available
A. *Prevention:* Early closure of lt-rt shunt
B. Gen advice
   1. Avoid strenuous physical exertion—to avoid chest pain/syncope
   2. Adequate fluid intake to avoid hyperviscosity
   3. Not to stay at higher altitude
   4. Avoid preg. (Surgical stabilization) (CC pills carry high risk of thrombosis)
   5. Avoid NSAIDS (because of bleeding atresis)
   6. *Phlebotomy:*
      • Advised in polycythemia and hyperviscosity
      • Can lead to anemia-CHF
      So give adequate iron supplementation
   7. Low dose O_2 to prevent polycythemia cont/nocturnal O_2 in all advanced cases
   8. *RV failure:*
      • Low salt diet, digoxin, diuretics (caution)
      • Adequate preload maintenance
   9. Chronic anticoag advised in some cases
   10. BB, Amiodarone, sotalol for arrhythmias
C. Drugs for ES
   1. *CCB:* Long acting -Nifedipine, Amlodipine
      Goal: To prevent increased rt - lt shunt by decreased PAP and PVR
      High dose: Nifedipine 180-240 mg/d
                   Amlodipine 20-30 mg/d
   2. Targeted therapy
      • Selective pulm vasodilators are ideal
   All drugs have both pulm and syst effect
   1. Prostanoids (prostacyclin Analogues)
      • *Epoprostenol:* IV only
                        2 mg/kg/min-up to 25–40 mg/kg/min
                        S/E - jaw pain, nausea, rash, flushing, diarrhea
      • *Treprostinil:* IV/SIC/oral/inhal
                        50–80 mg/kg/min
                        S/E-same
      • *Beraprost:* Oral
      • *I/o prost:* Inhalation only
      • *Selexipag:* Oral
   2. PDE-5 inhibitor:
      • *Sildenafil:* 200 mg TDS (up to 80)
                      Child 1–5 mg/kg/d in 4 divided dose
      • *Tadalafil:* 40 mg daily
   3. Endothelin receptor antagonist
      • *Bosentan:* 125 mg BD
                    Child 1–2 mg/kg/BD ⎤ Anti-inflammatory
      • Macitentan   ⎬ prevent fibrosis
      • Sitaxsentan   ⎦ reduces PVR
   4. Soluble guanylate cyclase stimulator
      • Riociguat
      • No inhalation
   5. Gene therapy
      Under trial
D. Role of surgical treatment
   • If PVR can be reduced by medical management to < gr 3 health Edwards class
                    ↓
           Surgical closure consideration
   • Balloon atrial septostomy in some patients
E. Heart lung transplant

5.15 FONTAN SURGERY

TYPES OF FONTAN

- RA to PA anastomosis
- RA to RV connection
- Intra atrial lateral tunnel
- Extracardiac conduit

Q.1 Current status of Fontan (Aug 94)
Q.2 Fontan Indication and follow-up (June 02)
Q.3 Failing Fontan: Mech and management (Dec 08)
Q.4 Fontan pre req Indi and complication (Dec 10)
Q.5 Criteria for selection for Fontan post op Compli (June 13)

- First performed in 1968

CONCEPT

Normal CV System Consists of 2 Circuits

- *Pulm and systemic:* Connected in series
- Driven by 2 synchronized pumps (vent)

Fontan Circulation

- No pump to propel blood into pulm arteries (syst veins are directly connected to PA)
- Postcapillary energy is harnessed to drive blood through the lungs

↓

Pulmonary impedance hampers venous return
↓
Creates a bottle neck

- Congestion upstream
- Restricted flow downstream

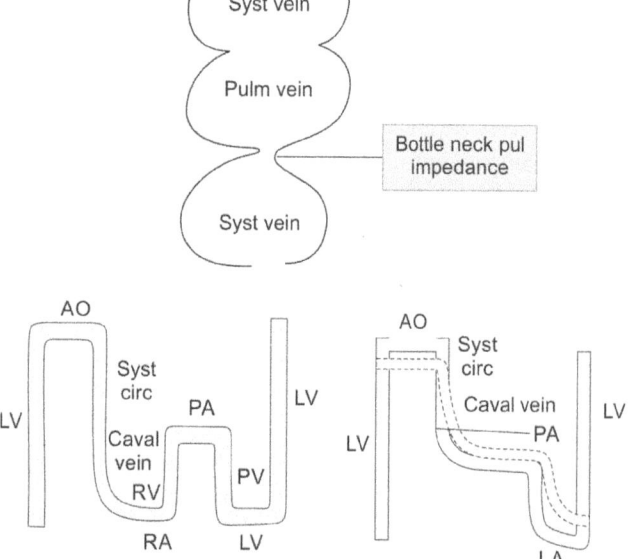

CARDIAC OUTPUT IN FONTAN

Determined by
- Presume just above and below bottle neck
- Resistance within bottle neck (Neoportal system)

↓

Body can tolerate only narrow window of increased pressure in syst veins (up to 20 mm Hg) and a small range of ventricular filling pressure

↓

Impedance in neoportal system remains critical determinant for CO

↓

LV although provide driving force to the circulation but it is not enough

↓

Additional suction force is also required (Which is not physiological)

↓

Ventricle no longer control CO

↓

Its role is restricted to pump the output allowed by fontan

↓

With time ventricle will detonate as a result of limited flow through bottle neck

↓

LVEDP increases

↓

Worsens systemic venous congestion

↓

Further reduce cardiac output

Factors determining impedance in Fontan bottle neck
- Syst vein-PA connection
- Pulm arteries
- Pulm capillaries
- Postcapillary venules
- PV to LA connections

Affected by
- Pulmonary hypoplasia
- Pulm art stenosis
- Pulm art distortion
- Loss or exclusion of large vessel or micro vessels
- Vasoconstriction
- Pulm vascular disease
- Collateral flow
- Turbulence and flow collision
- External compression

Bypassing Bottle Neck

Fontan fenestration
↓
- Improve cardiac output
- Reduce systemic congestion but
- Detriment in arterial saturation

Successful Fontan
- Only mid decrease in CO
- Only mid increase in systemic venous pressure
↓
No need for fenestration

Failing Fontan
- High resistance of neoportal system
↓
- Reduction in CO
- Raised venous pressure to intolerable level
↓
Fenestration needed
↓
Systemic desaturation

FONTAN AND EXERCISE

Normally during exercise, PVR falls due to vasodilatation and recruitment of segment.
RV output as well as systemic pressure also increased in Fontan, there is restricted ability to increase cardiac output
However,
- Most of Fontan patients enjoy near normal life
- 90% remains in NYHA 1-2 for decades

VENTRICLES IN FONTAN

- During fetal life and during palliation
↓
Single functioning ventricle is overloaded
(250-350% of normal for BSA)
Ventricular overgrowth
↓
Excessive hypertrophy (eccentric)
↓ Long-term
Spherical, dilated ventricle
Ventricular dysfunction
- Glenn procedure
↓
Volume load on ventricle decreases to 90% for BSA
↓
- Completion of Fontan
↓
Load further reduce to 50-80% for BSA
↓
Ventricle is overgrown and severely deprived
↓
This reduction in preload lead to increased arterial vasoconstriction-increases after load
↓
Systolic as well as diastolic dysfunction
↓
*Low preload also leads to vent remodeling

Decreased ventricular compliance and ⎤ (Disuse
Increased filling pressure   ⎦ Hypofunction)
↓
Increased pulm venous atrial pressure
↓
Further worsen CO
↓
*Diastolic dysfunction
↓
Further hamper the suction effect on bottle neck
↓
Adds to failing Fontan

Pulm Vasculature in Fontan

- *Fetal life:* Reduced pulm flow
- Initial palliation
- *Glenn shunt/BDCPA:* Reduced pulm flow
- Definitive Fontan

Only period where catch up pulmonary growth can occur
↓
However, syst to pulm shunt leads to mal disturbed underflow and overflow in pulmonary circuit
↓
Patchy pulm hypoplasia and varying degree of vascular disease
↓
Fontan operation
↓
Generate abnormal environment
- Long standing diminished flow
- Desaturation
- Increased collateral flow
- Substandard SVC and IVC mixing
- Lack of pulsatile flow
- Endothelial dysfunction
- Absence of period of high flow and high pressure with vessel recruitment as occur normally during exercise

↓
Further hamper growth
↓
Increased PVR

Failing Fontan circuit is characterized by
- Large spherical ventricle
- Hypertrophied wall
- Systolic and diastolic dysfunction
- Raised filling pressure
- Unresponsive to traditional treatment
- High and increasing PVR

    PLLE = protein losing enteropathy

- Treatment of failing Fontan
    Critical bottle neck = neoportal system

- Systems develop at advanced stage of failure
- Identification of failing Fontan before development of Ascites and PLE is essential to improve outcome
- Monitoring of function status, rhythm, biomarker, liver changes are essential to detect it early
- Aggressive therapy for rhythm and hemodynamic abnormality improve long term status

TARGET FOR TREATMENT
- Open up bottle neck (reducing impedance)
- Bypassing bottle neck (fenestration)
- Increasing pressure before bottle neck (Systemic venous pressure)
- Enhance run off after bottle neck (Ventricular suction)

- Increasing pressure before bottle neck:
Exercise:
    Increasing systemic venous pressure by 30 mm Hg
  - However chronically elevated pressure are poorly tolerated
    ↓
    Congestion, edema, ascites, lymphatic failure, progressive veno-venous collaterals with cyanosis

- Opening up bottle neck
  Reduction of impedance in neoportal system
  - *Modified Fontan:* Cavo-pulmonary connection
    ↓
    Improved surgical technique to keep impedance low in neoportal circuit
    (Older Fontan should be considered to conversion to modified Fontan when it fails)

- Regular exercise and adopted breathing
    ↓
    Lower pulm impedance by repeated vessel recruitment and vasodilatation
- *Other agents:* O_2 at altitude, sildenafil, bosentan, inhaled iloprost
- Pulling through bottle neck
  Ventricular suction
  Non lusitropic agent available that can lower ventricular filling pressure and increases suction effect
- Fenestration (bypassing bottle neck)
    ↓
  - In failing but "pink" Fontan result in degree of cyanosis that may not be tolerated
    ↓
    Difficult to achieve balance between (cyanosis and increasing CO + decreasing congestion) by fenestration
  - In others, fenestration increases CO and decreases venous congestion at cost of balanced cyanosis impossible to cause Fontan at birth as PVR is revised for several weeks

INDICATION

- Cardiac malformation and a single chamber
  - Dysfunctional heart valve
  - Absent or inadequate pumping chamber
- Tricuspid Atresia
- Pulm Atresia with IVS
- Hypoplastic left heart syndrome
- Double inlet ventricle

CRITERIA FOR SELECTION (10 COMMANDMENTS)

1. Age at operation 4–15 years
2. Pressure of normal sinus rhythm
3. Normal systemic venous connection
4. Normal RA size
5. Normal PA pressure (mPAP ≤15 mm Hg)
6. Low pulm vascular resistance (4 woods unit)
7. Adequate sized PA (PA dia ≥75% of aorta)
8. Absence of mitral valve insufficiency
9. Normal LVEF (≥60%)
10. Absence of complicating features from previous surgical treatment

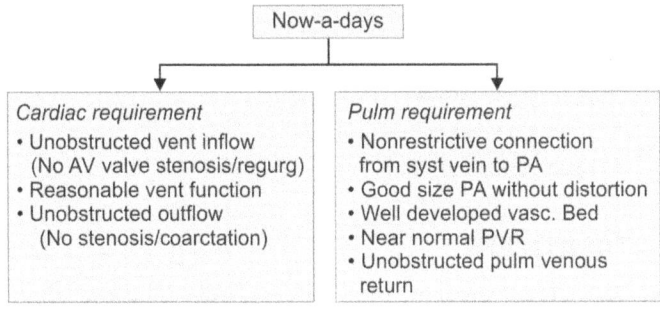

- Dilated RA can compress connection to pulm artery, compress pulm venous return from rt lung
- *Modified Fontan:* Patients with tunneled cavopulm anastomosis usually do not develop marked RAE
- Any abnormality (> mild stenosis or > mild regurgitation) of AV valve
  ↓
  Hamper pulmonary venous rupture
  ↓
- Chronic venous Congestion of liver and spleen
  - Sequestration of platelet—Thrombocytopenia
  - Increased bilirubin and liver enzymes
  - Liver cirrhosis
- Arrhythmias
  - SA node dysfunction
  - Junction rhythm
  - AV nodal block
  - SVT/VT
  - SCD
    ↓
  - Modified Fontan: Reduced SND from 40–25%
  - AF is more common in old classical Fontan
    1. Rapid tachycardia
       ↓
       Hemodynamic compromise
       ↓
  Need urgent conversion catheter ablation if required
- Ascites
  Due to
  - Increased RA pressure
  - Protein losing enteropathy
  - Hepatic dysfunction

FAILING FONTAN

Clues to failing Fontan
- Growth
  In general fontan: Shorter than normal population
  Failure to gain weight appropriately
  - Due to failing Fontan
  - Due to decreased CO
- Decreased exercise capacity
  - Due to abnormal pulm compliance or chronotropic incompetence
  - Common in single vent physiology/lateral tunnel repair
- Cyanosis
  - Mid cyanosis is always present in Fontan
    Due to
    - Pulm shunting
    - CS draining into LA
  - Resting SPO_2 <90% suggests
    - Intracardiac rt to lt shunt (residual)
    - Pulm veno-venous collaterals
    - Pulm AV malformations
      ↓
    Coil embolization of collaterals or catheter based occlusion of shunt improves condition
    4. Classic Glen to RPA-incomplete hepatic blood flow to the lung
       ↓
    Benefit from surgical treatment intervention to provide confluent PA and increased Hepatic flow to right lung
- Pathway obstruction and valve dysfunction
  Clues: Declining exercise tolerance
  Declining resting/exercise SPO_2
  Hepatomegaly
  Cardiomegaly
  Murmur
  - Old Fontan – atrio pulm connections
    ↓
    Develop marked RAE (2 degree to anatomic obstruction at the anastomosis)
    ↓

COMPLICATION OF FONTAN

Due to increased venous pressure and decreased cardiac output
- Worsening functional status and exercise tolerance
  - 90% of post Fontan remains in NYHA I-II
  - Have educational qualification equivalent to normal population
  - Participate in low-medium grade sports
    ↓
  - But if patient selection is not proper
    ↓
  - Progressive weight loss/inadequate gain
  - Progressive worsening exercise capacity
- Impaired systolic and diastolic function-heart failure
  Described earlier
- Impaired pulm circulation
  Described earlier

- Arrhythmias: Atrial dysrhythmias - MC
  Due to
  - Atrial dilatation (old circuits)
  - Atriotomy
  - Injury to sinus node or its supplying vessel
- Hypoxemia due to residual intracardiac shunts
  Normally Fontan are mildly desaturated
  <90% SPO_2 -search for shunts
- Protein losing Enteropathy

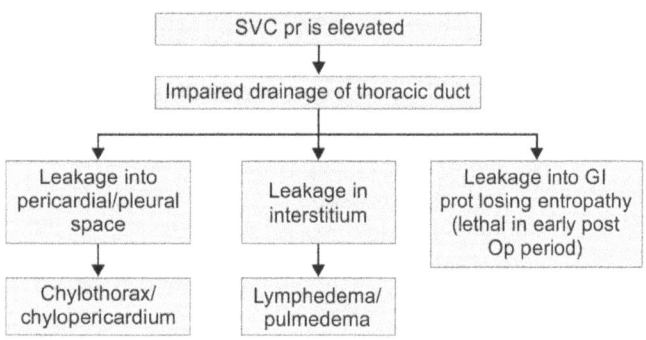

Impaired drainage of thoracic duct
↓
Interstitial lymphangiectasia
↓
Leakage of lymphocyte, chylomicron, serum protein (albumin and immunoglobulin)
↓
PLE
↓
Ascites, immunodeficiency, hypocalcemia

- PLE is long-term complication
- Incidence 0–5% (avg 3.5%)
- Very poor prognosis
  - 5 yr survival = 60%
  - 10 yr survival <20%

TREATMENT

- *Diet:* High protein, high calorie, high medium chain triglyceride fat low salt
- Cautious use of diuretic
- Albumin infusion on weekly/monthly basis
- Avoid stay at high altitude or long flight (hypoxemia induced pulm vasoconstriction can lead to PLE)
- Aggressive treatment of arrhythmia and valvular dysfunction
- Plastic bronchitis (rare 1–2%)

  Leakage of lymph into bronchus
  ↓
  Plastic bronchitis

- Late mortality
- Coagulopathies
  - Protein C, protein S, and antithrombin III defining
  - MC cause of sudden out of hospital death
  - Chronic multiple pulm microemboli lead to pulm vasc obstructive disease
- Sepsis

5.16 HYPOPLASTIC LEFT HEART SYNDROME

DEFINITION
It includes a group of cardiac malformations in which these occurs hypoplasia, stenosis or atresia of aortic valve with hypoplasia of LV and of ascending aorta
- Lack of normal development of whole lt side
  Right side is well developed
- Most malignant disease
  Easily identifiable by fetal ECHO
  Amenable for fetal cardiac intervention

HISTORY
- 1952—Lev introduced hypoplasia of aortic tract
- 1958—Nooran and Nadas used the term HLHS

INCIDENCE
- 0.016–0.036% of live births
- MC cause of death in 1st week
- 23% of deaths due to CHD in newborn are due to HLHS
- *Genetic syndrome:* Turner, Noonan, Holt Oram, smith-lemli-opitz syndrome; CATCH-22 syndrome
- Male predominance M:F = 2:1

EMBRYOLOGY
Basic Defect
- Reduction of either the inflow or outflow LV
- Developmental arrest occur soon after Septation of heart is complete

Probable Cause
1. Congenitally small, absent, or premature closure of foramen ovale
2. Displaced septum primum may obstruct normal shunting of IVC blood through Foramen ovale to LV limiting LV inflow
3. Malalignment of common AV valve (failure of dev of AV endocardial cushion)—limits ventricular inflow
   - Cong AS—Enlargement of LA
   - HLHS—hypoplastic LA
4. Failure of LV differentiation out its inflow and/or outflow tract portion

ANATOMY
- 85% of patients with HLHS - combination of atresia or stenosis of aortic and mitral valve
- 15%-common AV septal defect with common AV valve malaligned to rt resulting in LV hypoplasia
- Situs solitus
- Levocardy
- AV ventriculo art concordance
- RA dilated
- LA small with endocardial thickening
- IAS small in diameter, thickened and fibrous
- Variable size of opening in IAS
- TV is usually normal
- Pulm vein connects normally to LA
- RV dilated, hypertrophied and PA dilated
- Hypertrophied RV infundibulum and IVS
- PV morphologically normal
- MV is atretic or imperforated
- Hypoplastic annulus
- Hypoplasia of LV inflow and outflow tract
- LV myocardium is grossly hypertrophied with small LV cavity
- Infarction or ischemia of LV endocardium with endocardial fibroelastosis
- AV atretic or stenotic
- Variable degree of hypoplasia of Asc Ao
- Ao arch usually left sided
- Persistence of sporsy myocardium (embryonic pattern) and myocardial fiber disarray (like HCM) are present
- Anomalies of IAS: ASD secundum, ASD primum, aneurysm of septum primum

IAS intact in 10%
- When IAS intact with mitral atresia
  - PV drainage occurs via
    - Anomalous PV connection to syst vein
    - Persistent LSVC opening to LA
    - Unroofed coronary sinus, where LA communicates with CS directly

Underdeveloped LV and Ao (LV hypoplasia with atresia or severe AV stenosis) with intact IVS is (MC) form of HLHS

Coronaries
1. Hypoplastic Ascending So acts as common coronary artery receiving retrograde flow from ductus both coronary arteries
2. Ventriculo coronary circulation through myocardial sinusoids (persistence of embryonic channel connecting LV to coronaries)
3. Abnormal origin of coronaries from PR

HEMODYNAMICS

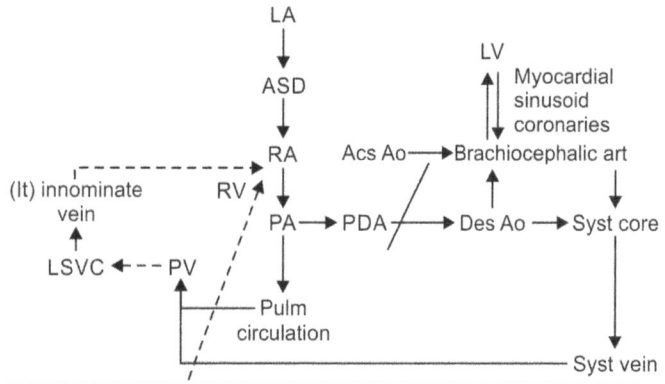

- Fetus tolerates anomaly well in utero
  After birth, as SVR increases and Ductus closes—marked reduction in systemic blood flow-circulatory shock–met acidosis
  Syst blood flow depends on
  - Interatrial communication (ASD present in 90%)
  - Adequate size and persistence of PDA
- LV is non-functional
- RV maintains both pulm and systemic circ
- Cerebral and coronary supplied through retrograde flow from PDA

C/F

- Newborn appears normal at birth
- Critically ill after 24 hrs of birth when ductus starts closing- mild cyanosis with respi distress due to pulm venous congestion
- Deep cyanosis when CO significantly reduces after ductal closure
- Weak peripheral pulses and cold extremity (vasoconstriction due to syst hypoperfusion)
- Dominant RV impulse (No impulse)
- S1 normal
- S2 loud and single (P2)
- Pulm ejection click
- 50%—no murmur; 50%—ESM at ULS border due to dilated pulm trunk
  - Some cases TR murmur +
  - Enlarged liver and basal rates - CHF
  - Some infant shows intermittent recovery due to variation in degree of ductal closure—finally they deteriorate and die

ECG

- NSK, RAD, PVH—always present; RAE—peaked P
- Mean QRS axis +90-+210
- *Left precordial leads:* No q and small R - indicates No LV force
  - qR in V1
  - *ST changes:* Particularly Tm Version in precordial

CXR

Globular heart (mod-marked cardiomegaly)–75-85%

ECHO

- Can be used by fetal ECHO
- After birth—Atretic/stenotic MV and AV
  - Thick walled small LV
  - Echo bright endocardium (fibroelastosis)
  - Small LA and LV
  - Hypoplastic Ao
  - Flow from LA-RA
  - Retrograde flow in Asc Ao and large PDA
  - Ao dimension increases beyond ductus
    Case taken to assess small restrictive ASD (require BAS)
  - RV function by echo (prereq for surgical treatment)

Cardiac Cath

Rarely done
- Obligatory lt - rt shunt at IAS level and rt-lt shunt at PDA level
- Systemic venous O_2 is low
- Rise in O_2 sats in RA, RV, PA
  Asc-Des Ao and PA sats are same
  RV pr = systemic; RVEDP increased
- RA and LA mean pr increased
- Selective injection of contrast in to RA and MPA helps in diagnosis of Aortic atresia

CT/MRI

Rarely dare

NATURAL HISTORY

Most malignant form of cong heart disease
- 95% infants die within 1st month of life
- 25% of cardiac death during 1st week

MANAGEMENT

- Presurgical medical management
  - Patient should be intubated and ventilated with O_2
  - Correction of metabolic acidosis
  - IV infusion of PGE1 temporarily improve HLHS by reopening ductus
  - Balloon atrial septostomy—to decompress LA to give temporing relief
  - Careful, genetic, ophthalmologic, and neurologic evaluation
- *Surgical:* Three options

1. Norwood surgery followed by Fontan type surgery
2. Hybrid surgery followed by fontan type surgery
3. Cardiac transplant

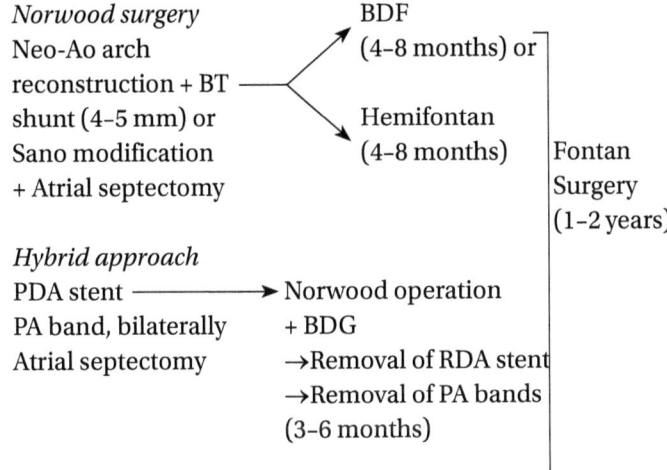

Norwood surgery
Neo-Ao arch reconstruction + BT shunt (4-5 mm) or Sano modification + Atrial septectomy

Hybrid approach
PDA stent
PA band, bilaterally
Atrial septectomy
→ Norwood operation + BDG
→ Removal of RDA stent
→ Removal of PA bands
(3-6 months)

Norwood Surgery

- Main PA is divided, distal stump is closed and ductus arteriosus is ligated
- Proximal PA connected to hypoplastic asc Ao and aortic arch
- PBF established by
  - BT shunt (rt sided)
  - Sano modification (RV-PA shunt)

- Atrial septostomy
  - Sano modification better than BT
    - Promote symmetrical growth of PA
    - Higher Ao diastolic pressure and higher coronary perfusion pressure then BT shunt
- Norwood procedure carries highest risk amongst cyanotic CHD-7-19%
- Between Norwood and 2nd stage surgery 4-15% patients die
- *Post Norwood*
  - Small dose diuretic
  - Digoxin
  - Captopril—after load reducing agent
  - Aspirin—to prevent stent thrombosis
  - Nutritional support

Hybrid approach—(preferred now-a-days)

Adv:

- Stable, balanced circulation without use of open heart surgery (without CPB)
- Delays open heart surgery until later in life when BDG or hemi fontan can better performed
- Mortality (surgery) = 2-5%

5.17 FETAL ECHO

ADVANTAGES
- Improves fetal outcome
- Early diagnosis of CHD allows anticipated management and prompt evaluation of genetic syndromes
- Timely referral of mother with affected fetus to tertiary care center
- Identify candidate for in utero cardiac intervention
- Prenatal detection of arrhythmia allows in utero treatment
- Helps in more specific family counseling

TIMING
- *9-10 weeks:* Possibly by TVS (only markers)
- *11-14 weeks:* Cardiac details not well appreciated may detect various marker of CHD
- *18-22 weeks:* Optimal timing
- *>30 weeks:*
  - Image acquisition difficult due to
  - Fetal rib shadowing
  - Fetal position
  - Maternal body habitus

MARKERS OF CHD
(First trimester)
1. Nuchal Fold thickness >3.5 mm
2. Presence of TR determined by PWD
3. Abnormal flow (absence of "a" wave or reversal of "a" wave) in ductus venosus Doppler

INDICATIONS
- Maternal indication
  - F/H/O CHD
  - Metabolic disorder (pku, DM)
  - Exposure to teratogens
  - Exposure to PG synthetase inhibitors (Ibuprofen, salicylic acid)
  - Rubella infection
  - Autoimmune disease (SLE, Sjogren)
  - Familial inherited disease (Ebs van creveld, Marfan, Noonan disease)
  - In vitro fertilization
- Fetal indication
  - Abnormal cardiac screening examination
  - Abnormal HR or rhythm
  - Extra cardiac anomaly (spina bifida)
  - Nonimmune hydrops
  - Nuchal Fold thickness >3.5 mm
  - Monochorionic twins
  - Unexplained severe polyhydramnios

When to Convert Routine Scan to Fetal ECHO
- Chamber asymmetry
- Altered cardiac axis
- Altered position of heart
- Enlarged fetal heart
- Arrhythmia

LIMITATION
- Operator dependent
- Technical limitation
  - Poor fetal positioning
  - Difficult due to maternal habitus
- Difficult to diagnose
  - Small VSD
  - As ASD vs PFO
  - Anomalies of PV
  - PDA

TECHNIQUE
Read ppt

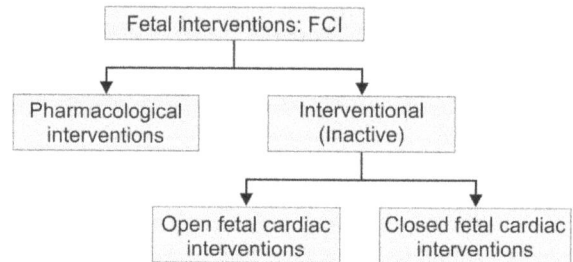

Pharmacological FCI
Indi
1. Fetal hydrops
2. Sustained tachyarrhythmias
3. Cardiac dysfunction

Mode of Administration
- Intravenous
- Transseptal
- Umbilical vein
- Maternal oral administration

Cardiac Arrhythmias
1. *Fetal tachyarrhythmias* (SVR/VT/AF)
   - MC indication for pharmacological FCI
   - Digoxin-mainstay of treatment
   Alternate—sotalol, Amiodarone, flecainide, propranolol

2. Fetal Brad arrhythmias
   - E.g., Sinus Brady, CHB, LQT, AV blocks
   - MC and 1 degree Indi for FCI is high grade AV block with VR <55
   - Atropine, Isoproterenol
   - AV block associated with
     - L-TGA, Heterotaxy, Autoimmune (anti Ro/La)
   - Autoimmune AV block can be treated with
     - Maternal dexamethasone and sympathomimetics
3. Other use of digoxin (efficacy unknown)
   - Fetal hydrops due to other str cardiac disease (Ebstein's, absent PV synd, premature, closure of ductus, cardiomyopathy)

Open Fetal Cardiac Intervention

- Any intervention in which uterus is opened surgically or accessed through surgical trach or 3 mm in dia
- Includes most fetoscopic procedures
- 1st reported - fetal pacemaker placement

Closed FCI

Mechanical intervention in which uterus is not opened or accessed with a post <3 mm in diameter

Fetal Aortic Valvuloplasty

- MC common FCI procedure
- Commonest Indi - HLHS: As
- Performed at 21–32 weeks gestation
- Insert needle in mother's and wall into uterine cavity under USA guidance
- Balloon advanced over guidewire

Compli

- AR
- Fetal Brady and AV block
- RV dysfunction
- Hemopericardium
- Fetal death
- Premature labor

Technical success - 75–80% for HLHS and As

Fetal-atrial Septostomy

- *Indi:* HLHS with restrictive ASD/IAS intact
- *Rationale:* Restrictive atrial communication reduces forward flow and increases reversal of flow into PV at time of atrial cont
  - This causes pulm congestion and dev of chronic pulm HTN

Predictors of success:
- Ratio of forward to reverse flow in PA
- Absolute velocities of reversal flow

New 1:
- High intensity ultrasound
- Noninvasive
- Ultrasound Freq 500 kHz to 10 MHz
- Causes localized tissue hyperthermia and damage at predictable depth without injuring surrounding tissue

Fetal Pulm Valvuloplasty

Indi:
- Pulm atresia with intact IVS
- Severe PS with intact IVS

Rationale

PA/PS with intact IVS—hypoplastic RV
- Decreased possibility of bivent repair in future and greatly affect 5-years survival

Fetal Pacing

- Cong heart block is responsible for fetal heart failure and hydrops with >80% mortality

Indi: Fetus who is premature to be delivered and refractory to medical treatment

5.18 OPERABILITY ASSESSMENT IN LT ≥ RT SHUNT

INTRODUCTION

- Pulm vasc disease is major risk factor for surgical management of patient with large post-tricuspid shunts as well as pretricuspid shunts
- Decision about whether to close or not depends on reversibility of PHT

PATHOGENESIS OF PV DISEASE

Precise mal not clearly understood
Left to rt shunt
↓
Increased PBF
↓
Shear stress/circumferential stretch
↓
Increases (endothelin-1) (No) decreases endothelial dysfunction; vasc remodeling; SMC proliferation; ECM: intravasc thrombosis
↓
Increase in PVR
↓
Inverted shunt: rt to lt
↓
Cyanosis

- Post-tricuspid shunt develops it earlier than pretricuspid
- Associated LV inflow and outflow obstruction potentiates PHT
- Children born at high altitude and who have Down's syndrome are especially at high risk (they develop PVOD early)
  Note: Presence of PHT is not similar to high PVD or PVOD
- All patients with unrestricted septal defect or AP window have severe PHT due to direct transmission of systolic pr
- Most of these PHT revert to normal within few months if operated early

↓

- Full blown Eisenmenger not only have severe PHT but also have irreversible PVD

↓

Do not benefit from shunt closure

DETERMINING OPERABILITY

Favorable outcome	Unfavorable outcome
C/F	
▪ Failure to thrive, repeated Respi tract inf, increases work of breathing	▪ No sign of failure
	▪ Fatigue, exertion syncope
▪ Pink, tachycardia, tachypnea, hemoptysis	▪ Cyanosis, clubbing
▪ MDM, S3	▪ No MDM/S3
CXR	
▪ Cardiomegaly with increased vascularity	▪ Normal heart disease, peripheral pruning
ECG	
▪ Deep Q in lateral leads (for post-tricuspid shunt only)	▪ No Q waves
ECHO	
▪ Lt → rt shunt, increased pulm	▪ Rt to lt shunt
▪ Venous return, persistence of LA and LVVO (for post-tricuspid only)	▪ Normal or decreased pulm ven return
Cath	
▪ PVR <6 wu/m²	▪ PVR > 9 wu/m²
▪ PVR: SVR < 0.3	▪ PVR: SVR > 0.5
• Acute vasodilator challenge	
• Indi: Baseline PVR 6–9 wu/m² and PVR: SVR 0.3–0.5	
• Decrease in PVR index of 20%	
• PVR: SVR decrease of 20%	
• Final PVR index < 6 wu/m²	
▪ Final PVR: SVR < 0–3	
• Lung Bx ≥ minimal role in assessing operability	

5.19 PERSISTENT LSVC

INTRODUCTION
Develop when there is failure of obliteration of left anterior cardinal vein

EPIDEMIO
- 0.5% of normal population
- Associated with 3-5% of all CHD

ANATOMY
Originates from (lt) innominate vein and (lt) IJV–descends down in front of aortic arch–drains into CS

When both RVSC and LVSC present–communication between them: left innominate vein (aka bridging vein)

HD
Venous return from LVSC is <1/5th of cardiac output
- No HD abnormality

C/F:
Nonspecific

ECG
Usually within normal limits

CXR
Increased width of the vascular pedicle on left border of mediastinum if detected in PA view—LSVC suspected

ECHO
- Dilated CS with anomalies LSVC connection
- CS seen in PLAX in AV groove seen in AP4C
- LSVC imagined from suprasternal view as a vertical str on left side of aortic arch
- Contrast ECHO helps

LSVC DRAINING TO LA
- LSVC passes inferior to left PA and drains to LA between atrial appendage and LSPV
- Associated with rt atrial or lt atrial isomerism
- *Associated with:* TOF
   Single vent
   Common atrium
   Complete AVCD
   Eisenmenger syndrome

EMBRYO
Absence of development of CS
↓
LVSC drain to LA

RAGHIB'S COMPLEX
- CS type ASD+
- Unroofed CS+
- LSVC drain to LA

HD
Acts like rt to lt shunt (desaturated blood draining into LA)
- No extra Hemodynamic burden
- Paradoxical embolism/abscess may occur

C/F
- Mild cyanosis from birth
- Otherwise infant is completely asymptomatic

INVESTIGATION
ECG-WNL: Atrial arrhythmia and superior axis present
- *CXR:* Increased width of vasc pedicle or lt border of mediastinum arouse suspicion of LSVC
- *ECHO:* Suprasternal view: LSVC viewed with venous type of flow besides Aorta [(laterally)-on it]
- Contrast ECHO is useful

Imp: Surgical importance when associated with other anomalies

IVC Interruption with Azygos vein Continuation
Communication between rt subcardinal and hepatic vein incorporates IVC to RA
↓
Failure of such communication
↓
Interrupted IVC
↓

- Anastomosis between rt subcardinal vein and supracardinal vein diverts IVC blood through Azygos vein to SVC-RA
- If similar anastomosis develops on lt side IVC- hemiazygos vein—LSVC-CS -RA

Frequently seen with—situs inversus + levocardia
   Visceral heterotaxy syndrome
   AVCD, DORV, TGA

C/F
Isolated IVC interruption asymptomatic

INVESTIGATION
CXR
Rt supracardiac border (near junction of SVC and RA) appear bulged—presence of dilated Azygos vein suspected

ECHO
- Hepatic portion of IVC absent in subcostal view
- Hepatic vein may confuse with IVC, hepatic vein ends in liver but IVC can be traced beyond it
- Entry site of Azygos vein to SVC can be imaged in suprasternal view
- Diagnosis established by cath
  Catheter inserted from FV enters IVC
- Azygos vein (appears that it has entered RA as—Azygos is posterior to PA) ≥SVC

ANOMALOUS IVC TO LA
- Mostly associated with levocardia with situs inversus
- Sometimes large Eustachian valve diverts blood to LA
- Anomalous venous drainage in spite of normal anatomy
- Cyanosis + clubbing: main only feature
- *Cath:* Catheter passed from FV-IVC- LA (SPO$_2$ are equal to systemic blood) -PV
  Catheter passed from upper limb passes normally to SVC-RA -RV -PA

ANOMALIES OF CORONARY SINUS
- Normally situated in AV groove
- Classified by Kirklin Barret Bayes
  - Type 1: Complete unroofed without LVSC
  - Type 2: Completely unroofed without LVSC
  - Type 3: Partially unroofed mid portion
  - Type 4: Partially unroofed terminal portion
- *Unroofed CS:*
  - Normal partition between CS and LA is absent
  - No HD consequences
  - No adverse HD consequences
  - Raghib's complex
- Hypoplasia, atresia or absence of CS
- *Stenosis of CS at opening to RA:*
  - Myocardial ischemia or infarction
  - CS blood finds alternate pathway for drainage (through LVSC-innominate vein—RVSC-RA)
- *Rare anomalies of CS*
  - CS draining into IVC
  - CS diverticulum—buries through rt and lt vent wall and may communicate with cavity

PERSISTENT DUCTUS VENOSUS
- Persistent ductus venosus connects portal vein to IVC
- Blood from portal vein bypass the liver

TOTAL ANOMALOUS SYST VENOUS CONNECTION
(1) Absence of RSVC, (2) Absent intrahepatic IVC; (Hemiazygos continues—LVSC-LA), (3) Hepatic vein connected to LA, (4) IAS absent, and (5) RA hypoplastic

HD
- LA receives all venous blood
- O$_2$ sats equal in all 4 chamber
- Unlike TAPVC—No increased PBF

5.20 INTERRUPTED Ao ARCH

DEFINITION

Complete anatomical separation of ascending aorta from descending aorta at variable location
- Also known as Steidele's complex

EPIDEMIO

- 1% of all congenital heart disease
- Isolated interruption of Ao Arch-rare
- Mostly associated with CHD
- M:F = 1:1
- Associated with 22q11 deletion and Digeorge syndrome

CLASSIFICATION

- *Abbot classified:* 2 types
- *Celoria and Patton classification:* 3 types
    1. *(43%)* → *Type A:* Interruption after normal branching (Distal to left subclavian)
    2. *(MC)-(53%)* → *Type B:* Interruption between left common carotid and left subclavian
    3. *(4%)* → *Type C:* Interruption between rt innominate and lt common carotid

Type B associated with VSD (coral-septal-malalignment type with sub aortic obstruction); Digeorge syndrome; 22q11

EMBRYOLOGY

- Maldevelopment of Aortic Arch
    - (Early) failure of formation or (later) regression of specific segments of Aorta
- Other hypothesis (flow theory)
    - Intrauterine decrease in aortic flow due to congenital defect—hypoplasia of aortic arch—regression of aortic segment
    - Type A: Due to atrophy of proxy dorsal Ao
    - Type B: Due to regression of left dorsal aorta or 4th Ao arch during 6th-7th week of intrauterine life

Associated Lesion

- Always associated with other defects
- Large VSD and PDA always present (survival depends on this)
- LVOT 0 is also seen in type B defect due to malaligned VSD
- 50% of type A defect IVS is intact, where large AD window is always present
- DORV, Truncus, TGA, ccTGA

HD

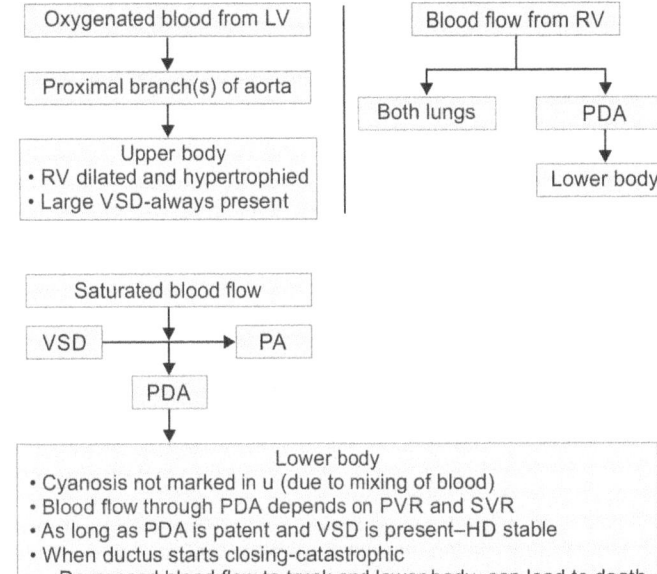

Subclavian steal when subclavian artery arise distal to interruption-decreased cerebral blood flow

C/F

- Neonate at birth: healthy
- After approx 24 hrs-when ducts starts closing—symptomatic.
    - Respi difficulties ⎤
    - Tachypnea   ⎬ CHF
    - Tachycardia   ⎦
    - Circulatory shock and severe acidosis
    - Differential cyanosis becomes apparent
- *Peripheral pulse:* Normal as long as ductus patent when duct close—LL pulse are diminished
- When branched (lt) pulse diminished—left subclavian arising distal to obstruction
- Carotids well felt and Brachial + Femoral weak—interruption proximal to both subclavian
- Weak lt arm and famorals with normal rt arm and carotid—type B interruption
- Cardiomegaly +
- RV impulse
- S1S2 normal
- No murmur
- No PDA murmur—because pulm trunk, ductus arteriosus and descending Ao behave as cont vessel

INVESTIGATION

ECG
RAD, RVH, RAE

CXR
- Cardiomegaly
- RA and RV enlargement
- MPA is prominent
- Pulm vascularity normal or increased
- Aortic knob absent
- Rib notching in elderly (depending on site of Obstruction and collateral flow)
  → ≥Origin of one subclavian distal to interruption produces contralateral rib notching
- SPO_2: Difference in SPO_2 between upper limb (Type B) Diff in SPO_2 between UL and LR (Type C)

ECHO
Subcostal view to visualize intra cardiac anatomy
- Suprasternal view to delineate ascending aorta and arch
- *In Type B:* Asc Ao divide into 2 branches that look like finger pointing upward
  - PA-PDA and Desc Ao are continuous and may confuse with Ao Arch
    (D/D is pulm artery branches and no bracheocephalic branch)
- *In Type C:* Antegrade flow in rt carotid, but retrograde flow in lt carotid
- Imp to delineate VSD, AP window and LVOTO

Cardiac Cath
- Avoided in many sick infants
- LV and RV angio helps to delineate aortic anatomy

CT and MRI
Best noninvasive modalities

PROGNOSIS
- Natural course of this anomaly is grave
- 50% infant dies during 1st week
- 3/4th dies by 1st month
- Only 10% survive up to 1st birthday

MANAGEMENT
- PGE, infusion (before 4 days of age) with intubation and O_2 administration
- Work up for Digeorge syndrome (i.e., hypocalcemia)
- Hyperventilation to be avoided ⎤ Avoided in
  → Causes respi alkalosis and tetany ⎬ Digeorge
  Citrated blood—chelates Ca^{++} -tetany ⎦ syndrome

Surgical Treatment
Primary complete repair of interruption and VSD closure (if simple VSD)

If complex VSD
↓
Initial procedure PA banding and repair of interruption
↓
Debanding and repair of other cardiac anomalies at later date

- Dacron patch ⎤
- 1° Anastomosis ⎬ Can be used to repair
- Vascular graft ⎬ interruption
- Venous homograft ⎦

Surgical mortality <10%

5.21 PA WITH INTACT VENT SEPTUM

DEFINITION

Characterized by complete obstruction of right ventricular outflow in presence of intact ventricular septum
- Survival depends on patency of ductus
- *Spectrum:*
  - Pulm atresia
  - Various degree of RV and tricuspid valve hypoplasia
  - Anomalies of coronary circulation
- Also referred as hypoplastic rt heart syndrome
- First described by John Hunter

EPIDEMIO

- 0.083 per 1,000 live births
- 3.1% of all critically-ill infants with CHD
- 10th most common CHD among neonates

EMBRYO

Presence of raphe in the memb that forms plane of valve and presence of well-developed pulm art—suggests that blood flow was patent previously—means that PA IVS develop late in development

Basic defect: Maldevelopment of endocardial cushion (large lateral cushion)
↓
Abnormalities of SLV
(Some authors thought it to be RV endocarditis in fetal period rather than cong. malformation)
Size of RV has imp surgical implication
- Anatomic abnormality

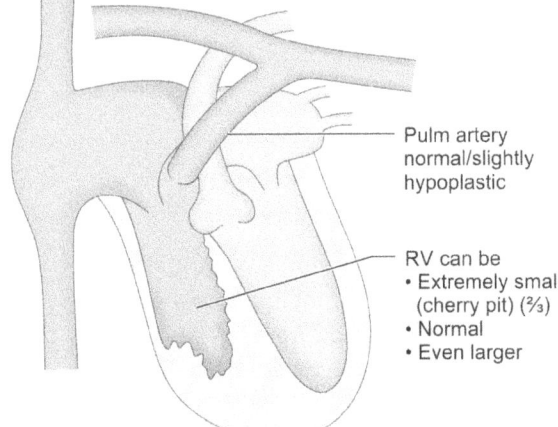

SPECTRUM (RVOT AND PULM VALVE)

▪ Pulm valve is atretic with 3 semilunar cusp completely fused and well developed RV	▪ Atretic infundibulum with severely hypoplastic RV

- *RV:* When RV is small—either inlet portion alone or inlet and trabecular portion are well developed (Bipartite RV)
- *TV:* Almost always abnormal
  - Functionally as well as morphologically
  - Strongly correlate with size of RV
  - Small RV- thick leaflet, abnormal chordec
  - Variable degree of TR
- *RA:* Always enlarged
  - ASD (80%)/PFO (20%) present in all cases (obligatory)
- *LA:* Dilated (receiving syst and pulm blood both)
- *LV:* Hypertrophied
- *Aorta-normal:* Always left sided arch
- *Myocardium:* Ischemia, fibrosis, Infarction, disarray endocardial fibroelastosis

Coronary cameral fistula
- Myocardial sinusoid ↓
- Persists as channel from RV—coro art ↓
- Retrograde flow from RV—coronary art (Due to increased RV systolic pr) ↓
- Coronary stenosis, coronary interruption ostial stenosis
- (If severe stenosis/interruption—coronary flow depends on RV: RV dependant coronary circulation)

CIRCULATION

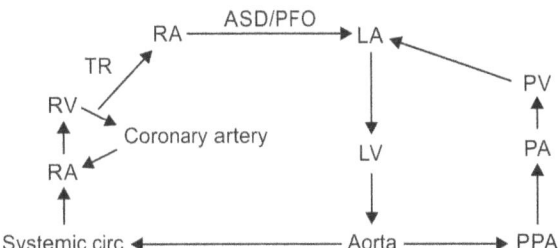

CLASSIFICATION

- Greenwood pathological classification old
  Based on size of RV
  - *Type 1:* PA with IVS, small volume thick walled RV and hypoplastic tricuspid orifice (More common 3/4th)
  - *Type 2:* PA with IVS; normal sized or dilated RV and TR
- Bull and delaval classification
  - Gr 1: Those with tripartite RV
  - Gr 2: Those with absent trabecular portion
  - Gr 3: Those with absent trabecular and inlet portion

- Milken classification (surgically oriented)
  Based on degree of RV hypoplasia
  - *Mild:* Adequate TV annulus
    Mildly hypoplastic RV cavity
    Well developed RVOT
  - *Mod:* Moderately hypoplastic TV annulus
    Moderately hypoplastic TV cavity
    Moderately hypoplastic RVOT
  - *Severe:* Severely hypoplastic TV annulus
    Severely hypoplastic RV cavity
    Severely hypoplastic RVOT
- Pulm valve abnormality divided into
  Catheter intervention possible
  - *Memb type:* Well developed PV, complete commissural fusion, RV infundibulum and trabecular portion normal, TV nearly normal; mild TR: No RV—coronary collateral
  - *Muscular type B:* Atretic PV, muscular atresia of infundibulum; hypoplasia of RV cavity, distorted TV, RV—dependant coronary circulation

PATHOPHYSIOLOGY

In Fetus
- All blood has to enter left heart via foramen ovale—large foramen ovale
- LV output and Ao blood flow increased
- Aortic isthmus as wide as aorta
- Normally
  - Large vol of blood (55–60%) of CO carried by ductus from PA-Ao
  - In PA-IVS 8–10% of CS is carried by ductus from Ao- PA

After Birth
- Fetal circulatory pattern maintained
- Mentioned on prev page
  Normal postnatal ductus closure results in profound hypoxemia and death

HEMODYNAMIC
- Obligatory RA–LA shunt
- Supra systemic RV pressure (if TV competent)
- *Circular shunt:* RV - sinusoid - coronary artery - coronary sinus - RA-RV
- *Sub systemic RV:* (If TV incompetent)
- LV is volume overloaded and less compliant
- Coronary flow is abnormal
  TA-counter clock depolarization
  PA-IVS - clockwise depolarization

C/F

Cyanosis

Immediately after birth
↓
After day or 2—cyanosis reopens with respiratory distress (due to ductal closure)
↓
Severe, hypoxemia, tachypnea, respi distress

CHF
From birth

Signs
Central cyanosis—in all infants
  Clubbing if survive >6 months
  Arterial pulse - normal
  JVP-raised (giant a and v wave: TR)
  Silent precardium
  LV impulse well felt
  No RV impulse
  S1S2- single and muffled
  Soft mid systolic murmur due to large flow in Ao
  High pitch cont murmur over left
  Sternal border (flow across closing duct)
  TR murmur

ECG
LV dominance with absent RV force - pathognomic (adult precordial pattern)
- LAD (30–90 degree)
- Clockwise depolarization
- RA enlargement

CXR
No characteristic appearance

ECHO
Well-developed LV, hypotrophied - normal RV
- Atretic PS as thick, immobile, dense line
- No visible/Doppler flow from RV–PA
- PDA and dilated coronary arteries; PFO/ASD Dilated RA; severe TR
- RV endocardium shows myocardial

Tricuspid z score
- Z measured Dia - mean normal dia
- SD of mean normal Dia

Z score ≥2.5—no risk of having RV dependent curc
Z score ≥2.5—high likelihood of achieving bivent repair

- D/D between functional pulm atresia and atretic PV
Detecting systolic flow across PV (systolic PR)
When PDA jet hits the valve
Or
Detecting forward flow across PV during positive pr ventilation

Cardiac Cath

- Must before definitive treatment
  - To search for coronary art abnormalities
  - To look for myocardial sinusoids
  - To look for ventriculo art communication
  - Trans catheter based intervention
- *Findings:*
  - RA mean > LA mean
- Suprasystemic RV
- Sub systemic RV pr in patient with TR
- SVC, IVC, RA, RV, RV sats are similar
- PV sats are high >95%
  PA O_2 sats ~ systemic O_2 sat
  PA IVS rare beyond 6 months of age
- *RV angio:* Size of RV defined, Severity of TR, (Goodale and lubin catheter—end hole z side hole)
- *Ao root angio:* Define origin and root of coronary art

CT/MRI

- Excellent tool
- Obliviate need for cardiac cath

Complication

- SCD
- CHF
- Angina
- Complications related to polycythemia
- Arrhythmia

Natural History

- Untreated—Grave prognosis
- 50% die within 2 weeks
- 85% due within 6 months
- Very rare

MANAGEMENT

- Medical
  - PGE1—as soon as diagnosis suspected
    - Prostin 0.05-0.1 μg/kg/min
    Grad Reduced to 0.01 μg/kg/min (once derived effect achieved)
    For small premat infants—prolonged course of PGE1 is required
  - PDA stenting (at some centers)
    - In patients with monaparatile RV, who are not candidate for BiV repair
    - PDA stenting done instead of BT shunt
    Less reliable
  - Balloon atrial septostomy can be done to increase rt to lt shunt
  - In patients with memb atresia of PV-laser assisted pulm valvotomy with balloon pulm valvuloplasty is an alternative
- *Surgical*
  Options are decided based on
  - Size of RV
  - Presence of RV dependant circulation

Options

- *Biventricular repair:* Ultimate goal whenever feasible; Possible only when there is adequate size of RV cavity with adequate RVOT is available
- *One and one half repair:* Done when RV size is borderline for BiV repair
- One vent repair (Fontan) used when
  - Monopartite RV
  - RV development coro circulation
- Cardiac transplantation

BiV Repair

First stage
- Transmular RV outflow patch and systemic to PA shunt
- For patient with well-formed PV and adequate infundibulum - closed transpulm valvotomy + left sided BT shunt
- Laser guided pulm valvotomy as alternative to closed valvotomy

FOLLOW-UP

- To monitor growth of RV
- Stable O_2 sats (>70%)
- Z score ≥2.5
- Cardiac cath within 6-18 months of initial surgical treatment (if patients can tolerate balloon occlusion of shunt-patient considered for BiV repair)
Second stage
BiV repair

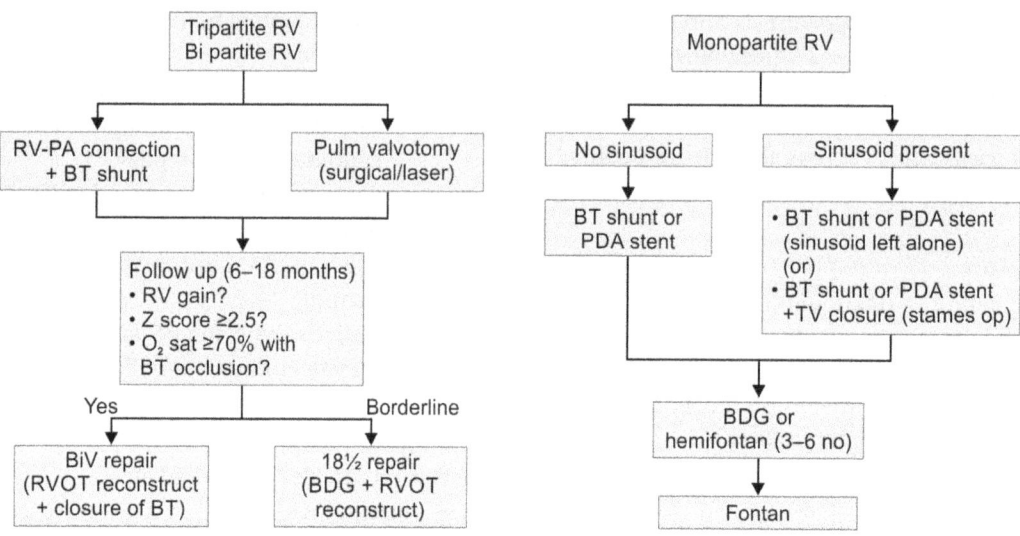

5.22 PULM ATRESIA WITH VSD

DEFINITION
Characterized by luminal discontinuity and absence of blood flow from earlier vent to PA in biventricular heart
- PBF derived totally from syst circulation in a complex manner
- Initially considered as type 4 truncus arteriosus (pseudotruncus)
- Also considered as extreme form of TOF (TOF-PA; VSD-PA; cTGA-PA-VSD)

EPIDEMIO
- 0.07/1,000 live births
- 1.4% of all CHD
- 20% of all TOF
- Associated with 22q11 deletion
  - Velo Cardio facial defect
  - Digeorge syndrome
- Associated with maternal diabetes
  - Phenylketonuria
  - Ingestion of retinoic acid
  - Ingestion of trimethadione

EMBRYO

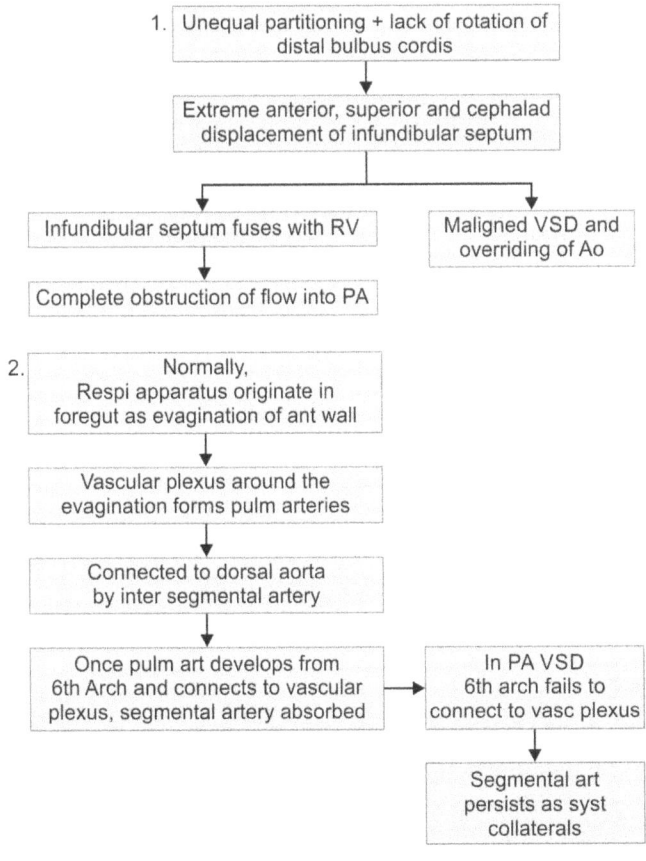

Note: If PA atresia develop after absorption of inter segmental artery pulm circ supported by bronchial art

Note: Ductus is usually absent as it has no fusion to perform If at all present-"vertical ductus"
- Which acts as collateral from aorta to pulm art
  Right Ao arch never seen in PA-IVS

ANATOMY
(Similar to TOF)
- Maligned nonrestrictive VSD
- Aortic override
- No continuity between RV and lumen of MPA or branch pulm art
- RV infundibulum is atretic

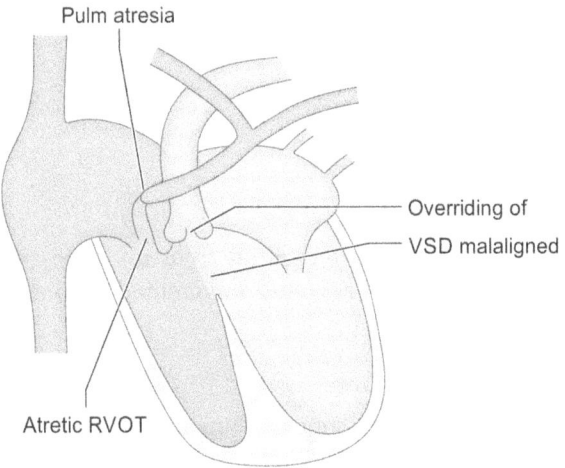

- In some cases infundibulum is developed and there is thick fibrous memb between infundibulum and pulm art
  - Right Aortic Arch 25-50%
  - AR can be present due to aortic dilatation
  - ASD association in 50%
  - RV usually hypertrophied and dilated
  - LA 2 LV is normal
  - Coronary art anomalies uncommon
  - Majority atrioventricular and ventriculo arterial concordance
  - MPA, central pulm arteries and hilar
  - *Artery:* May be present or absent
  - *Distal:* Pulm arteries always present
  - MPA is funnel shaped (wider end distally)
  - MPA absent in 5%

CIRCULATION

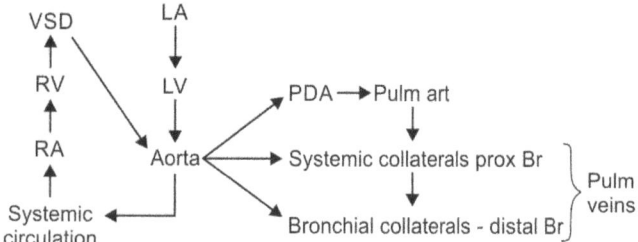

Rabinovitch described 3 types of systemic collateral arteries (SCA)

- *Type 1:* Bronchial artery branches entering lung parenchyma to form intrapulm anastomosis
- *Type 2:* Direct aortic branch connecting to hilar pulm artery
- *Type 3:* From major branch of Ao (Internal mammary, innominate or subclavian art) connects to hilar or lobat pulm art
  - Collaterals are commonly from descending thoracic Ao
  - Less common from subclavian/coronary (10%)
  - Very rarely from Abd Ao

Type of anastomosis:
1. Intrapulmonary
2. Extrapulmonary
3. Hilar

Note: When lung receive blood from multiple source-pulm art distribution becomes fragmented—arborization abnormally

CLASSIFICATION

- By congenital heart surgery nomenclature and database project (based on pulm circ)
  Type A: There is persistence of native pulm Ao
  - Pulm blood flow supplied by PDA
  - No MAPCAs present
  Type B: Both native pulm art and MAPCAs present
  Type C: No native Pulm Art
  - Pulm circulation supplied by MAPCA
- Somerville classification
  Based on type of branching of pulm art
  Type 1: Presence of both a main trunk and confluent pulm arteries
  Type 2: Main trunk absent
        Branches present (confluent or nonconfluent)
  Type 3: Main trunk and 1 branch absent
        Hilar arteries present
  Type 4: Main trunk and both branches absent
- Castaneda classification
  Based on anatomy of pulm circ
  Gr 1: Pulm circ by PDA; No MAPCA; patent MPA with confluent branches
  Gr 2: Pulm circ by PDA; No MAPCA
       Absent MPA with confluent patent branch PAs
  Gr 3: Pulm circ by MAPCA
       Hypoplastic hilar native PAs
  Gr 4: Pulm circ b, MAPCA
       No hilar native pulm art

PATHOPHYSIO

- Distribution of systemic and pulm blood flow depends on relative resistance offered by either circ
- Systemic art sats depends on relative proportion of blood flow to lungs
- PVR (total) is high
  - When PBF is unifocal—PVR can be calculated
  - When multifocal—impossible to calculate PVR: One segment of lung gets hypertensive flow and are having pulm art disease; another segment may have minimal blood flow with stasis thrombosis
  → Cyanosis from birth

C/F: Majority infant present as
- Mild cyanosis
- Asymptomatic
- Grow with poor weight gain

Some present as
- Mod-severe cyanosis ⎤
- Become hypoxic   ⎬ Indicate that PBF is duct dependent
- Irritable   ⎦

Childhood or adolescent
- Develop exertional dyspnea ⎤ Indicates good
- Easy fatigability   ⎦ collateral develop

Rarely infants present as ⎤ Indicates early
- Heart failure without   ⎬ developmental of cyanosis   ⎦ collaterals

SIGNS

- Mild to mod cyanosis (or severe) depending of PBF
- Clubbing-late infancy
- Pulse-normal; large vol-collaterals/PDA
- JVP-normal
- Precordium silent; no thrill
- S1-normal
- S2-single (A2)
- Loud aortic ejection click (dilated Ao)
- Cont murmur over chest and back (MAPCA)

ECG

RAE, RVH, RAD (100–180°)
   BiV enlargement may be seen
   [RVH differentiate PA with VSD from PA with IVS
   In PA with IVS -LVH without RV force]

CXR

Resembles TOF
- Coeur-en-sabot (most often found in PA-VSD than in TOF)
- Mild to no cardiomegaly
- MPA segment is concave
- Pulm vasc markings uneven—characteristic of collateral flow

ECHO

- Dilated RA, Hypertrophied RV, Large VSD with overriding of Ao, bind RVOT pouch or imperforate pulm value (seen as thick band)
- Absence of flow from either vent to pulm art
- Size, presence and integrity of prox pulm art and confluence
- Presence or absence of duct (PDA)
- *Associated anomalies:* ASD, AVCD, rt Ao Arch
- *Limitation:* Cannot delineate all collateral supply to lung

CT/MRI

- Shows intracardiac as well as pulmonary connection
- Useful when angiocardiography failed to show pulm artery or delineate collaterals

Cardiac Cath

- Mandatory before definitive surgical treatment
- *Findings:* RA mean pr normal
  Systemic RV pressure
  Ao pr-normal
  Syst Art desaturation
- *LV angio:* Maligned VSD with overriding
- Delineation of pulm blood supply

COMPLICATION

- Headache 2 degree to polycythemia
- Cerebral abscess
- Infective endocarditis
- Risk of syst Art embolize (like any other rt-lt shunt)

NATURAL HISTORY

Depends on PBF
  Miller suggested

Group 1 (50%):
- Infant with inadequate PBF
- Duct dependent
- Half of patients fall in this group
- Very short life span unless immediate surgical steps taken

Group 2 (25%):
- Hypoxia does not manifest until childhood
- PBF from collateral
- Become inadequate with growth
- Live up to 2nd–3rd decade

Group 3 (25%):
- Increased PBF
- Early development of collaterals
- Some present as CHF
- If they thrive crisis—live up to 3rd–4th decade

MANAGEMENT

- PGE infusion
  - As soon as diagnosis is suspected
  - To keep duct open additional study and surgical treatment
  - Alprostadil: 0.05–0.1 ug/kg/min
    ↓
    Once desired effect obtained
    ↓
    Dose reduce to 0.01 uh/kg/min
- Emergency cardiac cath/MRI to delineate anatomy of PA and collaterals
  - Surgical management

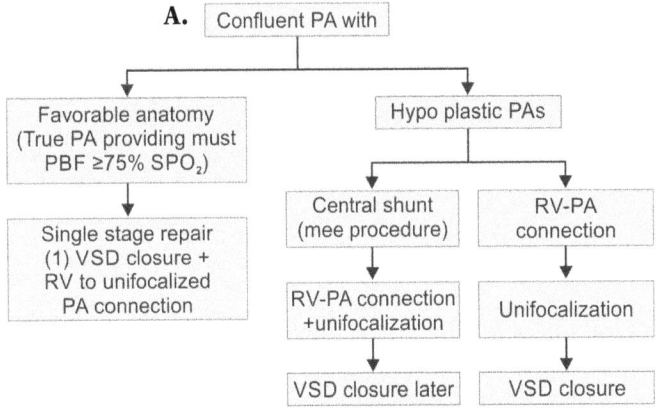

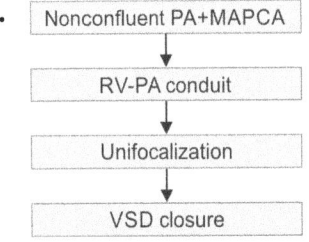

Principle: RV-PA connection must be established at earliest to allow tiny central PAs to enlarge during first year of life with improved distribution of pulmonary artery and improved development of alveolar units

Two ways:
1. Central shunt
2. RV–PA conduit

Central shunts:
- **MEE procedure:** Directly connecting PA to ascending aorta
- BT shunt is avoided
  - Difficulty to perform on small PA
  - Can develop stenosis

↓

Followed by unifocalization, RV-PA connection

↓

Followed by VSD closure

RV-PA connection:
- *Single stage repair:* When true PA provide most of PBF and SPO_2 >75%
  - If additional collateral found-occlude on table and check for Art SPO_2
  - If SPO_2 art remains >75%—coil embolization of collateral
  - *Good candidate:* Nakata index >200
  - *Procedure:* RV-PA connection + unifocalization + VSD patch closure

2. *Multistage procedure*
   Stage1: RV-PA conduit: (by homograft)
   - Cath after 3-6 months to identify PA size, identify collaterals and coil occlude

   Stage 2: Unifocalization: Aortopulmonary collaterals are divided from Ao origin and anastomosed to PA or conduit
   - Cath after 3-6 months to check for any stenosis in circuit and do balloon dilatation

   Stage 3: VSD closure +- Fenestration
   - If RV or 10–20% greater than syst pr then fenestration of age required (3-4 mm) ⎤ 1-3 years

POST OP FOLLOW-UP

- Freq. Follow-up
- Vahed conduit may degenerate

↓

Can be balloon dilated or may need to replace at later date

- Dysfunctional conduit or homograft can be replaced percutaneously with bovine jugular venous valve
- Survivor needs SBE prophylaxis for indefinite period
- Certain limitation of activity needed
- Majority patients remain in NYHA 1-2

5.23 CONGENITAL PULM AV FISTULA

DEFINITION
Congenital pulm AV fistula are direct communication between pulm arteries of varying size with pulm veins without going through pulm capillaries

INCIDENCE
- Not uncommon
- Congenital
- Often accompanied by hereditary hemorrhagic telangiectasia
- *Rarely acquired:* Cirrhosis of liver, schistosomiasis, metastatic CA of thyroid trauma, after palliative surgical treatment of cavo-pulm anastomosis
- *Associated:* Polysplenia, ASD

EMBRYOLOGY

In embryo 3rd–10th week
↓
Angiogenic cell appear from primitive mesenchymal cells
↓
Forms a cluster called blood islands
↓
Develop to form plexus of vessels by process of coalescence, resorption and separation
↓
Cells derived from neuroectodermal cells surround these primitive vessels to form smooth muscle cells
↓
Abnormality of this complex process of vasculogenesis is responsible for abnormal communications

PATHOLOGY

Types
- Localized or diffuse
- Single or multiple
- Small to large
- MC (70%)—present in lower lobe or right middle lobe
- Gross pathology is an enlarged and tortuous pulm artery or multiple pulm arteries entering into an aneurysmal sac
  ↓
  Equal size of tortuous vein or multiple veins emerge from it
- *Arterial walls* thin lined by endothelium, smooth muscle layer—disorganized and intimal larger is lost
- *Vein* emerging from it appears arterialized and thicker than normal
- *Aneurysmal sac* may consist of multiple communications
- Sometimes sac is very large and rounded with presence of thrombus
- Rarely direct communication between pulm artery segment and LA (due to complete incorporation of venous part of fistula into LA)
- Pulm AV fistula may be a part of gen vascular disorder and associated with other vascular abnormality e.g., HHT (Rendu-osler-weber syndrome)

HD
- Shunt from PA-PV
- Usually covers <½ of CO and does not alter amt of blood returning to lt heart
  So No volume overload
- It is veno-arterial shunt
  Systemic desaturation (SPO_2 75–85%)
  (Contrast to systemic AV fistula—where CO increases and significant HD abnormality)
- Flow through fistula located in lower lobes decreases when they are mechanically compressed as in preg/upright posture
- Inspiration and Müller maneuver increases flow through fistula: expiration and valsalva maneuvers have opposite effect

C/F
Depends on size and number
- Asymptomatic till adulthood
- Few with large shunt becomes symptomatic on infancy or childhood
- Mean age of presentation 39 years
- *Orthodeoxia platypnea:* Dyspnea in upright posture (due to gravitational pull more blood flows in fistulas located in lower lobe)
  Cerebral symptoms: Dizziness, diplopia, speech abnormality (due to paradoxical emboli) stroke, brain abscess
- Headache (polycythemia)
  Recurrent epistaxis, hematoma, hematemesis (mucosal hemangioma)
  Rupture of aneurysmal sac in bronchus—hemoptysis
- Rarely present with deep cyanosis
- Infective endarteritis

Signs

Pulse, BP, JVP-WNL
  Cyanosis and clubbing-common
  Classic triad: Cyanosis
              Clubbing
              Vascular bruit (syst murmur)
No cardiomegaly
S1S2 normal
No murmur over precordium
(50%)—cont murmur: Loud during systole as the major portion of flow through fistula is during systole) (increases with deep inspiration and Müller maneuver) (decreases with deep expiration and valsalva)

- *Hereditary—hemorrhagic telangiectasia:* Small Ruby lesion in face, skin, young, nail beds and on pressing blanching occurs)

INVESTIGATION

ECG
Normal

SPO$_2$
- O$_2$ desaturation in presence of normal clinical findings and normal ECG
- Desaturation limits even with 100% O$_2$ inhalation

CXR
Single or multiple well defined rounded or lobulated opacities in lung fields

ECHO
- Direct visualization of fistula not possible
- Contrast ECHO: Contrast appears in left sided chamber after several heart beats

Cardiac Cath
- Contrast injection in appropriate pulm artery shows the fistula which is dilated, elongated and tortuous
- Feeding artery and draining vein-well visualized
- Aortogram is necessary to discover possible syst. Arterial supply from systemic artery
- Mandatory to know size of the vessels before embolization or even surgery

CT/MRI
Can accurately delineate anatomy

PROGNOSIS
- Good
- Death due to extra cardiac cause
- With increasing age fistula increases in size
- When two large—give rise to respi problem and CHF
- *Large series:* 27% died in childhood/early adult
              12% alive but symptomatic
              37% alive and asymptomatic
              24% died from unrelated causes

COMPLICATION
- Polycythemia 2 degree to syst desaturation
- Paradoxical embolism
- Infective endarteritis
- Rupture of fistulous sac- hemorrhage
- Rarely CHF

MANAGEMENT
- No specific medical management
- Asymptomatic—observe
- Symptomatic—all need treatment
  - Catheter embolization—procedure of choice
    - Stainless steel coil
    - Detachable balloons
    - Vascular plug
  - Surgical excision
    (Lobectomy/wedge resection)
- Indication for surgical treatment is limited—because lesion is progressive
- Device management is preferred even in cases with thrombosis and embolism

5.24 ANEURYSM OF SINUS OF VALSALVA

SINUS OF VALSALVA

Pocket like space constructed by 3 aortic cusps and adjacent aortic wall that is somewhat dilated forming 3 bulges

End of sinus (that is most distal portion) is called sinotubular junction

ANEURYSM OF SINUS OF VALSALVA

- Thin walled out pouchings
- Protrude into adjacent cardiac chamber via either a direct connection or a "windsock" tract that extends from aneurysm

INCIDENCE

Rare congenital defect
- 0.1–3.5% of all CHD
- 5 times more prevalent in Asians because of higher incidence of supracristal VSD
- M>F = 4:1

EMBRYOLOGY

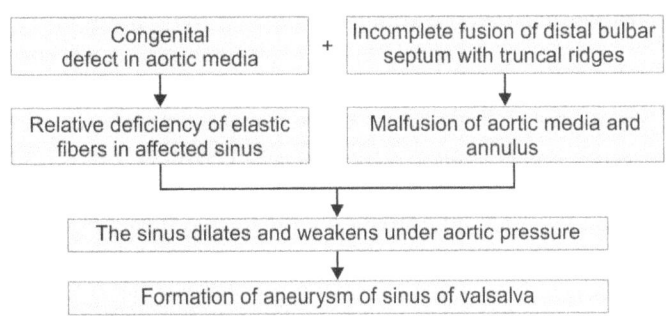

MC = right sinus of valsalva (80–85%)

2nd = noncoronary sinus (5–15%)

Rare = left sinus (because LCC embryologically is not derived from bulbar septum)

ETIOLOGY

Congenital/acquired
- Congenital/primary
  - Most common
  - Due to spontaneous genetic mutation
  - Associated with VSD (30–60%); BAV (15–20%); AR (40–50%) and PLSVC
- Acquired/secondary
  - Abrupt deceleration trauma
  - Infections—bact endocarditis syphilis and TB
  - Degenerative disease—cystic medical necrosis and atherosclerosis
  - Intensive physical activity—cause rupture

Weaken juncture between the media and the annulus fibrosis of Ao

More diffuse, involve more of the sinus, involve multiple sinus

CLASSIFICATION

A. *Sakakibara and Konno classification*
   - Based on site of origin
   - Four types
     Type 1: From left portion of right sinus
     Type 2: From central portion of right sinus
     Type 3: From posterior portion of right sinus
       3a: Ruptures into RA
       3b: Ruptures into RV
     Type 4: From right portion of noncoro-sinus

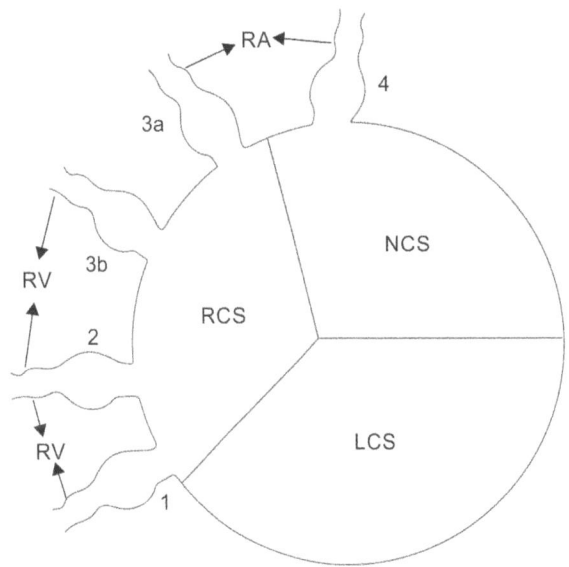

ASSOCIATED VSD

Type 1: VSD immediately below commissure of left and right semilunar cusps of the pulm valve, aneurysm rupture in RVOT

Type 2: VSD rests on crista supraventricularis

Type 3: VSD lies just below crista supraventricularis

Type 4: VSD rests on pars membranancea

Avg age of RSOV = 30 years
- Modified Sakakibara classification
  RSOV classified by anatomic location of protrusion site

  RV
  - Protrusion and rupture into RV just below PV
  - Penetration and rupture into or just below crista supraventricularis of PV
  - Penetration and rupture into RV adjacent to or at tricuspid annulus

  RA
  - Penetration and rupture into RA adjacent to tricuspid annulus
  - Protrusion and rupture in to RA
  - Other rare conditions (rupture into LA, pulm art, LV or other structures)

HEMODYNAMICS

A. *Unruptured*
- No significant HD changes
- Rarely causes distortion and obstruction of RVOT
- Can lead to AR

B. *Ruptured*
- HD depends on (1) amt of shunt and (2) cardiac chamber to which the aneurysm ruptures and (3) whether it develops acutely or subacutely magnitude of shunt depends on size of the fistulous opening

  PSOV
  ↓
  Increases pulm blood flow
  ↓
  Increased LA volume and flow
  ↓
  LV vol overload
  ↓
  CHF

  Acute rupture—sudden onset CHF -fatal
- If patient survives acute episode—HD gradually stabilize—ultimately CHF ensues

C/F

Three different ways
1. *Acute rupture*
   - Occur after unaccustomed exercise or trauma to chest wall
   - Chest pain—followed by dyspnea/orthopnea
   - Chest pain due to—rupture itself
     └─ Coronary insufficiency
   CHF gradually improve within some days because of compensatory mech
   ↓
   After a latent period (variable duration)
   ↓
   Again orthopnea, PND, dyspnea appears because heart fails to compensate cont vol overload
   ↓
   CHF
   ↓
   Death if not treated/closed

2. *Subacute rupture*
   - 1/3rd patients
   - Gradually becomes symptomatic (CHF)
   - No H/O acute episode

3. *Unruptured*
   - Asymptomatic
   - Angina may be present 2 degree to coro compression
   - Obstruction of RVOT and TR
   - Rarely AR
   - Rarely systemic embolic event
   - May lead to medically refractory VT from RVOT

Signs

1. *Ruptured*

   Murmur does not peak around S2 (D/D PDA)
   - Cont murmur-most characteristic finding
   - If rupture in RA; cont murmur is maximum along rt or lt sternal border and loud in systole
   - If rupture into body of RV—cont murmur is maximal at mid-low left sternal border, systolic part may be diminished due to fistulous tract compression by myocardium diastolic murmur is longer and louder
   - Rupture into PV near TV—may be associated with cont murmur over rt sternal edge
   - Rupture into RVOT—murmur in upper lt sternal border
   - Rupture into LV—EDM similar to AR

2. *Ruptured (peripheral finding)*
   - High vol or water hammer pulse due to aortic run off through aneurysm into low pr chamber
   - PP not increased in acute rupture—but after some days PP increases
   - JVP elevated with onset of CHF
   - LV apex forceful, heaving
   - Brisk para sternal heave due to RV overload
   - Thrill sometimes feels in large rupture
     - Cont thrill
     - Very superficial and well palpable on slightest touch

INVESTIGATION

ECG

Sinus rhythm
- LA or BAE
- Occasionally AV conduction defect
- LVH (due to overload)
- BiV hypertrophy
- In acute rupture—S.Tachy with nonspecific ST-T changes

CXR

Acute rupture: Signs of pulm venous HTN and pulm edema without cardiomegaly

Subacute Rupture: Cardiomegaly (all cardiac chamber may be enlarged)
- Pulm plethora
- Pulm venous HTN (prom upper lobe veins)

CT/MRI

To diagnose site of rupture

ECHO

- *Criteria*
  - Root of aneurysm be superior to the aortic annulus
  - Aneurysm be saccular in appearance
  - Aortic root is normal in size
- *Aneurysmal* dilatation of sinus of valsalva gives "wind shock appearance" in >50% cases
- Doppler (cw and color)
  - Cont turbulence detected
  - With high velocity
  - On color mosaic pattern
- TEE-better than TEE
- 3D ECHO—Exact site of rupture, size and shape of defect can be seen

Cardiac Cath

- Presence of step up in O_2 saturation in rt heart and filling of rt heart chamber by contrast media from asc aorta
- *Indi:*
  - Prior to trans cath closure
  - To know profile of rupture and its relationship with coro arteries
  - Coro angio

D/D
- PDA
- VSD with AR
- Coro AV fistula

COMPLICATIONS
- CHF-acute or progressive
- AI
- IE
- Angina and myocardial ischemia
- Heart block
- Aortic bronchial/aortic pulm fistula
- SCD
- Cardiac tamponade
- Rarely CVA

NATURAL HISTORY
- *In Asians:* 40–80% RSOV occurs in 3rd–4th decade
- Poor prognosis
  For Congenital sinus of valsalva-survival at 20 year is 95% (because rupture is uncommon up to age 20)
- Ruptured aneurysm due within 1 year after onset of untreated COD: CHF/IE (mean survival time = 3–9 years)

MANAGEMENT
- Medical care
  - Management of CHF
  - Treatment of endocarditis/prevention
  - Management of arrhythmia and myocardial ischemia
- Transcatheter treatment
  - Percutaneous closure of RSOV
    Amplatz duct occluder/amplatzer septal occluder
    C.I: associated VSD/AR
  - *Procedure:* Retrograde crossing with guidewire, snaring of wire from venous side to form a loop—provide stability, delivery of occlusion device from femoral vein-device deployed at site of rupture rather than at site of origin (to avoid aortic valve involvement)
  - Post-procedure Aspirin
- Surgical management
  - For all ruptured RSOV
  - For unruptured SOV if
    - Malignant arrhythmias
    - Obstruct coronary ostia or RVOT
    - Infected

5.25 SINGLE VENTRICLE

SYNONYMS
Univentricular heart, Holmes heart, cor triloculare biatriatum, DILV/DIRV

DEFINITION
All hearts with AV connections exclusively to one main ventricle chamber that is well developed (right or left or indeterminate)
- Small ventricle not receiving any AV value is termed: trabecular pouch, outlet chamber, rudimentary, nondominant, etc.

HISTORY
- Noticed as early as 1699 by chemineau
- Earliest report by Holmes in 1829
  - Taussig and Edwards started using term single ventricle: 1939
  - Clear definition by Van Praagh in 1965

EPIDEMIOLOGY
- Overall incidence = 1.1%
- 3.2% of all cyanotic heart disease
- M>F = 3:1
- 1.05% of all major congenital heart disease (India)

EMBRYOLOGY
- Normally Inlet portion of primitive ventricle tube forms LV and outlet portion for RV
- Abnormal development of this component is responsible for genetics of SV ↓
  This complex disease develops from time of acute bending of the cardiac loop
- Anatomical abnormalities

Ventricular Pattern
- LV pattern (dominant LV)
  - 65-75% cases
  - Smooth cavity with fine trabeculations
  - Majority of cases (90%) are l-loop
  - *Situs solitus:* Both AV valve open in SV
  - Ventricular septum does not extend up to crux
  [10% normally related GA connection known as Holmes heart]

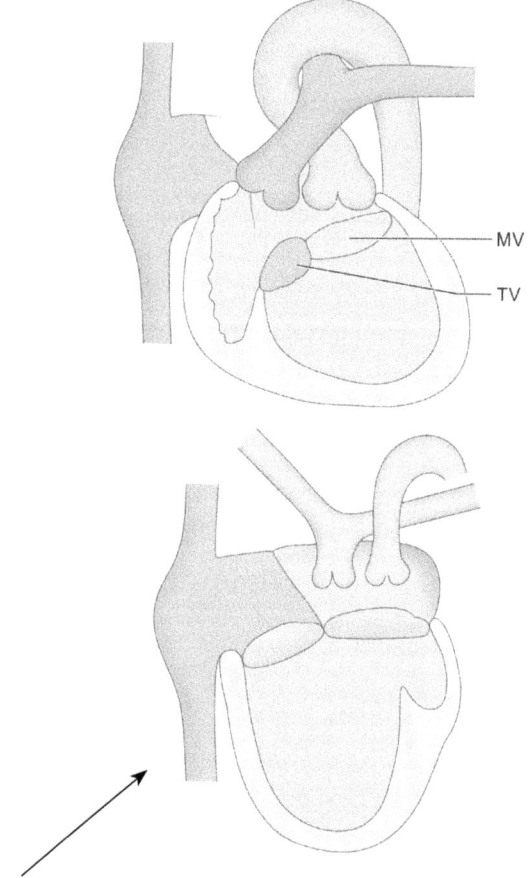

(90%) | Ao arise from rudimentary RV; communication between LV and rudimentary RV via VSD

- RV pattern (Dominant RV)
  - Trabecular cavity appears irregular with coarse trabeculations
  - 20-25%
  - d-looped
  - VSD extended up to crux; Infundibulum is always associated with RV
  - Both great arteries arise from RV

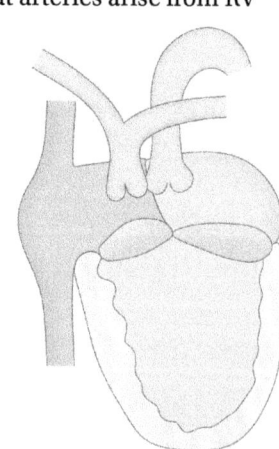

- Indeterminate type
  - 5–10%
  - Clear cut morphology of vent cavity is lacking
  - Often lacks any rudimentary chamber
  - Associated with Atrial isomerism/vent heterotaxy
  - Both great arteries arise from single chamber

AV CONNECTION
- Double inlet (both atria open in 1 vent)
- Single inlet (absence of rt or lt AV connection)
- Common AV valve

GREAT ARTERIES
- Concordant or discordant
- LV type = 90%—discordant
  10%—concordant (Holmes heart)
- RV type = Both from SV

BULBOVENTRICULAR FORAMEN
- Term used to describe VSD to well-developed LV heart with discordant great arteries

CORONARIES
- Usually abnormal
- LM from left postsinus
- RCA from postsinus

CONDUCTION DEFECT
Classification
- Van Praagh's
  Type A: DILV: Absence of RV sinus portion (MC)
  Type B: DIRV: Absence of LV sinus portion
  Type C: Double inlet vent of mixed morphology
  Type D: Double inlet vent of indeterminate morphology
- B. Types of DILV (based on GA relationship)
  - Normally related GA
  - d transposition (rt anterior aorta)
  - l-transportation (lt anterior aorta)
  - Inversus type (left posterior aorta)

HEMODYNAMICS
- Decided by
  - Mixing in main chamber
  - Presence or absence of PS
  - PVR
  - Functional status of single or main ventricular chamber

- Favorable streaming of 2 atrial inflow with little mixing is commonly seen in single LV inverted rudimentary chamber
- When subvalvular PS or PVR develop—mixing increase; cyanosis worsen
- When sub aortic stenosis—burden on SV increases resulting in early HF

Rule of thumb: Systemic SPO_2 > 85% and <75% are taken to represent increased and decreased PBF respectively

CLINICAL FEATURES
Three major clinical forms
1. Marked cyanosis
   Gradually develop hypoxic spells, restlessness and met Acidosis
   Critically ill when PDA closes
   Ultimately die if no intensive cure
   — Severe PS or Pulm atresia
2. Mild-mod cyanosis
   Asymptomatic course
   Retarded growth
   O/E: Normal pulse, quiet precordium, LV impulse, Single S2 (loud A2), ESM over UL sternal border occasionally long syst murmur over lower, sternal border due to flow across bulboventricular foramen
   — Mild-mod PS
3. CHF in early infancy
   High PBF
   Very symptomatic
   Refractory CHF may indicate
   Sub aortic obstruction or Interrupted arch.
   LV type impulse, visible
   Precordial pulsation, split
   Loud S2 and prominent
   Long ESM due to flow across
   lt AV valve retarded growth
   Subsequently develop
   Eisenmenger
   — High PBF with Sub aortic stenosis

ECG
Site of OC (outflow chamber) influence ECG
- Noninverted OC
  - Left axis deviation, LAE or BAE, LVH, stereotyped precordial QRS, large amplitude R
- Inverted OC:
  - Inferior or rt ward axis; PR prolongation, prominent R in right precordial leads, large biphasic RS (stereotyped) complex in mid-precordial leads, Absent Q in left precordium

- T inversion in left precordial—suggests sub Ao stenotic
- *Pre excitation:* LGH, WPW
- SVT (some cases)

CXR
- Visceral situs (gastric bubble and atrial situs (bronchial anatomy) can be ascertained
- Increased pulm vascularity if PBF increases
- Waterfall appearance: due to lifted RPA by dilated MPA that is not border forming due to malposition

ECHO
- Identifies visceral and atrial situs solitus
- Morphology of main and rudimentary chambers
- AV and ventricular connections
- Absence or presence (and degree) of sub arterial obstructions

Cardiac Cath
- Accurately measures vent pressures presence and degree of obstruction to PBF; calculation of PVR
- For SV, PA size should be adequate for repair with PAP <20 and PVR <4

MRI
Advised when ECHO/cath cannot delineate pulm anatomy or vent morphology

NATURAL HISTORY
- 57% survival at 1 year
- 45% survival at 5 years
- Small subset with protected pulm vasculature
- 90% survival at 10 years

MANAGEMENT
A. Initial medical management:
- Newborn with severe PS or PA Interrupted Ao arch. ⎤ PGE infusion (Lifesaving)

B. Surgical:
- Initial surgical palliative procedure:
  - *Purpose:* To make patient acceptable candidate for BDG or hemi fontan
    - No PS and large PBF—PA banding (Mortality high = 25%) (tolerate only if BVF large)
    - No PS and if bulbovent foramen is small DKS operation (Damus-Kaye-Stansel)
      - PA to Aorta anastomosis with rt sided BT
    - If PS/PA—BT shunt
      - PDA ligated after creation of shunt (Alternative to BT shunt = PDA stenting + BIL PA banding + Balloon atrial septostomy)
    - If PS + small/obstructed BVF
      - Enlargement of BVF via trans aortic approach

↓

Follow-up closely till second stage surgical treatment (for cyanosis; O₂ sats <75% or sighs of CHF)

↓

C. Second stage surgical palliative procedure
- Bidirectional Glenn at 3-6 month of age
- Hemi Fontan

↓

D. Definitive procedure
   Fontan surgical treatment at 18-24 months of age

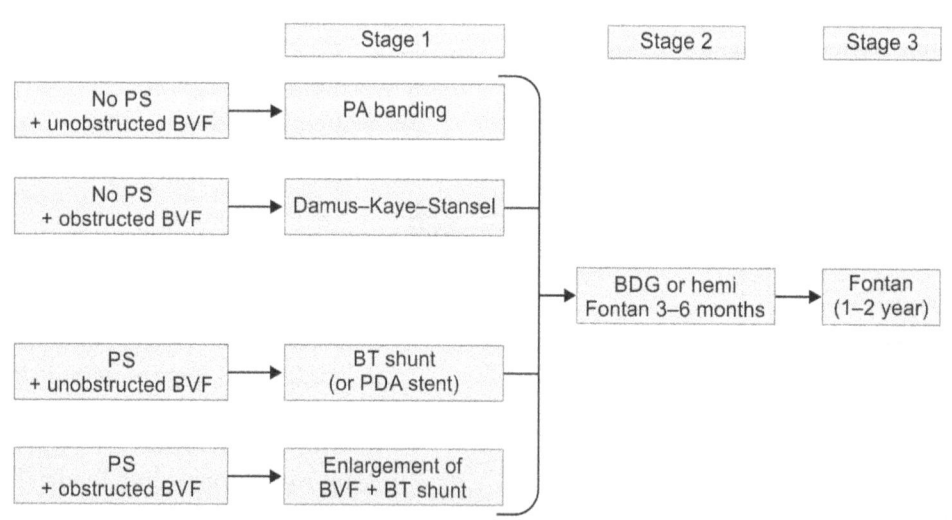

5.26 TOTAL ANOMALOUS PV CONNECTION

DEFINITION

When all PV are not connected to LA, the clinical condition is known as TAPVC
↓
All 4 veins from both the lungs join together to form a venous sinus or pulm venous confluence and then run in a single channel to join RA or systemic vein or both

HISTORY

- First described 1798 by Wilson
- TAPVC description by fridlowsky
- First successful repair by Müller 1957

EPIDEMIC

- 4–6/100,000 live births
- 1–3% of cases of CHD
- Associated with asplenia syndrome
- M:F = 1.1 (strong male predominance M:F = 4:1 in infra diaphragmatic type)
- India M:F = 2:1

EMBRYOLOGY

1. Lung bud arise as outgrowth from primitive foregut
   ↓
   Foregut is covered by super clinic venous plexus
   ↓
   Part of plexus around lung bud forms pulm vascular bed
   ↓
   Brain to cardiac and umbilical vein
2. Primitive venous channel develop from LA
   ↓
   Connects with pulm venous plexus
   ↓
   Subsequently connection between pulm venous plexus with cardinal and umbilical vein atrophies
   ↓
   4 separate pulm vein develop from venous plexus and joins common pulm vein
   ↓
   This incorporates into LA

TAPVC: Common PV fails to develop
↓
Pulm venous plexus unable to join LA
↓
Pulm venous plexus to cardiac vein connections persists
↓
Cardinal vein form SVC and IVC
↓
Pulm to systemic venous connection persists
↓

Note: (Indirect drainage is through persistence LVSC to innominate vein and then to right SVC or directly into RA or into IVC)

CLASSIFICATION

- Smith's classification
  - Supradiaphragmatic type
  - Infradiaphragmatic type
- Neil classification based on embryologic basis
- Burroughes and Edwards classification
  - Long
  - Intermediate
  - Short

Most popular
4. Darlings classification
   - *(55%) Type 1:* Supracardiac connection
     Common venous sinus joins SVC
   - *(30%) Type 2:* Cardiac connection
     Common pulm venous vein drains into coronary sinus or PV enters into RV separately
   - *(13%) Type 3:* Infracardiac connection
     Pulm veins drain into portal vein
   - *(2%) Type 4:* Mixed
     Combination of cell types
     Rt and lt PV drains into diff sites commonly associated with cardiac anomalies

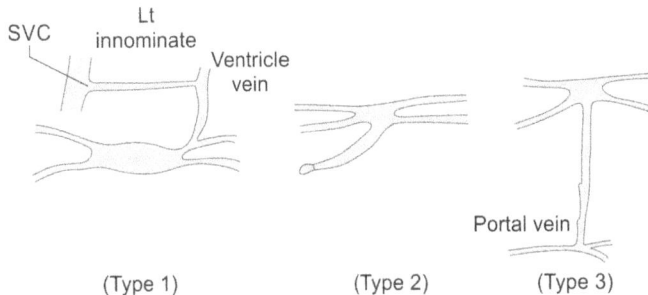

(Type 1) (Type 2) (Type 3)

ASSOCIATED ANOMALIES

- TAPVC—Isolated in 2/3rd of cases
- Remaining 1/3rd—PDA, TOF, HLHS, single ventricle, AV canal defect, TGA, cat's eye syndrome, polysplenia syndrome
- Usually associated with type 4

ABNORMAL ANATOMY

- *Supracardiac type:*

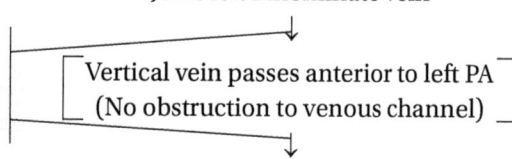

4 veins join to form a confluence
↓
Through left vertical vein
↓
Joins left innominate vein
↓
[Vertical vein passes anterior to left PA
(No obstruction to venous channel)]
↓
Drain into SVC

Note: When vertical vein passes between LPA and lt bronchus—it may compressed
(Known as hemodynamic vice)

- *Cardiac type:*

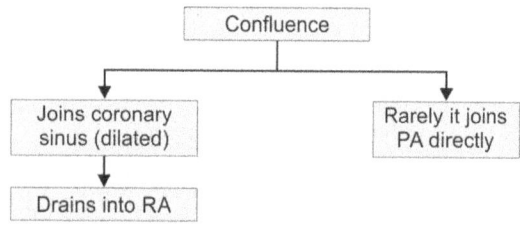

Rarely gets obstructed

Supracardiac may get compressed due to
- Abnormal course—extrinsic compression
- Intrinsic compression
- Obstruction at site of drainage
- Restricted ASD/DFO (acts as venous obstruction)

Infracardiac type: confluence
↓
Abnormal vascular channel
(vertical vein)
↓
Enter abd. through esophageal hiatus
↓
Terminate into portal vein near its origin
↓
Pulm venous blood then comes in hepatic vein-IVC-RA

Rarely it can join: Hepatic vein, or IVC directly
[Always associated with obstruction]
Obligatory shunt ASD/PFO has to be present

HEMODYNAMICS

Depends on
- Size of ASD/PFO
- Obstructive type is non obstructive
- Relative resistance of PVR and SVR

Unobstructive type
Supracardiac
(may get obstruction)
↓
Similar to ASD

Obstructive type
Infracardiac
- Discrete or diffuse
  1. At site of entry in diaphragm
  2. Or at joining to portal vein
  3. Portal circulation in liver acts as an obstruction to venous return
↓
Similar to MS

1. *Unobstructed type:*
RA receives entire venous return
↓
PA-LA shunt
(ASD/PFO size determines systemic blood flow)
↓
After birth, PVR decreases and RV compliance increases
↓
More blood directed to RV
↓
Pulm circ 5 times more than syst circ
↓
RV failure
↓
[Char: RAP and LAP are equal
−O₂ sats in all cardiac chambers are equal]
↓
As disease progress, PVR increases
↓
Increase systemic desaturation, so cyanosis becomes prominent

2. *Obstructive type:*
Obstruction to flow
↓
Pulm venous pr increases
↓
Increases capillary pr
↓
Interstitial and alveolar edema
↓
Infant becomes sick and die due to pulm edema
↓
Immediate relief to venous obst is only solution

C/F

Depends on
- Presence/absence of obst to pulm venous return
- PVR
  - Without pulm venous obstruction and low PVR

    (Similar to large ASD)
    - Dyspnea ⎤
    - Tachypnea. ⎬ During feeding—Indicates CHF
    - Diaphoresis ⎦
    - Mild cyanosis
    - Symptoms from 1st month of life
    - 80% die due to CHF before 1 year
    - Peripheral pulses will felt
    - Prominent precordial pulsation with RV impulse
    - Hepatomegaly (due to CHF)
    - S1 loud and single
    - S2 wildly—fixed split with loud P2
    - RV S3 present
    - ESM (3-4/6) one upper lt sternal border (due to pulm flow)
    - PSM (of TR)
    - MDM (flow across TV)

Few cases: Cont murmur over upper lt sternal border- indicates obstructive type of supracardiac TAPVC (flow across obstructed vertical vein)
  - Cont murmur can be heard in nonobst type also due to cont flow through venous confluence, vertical vein or innominate vein
- Without obstruction and high PVR
  - Symptoms of high flow disappear
  - Symptoms of low C.O. and cyanosis become more apparent
- With PV obstruction
  - Tachypnea ⎤
  - Tachycardia. ⎬ Within few hours of birth
  - Cyanosis (severe) ⎦
  - Death from pulm edema and RV failure within few days or weeks of life
  - Pulm edemas do not develop because of
    - Excessive pulm lymphatic flow
    - Alternate pulm bypass channel
    - Reflex arteriolar constriction

So pulm edema do not develop at cost of giving rise to pulm HTN and pulm obstructive vascular disease—RV failure
  - Minimal cardiac findings
  - Signs of PAH
  - No cardiac enlargement
  - Diffuse RV type apical impulse
  - S1 normal
  - S2 closely split, loud P2
  - Short systolic murmur at base due to dilated PA
  - Liver enlargement

ECG

Nonobstructed: ECG similar to large ASD RAD, RAG, RVH
- *Obstructed:*
  - Tall packed p(RAE) and RVH
  - qR in V1-V2 (RVH)

CXR

Nonobstructive
- RA and RV enlargement
- Lung fields plethoric

Pathognomic: "figure of 8", "snow man" or "cottage loaf" appearance: when left vertical vein connects with left innominate vein and then with left innominate vein and then with right SVC

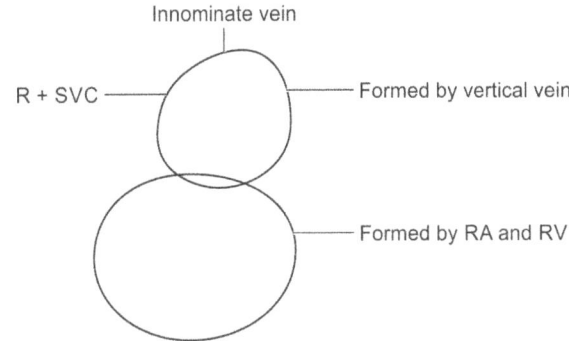

Cardiac Type
- Cardiomegaly
- Enlarged RA appendage

Obstructive Type
- Distention of pulm vein and lymphatics
- Interstitial edema
- Ground glass appearance of lung fields
- Occ.-kerley B lines
- Pulm edema—bat wing app

ECHO

Method of choice
Imp finding: not a single vein entering LA
- Feature of RVVO, RAE, RVH
- Common venous confluence can be imaged behind LA in SAR/suprasternal view
- Confluence can be traced joining systemic vein
- Rt to lt flow across ASD

- CS—dilated if confluence connected to it
- In infra diaphragmatic type, venous channel from confluence can be traced through diaphragm to portal vein
  (Nonpulsatile channel with continuous flow with direction away from heart)

CT and MRI

Not often used

Cardiac Cath

If echocardiography is in conclusive pathognomonic sign: Sats (45–92%) similar in oil chamber and great vessels

Selective pulm vein/artery angiograph
- If pulm vein can't be entered, PA angio done
- PA angio in levophase shows anomalous venous connection—Snowman's cardiac contar
- Angio directly into common venous channel with outline its course
- Infracardiac type
  Connection of common PV to portal vein is very characteristic and described as tree in winter
- When PV drainage occurs to CS positive angiographic picture in described as "golf ball appearance"

MANAGEMENT

- *Medical:*
  - Anti-congestive measure
  - Metabolic acidosis correction
  - Infant with severe pulm edema—intubated and ventilated
  - Some patient with pulm HTN—PGE, increases systemic flow by keeping duct open
  - *BAS:* If size of interatrial communication is small and immediate surgical treatment is not possible/not indicated
- Surgery
  - Obstructive type: Operated in newborn period soon after diagnosis
  - Nonobstructive type: between 4-6 months
    - No palliative surgical treatment
    - Definitive surgical treatment is necessary for all
    - *Aim:* Redirect pulm venous return to LA

Supra cardiac type: Large side-to-side anastomosis between common PV and LA

Cardiac type: Unroofing of coronary sinus to make communication between CS and LA

Infra cardiac type: Large vertical anastomosis between common PV and LA

Surgical treatment 5–10% (for unobstructed)
                20% (for Infracardiac)

COD-post op paroxysmal PHTN
    Pulm vein stenosis

FOLLOW-UP

- 6–12 monthly follow-up
- Pulm vein obstruction at surgical treatment anastomotic site develop within 6–12 month after repair
- Atrial arrhythmias
- Activity restriction unnecessary

5.27 TETRALOGY OF FALLOT

HISTORY
- First mention by Neil Stenson in 1671
- Described by Arthur Fallot in 1888
- Blue baby described by William hunter—1785
- BTT shunt—1945
- 1st total intra cardiac repair—Lillehei (1954) and Kirkin (1955)

DEFINITION
Four classical clinical abnormalities:
1. Stenosis of pulm Art—infundibular PS
2. Interventricular communication—nonrestrictive, peri-membranous, maligned VSD
3. Deviation of origin of aorta to the right-overriding of aorta
4. RV hypertrophy—almost always concentric

EPIDEMIC
- MC cyanotic heart disease encountered after infancy
- 5th most common heart defect
- 0.8% of all CHD
- 1 in 3,600 live births
- M:F = 1:1
- *Risk factors*
  - Recurs in families and siblings
  - Maternal DM (3 fold increased risk)
    Maternal phenylketonuria
    Maternal use of retinoic acid, Trimethadione

ASSOCIATION
- 22q11 deletion-CATCH 22
- Down syndrome
- Velo Cardio facial syndrome
- Goldenhar's syndrome
- Digeorge syndrome
- Poland's syndrome (absence of pectoralis major)
- Syndactyly
- Absent thumb and 1st metacarpal
- Brady dactyly with hypoplasia of ipsilateral hand
- Alagille syndrome
- CHARGE association
- VACTERL association

EMBRYOLOGY

Infundibular septum deviated anteriorly and cephalad and not aligned with trabecular septum
↓
Malalignment of infundibular septum
↓
Deviated infundibular septum encroaches on RVOT and causes infundibular RS and overriding of aorta
↓
Responsible for systemic systolic pressure in RV and concentric RV hypertrophy

ANATOMY
- RVOT obstruction
  - Infundibular (50%) ⎤ Pulm valve frequently
  - Valvular (20-25%) ⎦ Stenotic and bicuspid (40%)
  - Infundibular + valvular (20-25%)
  - Supravalvular and pulm art stenosis (rare)
- VSD
  - Maligned, nonrestrictive
  - Located in perimembranous septum with extension into infundibular septum
  - Fibrous continuity between Aortic and mitral annulus is preserved
- Overriding
  - Varies from 15-95%
  - Rt sided arch in 25%
- Coronary Anomalies
  - LAD from right coronary sinus (5%)
    → Coursing in front of infundibulum
  - Single coronary artery from rt sinus (4%)
  - Large conal branch from RCC (15%)
- Other
  - ASD (15%)/PFO (83%)
  - L-SVC (11%)
  - Additional VSD (5%)
  - Coexistence of TOF + AVSD (trisomy 21)
  - Rt sided ao arch (25%)
  - AR due to infective endocarditis, trauma and progressive aortic root dilatation LPA stenosis

MAPCA

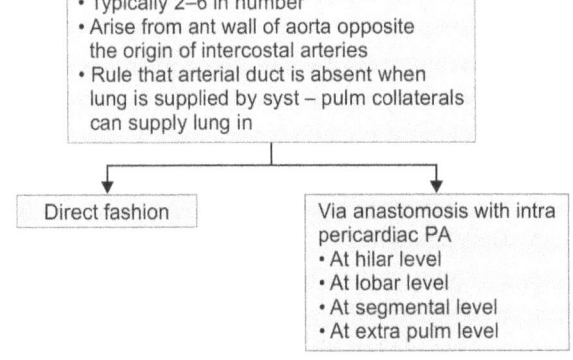

- Typically 2–6 in number
- Arise from ant wall of aorta opposite the origin of intercostal arteries
- Rule that arterial duct is absent when lung is supplied by syst – pulm collaterals can supply lung in

Direct fashion

Via anastomosis with intra pericardiac PA
- At hilar level
- At lobar level
- At segmental level
- At extra pulm level

Hemodynamics

Determined by
- Degree of obstruction to PBF
- SVR

↓

Determine direction and magnitude of shunt

Fetal circulation: Not affected
Fetus grow normally

Neonatal circulation:

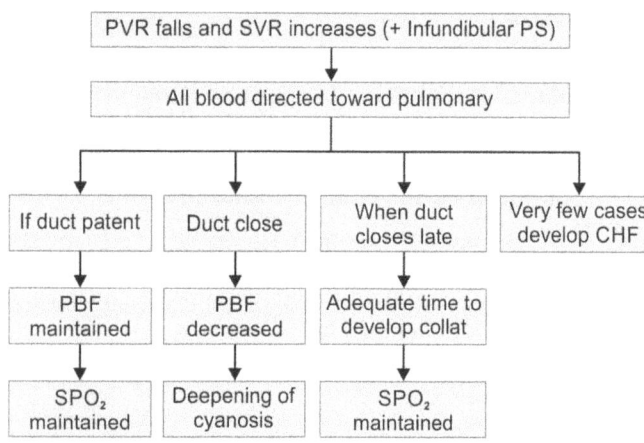

Four phase:
1. *Precyanotic phase:* Due to mild PS and low PVR
2. *Early cyanotic phase:* Blood flow to syst and pulm circuit is balanced
3. *Cyanotic phase:* Obstruction to RVOT increases and rt to lt shunt established
4. *Extremely cyanotic:* Severe PS or atretic PV; or PDA closes early

CLINICAL FEATURE

Three types
- Deep cyanosis with no murmur or faint ejection systolic murmur (severe RVOT obstruction)
- Mild-mod cyanosis with ejection syst murmur (less severe but significant RVOT obstruction)
- No cyanosis with prominent ESM (mild RVOT obstruction and good PBF) pink TOF
  - *TOF with mild PS*
    - Grows normally and asymptomatic till late childhood
    - Fatigability, breathlessness, weakness on exertion
    - Cyanosis on exertion
    - May develop CHF due to significant lt-rt shunt
    - Develop mild-mod cyanosis in childhood due to
      - Progressive increase in RVOT obstruction
      - Increased O_2 req. in growing child
      - Shift of predom Hb from fetal to adult type
  - *TOF with mod-severe PS:*
    - Symptomatic from beginning
    - Cyanosis from infancy
    - Cyanotic spell and exertion
    - Cyanotic spell depends on severity of RS
    - Growth retarded
    - Cyanosis from birth (TOF with PA)

Dyspnea

Isotonic exercise—fall in SVR-Increase veno-arterial mixing—rt to lt shunt—exercise induced hypoxemia and hypercarbia—stimulate respiratory center and carotid body—hyperventilation—perceived as dyspnea

Cyanosis

Due to dynamic infundibular spasm

Hypoxic Spells

- Dramatic and alarming feature of TOF
- Peak incidence 2nd and 6th month
- Few spells after 2 years of age
- Dare in adults
- Typically begins with stress of feeding, crying, bowel movement, awakening from long deep sleep
- Sometimes occur without precipitating cause
- Begin with progressive increase in rate and depth of breathing
- Results in paroxysmal hyperpnea, deepening cyanosis, limpness, syncope
- Occasionally convulsion, CVA and death

PATHOPHYSIOLOGY

- *Paul Wood Theory:* Dynamic RVOT obstruction caused by sympathetic stimulation—direct RV blood into the aorta

Accepted
- *Morgan's theory:* Vulnerable respiratory control mechanism, especially sensitive after prolonged deep sleep, react to sudden increase in cardiac output provoked by feeding, crying or straining

Cyanotic spells in: TOF, TGA with VSD with PS; severe valvular

PS with VSD: DORV with PS: single vent with RS

Sympathetic stimulation—HR and CO increases—venous return increases—rt to shunt increases (as there is fixed RVOT obstruction)—hypoxemia and hypercarbia—vulnerable respiratory center and carotid body overreacts—hyperpnea—further increased CB—vicious cycle

Infundibular contraction reinforces this pattern but does not initiate is

Accepted
- *Guntheroth theory:* Sleep sensitive respi center over react to this chemical stimuli
- *Young's theory:* Arrhythmias precipitate it
- *Kothari's theory:* Stimulation of mechanoreceptor present in RV cavity
  - Relief from spell
    - *Squatting:* Increased compression over abdominal aorta (Femoral arteries)—increased SVR and decreased CO and decreased venous return
    - Sitting with legs down underneath
    - Standing with legs crossed
    - Infant held in knee—chest portion
    - Lying down
  - Can lead to (repeated spells)
    - Brain damage
    - Mental retardation
    - Cerebral venous sinus thrombosis
    - Brain abscess
    - Cerebral embolism
    - Hyper nasal resonance or nasal speech

MANAGEMENT

Aim: Relieve pain and anxiety
Increase systemic vascular resistance
Increase PBF

- Infant should be picked up and held in knee—chest
- Most spells are self-limiting
- If no improvement in few mins—start O_2 and obtain IV access
  - IV bolus of colloid/crystalloid—increased intra-vascular volume—increased pro load and improve CO
  - IV/IM morphine (0.1-0.2 mg/kg) to relieve pain and anxiety (reduce endogenous catecholamine release—decreased HR and RR)
  - IV propranolol (0.015-0.02 mg/kg) or esmolol (0.5 mg/kg over 1 min)—lower HR and improve diastolic filling—improve CO
  - IV sodabicarb (1 mEq 1 kg)—only if there is worsening of acidosis despite above measures
  - *Unremitting cases:* IV vasoconstriction e.g.: Phenylephrine (0.005-0.001 mg/kg) or norepinephrine (0.05-1 µg/kg 1 min)
  - Rarely anesthesia, intubation and ventilation
  - *Very rarely:* Emergent surgical treatment intervention and mechanical circulatory support

Signs

Physical appearance
- Usually underdeveloped
- *Cyanosis:* Symmetrical; absent to severe
- *Arterial pulse:* Normal (irrespective of severity of PS)
- Brisk arterial pulse with wide pulse or
  - Large MAPCA
  - AR
- JVP-normal in height and wave form
- Prominent A wave seen in
  - Accessory tricuspid leaflet tissue partially occlude VSD—RV syst pressure is suprasystemic—RA pr increases
  - Systemic HTN—increased RVEDP—RA contracts forcefully
  - Acquired As or BAV

Inspection and palpation
- Precordial impulse is gentle (like impulse of a normal neonatal RV)
  - 4th and 5th ICS
  - Subxiphoid area
- LV impulse absent: underfilled LV
- Dilated right aortic arch
  - Impulse at rt sterno-clavicular junction
  - Aortic component of S2 palpable
- Pulmonary thrill
  - In cyanotic TOF

Auscultation:
- S1: Normal
- S2: P2 is soft or absent
- With pulm atresia—P2 absent

Trilogy: PS + RV hypertrophy + ASD/PFO (No VSD)
Counter clock associated AVCD + LAD
- Ao ejection click: Marker of severe PS
- ESM in pulm area—due to infundibular stenosis—3rd LICS
- Murmur of VSD
  When shunt is balanced-VSD silent
- Cont murmur
  - Sign of pulm atresia
  - MAPCA
- Diastolic murmur -AR

Adult TOF
Specific features
- Male predominance: 2:1
- Dyspnea—MC (95%)
- Cont murmur more common—over infra scapular and axillary area
- AR—7% (Infective endocarditis)
- Congenital BAV or prolapse of aorta RCC)
- Cardiomegaly—due to AR or PR, HTN, IE, large MAPCAs

ECG

P wave normal; PR interval normal
- QRS axis—same as that of healthy newborn

RAE in adult
RVH in adult/child

- Clock wise depolarization
- *RVH:* Tall monophase R in V1—abrupt transition to rs to V2
- Rs in V2-V6 (decreased PBF with underfilled LV)
- Small q and well-developed R in V5-V6 (balanced shunt)
- Deep q in left precordial and relatively tall R (lt-rt shunt)

CXR

Normal size of heart
- Boot shaped–coeur en sabot
  - Small underfilled LV that lies above horizontal IVS
  - Concentrically hypertrophied but nondilated RV which lies inf to LV
  - Concave MPA segment
- Pulm vascularity reduced
- Middle and outer 1/3rd of lung field displays paucity of vasc markings
- Lacy pattern of vascularity in severe TOF due to well-developed collaterals

ECHO

Investigation of choice
- PLAX: VSD; degree of override
- Basal SAX: RVOT and proximal pulm arteries
  - Degree of PS
  - Presence of PDA
  - Coronaries
  - Size and confluence of MPL, LPA, RPA

Cath

Less frequently done
    Kugelberg's classification for early surgical treatment repair

Indices to decide about transmular patch (Based on ECHO/Angio)
- Black stone/Kirklin index
- NAKATA index
- AAC Goon index
- Natio index

Management

- Recognize and treat hypoxic spells
- Oral propranolol (0.5–1.5 mg/kg every 6 hrs) to prevent hypoxic spells (while waiting for surgical treatment)
- Balloon dilatation of RVOT and PV (attempted to delay repairs)
- Relative iron deficiency should be detected and treated

Surgical

A. Palliative shunts:
Indication: to increased PAF
- Neonatal TOF and pulm atresia
- Infant with hypoplastic pulm annulus which require transmular patch for repair
- Child with hypoplastic PAs
- Unfavorable coronary anatomy
- Infant younger than 3–4 months
- Infants weighing <2.5 kg

Options

- BT shunt- classic (for >3 month age) subclavian art to I/L PA
  Modified (for <3 months) using Gore-Tax interposition shunt (lt sided for lt Ao arch)
- *Waterson shunt:* Ascending aorta and RPA
- *Dott's shunt:* Descending Ao and LPA

B. Complete surgery repair:
Indication
1. O_2 sat <75–80%
2. Symptomatic infant who have favorable RVOT and PA anatomy-primary repair anytime after 3–4 months
3. Asymptomatic, acyanotic or minimally cyanotic - many centers prefer surgical treatment by 1–2 yrs of age
4. Mildly cyanotic infants who had previous shunt-total repair at 1–2 years
5. Asymptomatic with coronary defects—after 1 year

Mortality: 2–3% during first 2 years
    At risk <3 month and >4 years
        Severe hypoplasia of RVOT and PA
        Multiple VSD, large MAPCD, Down syndrome

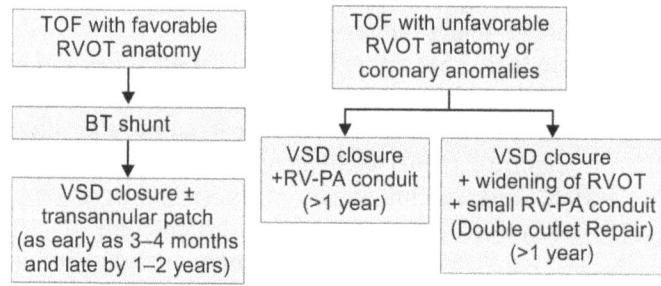

POST OP

Long term follow-up
- Every 6–12 months
- Check for residual RVOTO, residual VSD, PR, conduction disturbance, arrhythmias

- Residual RVOTO
  - Well tolerated immediate post-op
  - Due to inadequate relief of sub pulm obstruction or obstructed restrictive small PA
  - Present with murmur and raised RV presence
  - Long term—need for reoperation due to RV dysfunction and arrhythmias
- Residual or unrecognized VSD
  - Small 3-4 mm VSD—even if small it's poorly tolerated because of associated PR, noncompliant RV and unprepared LV for vol overload
- Significant PR
  - Well tolerated for decade or 2
  - Eventually RV dilatation and dysfunction
  - Require surgical homograft pulm valve
  - RV function best determined by MRI
  - PVR done when
    - RV regurgitation fraction ≥25% +
    - QOR more of following

- Criteria by Gera T
  - RVEDV ≥160 mL/m² (normal <108)
  - RVEDV ≥70 mL/m² (normal <47)
  - LVEDV ≥65
  - RVEF ≥45
  - RV OT aneurysm
  - *Clinical:* Ex intolerance, syncope, HF, QRS >180, VT
- Criteria by Lee et al.
  - RVESV ≥80
  - PVEDV ≥163
- Electrical problem
  - RBBB—almost all cases
  - Patchy vent fibrosis—increased risk of arrhythmias
  - Transient CHB-JET
- RV fibrosis
  - All TOF repair has RVOT fibrosis
  - Over half of patients also had patchy LV fibrosis
- RV dysfunction
  - Restrictive noncompliant RV
  - 28–67%

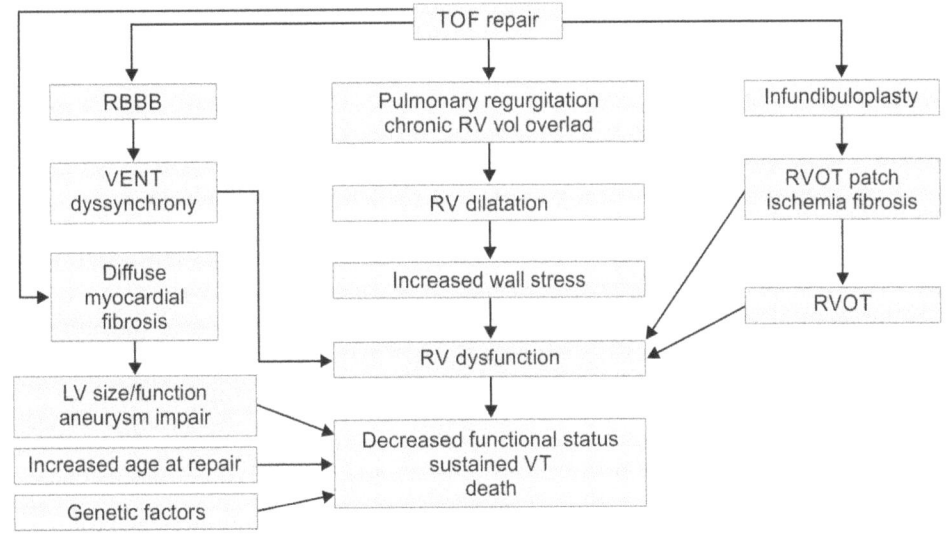

5.28 CYANOTIC CONGENITAL HEART DISEASE

TRICUSPID ATRESIA

Q.1 TA diagnosis and management
Q.2 Embryogenesis; C/F; investigation of tricuspid atresia

DEFINITION

Defined as genesis of morphological tricuspid valve including inlet portion of RV
  No communication between RA and RV

HISTORY

- First described by Kreysing 1817
- Tricuspid atresia term given by Schuberg (1861)
- First classification by Kuhne (1906) on basis of pulm blood flow
- Most popular classification
  Edwards and Burchell
- Fontan procedure was done for TA first in 1971

INCIDENCE

- 2.7% of all congenital heart diseases
- 1:15,000 live births
- M:F = 1:1 (if associated TGA → M>F)

EMBRYOGENESIS

Exact pathogenesis—not known
- Abnormal development of AV canal ⎤ During
- Failure of migration of AV orifice ⎥ 4th/5th
  in either ventricle   ⎥ week of
- Early fusion of endocardial cushion ⎥ intrauterine
  on rt side   ⎦
  ↓
  Give rise to tricuspid atresia

Genetics: Associated with
- Microdeletion of 22q11
- Trisomy 13, 18, 21
- Mutation on chromosome 3, 4, 8
- Inactivation of zfpm 2 gene
- Involvement of TGF β/BMP and NOTCH pathway

CLASSIFICATION

- Edward and Burchell (1949)
  - TA with normally related great arteries
  - TA with d-transposed great arteries
  - TA with l-transposed great arteries
  Given in Moss and Adams
- Tandon and Edward classification
  (Modified by Keith)
  Type 1: TA with related great arteries (70–80%)
      A: Pulm atresia + no VSD
      B: Pulm stenosis + restrictive VSD-MC
      C: No pulm stenosis + large VSD

  Type 2: TA with d-TGA (10–25%)
      A: VSD + Pulm atresia
      B: VSD + Pulm stenosis
      C: VSD + No pulm stenosis
  Associated with other anomalies
  - Coarctation of aorta
  - Interrupted aortic arch
  - Persistent LSVC
  - Juxtaposition of atrial appendage
  Type 3: TA with l TGA/cc-TGA (<10%)
- Clinical classification by Gasul
  Group 1: TA with diminished or normal PBF
  - Without TGA
    - With pulm atresia
    - With PS or subpulmonic stenosis
    - Without PS
  - With TGA
    - With pulm atresia
    - With PS
  Group 2: TA with excessive PBF
  - Without TGA
    - With AS or aortic atresia
  - With TGA
    - Without PS
- Neimberg classification
  - Five types
  According to the nature of tissue between RA and underdeveloped RV
  1. Muscular atresia—floor of RA is muscular-(MC)
  2. Membranous atresia—floor is formed by membranous tissue
  3. Valvular atresia—tiny imperforate valvular type tissue forms the floor
  4. Ebstein's form—the valvular tissue are attached to RV; forming atrialized RV
  5. Common AV canal with the valve sealing the RV entrance—extremely rare

HEMODYNAMICS

Depends on
- Consistent features with all TA
  - Absence of tricuspid valve
  - Enlarged and hypertrophied RA
  - Hypoplasia/underdeveloped RV
    - Absent inlet portion
  - Interatrial communication
    - OS.ASD (25%)
    - PFO (75%)
  - Systemic pulmonary communication
    - VSD (restrictive or nonrestrictive)
    - Uncommonly small PDA

VARIABLE FEATURES

Ventriculo-arterial relation
- Pulmonary flow
- Interatrial communication is obligatory
- VSD is the rule rather than exception
- Flow pattern in TA

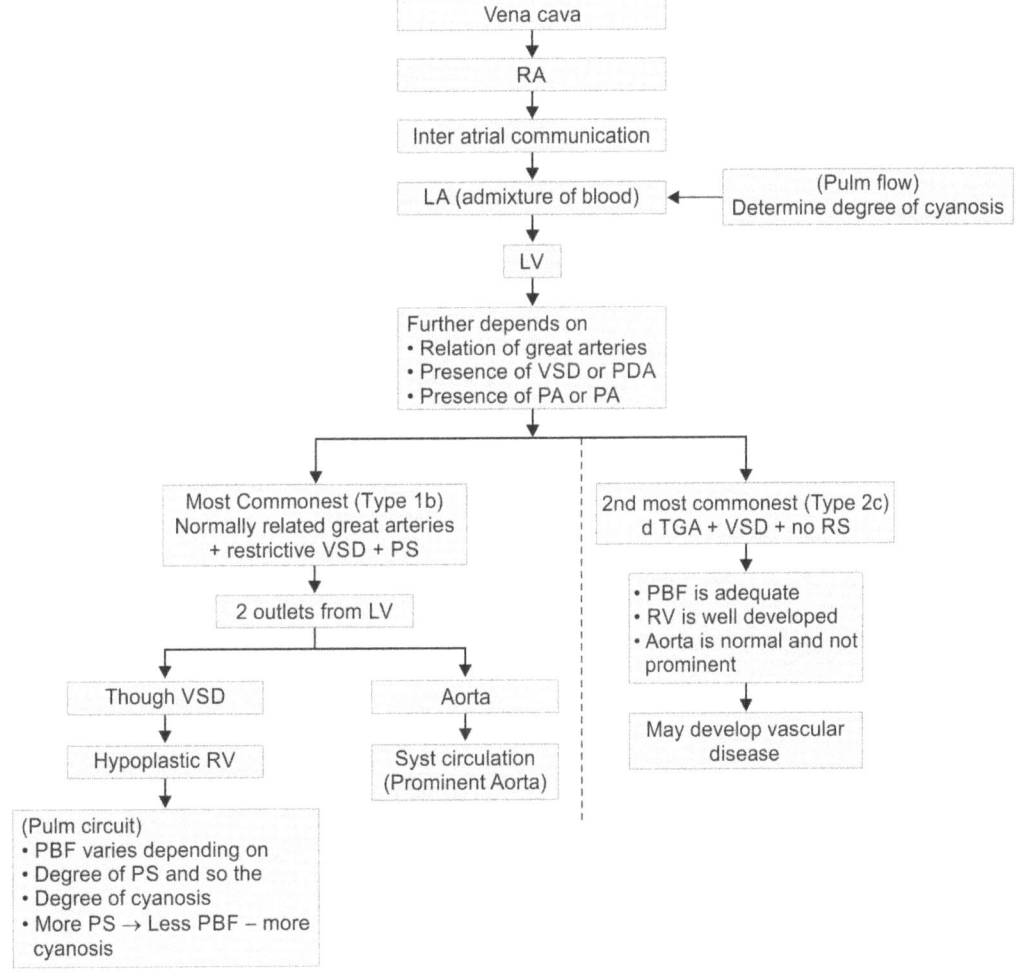

- Fate of VSD

    VSD is muscular
    ↓
    Becomes smaller with time
    ↓
    Child develop subpulmonic stenosis
    ↓
    Decreases PBF
    ↓
    Worsening of Cyanosis

- Alternative route to pulm circulation

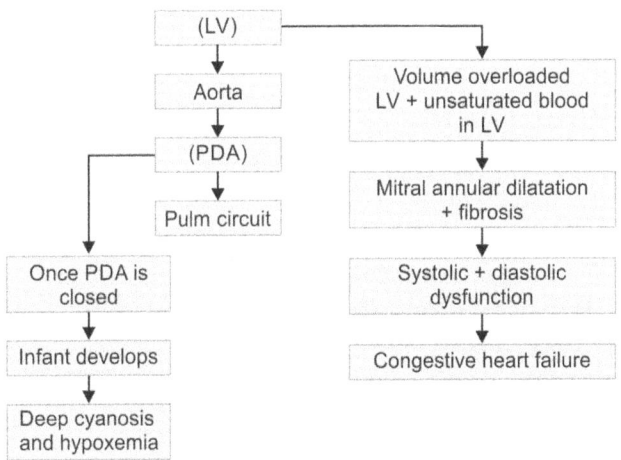

CLINICAL EVALUATION

Symptoms
- Cyanosis
  - Depends on PBF
  - Diminished PBF-more cyanosis
  - Due to
    1. Pulm atresia
    2. Pulm stenosis
    3. Restrictive VSD

  Cyanosis present since birth
  Cyanotic spells—PS more likely than PA
- Congestive heart failure
  - Progressive dyspnea
  - Feeding difficulty
  - Recurrent LRTI

  ↓

  Can be due to increased PBF (As PVR decreases after 2-3 weeks)
  Less cyanosis/no cyanosis
- Growth failure
- Others
  Headache ⎤
  Seizure ⎬ Infective endocarditis and brain abscess
  Neurological deficit ⎦

  Neurological deficit—intravascular thrombosis and embolic phenomena

SIGNS

Type 1b: TA + no TGA + restrictive VSD + RS
- Cyanosis
- Clubbing
- Normal volume pulse
- LV type apex
- RV impulse not palpable
- Raised JVP
- Single first heart sound (M1)
- Single second heart sound (A2)
  (Due to anteriorly placed prominent Aorta)
- Pan systolic murmur of VSD
- ESM in pulm area (PS)

Type 1a: TA + No TGA + PA + no VSD
- Cyanosis at birth
- Hypoxia (tachypnea) + acidosis
- Duct dependent circulation
- PDA closes-severe cyanosis
- Growth retardation
- Survival >1 year is unusual
- Raised JVP
- LV type apex
- RV impulse not palpable
- Single S1
- Single and loud S2
- Continuous murmur of PDA over left upper sternal border or infraclavicular area

Type 1c: TA + no TGA + large VSD + No PS
- At birth asymptomatic with mild cyanosis
- Symptomatic after 6-8 weeks of birth
  (Dyspnea + feeding difficulty + excessive diaphoresis)
  Due to increased PBF
- By 2-3 months of age, LVF and CHF
- LV apex
- No RV impulse
- Single S1
- Normally split S2
- LV S3 present
- PSM (due to VSD)
- Usually grow to childhood adolescent
  (Delayed milestones)
- After few years
- Easy fatigability; exercise intolerance; signs of pulmonary hypertension

Type 2C: TA + dTGA + large VSD + no PS
- Symptomatic from birth
- CHF (tachypnea, tachycardia, feeding difficulty)
- Minimal or absent cyanosis
- Subaortic stenosis—hypotension; severe CHF; severe acidosis
- Freq. respi tract infection; poor weight gain
- Peripheral and facial edema
- Low pulse volume
- Hepatomegaly
- Normal S1
- Single S2 (as aorta is anterior)
- Sometimes normally split S2
- LV S3
- Short ESM (RV out flow murmur)
- No PSM (large VSD)
- MDM (due to increased flow through mitral valve)

INVESTIGATION
- CBC—to know degree of polycythemia
- ABG—to know degree of acidosis/hypoxia
- ECG—sinus rhythm
  - May have atrial tachy/AF due to enlarged RA
  - Tall and peaked P wave (P congenital)
    Due to RA enlargement
  - If LA is also enlarged (high PBF)
    P is bifid in inferior leads
    P is biphasic in V1

- Left axis deviation or superior axis (-45° to -90°)
- rS in V1 and qR in V5-V6
  Suggest LV preponderance
- No RV forces in rt precordial leads
- T inversion in V5-V6 (older children)
- Signs of LVH

CXR

Depends on type
- With decreased PBF
  - Normal sized cardiac silhouette
  - Decreased pulm vascular markings (80%)
- With increased PBF
  - Cardiomegaly
  - Increased pulm vascular markings
- Common features
  - Prominent right border (RA enlargement)
  - LV enlargement
  - Prominent pulmonary (under developed MPA/PA)
  - Prominent ascending aorta
  - Rt sided arch: 5-8%

ECHO

(can also be diagnosed by fatal ECHO)

2D
- Absence of tricuspid valve (echodense band)
- Discordant ventricular cavity size (LV>RV)
- Nearly normal sized RV infundibulum
- Enlarged RA
- Enlarged and hypertrophied LV

Doppler
- Absence of any flow from RA-RV
- Flow across interatrial communication
- Presence of VSD
- Relation of great arteries
- Degree of PS

Limitation of ECHO
- Can't differentiate severe PS from PA
- Distal pulm artery not seen
- PVR cannot be assessed

TEE: provide details
- CoA
- AS/subvalvular AS
- Interrupted aortic arch
- Persistent LSVC

Cardiac Cath

- Necessary before surgery
- To estimate pulm artery pressure and PVR (for PA banding)
- For balloon atrial septostomy
- For sizing MPA and branch PA for Fontan surgery

Findings
- RA pressure always elevated (5-15 mm Hg)
- PA pressure is low (except high PBF situations)
- LV and RV pressure normal (for nonrestrictive VSD)
- Mostly LV pressure >RV pressure
- LV-Ao pullback gradient present
  (If sub aortic stenosis present)
- Saturation of LA, LV and RA are almost equal
- RA angiogram opacifies LA and LV
- LV angio: gives info about LV and RV size, site of VSD, relation of great vessels; degree of PS; PA, degree of As/subvalvular As; distal PA
- Angiogram also excludes CoA; persistent LSVC

CT/MRI

- Superior to ECHO
- Can be recommended before surgical correction if any doubt

PROGNOSIS

Depends on
- Size of interatrial communication
- Relation of great arteries
- Pulm blood flow
  - Size of VSD
  - Degree of PS/PA
  - PVR
  - Patency of PDA
    - Overall 9 out of 10 due before 10 years
    - Rarely they reach 3rd decade
    - Worse prognosis for high PBF group
    - Worse prognosis for d TGA group

Usually due before 6 months of age

MANAGEMENT

- Initial medical management
  - Prostaglandins (PGE1)
    - To maintain patency of PDA
    - In neonates with severe cyanosis
  - Management of CHF
    - Digoxin/diuretics/vasodilators

- Prevention of bacterial endocarditis or thromboembolic events
- Infants with TA + normally related great arteries + adequate PBF through VSD
  ↓
  Close observation for hypoxia which may develop when VSD tends to reduce in size
- Infants
  Palliative procedures (*Stage 1*)
  (Before definitive fontan like surgery can be performed)
- In patients with cyanosis at birth
  Increased PBF by
  - Systemic to pulm shunt
    BT shunt (branch of subclavian/carotid anastomosed with RPA)
    DKS (Damus-Kaye-Stansel) + shunt
    For infants with TA + TGA + VSD
    DKS—MPA is transected just below its bifurcation into RPA and LPA—distal end is sewn up—prox end is Anastomosed with aorta (end to side)
    - So blood from LV enters aorta via MPA stump
    Systemic to pulm shunt is done to maintain PBF
  - BDCPA (bidirectional cavo-pulmonary anastomosis) in older Infants
  Note: Shunts done on RPA to avoid distortion of central PA
  - Shunt size should be <3.5 mm to avoid LV volume overload and myocardial dysfunction
- In patients with unrestricted PBF
  - PA band (caution: it may accelerate VSD clause)
- Preservation of myocardial function
  - Prevent LVVO by using relatively small sized syst to pulm shunts (<3.5 mm for neonates)
  - Avoid LV hypertrophy by reliving LV outflow obstruction
- Rashkind procedure (balloon atrial septostomy)
  - To maintain adequate interatrial communication (when it is found to be inadequate by ECHO)

*Follow-up after stage 1 Palliative procedures
- *Watch for cyanosis:* (SPO$_2$ <75%) should be investigated by cardiac cath/MRI
- *Poor growth:* Indicate large PBF tightening of PA ban should be considered

Stage 2 at 3-6 months
- BDG (bidirectional Glenn shunt)
  Also known as bidirectional cavo-pulmonary anastomosis (BDCPA)
  - End-to-side SVC to RPA anastomosis
  - Done by 2.5-3 months (by this time PVR is sufficiently low to allow passive venous flow
  - IVC blood still bypasses lungs (IVC-RA-LA)
- *Hemi fontan surgical treatment:*
  - Incision made in RAA and SVC
  - Connection is made between this opening and central PA
  - Interatrial baffle placed to direct SVC blood to PA
  - *Disadv:* Chances of damage to sinus node/sinus nodal artery

Follow-up after stage 2 procedures
- Remarkable improvement in SPO$_2$ (>85%)
  Desaturation can be due to
  - Opening of venous collaterals which decompress upper body
  - Development of pulm AV fistulas (due to lack of hepatic inhibitors factors—because IVC blood is not entering pulm circulation)
  Long term Aspirin may prevent this
- SPO$_2$ <75% → proceed with Fontan surgical treatment
  - Cardiac cath to find the cause
    (Persistent LVSC-coil closure)
- Transient HTN:
  1-2 weeks post op
  May use ACE inhibitor
- Cardiac cath after 12 months of stage 2 check for risk factors (≥2 high risk)
  - Mean PAP >18 mm Hg or PVR >2 u/m^2
  - LVEDP >12 mm Hg or LVEF <60%
  - Distorted PAs 2 degree to orev shunt
  - AV valve regurgitation

Stage 3 Modified Fontan (at 2 years of age)
- After BDG shunt
  - Cavocaval baffle or lateral tunnel with fenestration
    Benefit
    - Decompression of syst venous circulation
    - Augment cardiac output
    Drawback
    - Systemic desaturation
    - Possibility of paradoxical emboli
    - Need to close with device later on
  - Extracardiac conduit with or without fenestration
- After Hemifontan
  - Intra atrial baffle removed
  - Lateral tunnel is created to direct IVC blood to SVC—PA communication

5.29 TGA

DEFINITION

Aorta arise entirely or in large part from RV and PA arise entirely or in large part from LV-creating ventriculo arterial discordant connection

(Also known as d-TGA: 'd' indicates d-bulbovent loop that places aorta right and anterior to PA)

HISTORY

- First description: 1797
  - Term given by Ferre 1814
  - Major advance in treatment: Balloon atrial septostomy 1966 by Rashkind and Miller for 1st time
  - Arterial switch operation—Jatene et al. (1975)

EPIDEMIO

- 5–8% congenital heart disease
- 25% of naturally occurring death from CHD in 1st year
- 1 in 2,300 to 1 in 5,000 live births

Association: Infant of diabetic mother or prenatal exposure to sex-hormone therapy

M>F = 4:1

EMBRYOLOGY

[Theory of conal inversion]—most accepted

Normally: Sub aortic conus is absorbed and subpulmonic conus persist that moves anterior

↓

In TGA: Sub aortic conus persists

↓

Brings aorta anteriorly to connect PV (ant-vent) and subpulmonic conus absorbed

↓

Pulm valve remain posterior with continuity to mitral valve and pulm art arise from LV

PATHOPHYSIOLOGY

- *Complete TGA:* Situs solitus; d-loop; concordant AV connection; but ventriculoarterial discordance
- *Simple TGA:* TGA with intact IVS and no other significant associated lesion
- *Complex TGA:* Large VSD, large PDA and significant LVOTO, hypoplasia of RV, PA, or TA

ANATOMY

- *RV:* Thicker than normal; increased thickness with age
- *LV:* When IVS is intact—LV thickness remain static after birth—within few weeks
- LV wall has less than normal thickness—become thin walled by 2-4 months of age
- *VSD:* LV wall thickness remains well within the normal limit during first year of life
- *LV:* Cavity is ellipsoid shaped at birth—soon becomes banana shaped
- *RV:* Ultimately RV function deteriorates in face of systemic circulation
- *Pulm vasc:* PVD starts in early infancy in TGA with VSD, by end of 1 year most of infants have > grade 3 changes of health Edwards classification
- *Coronary art:* 90% cases—arise from 2 separate cusp
  - RCA accompanies morphological RV and ⎫
  - LCA accompanies morphological LV ⎭ Concordance

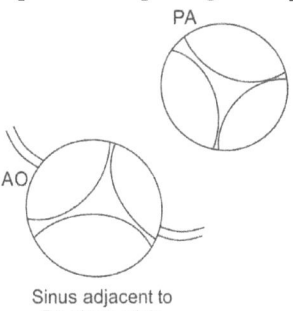

Sinus adjacent to PA gives origin To coronaries

Anomalies: LCx from RoA (16%); single RCA (4%), single LCA (2%), inverted coronaries; intramural coronaries

SA nodal artery from RCA—surgical imp

Association: 50%—no other anomaly except PFO/PDA

- VSD in 40–45% (1/3rd are small)
- VSD + LVOTO in 10%
- Isolated LVOTO 5%0

VSD: Most common associated anomaly

(Perimemb—33%; malaligned—30%; muscular → 7%; AV canal 5%; outlet 5%)

Subaortic stenosis: Caused by anterior malalignment of infundibular septum is associated with aortic arch hypoplasia, coarctation or interruption of arch

LVOTO: Product subpulmonary obstruction

May be due to fibrous memb, ⎫
fibromuscular ridge, accessory ⎬ Fixed LVOTO
mitral leaflet tissue ⎭

SAM of mitral valve ⎤ Dynamic LVOTO

Other anomalies: PDA 50%—close by 1 year

(Large PDA associated with increased incidence of PVD)

- Mitral valve abnormality 20–30%

  Partial or complete cleft of AM4, straddling of MV, abnormal papillary muscle

PATHOPHYSIO

Circulatory pathway

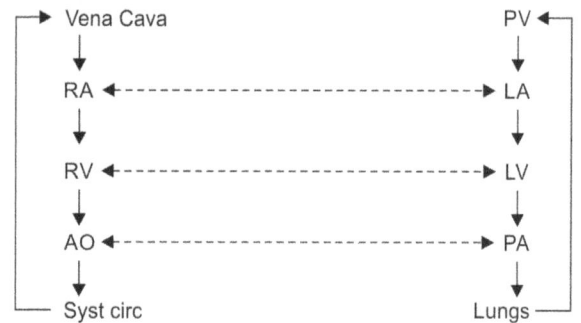

Effective syst flow: Amount of oxygenated blood passing from pulm circulation to syst circ through inter circulatory shunt
Effective PBF: Amt of deoxygenated blood passing from syst circ to pulm circ through inter circulatory shunt

Effective syst flow and effect PBF are equal
Survival depends on this

Depends on size of anatomical communication and total blood flow to pulm circuit

- When IVS in intact and duct
- Duct closes → severe hypoxemia
- 2° to in adequate mixing at

- When PVR is less
- High total PBF
- Mainatin syst O_2 sats

C/F

Male preponderance
- Cyanosis from 1st day of life in >90%
- Delayed onset of mild cyanosis with CHF—in TGA with nonrestrictive VSD or large PDA
  (Reverse diff cyanosis in TGA + PVD + large PDA)
- Necrotizing enterocolitis due to reduced mesenteric circ
  Spont closure of PDA—severe cyanosis
  When VSD + PDA—PVR increases—CHF improve at cost of cyanosis
  Severe BS/pulm atresia—intense neonatal cyanosis
  Dynamic sub pulm stenosis—responsible for hypercyanotic spells

MODES OF PRESENTATION

- Predom cyanosis; (TGA with intact IVS/small VSD and poor intercirculatory mixing)
  - Cyanosis from birth—no CHF—metabolic acidosis due to hypoxia and critically ill
- Predom CHF (TGA with large VSD/PDA and good intercirculatory mixing)
  - PVR occur early
  - Decrease PBF
  - CHF improve
  - Cyanosis worsens
- Tachypnea, tachycardia, restlessness hepatomegaly } Even on 1st day of birth
- Cyanosis not evident
- *Relatively asymptomatic:* TGA with VSD and mild LVOTO) balanced mixing
  - Asymptomatic for week or more
  - No cyanosis
  - No murmur

EXAMINATION

- S1 normal
- S2 loud A2 (because of ant position of Ao)
  PA impulse is absent (even if its dilated—Post PA)
  → S2 loud and single
  Pulm ejection click
  Syst murmur—usually not heard (except LVOTO)
  VSD—silent at birth; murmur appear after PVR falls—subsequent increase in PVR
  Shorten murmur—disappear when PVR high
- Murmur of PDA is systolic (not continuous)
  Flow from Ao—PA occur only during systole

ECG

- NSR, RAD, RVH—more marked with intact IVS
- BiVH—indicator of nonrestrictive VSD with vol overload of LV
- LAD—TGA with AV canal defect

CXR

- In neonatal—normal
- As PVR fails—oval or "egg on side" appearance mild cardiomegaly with narrow pedicle
- Increased pulm vasc masking
- Prominent pulm vasc margin—when large VSD with low PVR
  - Sometimes pulm vasc margin when large VSD with low PVR
- Sometimes pulm vascularity more marked on rt side due to rt ward flow of MPA
- rt Ao arch –8% (overall)
  - 15% (when TGA + VSD + PS)

ECHO

Method of choice for diagnosis
- Diagnosis based on demonstrating AV and ventriculo arterial relationship
- *Based PSAX:* Double circle with Ao anterior and rt of MPA
- PA and Ao distinguished by their branching pattern
- Color flow show VSD, LVOTO, prox coro abnormality
- Fetal echo can diagnose by 15 weeks of gestation
- ECHO can guide balloon atrial septostomy

Cardiac Cath

Not done routinely
- Can be done during BAS (neonate with poor mixing are candidates for BAS)
  Also in complex TGA (to know PAP, PBF, PVR)
- Distinguishing features of transposition physiology is that O_2 sat in pulm art is always higher than in Ao (however with large intracardiac mixing, sats may be similar)
  Angio may reveal ventriculo arterial discordance
  No and size of VSD, LVOTO
  Small peak syst pr diff (<20 mm Hg) between MPA and LV suggests high pulm flow and functional stenosis at PV.

NATURAL HISTORY

- *TGA and IVS:* 80% alive at 1st week but only 17% at 2 months and 4% at 1 year
  - Better survival with true ASD or adequate inter circulatory communication achieved by BAB
    75% survival at 6 months
    65% survival at 1 year
- *TGA and VSD:* Early survival is higher
  90% at 1 month; 40% at 5 months, and 30% at 1 year
  - Large PBF reduces survival
  - Obstructive PVD increases survival at 40% at 1 year
- PDA increases risk of early death
  Small duct (<3 mm)—no impact
- *TGA + VSD + LVOTO:* Early survival is better
  70% at 1 year and 30% at 5 year
  Complication: Inter current infection, polycythemia and increased viscosity

MANAGEMENT

Simple TGA → Aso (1-3 weeks) (Arterial switch)
TGA with other simple defect → Aso (1-3 wks) + Repair of other defect (PDA/VSD/dynamic CV mid PS)
TGA + VSD + severe PS → Shunt → 1. VSD-Ao Operation ± tunnel + Rastelli (1-2 yr)
2. REV procedure (>6mths)
3. Nikaidoh procedure (>1 year)

TGA + large VSD → Initial → Damus-Kaye-Stansel + sub aortic stenosis BT shunt (±) +VSD closure + RV-PA connection (1-2 years)

- *Medical:* To stabilize patient before emerg. Cardiac cath
  - Correction of metabolic acidosis; correction of hypoglycemia
  - PGE1 infusion (to improve arterial O_2 sats)
  - O_2 for severe hypoxia—lower PVR and increased PBF
  - Rashkind procedure (Balloon atrial septostomy)
    - To have some flexibility in planning surgery
  - Treatment of CHF with diuretics and digoxin
- *Surgical:* Switching of rt and lt sided blood at 3 level
  1. Atrial level (senning or mustard op)—rarely performed
  2. Vent leve (Rastelli op)
  3. Arterial level (arterial switch)—procedure of choice
  DKs + Rastelli performed for TGA + VSD + sub Ao stenos
  Arterial switch: Procedure of choice
  - Coronaries transplanted to PA and
  - Prox end of great artery—anatomic correction

COMPLICATIONS

Infrequent
- Coronary art obstruction
- Supravalvular PS at anastomotic site (~12%)—(MC)
- Neoaortic valve regurgitation and supra valve stenosis

REQUIREMENT

- LV pr—LV that can support syst circulation must be present—ASD should be performed early in life (1-3 weeks)

Two stage switch
When ASD not done in early life and LV pr is low
↓
PA banding for 7-10 days before surgery
↓
LV pr >85% of RV PV
↓
Switch operation

5.30 SEGMENTAL APPROACH

INTRODUCTION

Segmental approach by Richard van Praagh
Three segments
1. Atrial segment
2. Ventricular segment
3. Great vessel segment

Three communications
1. Venoatrial communication
2. Atrioventricular connection
3. Ventriculo arterial connections

DETERMINE VISCERAL SITUS

- Situs refers to spatial arrangement of viscera
- Three types
  1. S-solitus (normal arrangement)
  2. I-inversus (mirror image arrangement)
  3. A-Ambiguous
  When visceral position does not confer either to solitus or inversus—condition is called situs ambiguous or visceral heterotaxy
- Liver centrally placed
- Lungs and bronchi are symmetrical
- Position of stomach is abnormal
- Spleen location determines heterotaxy
- When spleen absent (asplenia)
  - Either side of midline resembles right side: Rt isomerism (aka B/L rt sidedness or IVC mask syndrome)
  - Both lungs trilobed
  - Bronchi short, straight and symmetrical
  - Central liver with 2 rt lobe (mirror image)
  - Absence of spleen—Howell Joley bodies, Heinz bodies and target cells seen in peripheral blood
  - Neonate susceptible for bacterial infection and septicemia
  - Both atria appears as RA
  - With B/L SVC and B/L SA node
  - Common in males
  - Associated with complex cyanotic CHD
  - With decreased PBF
    (e.g., bilocular heart with complex transposition, TAPVC, complex AVCD, common atrium, single vent)
  - Associated with midline defect such as tracheo-esophageal fistula, cleft lip/palate, horseshoe kidney, meningomyelocele, etc.

- Polysplenia (both side resembles left side)
  - Known as left isomerism/B/L left sidedness
  - Both lungs bilobed
  - Long and more horizontal bronchi
  - Central liver
  - Multiple small spleen (splenunculi) or both sides
  - Both atria resemble LA with B/L absence of SA node
  - Associated with PAPVC, IVC interruption with Azygos or hemiazygos continuation
  - Common in females
  - Associated with complex CHD with increased PBF and CHF
    - *ECG*—superior P axis (due to absent SA node)
    - *Extra cardiac:* Biliary atresia, esophageal atresia and other midline defect

CARDIAC POSITION AND ORIENTATION

Depends on position of heart in chest and orientation of its apex

1. Location of heart in chest
   Levoposition: To the left
   Dextroposition: To the right
   Meso position: In center
2. Orientation of apex
   Levocardia: Apex directed to left
   Dextrocardia: Apex directed to surgical treatment
   Mesocardia: Apex oriented inf in medline
3. Atrial situs

RA	LA
Triangular, broad based anterior appendage	Narrow fingerlike post appendage
Septum secundum lies on RA Side	Septum primum lies on LA side
Crista teriminalis and Eustachian valve	Smooth with flow trabeculations

How RA/LA Decided?

- Entry of IVS
  In whichever atrium IVC enters—its RA
- Same thing not true for SVC/PA
- By atrial appendage
  - Long and narrow base—LA appendage
  - Short and broad base—RA appendage

Congenital Heart Diseases

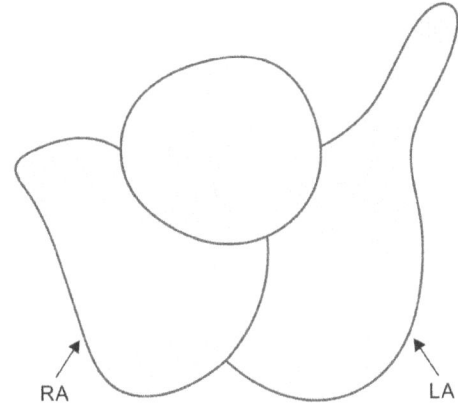

Atrial situs
- Solitus = Normal atrial position → "S"
  rt on rt and lt on lt
- Inversus = RA on lt side and → "I"
  LA on rt side
- Ambiguous = Both are LA or → "A"
  Both are RA

VENTRICULAR LOOPING

How to decide RV/LV?
- By AV valve
  - MV is always superior
  - TV is always inferior (apically)
  ↓
  Whichever ventricle receives TV → RV
- Moderator Band (in mid vent level)
  Note: Thin strands of chordae found in LV also but they are thin and near to apex
- Vent with 2 wall differentiated pap muscle is morphological LV
- LV finely trabeculated/RV coarsely trabeculated

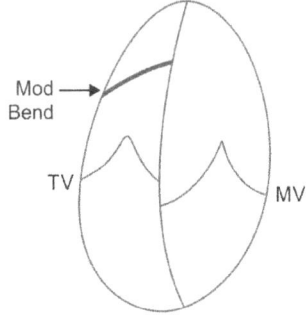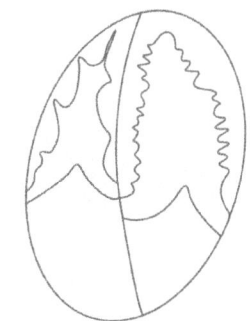

D loop = LV on left side and RV on right side – "D"
L loop = LV on right side and RV on left side – "L"

ATRIOVENTRICULAR CONNECTIONS

Concordant = normal connections
  RA → RV and LA → LV
Discordant: RA → LV and LV → RV
Univentricular AV connections
- Absent AV connections
- Common AV valve
- Double inlet connections

GREAT VESSEL SITUS

How to decide
- Vessel which go superiorly—aorta
  Posteriorly—PA
- Vessel which bifurcates—PA
  Gives branches—aorta
- Vessels which give coronaries—aorta

Situs/relationship

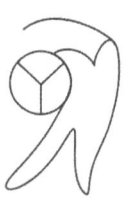 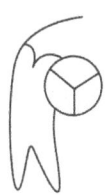

Normal relation of great arteries | Inverted relation of great arteries
↓ | ↓
Pulm valve superior and the left | PV superior and to the right
↓ | ↓
"S" solitus | "I" inversus

Aorta anterior and to rt = D malposition - "D"
Aorta anterior and to left = L malposition - "L"

VENTRICULOARTERIAL CONNECTION

- *Concordant:* Aorta from LV and PA from RV
- *Discordant:* Aorta from RV and PA from LV
  Double outlet
  Common arterial trunk
  So segmental analysis
  Normal = S, D, S
  Situs inversus dextrocardia= I, L, I
  D-TGA = S, D, D
  D-TGA with situs inversus = I, L, L
  L-TGA with situs solitus= S, L, L

SECTION 6

Endocrine System

6.1 ADRENAL AND CV DISEASE

ADRENAL GLAND CORTEX

- Zona glomerulosa → Aldosterone
- Zona fasciculata → Cortisol and some androgenic steroid
- Zona reticularis → Cortisol and androgens

Cushings
- Excessive control secretion due to
  1. Excessive secretion by adrenal gland → Cushing syndrome
  2. Excessive secretion of ACTH by pituitary → Cushing disease
  3. Excessive ectopic ACTH production by SCC lung, medullary CA thyroid and other adero CA.

MECH

Cortisol
↓
Binds 10 monomeric receptor in cytoplasm
↓
After binding, receptor dissociate from this complex
↓
Enters nucleus and serve as transcription factor

- Several cardiac gene contain glucocorticoid response element in their promoter regions
  1. Voltage gated K^+ channel
  2. Protein kinases which serve to phosphorylate and regulate voltage gated Na^+ channels

CV EFFECTS

1. HTN
2. Abnormal glucose metabolism
3. Hyperinsulinemia
4. Altered clotting
5. Altered plt function

} Accelerate atherosclerosis

HTN due to
- Change in vascular reactivity
- Increased SVR
- Impaired no mediated vasodilatation

6. Increased Sr Glucose level and insulin resistance
   Promote pro inflammatory cytokines (TNF alpha and IL6)
7. Cortisol excess can promote inflammation
8. Excess androgen production atherosclerosis

} Also promote atherosclerosis

9. Cerebrovascular disease
10. Peripheral vascular disease
11. Coro art disease
12. MI
13. CHF
14. Hypertrophy and impaired contractility
15. DCMP
16. Increased coro art calcification and plaque volume

} Increased CV mortality

17. Marked muscle weakness due to cortisol induced myopathy

} Markedly limit Ex. capacity

ECG

Duration of PR interval inversely proportional to adrenal cortisol production rate (May be due to effect on SCN5A or direct effect on voltage gated K^+ channel)

Carry complex: Cushing syndrome
↓
AD
Q2 region of chr 17

Cardiac myxoma
Pigmental dermal lesion (No cafe au lait)

MANAGEMENT

A. Transsphenoidal surgery for ACTH secreting tumor
   - Unilat adrenalectomy for adrenal adenoma/CA
   - Bilat adrenalectomy
   - Adrenal enzyme inhibitor: ketoconazole
B. Hyperaldosteronism (Conn's syndrome)
   - Sodium retention
   - HTN
   - Increased renal loss of K^+ and Mg^{++}
   - Decreased arterial compliance
   - Increased SVR
   - Alter symp and para symp neural regulation
   - Cardiac hypertrophy
   - Diastolic dysfunction
   - May promote AF
C. Addison disease: Acute addison crisis
   - Hypovolemia
   - Hypotension
   - Acute CV collapse due to renal sodium wasting, hyperkalemia and loss vasc tone

CAUSE

- B/L loss of adrenal function on an autoimmune basis due to infection, hemorrhage or metastatic malignancy
- Inborn error of steroid hormone metabolism
- HPA axis suppression

C/F

Noncardiac
- Increased pigmentation
- Abd pain with Nausea/vomiting
- Weight loss

Cardiac
- Tachycardia
- Hypotension
- Loss of autonomic tone
- Electrolyte abnormality
- Low diastolic pr (<60 mmHg) along with orthostatic changes

Newly diagnose, untreated addison → reduced LV
Eb dimension and Es dimension

Cardiac atrophy seen in
1. Addison's disease (teardrop heart)
2. Na^+ deficient diet
3. Malnutrition caused by anorexia
4. Astronauts after prolonged space flight

6.2 AMIODARONE AND THYROID FUNCTION

AMIODARONE-IODINE RISK ANTIARRHYTHMIC

- 30% iodine content by weight
- Structured similarly to levothyroxine

↓

Leads to thyroid abnormality in as many as 60% patients treated

MECH

Amiodarone
↓
Inhibits 5-mono deiodination of T4 in liver
↓
Decreased serum T3 and increased serum T4 level
Scrum TSH remains normal initially
↓
With prolonged treatment, T4 synthesis and release from thyroid gland can be inhibited
↓
Producing rise in TSH level
↓
Can progress to overt hypothyroidism

A. Hypothyroid
- 15–30% of amiodarone treated patient have hypothyroid
- Effect on thyroid function does not depend on dose
- Can occur any time after initiation of treatment
- Can occur up to 1 year after discontinuation of treatment
- Check thyroid function every 3 months

B. Thyrotoxicosis
- 10% prevalence
- Sudden onset
- Can occur shortly after initiation, during treatment and up to 1 year poststopping

C/F
- Vent irritability
- Decreased warf dose requirement
- Return or worsening of obstructive physiology of HCM

PATHOGENESIS

Two forms

Type 1: In patient with preexisting thyroid disorder common in iodine deficient areas

Type 2: Identified as a form a thyroiditis mediated by pro-inflammatory cytokines

   Primarily destructive process causing release of pre-formed thyroid hormone

   Also with low to absent radioiodine uptake

Hyperthyroidism: 8 fold increased risk of MACE

MANAGEMENT

Discontinue amiodarone: Important issue
- No evidence of stopping treatment hastening resolution of chemical hyperthyroidism
- Certain patient require amiodarone for arrhythmia—life saving
- Most of the patients have amiodarone retention in body in lipid soluble stores in excess of 6 months

Dronedarone:
- Noniodinated antiarrhythmic
- Do not alter thyroid function

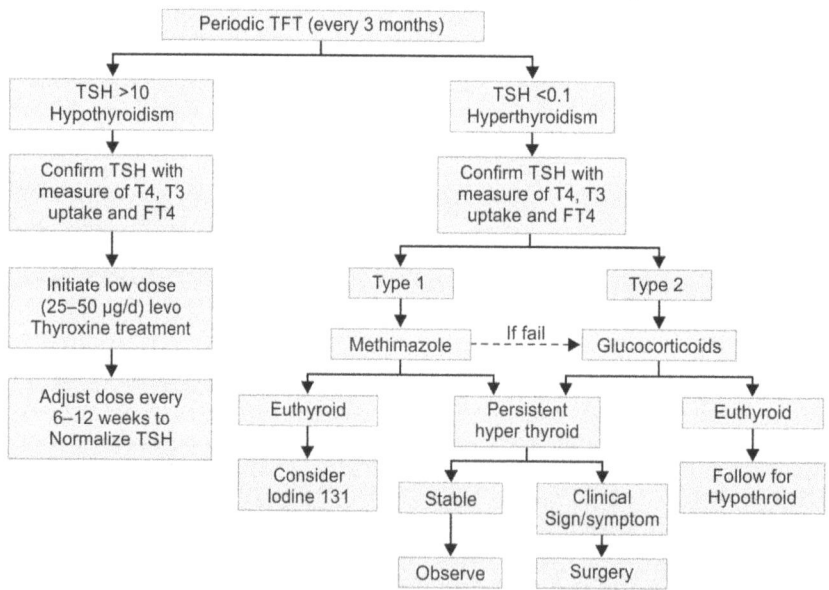

6.3 ENDOCRINE DISORDER AND CV DISEASE

GROWTH HORMONE IN CV DISEASE

Excessive hGH before fusion of bony epiphysis → Gigantism
Excessive hGH after fusion or maturity → Acromegaly

MECH OF ACTION

- Via hGH receptor on heart
- Via stimulation of synthesis of insulin like growth factor IGF1 which acts on IGF receptor.

CV MANIFESTATION

- Acromegaly is relatively uncommon
- Markedly increased mortality and mortality from CV disease
- Markedly shorten life expectancy
- <20% survive beyond 60 years
- Cause of death
  - Neoplasia from GI tract
  - Colon polyp
  - Colon CA
  - Pulm disease
    HTN
    Cardiomegaly ⎤ Also limits survival
    CHF
    CVA
- CV effects depend on
  - Age
  - Severity
  - Duration of the disease
- Recently diagnosed (<5 years)
  - No significant abnormality
  - ECHO shows increased LV mass index
  - CI also increases
  - Systolic function—stroke index increases
  - SVR increases by 20%
  - Diastolic function—normal
- Longer duration
  - LV dysfunction and cardiomyopathy
  - Global LVDD
  - Cardiac hypertrophy
  - Regional strain abnormalities

Overall

Various cardiac risk factors in patient with acromegaly
- HTN (20–40% patients)—mech not understood
- Insulin resistance
- Diabetes mellitus
- Dyslipidemia
- Significant CAD—11%
- Dilated coronaries in most cases
- Atherosclerosis and IHD are unlikely to account for marked BiV hypertrophy, CHI, and CV mortality
- 2/3rd patient have ECHO LVH ⎤ Even in absence
- RV mass increased   of HTN suggesting deleterious effect of hGH and IGF-1
- Increased prevalence of VHD
  - Progressive MR
  - Dilatation of Ao root
- Defect in cardiac conduction system
- Heart failure (treatment can prevent this)

Histology

Hypertrophy without increase in cell number
- Interstitial fibrosis
- Inflammatory infiltrates
- Apoptosis (IGF-1 promoted)

ECG

- Left axis deviation
  - Septal Q wave
  - ST-T depression
  - Abnormality QT dispersion   in 50% of patients
  - Conduction system defect
  - Dysrhythmias
    - APC/VPV
    - SSS   4 fold increased
    - SVT   risk of arrhythmias
    - VT
  - In patients with long standing acromegaly
  - Arterial initial thickness increases
  - Respond to lowering hGH
- Growth hormone promotes Na$^+$ retention and volume expansion and has potential antidiuretic effect
- ARB/ACEF causes paradoxical increase in BR in patients with acromegaly
- Increased serum insulin contribute to urinary Na$^+$ retention, impaired endothelial dependent vasodilatation, decreased no production and increased sympathetic activity.

DIAGNOSIS

- Serum hGH level >5 ngm/dL
- Serum IGF-1 level >300 mzu/mL (measured 1 hour after 100 g glucose load)
- Fasting hGH level > ng/mL
- MRI pituitary for macroadenoma (99% cases)

TREATMENT

- Transsphenoidal surgery with resection
- Octreotide-somatostatin analog
- Radiotherapy in older patients
- Dopamine/serotonin receptor agonist in younger patients
- Pegvisomant-GH receptor antagonist

6.4 PARATHYROID DISEASE

INTRODUCTION
Can produce CV disease in 2 ways
1. Change in secretion of PTH
2. Change in Sr Ca^{++} level

PTH
- Bind to its receptor-increased intracellular cAMP level- alter spontaneous beating rate of neonatal cardiac myocyte
- Can also alter Ca^{++} influx-alter cardiac contractility in adult cardiac myocyte
- PHTrP synthesized in variety of tissue (including cardiac myocyte)-stimulate accumulation of cAMP and contractile activity as well as regulate L-type Ca^{++} channels

A. Hyperparathyroidism
CV effect of hypercalcemia
- Increased contractility
- Shortening of vent –APD (due to change in phase-2 and blunting of T wave)
- Changes in ST segment
- QT interval shortened
- Decreased PR interval
- Pathological changes in myocardial interstitium and conduction system
- Calcific deposit in valve cusp and annuli
- LV cyst function maintained
- Severe/chronic disease can impair diastolic function

B. Hypocalcemia
- Prolong phase 2 of APD—QT prolongation
- Impair cardiac contractility

C. Vitamin D
- Low level of Vitamin D associated with all case and CV mortality increases

THYROID AND HEART DISEASE
Cellular mechanism of thyroid hormone action on heart

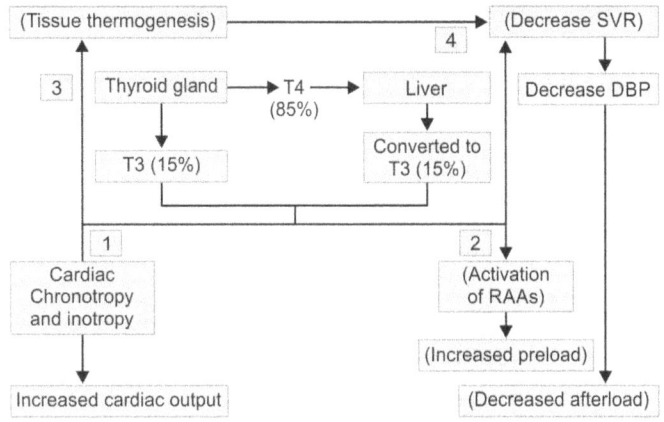

Cardiac myocyte can't metabolize T4 to T3

T3
↓
Birds to transporter protein of MCT and OAT family on cell surface transporters
↓
Enter cytosol and binds to thyroid hormone receptor
↓
Enters nucleus and birds to thyroid hormone response element in promoter region of specific gene
↓
Activate or repress gene expression

Thyroid hormone regulation of cardiac gene expression

Positively regulated	Negatively regulated
1. α-myosin heavy chain	1. β-myosin heavy chain
2. Sr Ca^{++} ATPase	2. Phospholamban
3. Na^+-K^+ ATPase	3. Na^+-Ca^{++} exchanger
4. Voltage gated K^+ channel	4. Monocarboxylate transporte of SIO
5. ANP and BNP	5. Thyroid hormone receptor α
6. Malic enzyme	6. Adenylyl cyclase type 5, 6
7. Beta adrenergic receptor	7. Guanine nucleotide binding protein Gi
8. Guanine nucleotide-binding protein Gs	
9. Adenine nucleotide transporter 1	

- Human vent mainly express Beta myosin
- SERCA (sarcoplasmic reticulum Ca^{++} ATPase)
- Determine magnitude of myocyte calcium cycling: Reuptake of Ca^{++} in early disable determine rate at which LV relaxes (IVRT)
- Phospholamban inhibit SERCA 2 activity
- Inotropic agents that enhance cardiac contractility through increase in cAMP do so by phosphorylation of phospholamban (phosphorylation discontinue inhibitory effect)

↓

Thyroid hormone inhibit expression of phospholamban and increases phosphorylation phospholamban

↓

Most of cardiac action of thyroid hormone is regulated by SERCA-phospholamban system

↓

This explains why diastolic function varies inversely across entire spectrum of thyroid disease

↓

Even mild subclinical hypothyroidism has diastolic dysfunction

↓

CV changes with thyroid diseases

	Hypo	Hyper
1. SVR	increases	decreases
2. HR	decreases	increases
3. CO	decreases	increases
4. Blood vol	decreases	increases

- T3 regulate cardiac inotropy and chronotropy through direct and indirect mechanism
- T3 increases myocardial O_2 consumption and tissue thermogenesis
- T3 decreases SVR
- Increase in pl volume coupled with increase in erythropoietin leads to increase in blood volume and rise in cardiac preload
- Lower SVR + increases preload → increases output HTN
- Arterial compliance also fall in hyperthyroidism, explaining why
  MAP and DBP is low and systolic pr increases

↓

Combination of increases CO and decreases vasc compliance leads to syst HTN (up to 30% patients)

HYPERTHYROIDISM

- Decrease cyst vasc resistance—decreases afterload increased
- Increase in pl vol and blood volume—increases afterload CO
- Increased CO + decreased vasc compliance → HTN
- Palpitation due to tachycardia caused by increased symp tone and decreased para symp activity
- Normal diurnal variation of HR is blunted and increased HR during exercise is exaggerated
- Poor exercise tolerance and capacity/exertional dyspnea
- Due to
  • Skeletal and respi muscle weakness
  • Low SVR and increased preload reduces cardiac function reserve → submaximal ex. capacity

Beta blockers ←
- Angina like pain: Due to increased workload, increased CO and increased myo O_2 demand

Calcium channel blockers ←
- Syndrome of chest pain with ischemic ECG changes due to vasospasm mainly in young females

Treat ←
- Cerebrovascular ischemic symptoms Hyperthyroid
  • Moyamoya disease
  • Anatomic occlusion of terminal portion of ICA

Treat ←
- Pulm HTN
  Hyperthyroid: Can lead to RV dysfunction
- Atrial fibrillation
  • 2–20% (15% in patients >70 years)
  • MC is sinus tachy
  • Treatment-beta blockers (Propranolol, Atenolol, metoprolol, esmolol)
  • Digitalis may help (but its clearance is increased in hyperthyroid + sensitivity of drug is decreased due to up regulation of Na^+-K^+ ATPase pump + decreased parasympathetic tone

  ↓

  Higher dose is required
  • Anticoagulation as per CHADS2 VASC score
  • Treat hyperthyroidism
  • Restoration of T2, T4 level results in reversion to sinus rhythm in 2/3rd of patients in 2–3 months
  • Electric cardioversion: >90% patients revert to SR and remain in SR
- Heart failure
  Mech
  • Increased CO and contractility ⎤ HF
    ◆ Increased resting HR ⎦
  • High output failure is not appropriate term because although resting CO is 2–3 times normal, exercise intolerance does not appear to be due to cardiac failure (its due to skeletal mu weakness/PH)

- High output state → leads to increased Na$^+$ reabsorption—fluid overload
- PAP increase in hyperthyroid—increased JVP, hepatic congestion, peri edema (RV fail)
- Long standing tachycardia and AF
- Hyperthyroid cardiomyopathy

DOE, orthopnea, PND, peri edema, increased JVP, S3
+
Failure to increase LV EF with exercise
↓
Hyperthyroid cardiomyopathy

Treatment- low dose BB + standard treatment of HF
Correction of hyperthyroidism

HYPOTHYROIDISM

- Subtle changes
- O/E
  - Mild bradycardia
  - Narrow pulse pr
  - Diastolic HTN
  - Relatively quiet precordium
  - Reduced intensity of apical impulses

INVESTIGATION

1. Increased total and LDL chol (Due to decrease in biliary excretion, decrease in LDL receptor number)
2. Ck level increase by 50% to 10 fold
   Decreased in up to 30% of patients
   (More than 96% is CKMM)

ECG

Sinus brady
- Low voltage
- Prolongation of APD
- Prolonged QT interval—predispose to vent arrhythmias

ECHO

Pericardial effusion
  May be cardiac tamponade
CV risk
- Increased risk factors for atherosclerosis (HTN, hypercholesterolemia, increased homocysteine)

- Decreased CO
- Decreased contractility

PET has shown energy inefficiency of hypothyroid myocardium (O_2 cos of work primarily because of increased SVR and after load)

- Blood volume
- Increased HR
- Noninvasive studies have suggested abnormality in perfusion -
       >suggestive of myo ischemia
       ↓
Improve with treatment of hypothyroidism

Hypothyroid treatment and coexisting CAD
- Patients younger than 50 years with no HIO heart disease
  - Generally possible to initiate full replacement dose of levothyroxine (100–150 μg/d) without concern for cardiac effects
- Known CAD and hypothyroid
  - UA, LMCA, TVD → PCI/CABG followed by thyroid hormone replacement in post op period (full dose)
  - Patients with SIHD in whom revasc is not indicated
    - Low dose levothyroxine (12.5 μg) and stepwise increases (12.5–25 μg) every 6 to 8 weeks until serum TSH levels normalize
    - Thyroid hormone replacement decrease SVR and decreased afterload—decreased clinical sign of ischemia
    - Beta blocker as concomitant therapy
- Patients who are at risk but no clinical findings
  - Low dose thyroxine 25–50 μg/d and increases by 25 μg every 6-8 weeks until serum TSH is normal hypothyroid-related myalgia—nonspecific muscle symptoms, cramping, variable ck levels. Hypothyroid-related myopathy-impaired endurance with elevation of ck levels. Hypothyroid-related Hoffmann syndrome-impaired function, pseudohypertrophy, marked elevation in ck levels. Statin-induced myalgia—muscle ache, weakness without ck elevation. Statin-induced myopathy. Statin-induced myositis-symptoms +ck elevation. Statin-induced rhabdomyolysis.

6.5 PHEOCHROMOCYTOMA

INTRODUCTION

- Benign tumor arising from neuroectodermal chromaffin cells
- Usual location: Within adrenal medulla/abdomen
- May arise anywhere within plexus of sympathetic adrenergic nerves
- Majority arises as U/L adrenal mass
- 10% familial, 10% B/L; 10% extra adrenal
- Syndromic associated
  - MEN2B:
    - Coexist with medullary CA thyroid
    - Mucosal neuromas (lips/tongue)
    - Mutation in RET proto oncogene
  - Occasionally associated with hyperparathyroidism
  - Associated with neurofibromatosis
  - VHL syndrome; cerebellar/retinal angiomas

C/F

Headache, palpitation, excessive sweating, tremulousness, chest pain, weight loss, and other constitutional syndrome

- Episode HTN
- Parodically association orthostatic hypotension in morning

CV Effect

- Increases SVR
- Increases CO (minimally)
- Increases HR
- LVH and repolarization abnormality
- Vent and atrial ectopics
- SVT
- Impaired LV function and CM pathy

MECH OF CM PATHY

- Increased LV work and LVH from associated HTN
- Adv effect of excess catecholamines on myocyte str and contractility
- Changes in coro art (thickened media)
- Catecholamine stimulates tachycardia

DIAGNOSIS

- 24 hour urinary metanephrines ← most reliable
- Provocative test
  - Aim to increase plasma cortisol level in patient with episode disease
- Clonidine suppression test
  - Safe and suppress pl norepinephrine by >50% in patients with essential HTN but not in patients with pheochromo
- CT highly sensitive
- MRI highly specific
- Elevated surgical level of dopamine → malignant transformation; tumor arising in extra adrenal site

TREATMENT

Surgical removal

- Preop pharmacological management
  - 7–14 days of α blockade (prazosin/phenoxybenzamine)
  - B-blockade only after α blockade
  - If SVT ≥ β1 selective BB (atenolol) preferred
- IV phentolamine/nitroprusside may be required to treat episode HTN during surgery
- Post op: Large vol of crystalloid to maintain BP and prevent hypotension
- Metyrosine can be used to decrease catechol syn and improve CV S/S

SECTION 7

Heart Failure

7.1 LEFT VENT REMODELING

INTRODUCTION

Neurohormonal activation
Hemodynamics alteration
Epigenetic
Genetic factor
Comorbid condition
↓
Influences LV remodeling

GENETIC FACTORS

Index event

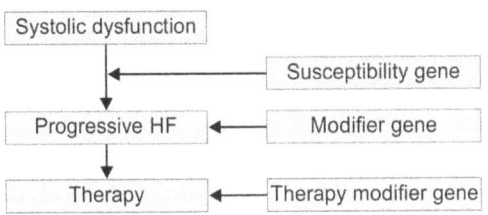

OVERVIEW OF LV REMODELING

A. Alteration in myocyte biology
   - Excitation
   - Myosin heavy chain gene expression
   - Beta-adrenergic desensitization
   - Hypertrophy
   - Myocytolysis
   - Cytoskeletal proteins
B. Myocardial changes
   - Myocyte loss (necrosis, apoptosis, autophagy)
   - Alteration in ECM (matrix degeneration myocardial fibrosis)
C. Alteration in LV chamber geometry
   - LV dilatation
   - Increased Sphericity

- LV wall thinning
- Mitral valve incompetence

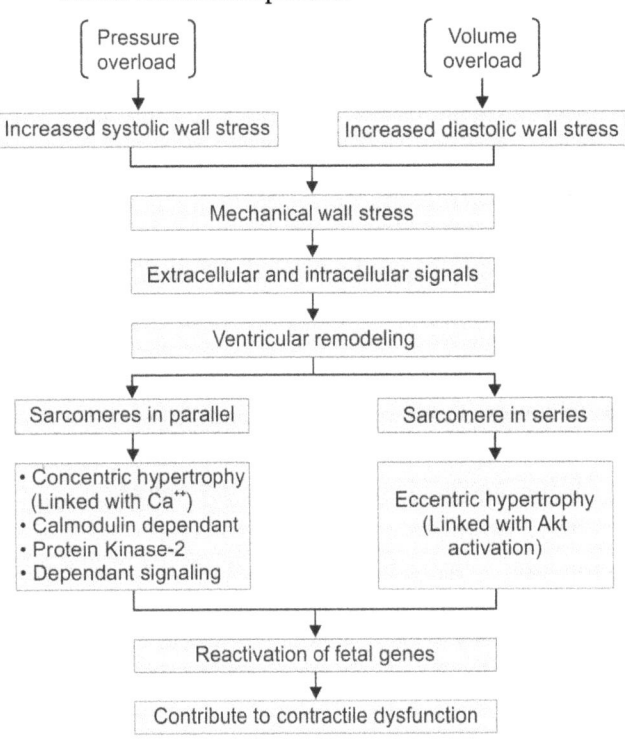

A. Alteration of myocyte biology
   ↓
   a. Decreased alpha-myosin heavy chain gene expression
   b. Increase beta-myosin heavy chain expression
   c. Progressive loss of myofilaments in cardiac myocyte
   d. Alteration in cytoskeletal protein
   e. Alteration in excitation contraction coupling and energy metabolism
   f. Desensitization of Beta-adrenergic signaling
   ↓

HYPERTROPHY AND MYOCYTOLYSIS

1. Cardiac myocyte hypertrophy
   Pr. Overload – conc. Hypertrophy
   Vol. Overload – Ecc hypertrophy
   ↓
   See chart on prev. page
   Stimulation for genetic reprogramming
   ↓
   - Mechanical stretch/strain
   - Neurohormone (NE, angiotensin 2)
   - Inflammatory cytokines (TNF alpha Il-6)
   - Other peptides (ET)
   - ROS (superoxide, No).

Early Stage of Hypertrophy

- Increase in number of myofibril and mitochondria
- Enlargement of nuclei and mitochondria
- Myocyte larger than normal
- Cellular organization preserved

As hypertrophy continues
- Increased number of mitochondria
- Addition of new contractile elements
- Disruption of cellular organization
  (Enlarged nuclei, multilobulated memb, displacement of adjacent myofibrils) preserved Z band.

Late Stage

Loss of contractile element (myocytolysis)
- Marked disruption of Z band
- Dilation and increased tortuosity of T tubule

2. Altered excitation-contraction coupling
   Impaired contraction and relaxation of failing heart at higher heart rate
   ↓
   Depressed force-frequency relationship
   ↓
   Secondary to Decreased amplitude of intracellular Ca^{++}
   b. Prolonged decline of Ca^{++} transit
   c. Increased diastolic Ca^{++} level

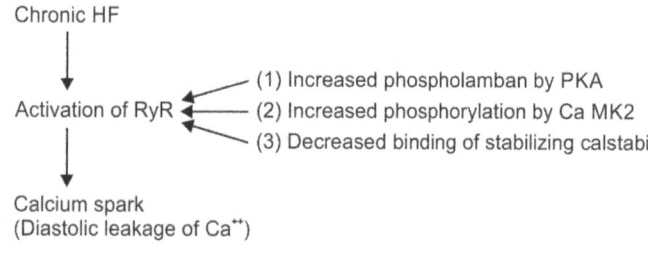

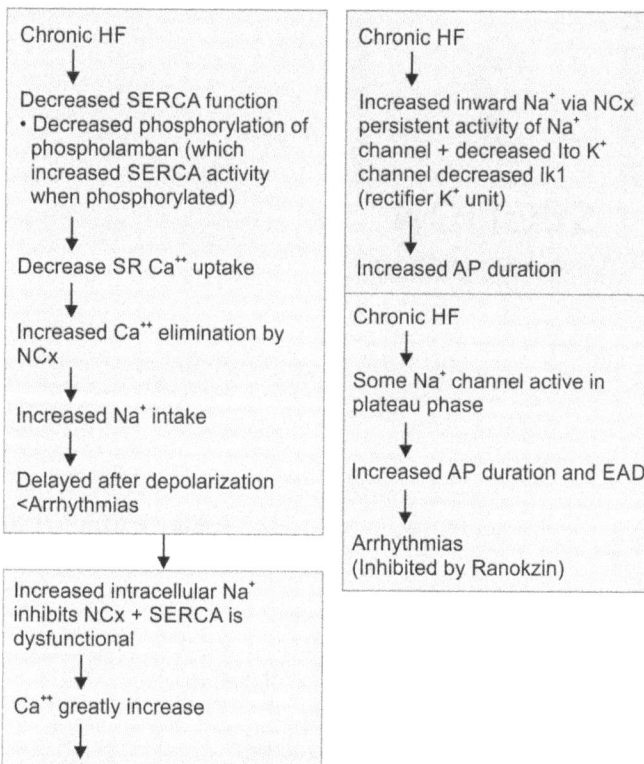

3. Abnormality of cytoskeletal and regulatory proteins

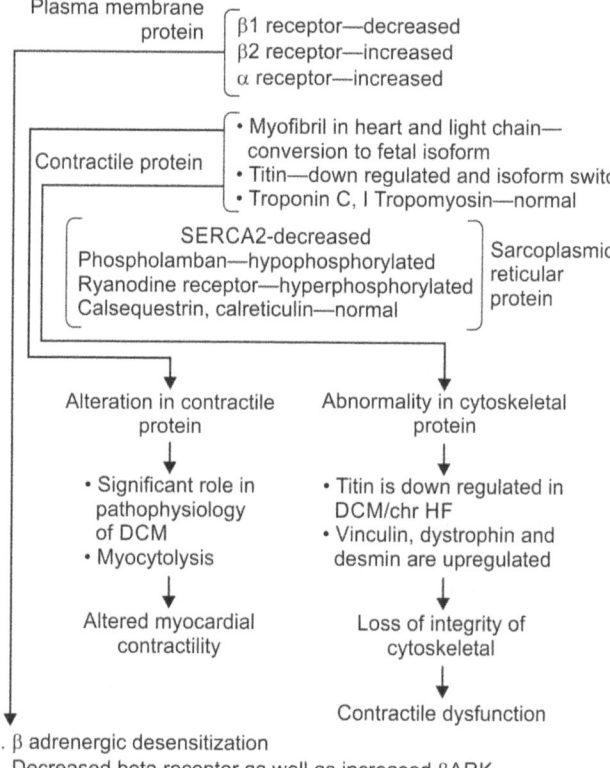

4. β adrenergic desensitization
   Decreased beta receptor as well as increased βARK
   (β associated receptor kinase) - will increase β arrestin
   ↓
   Beta arrestin desensitize both β1 and β2 receptor

DESENSITIZATION OF BETA RECEPTOR

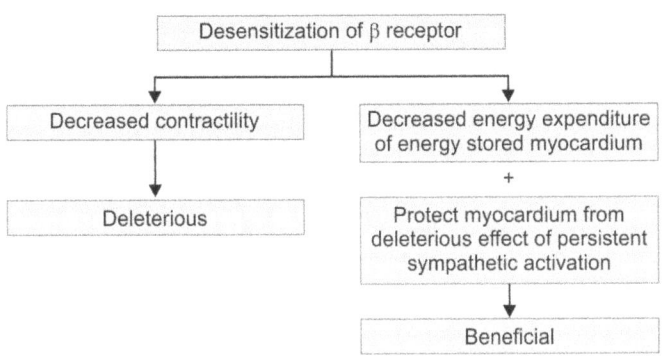

A. Myocardium changes
- *Necrosis*
  - Loss of plasma memb integrity
  - Depleted cellular ATP
  - Cell swelling and rupture
  - Swelling of mitochondria

Causes

Ischemia, myocardial injury, toxin, infection, inflammatory

Neurohormonal activation, excessive

Stimulation with angiotensin 2, ET or TNF

↓

Release of intracellular protein

↓

Intense inflammatory reaction

↓

Fibrotic scar

↓

Hamper ventricular function

- *Apoptosis:* (Programmed cell death)
  Mediated by 2 pathways

DEFINITION

It is a pathway of cell death induced by tightly regulated intracellular process which leads to degradation of cells own DNA and nuclear cytoplasmic protein by enzymatic action.

B. Initiation Phase

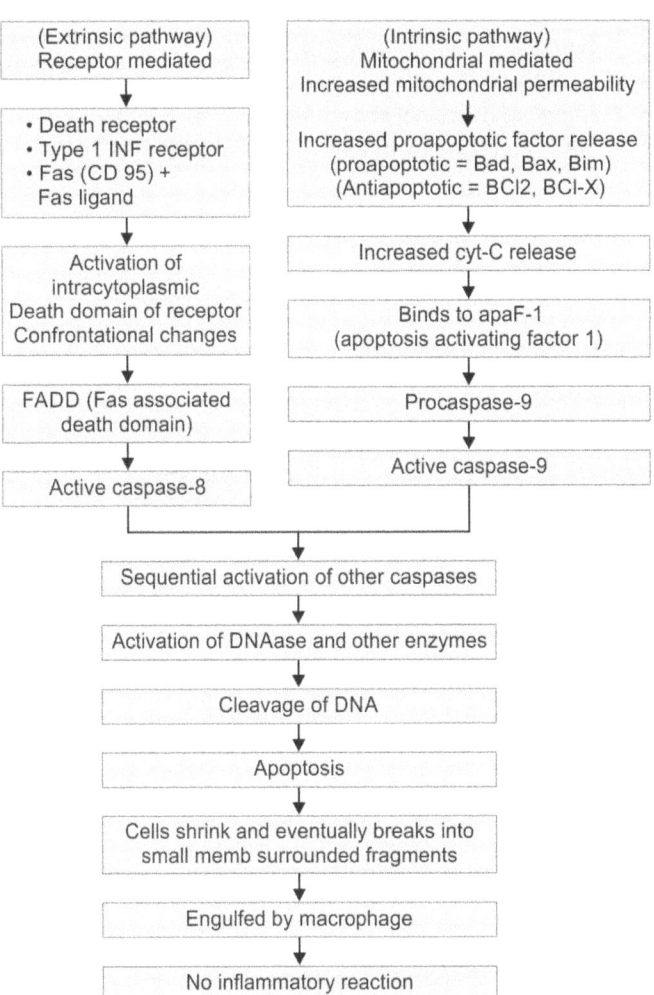

*Apoptosis likely to play important role in heart failure
Acute ischemia /DCM - apoptosis can be triggered inappropriately

- *Autophagy:* Homeostatic cellular process of sequestrating organ cells, proteins and lipids in double membrane vesicle inside the cell (autophagosome)

↓

Contents are subsequently diverted to liposome for degradation

- Change in extra cellular Matrix
  ECM consists of basement membrane, fibrillar collagen network that surround myocyte, proteoglycan, glycosaminoglycan and matricellular protein
  (Major type of collagen in heart = type 1 and 3
  1:3-1:9:1

Heart failure
↓
- Change in fibrillar collagen synthesis
- Collagen degradation
- Change in degree of cross linking
- Loss of collagen strut that connect myocyte
↓
Structural change in heart
↓
LV remodeling

CARDIAC FIBROSIS

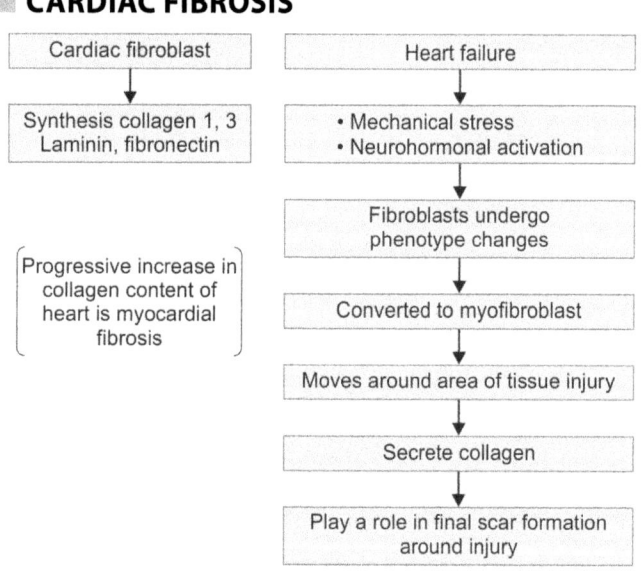

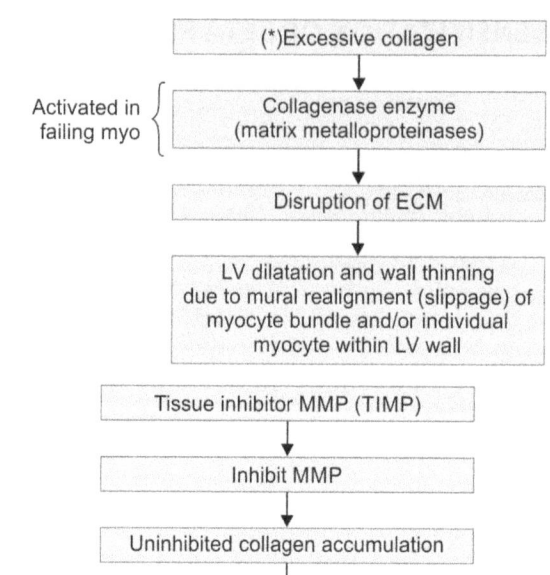

C. Alteration in LV structure

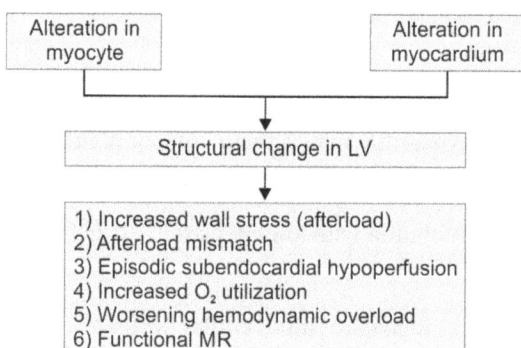

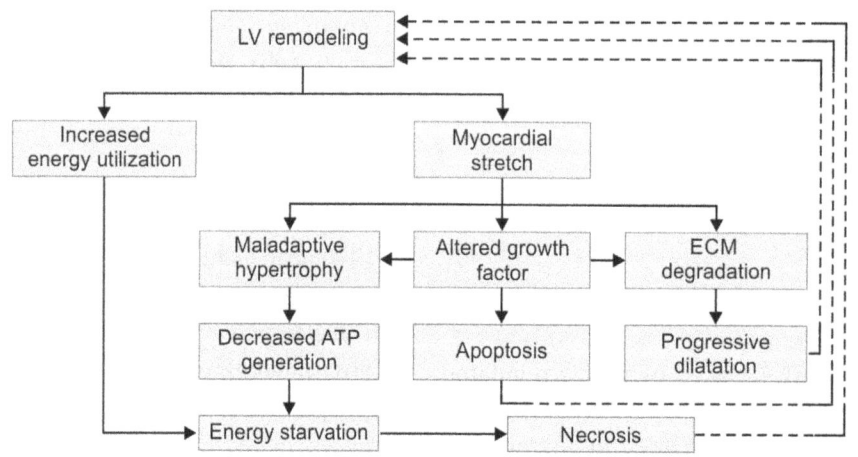

In heart failure,
    Energy requirements increased
    ATP concentration, creatine kinase activity decreased
         ↓
    Leads to energy starvation

■ REVERSIBILITY OF LV REMODELING

Better referred as reverse remodeling

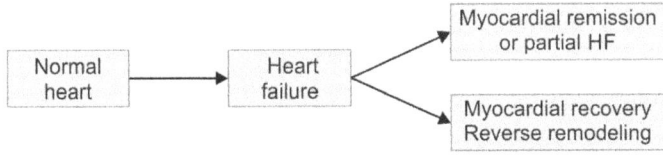

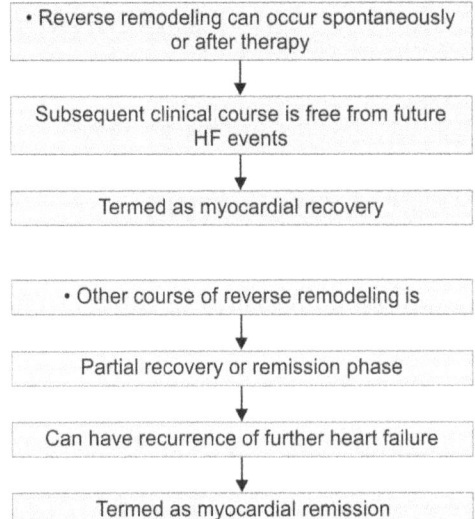

7.2 MECHANICAL CIRCULATION SUPPORT

Q.1 Types of mech VAD, Indi and physio impact (Dec 12)
Q.2 Mechanical support in cardiogenic shock (Dec 14)

MECHANICAL CIRCULATION SUPPORT DEVICE

- Mechanical pump designed to assist or replace the function of either LV or RV or both ventricles.

Characteristics

- Location of pumping chamber
- Specific ventricle supported
- Pumping mechanism
- Indicated duration of support
  Temporary (days-weeks); long term (months - years)
  Short term Extracorporeal/paracorporeal
  Long term intracorporeal (Implanted).

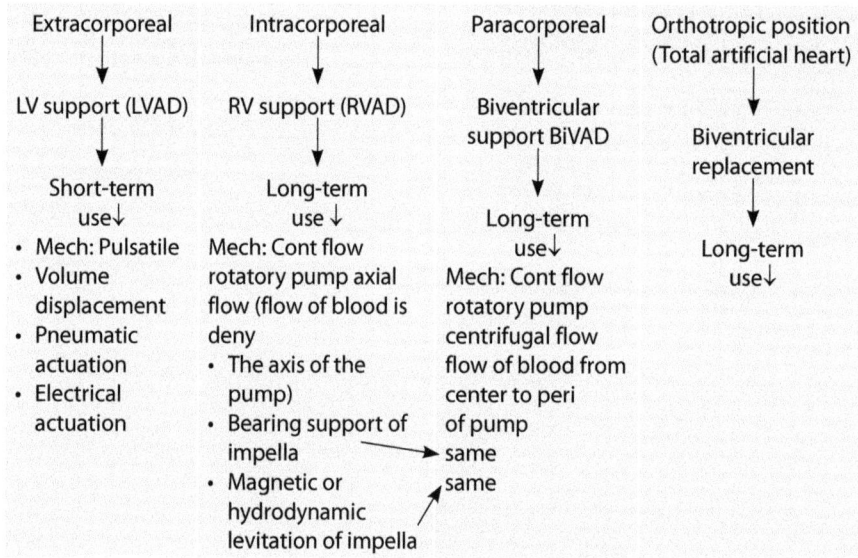

Mech Circulatory Support

A. Surgical implanted MCS
  - Extracorporeal pulsatile
  - Implantable cont flow
  - Implantable pulsatile
B. Percutaneous MCS
  - LA to femoral - Tandem heart
  - LV to Ao-impella
  - ECMO
  - IABP.

INDICATION

Three indication are approved by USFDA

A. Bridge to recovery
- Acute cardiogenic shock/decompensated heart failure that is refractory to OMT
- Expectation that myo injury is reversible and myocardial function will recover during a short period of MCS
- Most common indication
  E.g., AMI
     AC myocarditis
     Postcardiotomy cardiogenic shock resulting from ischemic stunning

Possible devices
(1) IABP (2) ECMO (3) VAD (4) ECLS (extra corporeal life support)
  ↓
Can be continued as
- Implantation of long term VADs (Bridge to bridge)
- Bridge to transplant

B. Bridge to transplant
- Patients with cardiogenic shock/decompensated heart failure that is refractory to OMT and unlikely to recover
  E.g., Long standing ischemic CMP
       Valvular cardiomyopathy
       Idiopathic cardiomyopathy
       Severe acute MI or myocarditis
Implanted in patients who are on long term inotropes
  (or) not on inotropes but symptomatic at rest
  (and) in whom hemodynamics are stable and end organ function is preserved

C. Destination therapy
- Permanent alternative to transplant
- Patients with chronic refractory symptoms of advanced heart failure that result from irreversible forms of either nonischemic or ischemic cardiomyopathy and who are ineligible for transplant

REMATCH trial: LVAD therapy reduce mortality by 50% and experience better QOL

CRITERIA FOR DT

- Ineligible for transplant
- Significant function limitation (NYHA 3-4) despite use of OMT
- LVEF <25%
- Peak VO_2 <14 mL/min/kg
- On IV inotropes >14 d or IABP >7d

PATIENT SELECTION

No absolute hemodynamic criteria

- Patients presenting with AMI – despite OMT
  - Cardiac index <1.8-2.2 l/min/m²
  - SBP <90
  - PCWP >20
  - RAP >18-20
  - Poor tissue perfusion (oliguria, rising creat and liver transaminase, mental status change, cool extremity)
- Chronic advanced HF – Inspite of OMT
  - Resting tachycardia
  - Progressive organ dysfunction
  - Persistent HF symptoms leading to limited function capacity and poor QOL
- Patients who required inotrope therapy or who do not tolerate inotrope therapy as a result of refractory vent arrhythmias

or

Those who have life threatening coronary anatomy and unstable angina not amenable to re vascularization and who are retreat of death

↓

Both can be considered for MCS even if they do not follow hemodynamic parameters

Renal function greatest risk of morbidity/mortality with use of MCS is renal dysfunction

Can be 2° lo

- Decreased perfusion to kidney in cardiogenic shock
- Nephrotic drugs (ACEI)
- Over activity of RAAS/SNS
- Non cardiac comorbidity (DM)
  - AC onset of renal dysfunction is not a contradiction.

PULMONARY FUNCTION

<50% of predicted FVC, FEV or dlco → should undergo HRCT

- SPO_2 <92% on RA – ECHO to rule out rt to lt shunt (ASD/PFO) – if negative – spiral CT or nucleotide scan to r/o thromboembolic disease

PVR >6 woods unit-relative contraindication of MCS

Peri op hypoxia 2° to significant underlying lung disease also contribute to pulm vasoconstriction leading to RV failure – indication for VAD.

HEPATIC FUNCTION

- Portal HTN with liver cirrhosis -contraindication
- Significant alcohol use- contraindication
- Check for previous HBV/HCV inf
- Bilirubin and transaminases >3ULN → risk factor for adverse outcome.

RV FUNCTION

RV dysfunction – major contributor to mortality and morbidity

Need for BiVAD support is associated with worse survival with both short term and long term MCS

RV Failure is prominent factor leading to renal dysfunction after LVAD

Pre-op optimization of RV function with a goal
RAP <15 mm Hg is important in reducing need of post of RV support
Higher LAP/PCWP at time of implantation

Greater benefit to RV and PAP when LV is totally unloaded and LAP falls

Recovery of RV function however may lag for several days (because total decomposition of LV significant allows significant shift of IVS towards LV, with further distention and dysfunction of RV).

COAGULATION

- Coagulopathy is significant risk factor
- Abnormal INR is in absence of war form is poor prognosis factor

Lead to significant periop bleeding, require multiple transfusion, increased PVR, RV failure, decline in RFT, HD instability and multi organ failure

Screening test: INR, PT, PTT, platelets plt aggregation study, HTT assay.

NUTRITION

Important contribute to overall outcome
- Sr albumin <3.3 → risk factor for mortality
  → increased risk 6.6 fold
  Poor wound healing
  Increase risk of infection
  Impaired T-cell function
- BMI <22 or >36-risk for peri operative compli
  - Cachexia-more risky
  - Can be treated with oral nutritional supplement or enteral feeding

  Other
  - Significant aortic, mitral or tricuspid valve disease
  - CAD
  - Atrial and vent arrhythmias
  - Intracardiac shunts.

DEVICE AND OUTCOME

A. Temporary mechanical circulatory support
- ECLS (extracorporeal life support) or ECMO (extracorporeal membrane oxygenation)
  - *Mech:* Continuous flow rotatory pump with centrifugal design
  - *Method of placement:* Percutaneous or operative placement
  - *Vent supported:* Venous arterial configuration

  Partial unloading of RV and LV by reduction in preload with oxygenation of blood
  Full support 4-6 l/min
  Barlett and colleague → survival in adults was improved by using ECLS as a bridge to placement of long term device

- Tandem heart PVAD (Paracorporeal VAD)
  - *Mech:* Cont flow rotatory pump with centrifugal design (bearing support of impeller)
  - *Method of placement:* Percutaneous placement
    - Require trans-septal placement of cannula for LA drainage
    - Arterial return to Femoral artery
  - *Vent supported:* LV

  Partial support 2-4 l/min
  Thide 8 colleague – reported more effective improvement in cardiac index as well as other hemodynamic and metabolic variables

- Impella
  Mech: Cont flow rotatory pump with micro axial design
  Method: Percutaneous via femoral artery or operative placement via aorta or axillary depending on dense size
  Inflow from LV and outflow in asc Ao

  Support: LV
  - Partial support (1-3L/min) for impella 2.5
  - Full support (3-5L/min) for impella 5
  - Cardiac index was significantly increased in patients with impella 2.5 compared with IABP
  - In comparison with an IABP, these device provide a much larger increment in cardiac output and superior LV unloading

- IABP
  Mech: Counterpulsation
  Method: Percutaneous via femoral artery or operative placement
  Support: Reduction of LV afterload
  Partial support
  Shock 2 trial: IABP did not reduce 30 d mortality in patients with acute MI complicated by cardiogenic shock

B. Device for long term MCS
- *VAD:* Thoratec heart mate 2
  Most evaluated device

SURGICAL IMPLANTED MCS

Type of pump	Flow char		Device
1. Axial flow	• Outflow parallel to axial rotation • Flow rate 3–7 L/min • Less sensitive to Pre and afterload		• Heart mate 2 • Jarvik 2000 • IN cor heart assist
2. Centrifugal flow	Outflow perpendicular-HVAD to axial rotation • Flow rate 0–10 L/min More pulsatile waveform • Low risk of suction events • Sensitive to pre and after load		heart mate 3
3. Mixed design	• Outflow follows Axial rotation		MVAD
Device Thoratec PVAD	Mech pulsatile vol displace	Vent support rt/lt/BiV Paracorporeal pump position	Indi BTT or BTR
Thoratec IVAD	Pulsatile vol displace	rt/lt/BiV implantable pump requiring preperitoneal pocket	BTT
Heartmate 2	Cont flow Rotatory pulm Axial design (Bearing support pocket of impella)	LV require pre-DT peritoneal	BTT

TRIALS

- Heartmate 2 pivotal trial: significant improvement in function status and QOL at 3 and 6 months
- Heartmate 2 DT pivotal trial: greater than 4 fold increase observed in the percentage of a heart mate 2 patients who successfully reached 1° endpoint (composite of survival to 24 months without disabling stroke or need to repair or replace device)
  - Less adverse event amongst heart mate 2 patients with less sepsis, less device related infection, rt sided heart failure, renal failure and rehospitalization
  Revolutionary cont flow technology introduced with heart mate 2 and it proved survival and reduction in major adverse events
  INTERMACS: Integrated registry for mechanically assisted circulatory support)
  - Compared with pulsatile flow devices, cont flow technology demonstrated equal efficacy regarding HD support, improve renal and hepatic function, rates of heart transplantation and overall survival
  - Incidence of major events contributing to fatalities such as stroke, infection and device malfunction was significantly lower
- HVAD: (heartware VAD)
  Mech: Cont flow rotatory pump with centrifugal design (magnetic levitation; no bearing)
  Support: LV implantable pump with intrapericardial placement
  No preperitoneal pocket required
  Trials ADVANCE: Noninferiority of HVAD
  - HVAD approved by USFDA for BTT
- Total artificial heart (syncardia cardiowest TAH-t)
  Mech: Pulsatile volume displacement
  50 cc and 70 CC models
  Patient tethered to portable drive unit
  Support: Bivent orthotropic placement with removal of both vent
  Approved for BTT and DT
  Trial: Overall 1 year survival rate was 70%

FUTURE

- Heart mate 3
  - Implantable continuous flow rotatory pump with centrifugal design intended for long term MCS
  - Small and design for intrapericardial placement
- MVAD
  - Small implantable cont flow rotatory pump with axial design
  - Use hydromagnetic levitation of impera that eliminates need of integrated bearing for impeller support
- Wireless MCS system
- Concept of small partial MCS device being developed for patients with less advanced HF to reverse HF symptoms with only limited assist of cardiac function
  E.g., synergy
  C-pulse
- For pediatric field
  - Miniaturized ECLS system / PUMPKIN
  - Jarvik 2000 VAD   / trial

[Mechanism of LVAD]

Two type:
1. Axial flow
2. Centrifugal flow

LVAD
↓
Continuous ventricular unloading (systole and diastole)
↓

- Transform Pr. Volume from its typical trapezoid shape to one resembling triangle
- Shift Pr. Volume loop leftward towards lower LVEDV and pressure

↓

Reduce stroke work (the area within pressure volume loop) and myocardial oxygen consumption (correlated to pressure volume area = the area within pr volume loop + diastolic portion of pr volume loop + end systolic pr volume relationship

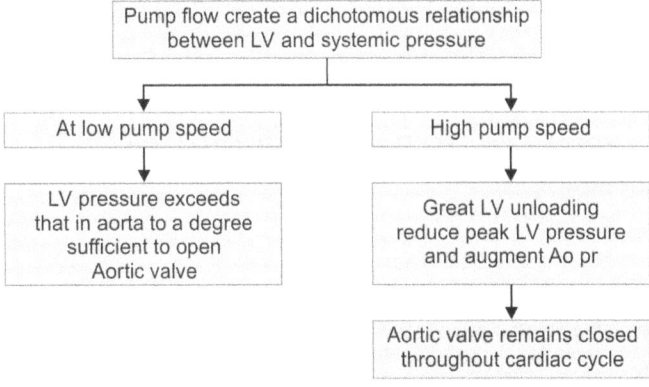

MONITORING OF PATIENTS ON VAD

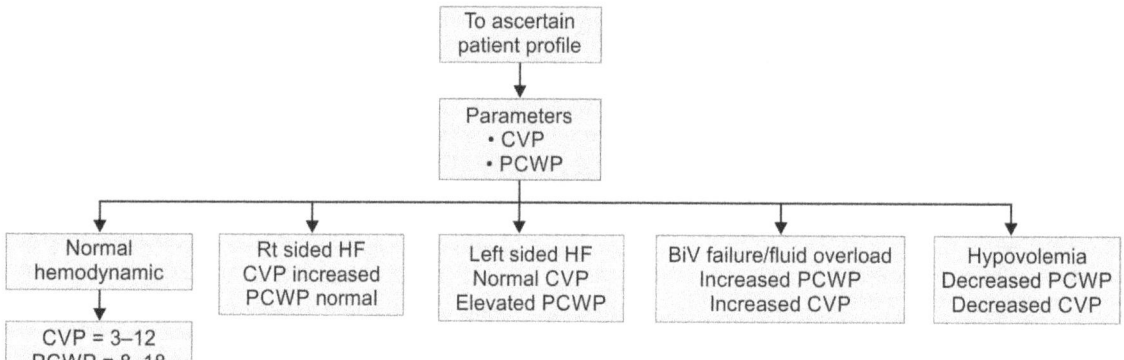

- Patient with left sided failure = benefit by increased pump speed
- Congestion or BiV failure: increased volume removal with augmented diuretic therapy
- Hypovolemia on VAD-fluid resuscitation
  ↑
  > One must rely on right heart catheterization and ECHO to adjust pump speed and achieve optimal pump mechanics
  > (no invasive parameters like pressure volume loop is required)
- Echocardiographic ramp test
  - Pump speed increased by series of fixed increments over a set of period of time to determine volume unloading
  - *Parameters:* Septal repositioning, presence and severity of MR, frequency of AV opening and change in LVEDP
  - Heart mate 2 found linear relationship between pump speed and LVEDP at all speed
  - HVAD appears to provide minimum unloading until AV is closed; after which there is rapid unloading
  ↓

Reason: subdiaphragmatic position of heart mate 2 pulls the apex inferiorly, whereas inter cardiac position of HVAD pushes apex upwards.

TRIALS OF DT (DESTINATION THERAPY)
- REMATCH
- INTrEPID
- Heart mate 2 DT trial
- Early vs. late HM2 BT
- HM2 post approval
- ENDURANCE
- ROADMAP
- INTERMACS-7th annual report
- MOMENTUM-3.

ADVERSE EVENTS WITH LVAD
- Those intrinsic to pump
  Pump malfunction, controller faults, driveline faults, short to shield malfunction)
- Patient related (develop due to inability of native heart)
  Arrhythmias valvular insufficiency, RV failure
- Pump patient interface
  Infection, stroke, pump thrombosis, acquired Von-Willebrand disease.

Contraindications
- Uncontrolled sepsis
- Aortic incompetence-needs to be treated before implantation of VAD
- Severe MS-should be also be treated before VAD
- Preexisting mechanical prostatic valve-need to change to bio prosthetic valve
- Hypercoagulable state
- Aortic aneurysm
- Bleeding diathesis
- PFO and ASD need to be closed (to prevent right to left shunting and paradoxical emboli)
- Multi organ failure
- Metastatic tumors.

Predictor of Poor Outcome
- Age
- RV failure
- V.O <30 mL/h
- CVP >16 mm Hg
- Receiving mechanical ventilation
- Cachexia syndrome
- PT <16 sec
- Reoperation

Echo-Doppler Assessment

- Position of inflow cannula at LV Apex
  - If angled toward septum-inflow obstruction
  - If velocity across inflow of cannula >2m/s - obstruction of cannula should be suspected (thrombus)
- Adequate LV decompression
- Aortic valve (AR)
- Doppler evaluation of inflow and outflow cannula
- RAMP test.

ECHO FOR LVAD

A. Peri op period (TTE/TEE)
- LV size and function: 3D >2D biplane sympson method LVEF <25
- LVIdD and LVEDV — qualify for destination
- Intra cardiac clot, contrast ECHO (not an absolute C-I)
- RV assessment: 3D ECHO
- Valve abnormality: MS can hamper cannula inflow
  - Determine need for AVR
    - As do not affect LVAD
    - AR effect function of LVAD
      - VC >0.3 or jet width/LVOT ratio >46% determine severity
    - MR usually improve after LVAD
- IAS to look for shunt-PFO/any shunt needs to be closed
- IVS to look for shunt
- Assess for prosthetic valve
- Assess for aortic disease

B. Periop ECHO (TEE)
- Reconfirm all findings
- To check for presence of air in circuit
  - LA, LV, inflow cannula, Ao root, Asc Ao, outflow cannula, coronary ostia
  - AC RV dysfunction/TR suggest emboli to RCA
- Initial LVAD initiation
  - Inter atrial shunt - desaturation (rt-lt shunt)
  - AV opening and degree of AR
  - RV dysfunction (High speed - LV become small-Septon shift - distort RV geometry/TV annulus/TR)
  - RV dysfunction at low pump speed - BiV support
  - Inflow and outflow cannula evaluation

C. After LVAD implantation
- LV size and function
- Diastolic function
- RV size and function
- IVS position
- Total cardiac output
- IAS position
- Ao valve
- MV/TV
- Inflow cannula
- Outflow cannula
- RAMP test.

7.3 POTENTIAL NEW THERAPIES FOR HF

VASODILATING AGENTS

A. Serelaxin

Relaxin first identified as major hormone of pregnancy
Serelaxin (recombinant hyman relaxin-2)
↓
Systemic and renal vascular effect
↓
Beneficial for cardiac preconditioning, beneficial effect on ischemia, inflammation, fibrosis, and apoptosis

Trial: RELAX-AHF: Demonstrated efficacy of serelaxin in improving dyspnea

Associated with improvement in signs of congestion, decrease in-hospital worsening heart failure, shorter length of stay, decreased cardiovascular and all-cause mortality.

B. Other Natiuretic peptide:
- *Urodilatin:* Modified pro ANP
  - Synthesized and secreted from distal tubules of kidney
  - Increased Camp level
  - Regulate renal Na^+ and H_2O homeostasis
- *Ularitide:* Synthetically produced urodilatin
  - Beneficial effect on hemodynamic and symptom relief
  - TRUE-AHF trial: enrolling patients
- Chimaric natriuretic peptide
  - Molecule engineered to combine beneficial aspects of different natriuretic peptides into single molecule with attempt to minimize potential negative side effect
    i. CD-NP: Beneficial effect of CNP + DNP
       CNP = venodilator primarily
       DNP = significant natriuretic
       Cenderitide

C. Neurohormonal antagonist
- *Direct Renin Inhibitor:* Aliskiren
  - Approved for treatment of HTN
    ↓
    Reduces SVR
    ↓
    Increases cardiac index
    Trial: ASTRONAUT Trial

- *Endothelin:* Receptor antagonist
  - Blocks the action of Endothelin-1 (ETA and ETB receptor)
    i. *Tezosentan:* Non-selective ETAB antagonist
       Trial: VERITAS-Tezosentan did not alleviate symptoms or decrease worsening of HF at 7 days
       Under development
       ↓
- Angiotensin 2 type 1 receptor beta-arrestin biased ligand
  Agonize favorable beta-arrestin pathway + antagonize angiotensin 2 signaling

D. Soluble Guanylate cyclase activator
  Cinaciguat: vasodilator
  MOA like nitrate – activates guanylyl cyclase shown to improve hemodynamics, at high dose it is associated with hypotension
  ↓
  Studies terminated

Inotropic Agents

A. Cardiac myosin activator (omecamtiv mecarbil)

Increased transition from weakly bound to strongly bound state of myosin head
↓
Necessary for initiation of power stroke
↓
Unlike current inotropes — Can increase LV ejection time without altering rate of LV pressure development
↓
Increased stroke volume and CO without increasing Intracellular Ca^{++}

Trial ATOMIC AHF (underway)

B. Stress copin or urocortin-2
- Peptide hormone of corticotrophin releasing factor family
- Binds to CRH-type 2 receptor (highly expressed in myocardium and vasculature
- Shown to improve cardiac output, heart rate and LVEF; while decreasing svr

C. Istaroxime:

MOA (1) Stimulation of membrane NA^+-K^+ ATPase

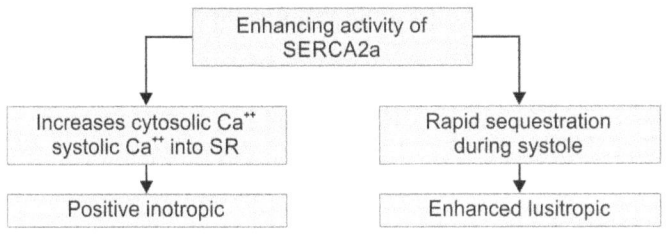

HORIZON HF-Addition of istaroxime to standard regimen – lowered PCWP and HR and Increased CO/SBP

- No change observed in neurohormones, renal function and trop 1 level

Renoprotective Agents

Adenosine-A1 Receptor Antagonist

Increased RBF and enhance dieresis without activating tubuloglomerular feedback

Rolofylline: Highly selective Adenosine-A1 receptor antagonist

Phase 2 PROTECT trial failed to show any clinical benefit.

7.4 PATHOGENESIS OF HEART FAILURE

HEART FAILURE

- Progressive disorder
- Initiated after index event
  - Damage heart muscle-loss of functioning cardiac myocyte
  - Disruption of ability of myocardium to generate force-prevent heart from contracting normally

Index event

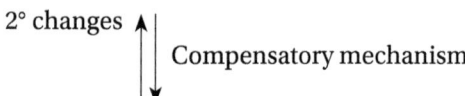

2° changes ↑↓ Compensatory mechanism

Progressive heart failure

INDEX EVENT

- Abrupt onset-MI
- Gradual onset-pressure/volume overload
- Hereditary-genetic cardiomyopathies

↓

- Damage heart muscle-loss of myocyte
- Decrease contractile function

↓

Decline in pumping capacity

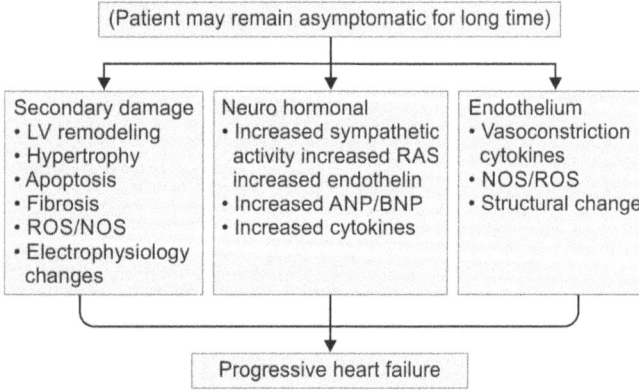

LV REMODELING

Sustained activation of neuro hormonal and cytokine system leads to series of end organ changes within myocardium, collectively known as LV remodeling.

Neurohormonal Mechanism

Compensatory Mechanisms

- Activation of adrenergic system
- Activation of renin-angiotensin system

↓

- Maintain cardiac output
- Increase water and salt retention
- Peripheral arterial vasoconstriction
- Increased contractility

- Inflammatory mediators responsible for cardiac repair and remodeling

A. Activation of sympathetic nervous system

Heart failure
↓
Decrease cardiac output
↓
Activation of sympathetic nervous system
(occur early in course of HF)
↓
Accompanied by concomitant decreases in parasympathetic tone

Normally

- High pressure carotid sinus and Aortic arch baroreceptor
- Low pressure cardio pulmonary mechanoreceptor
- non-baroreflex peri-chemoreceptor
- muscle metabo-receptors

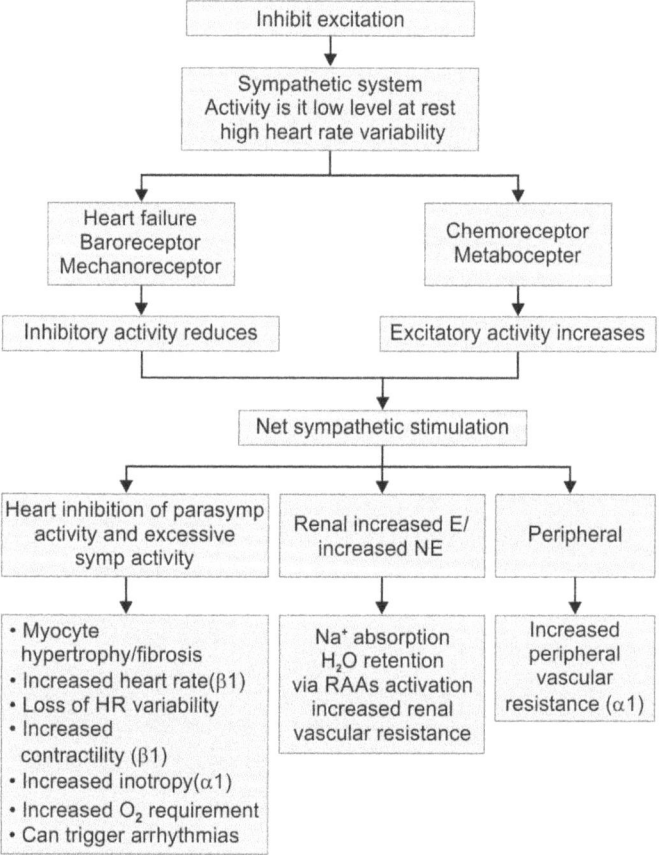

In advanced HF, circulating level of NE are 2 to 3 times higher
↓
This plasma level of NE can predict mortality in HF
↓
Coronary sinus NE is even higher than arterial NE

However,

Severe heart failure
↓
NE levels are low
↓
Reason unknown
Possibly

- Exhaustion phenomena
- Decreased activity of myocardial tyrosine hydroxylase

Withdrawal of Parasympathetic Activity
↓
- Increased sympathetic
- Activity decrease No levels
- Increased inflammation
- Worsening LV remodeling

INNOVATE HF
NETAR-HF — examine the effect of vagal stimulation on LV structure and clinical status of patients with NYHA 3 HF

B. Activation of RAAs
- Later in HF

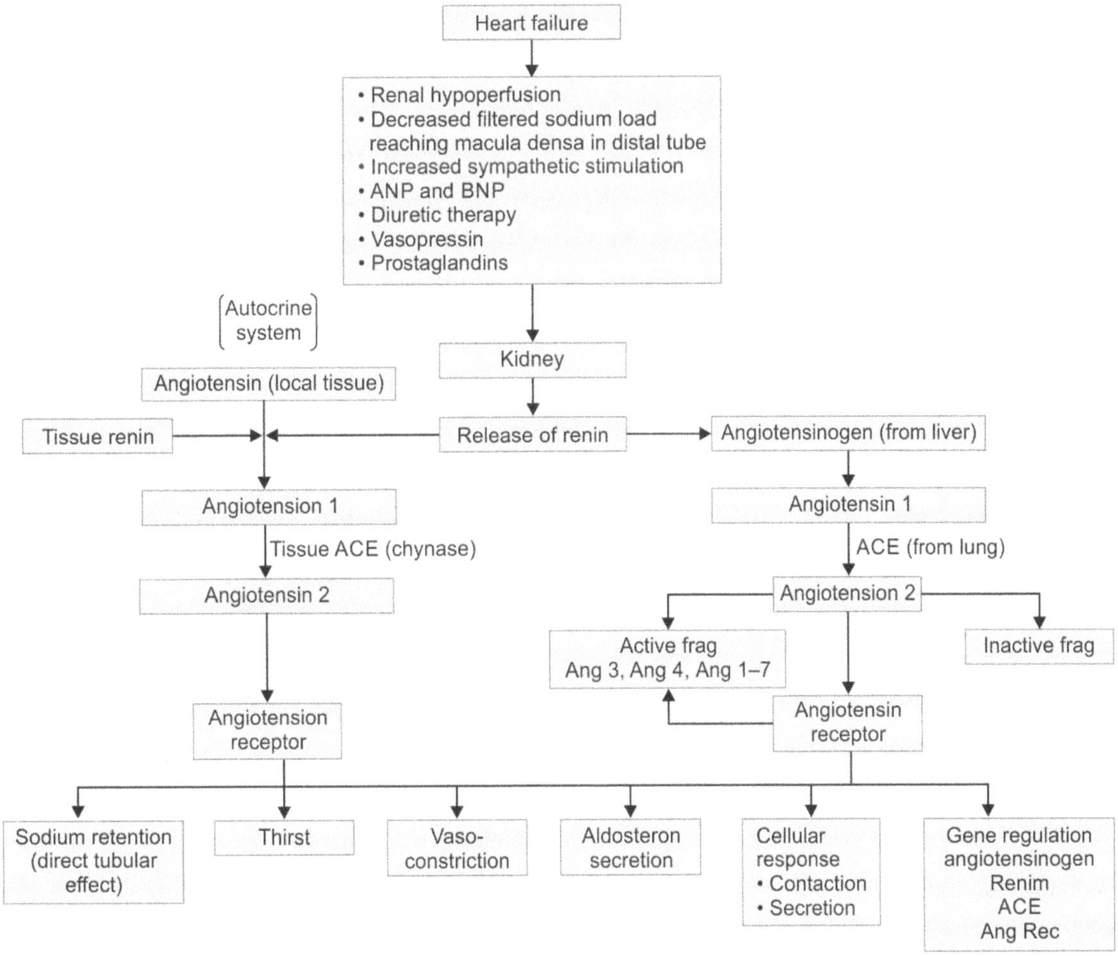

ANGIOTENSIN RECEPTORS

- *AT1:* Predominant receptor in vasculature
  - Most abundant in nerves in myocardium
  - Activation-vasoconstriction, cell growth, aldosterone secretion, catecholamine release
- *AT2:* Most abundant in fibroblast and interstitium in heart
  - Activation-vasodilatation, inhibition of cell growth, bradykinin release, natriuresis

  (AT1) receptor levels downgraded in failing heart

Sustained expression of angiotensin 2
↓
1. Worsening neurohormonal activation by enhancing release of NE from sympathetic nerve endings
2. Fibrosis of kidney, heart and other organs
3. Stimulating zona glomerulosa of adrenal cortex to produce aldosterone
↓
Sustained expression
↓

- Hypertrophy and fibrosis within vasculature and myocardium
- Endothelial cell dysfunction
- Beta receptor dysfunction
- Inhibition of NE uptake
  Worsen heart failure

C. Oxidative stress

HF
↓

- Mechanical strain of myocardium
- Neurohormonal activation
- RAAS activation
- Inflammatory cytokines (TNF-α, IL-1)
↓
Increased production of ROS and/or Reduce antioxidant capacity
↓
Oxidative stress

D. Neurohormonal Alteration of renal function

THREE THEORIES

1. Foreword failure: sodium retention 2° to inadequate renal perfusion
2. Backward failure: Increased venous pressure favors exudation of salt and water form intravascular to extravascular compartment
3. Decreased effective arterial blood volume
   Despite increase in blood volume in heart failure, inadequate CO is sensed by baroreceptor leads to compensatory neurohormonal change that resembles acute blood loss related changes
   Ongoing XR-1 trial: Using implantable baroreceptor stimulation device to decrease sympathetic activation in patients with symptomatic heart failure

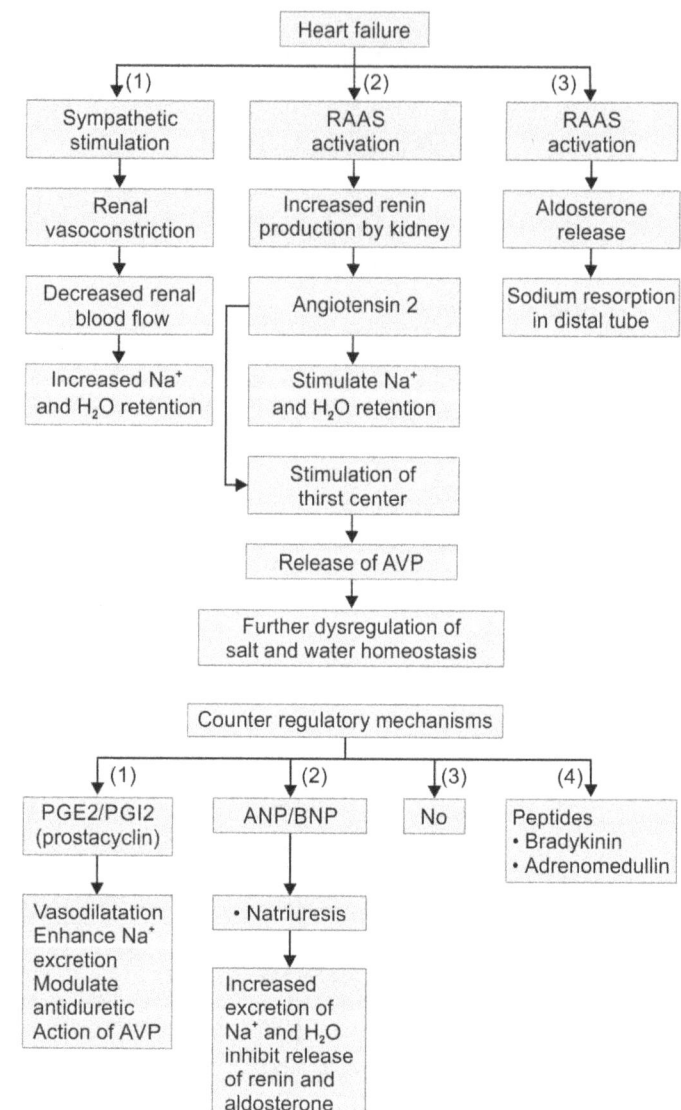

NATRIURETICS PEPTIDES

Five peptides
   ANP-from atria - secreted in short bursts 2° to acute change
   BNP-from ventricles - secreted in response to chronic increase in atrial/vent pressure
   CNP-from vasculature
   DNP (Dendroaspis Natriuretic peptide)
   Urodilatin

Released in response to
- Wall stress
- Neurohormones (angiotensin 2, ET-1)
- Physiologic factors (age, sex, renal function)

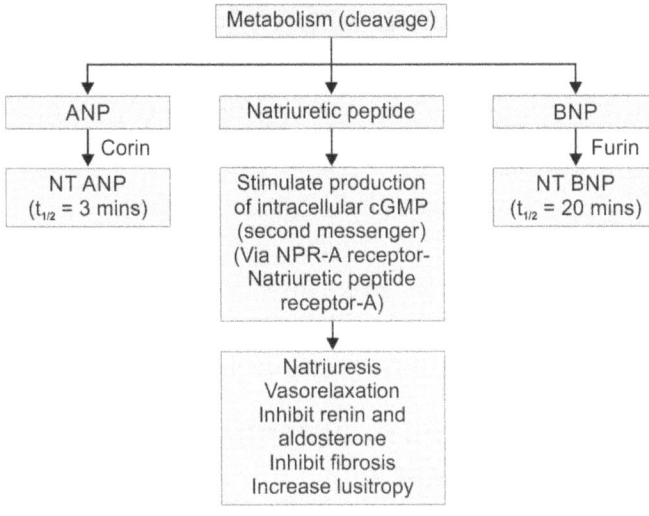

NEPRILYSIN

Natriuretic peptide
↓
Degraded by neprilysin
(Neutral endopeptidase)
↓
Neprilysin Inhibitor poterit rate
Renal protective effect of ANP/BNP

E. Neurohormonal Alteration of peripheral vasculature

Heart failure
↓
Complex interaction between autonomic nervous system and local autoregulatory mechanism
↓
Preserve circulation to brain and heart at cost of decreasing blood flow to skin, skeletal muscle, splanchnic organs and kidneys

VASOCONSTRICTORS

- Norepinephrine (most potent)
- Endothelin
- Angiotensin 2
- Neuropeptide Y
- Urotensin 2
- Thromboxane A2
- aVP.

VASODILATORS

- NE – central alpha 2 stimulation
- Epinephrine – beta 2 stimulation
- Dopamine
- NO
- PGE2/Prostacyclin
- Bradykinin.
- Adrenomedullin
- Apelin.

NO 3 Isoforms

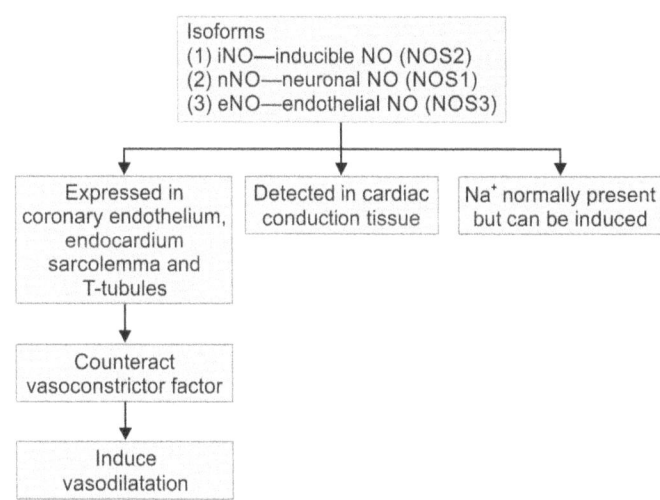

In heart failure, endothelium NO mediated vasodilatation is impaired (due to decreased expression of NOS3

ADIPOKINES

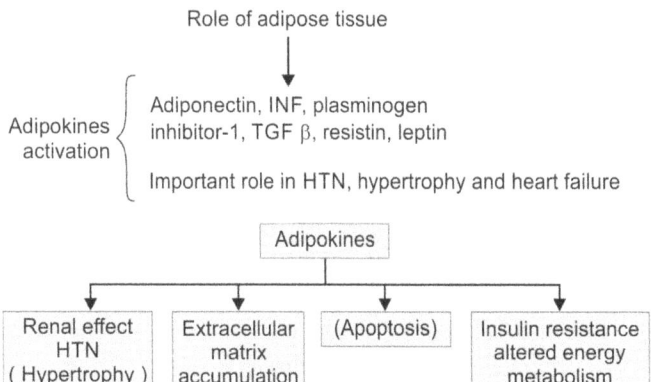

7.5 SARCOLEMMA CONTROL OF CALCIUM AND SODIUM

CHANNELS

- Ca^{++} and Na^{++} channels are highly selective
- However, nonphysiologic ion can permeate Ba^{+2} and Sr^{+2} can permeat Ca^{++} channel Li^+ can permeate Na^+ channel

Structure

(Both Ca^{++} and Na^{++} channels)
- Four transmembrane domain (1 to 4)
- Each domain has 6 transmembrane helices (S1 to S6)
- Auxiliary sub unit ($\alpha 2\delta, \beta$ and r)

1. Ca^{++} channel
   Types: 2 types of Ca^{++} channel
   L-type and T-type
   (–)T (transient) type channel open at a more negative voltage; have short burst of opening and do not interact with conventional Ca^{++} antagonist drug

Measurable no of T-type channel present in
- Neonatal vent myocyte
- Purkinje fiber
- Some atrial fiber

In adult vent myocyte L-type Ca^{++} channel predominates
   (–) L type (Long lasting) channel
   • Concentrated in T-tubules
   • Responsible for activation of RyR
   • Inhibited by Ca^{++} channel blocker
   • Rapidly activated during AP
   • Inactivated by local (Ca^{++}) SR release and voltage mediated inactivation

$$\beta\text{-adrenergic stimulation} \\ \downarrow \\ cAMP \\ \downarrow \\ pKA \text{ (Phoshorylase kinase A)} \\ \downarrow \\ \text{Phosphorylation of } Ca^{++} \text{ channel} \\ \downarrow \\ \text{Shifts activation to more negative voltage and increase open time of channel} \\ \text{Greatly increase ICa} \\ \downarrow \\ \text{Increase } Ca^{++} \text{ load of SR and cell as well as increased SR } Ca^{++} \text{ release}$$

2. Sodium channel: (Voltage gated)
$$\text{Depolarization} \\ \downarrow \\ \text{Activates INa} \\ \downarrow \\ \text{Rapid activation and rapid inactivation} \\ \downarrow \\ \text{Responsible for phase 0 of AP}$$

INaL-LATE SODIUM CURRENT

- Responsible for persistent influx of Na^{++} throughout plateau phase of AP

$$\text{Under pathophysiological condition} \\ \downarrow \\ \text{INaL is significantly increased} \\ \downarrow \\ \text{Acquired LQTS syndrome}$$

Ca^{++}/CALMODULIN-DEPENDENT PROTEIN KINASE 2

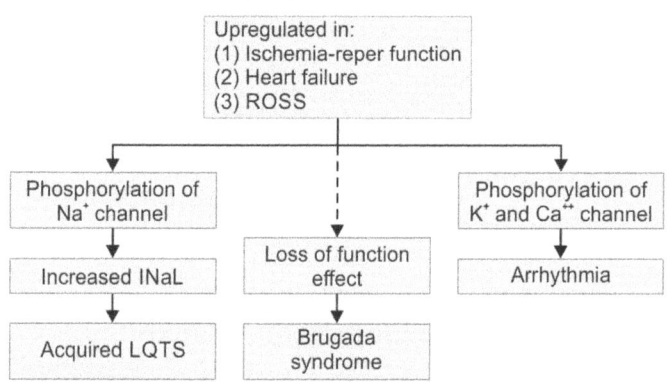

PUMPS

Amount of Na^+ and Ca^{++} entering cell must be expelled to maintain steady state

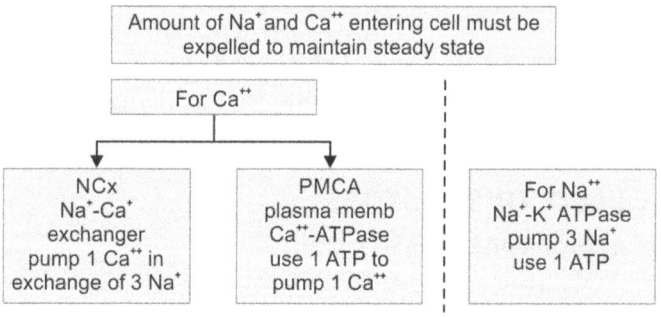

1. NCx pump
   NCx is reversible
   ↓
   When ICa is smaller or I[Na]I is too high or SR Ca^{++} release is small (occur in heart failure)
   ↓
   NCx can continue to bring Ca^{++} into cell even during action potential
   ↓
   Partially compensate for ICa or SR Ca^{++} release

So overall
Ca^{++} removal from cytosal occur by
1. SERCA : 70–75%
2. NCx : 20–25%
3. PMCA : ≤1%

In heart failure SERCA is down regulated and NCx up regulated

BOWDITCH/TREPPE PHENOMENA

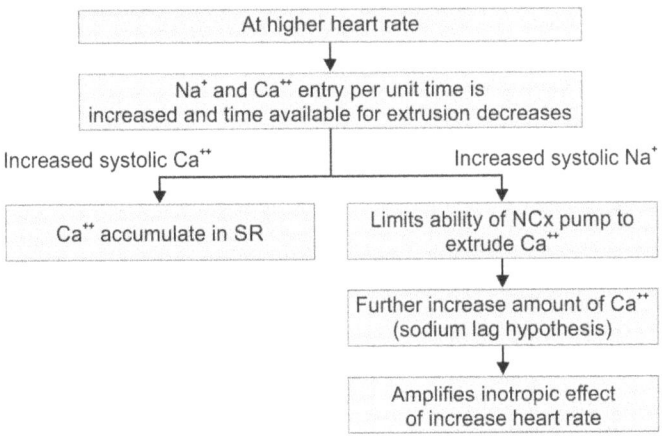

2. Na^+-K^+ ATPase pump
   Transport 3 Na^+ out
   2 K^+ in
   Uses 1 ATP
   - Inhibited by phospholamban (SERCA)

SYMPATHETIC

Stimulation → when phospholamban is phosphorylated
↓
-Na^+-K^+ ATPase activated
↓
Can cope up with higher systolic
Na^+ concentration during increased heart rate

Digitalis glycoside
↓
Inhibit Na^+-K^+ ATPase
↓
Increase systolic Na^+ concentration
↓
Limits ability of NCx to extrude Ca^{++}
↓
Promotes contraction
Too much inactivation
↓
Excessive Ca^{++}
↓
Arrhythmogenic

7.6 HEART FAILURE

DEFINITION
Heart failure (HF) is a complex clinical syndrome resulting from structural and functional impairment of ventricular filling or ejection of blood.
- HFpEF defined as LV ejection fraction of 50% or greater
- HFrEF defines as LV ejection fraction below 40% (35%).

STAGES OF HF
ACC/AHA staging
NYHA functional Class

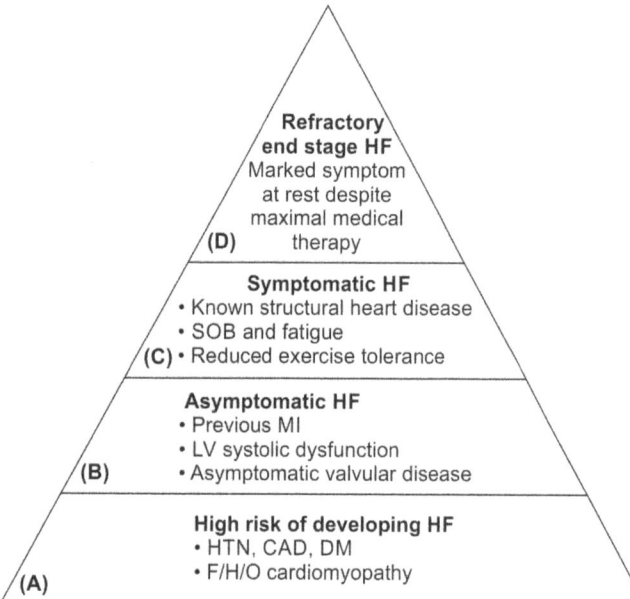

NYHA class
- No limitation of physical activity
  Ordinary physical activity does not cause symptoms of HF
- Slight limitation of physical activity
  Comfortable at rest. Ordinary physical activity causes symptoms of HF
- Marked limitation of physical activity comfortable at rest. Less than ordinary activity causes symptoms of HF
- Unable to carry on any physical activity without symptoms of HF or symptoms of HF at rest.

SYMPTOMS
S/S- shortness of breath at rest/exercise

- Dyspnea
- Fatigue
- Tachypnea
- Cough
- Orthopnea
- PND
- Decreased exercise activity
- Nocturia
- Weight loss/gain
- Peripheral edema
- Increasing abdomen capacity
- Loss of appetite

Past history of:
- Heart failure
- Cardiac disease (CAD, VHD, CHD)
- Risk factors (DM, HTN, obesity)
- Systemic illness that can involve heart (Amyloidosis, sarcoidosis, inherited neuromuscular disease)
- Recent viral inf/ HIV inf
- F/H/O heart failure
- Environmental – exposure to cardiotoxic substance
- Non cadiac illness – Anemia. Hyperthyroid, AV fistula

O/E
Tachycardia
    Tachypnea
    Narrow pulse pr
    Pulsus alternans
    Cool extremity
    Elevated JVP
Ansc: Rale/rochi/wheeze
    Leftward displaced apical impulse
    Parasternal lift

S3/S4	Pedal edema
TR/MR	Anasarca
Hepatomegaly	Presacral edema
Ascites	chr. Venous statis changes

CARDINAL SYMPTOMS
- Worsening dyspnea – associated with filling pr
- PND- highly reliable indicator
- Fatigue – cardinal feature – related with reduction in cardiac output
- Rales heard >1/3rd of lung
- S3-suggest increased vent filling pr – prognostic marker
- Ascites (mod-massive)
- Orthopnea (requiring >2 pillow)
- Hepatomegaly (>4 finger beyond costal margin)
- Hepatojugular reflux
- JVP ≥12

CATEGORIZATION OF HEART FAILURE
Congestion at rest?
(orthopnea, elevated JVP, pulm rates. S3 gallop, edema)

		No	Yes
Low perfusion At rest?	No	Warm and dry	Warm and wet
(Narrow pulse Pr, cool extremity hypotension)	Yes	cool and dry	cool and wet

Biomarkers

Braunwald suggested 7 categories

1. Inflammation
   - CRP
   - TNF
   - Fas
   - IL-1, 6, 8
2. Oxidative stress
   - Oxidized LDL
   - Myeloperoxidase
   - Urinary biopyrin
   - Pl. Malondialdehyde
3. ECM remodeling
   - MMP
   - TIMP
   - Collagen propeptides
   - Propeptide procollagen 1
   - Plasm procollagen 3
4. Neurohormone
   - Norepinephrine
   - Renin, angiotensin, aldosterone
   - Arginine vasopressin
   - Endothelin
5. Myocyte injury
   - Cardiac specific Trop I and T
   - Myosin light chain kinase
   - Heart type fatty acid binding
   - cKMB
6. Myocyte stress
   - BNP/NT pro BNP
   - Mid regional adrenomedullin
   - ST 2
7. Others
   - Chromogranin
   - Galectin 3
   - Osteoprotegerin
   - Adiponectin.

7.7 SURGICAL MANAGEMENT OF HF

CORONARY ARTERY REVASCULARIZATION

Ischemic Cardiomyopathy

Term used to describe the myocardial dysfunction that arise 2° to occlusive or obstructive CAD.

Selection of Patients for Revasc

- STICH Trial
- Veterans administration cooperative study
- European coronary surgery study
- Coronary art surgery study
  Excluded patients with HF
  Peri op risk in patients with severe LV dysfunction = 2–10%

Marker

Availability of targets
  Viability of myocardium
  RV dysfunction
  Advanced HF symptoms
  LVEDP increases
  Comorbidity
  PVD
  COPD
  STS score can predict risk of death
Predictor of death
- Age >70 years
- Significant PAD
- LVEDP >25 mm Hg.

CABG Patch Trial

- High mortality (4.8% vs. 1.3%) in mild HF patients
  For cardiogenic shock after MI, result of emergent CABG is poor but still better than medical management.

SHOCK Trial

Mortality rate post CABG
  30 d 47% (56% with OMT)
  6 m 50% (63% with OMT).

STICH Trial

- Peri op mortality was 4% in medical management + CABG arm, which was 1% in medical treatment group – No statistically significant diff
- Significant diff between CABG and medical management in terms of composite end points of CV death, death from any cause with hospitalization for CV events
- LVEF <35% and LM stenosis >50% is associated with survival advantage over MED through 10 years of follow-up

A. Valve surgery in patients with LV dysfunction:
- MVR has been shown to be safe with low operative mortality and associated with significant reversal of LV remodeling as well as improvement in NYHA functional class
- Reverse remodeling has also been shown in various studies

Indication (ESC/EACTS 2012)
- Severe MR undergoing CABG & LVEF >30%
- Moderate MR undergoing CABG
- Symptomatic patients with severe MR and EF <30%
- Severe MR LVEF >30 who remain symptomatic despite OMT.

RESTORE MV

- 30 d mortality was 14.1%
- Significant improvement in LVEF and NYHA class with reduction of LVED dimensions
- Increasing age and renal disease were associated with decreased survival.

CONCLUDE

There is currently no evidence that elimination of mitral insufficiency in HF patients conveys a survival benefit

RECURRENCE

Multiple studies – 30–40%
With flexible ring 9–5%
With non flexible ring 2–5%
- AVR can be performed safely

Albeit at higher operative risk in patients with severe LV dysfunction and heart failure – better clinical outcome than that achieved with current medical therapy.

B. Left ventricular reconstruction
Goals:
- To remove or to exclude the infracted segment to restore an elliptical vent chamber
- Diminished remote wall stress to promote helical fiber orientation
- Increased thickening of akinetic or dyskinetic portion of chamber to reduce ESV
- Eliminate residual ischemia

E.g., SVR (surgical vent reconstruction) or Dor procedure
- Reserved for patients with large anteroapical infarct involving the apex, anterior wall, and septum with LV remodeling

Trials
- *RESTORE:* Reconstruction resulted in significant increase in LVEF
- *STITCH-(SVR portion):* No significant diff was found in 1° outcome variable of death from any cause or hospitalization for cardiac cause

C. Passive cardiac support device
- Developed out of original observation with dynamic cardiomyoplasty
- Benefit of dynamic cardiomyopathy derived from passive gridling of the muscle wrap, which limits vent dilatation. Cardiac support devices has failed till date to show any benefit.

D. Cardiac transplant

E. Device based autonomic modulation
- Vagus nerve stimulation
- Spinal cord stimulation
- Baroreceptor activation
- Renal symp denervation.

REFRACTORY HF
Device and Surgery

A. Implantable device
CRT/ICD/CRT-D

B. Percutaneous Therapy
- PTCA
- IABP
- Assist device
  - IMPELLA; Tandem heart
- Percut MI repair/ TAVI
- Percut reshaping device like vent positioning in dilated heart with aneurismal segment
- Percut stem cell delivery

C. Surgical treatment
- CABG
- MV repair or replace
- LV reshaping surgery
- Stem cell
- LVAD
- Cardiac transplant

D. Other
- Ultrafiltration
- CPAP.

7.8 CARDIOPULMONARY EXERCISE TEST

INTRODUCTION

- NYHA criteria or (6 min walk test) are subjective and insensitive measure of functional capacity
- Does not discriminate between cause of impaired exercise capacity (e.g., cardiac, pulmonary, orthopedic)

↓

When more precise information is needed, cardiopulm exercise testing is used

↓

EXERCISE INTOLERANCE IS PRIME SYMPTOM OF HEART FAILURE

CPx can be performed using
- Treadmill
- Cycle cryometer

Parameters to be Measured

- Oxygen uptake (VO_2)
- Expiratory ventilation (VE)
- Carbon dioxide output (VCO_2)

Expressed as ratio of their slope

↓

Gives analysis of gas exchange at rest, during exercise and in recovery phase

(Fick's principle)

↓

$VO_2 = CO \times \Delta PO_2$

$VO_2 = CO \times [O_2$ content art $-O_2$ content venous$]$

— strong prognostic value

VE/VCO_2 slope expression of efficacy of pulm CO_2 clearance during exercise

Has prognostic value

Use of CPX

1. Monitoring effect of various therapy on functional status (Not standard)
2. Before heart transplant
   - $VO_2 <14$ mL O_2/kg/min – poor prognostic threshold
   - $VO_2 <10$ mL O_2/kg/min – poor prognosis
   - $+VE/VCO_2$ slope $\geq 45°$ – poor prognosis

7.9 CARE OF PATIENT WITH END STAGE HEART DISEASES

DEFINITION

Advanced Heart Failure

Defined as significant symptoms, end organic compromise, or severe functional limitation from HF despite OMT and device therapy.

Data

⌈ LVAD buys 2 to 8 years ⌉
⌊ And Transplant buys on san avg 15 years ⌋

Data from Companion—
- Quarter of people with advanced HF die of problems not related to HF
- 3/4th patients eventually die of prog HF or SCD
- Life expectancy of patients with chronic HF = 10-20 years
  - Age 65-74: Cardiac conditions common ⌉
  - Age > 75 years: Dementia and osteoporosis common   Reason for Hospital adm.
  - Age > 85: Three or more noncardiac-related comorbidities Dominate ⌋

Frailty
- Char by: weakness, fatigue, weight loss, slow gait speech
- Present in ¼ th-½ of patients with HF (elderly)
- Associated with death within 12 years
- Related to exercise intolerance.

Sarcopenia

Muscle wasting of frailty and
   That of HF is equivalent both
   May improve with RAAs blockade.

Other

Cognitive impairment
Vascular dementia.

MANAGEMENT OF END STAGE HEART DISEASE

Management strategy needs to integrate plans to assist in medication compliance, dietary sodium management, assessment of volume status and titration of diuretics.

A. Medical management
- Optimized blockade of RAAs and SNS
- Hypotension and renal dysfunction may limit medication use
- No data about what to continue and what to discontinue
- Approach other than 100p diuretic are considered appropriate for management of vol. Status
- Nocturnal hypoxia contributes significantly to hypoxia and in turn to increase PAP
- Use cPAP or nocturnal O_2
- Improve vol status; symptoms; QDL
- Aggressive control of oral fluid and Na^+ intake
- Limit oral intake to 1 L/day
- Addition of aldosterone antagonist.

B. Symptoms management
- *Pain:*
  - Prevalence as high as 84%
  - NSAIDS associated with worsening renal function and fluid status → patients are advised to avoid OTC drugs
  - Nonacetylated salicylates are effective
  - Opioids are safe for pain as well as alleviating dyspnea
  - Morphine should be avoided for chronic use
  - Fentanyl/methadone can be used
  - Heat or cold therapy and physical therapy should be considered whenever feasible

  Topical capsaicin, topical NSAIDS and topical salicylates
- Dyspnea
  - Sodium and fluid restriction along with diuretics
  - Dyspnea present in HF patients even when euvolemic and related to skeletal myopathy associated with HF syndrome
  - Thigh muscle stretching reduces dyspnea and fatigue
  - Exercise therapy also reduces sensation of dyspnea
  - Opioids reduce responsiveness of respi center and reduce anxiety

  - Opioids increases HF patients exercise tolerance, thereby resulting in decrease in respi effort and decreased sensation of dyspnea
  - Morphine also reduces preload: appropriate for acute management
  - Nitrates reduce LVEDP and may reduce dyspnea and improve ex tolerance
- O_2 supplementation when dyspnea related to hypoxia
- Anxiety and depression
  - For patients with OSA – cPAP reduces anxiety and depression (as it reduces NE/E level associated with OSA)
  - Sertraline safe in mod HF
  - Paroxetine effective as antidepressant
  - SSRI causes vol. overload and hyponatremia in elderly → so Na^+ and vol status must be monitored during its use

- TCA, nortriptyline and desipramine are safe but higher doses cause orthostatic hypotension and prolong QTe
- GI symptoms
  - HF – Intestinal edema, ascites and hepatic congestion–early satiety
  - Optimizing fluid status and treating sleep apnea - decreased early satiety
  - Beta-blocker and ACEI counter the cachexia in patients with HFrEF by reducing neurohormonal and immune dysfunction
- Fatigue
  Due to increased CD, elevated neurohormones and inflammatory cytokines; deconditioning, sleep impairment, depressing-anxiety
  - Fluid and Na^+ restriction decreases fatigue as well as decreased edema and dyspnea
  - Anemia: Erythropoietin/iron
  - Opioid, caffeine and other stimulants can improve exertional fatigue

C. End of life care.

7.10 CONTRACTILE CELL AND PROTEIN

Q.1 Microanatomy of contractile cell and protein. Ca^{++} ion fluxes in cardiac contraction and relaxation cycle
(June 14)

Q.2 Excitation contraction coupling.

Contractile cells
Ventricular myocardium
↓
(Myocyte)

- Main contractile cell
- Compromise 75% of total vent myocardium
- Approx 1/3rd number of all cells
- Vent myocyte = Brick shaped
- Atrial myocyte = small and spindle shaped
- Light microscopy = cross striation
  → Bounded by sarcolemma
  → Filled with myofibrils
    ↓ Contractile element
    Invaginate to form
    Extensive tubular network (t tubule)
    That extends extracellular space
    Into the interior of the cell.

STRUCTURE OF MYOCYTE

- ½ of myocyte is formed by myofibrils
- 1/3 rd - ¼ th by mitochondria
  - Located between myofibrils
  - Immediately beneath sarcolemma
  - Generate ATP
- Sarcoplasmic reticula
  - Critical for Ca^{++} cycling
  - Type of endoplasmic reticula
- Nucleus
- Cytoplasm.

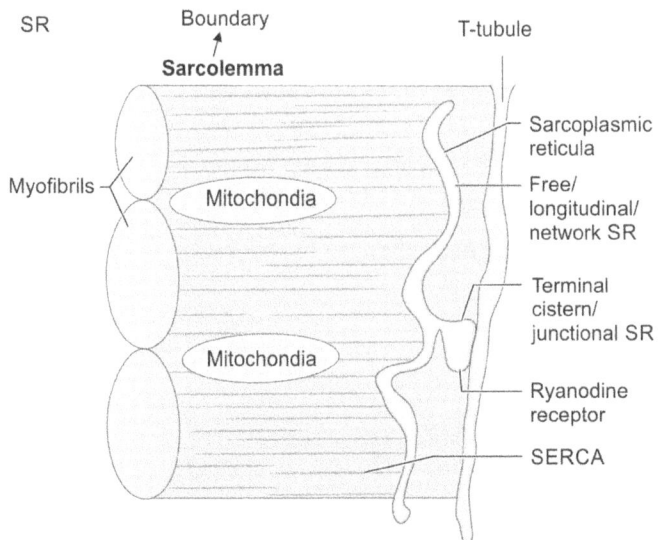

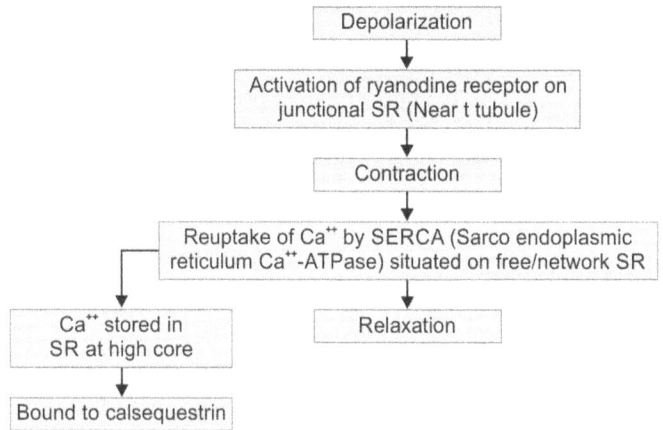

MITOCHONDRIA

- One went myocyte contain 8,000 mitochondria
- Outer and inner mitochondrial membrane
- Int member is crumpled-large surface area
- It contains enzymes of TCA cycle
  ↓
  Forms ATP

Mitochondrial $Na^+ - Ca^{++}$ transport

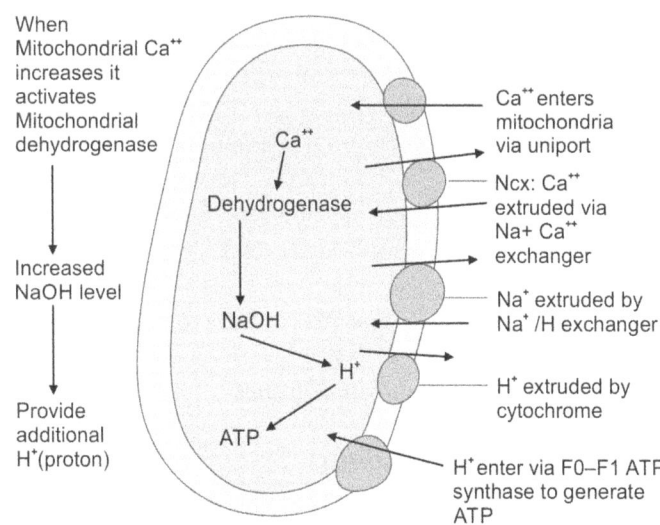

So, Ca^{++} uptake is energy dependent

H^+ (proton) which can be used to generate ATP is used here to extrude Na^+ and Ca^{++}

During Ca^{++} overload mitochondrial dehydrogenase gets activated-provide additional H^+

Chronic Ca^{++} overload

(1) Ca^{++} uptake occurs at the cost of ATL

(3) Elevated Ca^{++} increases mitochondrial permeability
↓
Matrix content released to cytosol
↓
Can induce (1) apoptosis and cell death
(2) ROS and necrotic cell death.

CONTRACTILE PROTEIN

Two chief contractile protein: Actin (Thin filament)
Myosin (thick filament)

Role of actin

Thin Filament

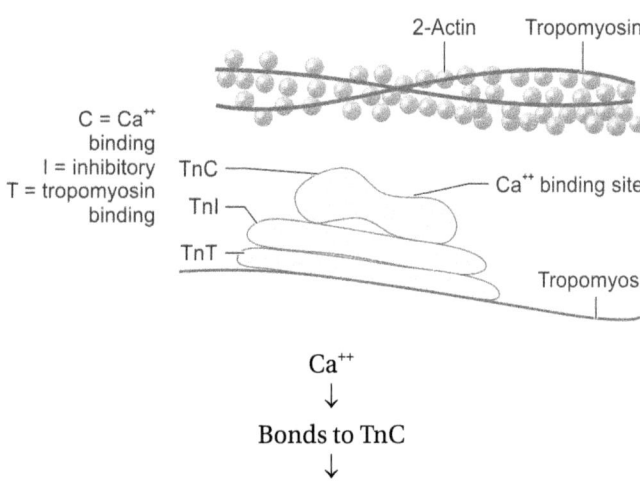

Ca^{++}
↓
Bonds to TnC
↓
Confrontational changes (tropomyosin roll deeper into thin filament and active site of actin is exposed)
↓
Removes inhibition exerted by troponin complex
↓
Myosin head binds to active site on actin filaments (known as cross-bridge cycle)
↓
Myosin pulls actin towards center of sarcomere
↓
Contraction ensues

Strong and Weak Binding

- Ca^{++} binding to TnC – strong binding of actin myosin
- Binding of ATP to myosin head- makes cross bridges weak (even when Ca^{++} is high).

Role of Titin in Contraction

- Giant Molecule
- Largest protein yet described
- Extraordinary long and flexible myofibrillar protein
- Connects thick filament to z line
- Extends from z line but stops just short of m line
- Provides elasticity to contracting myocyte

Two segments
1. *Anchoring segment:* In extensible
2. *Elastic segment:* Extensible

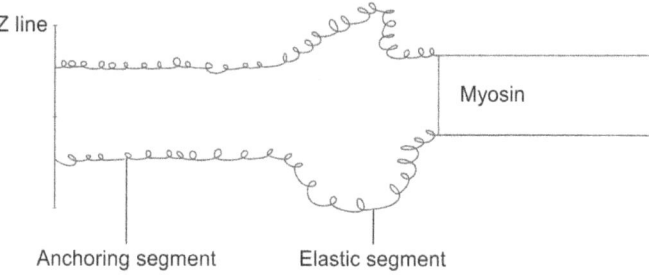

FUNCTION

- Tethers the myosin molecule to z line
  Stabilizing contractile system
- Elasticity contribute to stress strain relationship of cardiac and skeletal muscle
- Stretched elastic segment during diastole contracts more vigorously in systol to maintain CO
- May transduce mechanical stretch into growth signal
  ↓
  Stretched Titin transmit signals to MLP protein attached at terminal part of Titin (near z line) ⎫ Defective
  ↓   ⎬ in protein
  MLP transmits signal responsible for myocyte growth (volume overload state) ⎭ with DCMP

ROLE OF MYOSIN

Rayment Model

Base of head or neck changes configuration in response to ATP.

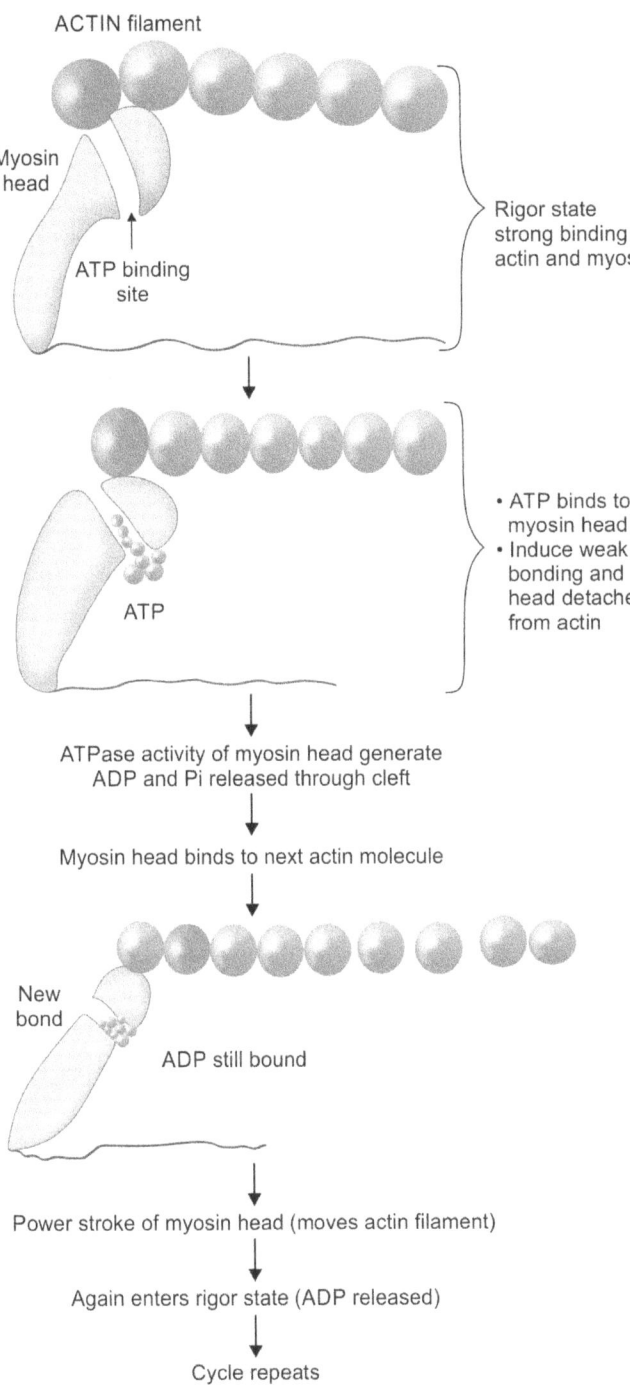

Each actin unit has two actin filaments
Each myosin unit has two myosin filaments

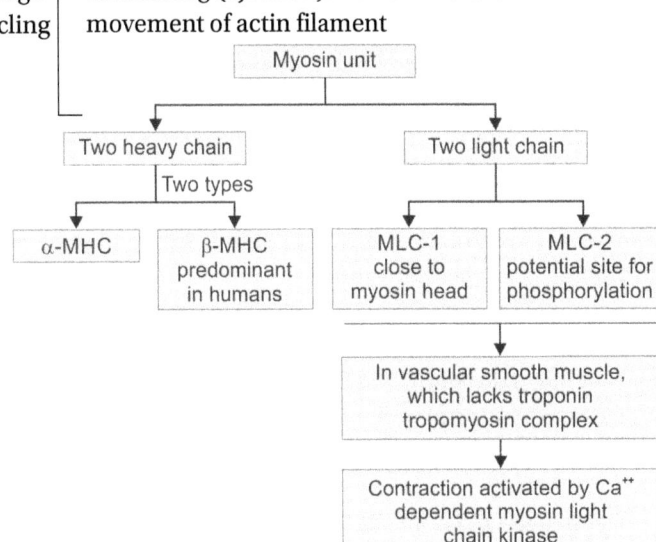

Defect in myosin and myosin binding protein G
↓
Responsible for familial hypertrophic cardiomyopathy

ROLE OF FRANK STARLING RELATIONSHIP

Besides Ca^{++} other major factor influencing the strength of contraction is sarcomere length at the end of diastole
↓
More the diastolic length, more the strength of contraction
↓

Reasons

- Increasingly optimal overlap between actin and myosin filament
- Substantial increase in myofilament Ca^{++} sensitivity with increase in sarcomere length
- Decreasing interfilament spacing as the heart muscle is stretched
  - Change in diastolic length (preload) is the cause of altered contractile strength-Frank Starling effect
  - Conditions were strength of contraction increases independent of sarcomere length (e.g., Increasing Ca^{++} transit) – referred as positive inotropic state or enhanced contractility.

7.11 DEVICE FOR MONITORING AND MANAGING HF

Q. Device for monitoring and managing heart failure (June 14)
Q. CRT (June 04)
Q. CRT-current evidence and guidelines (June 15)

■ VENTRICULAR DYSSYNCHRONY AND CRT

Abnormality in HF (in conduction system)

Bundle branch block-alter timing and pattern of ventricular contraction-already feeling heart placed at further mechanical disadvantage

- Sub Optimal vent filling
- Reduction in LV contractility
- Prolonged duration of MR
- Paradoxical septal wall motion

These mechanical manifestation of altered vent conduction is Termed vent dyssynchrony

Defined as QRS duration (>120 msec) on surface ECG

In short

Conduction disturbance (QRSd >120 on surface ECG) + mechanical manifestation of altered vent conduction

Incidence: approx 1/3rd of systolic heart failure
Increase mortality

■ RANDOMIZED TRIALS OF CRT

1. *MUSTIC:* Multisite stimulation in cardiomyopathy
2. *MIRACLE:* Multicenter in sync randomized clinical evaluation
3. MIRACLE ICD
4. CONTAK CD
5. *CARE HF:* Cardiac resynchronization in HF
6. *COMPANION:* Comparison of medical therapy, pacing and defibrillation in HF

1. *MUSTIC*
   - Designed to evaluate safety and efficacy of CRT In patients with advanced HF
     a. 58 patients
        - NYHA 3 HF
        - HSR and QRSs >150 } CRT pacing vs. no pacing
     b. • 37 patients
        • AF and slow VR } BiV pacing vs. VVIR
        ↓

   One degree endpoint were exercise tolerance as assessed by measurement of peak VO_2, or 6 min walk test and quality of life
   ↓ ↓

   Result from NSR Arm provided strong Evidence of benefit (Significant improvement In qualities of life And NYHA functional status)

   AF arm also showed similar improvement (magnitude of benefit was slightly lower)

2. *MIRACLE* first perspective, double blind, randomized parallel controlled trial

   One degree end points: NYHA class, quality of life and 6 min walk

   Two degree endpoints: Composite clinical response, CPAX performance, cardiac str and function, measures of worsening HF, morbidity and mortality
   ↓

   CRT significantly improved NYHA class, quality of life and 6 min walk performance, TMT ex. Time peak VO_2 and LVEF

   Also provide % reverse LV remodeling with chronic CRT (decreased LVEDV and decreased LVESV; decreased LV mass, Increased EF; decreased MR flow and improve MRI

   (Results of this trial led to US-FDA approval of In sync system in August 2001)

3. *MIRACLE-ICD*
   - Assessed safety and efficacy of combined CRT-ICD
   - HF patent with indication for ICD benefits as much from CRT as do patients without an indication for an ICD

4. *CONTAK CD* did not met 1° end point of reduced hospitalization for HF, all cause mortality, vent arrhythmias requiring defibrillation therapy

   Although trends were in direction favoring improved outcome with CRT

5. *CARE HF*

   Risk for death from any cause or unplanned hospitalization for major cardiac events (1 degree endpoints) were significantly decreased with CRT

6. *COMPANION* (Medical treatment vs. CRT)
   - NYHA class 3 and 4 heart failure and no indication for device
   - Combined end point of mortality and hospitalization for HF was reduced in patients receiving CRT and CRT-ICD
   - CRT also improve exercise tolerance

7. *2005 guidelines:* Recommend CRT for patients with LVEDP ≤ 75%, SR, NYHA 3 or ambulatory 4 symptoms despite recommended OMT

8. *MIRACLE ICD 2:* Suggested such a benefit in small cohort of NYHA class 2 subject

9. RCTS of CRT in patients with NYHA 1 and 2 class

REVERSE: Significant benefit of CRT in improvement in LV structure and function and in HF morbidity. Relative risk reduction in time to 1st HF hospitalization
- First large RCT to demonstrate potential for CRT to slow progression of disease through reverse remodeling in patients with NYHA 1 and 2 HF patients.

MADIT-CRT

- Prophylactic CRT + ICD vs. ICD alone
- 18-20 patients
- Both ischemic and non-ischemic group showed benefit with CRT
- Greater benefit noted in women with QRS >150
- Patients benefit most having LBBB
- Led to FDA approval expansion of indication for CRT to NYHA class 2 or ischemic class 1 with LVEF <30% and QRSd >130 and LBBB

RAFT (only class 2 patients)
  1st to show mortality benefit of ICD-CRT over ICD alone

10. 2012 ACC/AHA

Class 1: NYHA 2, 3 or ambulatory 4, LVEF ≤35%, NSR, LBBB, QRSD ≥150

Level of evidence
A. For class 3 and 4 NYHA
B. For class 2 NYHA

Class 2a
- Non LBBB pattern with QRS ≥150 (NYHA 3/4)
- QRSd 120-149 (NYHA 2, 3, 4)
- AF & LVEF ≤35%
- LVEF ≤35% and undergoing PPI with anticipated req -for significant vent pacing

Class 3: NYHA class 1 or 2 with non LBBB pattern and QRSD <150
- Whose comorbid condition and/or fraility limit survival with good function capacity to <1 year
  PROSPECT trial Did not support use of ECHO measures of dyssynchrony as selection criteria for CRT in patients with QRSD >120 msec

CRT indication
- LVEF ≤35%
- Sinus rhythm
- LBBB with QRSd >120
- NYHA 2, 3, and 4 campulatory
- On OMT

Nonresponders
Factors associated
- Suboptimal LV lead placement
- Suboptimal AV and LV timing

- Ventricular scar
- Progression of heart failure disease

MIRACAL-EF: Evaluating CRT on morbidity and mortality in patients with NYHA 2 and 3 and LVEF 36-50% and QRSD <130 and LBBB.

CURRENT ROLE OF ICD AND HF

RCTs of ICD

- MADIT-2 (Multicenter automatic defibrillator implantation trial 2)
  - To assess survival benefit of ICD in post MI patient with reduced CF (<30%)
  - No arrhythmias marker for inclusion
  - Mainly class 2&3 patients (NYHA)
  - Class 4 patients were excluded
    Result: Survival benefit observed in MADIT 2 begun approx 9 months device implantation
  - HF with mild to mod symptoms and mod-severe reduction in LVEF may benefit the most
- DEFINITE (Prophylactic defibrillator implantation in patients with non-ischemic DCM)
  - First randomized trial of 1 degree prevention with an ICD in patient with non ischemic DCMP
  - Included patients with EF <30%; HIO symptomatic heart failure; presence of ambient Arrhythmias defined as episode of NSVT or at least 10pvc per 24 hours during holter monitoring

ICD vs. OMT

Result ICD-non significant 35% reduction in death from any cause and significant reduction in risk of SCD by 80%
  - Subgroup (NYHA 3) all cause mortality significantly decrease in ICD arm
- SCD HeFT (SCD – heart failure trial)
  - NYHA class 2/3 with LVEF ≤35 (due to ischemic or nonischemic causes)
  - ICD vs. Amiodarone vs. placebo

Result: ICD associated with statistically significant (23%) reduction in all-cause mortality aa compared to placebo. Mortality in Amiodarone arm was not significantly different than placebo

Similar degree of ICD benefit in ischemic and non-ischemic arm
- *Prophylactic ICD in HF* (Indications)
  2013 ACC/AHA-class 1 recommendation
  LDE (A) ICD for 1 degree prevention of SCD in selected patients with HFrEF; 40 days post MI with LVEF <35% and NYHA 2 or 3; on GPMT; expected to live <1 year.
  LDE (B) ICD for 1 degree prevention of SCD patients with HFrEF; 40 days post MI; LVEF <30 and NYHA 1: on GDMT; Expected to live <1 year.

7.12 MYOCARDIAL O_2 UPTAKE

INTRODUCTION

O_2 uptake increased by
- Increased wall stress
- Increased after load
- Increased preload
- Beta-adrenergic stimulation
- Any increase in ATP requirements
- Increased heart rate.

PRACTICAL INDEX FOR O_2 DEMAND

- Double product
- SBP x heart rate

A. Work of the heart

1. External work = pressure x volume
- Done by the heart with stroke volume being the volume moved against arterial blood pressure
- Volume work (associated with increased stroke volume) requires less oxygen)
- Pressure work (associated with increased pressure requires more oxygen
  So, minute work = SBP × HR × SV

2. Internal work (Potential energy)
   That is energy generated with each contraction cycle but not converted to external work

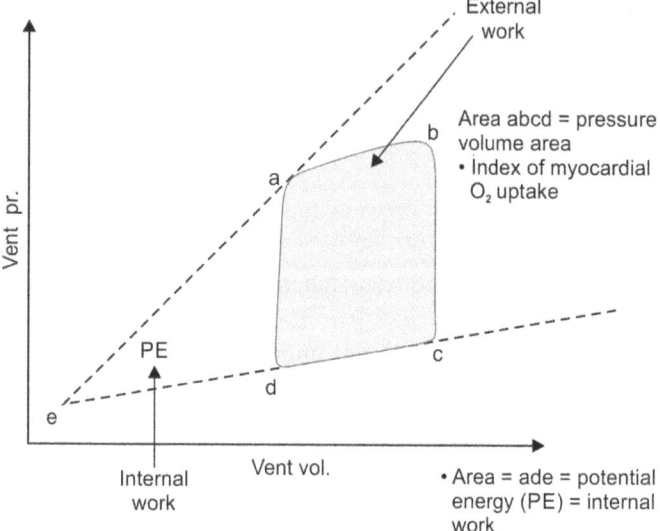

3. Kinetic work
- Component of work required to move blood against the after load
- <1% of total
- In As – kinetic work increase sharply as the CSA of Ao narrows.

  Whereas pressure work increases as the gradient across the aortic valve rises.

7.13 FRANK STARLING RELATIONSHIP

INTRODUCTION

Starling 1918: "Within the physiological limit, larger the volume of the heart, the greater the energy of its contraction and the amount of chemical change at each contraction".

Frank 1895: Better the initial LV volume, the more rapid rate of rice the greater the peak pressure reached and faster the rate of relaxation

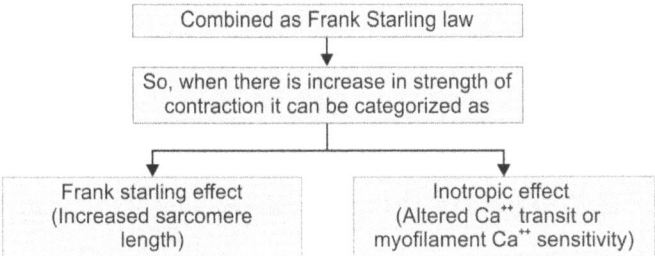

ANREP EFFECT

(abrupt increase in afterload)
Abrupt increase in Ao pressure
↓
Ejection is limited
↓
EDV tends to increase
↓
Increases force and pressure at next beat (Frank Starling)
↓
However these is slower adaptation that takes seconds to mins
↓
This slow force response or adaptation is referred as Anrep effect

WALL STRESS (LAPLACE'S LAW)

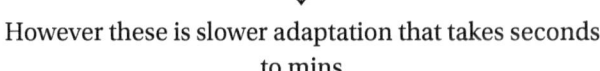

- Develops when tension is applied to a CSA
- Unit of wall stress is force per unit area

From above equation
- Larger LV size and radius – higher wall stress
- Greater pressure developed by LV-higher stress
↓
Any of these 2 mechanisms
↓
Increase myocardial O_2 uptake
↓

- Hypertrophy (compensatory) can compensate for increased LV size and intracavitary pressure
- In congestive heart failure, heart dilates
↓
Increase wall stress
↓
Additionally EF and stroke volume is low in heart failure
↓
Radius/size of LV remain too large throughout cardiac cycle
↓
Both end diastolic and end systolic wall stress are higher
↓
Reduction in heart size decreases wall stress and improves LV function
↓
Wall stress, preload and after load
↓
Preload now defined more exactly as wall stress at end diastolic and therefore at maximal resting length of sarcomere
↓
After load defined as wall stress during LV ejection
- Measurement of wall stress in vivo is difficult because use of LV radius neglects the confounding influence of complex LV anatomy.

PEAK SYSTOLIC WALL STRESS

Three components
1. Peripheral resistance
2. Arterial resistance
3. Peak intra ventricular pressure.

SBP can be used as indirect approximation for measuring after load clinically.

MEASUREMENT OF WALL STRESS

- Strain imaging
- Aortic impedance calculation (invasive)
  AI = Aortic pressure/Aortic flow
  Factors reducing aortic flow (As, high arterial BP, loss of aortic compliance)
  ↓
  Increases impedance and after load

In LV failure aortic impedance is augmented not only by peripheral vasoconstriction but also by decrease in Aortic compliance.

HEART RATE AND FORCE FREQUENCY RELATIONSHIP

Treppe or Bowditch Effect

Increasing heart rate
↓
Progressively enhancing force of contraction
↓
Known as Bowditch staircase phenomena
↓
Negative staircase effect = decreased heart rate
↓
However at higher heart rate
↓
Force of cont progressively decreases
(Due to change in Na^+ and Ca^{++})
↓

High heart rate
↓
More Na^+ and Ca^{++} entry per unit time
And less time for extrusion of these ions
↓
(Higher cellular Na^+) and cellular + SR Ca^{++} conc
↓
Increased SR Ca^{++} increase release of Ca^{++} during AP
↓
Increase in contractility
↓
Reduce efficacy of NCx in extruding Ca^{++} – further gain in SR and cellular Ca^{++} [Na^+ lay hypothesis]
↓
New steady state achieved
(Ca^{++} extrusion via NCx match the amount of Ca^{++} influx)

7.14 CARDIOVASCULAR REGENERATION AND GENE THERAPY

Q.1 Gene therapy in IHD (Jan 2000)
Q.2 VEGF gene therapy in patients with severe CAD (Dec 03)
Q.3 Stem cell therapeutics in CV disease (June 04) (Dec 08)
Q.4 Design an investigation protocol to test the efficacy of stem cell therapy in CHF
Q.5 Current status of gene therapy and stem cell transplantation in CV disease (Dec 13)
Q.6 Stem cell in CV disorder (June 15)
Q.7 Principle of cell and gene based cardiac regeneration therapy. Cell and gene delivery system. Clinical trials of gene therapy (5+3+2) (June 17)

CELL THERAPY

Repopulate damaged areas within the heart with new cells.

GENE THERAPY

To repair the compromised cardiac myocyte in failing heart.

Goal

To improve the function of failing cardiac myocyte by modulating the expression of specific genes
↓
In other words, gene therapy repair the compromised cardiac myocyte in failing heart

Basic Principle

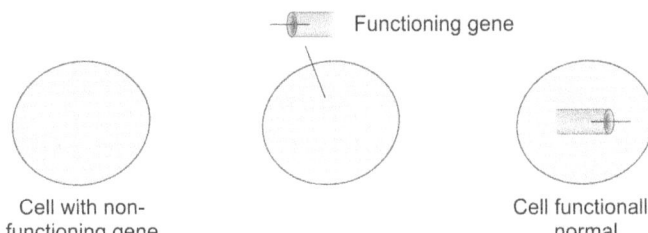

Molecular Targets

A. Targeting beta adrenergic system
- Regulation of g protein coupled receptor kinase 2(GRK2)- link to beta AR signaling abnormality
  Therapy to manipulate beta AR can enhance function
- Activation of adenylyl cyclase

B. Targeting Ca^{++} homeostasis
- Decreasing SERCA2a-improved cardiac function
- Inhibition of phospholamban
- Inhibition of phosphatase 1 – increased phosphorylation of phospholamban-inhibit SERCA
- S100- implicated in intracellular Ca^{++} regulatory activity
- SERCA2a PVT in parallel with level of small ubiquitin like modifier type 1 (SUM01).

GENE DELIVERY SYSTEM

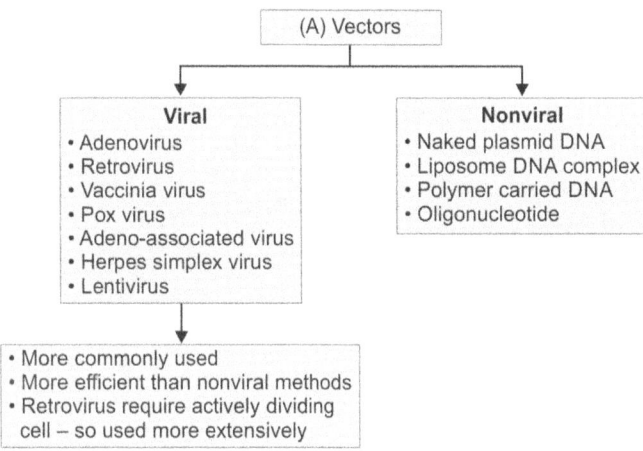

B. Delivery techniques
- Direct myocardial injection
  Pros
  - Simple and safe
  - High density gene transfer
  Cons
  - Small area of gene expression
  - Multiple injection sites needed
  - Acute inflammatory response at injection site
- Intracoronary injection and retrograde infusion through coronary sinus
  Pros:
  - Deliver gene globally across myocardium
  - More homogeneous distribution
  Cons:
  - Delivered in systemic circulation
- Aortic cross clamp-LV cavity infusion
  Cons:
  - Need open heart surgery
- Cardiopulmonary bypass perfusion and closed loop system
  Pros:
  - Separate coronary circulation from systemic circulation
- Epicardial painting
- Electroporation

Use in Cardiovascular Disease

A. For Coronary artery disease
- For patients suffering from severe angina pectoris despite OMT and no longer treatable with PCI or CABG
- For therapeutic angiogenesis (experimental)

Molecular Targets
- VEGF (vascular endothelial growth factor)
- FGF (fibroblast growth factor)
- Hepatocyte growth factor
- Platelet derived growth factor
- Hypoxia inducible factor

B. For heart failure
- For resistant heart failure
  Molecular targets
  - SERCA 2a
  - Stromal derived factor 1
  - Adenylyl cyclase-6
  - β-AKK(C⁺) carboxyl terminal peptide for GRK2
  - S100 A1
  - PVALB- parvalbumin.

Effects
Decreased HF symptoms; Increased functional status; reversal of negative LV remodeling; improve QOL

C. For Arrhythmias
- Vent Arrhythmias refractory to treatment
- VT storm
- Reentrant Arrhythmias
  Molecular targets
  - KCNH2, SCN4A
  - Connexin-32, 40, 43
  - SERCA2a
  - Adenylyl cyclase 1 and 6
  - kir 2-1

Effects: Prolongs refractory period, Reduced VT inaudibility; improve conduction and reduced arrhythmia susceptibility.

Trials
- *1st trial (2007) CUPID:* (Ca^{++} up regulation by percutaneous administration of gene therapy)
  - 12 month follow-up – study group exhibited reduced signs and symptoms of HF, improved functional status, biomarker profile and LV function
  - Significant decrease in CV everts, HF related hospitalization, death or requirement of LVAD
  - No increase in adverse event
- Two other trials involving SERCA2a are currently recruiting patients
  - 1st-in patients with advanced HF
  - 2nd-investigating impact of SERCA2a on cardiac remodeling parameter in patients with severe HF
- *Another trial:* Examining effect of SDFI injection directly into myocardium of patients with IHD
  - Found to be feasible and safe

Goal: To repopulate areas of damaged myocardium with cells capable of engraftment and tri lineage differential into cardiac myocyte, VSMC and endothelium.

STEM CELL THERAPY

Goal
To replace permanently lost cardiac myocyte improve function.

Principle
Three fundamental principles
1. Multipotent cardiac progenitor cells exists in embryonic mammalian heart
2. There is formation of limited number of new heart cells after birth
3. Some vertebrates such as newts, zebra fish and neonatal misc can regenerate myocardium following experimental injury.

HOW CELL THERAPY EVOLVED

Approach to find effective cell based therapy have evolved considerably
- 1st major attention shifted from embryonic/pluripotent stem cell to source of adult cells that have capacity for cardiac repair
- 2nd many other facets of cell based therapy have potential to contribute to success of the approach. These includes antifibrotic effect, neovascularization, and stimulation of endogenous CSC
- 3rd attention paid to advancing practical aspect of cell delivery through development of effective delivery system.

Classification of Stem Cells
- Somatic stem cells
  - Self renewable cells present in virtually all organs of body

- Limited differentiation capacity
- Multipotent or unipotent
- Embryonic stem cells
  - Pluripotent
  - Derived from preimplantation embryos
  - Totipotent cells derived from embryos before differentiation of trophectoderm and inner cell mass (i.e., Morula cell)
- Induced pluripotent stem cell
  - Capable of indefinite expansion
  - Differentiate into ectodermal, mesodermal and endodermal cells
  - Generated from somatic cells by biogenetic engineering
- Endogenous cardiac stem cells
  - Potential to differentiate into all 3 cardiovascular stem type Cardiac myocyte, endothelial cells and smooth muscle cells
  - Express c-kit.

CELLS USED FOR CARDIOVASCULAR THERAPEUTICS

BAMI Trial

SCIPIPO trial In ischemic CM it improved EF and decreased infarct size

1. Autologous whole bone marrow cell
2. Mesenchymal stem cell
3. Skeletal myoblast — 1st generation
4. Endothelial precursor cells
5. Cardiac stem cell (c-kit positive) — 2nd generation
6. Mesenchymal precursor

Mechanism of stem cell therapy
Stem cell delivery

Intravenous/Intracoronary/Intramyocardial inj.
↓
Numbers of endogenous factors enhance stem cell mobilization to the injury area

Cell homing:
- Stem cell factor-clit
- Stromal derived factor-1 (SDF-1)
- SDF-1-CXCR4 complex

↓
Recruit large number of progenitor cells
↓
Various pharmacological factors as well as non-pharmacological factors (diet, exercise) Can also promote cell homing
↓
Differentiation into mature cell

CLINICAL APPLICATION

- IHD
  - Acute MI - therapy prevents remodeling
  - Chronic ischemic myocardium-reverse remodeling
  - Hibernating myocardium
  - Intractable angina pectoris
- Idiopathic DCM
  - Ongoing POSEIDON-DCM trial
- Congenital heart disease
  - Children with cardiomyopathy
  - Regenerative strategy involving tissue valve regeneration and the constitution of biological patches – potential to treat CHD.

TRIALS

- *Osiris:* Allogeneic MSC in Ac MI
- *C-CURE:* Cardiopoietic MSC in ischemic CMP
- *Mesoblast:* Mesenchymal precursor cell in ischemic CMP
- *TAC-HFT:* Autologous MSC in Ischemic CMP
- *POSEIDON-DCM:* Autologous vs. Allogeneic MSC in DCMP
- *BAMI:* Autologous whole BM in Ac MI
- *CD34:* $CD34^+$ endogenous precursor cell in angina pectoris.

7.15 HFrEF MANAGEMENT

INTRODUCTION
- *Incidence:* F < M
- *Prevalence:* M = F (because of longer life expectancy)
  (HFrEF = EF <35%)   (HFpEF = EF >50%)
  (35–50 = gray zone)

ETIOLOGY

A. Myocardial disease
B. Coronary art disease
   - Infarction
   - Ischemia
C. Chronic pr overload
   - HTN
   - Obstructive valvular disease
D. Chronic vol overload
   - Regurgitation valvular disease
   - Intracardiac shunt
   - Extracardiac shunt
E. Disorder of rate and rhythm
   - Chr bradyarrhythmias
   - Chr tachyarrhythmia
F. Nonischemic DCM (20–30%)/Idiopathic
   - Familial/genetic disorder
   - Excess alcohol
   - Infiltrative disorder
   - Viral infection
   - Toxin/drug induced
   - Chemotherapy induced
   - Metabolic disorder
G. Pulm disease
   - Cor pulmonale
   - Pulm vasc disorders
H. High output state
H1. Metabolic disorder
   - Thyrotoxicosis
   - Nutritional (Beriberi)
H2. Excessive blood flow treatment
   - Chr Anemia
   - Syst AV shunting

PROGNOSIS
- Women with HF had better prognosis
- However women had greater functional incapacity for some degree of LV dysfunction.

Prognosis Variables
A. *Demographics:* Age, gender, race
B. *Etiology:* CAD, idiopathic DCM, valvular heart disease, myocarditis, hypertrophy, alcohol, anthracycline, amyloidosis, hemochromatosis genetic factors
C. *Comorbidity* HTN, DM, 9 HTN, sleep apnea, obesity, renal dysfunction, COPD
D. *Clinical assessment:* NYHA class, syncope, angina, systolic versus diastolic function
E. *Hemodynamics:* LVEF, LVEDP, RVEF, PAP, JVP, PCWP, CI, exercise hemodynamics
F. *Exercise testing:* Metabolic assessment, BP response, heart rate response, 6 mm walk test, peak VO_2, VE/VCO_2 curve, O_2 uptake slope
G. *Metabolic:* Sr Na^+, thyroid dysfunction, Anemia, acidosis/alkalosis
H. *CXR:* congestion, cardiothoracic ratio
I. *ECG:* Arrhythmia, voltage, QRS width, QT interval, SA-ECG, HR variability
J. *Biomarkers:* NE, PRA, AVP, Aldosterone, ANP, BNP, proBNP, endothelin, TNF, STNFR-2, Galectin-3, cardiac troponin, hematocrit
K. *Endomyocardial biopsy:* Inflammation, degree of fibrosis, degree of cellular disarray, infiltrative process

- Age strongest and most consistent risk factor for prediction of worse outcome in HF
- Strong inverse correlation between survival and biomarkers-NE, renin, angiotensin, Aldosterone, AVP, ANP, BNP, NT pro BNP, endothelin-1
- Inflammatory markers (TNF, STNF, receptors, CRP, Galectin-3, Pentraxin-3 and soluble ST2) also has inverse correlation with survival
- Markers of oxidative stress (oxidized LDL, uric acid) also associated with worse outcome
- Cardiac troponin increased in non-ischemic DCMP- denotes worse Prognosis
- Low Hb/hematocrit – worse outcome, worse symptoms and function class, greater risk of hospitalization and decrease survival
  (Correction of Anemia by IV iron improves function class)
  (FAIR-HF trial)
  (Correction of anemia by erythropoietin along with darbepoetin alpha) (Red HF trial)
  No significant difference found

RENAL INSUFFICIENCY IN HF
- Marker of poor prognosis
- Not clear whether impairment is due to worsening HF or impaired renal function leads to worsening HF
- Majority of HF patients had some degree of renal dysfunction
- 50% increased relative mortality risk
- Similar findings observed in ADHERE study.

APPROACH TO PATIENT

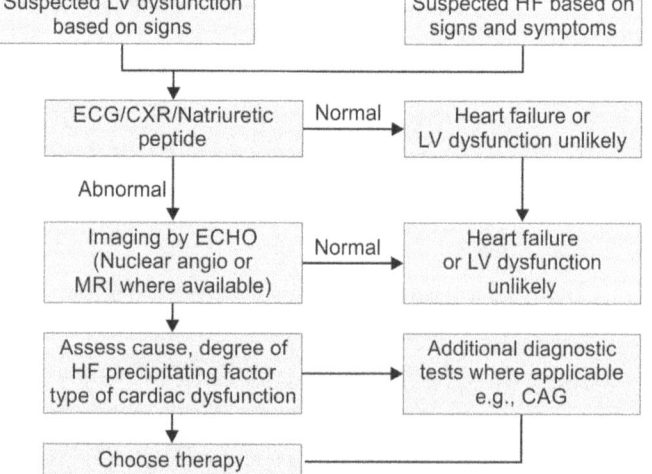

Framingham diagnostic criteria		
Major criteria	Minor criteria	Major/minor
• PND/orthopnea • Neck vein distention • Rales • Cardiomegaly • Ac pulm edema • S9 gallop • Increased venous pr >16 cmH$_2$O • HTR	• DOE • Night cough • Pl Effusion • Ankle edema • VC decreased by 1/3rd • Tachy (>120) • Hepatomegaly	• Weight loss >4.5 kg in 5d response to treatment

NHANES CRITERIA

History: Dyspnea on hiking on hill	1
Dyspnea when walking at ordinary pace	1
Do you stop for breathing when walking at ordinary place?	2
Do you stop for breathing after walking 100 yards on ground?	2
Examination: Heart rate 91–110/min	1
>110/min	2
JVP >6 OM H$_2$O	1
With hepatomegaly/edema	2
Rales Basilar rales	1
More extensive	2
CXR: Upper zone flow redistribution	1
Interstitial fluid	2
Interstitial fluid + effusion	3
Alveolar fluid + pl fluid	3

ALGORITHM FOR DIAGNOSIS

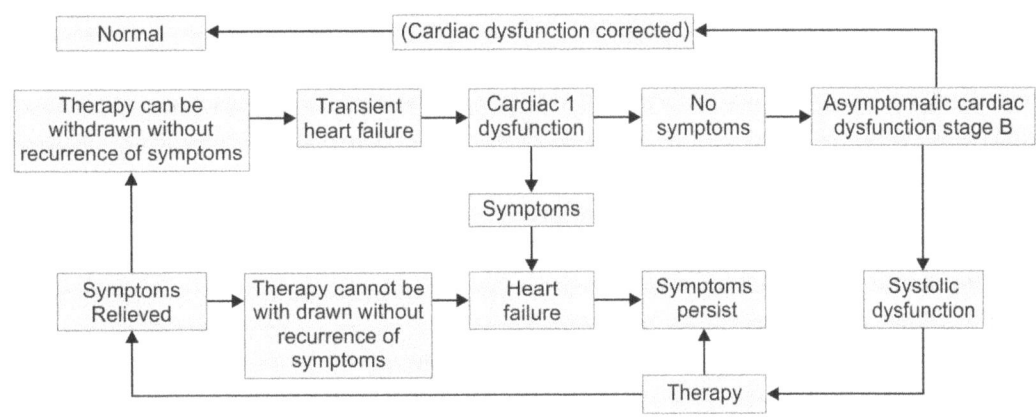

MANAGEMENT

Goal

Reduce symptoms
- Prolong survival
- Improve quality of life
- Prevent disease progression.

Braking Phenomena	NYHA 1	NYHA2	NYHA3	NYHA 4
	Asymptomatic LV dysfunction	Symptomatic HF	Worsening HF	End stage HF
ACE 1	Indicated	Indicated	Indicated	Indicated
ARB	Indicated (if ACE tolerant) →	Same ———— →	Same ———— →	Same
Diuretics	Not indicated	Indicated if fluid retention	Indicated	Indicated
β-Blocker	Post MI indicated	Indicated	Indicated	Indicated
Aldosterone antagonist	Recent MI	Indicated	Indicated	Indicated
Cardiac glycoside	1. For rate control in AF 2. When improved from HF and in sinus rhythm	Same	Indicated	Indicated
CRT	May be considerable	Indicated	Indicated	Indicated
ICD	Indicated		Indicated	Not indicated

Management of stage A HF-prevention of HF by treating risk factors (HTN, DM, dyslipidemia)
Management of stage B, C, D HF-depends on NYHA class

A. General measures
   - Identify and correct condition underlying
   - Aggressively treat Comorbidities DM/HTN
   - Treat creative provocative factors
     (Dietary indiscretion, medication discontinuation and nonadherence to treatment, MI, arrhythmias, infection, anemia, NSAIDs, alcohol consumption pregnancy, worsening hypertension, acute valvular insufficiency)
   - Stop smoking and limit alcohol
   - Extreme temperature and heavy physical exertion to be avoided
   - Daily weight and fluid status check
   - Vaccination to those patients who are at high risk of pneumococcal pneumonia and influenza
   - Educate patient and family
   - Routine modest exercise is beneficial
     - For euvolemic patients-Isotonic exercise like walking or riding stationary bicycle is useful
     - For patients who had HF episode in past weeks exercise training is not recommended
   - Diet sodium restriction (2 mg/d)
     - Fluid restriction for hyponatremia patients or for patients whose fluid retention is difficult to control in spite high dose diuretic and Na^+ restriction
     Calorie supplementation for advanced heart failure and unintentional weight loss
B. *Management of fluid retention*
   - Diuretics-loop:
     - Thiazide
     - Potassium sparing
   Loop diuretics: Negative Na^+ and water balance
     - Decreased cardiac filling pr - decreased wall stress and endocardial ischemia
     - Improve myocardial function
   Loop diuretic increased Na^+ excretion up to 20-25% of filtered load of sodium
   Thiazide increased only by 5-10%
   Aquaretics: Drugs which increase water excretion
     - Demeclocycline
     - Lithium
     - Vasopressin V2 receptor antagonist.

Available Drugs

Loop Diuretics
- Furosemide: 20-40 mg OD/BD (max 600 mg)
- Bumetanide: 0.5-1 mg OD/BD (max 10 mg)
- Torsemide
- Ethacrynic acid

Thiazide Diuretic
- Hydrochlorothiazide - 25 mg OD/BD (max 200 mg)
- Chlorothiazide-(250-500 mg OD/BD)
- Chlorthalidone-(12.5-25 mg OD)
- Indapamide-2.5 mg OD (max 5 mg)
- Metolazone-(2.5-5 mg OD) (max 20 mg).

Potassium Sparing
- Amiloride-12.5-25 mg OD
- Triamterene-50-75 mg BD

AVP Antagonist
- Tolvaptan 15 mg OD (max 60 mg)
- Conivaptan 20 mg IV - 20 mg/d infusion
- Satavaptan.

Sequential Nephron Blockade
- Metolazone 2.5-10 mg once + loop diuretic
- Hydrochlorothiazide 2.5-100 mg + loop diuretic
- Chlorothiazide 500-1000 mg + loop diuretics.

LOOP DIURETICS

MOA: Reversibly inhibit $Na^+- K^+ -2Cl^-$ symporter
On apical membrane of epithelial cells in thick ascending loop of henle.

Pharmacokinetic

Bound extensively to plasma protein
Delivery to tubule by filtration is limited
However secreted efficiently by organic acid transporter in proximal tubule gain access to target site (so efficacy of loop diuretics depends on efficient renal plasma flow and efficiency of organic acid transporter in prox tubule
Bioavailability: Furosemide-40-70%
   Bumetanide >80%
   Torsemide
Inhibit absorption of Na^+ from loop of Henle - reduce driving force for H_2O reabsorption

$Na^+ - H_2O$ excretion
- Also increased excretion of Mg^{++}, K^+, Ca^{++}
- Also access venodilator and reduce RAP and PCWP within minutes when given intravenously (due to release of vasodilatory prostaglandins)

Thiazide Diuretics

MOA: blocks $Na^+ Cl^-$ transporter in critical portion of ascending loop of Henle and DCT

↓

Prevent maximum dilution of urine

↓

Decrease kidney stability to increase free water clearance

↓

Contributes to hyponatremia

↓

Also increases Mg^{++} excretion

Ca^{++} absorption increases hypercalcemia.

Mineralocorticoid Antagonist

Spironolactone and Eplerenone

↓

Act on distal nephron to inhibit Na^+/K^+ excretion at the site of aldosterone action

↓

→ Spironolactone had antiandrogenic effect- causes gynecomastia or impotence

↓

→ Eplerenone developed to overcome this side effect

→ Administered in HF to antagonize RAAS system rather than diuretic action

Potassium Sparing

Triamterene and Amiloride
- Mild increase in NaCl excretion
- Antikaliuretic property
  Blocks Na^+ reabsorption in late distal tubule and collecting duct
  However Na^+ retention occur mainly in proximal tubule in HF Amiloride alone cannot generate net negative balance for Na^+

Carbonic Anhydrase Inhibitor

(Acetazolamide)

↓

Near complete loss of $NaHCO_3$ Absorption in proximal tubule

↓

Can be used in HF as temporary administration to correct the metabolic alkalosis that occurs due to "contraction phenomena" in response to other diuretics.

Vasopressin Antagonists

V1a antagonist – blocks vasoconstricting effect

V2 antagonist – inhibit recruitment of aquaporin channels in apical memb of collecting duct epithelial cells

↓

Decreased ability of collecting duct's water reabsorption

Diuretic for HF

Indi:
- E/O volume overload
- H/O fluid retention
- Always used in combination with neurohormonal antagonists that is known to prevent disease progression

Moderate to severe symptoms or renal insufficiency-loop diuretics required

↓

Once patient achieved adequate diuresis

↓

Document 'dry weight'

↓

Daily monitoring of weight

Complications

- Electrolyte and metabolic disturbance
- Volume depletion
- Aldosterone antagonists associated with hyperkalemia
- Hypomagnesemia, metabolic alkalosis, hyperglycemia, hyperlipidemia, hyperuricemia
- Hypercalcemia with thiazide Diuretics
- Hypotension
- Decreased exercise tolerance excessive Diuretics
- Increased fatigue
- Impaired renal function
- Increased neurohormonal axis activation
- Ethacrynic acid-ototoxicity.

DIURETICS RESISTANCE

Mech

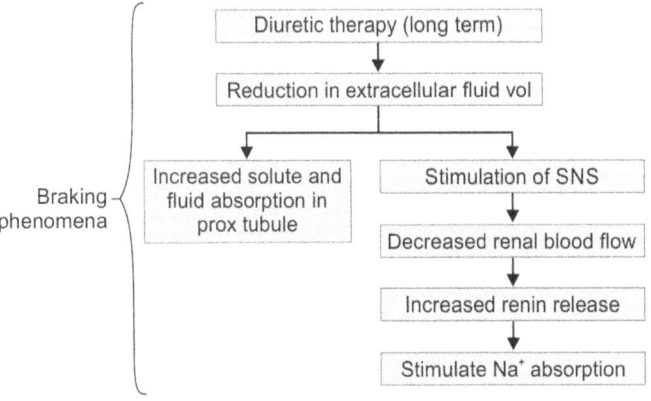

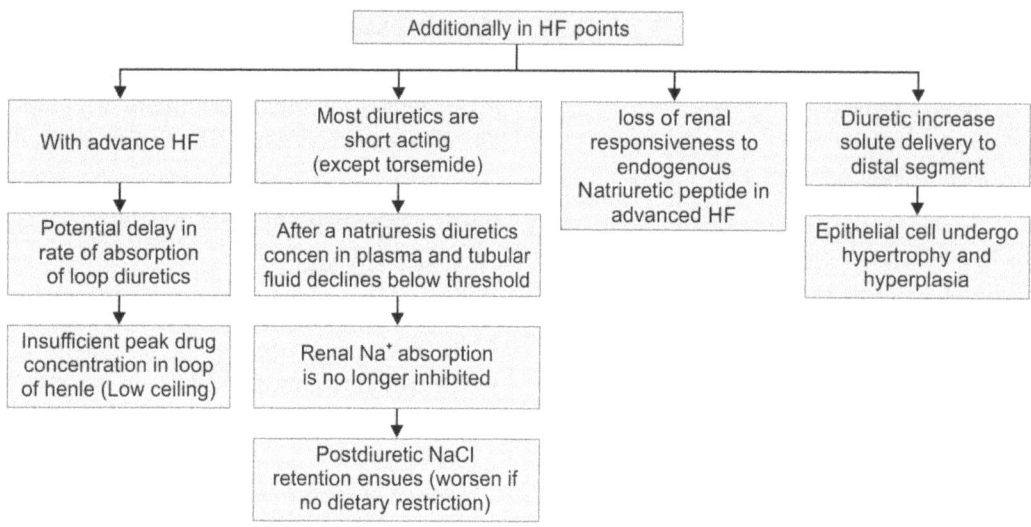

Shifts dose response curve to rt (even with IV)

Additionally:
- Abrupt decline in cardiac/renal function lead to
- Noncompliance with treatment diuretic resistance
- Cardiorenal syndrome.

Definition

Patients with HF considered to be resistant to diuretic drug when moderate dose of loop diuretic do not achieve derived reduction in extracellular fluid volume.

Management

- Coadministration of two different class of diuretics
  E.g., Diuretic (loop) + hydrochloro (thiazide)
  loop diuretic + (metolazone)
    - Longer half Life
    - Prevent post diuretic NaCl retention
    - Inhibit Na^+ transport along the proximal tubule (as most thiazide diuretic are also carbonic anhydrase inhibitor)
    - Inhibit NaCl transport in distal tubule

Initially add thiazide without altering loop diuretic dose
↓
Once desired fluid loss is achieved
↓
Switch to three times a week thiazide to avoid excessive diuresis

- Administration of loop diuretic by cont infusion
  ↓
  - Avoids post diuretic NaCl retention
    Dose: Trial did not show significant difference between IV bolus and IV infusion
- Device based therapy for fluid overload
  - Extracorporeal ultrafiltration
    - For patients who become resistant to diuretic
    - Remove salt and water isotonically
  - Cont hemofiltration
  - Cont hemodialysis
  - Cont hemodiafiltration
    RAPID CHF trial (ultrafiltration vs. Diuretics)
    UNLOAD trial (ultrafiltration vs. Diuretics)
    ↓

Two treatment where found to be similar in ability to relieve dyspnea ultrafiltration was associated with significant greater fluid loss over 48 hours and lower rate of rehospitalization within 90 days
CARESS evaluated role of UF in CRS patient
↓

UF resulted in similar weight loss but increase in creatinine levels compared to standard case and was associated with more severe adverse events

C. *Prevention of disease progression*
1. *ACE inhibitors*
   MOA:
   - Inhibit conversion of angiotensin 1-2
   - Induce a regulation of bradykinin (further enhance effects of angiotensin separation)

   Action:
   - Stabilize LV remodeling
   - Relieve symptoms.

- Prevent hospitalization
- Prolong life

How to Start?

- Optimal dose of diuretic has to be achieved before ACE inhibitor (fluid retention reduces effect of ACEI)
- Start with low dose
- May required to decrease dose of diuretic duration initiation to prevent hypertension
- Doubling dose even 3 to 5 days until maximum effect achieved
- BP, renal function and K^+ should be evaluated within 1 to 2 weeks a
- Abrupt withdrawal may lead to rebound hypertension and worsening of clinical status.

Trials

SOLVD, SAVE, TRACE-Asymptomatic patients with LV dysfunction are less likely to develop symptomatic HF and to require hospitalization for HF when treated with ACEI.
   Benefit greatest in patient with most severe HF.

CONSENSUS 1-larger effect than SOLVD
V-HeFT-2-ACEI history of HF through mechanism other than vasodilatation-subject treated with enalapril had significantly lower mortality than subjects treated with vasodilatory combination.

Complications

1. Hypertension
2. Mild azotemia
3. Renal dysfunction
4. Potassium retention
5. Kinin potentiation-nonproductive cough, angioedema
2. ARBS
- As effective as ACEI
   Trails CHARM alternative: Candesartan reduced all cause mortality
   Val-Heft similar findings with valsartan
   ELITE 2-compared ACEI & ARBS
- Losartan was not associated with improved survival in elderly patients with HF (compared to captopril)
- But better tolerated

ACE + ARB
- VALIANT valsartan non-inferior to captopril
- Combination of valsartan + captopril produced no further reduction in mortality
- CHARM-added Trial: No beneficial effect of ACEI + ARBS
- Val Heft No additional effect with ACEI + ARB

3. Beta blockers
   MOA:
   - Antagonize beta-1, beta-2 and alpha1 receptor activity
   - In HF it antagonize deleterious activity of sustained activation of sympathetic nervous system

   Choice: beta blockers shown to be effective
   - Bisopropol ⎤ competitively block beta-1
   - Metoprolol ⎥
   - Carvedilol ⎦ completely block alpha1, beta-1, beta-2

Given with ACEI

- Reverse LV remodeling
- Relieves symptoms
- Prevent rehospitalization
- Improve survival.

How to Start?

- Start in low dose
- Should be increased after 2 weeks (ACEI in 3-5 days)
- Imp to optimize dose of diuretic before beta blocker (Reason: abrupt withdrawal of alpha action by betablockers can lead to worsening of HF)

   If HF worsens, it occurs in 3-5 days (need to increase dose of diuretic)
   ↓
- Even in patients receiving low dose ACEI beta blocker addition produce greater symptomatic relief and improves survival
- Beta blocker can be safely started before discharge and it is well tolerated by majority of patients with HF.

Trials

- MDC: Metopolol in DCM: first trial with beta blocker
- *CIBIS-1 Trial:* First trial performed with Bisoprolol-non significant risk reduction for mortality at 2 years
- *CIBIS-2:* Bisoprolol reduced all cause mortality, SCD, HF hospitalization and all cause hospitalization
- *CIBIS-3:* Beta blocker was non inferior to ACEI Overall safety of both were similar
   Current guideline continue to recommend starting with ACEI and subsequent addition of Beta blocker
- Cardinal studied extensively
   - COPERNICUS trial
   - CAPRICORN Trial
   - COMET trial (carvedilol vs. Metoprolol)
   Carvedilol is non inferior
- Nebrivolol (selective beta receptor blockers)
   Trail SENIORS-significantly reduce composite outcome of death and CV hospitalization but did not reduce mortality

S/E

- Problem of fluid retention
- Gen fatigue or weakness
- Bradycardia/heart block
- Combined alpha + beta blocker – vasodilatation side effect

Caution

- Continuation of beta blocker during acute episode is safe but dose reduction is needed
- Do not continue in patients with asthma + active bronchospasm
4. *Aldosterone antagonist*
   (Spironolactone)(Eplerenone)
   ACEI- transiently decrease aldosterone release but with chronic therapy
   There is rapid return of aldosterone to level similar to those before ACEI

Aldosterone Antagonists
- Not recommended for asymptomatic HF
- Recommended for NYHA 2-4 with low EF and who are receiving ACE + beta blocker + diuretic.

SPIRONOLACTONE

Start at 12.5-25 mg – uptitrate to 25-50

Eplerenone
Start at 25 mg/d – uptitrate to 50/d
- Avoid K^+ supplement and K^+ containing diet with aldosterone Antagonist

Trials: RALES: Spironolactone in HF
        EMPHASIS HF: Eplerenone in HF
        EPHESUS-Eplerenone post MI

S/E:
- Life threatening hyperkalemia
- Not recommended for cr >2.5 or K^+ >5.5 mmol/L
- Painful gynacomastia with aldosterone
- *IVABRADIN*
  MOA: Blocks cardiac pacemaker if current that controls spontaneous diastolic depolarization of SA node
  - Blocks If channel in concentration dependent manner
  - Blocks If channel by entering channel pure from intracellular side-can only block channel when its open
  - More effective at higher heart rate (If blocking is related to frequency of opening of channel)
    Approved antianginal drug in Europe
  Trial:
  - SHIFT Ivabradine reduced primary composite end point of CV death and HF hospitalization

- BEAUTIFUL Trial - did not meet 1° end point of reducing CV death, MI or HF hospitalization
  The drug was well tolerated
- *Renin Inhibitor* (aliskiren)

RAAs escape: AECI and ARBS provoke compensatory increase in renin and downstream intermediateries of RAAs system
Attenuation of effect of ACEI/ARB
↓

MOA: Aliskiren binds to active site of renin

Trial

ALOFT
   ASTRONAUT: No significant difference in 1° end point of CV death or HF rehospitalization
   ATMOSPHERE: Evaluating efficacy and safety of Aliskiren alone and Aliskiren+ enalapril.

S/E

Hyperkalemia
   Hypotension
   Renal impairment.

Algorithm HF Diagnosis Confirmed

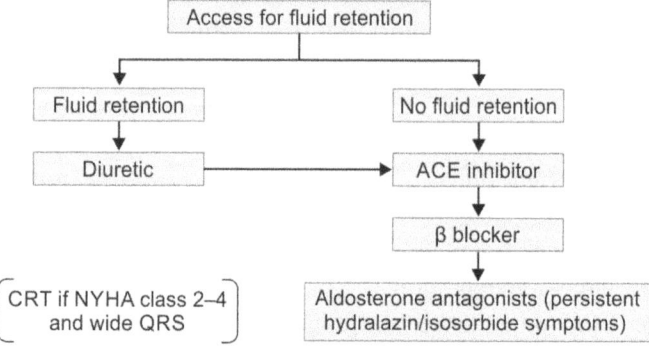

CARDIAC GLYCOSIDE

(Digoxin) and (Digitoxin)
Digoxin is most commonly used and tested in placebo controlled trial
- Recommended for patients with symptomatic LV dysfunction who have concomitant AF and
- Should be considered for patients who have signs or symptoms of HF while receiving standard therapy

MOA:
- Inhibit $Na^+ - K^+$ ATPase pump
         ↓
  Increased intracellular Ca^{++}
         ↓
  Increased contractility (inotropy)

- More likely mechanism
  ↓
  Sensitive $Na^+ - K^+$ ATPase activity in vagal afferent nerve
  ↓
  Increased vagal tone
  ↓
  Counter balance increased activity of adrenergic system in HF
- Inhibit $Na^+ - K^+$ ATPase in kidney
  ↓
  Blunt renal tubular resorption of sodium.

Trials
- RASIANCE ⎤ Provide strong support for
- PROVED ⎦ clinical benefit of digoxin
- DIG (Digoxin investigator group) Trial strong Trent towered a decrease in death 2° to progressive pump failure. Mortality was directly related with Sr. Digoxin level Level between 0.6 and 0.8 mg/mL were associated with decreased mortality.

S/E
- Arrhythmia (including heart block) and ectopic Reentrant tachy
- Neurologic complains such as visual disturbance, disorientation, confusion
- Gastrointestinal symptoms such as anorexia, nausea and vomiting
  - Overt toxicity – digoxin level >2.0 mg/mL
  - May occur at lower level in (1) hypokalemia (2) Hypomagnesemia
  - Oral K^+ administration is often useful for atrial atrioventricular junctional or ventricular ectopic rhythms
  - For potentially life threatening dig toxicity, antidigoxin immuno therapy using Fab frag.

7.16 HFpEF

INTRODUCTION
- More likely to be older and female
- Systemic HTN is most common cause
- IHD is less common compared to HFrEF
- Has normal LVEDV and normal near EF and LSV
  Exhibit concentric remodeling of either LV chamber and or cardiomyocyte
- Standard HF treatment has not been found to reduce morbidity or mortality associated with

HFpEF
Substantial number of patients more than 50% in many studies who are diagnosed or hospitalized with HF have heart failure with preserved ejection fraction (HFpEF).

Natural History
Mortality
Five year survival rate less than 50% (all HF patients)
- Lower mortality in HFpEF
- Annual mortality 5 to 10%

Mode of Death
>70% cardiovascular deaths
- >20% due to HF
- >35% due to SCD

30% noncardiovascular 15% in HFrEF.

Morbidity
Readmission rate 50% at 6 months
- Conversion from HFpEF to HFrEF is uncommon
- Associated with incident injury (example MI).

PATHOPHYSIOLOGY
Basic Changes
- Altered LV relaxation and filling
- LV structural remodeling
- Altered LV geometry
- Changes in LV and vascular compliance.

Mechanism Contributing to Pathophysiology of HFpEF
A. *LV structure:*
   - Concentric remodeling and hypertrophy

B. *LV function:*
   - Systolic and diastolic function
   - Increased after load and increased filling pr
   - Dyssynchrony, dyssynergy
   - Ischemia
   - Chronotropic incompetence
   - Arrhythmias (SVT and VT)
   - Increased LA volume and stiffness decreased LA reservoir function
   - Arterial stiffening, endocardial dysfunction

C. *Cardiomyocyte:*
   - Abnormal Ca^{++} homeostasis
     (Increased diastolic Ca^{++} or decreased rate of reuptake- incomplete relaxation)
     (Deficit SERCA and Na^+ Ca^{++} exchanger activity)
     (Defective phospholamban calsequestrin)
   - Energetics
     (Decreased ATP or increased ADP slows actin-myosin cross bridge release)
   - Proteins regulating cross bridge formation
     Troponin C and troponin I complex
   - Cytoskeletal protein
     Increased microtubule density- increased diastolic stiffness
     Increased noncompliant titin increased diastolic stiffness

D. *Extracellular matrix:*
   - Collagen str, geometry, content, Type 1/3 rate
   - Collagen homeostasis-synthesis and post synthetic processing
   - Basement memb protein
   - Bioactive proteins peptides MMP/TIMP/SPARC
   - Fibroblast structure

E. *Extracardiac:*
   - LV-RV interaction and pericardial constraint
   - Peripheral muscle dysfunction
   - PAHTN
   - Neuro hormonal activation
   - Comorbid condition.

LV RELAXATION
- Active, energy dependent process
- Begins with decay of force generation capacity (from completion of ejection phase of systole through isovolumic relaxation and rapid filling).

In HFpEF

Relaxation and recoil are abnormal at rest as well not enhanced during exercise

Filling can only be maintained by increasing LA pressure
↓
HFpEF has longer dp/dt (peak rate of pressure fall)
↓
Relaxation rate is decreased
↓
HFpEF: Elastic recoil of material annular tissue (which determine long axis lengthening rate) also decreased
↓
Elastic recoil is impaired

Role of Hemodynamics

Aging   Systolic hypertension
↓
Increased age related vascular stiffness
↓
Alters timing of reflected pressure waves in the vascular tree
↓
Reflected waves arise in late systole rather than diastole
↓
                              Acute increase in BP
                              during rest or exercise
Increased LV pressure in late systole
↓
Impair LV relaxation and LV relaxation rate
↓
Decreased LA-LV gradient decreased early filling and increased LV diastolic and pressure

Role of Dyssynchrony and Dyssynergy

Synchrony: Timing of relaxation of different myocardial segment

Synergy: extend to which myo segment relax

Dyssynchrony ⎤
Dyssynergy   ⎦ Impair global LV relaxation

LV Diastolic Stiffness, Compliance and Distensibility

How to Measure?

- Can be described by diastolic pressure volume relationship.
- Should be obtained after relaxation is complete and slow feeling great (so viscous effect are not present)
↓
- Approximated using points obtained in late diastole
↓
Resultant diastolic pressure volume relaxation relation PPVR is nonlinear and can be approximated by an exponential function
- *LV stiffness*-(*definition*) – Ratio of LV diastolic pressure and LV diastolic volume (LV dp/dv) at any given diastolic volume
- *LV complaints* is reciprocal of stiffness
- *Diastolic distensibility* (*definition*) End diastolic pressure required to distend the LV and EDV
(HFpEF)
Reduced distensibility indicated by normal or reduced LVD and Elevated LVDP

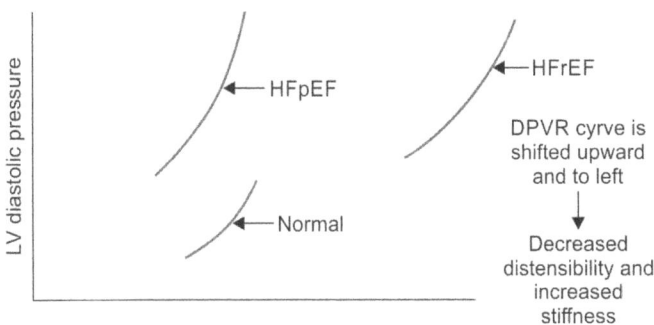

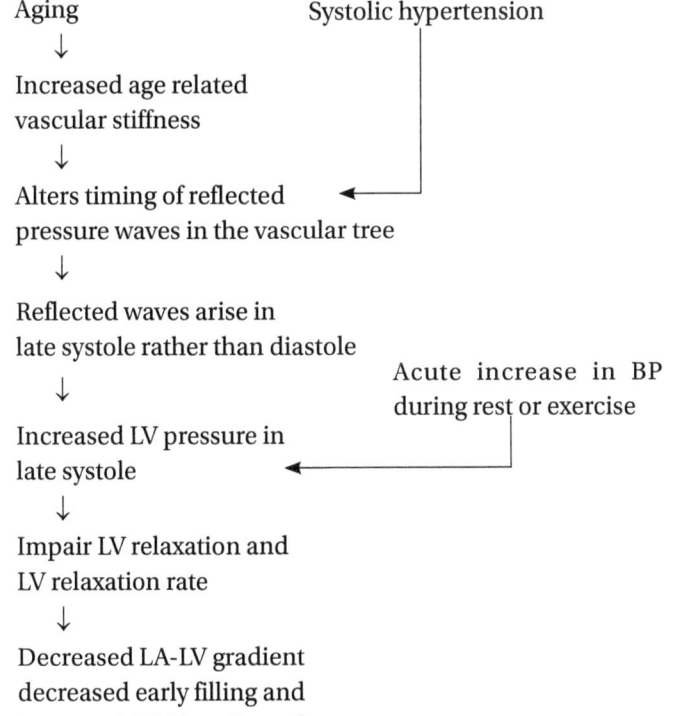

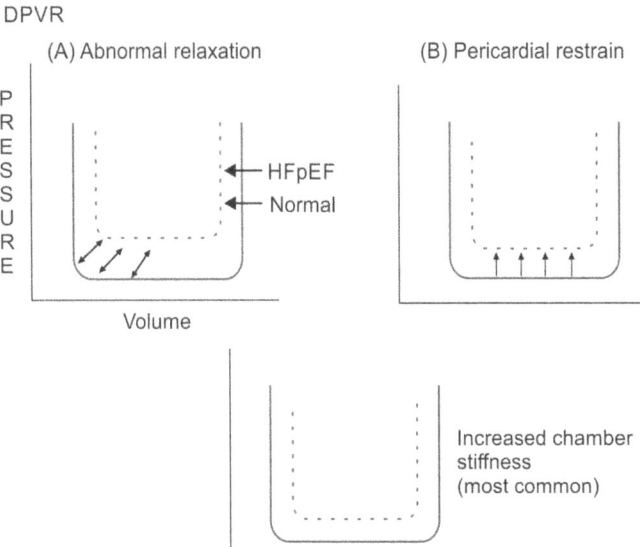

Determinants of DPVR

- Presence of LV and cardiomyocyte concentric remodeling and hypertrophy
- Changes in material properties of myocardial muscle itself (stiffness)

Diastolic stiffness determined by
Stress and strain relationship
↓   → Increase in length
Distending force

LVDPVR affected by
- Factors that influence ECM
  Fibrillar collagen, cellular structure and processes at cardiomyocyte level such as Ca^{++} homeostasis and energetics and myofilament and cytoskeletal protein (Titin).

Extracellular Matrix
Myocardial collagen network:
- Endomysial fiber surrounding individual myocyte and capillaries
- Perimysial fiber- intervene muscle bundles
- Epimysial fiber- form Matrix adjacent to epicardial and endocardial
  ECM structure is dynamic and regulated by physical neuro hormonal and inflammatory mediators
  In HFpEF ECM collagen content is increased
  ↓
  Increased diastolic stiffness
  ↓
  Diastolic dysfunction

Myofilament and extra myofilament protein number of factors including titin Isoform switches and titin phosphorylation affect diastolic stiffness.

CLINICAL FEATURES OF HFpEF

Signs and symptoms of HF

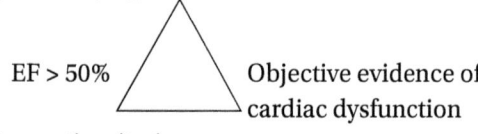

EF > 50%   Objective evidence of cardiac dysfunction

Diagnostic criteria
By heart failure society of America

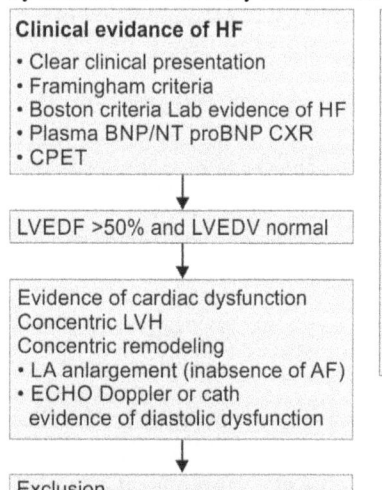

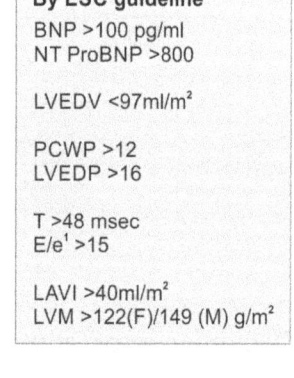

C/F are same for HF
Dyspnea at rest/exertion, decreased exercise tolerance, orthopnea, PND, peripheral edema, pulm congestion apparent on radiograph

| Displaced LV apex pulses alternans | Presumed to be exclusive to HFrEF |

Note: None of symptoms/signs or CXR findings can be used to distinguished HFpEF and HFrEF

CAUSES

Biomarkers
HFEPF have smaller LV cavity and thicker LV walls -their end-diastolic wall stress is much lower than in patients with HFrEF low BNP and NT Pro BNP levels.

Demographic
- HFpEF increase with age; more in women
- HTN present in 80 to 90%
  - Obesity in 30 to 50%
  - Diabetes in 20 to 30%
- AF in 20 to 30%
- Prevalence of renal disease high
  - Prevalence of CAD 20 to 40%.

Rare Causes of HFpEF
- Sleep apnea, pulm HTN
- Hypertrophic cardiomyopathy
- Infiltrative cardiomyopathy e.g., Amyloidosis
- Valvular disease
- Constrictive pericarditis
- Radiation induced heart disease.

Acute Decomposition in HF
- Result from increased feeling pressure with or without significant changes in LV diastolic volume
  +
- Increased LV diastolic volume and pressure can result from increase in total intra vascular volume or shift of intravascular volume due to splanchnic vasoconstriction.

Mech
- Worsening diastolic dysfunction
- Increased neurohormonal activation
- Poorly controlled comorbid disease
- HTN, DM, myocardial ischemia
- atrial Arrhythmia
  All patients admitted with ADHF → 50% had HFpEF

CLINICAL ASSESSMENT OF CARDIOVASCULAR FUNCTION AND STRUCTURE

- ECHO
- MRI
- CT

A. LV structure
- LV volume >90% patient with HFpEF have normal LV chamber dimension, area and volume
- LV mass increased and reaches criteria for LV hyper trophy in 30 to 50% patients with HFpEF Associated with coarse prognosis
- LV geometry ratio of mass to volume (m/v) or wall thickness to internal dimension (relative wall thickness) describe LV geometry
- When mass or thickness is increased relative to (or out of proportion to) volume or dimension Termed concentrate remodeling
- Concentric remodeling associated with 20 to 30% cases of HFpEF even in absence of LV hypertrophy
- Associated with 25% higher risk of HF events

B. *LV function:*
- *Diastolic properties*
  HFpEF-delayed and slow relaxation
  Decreased elastic recoil
  Slow and incomplete early filling
  Increased filling during atrial cont
  Decrease distensibility.

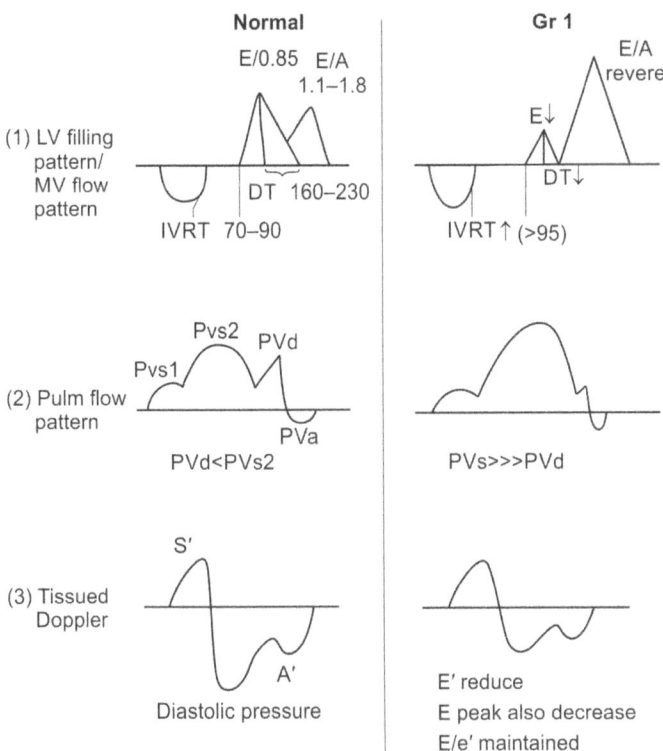
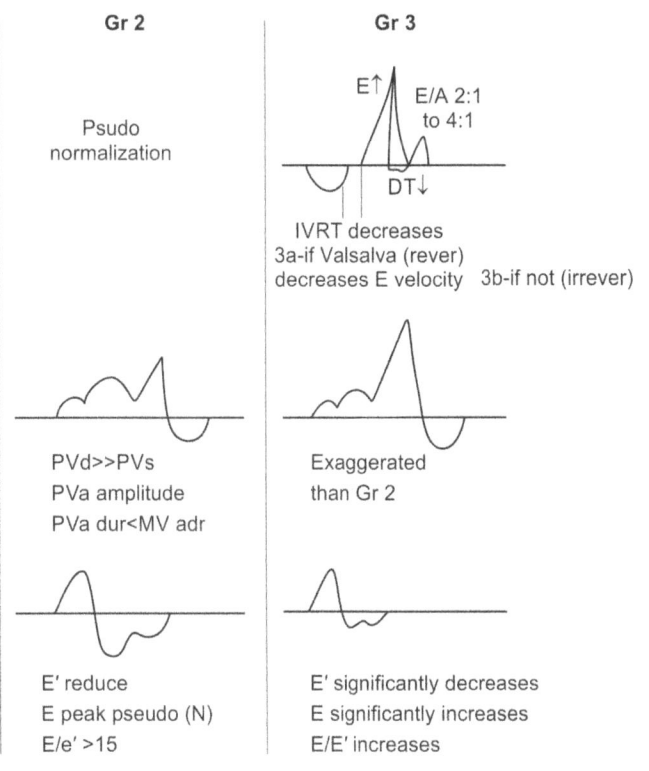

- *Diastolic pressure:*
  - Important for diagnosis, predicting prognosis and directing therapy
  - Direct measure invasive
  - Indirect measure noninvasive ECHO
  - Pseudo normalization and restricted filling pattern (Gr 2) indicates presence of both diastolic dysfunction and elevated LA pressure
  - Impaired relaxation pattern (Gr1) indicates diastolic dysfunction without marked elevation of LA pressure
  - ECHO measures that may reflect diastolic filling pressure includes
  - Peak RV systolic pressure (TR jet velocity)
- LA volume
- Depends on product of diastolic pressure and time
- Increased LA volume ⎤
- Abnormal diastolic dysfunction gr ⎬ Highly associated with prevalent-poor in HFpEF prognosis
- Increased RVSP ⎦
  Most commonly used and easily interpretable measure of E/e' ratio
  E/e' >15 – elevated PCWP (LAP)
  E/e' <8 – normal LAP
  (E/e' average should be measured)
- Abnormal diastolic dysfunction– 60 to 70% of HFpEF (I pressure and CHARM studies)
- LA enlargement in 66%

- Either DD Gr 2-3 or LAP → 85%
- Abnormal filling pattern + progressively worsening abnormalities of LV filling pattern (impaired relaxation-pseudo normalization-restricted filling) indicates subjects with progressively increased risk of mortality
- DD correlate with impaired exercise capacity in patients without MI. LVEF does not
  Stage of DD is strong predictor
- *Systolic property*
  HFEPF:
  - Normal EF
  - Normal dp/dt Max
  - Stroke volume
  - Preload recruitable stroke work
  - *LV end systolic elastance*
  - Increased in hfps ⎤ Coupling of LV and
  - Arterial elastance also increases ⎦ arterial system is nearly optimal to convert energy of contraction to SV

  [In HFrEF systolic elastic decreases ⎤ Benefit by
  and arterior elastance increases ⎦ vasodilatation

  HFpEF doesn't benefit by vasodilatation
  - Global LV performance normal in HFpEF
  - Abnormal parameters
    - Midwal shortening reduced
      - Appears to be offset by concentric remodeling or hypertrophy
    - Reduced LV longitudinal shortening velocity
    - Strain and strain rate decreases
    - Reduced apical systolic torsion
      ↓

Enhanced circumferential shortening offsets impact of these regional abnormalities

Impaired exercise capacity in HFpEF
- Decrease ability to augment indices of LV chamber systolic function and contractility during exercise
- Abnormalities of diastolic function
- Chronotropic incompetence
- Decreased response to SNS and RAAS stimulation
- Exaggerated increase in after load.

THERAPY

No treatment has been shown to significantly reduce morbidity and mortality

RCTs
- *DIG trial*
  Digitalis did not reduce CV mortality or HF related hospitalization
- *CHARM trial* (candescartan)
  - No impact on mortality
  - 1° and CV death or HF related readmission showed significant difference only after adjustment
- *PEP-CHF* (Perindopril)
  - No significant difference in mortality of readmission
  - Post hoc analysis showed minor benefit given by reduction in HF related hospitalization
- *I-preserve* (irbesartan)
  No effect of irbesartan
- *SENIORS* (Nebrivolol)
  - Study failed to draw any conclusion about role of beta blocker in HFpEF
  Several novel approaches decrease phase 2 trial
  - Spironolactone-TOPACT trial
  - ARNI-PARAMOUNT-HF trial
  - Sildenafil-RELAX trial.

MANAGEMENT

Three main components
1. Reduction and prevention of pulm venous congestion
   - Fluid and Na^+ restriction
   - Judicious use of diuretic and nitrate
   - Selective application of neuro hormonal modulation
2. Aggressive treatment of antecedent and comorbid disease (BP, DM, renal dysfunction and ischemia)
3. Optimization of cardiac function status
   - Prevent excessive tachy or Brady
   - Match HR to metabolic needs
   - Maintain/restore NSR
   Control vent response rate during atrial arrhythmias
- Non Pharmacological measures
  - Diet and lifestyle
  - Avoidance/reversal of obesity
  - Exercise
    - Adherence to medications
  - Daily monitoring of weight
  - Close medical follow up
- Treatment of comorbid condition
  - HTN goal BP <140 to 190 mm Hg
  - Diabetes
  - *Obesity:* BMI is important indicator of outcome
  - Treat USA
  - cKD
  - Anemia
- Pharmacological and device based treatment

RAAs antagonists
- Manage HTN
- Reverse LVH
- Preserve renal function in diabetics
- Device based treatment is being developed

■ Remote monitoring system
- COMPASS HF studied implantable hemodynamic monitor
  ◆ Measured estimated pulm art diastolic pressure (Approximates PCWP in absence of pulm vascular disease)

  Results:
  1. HFpEF demonstrated significantly increased filling pressure even in compensated state
  2. Pressure increases further when they become decompensated
  3. Both baseline pressure and change from baseline pressure predicted outcomes
     Modifying treatment based on data obtained from remote monitoring prevent and increase in HF events
- CHAMPION trial
- LAPTOP-HT trial

■ Neurohormonal modulation
- Renal artery deenervation
- Implantable baroreceptor or vagal stimulation

] Decreased BP and activation causes regression of LVH and improve diastolic function

7.17 ROLE OF Ca^{++} IN CARDIAC CONT. RELAX CYCLE

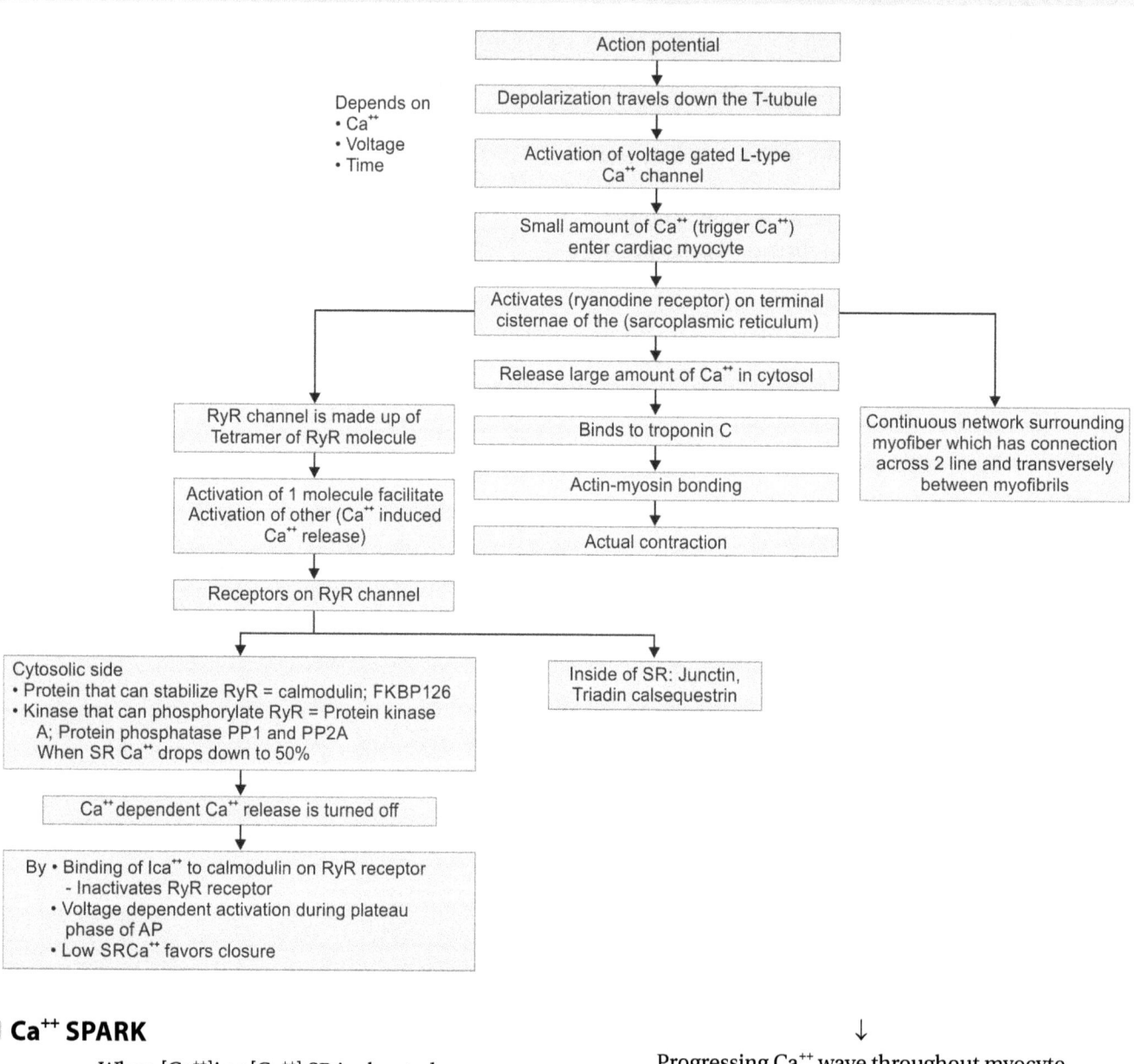

Ca^{++} SPARK

When [Ca^{++}]i or [Ca^{++}] SR is elevated
or
When RyR is sensitized (by oxidation of stabilizing calmodulin)
↓
Spontaneous local Ca^{++} release (spark)
↓
Sufficient enough to activate next junction 1–2 um away
↓
Progressing Ca^{++} wave throughout myocyte
↓
Can activate Na$^+$/Ca^{++} exchange
↓
Generate action potential
↓
Arrhythmia
↓
Phospholamban inhibits SERCA

REUPTAKE OF Ca^{++} INTO SR

Reuptake starts as soon as [Ca^{++}]
Begins to rise
↓
[Ca^{++}]i activates calmodulin and
β-receptor   dependant kinase
↓   ↓
Protein kinase A → Phosphorylation of "Phospholamban"
cAMP   (inactive form)
↓

↓
Release of inhibitory effect on SERCA
(sarc endoplasmic reticulum Ca^{++} ATPase)
↓
Activated SERCA
↓
Uptake 2 molecules of Ca^{++} at the cost of 1 ATP
↓
Ca^{++} transferred back to calsequestrin and calreticulin
(Ca^{++} storing protein) near junctional reticulum

7.18 ADRENERGIC SIGNALING SYSTEM

A.

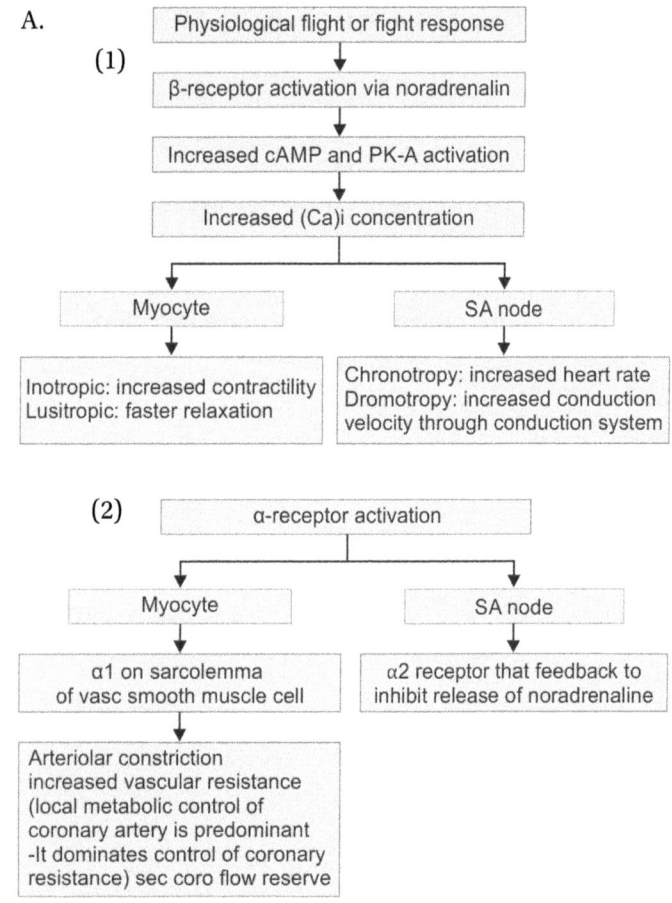

B. G-protein receptor system

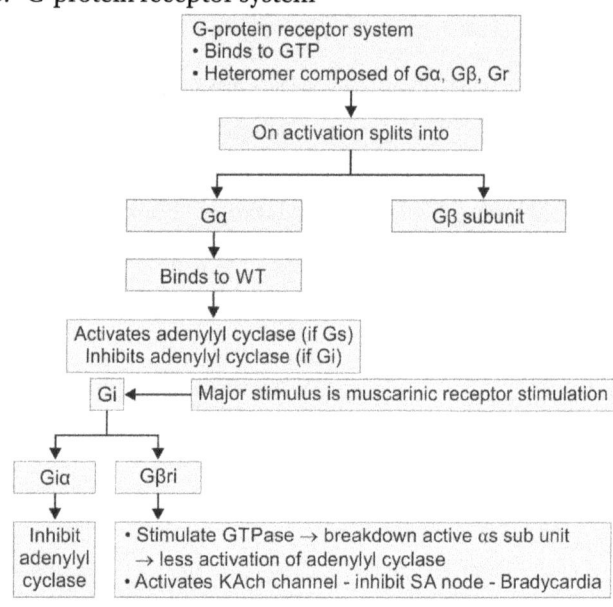

C. Adenylyl cyclase
- Transmembrane enzyme

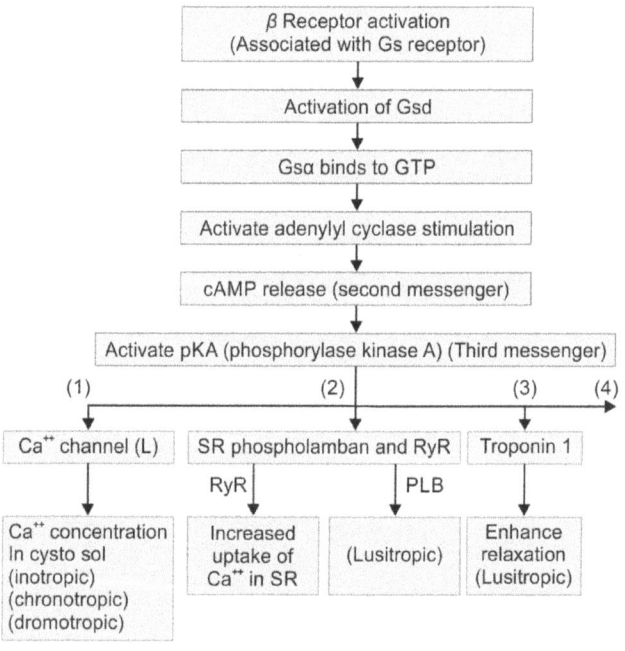

pKA also phosphorylase PLM small
PLB like protein that regulate Na⁺
K⁺-ATPase pump
Phosphorylated PLM
↓
Release of inhibitory activity on Na^+-K^+ ATPase pump
↓
Limits the rise of Na^+ concentration during sympathetic stimulation

Non-cardiac beta receptors are mainly beta-2

β-receptor
- 2 subtypes
- 1 (80%) predominates in heart
- 2 (20%)
  - Linked to both Gs and Gi
  - Linked to G portion stimulatory unit (Gs)
- Strength of Gs is lessened in heart failure
- Gi is augmented in heart failure

Sensitivity of receptors

α1 - Isoproterenol > epinephrine = norepinephrine
β2 - Isoproterenol > epinephrine > norepinephrine
α1 - Norepinephrine > epinephrine > isoproterenol

D. *Beta-receptor desensitization*:

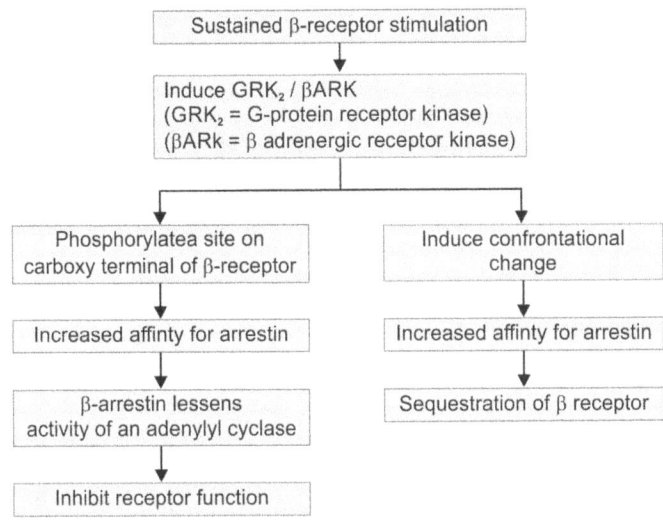

E. Calcium calmodulin dependent kinase II (CaMK II)- (chronic activation in heart failure)

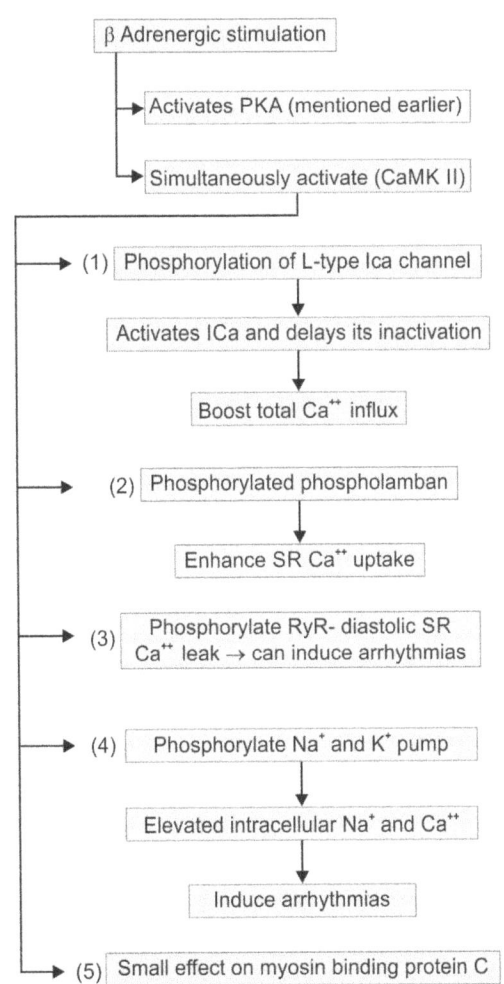

CHOLINERGIC AND NITRIC OXIDE SIGNALING

(M2) receptor ← Neuregulins: Growth factor that maintain
↓ Activity of muscarinic receptors
G-protein
Coupled receptor
↓
Activation of Gi
↓
Inhibit adenylyl cyclase
↓
Negative inotropy and Neg. chronotropy

Vagal: Highest vagal innervations in SA and AV
↓ Lower in atrial myocardium
Lower in vent myocardium
Stimulation - Activate M2 receptor
↓
Activation of coupled Gi
↓
Activation Ach activated K^+ current
↓
Increase K^+ conductance
↓
More negative diastolic potential
In pacemaker cell
↓
Hinders rate of diastolic depolarization

cGMP: Mainly negative inotropic effect
(Contrast to cAMP)
cGMP
↓
Activate Protein kinase G
↓
Modulation of Ca^{++} entry through
L-type Ca^{++} channel
↓
Negative inotropic effect

Phosphodiesterase 7 isoforms
- PDE1 and PDE3 – break down both vAMP and cGMP
- PDE4 → cAMP specific
- PDE5 → cAMP specific
↓
Inhibition by sildenafil can inhibit excess LV growth in response to aortic constriction

NO 3 isoenzyme form
NOS1 (nNOS – neuronal NOS)
NOS2 (iNOS – inducible NOS)
NOS3 (eNOS – endothelial NOS)

7.19 ACUTE HEART FAILURE

INTRODUCTION
MC cause for hospitalization in patients >65 years age.

DEFINITION
New onset or recurrence of symptoms and signs of heart failure requiring urgent or emergent therapy and resulting in seeking unscheduled care or hospitalization.

HFpEF:
More likely to be older
    Female
    H/O HTN
Less likely to have underlying CAD
In hospital mortality lower
Port discharge rehospitalization rates
Are similarly high

} As compared to HFVEF

PATHOPHYSIOLOGY OF ACHF
"AHF is not a single disease
    Its heterogeneous clinical syndrome"

AHF occur due to interaction of substrate (underlying heart condition), initiating mechanism or trigger and amplifying mechanism

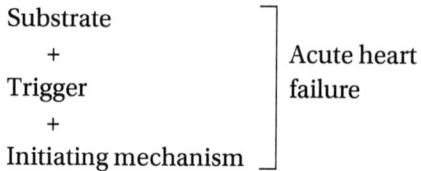

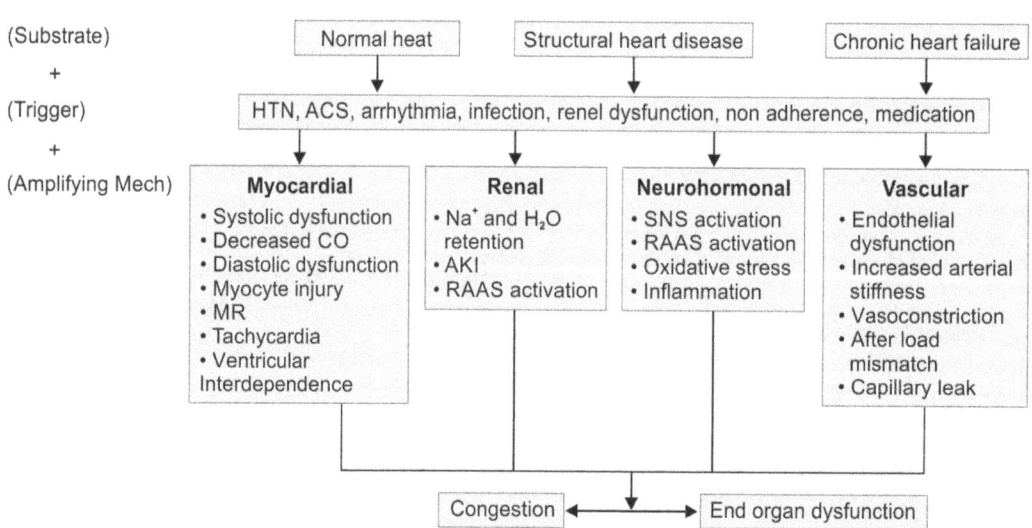

Hemodynamic congestion
- High LV diastolic pressure Without overt clinical sign
- May persist even after Treatment → high risk of rehospitalization
- Contribute to progression of heart failure (via its Positive action on SNS Activity, RAAS activity and Increasing wall stress)

Clinical congestion
- Signs and symptoms of congestion: edema, rates, Elevated JVP
- May resolve with treatment

CONGESTION

Two types:
1. *Clinical congestion:* clinical signs and symptoms Improves with treatment
2. *Hemodynamic congestion*
   - Defined by reused LVEDP
   - No overt clinical sign
   - May not improve with treatment
   - Lead to high risk of rehospitalization

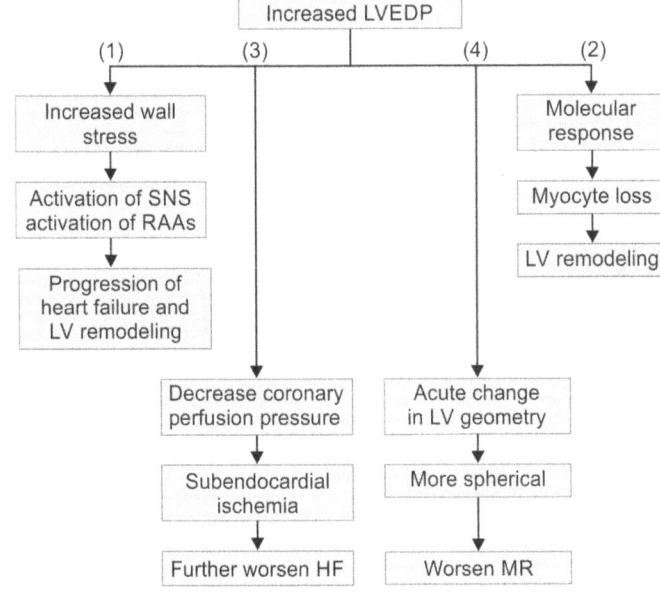

→ *Amplifying mechanisms for AHF*

A. *Myocardial function*

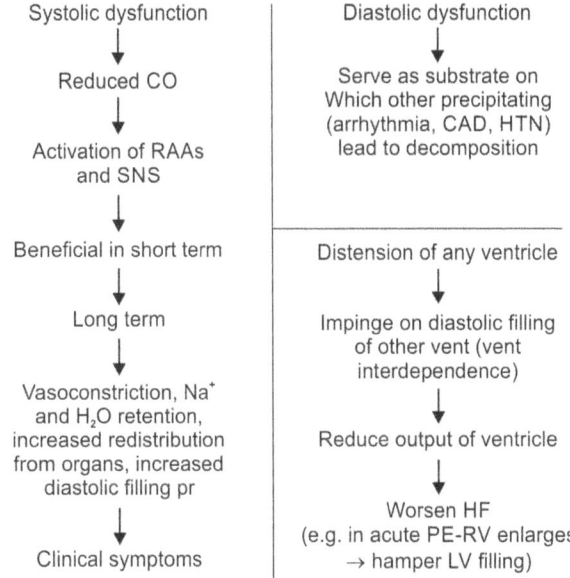

B. *Renal mechanism*
   Kidney plays 2 roles:
   1. Modulates loading condition of heart by controlling intravasc volume
   2. Responsible for neurohormonal output (RAAs)

Risk factors:

Age	Neurohormonal activation
Comorbid activation	SNS activation
	Central venous congestion
Increased GFR	Arterial underfilling
DM	
HTN	

Strongest predictor of worsening renal function → raised central venous pressure

Biomarkers: Sr creatinine
Cystatin C
NGAL (Neutrophil gelatinase associated lipid)

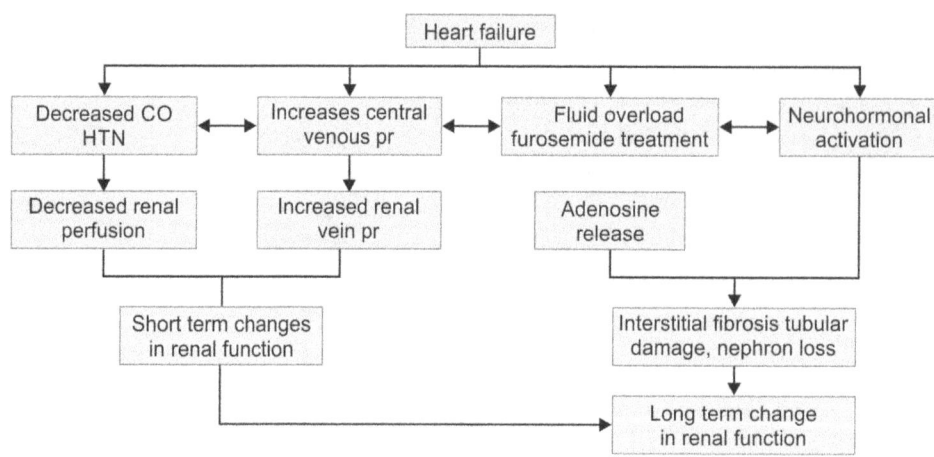

C. *Vascular mechanism*

Abnormal endothelial function → vasoconstriction

Arterial stiffness → increased cardiac loading condition

Peripheral vasoconstriction → Redistribution of blood → pulm edema

Elevated vasoconstriction → Reduce renal function → fluid retention

Pulm vasoconstriction → worsening of pulm edema and dyspnea

Increased vascular impedance → afterload mismatch

D. *Neurohormonal and inflammatory mechanism*:
- Increased pl. Conc of norepinephrine, renin, aldosterone, endothelin-1
  ↓
  Vasoconstriction, fluid retention
  ↓
  Myocardial ischemia and congestion
- Proinflammatory cytonic (TNF α, ILC)
  ↓
  Negative inotropic effect
  Increasing capillary permeability
  Inducing endothelial dysfunction

EVALUATION

Steps

1. Early diagnosis of AHF
2. Prompt treatment of life threatening conditions (shock, respi Failure)
3. Identify any trigger and treat
4. Risk stratification → proper level of care
5. Definitive treatment

At least 4 liter of extracellular fluid is accumulated to produce clinically detectable edema

Simplified Classification

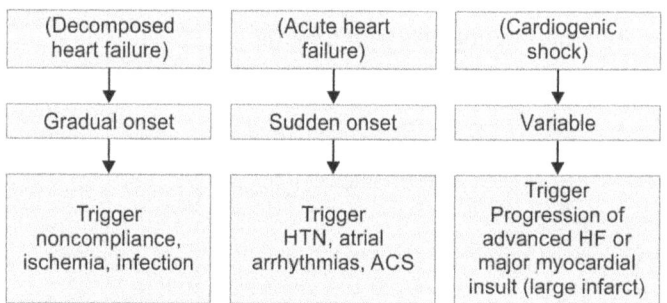

Signs and Symptoms of AHF

Predominant Vol Overload Related

- Dyspnea, orthopnea, PND
- Nocturnal cough, wheezing
- Foot and leg disconnect
- Abdominal discomforting bloating
- Early satiety
- Rales, Pl-effusion
- Peripheral edema
- Ascites, rt upper quadrant pain/discomfort hepatomegaly, splenomegaly
- Increased weight
- Increased JVP, HJR, S3

Predominant Related to Hypoperfusion

- Fatigue
- Altered mental states
- Dizziness, drowsiness
- Confusion, decreased
- Concentration
- Cool extremity
- Pallor, dusky skin discoloration
- Hypotension
- Narrow pulse pr
- Pulsus alternans

Other Signs and Symptoms

Depression, sleep disturbance, Palpitation

Orthostatic hypotension (hypovolemia) syst and diastolic murmur

Diagnose Testing

- *Biomarkers:* BNP and NT-proBNP
  Natriuretic testing in diagnosis of Acute dyspnea — Class 1 Indication
- Renal function
  BUN more directly related to AHF then creatinine
- CXR
- ECG
- ECHO

Clinical Triggers

Discussed already

Risk Stratification

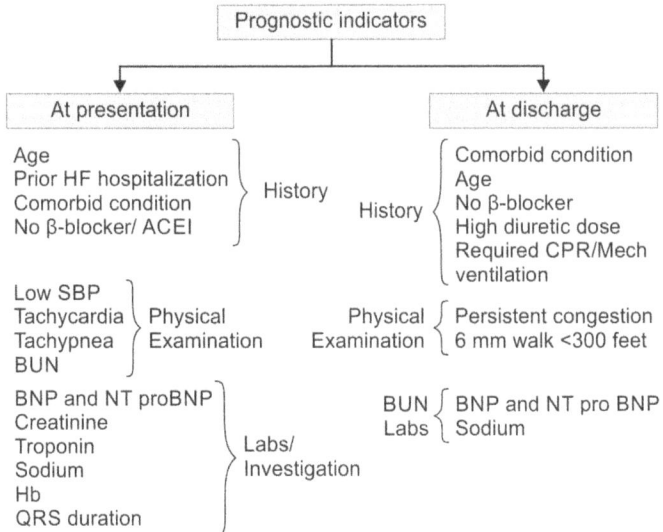

Management of AHF

Phases

A. Urgent/emergent case:

   Goal: 1. Early diagnosis
- 2. Prompt treatment of life threatening condition
- 3. Identify trigger and treat
- 4. Prompt symptom relief
- 5. Definitive treatment

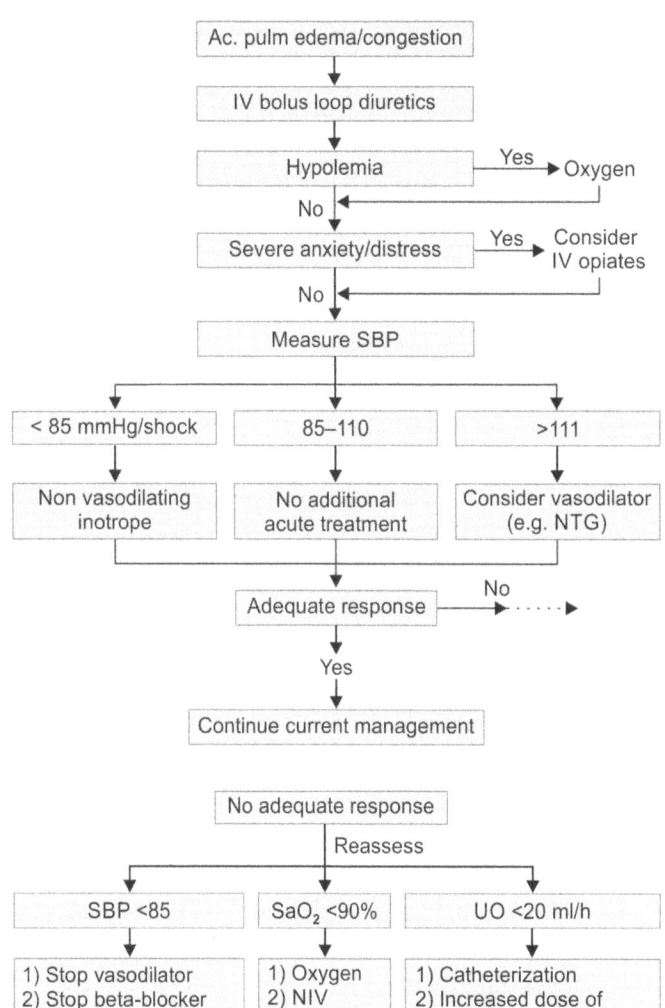

Cardiogenic Shock

Characterized by marked hypotension (SBP<80) lasting more than 30 mins, associated with severe reduction of cardiac index (usually <1.8L/min/) in spite of adequate LV filling pressure (PCWP >18) resulting in organ hypoperfusion

B. *Phase 2: Hospital care*
- Monitoring daily weight, intake-output vital signs, orthostatic BP, daily assessment of signs and symptoms, Daily electrolyte and renal function
- ECHO if not done recently
- Evaluation for myocardial ischemia if clinically indicated
- Daily sodium restriction (up to 2 gm/d)
- Fluid restriction (1.5-2L/day)
- Venous thromboembolism prophylaxis

- Withhold ACE inhibitor/mineralocorticoid receptor antagonist if renal function deteriorate
- Beta-blocker-reduce arrhythmias
  Reduce rehospitalization
- Educate patient about heart failure, monitoring daily fluid balance, daily weight, self-adjustment of diuretics, salt restriction etc.

C. *Phase 3: Predischarge planning*
- Optimize chronic oral therapy
- Preventing readmission
- Persistent clinical congestion at discharge is associated with high risk of rehospitalization (EVEREST study)
- Elevation of predischarge BNP associated with high readmission
- Evaluation of simple tools (function capacity)
  - 6 MM walk test
  - Climbing, flight of stairs or walking down corridor
- Criteria for discharge:
  - Near optimal volume status
  - All exacerbating factors treated
  - Intravenous-oral diuretics
  - Patient and family educated
  - LVEF documented
  - Near optimal pharmacotherapy achieved (ACEI + beta blocker)
  - Follow up after 7 days.

SPECIFIC THERAPIES

A. *Diuretic*:
  - For volume overload in patients with AHF
  - Rapid symptoms relief
  - Furosemide/Torsemide/Bumetanide/Ethacrynic acid
  - Initial dose = 2–5 times output dose (for patients on chronic oral diuretic therapy)
    ↓
    Double if no relief
    ↓
    Continuous infusion (if no relief)
    (If diuretic resistance)

S/E
- Electrolyte imbalance
- Activate neurohormonal system
- Increased risk of renal worsening
- Decreased survival

DOSE Trial
First large randomized trial
- BD vs. Infusion
- Low dose IV (equal to outpatient oral dose) vs. High dose IV (2.5 times oral dose)
  ↓

High dose associated with greater relief of dyspnea and net fluid loss at 72 hours
But high dose associated with transient increase in creat, which resolve at time of (o)
No significant difference between low dose vs. high dose
No significant difference between bolus IV infusion.

Diuretic Resistance
↓
- Thiazide diuretic (Blocks distal tubule)
- Chlorothiazide (500 to 1000) IV
- Metolazone (2.5 to 10 mg) oral given before loop diuretic
  *NSAIDS greatly reduce efficacy of diuretic.

Dose
- *Mod overload* Furosemide 20–40 mg
  Or Butamide 0.5–1
  Or Torsemide 10–20
- *Severe overload* Furosemide 40–160 (or 5–40 mg/h inf)
  Bumetanide 1–4 mg (0.5–2 mg/h)
  Torsemide 20–100 mg (5 = 20 mg/h)
  Ultrafiltration
- *Refractory to* -Add hydrochlorothiazide 25–50 BD
  Loop diuretic Or Metolazone 2.5–10 mg/d
  Or Chlorothiazide 250–500 IV

B. *Vasodilator*
- In absence of heart failure
- Nitroglycerin –20 µg/min –40–200 µg/min
  Isosorbide dinitrate
  Nitroprusside -0.3 µg/kg – 0.3–5 µg/kg/min
  Nesiritide – 2 µg/kg bolus – 0.010–0.030 µg/kg/min
- Caution with nitroprusside – in patient with active MRI
  Trial ALARM-HF registry: AHF patients treated with diuretic and vasodilator had significantly better in hospital mortality

C. *Nitrates*
- Potent vasodilators
- Rapid decreases in pulm venous and ventricular filling pressure - improve congestion
- At slightly higher dose, they are also arteriolar dilator - decreased after load and increased CO

- Relatively selective for epicardial as compared to intramyocardial coronaries.

D. *Nesiritide*
- Recombinant human BNP
- Potent vasodilatation in venous and arterial vasculature- significant decrease in venous pr and vent filling pr - mild increase in CO
- May be used for acutely decompensated HF who have dyspnea
- Should not be used to replace diuretic, enhancing diuretic, protecting renal function or improving survival
- Dose = 2 µg/kr - 0.01 µg/kg/min
- Trial:
  1. VMAC (vasodilatation in management of acute heart failure) - nesiritide may be associated with increased risk of worsening renal function as well as increased mortality
  2. ASCENO-HF No diff between nesiritide and placebo. Use of nesiritide was not associated with worsening RFT but was associated with increase in rate of hypotension

  MOA: Nesiritide - guanylyl cyclase linked natriuretic peptide (NPRA and NPRB) - cGMP mediated vasodilatation t1/2 = 18 mins
  Did not improve urine output or renal function

E. Inotropes/Inodilators
  DoBu: 1-2 µg/kg/min - 2-20 µg/kg/min
  Dopa: 1-2 µg/kg/min - 5-20 µg/kg/min
  NE: 0.2-1.0 UG/KG/MIN
  Milrinone: 25-75 µg/kg bolus -0.10-0.75 µg/kg/min
  Levosimendan: 12 µg/kg -0.1-0.2 µg/kg/min
  Indicator = increased CO through c-AMP mediated inotropy
  And reduce PCWP through vasodilatation

Problem

Even short term use of IV inotropes is associated with significant side effects such as hypotension, atrial or vent arrhythmia, increased in hospital and long term mortality
- Use should be limited to patients with dilated ventricle and low EF who presents with low BP (<90) or low measured cardiac output in presence of signs of congestion and organ hypoperfusion
- Should be stopped as soon as adequate organ perfusion restored
- Used in cardiogenic shock as temporary therapy to prevent hemodynamic collapse.

DOBUTAMINE
- Evidence that It increases mortality
- Many improve renal function with low dose dobutamine (1-2 µg/kg/min)
- Tachyphylaxis if used >48 hours
- Preferred inotrope in patients with significant renal dysfunction
- Concomitant use of beta-blocker - competitive antagonism of effect of dobutamine.

DOPAMINE
- Precursor of NE
- Agonist of both adrenergic and dopaminergic receptor
- Rapid release of NE - can case tachycardia as well as atrio-vent arrhythmias
- High dose can cause vasoconstriction → precipitate heart failure and poor perfusion

MILRINONE

PDE 3 an inhibitor
  Inhibit degradation of cAMP
                ↓
  Increased inotropy, increased chronotropy and increased lusitropy

Dose: 25-75 µg/kg bolus over 10-20 mins
       Infusion started at 0.1-0.25 µg/kg/min
       Elimination t1/2 = 2-5 h
       Pharmacodynamics t1/2 = 6 hrs

Ultrafiltration for AHF
- To remove excess H_2O and Na^+
- Use of ultrafiltration is uncertain
- UNLOAD trial - patients receiving ultrafiltration demonstrated a greater reduction in body weight at 48 hours - but no improvement in dyspnea or renal function
- CARRESS trial-ultrafiltration resulted in similar weight loss as diuretic but resulted in increased creat level and was associated with more serious side effect
- AVOID-HF will further evaluate role of ultrafiltration in management of AHF.

HYPERTONIC SALINE
- SMAC HF study
- Shorten length of stay, increased creat clearance, decreased readmission and improve survival
- Larger trials are needed.

7.20 CARDIAC TRANSPLANT

Q.1 Diagnosis and management of rejection after cardiac transplantation
Q.2 Long term result of cardiac transplant
Q.3 Discuss role of lipids in heart transplant patient
Q.4 Indication and limitation of cardiac transplant
Q.5 ECHO in cardiac transplant assessment
Q.6 Physiology of transplanted heart.

TECHNIQUES

Biatrial Approach
1. Standard technique
   - By lower and shumway preserve recipient atria
   - Standard LA anastomosis with separate bicaval anastomosis
   Bicaval anastomosis

Bicaval Approach
2. Total orthotopic heart transplant
   - By Webber and Neely
   - Five anastomosis: SVC, IVC, PA, PV, and AO

Biatrial anastomosis result in:
- Abnormally enlarged atrial cavity
- Distorted atrial geometry - AV valve insufficiency
- Bradyarrhythmias
- Increased need for pacing

Bicaval anastomosis results in:
- Narrowing of SVC and IVC → makes biopsy for surveillance difficult
- Prolonged technique and ischemic time.

PHYSIOLOGY OF TRANSPLANTED HEART

Physio
1. Less atrial contribution to stroke volume
EP
2. High Resting heart rate 95-110
3. Acceleration of heart rate during exercise is Slower (denervated heart)
ANS
4. Diurnal changes in BP is abolished
5. Diastolic dysfunction is very common (because myocardium is stiff from some degree of rejection)
6. Denervated heart
   1. Electrical activity cannot cross suture line
      - Recipient atrial activity present but not conducted
      - Donor atrium denervated but source of electrophysiologic response
   2. Loss of SNS, PNS innervation
      - Vagal stimulation has no effect
      - No reflex tachy in response to hypovol
   3. ECG has 2p waves
   4. Indirect sympathomimetic agents: no effect (Anticholinergic, anticholinesterase, ephedrine)
   5. Direct acting sympathomimetics work (Isoproterenol, NE, Epinephrine, phenylephrine, dopamine)

INDICATIONS

1. Cardiogenic shock requiring LV assistance device (<30 d)
2. Refractory HF with cont murmur inotropic infusion
   - Progressing symptoms with maximal therapy
   - NYHA 3 and 4 with poor 12 month prognosis
3. Life threatening medical and device interventions
4. Refractory angina in spite of OMT and unsuitable anatomy for revascularization

CONTRAINDICATIONS

Absolute
1. Age > 65-70
2. Systemic illness that limits survival
   Neoplasm, HIV/AIDS. ALE or sarcoid with multisystem involve, any systemic process with high probability of recurring in transplanted heart
3. Fixed PHTN
   PVR >5 woods unit
   Tans pulm gradient >15 mm Hg

Relative
1. PAD not amenable to treatment (ABI >0-70)
2. Asymptomatic carotid stenosis >75%
3. DM with end organ damage
4. Severe lung disease
5. Systemic infection making immune suppression risky (HIV, Hep B, conv)
6. Psychosomatic impairment
   - Antisocial personality disorder
   - Medication non-compliance
   - Drug or alcohol addiction
   - Cigarette smoking
   - Inability to rely on alternative caregivers in the event of patient impairment

CANDIDATE SELECTION

Does the patient have a <1 year life expectancy?
- Cardiogenic requiring mechanical support or high dose inotrope/pressure support
- Stage is refractory failure symptoms despite maximal therapy
- Recurrent arrhythmias despite maximal intervention and ICD
- Refractory angina without potential revasc

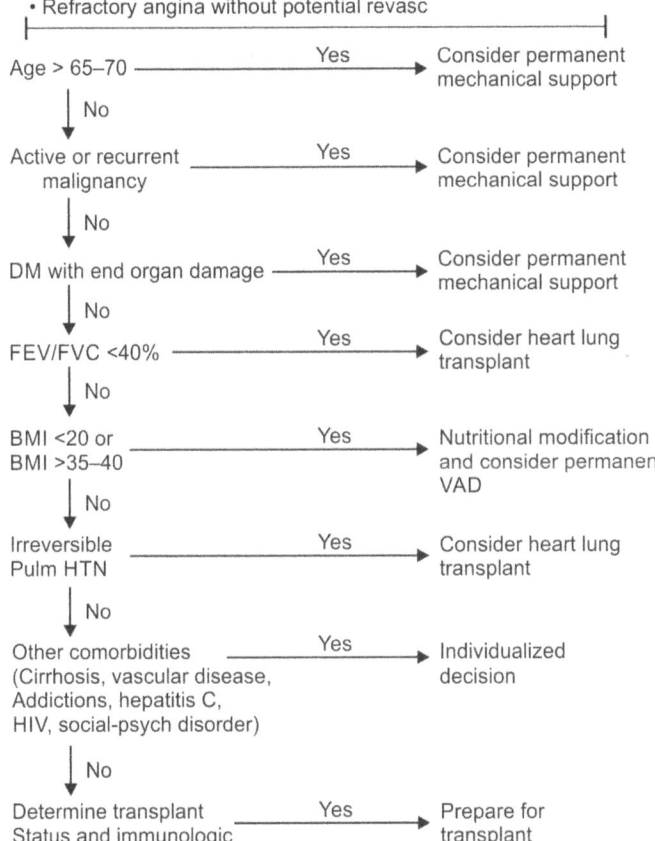

EVALUATION OF RECIPIENT

- Cardiac cath
- Cardio pulm test
- Labs: BNP, CBC, LFT, coag profile, TSH, HIV, Hepatitis, CMV, IgG, VDRL, PRA (Panel of reactive antibodies), ABO and Rh, CXR, PFT, ECG, ECHO
- Substance abuse history and evidence of abstinence for at least 6 months
- Mental health evaluation and social support
- Financial support.

CARDIAC DONOR-EXCLUSION CRITERIA

- Age >55 years
- Serotve (HIV, HBV, HCU)
- Systemic infection
- Malignant tumor with potential mets (except 1 degree brain tumors)
- Systemic comorbidities (DM, collagen vasc disease)
- Cardiac disease/trauma
- CAD
- Allograft ischemic time considered to be > 6 hours
- LVH or LV dysfunction or ECHO.

MATCHING DONOR AND RECIPIENT

- Because ischemic time during cardiac transplant is crucial, donor recipient matching is based on non-HLA typing
  - The severity of illness
  - ABD typing and matching
  - Response to PRA (rapidly measured anti HLA ab)
  - Donor weight to recipient weight (must be 75%)

POSTOP

Immunosuppressive agents to be started on day of surgery
- Corticosteroid
- Calcineurin inhibitors: Cyclosporine and tacrolimus
- Antiproliferative agents: Azathioprine, mycophenolate mofetil
- Sirolimus
- Everolimus

P. Jirovecii prophylaxis within 1st week of transplant

If patients or donor is CMV positive - Ganciclovir started on post op day 2

Endomyocardial biopsy on post op day 4 and steroid can be begin to toper if there is no rejection greater than gr zb

Anticoagulation started if heterotrophic transplant is performed

ECG obtained 3-4 times a day

Long term
- Endomyocardial biopsy
  Once a week for first month
  Monthly × 3 months
  3 monthly for 1 year
  4 monthly in 2nd year
  And 1-2 times per year thereafter
- Regular check of cyclosporine level
- ECHO as adjunct to endomyocardial biopsy
- Cardiac cath performed annually for CAV

POSTOP COMPLICATIONS

A. *Surgical*
   - Aortic pseudoaneurysm or rupture at puncture site
   - Hemorrhage pericardial effusion due to bleeding coagulopathy

B. *Medical*
   - Severe TR-due to biotin induced trauma
   - RV failure (pulm art compression, pulm HTN)

- LV failure (ischemia, operative injury, acute rejection)
- Coagulopathy induced by CPB

C. *Rhythm disorder*
- Asystole
- CHB
- Sinus node dysfunction with bradyarrhythmias
- AF
- VT

D. *Respi failure*
- Cardiogenic pulm edema
- Non cardiogenic pulm edema
- Infection

E. *Renal or hepatic insufficiency*
- Drugs
- CHF

F. Rejection

Hyperacute
- Caused by preformed antibodies against donor endothelial antigens
- Within minutes to hours
- PRA screening is best method to avoid

Acute
- Most common form
- Occurs at least once in 50% of transplant recipients
- Half of episodes occur in first 2–3 months
- Rarely observed beyond 12 months
- Cell mediated rejection

Acute humoral rejection
- Antibody mediated
- Days to months after transplant
- Manifest as graft dysfunction or hemodynamic abnormalities in absence of cellular rejection on biopsy
- More difficult to treat than acute rejection
- Carries worse prognosis

Chronic rejection
- Late graft failure
- Irreversible deterioration of graft function
- Months to years after transplant
- Mediated by antibody or as a result of progressive graft loss from ischemia
- Char by intimal thickening of graft vasculature
- Luminal occlusion of graft vasculature (Referred as CVA or transplanted CAD)

Grades of rejection
0-R: No rejection
1R (mild): Interstitial and/or perivascular infiltrate with up to
One focus of myocyte damage
2R (mod): 2 or more foci of infiltrate with associated myocyte damage
3R (severe): diffuse infiltrate with multifocal myocyte damage+ or- edema+ or- hemorrhage vasculitis

G. Infection

2 peak infection period:
  1st 30d post op: Nosocomial infection related to indwelling cath and wound infections
  2nd 2–6 months: Opportunistic infections related to immuno suppression

Opportunistic infections
1. *CMV:* Most common
   - Fever, malaise, anorexia
   - Severe inf affects lung, GF tract, retina
   - If donor positive and recipient negative
   - IV ganciclovir/foscarnet x 6 weeks
     Followed by oral acyclovir
2. *Toxoplasma Gondii:* Encephalitis, myocarditis
   Treated with pyrimethamine and sulfadiazine
3. *P. Jirovecii*
   Prophylaxis: TMP/sulfa (highly selective)
   Treatment: Dapsone and pentamidine
4. *Aspergillus*
   Treatment IV amphotericin

H. Malignancy
- 1000 fold increase in prevalence of malignant donor
- MC-post transplant lymphoproliferative disorder
   - Type of non-Hodgkin's lymphoma
   - Believed to be related to EBr
   - Treatment: Immunosuppressive reduction, acyclovir and chemotherapy
- Skin cancer- common with azathioprine use
- Any malignant tumor present before transplant carries risk of flare up due to immunosuppression

I. *Hypertension*
75% patients treated with cyclosporine and corticosteroid develops HTN

J. *Dyslipidemia*
- 80% patients develop dyslipidemia due to immunosuppression medications
- Treated aggressively with statin, fibrate to prevent accelerated transplant coronary vasculopathy risk.

RISK MARKERS FOR POOR OUTCOMES

- Age <1 year and >65 years
- Ventilator used at time of transplant
- Elevated PVR
- Underlying pulm disease
- Diffuse atherosclerotic vasc disease
- Small BSA
- Need for inotropic support pre transplant

- DM
- Ischemic time > 4 h for transplanted heart
- Sarcoidosis or amyloidosis as reason for transplant.

CARDIAC ALLOGRAFT VASCULOPATHY

- Long-term complication of transplant
- Annual incidence 5-10%
- After 1st pot op year it becomes increasingly important cause of death
- As early as 3 months post-transplant
- Angiographic detection in
  20% of grafts at 1 year
  40-50% of grafts at 5 year.

Reason

- Neointimal proliferation of vascular SMC (Generated process)
- Char by - concentric narrowing that affects entire length of coro art from epicardial to intramyocardial segment
- Rapid tapering, pruning and obliteration of third-order branches.

C/F

myo infarct/ischemia, HF, vent arrhythmia, sudden death
No angina as heart is denervated.

Risk Factors

- Increased HLA mismatch
- Increased number and duration of rejection episodes
- CMV infection
- Donor/recipient factor (age, sex, pre transplant diagnosis)
- Related to surgery (ischemia reperfusion injury)
- Smoking, obesity, DM, dyslipidemia, HTN → also contributes.

MONITORING

Done on Annual Basis:
- CAC-limited role as it affect concentrically entire length
- IVVS is most sensitive imaging technique
- Increase intimal thickness of at least 0.5mm in 1st year post transplant is Reliable indication for development of CAV na 5 year mortality

DSE: High sensitivity (83-95%)
     Specificity (53-91%)

Treatment sirolimus and everolimus has shown promising result in CAV treatment

* Selective involvement of engrafted vessel and sparing of native vessel suggests – immunologic difference between the host and recipient vessel might contribute to pathogenesis of the disease
* ECS is transplanted artery express MHC antigen than can engender an allogeneic immune response by host T cell - release of cytokine INFr1
- Recruit leucocyte by increasing adhesion molecule
- Vasculopathy (diffuse plaque formation)

7.21 DEVICES FOR MONITORING HF

INTRODUCTION

- Provide substantial physiologic information about patients with HF
- Information useful for evaluating HF clinical status and or in predicting episodes of HF decompensation.

A. ICD and CRT
   - Can provide information on atrial rate, rhythm, vent rate rhythm patient activity level heart rate variability intrathoracic impedance (in some devices) measure of lung wetness
   - May also provide trend about activity present, providing an objective record of numbers of hours per day that patients are physically active-declining trend of activity provide due to worsening exercise tolerance disease progression or decompensation
   - Decrease in HRV indicates increased sympathetic and decreased parasympathetic tone-associated with worsening of HF
   - Intra thoracic impedance indirect measure of fluid content in lungs-ICD/CRT can measure this impedance can predict hospitalizations
   - -Measurements of LV filling pr direct measure of fluid content in lungs
   - Trials suggested superiority of measurement of intra thoracic impedance over daily weight monitoring

   →PARTNER HF trial: Patients with positive combined HF device diagnostic score had 5.5 fold increase risk of hospitalization within one month of assessment
   →DOT-HF: Trade increase in output HF clinic visit and an expected increase in HF hospitalization with positive device assessment
   Till date no RCT has demonstrated reduction in HF re hospitalization on basis of this technology

B. Implantable hemodynamic monitors
   - Under investigation
   - Allow cont or intermittent assessment of hemodynamics
   - Focused on intracardiac or Pulmonary artery pressure measurement.

CHAMPION TRIAL

- Daily measure of PAP with standard care versus standard care alone
- Most pressure based medication changes involved diuretics and long acting nitrates
- Over 6 month period fewer HF hospitalization occurred in the treatment group then in control group (significant)
    E.g.: Implantable LA pr monitoring system
    Used similarly to how diabetic individual self-titrate insulin with use of glucometer.

7.22 BIOMARKERS AND NATRIURETIC PEPTIDES

CATEGORIZATION OF HEART FAILURE

Congestion at rest?
(orthopnea, elevated JVP, pulm rates. S3 gallop, edema)

	No	Yes
Low perfusion at rest? No	Warm and dry	Warm and wet
(Narrow pulse Pr, cool extremity hypotension) Yes	Cool and dry	Cool and wet

BIOMARKERS

Braunwald suggested 7 categories:

1. Inflammation
   - CRP
   - TNF
   - Fas
   - IL-1, 6, 8
2. Oxidative stress
   - Oxidized LDL
   - Myeloperoxidase
   - Urinary Biopyrin
   - Pl. Malondialdehyde
   - BNP/NT pro BNP
3. ECM remodeling
   - MMP
   - TIMP
   - Collagen propeptides
   - Propeptide procollagen 1
   - Plasm procollagen 3
   - Adiponectin
4. Neurohormone
   - Norepinephrine
   - Renin, angiotensin, aldosterone
   - Arginine vasopressin
   - Endothelin
5. Myocyte injury
   - Cardiac specific Trop I and T
   - Myosin light chain kinase
   - Heart type fatty acid binding
   - cKMB
6. Myocyte stress
   - Mid regional adrenomedullin
   - ST 2
7. Others
   - Chromogranin
   - Galectin 3
   - Osteoprotegerin
   - Adiponectin

NATRIURETIC PEPTIDE

(Also read from prev chapter)
- Useful for HF diagnosis
    Estimation of HF severity
    Monitoring management strategy
- T1/2: BNP = 20 mins
  NT ProBNP = 90 mins
- Natriuretic peptide level
  - Tend to increase with worsening NYHA class
  - More in HFrEF
  - Higher in acutely decompensated HF

- Also increased in valvular heart disease, pulmonary HTN, IHD, atrial arrhythmias and pericardial process such as constriction
- Other factors
  - Age
  - Renal failure
  - Hyperdynamic state
  - Sepsis
  - RV dysfunction (pulm emboli)
  - Aortic dissection

Obesity strongly associated with lower than expected BNP.

Trials

- *BNP (Breathing not properly):* BNP >= 100 was found to be highly accurate to diagnose acute decompensated HF
- *PRIDE:* NT Pro-BNP >900 was found to be comparable to BNP >100
- ICON (International collaborative of NT-pro BNP study)
  - Age stratification improved PTV of NT-pro BNP
  - NT-pro BNP <300 pg/mL was useful for exclusion of acutely decompensated heart failure

Prognostic IMP

- Serial BNP is more valuable than single BNP
- In patients with acutely decompensated HF who do not show robust reduction in BNP or NT-proBNP by time of discharge
  Tend to have higher morbidity and mortality
- BNP or NT proBNP decrease of 30% or more by hospital discharge is preferable.

Cut-off Value

- For execution of acute HF: BNP < 30–50
  NT ProBNP <300
- For identification of acute decompensated HF
  BNP $\geq$100 pg/mL
  NT ProBNP $\geq$900 pg/mL
- Multiple cut point
  BNP <100 – > to exclude
  BNP 100–400 – gray zone
  BNP >400 – to rule in.

Hemostatic System

8.1 ANTIPLATELET DRUGS

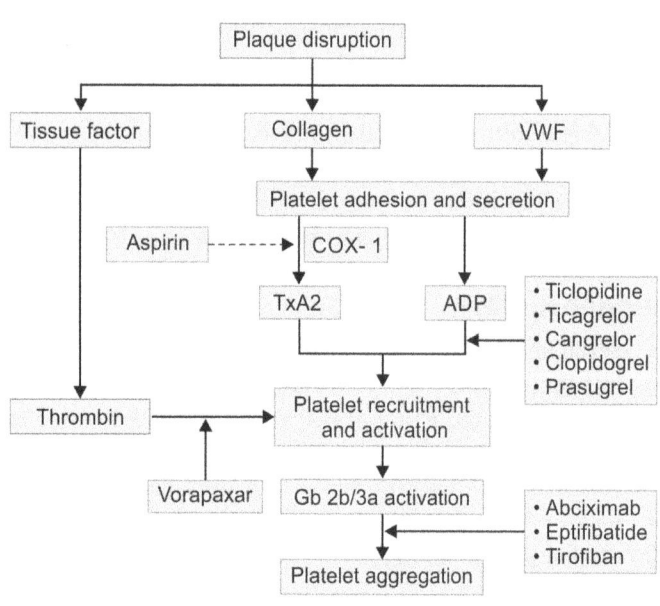

ASPIRIN

MOA

Irreversible inhibitor of COX-1 (critical enzyme in synthesis of TαA2)

At high dose (~1 gm/d) also initiates COX-2 (in endothelial cell COX-2 initiate synthesis of prostacyclin)

Indication

- For 2° prevention
- For 1° prevention—controversial
  → No longer recommended for 1° prevention Unless baseline CV risk is at least 1% per year and 10% at 10 years

Dose

75–325 mg OD

S/E

- (MC) GI side effects
  Dyspepsia to erosive gastritis and peptic ulcer
- Major bleeding—1–3% per year
  Eradication of *H. Pylori* and PPI
- Bronchospasm due to aspirin allergy
  - 0.3% of gen population
  - Common in patients with asthma
- Overdose associated with hepatic and renal toxicity

Aspirin Resistance

- Clinical resistance defined as failure of aspirin to protect against ischemic event
- *Biochemical def:* Failure of drug to inhibit TxA2 and/or AA induced plt aggregation

Mech

- Poor adherence
- Reduced or delayed absorption
- TxA2 generation via other pathway
- Increased activity of TxA2—independent pathway of plt activation
- Use of concomitant meds that interfere with Aspirin action
- Pharmacogenetic factor

Investigation
- Measurement of TxB2 (stable metabolite)
- Assessment of AA induced plt aggregation

THIENOPYRIDINES

Ticlopidine, Clopidogrel, Prasugrel
- *MOA:* Selectively inhibit ADP induced plt aggregation by blocking P2Y12 irreversibly
- *Pharmac:*
  - Ticlopidine and clopidogrel: Pro drug
  - Need metabolic activation by hepatic cyt P450
- *Prasugrel:*
  - Also pro drug
  - Onset of action more rapid
  - Greater and more predictable inhibition of ADP
  - Dependent patient aggregation
  - All absorbed Prasugrel undergo activation (c.f. clopidogrel – 15% only)
- Ticlopidine rarely used due to myelosuppression

Indication

- Decreased risk of CV death/MI/stroke
- Marginally more effective than aspirin
- Combi of aspi + clopi recommended for at least 4 weeks after BB and at least 1 year after DES
- Combi also useful in UA
- Prasugrel decreases CV death, MI and stroke as well as stent thrombosis as compared to clopidogrel on increasing bleeding risk

  Prasugrel should be avoided in older patients (>75 years)
  - And GI in patients with prev stroke/TIA
  - And caution in patients with weight <60 kg and renal Impairment

  ↓
  - Patients >75 year and/or weight <60 kg → 5 mg daily

S/E

Ticlopidine
- GI side effects
  - Bleeding
  - Neutropenia
  - Thrombocytopenia
  - TTP

No longer used because of myelosuppression

Clopidogrel and prasugrel: GI and hematological S/E are rare

Clopidogrel Resistance

Due to genetic polymorphism in CHP enzyme

1. Most imp = CYP2C19
   - Loss of function CYP2C19 * 2 allele exhibit reduced platelet inhibition and high rate of CV events
   - 50% Asians carry loss of function allele
2. Polymorphism in ABCB1—impaired absorption
3. Polymorphism in CYP3A4—decreased metabolic activation of clopidogrel
4. PPI inhibit CYP2CL5—decreased effect
5. Atorvastatin, competitive inhibitor of CYP3A4 reduce clopidogrel effect

⎫ Do not affect Prasugrel

There is no indication for clopidogrel resistance testing

TICAGRELOR

- Reversible inhibitor of P2Y12
- Does not require metabolic activation
- Rapid onset and offset of action
- Greater and predictable action
  - *Dose:* 180 mg loading
  - *S/E:* Bleeding
    Dyspnea (up to 15%)
    Asymptomatic vent pauses

Gp2b/3a Inhibitors

- Gp2b/3a is most abundant receptor
- Binds to fibrinogen and under high sheer stress binds to VWF

↓

Induce plt aggregation

Abciximab	Eptifibatide	Tirofiban
Humanized monoclonal antibody	Cyclic KGD containing heptapeptide	Nonpeptide RGO mimetic
Not specific for Gp2b/3a	Specific 2.5 hour	Specific 2 hour
Short t½ (min)	Short (sec)	Short (sec)
Plt bound t½ is long (days)		
No renal clearance	Yes	Yes

- Abciximab also inhibit alphavbeta3 receptor and alphambeta2—anti-inflammatory and antiproliferative property

S/E
Bleeding
Thrombocytopenia: 5% with abciximab
1% with Epti/tiro

■ NEWER ANTIPLATELETS

Cangrelor
Parental reversible P2Y12 inhibitor
- $t_{1/2}$ = 3-6 mins
- Plt function recovers in 60 mins if stopped
- Little or no advantage

Vorapaxar
Orally active inhibitor of PAR-1 (major thrombin receptor on plt)
- Decreased risk of CV death/MI/stroke but increased (doubled) risk of ICH
- Now licensed for patient with younger than 75 years, no prev h/o stroke/TIA and weight >60

■ ANTICOAGULANTS

Heparin
- Derived from porcine intestinal mucosa
- *MOA:* Activates antithrombin and accelerate rate at which it inhibits clotting factors (esp. thrombin and factor alpha a)

1. Heparin
↓
Binds to serpin on antithrombin via unique pentasaccharide sequence
↓
Conformational changes in reactive center loop of antithrombin
↓
Enhance rate of inhibition of F alpha a
↓
To inhibit thrombin heparin serve as template that binds thrombin and antithrombin simultaneously
↓
Bring both close together
↓
Covalent thrombin-anti thrombin complex
↓
Inhibit thrombin

2. Heparin
↓
Release of TFPI from endothelium
↓
Antithrombotic activity of Heparin

- Heparin has equal capacity to promote inhibition of factor alpha an 8 thrombin (1:1)

Pharmacology
- Binds to endothelial cell
↓
Dose dependent clearance
(at low dose, rapidly binds to endothelium and have short half-life)
(at high dose, once endothelium is saturated clearance is slower – longer $t_{1/2}$)
- $t_{1/2}$ range from 30-60 mins with bolus IV dose of 25 and 100 u/kg
- Also binds to plasma protein - reduce anticoagulant activity of heparin
- Activated Endothelium release VWF
- Activated platelets also release PF4

Heparin binds to these
↓
Reduce anticoagulant activity

Because this plasma protein level vary from person to person
↓
Anticoagulant response to heparin is highly variable

Monitoring Effect
- *aPTT:* 2-3 fold increase in aPTT
- *Anti alpha a level:* Therapeutic range = 0.3-0.7 u/mL
  25% patients with VTE are heparin resistant
  - Require >35,000 Iu/day to achieve therapeutic aPTT
  - Imp to measure anti alpha a level
  - Many have therapeutic anti alpha a level

Reason for Discrepancy
Elevated plasma level of fibrinogen and factor 8 (both acute phase reactants) shorten aPTT but have no effect on anti alpha a levels
Patients with cong or acquired antithrombin deficiency and those with elevated level of heparin binding protein also require high dose

Dosing
- For prophylaxis
  - Fixed dose 5000 s/c 2-3 times daily
  - No monitoring

- Therapeutic dose
  - *For ACS:* 70 μ/kg bolus—infusion at 12–15 μ/kg/h
  - *For VTE:* 80 μ/kg bolus—infusion at 18 μ/kg/h

Limitation
- Pharmacokinetic limitation
  - Poor bioavailability due to limited absorption of long heparin chains
  - Dose dependent clearance
  - Variable anticoagulation effect
  *Biophysical limitation
  - Reduced activity in vicinity of platelet rich thrombi – neutralized by PI4 released plt
  - Limited activity against F alpha a incorporated into prothrombinase complex and thrombin bound to fibrin – reduced capacity of heparin. Antithrombin complex to inhibit F-alpha a bound to activated platelet and thrombin

S/E
- Bleeding
  Treatment:
  - Protamine sulfate
  - Polypeptide isolated from salmon sperm
  - Binds heparin with high affinity to form complex that undergo renal clearance
  - 1 mg of IV protamine neutralize 100 V heparin
- Thrombocytopenia
  - HIT
  - Antibody mediated process
  - IgG subtype of antibody against heparin-PF4 complex
  - Same antibody binds to platelet Fc receptor
    - Such binding activates platelet
    - Release microparticles
    - Procoagulants

Features
- *Thrombocytopenia:* Plt = <100,000 decrease in plt count by >50%
- *Timing:* 5–14 days after heparin
- *Type:* More common with UFH
- *Type of patient:*
  - More common in surgical patient
  - More come in females
- *Thrombosis:*
  - Venous thrombosis > arterial thrombosis
  - Skin lesion at heparin inj. site

Type 1:
- Early (within 4 days)
- Mild within in plt (rarely < 1L)
- Typically recover in 3 days despite cont UFH
- Nonimmunologic mech
- No major clinical sequelae
- Associated with high dose IV hep.

Type 2:
- Substantial fall in plt
- Typical onset 5–14 d
- Occurs with any dose, any route
- Immunologic mech
- Rarely causes bleeding
- Life threatening thromboembolic episodes

Diagnosis
High-cost ELISA
- Detect antibodies against heparin—PF 4 complex rapid and simple low sensitivity
- Platelet activation assay (PAA)
- Most specific
- Serotonin release assay (SRA)
- Heparin induced plt activation (HIPA)

Management
- Stop all heparin
- Alternative anticoagulation; bivalirudin, fondaparinux, argatroban, lepirudin
- DO NOT give plt transfusion
- DO NOT give warf

↓

Patients with HIT – thrombosis – consumption of protein C – skin necrosis
- Evaluate for thrombosis (esp. DVT)
- Osteoporosis
  - Heparin – bone resorption by decreased bone formation and enhancing bone resorption
  - 30% patients
  - 2–3% had vertebral column
- Elevated level of transaminase
  - Unknown mech
  - Modest elevation
  - Returns to normal once drug stopped

LMWH
- Smaller fragments of heparin
- Mean mol. Wt. = 5,000 (1/3rd of UFH)

MOA
By activating antithrombin
- Catalyze inhibition of F alpha a more than UFH
- Less antithrombin activity
  Aniti alpha a – anti 2a = 2:1 to 4:1

Pharmacology
- SC/IV
- Shorter chain binds less avidly to endothelial cell, macrophage and pl. protein
  ↓
  No rapid clearance
  ↓
  Longer $t_{1/2}$ (approx 4 h)
  90% bio availability
  More predictable dose response
  Resistance to LMWH is rare

Monitoring
- Do not require monitoring
- Can measure anti alpha a level
- Prophylactic dose → anti alpha a level target 0.2–0.5
  Therapeutic dose → anti alpha a level target 0.5–1.2
  (For Heparin anti alpha a level target 0.3–0.7)
  When to measure—3–4 h after LMWH

Situations that may require LMWH monitoring
- Renal insufficiency
- Pregnancy
- Obesity
- High risk patient (patient with prosthetic valve who are given LMWH for prophylaxis)

Dose
- *For prophylaxis*
  - 4,000–5,000 U s/c daily or
  - 2,500–3,000 U s/c twice daily dosing
- *For treatment*
  - Unstable angina
    s/c BD 100–120 U/kg
  - Reduce in renal impairment
  VTE
  - 150–200 U/kg once a day or
  - 100 U/kg twice daily

S/E
- Bleeding
- Thrombocytopenia
  - 5-fold lower than LMWH
  - LMWH binds lens avidly in plt ant less release of PF4
  - LMWH not used to treat HIT—because most of antibodies have cross reactivity
- Osteoporosis

FONDAPARINUX
- Synthetic analogue of antithrombin binding polysaccharide
- Not approved for ACS in USA
- Approved in Europe and Canada
  - Mol wt = 1,728
  - Binds only to antithrombin and inhibit F alpha a
  - Too short to bind to thrombin

Pharmacology
- No binding to endothelial cell/plasma prot
- Complete bioavailability after S/C injection
- Clearance is independent of dose
- $t_{1/2}$ = 17 h
- s/c OD dosing
- CI in patients with oral <30
- Predictable anticoagulation response

Dose
- For prevention 2–5 mg daily
- For treatment LVTE 7.5 mg OD
  - For wt <50 kg → 5 mg OD
  - For wt >100 → 10 mg OD
  As effective as LMWH/VFH for treatment of DVT/PE
- For treatment (ACS)
  - 2.5 mg OD
  - No diff in rates of CV death, MI /stroke
  - Rate of major bleeding was 50% less
    ↓
    If patients undergoing PCI → risk of catheter thrombosis unless adjunct heparin given
  - Although fondaparinux can induce formation of HIT antibody—HIT does not occur
    ↓
    This paradox reflects that HIT requires heparin chain of sufficient length to bind multiple PF4 molecules. Fondaparinux is too small to do so

S/E
- Bleeding
- No antidote
- Recomb. of 8a has shown to reverse anticoagulant effect on fondaparinux

PARENTERAL DTI
- *Lepirudin*
  - Bivalent DTT
  - Interact with active site of thrombin and exotic 1 (substrate binding site)

- Cont IV infusion
- S/C for thromboprophylaxis
- plasma $t_{1/2}$ = 60 mins
- Renal clearance
- Antibody against drug develop in high proportion of lepirudin treated patient
  - Monitored with aPTT—not ideal because clotting time plateaus with higher conc
  - ECT provide better index of lepirudin dose
- *Argatroban:* Univalent DTI
Safer than lepirudin for patients with HIT and renal impairment
- *Bivalirudin*
  - Bivalent thrombin inhibitor
  - $t_{1/2}$ = 25 mins (shortest of all PTI)
  - Partially excreted by kidney
  - Monitored with ACT
  - With lower dose—can be monitored with aPTT
  - Adv. less bleeding

WARFARIN

- Water soluble vit K antagonist
- Initially developed as rodenticide
- Interfere with synthesis of vit K dependent clotting factors 2, 7, 9, 10
- Also inhibit synthesis of vit K dependent anticoagulant prot C and S

MOA

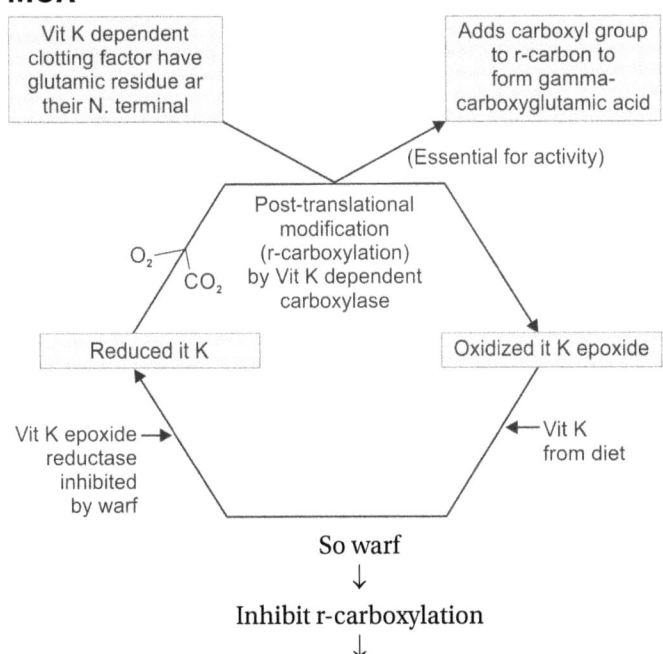

- Antithrombotic effect of warf require reduction in function level of factor x and prothrombin ($t_{1/2}$ of this factors are 24 and 72 hours respectively)

Pharmacology

- WARF = racemic mixture of r and s-isomers
- Rapidly and completely absorbed
- Peak approx 90 min after administration
- Plasma $t_{1/2}$ = 36-42 hours
- 97% bound to albumin
- Warf accumulate in liver
  ↓
  2 isomers metabolized via separate pathway
  ↓
  More active s-isomer metabolized by CYP2C9
  ↓
  Patient with one variant allele (CYP2C9*2/CYP2C9*3) require 20-30% lower maintenance dose
  ↓
  Patient who are homozygous for these alleles require 50-70% less dose than do patient with wild type CYP2C9*1 allele (less common in Asians)
- Warf interfere with vit K cycle inhibiting C1 subunit vit K epoxide reductase (VKORCI)
  ↓
  Polymorphism in VKORCI can influence anticoagulant response
  ↓
  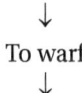
  To warf
  ↓
  - VKORCI variants more prevalent than CYP2C9
  - Asians have high prevalence of VKORCI
  - warf dose req
    - 25% less with heterozygotes
    - 50% less with homozygotes
- Dietary intake of vit K, drugs and various disease state also influence anticoag effect of warf

Monitoring

- PT INR = (patients PT/mean normal PT) × International sensitivity index range from 1.0-1.4
- Every lab should establish mean normal PT with each batch of thromboplastin reagent
- Maintain PT INR between 2-3
  For mechanical MVR 2.5-3.5

Dose

Depends on PT INR
- Concomitant treatment with parenteral anticoag × 5 days

- Minimum and should be continued until INR is therapeutic for 2 consecutive days

S/E

- *Bleeding*
  Treatment:
  - Asymptomatic + INR 3.5–9
    - W/H warf until INR return to therapeutic range
  - If patient at high risk for bleeding
    - S/L vit K
      - 1–2.5 mg for INR 4.9–9
      - 2.5–5 mg for INR >9
    - Oral vit K produce more rapid reversal of INR—helpful of INR is excessively high
  - Patients with serious bleeding
    - 10 mg vit K IV
    - FFp
  - For life threatening bleeding/if patient cannot tolerate volume load (FFP)
    - Prothrombin complex concentrate
- *Skin necrosis*
  - Rare
  - 2–5 d after initiation of treatment
  - Well demarcated erythematous lesion on thigh, buttocks, breast or toes
  - Center of lesion becomes prog necrotic
  - Biopsy shows thrombi in microcirculation
  - Occur in patients with cong/Acq def of prot C/S
    ↓
    Warf further reduce protocols
    ↓
    Anticoagulant activity of prot C/S lost before warf antithrombotic activity starts
    ↓
    Procoagulant state trigger
    Thrombosis in microvasculature

Treatment

- Discontinue warf
- Reversal with vit K
- Alternate anticoagulation heparin/LMWH
- Prot C concentrate – accelerate healing
- FFP
- Skin grafting
- *Prevent:* Overlapping treatment with parenteral anticoagulation when initiating warf
- *Fetal embryopath:*
  - Nasal hypoplasia and stippled epiphyses
  - Highest with warf administration in 1st trim freq

FIBRINOLYSIS

Approved fibrinolytics

Streptokinase/antistreptase/urokinase/
Rt PA (alteplase)/
Tenecteplase/reteplase

Recombinant rt PA

MOA

Converts proenzyme plasminogen – plasmin
- 2 pools of plasminogen
- Circulating plasminogen and fibrin-bound plasminogen urokinase/streptokinase
  - Nonspecific fibrinolytics activates both
  - Fibrin specific lytic agents activate fibrin bound plasminogen
  - Alteplase/reteplase/Tenecteplase

STREPTOKINASE

- Not an enzyme
- Do not convert plasminogen to plasmin directly
- Forms 1:1 complex with plasminogen
  ↓
  Conformational change in plasminogen
  ↓
  Expose its active site
  ↓
  Convert additional plasminogen to plasmin
  ↓
  Activate both force and fibrin band plasminogen
  ↓
  Plasmin degrade fibrin in occlusive thrombus as well as induce systemic lytic state

Dose

1.5 MV over 30–60 mins

Problem

- Antibody against it can be form in patient who had received it previously or patients with prev streptokinase inf reduce effectiveness
- Allergic reaction (5%)
- Transient hypotension (due to plasmin mediated release of bradykinin

ANISTREPLASE

- Streptokinase mixed with equimolar amt of lys-plasminogen (plasmin cleared from plasminogen)
- $t_{1/2}$ 100 min – single bolus dose

UROKINASE
- Derived from fetal kidney cell culture
- Directly converts plasminogen – plasmin
- Produce lytic state
- Nonimmunogenic
- No allergic reaction

ALTEPLASE
- Recombinant form of tPA
- Interaction with fibrin is mediated by finger domain and to a lesser extent by second kringle domain
- Fibrin specificity is limited because like fibrin, (DD) E also binds to alteplase with high affinity
- Plasmin generated on fibrin surface results in thrombolysis, whereas plasmin generated on surface of circulating DD (E) degrades fibrinogen
- Significant lower mortality with alteplase than streptokinase

TENECTEPLASE
- Genetically engineered
- Longer $t_{1/2}$ than tPA
- Resistant to inactivation by PAI-1
- Affinity to DD (E) is significantly lower
- Higher fibrin specificity

RETEPLASE
- Single chain variant
- Lacks finger domain, kringle domain and epidermal growth factors
- Binds fibrin more weakly (because it lacks finger domain)
- At least as effective as streptokinase
- Not superior to tPA

NEWER
- *Desmoteplase*
  - Recombinant form
  - Full length plasminogen activator
  - Isolated from saliva of vampire bat
- *Alfimeprase*
  - Truncated form of fibrolase
  - Isolated from venom of southern copperhead shake

Disappointing clinical studies

8.2 HEMOSTASIS/THROMBOSIS/FIBRINOLYSIS

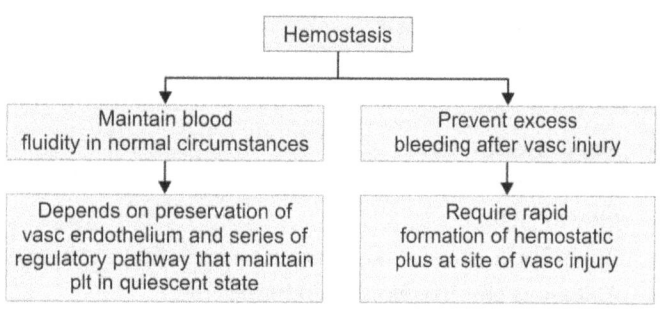

- *Arterial thrombi:* Form on top of disrupted atherosclerotic plaque
- *Venous thrombi:* Usually forms in valve cusp in deep vein of calf or where there is blood stasis.

Sluggish blood flow
↓
Decreased O_2 supply to vascular valve cusps
↓
Hypoxemia induces endothelial cells lining valve cusp to express adhesion molecule
↓
Tether leukocyte and micro particles onto its surface
↓
Induce coagulation

- Web of DNA released from activated neutrophils (called Neutrophil extracellular Traps—NETs) also contribute to thrombosis by providing scaphold that binds platelet - promote their activation and aggregation
- *Arterial thrombi:* Rich in platelet due to high sheer stress (Appear white)
- *Venous thrombi:* Few platelets and mostly fibrin and trapped RBC (appear red)

Recent evidence: Addition of low dose rivaroxaban to DAPT reduce recurrent ischemic event and stent thrombosis in patient with ACS

HEMOSTATIC SYSTEM
Major Components
- Vascular endothelium
- Platelets
- Coagulation and fibrinolytic system

Vascular Endothelium
- Inhibit platelet
- Suppress coagulation
- Promote fibrinolysis

A. *Platelet Inhibition:*
1.   Prostacyclin 2 No
            ↓

Potent vasodilator   Inhibit platelet activation and aggregation

2. CD39 (memb associated ecto-ADPase)
↓
Decreased plt activation by degrading ADP

B. *Anticoagulation activity:*
1. Heparan sulfate on endothelium
↓
Binds circulating antithrombin and enhance their activity
+
Also binds tissue factor pathway inhibitor (TFPI)
↓
Inhibition of coagulation

Note: Heparin and LMWH displace GAG bound TFPI from vasc endothelium – released TFPI may contribute in anticoagulant activity of these drugs)

2.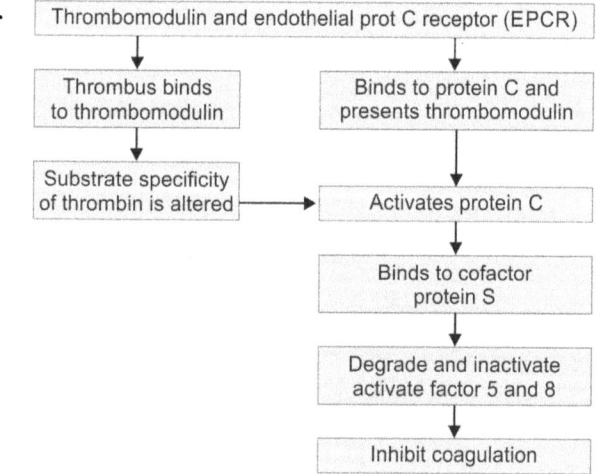

C. Fibrinolytic activity:

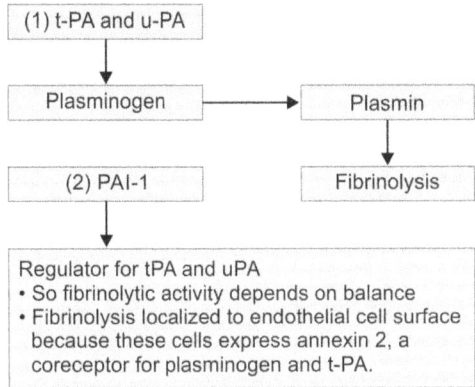

PLATELETS

- Anucleat cells – limited capacity to synthesize prot
- Life span 7–10 d
- Thrombopoietin = Glycoprotein synthesized in liver and kidneys, regulate megakaryocyte proliferation and maturation as well as platelet production
- VWF synthesized by endothelial cell and megakaryocyte
- Stored in weibe/palade bodies
- When released, most enters circulation
- VWF released from albuminal side of endothelial cells, accumulate in subendothelial matrix.

A. Adhesion

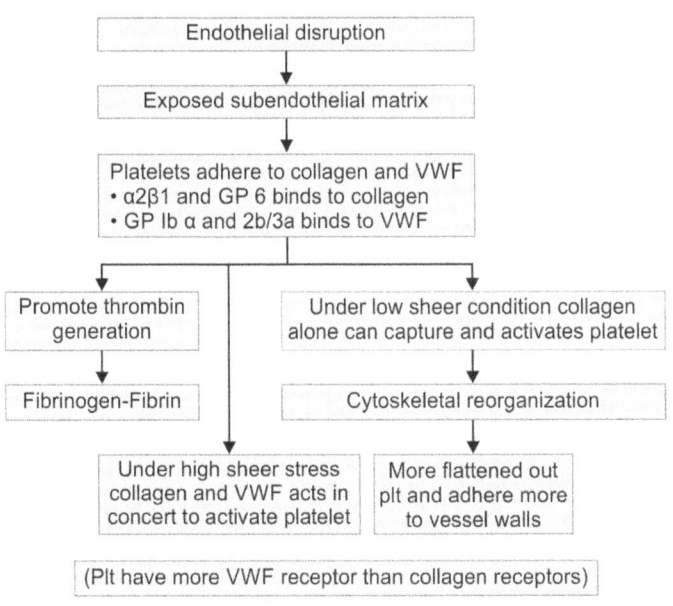

B. Activation:

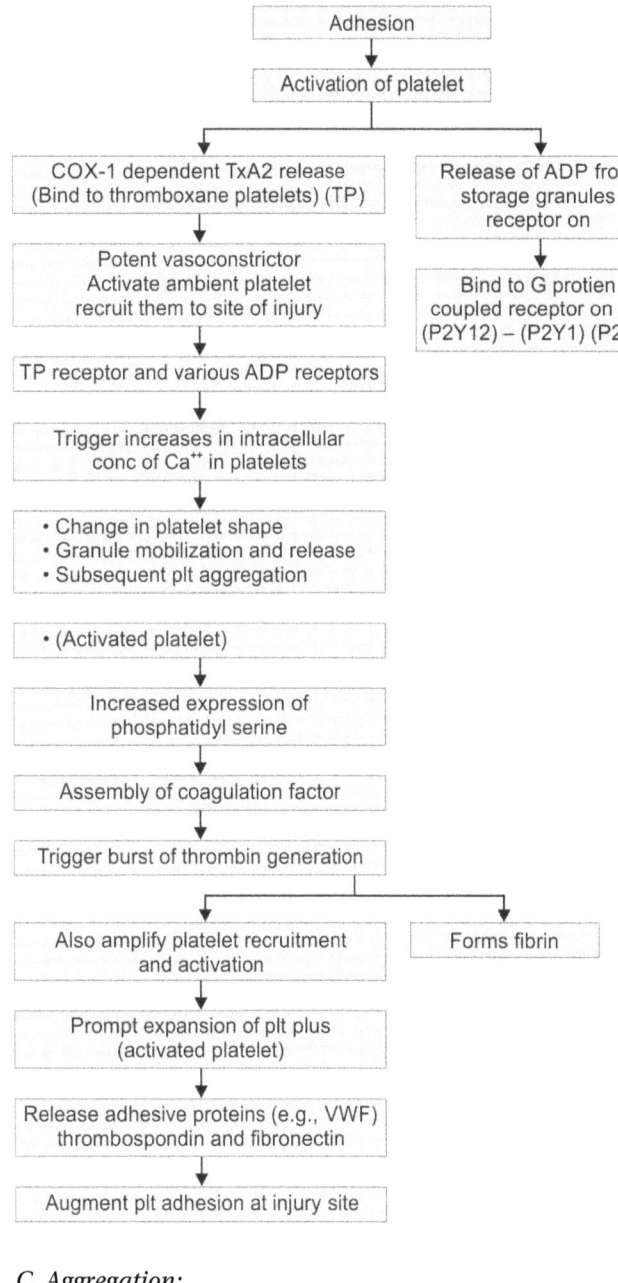

C. Aggregation:

Links platelets to each other to form clumps (Gp2b, 3a mediates this)
↓
Once bound to Gp2b/3a
↓
Fibrinogen and VWF induce outside-inside signals that augments platelets activation
↓
Activation of additional Gp2b/3a receptor
↓
Positive feedback loop

COAGULATION

A. Extrinsic Tenase
- Rupture of atherosclerotic plaque
- Denuding injury to vessel well

↓

Expose tissue factor expressed by
by subendothelial fibroblasts and SMC

↓

Serve as a receptor for factor 7 and activates it 7 a

↓

Factor 7a binds to tissue factor
in a calcium dependent fashion
to form extrinsic tenase complex

↓

Activates factor 10 and 9

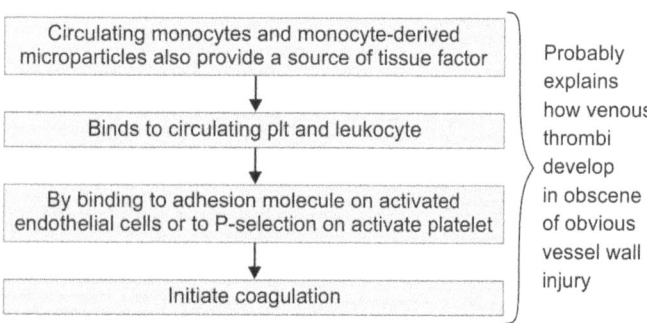

Probably explains how venous thrombi develop in obscene of obvious vessel wall injury

B. Intrinsic Tenase:

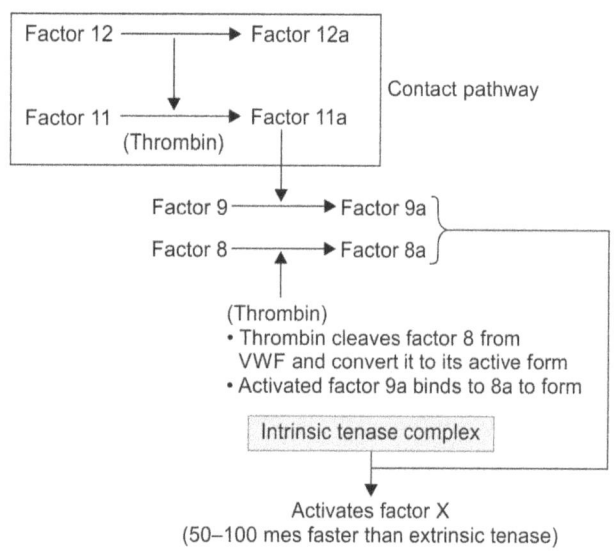

C. Prothrombin

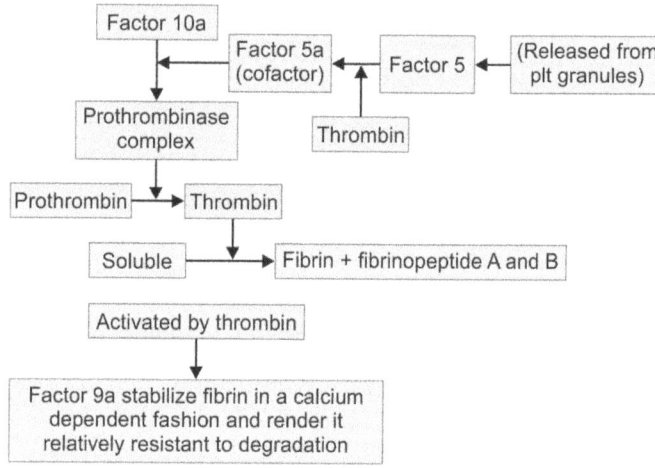

Note: In general,
- Coagulation occurs through action of discrete enzyme complex composed of a vit K dependent enzyme and nonenzyme co-factor (all assemble on anionic phospholipid membrane) in Ca^{++} dependent manner.
- Each enzyme complex activate vit K dependent substrate that become the enzyme component of subsequent complex
- These complex generate small amt of thrombin that feedback to amplify its own generation by activating non enzyme cofactor and plt

D. Contact pathway:
Includes factor 9, prekalikrein and high molecular weight kininogen (HMWK) is also important

↓

Coronary catheters and other blood contacting medical devices (mech value) trigger clotting through this mechanism.

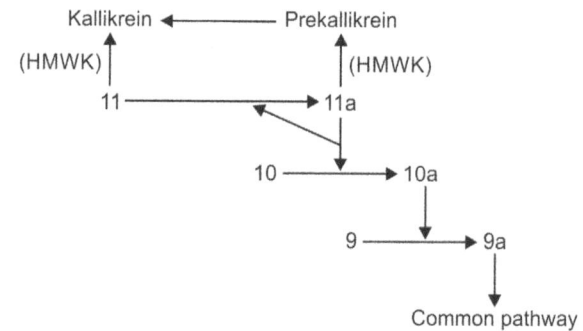

FIBRINOLYTIC SYSTEM

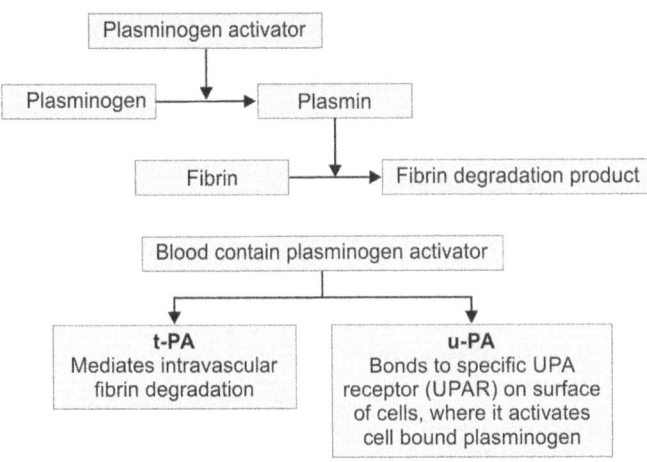

Regulation of Fibrinolysis

At 2 levels
1. PAI (inhibit plasmogen activator)
2. Alpha 2 antiplasmin (inhibitor plasmin)

PAI-1 (from endothelial cell)-Inhibit both tPA and uPA

PAI-2 (from monocyte and placenta) → inhibit only uPA

*Thrombin activated fibrinolysis Inhibitor (TAFI)

Modulates fibrinolysis—Link between coagulation and fibrinolysis

8.3 HYPERCOAGULABLE STATES

THROMBOSIS THRESHOLD

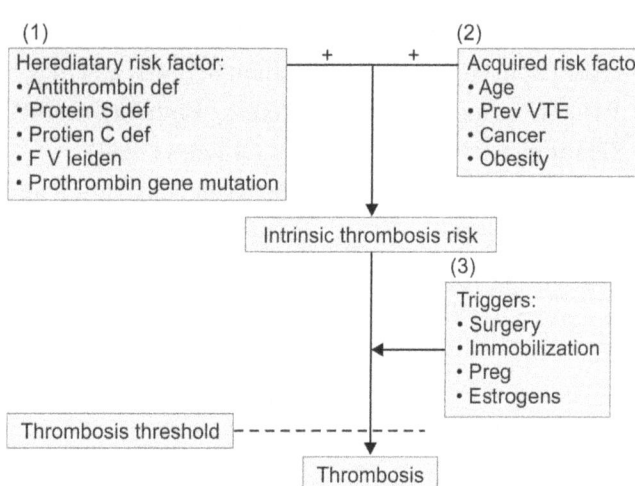

CLASSIFICATION OF HYPERCOAGULABLE STATES

Hereditary	Acquired	Mixed
Loss of function – Antithrombin def – Protein C def – Protein S def	Advanced age Obesity Prev VTE Cancer	Hyperhomocysteinemia
Gain of function – Factor V Leiden – Prothrombin gene mutation – Elevated factor VII, IX, and XI	Surgery Immobilization Preg, Purpurium Drugs-HRT	

All associated with increased risk of VTE

INHERITED

- Factor V Leiden (AD)
    - mc inherited thrombophilia
    - 5% of population (American whites)
    - Rare in Asians
    - Point mutation
    - Results in synthero of factor V G/n residue in place of avg residue at position 506
        ↓
        Resist rapid proteolytic and persist 10 times longer in time of activated
    Protein C
    - 5 fold increases risk for VTE
    - Absolute risk for VTE is low (yearly 0.1-0.3% subjects)
    - (Δ):
        ◆ Activated protein C assay
        ◆ Ratio of a PTT after addition of protein C divided by that determined before its addition
        ◆ Genetic testing using PCR
- Prothrombin gene mutation
    - Second mc (3% in whites) (*rare in asian*)
    - *a to A nucleotide transition* at position 20210 in 3 region of prothrombin gene
    - *Elevated level of prothrombin → increased thrombin generation*
    - Limit in activation of factor Va by activated protein C
    - Risk of VTE similar to factor V Leiden
        (Δ): *Genetic screening after PCR amplification*
- *Elevated level of 8,9,10:*
    - Also association risk of arterial thrombosis and mL
    - Genetic mean probably contribute
        (Δ): *Assessment of factor level*
- Antithrombin deficiency
    - Rare (hereditary and acquired)
    - 1 in 2,000 people
    - Can be due to (1) *decreased synthesis of normal protein in liver* or (2) *Synthesis of dysfn protein*
    - homozygous → embryonic lethality
        → Acquired antithrombin def:
        ◆ *Decrease synthesis:*
            – Severe hepatic disease
            – pt on L-asparaginase
        ◆ *Increased consumption*
            – Extensive thrombosis
            – MC
            – Severe septic
            – Disseminated malignancy
            – Heparin treatment
            – Prolonged Ecmo
        ◆ Enhanced clearance
            – Nephrotic syndrome
        (Δ) - *Antithrombin level and its activity*
            – Decreased level and decreased activity → Decrease synthesis
            – Normal level and decreased activity → Dysfunctional protein
- Protein C deficiency
    (Ref. Protein C pathology in endothelium)
    - Both *inherited* and *acquired*
    - 1 in 200 adults
    - AD (Heterozygous deficiency)
    - *Homozygous* deficiency can also occur → *Purpura fulminans* caused by *widespread thrombosis*

- Inherited deficiency: due to
  → *decreased synthesis* of protein
  → *dysfunctional* protein synthesis
- Acquired deficiency:
  1. *Decrease synthesis:* liver size|warf
  2. *Increased consumption:* severe septic, DIC
- (Δ) Same as antithrombin (level and activity)

- **Protein S def:**
  - Acts as cofactor for prot C
  - May directly inhibit prothrombin activation because of its capacity to factor Va and Xa
    - Inherited or acquired
    - *Inherited* due to
      1. Reduce synthesis
      2. Synthesis of dysfunctional protein
  - *Acquired:*
    - Decreased synthesis: liver disease | warf | L-asparaginase
  - Increased consumption: DIC
  - Increased clearance: Nephrotic
  - (Δ): measure both free and bound form

    ↓   ↓
    40%   60%
            bound to
        complement component

- **Other hereditary disorders:**
  - *Polymorphism in gene encoding for (EPCRS)* Endothelial Protein C receptor
  - Polymorphism in factor XIII
    ↓
    More rapid activation by thrombin
    ↓
    Small reduction in risk for VTE, MI, and Stroke

8.4 NOACs

RELY TRIAL
(RECOVER, RECOVER2, REMAP, RESONAT)

DABIGATRAN
- MOA – Direct thrombin inhibitor
- Pharma C
  - Absorption: Rapid
  - Metabolism: Hepatic
    - Rapidly and completely hydrolyzed to active form by Pl. and hepatic esterase
  - Excretion: Renal (80%)
  - $t_{1/2}$ 8–15 h
  - Onset of action 1–3 hours
  - Antidote – none

Contraindication
- Hypersensitivity to Dabigatran
- Active bleeding

Worsening/Precaution
- Bleeding tendency
- Renal impairment
- Planned invasive procedure
- P-gp inhibitors (azithromycin, clarithromycin, amiodarone, quinidine, ritonavir, verapamil)

Indi
- Non valvular AF-decreased risk of stroke and embolization
- Treatment of DVT and PE-(undergoing review for this indi)
- Reduce recurrence of DVT and PE

Dose
- 150 mg BD for Cr CL >30
- 75 mg BD for Cr Cl 15–30
- CI in patients with CrCl <15
  - ROCKET-AF Trial (EINSTEINE DVT, EINSTEINE PE)

RIVAROXABAN
MOA

Oral function alpha a inhibitor

Phramac
- Absorption – rapid
- Metabolism – Hepatic (33%) via CYP3A4/5
- Excretion – Renal (66%) Feces (28%)
- $T_{1/2}$ 7–11 h
- Onset of action – 2–4 h

S/E
- Pruritus (2%)
- Bleeding (6% if used for DVT prophylaxis) (21% if used for AF)
- Thrombocytopenia
- Increase in liver enzymes

Contraindication
- Hypersensitivity to rivaroxaban
- Active bleeding
- CrCl <15
- Severe hepatic impar

Drug Interaction
- PGP inhibitor/induces

Indi
- Non valvular AF
- DVT/PE prophylaxis
- Treatment of DVT/PE-approved
- Reduce recurrence of DVT/PE

Dose
- Non valvular HF: 20 mg OD for CrCl >50
  15 mg OD for CrCl 15–50
- Prophylaxis of DVT/PE: 20 mg OD
  35 d for hip and 12 d for knee replace
- Treatment of DVT/PE: 15 mg BD × 21 d – 20 mg OD × 21 d ARISTOTAL Trial (AMPLIFY EXT)

APIXABAN FACTOR ALPHA A INHIBITOR
- *Pharmac:*
  - Absorption – rapid
  - Metabolism – 15% liver metabolism
  - Excretion – 1° biliary/fecal (45–55%)
  - Renal (27%)
  - $T_{1/2}$ 8–15 h
  - Onset of action – 1–2 h

Indi
- Nonvalvular AF
- Prophylaxis of DVT
- Reduce recurrence of DVT/PE

Contraindicated

In patients with severe hepatic impairment

Dose

- (Nonvalvular AF)
  - 5 mg BD
  - 2-5 mg BD if
    1. 2 or more of these (age >80, wt <60, cr >15)
    2. Coadminister with ketoconazole/itraconazole/ritonavir
  - No data for CrCl <15
  - Patient on HD - 5 mg BD
    - 25 BD (if age >80 or at 60)
- Prophylaxis of DVT
  - 2.5 BD (1st done 12-24 h after surgery)
  - for 35 d post hip replace and 12 d post knee replace
- Treatment of DVT/PR
  - 10 mg BD × 7 d - 5 mg BD

EDOXABAN-ENGAGE –AF TRIAL

Pros of NOACs

- Lower incidence of IC bleed compare to warf
- Lower incidence of major bleed compare to warf
- Lower incidence of ischemic bleed compare to warf
- Lower overall mortality
- No mortality of PT-INR
- Shorter $t_{1/2}$ - easy periop management
- Fewer drug interaction

Cons

- High cost
- High incidence of GI bleed (Dabigatran)
- Possibly increased incidence of MI (Dabigatran)
- Renal monitoring and dose adjustment required
- No specific antidote

NOACs REVERSAL

Nonspecific reversal

- Administration of coagulation factor concentrates E.g.
  - Inactive prothrombin complex concentrate (octaplex, beriplex)
  - Activated prothrombin complex concentrate (FEIBA)
  - Recombinant activated factor 7

  Less beneficial and less logical
- Specific antidotes
  - Idarucizumab
    - Drug specific antidote (Dabigatran)
    - REVERSE AD trial
    - Antidote to dabigatran
    - All patients received 5 gm idarucizumab
    - Anticoagulant activity measured using dilute TT and ECT (Ecarin clotting time)
    - Reversal within minutes
    - Time taken to stop bleeding - 3-5 h
    - Drawback of trial: No comparator group
  - Andexanet alfa
    - Class specific antidote (rivaroxaban and apixaban)
    - 2 phase 3 trials shown good efficacy and safely
    - ANNEXA-4 ongoing phase 3 trial
  - Ciraparantag
    - Universal antidote
    - Phase 2 trial ongoing

	Idarucizumab (drug specific)	Andexanet alfa (class specific)	Ciraparantag (universal)
Reversal	Dabigatran	Apixaban	All
Fas		Rivaroxaban	
		Edoxaban	
MOA	Monoclonal antibody that binds dabigatran with high annifity (350 times more than Thrombin)	Decay F alpha a molecule that binds F alpha inhibitor anticoagulant restoring function of endogenous F alpha a for apixaban	Binds to anticoagulant via non-covalent hydrogen bonds and change interaction
Studied dose	• 5 mg IV as 25 mg • Boluses 14 min apart	• 400 mg bolus + 480 mg • Infusion over 2 h • For rivaroxaban/edoxaban • 800 mg bolus + 960 mg • Infusion 2 hrs	100–300 mg IV single dose
Onset of action	<5 min	<2 min	5–10 min
$T_{1/2}$ elimination	• *Diphasic:* Initial – 45 mm • Terminate 10 hrs	1 hr	24 hr

Contd...

Contd...

	Idarucizumab (drug specific)	**Andexanet alfa (class specific)**	**Ciraparantag (universal)**
Elimination	Renal	Not reported	Renal
Storage	Refrigerated	Refrigerated	Room temp
Status	Licensed by US, Canada and European	Phase 3 trial	Phase 2 trial
Approved	Reversal of dabigatrean	N/A	N/A
Indi	In patients with life threatening/need for surgical surgery		
Comment	No effect on F alpha inhibitor	• Also reverse enoxaparin • No effect on dabigatran	Binds to all NOACs, UFH, LMWH, fondaparinux

SECTION 9

Hypertension

9.1 PRACTICAL CLINICAL APPROACH TO EVALUATION AND MANAGEMENT OF AMBULATORY HYPERTENSIVE PATIENTS

INTRODUCTION

JNC-8 not sanctioned by NHLBI or any professional organization and thus does not constitute an official US HTN guideline.

INITIAL EVALUATION

- *Office BP:* HTN is diagnosed if the avg of multiple offices seated BP is 140/90 or higher and patient has electrocardiographically (or ECHO) confirmed LVH or other e/o HTN induced target organ damage.
- *Home/AmBP:* In absence of target organ damage or very severe office BP (>180/110), home or AmBP is important
  - Home or AmBP should be considered to detect masked HTN which is an indication for treatment, if office BP in preHTN range (120–139/80–89) in patients with DM, cKD who have high prevalence of masked HTN and in patients who have high prevalence of nocturnal HTN.
  - HTN diagnosed if home BP or daytime AmBP is 135/85 or higher or avg. 24 hours BP is 130/80 mm Hg or higher.
- *Global risk CV assessment*—most HTN patients have additional risk factor, e.g., Dyslipidemia, statin therapy, met synd, frank DM, cKD, cig smoking.
- *2° HTN:* Screening indicated in patients with early onset HTN (<30 years) and in all patients with truly resistant HTN, adrenal incidentaloma, or specific clues detected on routine initial evaluation (unprovoked hyperkalemia).

MANAGEMENT

- *Lifestyle modification*
- *BP treatment goal:*
  - Most current guidelines:
    - Mean office BP <140/90
    - Mean home BP <135/85

For elderly HTN: Seated BP of 155 mm Hg may be appropriate target for frail 70-year-old patients with marked orthostatic and post prandial HTN. Whereas home seated BP of 130 mm Hg may be appropriate for vigorously healthy 85-year-old patient whose chief concern is to avoid disability stroke

  - Symptomatic KH has to be avoided when treating older patients with long standing DM in whom autonomic neuropathy has developed
    - Nonproteinuric cKD—goal 140/90 mm Hg
    - Proteinuric cKD—goal 130/80 mm Hg
  - AmBP at least once with stage 3 or higher cKD because masked and nocturnal HTN will be present in most
- *First line treatment*
  1. CCB
  2. ACE/ARB
  3. Thiazide

Amlodipine as preferred CCB

- *Low dose combination*
  - Any 2 or 3 of first line anti HTN agent for all patients with HTN'
  - High dose should be avoided
  - BP control is more imp rather than class of anti HTN
  - Adherence best for ARB; Intermed for ACEI/CCB; least for BB and Diuretics

- *Resistant HTN*
  - Rule out pseudo resistance
  - Best add on drug is mineralocorticoid receptor antagonist and vasodilating beta-blockers

INDICATIONS FOR AmBP
- White coat HTNs
- White coat effect (pseudoresistance)
- Masked HTN
- Nocturnal HTN
- Secondary HTN – OSA, endocrine HTN, cKD
- Resistance HTN
- Syncope
- OH or postprandial hypotension
- Assessing response to treatment
- BP variability
- Pediatric HTN ⎤ White coat HTN
- Pregnancy ⎦ is common

Expanding trial

Evidence of benefit by treating preHTN
- CAMELOT trial
- PAHRAO trial
- TROPHY trial

Pathophysio of PreHTN

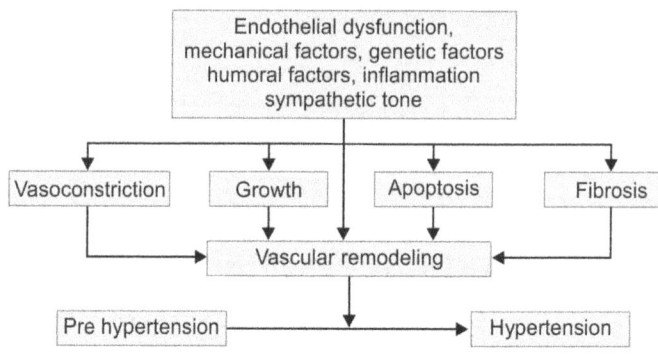

9.2 BP IN ACUTE CVA

RECOMMENDATIONS FOR DECREASED BP IN AC CVA

- Concept of permissive HTN for first 24 hours to maintain cerebral perf pr
  - Do not treat HTN in first 24 hours unless HTN is extreme (SBP >220; DBP >120)

  Or

  Patient has concomitant medical disease that needs treatment'
  - CAD (active ischemia)
  - HF
  - AOD
  - Hypertensive enceph
  - ARF
  - Preeclampsia eclampsia
- When treatment indicated—cautious lowering of BP
  - Approx 15% during 1st 24 hours
- For patients with eligibility for lytic treatment
  - Decreased BP below 185/110 mm Hg
  - And maintain <180/105 after lysis
  - Forthcoming trial (ENCHANTED) is evaluating role of intensive BP control (130-140 SBP)
  - Which drug
    - Labetalol
    - Nicardipine
- *For acute hemorrhagic stroke*
  INTERACT 2 and 2 trials
  - Class 1—ICH presenting with SBP 150-220 - acute lowering to 140
  - 2b—ICH with SBP >220 - aggressive BP reduction

9.3 APPROACH TO PATIENT WITH CHEST PAIN

COMMON CAUSES OF AC CHEST PAIN

- Cardiac
  - Angina
  - Rest or unstable angina
  - AMI
  - Pencarditis
- Vascular
  - Aortic dissection
  - Pulm embolism
  - Pulm—HTN
- Pulmonary
  - Pleuritis/Pneumonia
  - Tracheobronchitis
- Gastrointestinal
  - Esophageal rupture
  - Peptic ulcer
  - Esophageal reflux
  - Gall stone
  - Pancreatitis
- Musculoskeletal
  - Costochondritis
  - Cervical disc disease
  - Trauma/strain
- Infection
  - Herpes zoster
- Psychological
  - Panic disorder

SHORT TERM RISK FOR DEATH/NONFATAL MI IN PATIENT WITH UA

- High risk
  - Accelerating tempo of ischemic symptoms in prior 48 hrs
  - Prolonged ongoing (>20 min) pain at rest
  - Pulm edema
  - New onset or worsening of MR murmur
  - S3 or new onset or worsening rales
  - Hypotension/poradycardia/tachycardia
  - Age >75 years
  - Angina at nest with transient ST changes (>0.05 mv)
  - BBB, new or presumably new
  - Elevated JNI, TNT or CHMB

INDICATION AND CONTRAINDICATION FOR EXERCISE ECG IN EO

Requirement for Performing Exercise Testing

- 2 sets of cardiac enzymes at 4 hours inter should be normal.
- ECH at time of arrival and pre-exercise 12 level show no significant abnormality
- Absence of rest ECH abnormality that will preclude accurate assessment of exercise ECH
- From adm to 2nd enzyme: pr is asymptomatic, lessening chest pain, persistent atypical symptoms
- Absence of ischemic chest pain at time of exercise testing

Contraindication

- New or evolving abnormality on rest testing
- Abnormal cardiac enzyme levels
- Inability to perform exercise
- Worsening or persistent ischemic chest pain symptoms from adm to the time of exercise
- Clinical risk profiling indicates need for CAG.

9.4 CENTRAL Ao Pr

TECHNIQUES

- Applanation tonometry
  - Carotid pr used as a surrogate marker of central pr
  - Carotid pr wave forms recorded by applanation tonometry and scaled to brachial art mean diastolic pr
  - *Principle:* Mean and diastolic pr do not vary significantly
  Throughout arterial system
  - *Disadv:*
    - High operator dependency
    - Inability to obtain good wave form in obese
    - Possibility of minor amplification between aorta and carotid → misinterpretation
- Pulse wave analysis
  - Pr wave forms recorded from peripheral site (radial) and correspondingly central Ao pr derived using computerized function
- Blind identification
  - Novel method
  - Estimate central Ao pr waveform using peripheral art pr waveforms with data specific methods

IMP

- Central BP more relevant than peripheral BP
- Central BP more closely related to adv CV outcome and end organ damage
- Late syst augmentation of central pr – increased LV mass index, carotid atherosclerosis, vascular hypertrophy, diameter of Asc Ao in marfan
- *Trials:* STRONG – heart study: CAFE study; anglo-cardiff collaborative trial-2

9.5 DEVICE BASED TREATMENT FOR HTN

INTRODUCTION
- Renal denervation
- Baroreceptor activation
- *Median nerve modulation*
  - E-coin – implanted in forearm – stimulates median nerve – send impulse to multiple areas of brain – decreased SNS – decreased BP
  - Pivotal trial showed encouraging result

  Fall in BP both in office and AmBP readings

- *Central arteriovenous coupler treatment for resistant HTN*
  - Small fistula created between iliac art and vein with controlled shunt flow creating a low resistance vascular bed – SVR decreases – BP decreases
  - Study of 40 patients and 40 control: AV fistula group showed significant BP decrease at 6 months
  - Problem: 1/3rd of patients with AVF developed ipsilateral venous stenosis.

9.6 DIAGNOSIS AND INITIAL EVALUATION

INTRODUCTION

Three goals:
1. Measurement of BP
2. Assessment of patients CV risk
3. Detection of 2° forms of HTN

Measurement of BP

- *Office BP*

	SBP	DBP
Normal	<120	<80
PreHTN	120–139	80–89
Stage 1 HTN	140–159	90–99
Stage 2 HTN	≥160	≥100

- 2 or more readings taken at 2 or more office visit
- BP should be measured twice after 5 mins rest
- Seated in chair with back support
- Arm base and at heart level
- Tobacco and caffeine should be avoided 30 mins
- BP should be, measured in both arm and after 5 mins of standing

2011 guidelines:
- BP >140/90 – take 2nd measurement
- If diff between 1st and 2nd – 3rd measurement
- Record lower of last 2 BP measures
- Home or AmBP is recommended

- *Home and AmBP monitoring*
  - Provide clear picture
  - Predict CV events better than office BP overcome many errors (physician's error and white coat HTN)
  - *Home BP:*
    - 2 readings (1 in morning and 1 at night)
    - 4 consecutive days (preferably 7)
    - 1st day's reading discarded (falsely elevated)
    - HTN diagnosed when any home BP ≥ 135/85
    - Wrist monitors are inaccurate and not recommended
    - Not appropriate in patients with AF and extra systole
  - *Ambulatory BP*
    - Predict fatal and nonfatal MI + stroke
    - Recommended normal value include an avg of daytime pr <135/85 and nighttime <120/70 mm Hg and 24 hour pr <130/80
    - At least 2 measurements per hour should be taken during patients working hours. Average value of 14 measurements during that time confirms diagnosis

White coat HTN If AmBP daytime pressure is <135/85 and there is no target organ damage despite continuously high office readings; this patient has white coat hypertension
- Caused by transient adrenergic response to BP measurement
- Common in older patients
- In untreated patients with white coat HTN, long term risk is equal to normotensive person
- Treated patient with higher office BP and normal AmBP are at higher risk

Suspect white coat HTN is following criteria:
- Office BP >140/90 on 3 separate visit
- 2 measurements made each visit
- At least 2 out of office readings below 140/90
- No e/o target organ damage

One easier approach: Office automated BP measurement
- Patient in quiet room
- No medical personnel
- 6 readings taken
- Avg of last 5 readings >135/85 – HTN

White coat aggravation: White coat reaction superimposed on milder level of out-of-office HTN

- *Masked HTN*: Office reading sometimes underestimates out of office BP (Because of sympathetic over activity in daily life caused by job or home stress, tobacco use or other adrenergic stimuli)
- *Other uses of AmBP*
  - To diagnose *natural HTN*
    - Nocturnal HTN increases HD load CVS and predicts CV outcomes better than either daytime ambulatory BP or office BP
    - Common amongst patients with Ckd (Because of increased CO and Increased SVR
    ↓

Increased pl vol during supine	Failure to suppress increased vasoconstrictor drive during sleep because of persistent excitatory stimuli by diseased kidney

CV Risk Stratification

Minimum lab tests required: Blood electrolytes
- FBS
- Sr creat
- Lipid profile
- Hematocrit
- Spot urine analysis

- Urine alb: or ratio
- 12 lead ECG

Factors influencing prognosis
- *Risk factors for CV disease:*
  - Increased SBP and DBP
  - Increased PP
  - Age men >55; women >65
  - Smoking
  - Dyslipidemia (LDL >115)
  - FBS (102-125) or abnormal GTT
  - F/H/O CV disease (premature)
  - Abnormal obesity
  - DM
- *Established target organ damage:*
  - *CNS disease:* Ischemic stroke, cerebral hemorrhage, TIA
  - *Heart disease:* MI, angina, HF, coronary revasc
  - *Renal disease:* Diabetic nephropathy, renal impairment
  - *PAD*
  - *Advanced retinopathy:* Hemorrhage or exudates, papilledema
- *Subclinical target organ damage:*
  - LVH
  - Carotid IMT or plaque
  - Low eGFR
  - Microalbuminuria
  - ABI <0.9

Emerging methods to improve CV risk stratification in HTN
- *BP variability* - conflicting evidence
- *HR variability* - conflicting evidence
- *Non-invasive measurement of central aortic pr by pulse tonometry:*
  - Central Ao pr wave is sum of pr wave generated by LV and reflected waves from periphery
  - When large conduit artery are healthy and compliant—reflected wave merge with incident wave during diastole
  - When conduit art stiff - reflected and incident wave merge in systole - augment SBP - increased LV after load and decreased coronary flow
  - Sphygmocor-uses brachial art BP and generalized transfer function (software) to convert radial wave form to derive central ao pr waveform
  - FDA approved
- Pulse tonometry provides measure of
  - Aortic stiffness
  - Pulse wave velocity
  - Augmentation index
- *Erectile dysfunction:* >50% of men with HTN and independently predict fatal and non-fatal CV events

HYPERTENSIVE HEART DISEASE

- HTN patients have more unrecognized MIs and silent ischemia
- Patients with Ac MI often have preexisting HTN
- Electro cardiographic LVH present in 5-10% of HTN patients
- ECHO LVH is present in 30% of patients with HTN
- ECHO LVH is present in 90% of uncontrolled HTN
- Cardiac MRI is even more sensitive

LARGE VESSEL DISEASE

- Ao dissection
- Ao aneurysm
- PAD

CEREBROVASC DISEASE

- HTN major risk factor for stroke and dementia
- HTN accounts for 50% of stroke
- In HTN patients
  - 80% stroke are ischemic
  - 20% stroke is hemorrhage

CKD

- Small scarred kidney (Hypertensive Nephrosclerosis) likely resulting from chronic exposure of renal parenchyma to excessive pressure and flow
- *Markers:*
  - Urinary albumin excretion
  - Decreasing eGFR
  - Micro albumin
    - Ur Alb to Cr ratio
    - 30-300 mg/gm
- Most patients with HTN associated Ckd die of heart attack or stroke before renal function deteriorate sufficiently to require hemodialysis

9.7 HTN IN PREGNANCY

INTRODUCTION
- Major cause of maternal fetal morbidity and mortality
- Four categories of HTN:
  1. Eclampsia
  2. Chronic HTN
  3. Chronic HTN with superimposed preeclampsia
  4. Gestational HTN
- *Preeclampsia:* Severe progressive multisystem disorder diagnosed by any one of the following
  - BP of 160/110 mm Hg or higher despite bed rest
  - Thrombocytopenia
  - Proteinuria
  - Impaired liver function
  - Progressive renal insufficiency
  - Pulmonary edema
  - New onset cerebral or visual disturbance:

Pathologic mech endothelial dysfunction causing abnormality remodeling of placental spiral art

Diagnostic criteria for preeclampsia:
- BP >140/90 on 2 occasion at least 4 hour apart after 20 weeks of gestation in a women with previously normal preg
- ≥160/120 – HTN can be confirmed within short interval (minutes) to facilitate timely antihypertensive therapy (and) – Proteinuria (≥300 mg/24 hours urine collection or prot-creat ratio ≥0.3) (or) in absence of proteinuria; new onset of HTN with new onset of any of the following:
  1. Thrombocytopenia (plt < 1 LaL)
  2. Renal insufficiency (S. cr > 1.1 mg/dL or doubling of Sr. Cr in absence of other renal course)
  3. Impaired liver function
  4. Pulm edema
  5. Cerebral or visual symptoms

- *Chronic HTN:* SBP ≥140 or DBP ≥90 before prog or diagnosed before 20th week of gestation
- *Gestational HTN:* BP elevation after 20 weeks gestation in the absence of the additional systemic features listed in above table (BP normalize by 12 weeks postpartum)

*RISK FACTORS
- Material age <20 or >35
- Positive personal or F/H of gestational HTN
- Preexisting HTN
- Obesity
- Diabetes
- Antiphospholipid antibody
- Nulliparity
- Fetal triploidy
- BMI >35 kg/m^2
  —preeclampsia is a risk for peripartum cardiomyopathy

*MANAGEMENT
- Gestational HTN or chronic HTN
  - Monitored closely for development of preeclampsia
  - Serial BP measurement twice a week
  - Weekly assessment of plt count, liver enzyme, and proteinuria
  - No salt restriction or wt reduction
  - Anti HTN medication is not recommended for stage 1 gestational HTN
  - Medication reserved for stage 2 (BP >160/110) IV MgSO$_4$ is not reliable anti HTN but it prevents seizure in the setting of eclampsia or severe preeclampsia
  - IV labetalol is DOC (compared to hydra it carries lower risk of overshoot hypotension—which can impair fetal blood flow and does not cause reflex tachycardia
- Only cure for preeclampsia is delivery which removes diseased placenta
  - *Low dose aspirin:* Recommended in reducing risk for preeclampsia in women with P/H/O preeclampsia
- For women with stage 2 HTN during preg but without severe preeclampsia/eclampsia
  - Oral drug therapy
  - Labetalol
  - Alpha methyldopa
  - Nifedipine

  Conventional DOC is alpha methyl dopa—poorly tolerated and cause postpartum depression
- Delivery soon after maternal stabilization is recommended irrespective of gestational age in following situations
  - Uncontrolled severe HTN
  - Eclampsia
  - Pulmonary edema
  - Abrupt placenta
  - DIC
  - Fetal distress
  - IV NTG is DOC when pulm edema present with preeclampsia
- Postpartum BP should be measured × 72 hours in hosp and again on output basis 7-10 d after delivery
  - All BP drugs are secreted in breast milk but in low conc
  - Propranolol and nifedipin secreted in high conc
  - Should be avoided during lactation

9.8 SYSTEMIC HTN: MANAGEMENT

NONPHARMACOLOGICAL MEASURES
Lifestyle Modification

A. Dietary Interventions:
  1. Mediterranean diet
  2. DASH diet

- *Mediterranean diet*
  - No uniform definition
  - Diets which are higher in fruits (esp. fresh fruits), vegetables (emphasizing root and green variety), whole grain (cereals, breads, rice or pasta) and fatty fish (risk in omega-3 FA)
  - Diet lower in red meat, had lower-fat or fat-free dairy product substituted for higher fat dairy products; has oils (olive or canola) nuts (walnuts, almond or hazelnut) or margarines blended with rapeseed or flaxseed oil in lien of butter and other fats
  - Moderate in total fat (32–35% of tot calories)
  - Relatively low in transfat (9–10% of tot calories)
  - High in fiber (27–37 gm/d)
  - High in PUFA (esp. omega 3 FA)

  PREDIMED study: Showed overall benefit in CV outcome in dietary intervention group in terms of decreased stroke rate; an end point closely associated with BP
  - BP data not yet available
  - Mediterranean diet correlated with improvement in numerous biomarkers associated with CV benefits (ranging from BP to inflammatory effects as measured by CRP)
  - *Recent ACC/AHA guidelines:* Strength of evidence considered being low regarding consumption of mediterranean diet vs low-fat dietary pattern

- *DASH diet*
  - High in vegetables, fruits, low-fat dairy products, whole grain, poultry, fish, and nuts. And low in sweets, sugar sweetened beverages, red meat, saturated fat, total fat and chol rich in potassium, magnesium, calcium as well as protein and fiber
  - DASH dietary pattern—lowers SBP by >5 mm Hg in adults with moderate HTN
  - *2013 ACC/AHA guidelines*: Consider strength of evidence of high for DASH diet in controlling HTN

- *Sodium restriction*
  - Reducing salt intake reduces BP
  - For adults 30–80 years with/without HTN reduction of sodium intake by approximately 1 gm/d lowers SBP by 3–4 mm Hg

- K^+ *intake*
  - American society of HTN recommended K^+ intake 4–7 gm/d
  - ACC/AHA 2013: Strength of evidence is insufficient to establish relationship between increased dietary K^+ and altered risk for CAD, BP, HF and CV mortality

- *Carbohydrate diet*
  - *Omni heart:* Showed that exchanging dietary carbohydrate for either protein or MUPA lowers BP
  - *2013 ACC/AHA:* Insufficient strength of associated to make any recommendation

- *Moderation of alcohol consumption:* ACC/AHA 1 drink/day for females; 2 drinks/day for male

- *Sugar sweetened beverages*
  PREMIER study: Reduction in sugar-sweetened beverages by 1 serving/day resulted in 2 mm Hg decrease in BP
  - Direct relationship between fructose and glucose intake with BP
  - *Overall*: (Read from other note of Ath.)
    - Fruit and 100% juice ≥2 cups/day
    - Vegetables including juice/sauce ≥2.5 cups/day
    - Wholegrain ≥3 oz/day; dietary fiber ≥2 gm/d
    - Foh and Snell form ≥7 oz/week
    - Sugar <36 oz/week (beverages) <125 oz/week (sweets and bakery dessert)
    - Saturated fat <7%
    - Trans fat <1%
    - Little or no salt

  ACC/AHA

B. Obesity/overweigh
- Association of BMI with development of HTN
- Association of visceral adiposity with HTN
  ↓
  Control of body weight eliminates a great amount of morbidity associated with HTN

C. Physical activity
- Insufficient activity linked with CV risk
- Physical activity also influence body weight and obesity
  - It reduces CV mortality
  - Various people react differently
  - Some may develop HTN during exercise
  - Occasionally hypertensive patient develop symptomatic
- Hypotension post exercise—need reduction of dose of anti-hypertensive

- *NHLBI recommendation:* Aerobic physical activity: 3-4 session a week lasting 40 mm per session
- *ACC/AHA:* Aerobic physical activity reduces BP by 5 mm Hg in adult with or without HTN

D. Cigarette smoking
- No evidence of association between smoking and BP
- But smoking cessation decreases CV risk overall
- So smoking cessation is recommended

Antihypertensive Drugs

First line drugs
1. Calcium channel blockers
2. RAAS inhibitors (ACEI or ARBs)
3. Thiazide type diuretic

A. Calcium channel blockers
- Well tolerated
- No monitoring required
- Safe and effective in many large RCTs
- Also has some antianginal and antiarrhythmus effect
- Provide more protection against stroke than other anti-HTN drugs

MOA—Blocks opening of voltage gated L-type Ca^{++} channel in myocyte and vasc SMC
- Peripheral arterial dilatation – lower BP (Dihydropyridine > Diltiazem > Verapamil)

Clinical use
- *Amlodipine:* Best studied
- *ALL HAT:* Amlodipine was equally effective as chlorthalidone and lisinopril in protecting against non-fatal events, stroke, and death. But less protection against HF
- *Adv. of Amlodipine:* Predictable dose dependent potency, once daily dosing, tolerability and cost
- High salt diet or concurrent NAIDS therapy does not compromise effectiveness of CCB
- They have some diuretic effect
- *ASCOT; ACCOMPLISH* - Amlodipine + ACEI is one of the most effective drug combination for preventing CV complication of HTN
- Dihydropyridine (Amlodipine) has less reno protective effect compared to AECI/ARB in patients with cKD (Amlodipine is not the 1st line treatment)
- It may be used as adjunctive

S/E
- Dose dependent ankle edema
  - More common with 10 mg amlodipine
  - *Vasogenic edema:* Arterial dilatation
- Can response to concomitant use of AACE/ARB— balanced arterial and venous dilatation
- *Gingival hyperplasia*
  - Rare
  - Reversible if detected early
  - Can lead to serious dental problem

Contra indi:
For non-dihydropyridine CCB:
- AV block (Gr 2 or 3; trifascicular block)
  - Severe left vent dysfunction
  - Heart failure

B. ACEI/ARBS/Direct renin inhibitor
- ONTARGET—comparable effect of AECI and ARB to reduce CV event and preventing deterioration of renal function in high risk HTN patients
- ARB provide slightly more protection against stroke
- Dual RAs blockade

  ACEI + ARB ⎤ Contraindicated
  ACEI + DRI ⎦

MOA ACEI: Block conversion of angiotensin 1-2
- ARB: Block AT 2 receptors
- Both increases pro renin level-harmful
- Aliskiren: Direct renin inhibitor

Clinical use
- ACEI-ALLHAT:
  - ACEI monotherapy is equivalent to amlodipine monotherapy and chlorthalidone monotherapy
  - Slightly less stroke prevention with ACEI
  - ACE less effective in older patients with low renin HTN
    - → but they are quite effective in these group when combined with low dose diuretic/CCB

Meta-analysis: Better protection against HF than CCB ARB
- Same benefit as ACEI
- Less cough
- ACEI/ARB = superior renal protection than others (No study on aliskiren)

S/E:
Dry cough (ACEI) (Because ACEI block degradation of bradykinin - activates nociceptive sensory fibers in lung - cough)
- Angioedema

Contraindication
- Pregnancy
- Angioedema (with ACEI)
- Hyperkalemia (seen in patients with cKD or DM with type 4 RTA)
- B/L renal art stenosis

Note:
- In patients with stage 3 cKD, with initiation of ACEI/ARB -30% elevation in S. Gr is expected

- If Gr increases >30%—reduce dose/temporary discontinue treatment

ON TARGET: Showed serious side effect with combination of ACE + ARB

COOPERATE: Which showed supporting evidence for ACE + ARB, was retracted from publication in lancet)

C. Diuretics
- One of the 3 first line drug (JNC 7 and 8)
- ACC/AHA/CDC continues to recommend it as best choice
- *MOA*:
  - With initiation – contraction of blood vol causes fall in BP
  - With continuation – blood volume restored – anti HTN effect continues through opening of ATP sensitive K⁺ channel – vasodilatation
- *Loop diuretic:* Blocks Na^+-K^+-$2Cl^-$ in thick ascending loop of Henle
- *Thiazide and thiazide like:* Block Na^+-Cl^- co transporter in DCT
- Spironolactone and eplerenon: prevent aldosterone from activating mineralocorticoid receptor
- *Triamterene and amioloride:* Block ENaC directly because less Na^+ is presented to Na^+-K^+-ATPase on luminal side of DCT

*Clinical use
- *ALLHAT – Diuretic equivalent to ACEI/CCB
- *ACCOMPLISH-ACEI + CCB yielded better outcome than ACEI + diuretic
- Chlorthalidone rather than hydrochlorothiazide
- Chlorthalidone better than HCTZ (post HOC analysis of MRFIT)
- 25 mg chlorthalidone ≅ 50 mm HCT2
- Loop diuretic less effective in BP lowering (should be reserved in HTN with cKD)
- Diuretic enhance potency of other class of antihypertensive

S/E:
- Aggravate glucose intolerance
- Hypokalemia, hypomagnesemia
- Precipitate gout
- Increased lipid level with increased hepatic triglyceride context
- Hypercalcemia (Thiazide)
- Rarely photosensitive dermatitis
- More likely to cause erectile dysfunction as compared to ACEI/CCB
- Thiazide induced hyponatremia

Add-on Drugs for Difficult HTN

1. *Low dose aldosterone antagonist*
   - Spironolactone 12.5–100 mg/d
   - *ASCOT trial:* Used spironolactone as 4th line therapy
   - *Eplerenone:* More specific antagonist avoids sexual side effects of spironolactone (painful gynecomastia, erectile dysfunction, nonmenstrual uterine bleeding)

2. *Beta-blockers*
   - Vasodilators beta-blockers—labetalol, nebivolol, carvedilol
   - Standard beta-blockers—metoprolol, atenolol are not

MOA: Initiation BP changes little because compensatory increase in PVR offset fall in CO

Over time: BP falls progressively as peripheral vasculature relaxes
1. Decrease in CO (beta 2 receptors)
2. Decreased renin release (beta 2 receptor)
3. Decrease norepinephrine release (beta 2 receptor)
   - Metoprolol, atenolol, bisoprolol are cardio selective at low dose
   - Selectively lost at high dose
   - Carvedilol and labetalol also blocks alpha receptors
   - Nebivolol stimulates endogenous production of NO

Clinical use:
- Weak antihypertensive
- Provide stroke prev (Inferior to ACEI, ARB, and CCB diuretic)
- Modest protection against CV events but do not reduce all-cause mortality
- Increased risk of DM, (esp. beta-blocker + diuretics)

S/E: Fatigability, impair cardiac conduction, acute bronchospasm in patients with asthma, promote weight gain

3. *Alpha-adrenergic blocker*

MOA
- Causes peripheral vasodilatation
- By increasing blood flow in skeletal muscle alpha-blocker sensitivity
- Prazosin, doxazosin, terazosin and IV phentolamine selective alpha-blocker
- Phenoxybenzamine block – alpha 1 + alpha 2

Clinical use: Phenoxybenzamine – drug of choice for pre op management of pheochromocytoma
- After alpha blockade, beta-blocker should be added to block otherwise excessive reflex tachy
- Should not be used as monotherapy

S/E: Propensity to cause fluid retention leads to—tachyphylaxis unmask/exacerbate HF

4. *Central sympatholytic*
   *MOA
   1. Stimulation of post synaptic alpha 2 receptor and imidazole receptor in CNS – lower central sympathetic outflow
   2. Stimulation of presynaptic alpha 2 receptor in peripheral sympathetic nerve terminal – feedback inhibition of NE release
   Clinical use - Potent antihypertensive
   S/E: Troublesome CNS side effects rebound HTN
5. *Direct vasodilatation* (minoxidil, hydralazine)
   - *MOA:* Opening vascular ATP sensitive K+ channels
   - *Use:* Both induce reflex symp activation and tachycardia
     - Hydralazine + nitrate – useful for hypertensive HF
     - Minoxidil for cKD and profound HTN

PERCUTANEOUS INTERVENTIONS FOR MANAGEMENT OF BP

- Renal denervation
- Carotid Baro receptor activation

EVIDENCE BASED APPROACH TO HTN

A. *Patient with prehypertension:*
   TROPHY: ARB: 12% reduction in HTN incidence
B. *HTN patients in general*:
   - *FEVER:* CCB + D 27% decrease in CV events
   - *ELSA:* CCB + D vs BB + D: NS diff
   - *NORDIL:* CCB (DLT2) + ACEI vs BB + D: NS diff
   - *CADPP:* ACEI vs BB + D: NS diff
   - *CONVINCE:* CCB + D vs BB + D: NS diff
   - *ASCOT:* ACEI + CCB vs BB + D – 16% CV event reduction
   - *ACCOMPLISH:* ACEI + CCB vs ACEI + D – 21% CV event reduction
   - *ALLHAT:* D + BB vs ACEI + BB – NS diff
   - *ALLHAT:* D + BB vs CCD + BB – NS diff
   - *ONTARGET:* ACEI + ARB vs ACEI or ARB – NS diff in CV events, hypotension, renal impair

C. *HTN in elderly*
   - *HYVET:* ACEI + D vs placebo –34% reduction in CV events
   - *SCOPE:* ARB + D vs D + placebo –28% reduction in stroke
   - *SHEP:* BB + D vs placebo –36% reduction in stroke
   - *Syst EVR and syst chira:* ACEI + CCB vs placebo –31 and 37% decrease in CV events
   - *STOP* BB + D vs placebo – 40% decrease in CV events
   - *STOP2* ACEI or CCB vs BB + D – NS diff in CV events
     - Any Bp lowering regimen reduces CV events in elderly HTN patient
     - Benefit of treatment includes: fewer coro events, stroke, HF event and deaths
     - Intensity of BP reduction in elderly patient must be weighted against increased risk for hypotension which can precipitate falls and ischemic events
     - Office SBP treatment target below 150 mm Hg
     - AmBP is key to detecting post prandial hypotension and orthostatic hypotension
     - Management of post prandial hypotension is challenging freq. small carbohydrate meals, caffeine with meals and liberalized salt intake fludrocortisone may be added

D. *HTN with LVH*
   - *LIFE:* ARB + D vs BB + D – 37% CV mortality
   - ARB superior for regression of LVH
   - Beta-blockers are least effective

E. *HTN in patient with DM*
   - *ADVANCE:* ACEI + D vs placebo – 18% decreased CV risk
   - *ALTITUDE:* DRI + ACEI/ARB vs placebo + ACE/ARB –NS differs in CV + renal events
   - *ACCORD:* More intense 3-4 drug vs less intense (2-1 drugs) NS diff in CV + renal events

F. *HTN in patients with diabetic nephropathy*
   - *IDNT:* ARB vs placebo – 20% less renal impair
   - *IDNT:* ARB vs CCB –23% less renal impair
   - *RENAL:* ARB vs placebo – 16% less renal impair

9.9 HYPERTENSION: MECHANISM AND DIAGNOSIS

BLOOD PRESSURE VARIABILITY AND ITS DETERMINANTS

Behavioral Determinants

- *Smoking:* Nicotine in cigarette smoke transiently increases BP by 10-20 mm Hg
- *Alcohol:*
  - Moderate alcohol (1-2 drink/day) - Low risk of HTN
  - Heavy drinker (≥3 drinks/day) - High risk of HTN
- *Caffeine:* Small transient increase in BP
- *Coffee:* Risk of development of HTN does not increase with coffee consumption
  - It increases when caffeine is consumed in diet sodas
  - So coffee may contain protective antioxidant phenol
- *Physical activity:* Increased risk of HTN
- *Diet low in fresh fruits:* Increased HTN
- Excessive consumption of sodium and calories
  - Most important behavioral determinants of HTN
- *Dietary K^+ intake:* Reduce BP

Genetic Determinants

- BP higher in families
  - Higher in monozygotic twins
  - Higher among biological than among adopted siblings
- *Salt wasting syndrome:* Mutations in 20 salt-handling genes cause ultra-rare monogenic form of severe early onset hypotension
- Pediatric salt wasting = Bartter and Gitelman
- HTN can also be inherited as Mendelian traits

Mechanism of 1° (Essential) HTN

A. Hemodynamic subtypes: Three distinct subtypes
1. Systolic hypertension in teenage and young adults
   - ISH is main type in young adults
   - 17-25 years of age
   - Very hemodynamic abnormality = increased cardiac output and stiff aorta

   Both reflecting sympathetic over activity
   Affects only 2% of young women
   While 25% of young men
   May predispose to diastolic HTN in middle age
2. Diastolic HTN in middle age
   - Typically 30-50 years of age
   - 2 patterns
     1. Isolated diastolic HTN ⎤ Classical
     2. Combined systolic-diastolic HTN ⎦ essential HTN

   More common in men
   - Without treatment isolated diastolic HTN - progress to combined systolic-diastolic HTN

- *Baseline HD abnormality:* Elevated SVR with an inappropriately normal CO
  - Decreased renal perfusion pressure
  - Impair kidney's ability to execute NaH
  - Expansion of pl volume
  - Autoregulatory reaction of vascular SMC + Increased Neurohormonal drive
    - Vasoconstriction
    - Hypertension
3. Isolated systolic HTN in older adults:
   - After age of 55 ISH predominates (SBP > 140 and DBP <90)
   - SBP rises progressively with age
     While DBP rises up to age of 55 and then falls prog
   - Resultant widening of PP indicated stiffening of central aorta and a more rapid return of refracted pulse waves from the periphery, augmenting SBP
   - Stiffening occurs due to increased collagen deposition in aortic walls
   - So, ISH is exaggerated form of age dependent stiffening process
   - More common in women
   - Associated with HFPEF
   - Most causes arise de novo (and not burnt out diastolic HTN patient). However more than 50% of patient with IDH will develop ISH

   (Multitude of neurohormonal, renal and vascular mechanism interact to various degree in contributing this subtypes of HTN)

B. Neural mechanism:

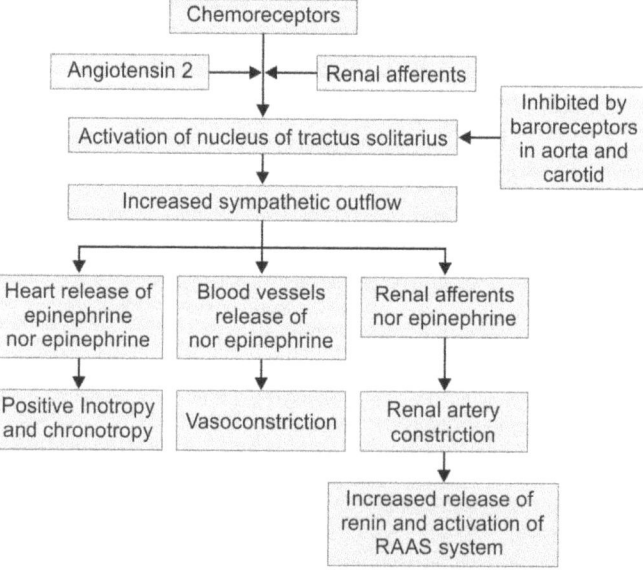

- Carotid Baroreceptor Pacemaker:
  - Rheos system
  - Surgically implanted
  - Patient under GA
  - Electrode wires implanted around carotid sinus nerves in the neck and connected to pacemaker generator placed in s/c space in chest
  - Electrical stimulation of carotid sinus nerve sends afferent signal to brain stem – interpreted as rise in BP – evoking reflex reduction in BP
  - Afferent arm of this reflex
    - To heart – slows heart rate
    - To peripheral circulation – decreased SVR
    - To kidney – decreased renin release and Na^+ excretion

  Data regarding usefulness of barrow receptor pacemaker is kikins
- Rheos pivotal trial
  - Randomized double blind placebo controlled trial patients with drug resistant HTN
  - 265 patients
  - Group A immediate initiation of B/L Carotid receptor pacing
  - Group B delayed initiation of B/L Carotid pacing until 6 month visit
  - No difference at 6 or 12 months in 1° and points of percentage of subject in whom SPB decreases by at least 10 mm Hg
  - Post noc analysis showed 42% patient in group A and 24% in group B achieved SBP ≤ 140 mm Hg at 6 month follow up we just 50% of both groups achieve SBP control of 12 month
  - Small initial decrease in GFR noted
    *More resher is need to determine efficacy and safety of device and improvement by additional techniques
    *Aortic baroreceptor, which are not inhibited with device can offsetting erotic baroreceptor response improve BP control and need further trials
- *Barostim Neo*
- 2° gen minimally invasive
  U/L carotid nerve pacing
  - Encouraging preliminary report
- Catheter based renal denervation
  - Renal sympathetic nerve causes renal vasoconstriction and vascular hypertrophy via alpha one receptors simulates renin release via beta one receptor and stimulates renal Na^+ H_2O absorption via alpha one receptor

Symplicity HTN 2 trials
- Catheter inserted into renal artery with patients under conscious sedation and 4 to 6 discrete low proper RF treatment were applied along intraluminal length of both arteries – goal was to cause thermal destruction of renal nerves situated on adventure surface of renal arteries
- Office based BP fall dramatically by 32/12 mm Hg

Smaller studies

Adv of renal denervation
- Improvement in glycemic control
- Sleep apnea improve
- Improve QOL
- Regression of LV mass
- Reduction in central aortic stiffness
- Adjunctive treatment of RF

Adjunct benefit derived by destruction of renal afferent nerve
- Symplicity HTN 1 showed impressive reduction in office BP: ABP was not assessed
- Symplicity HTN 3 did not show any significant reduction in office/AMBP 6 months post procedure compared to sham procedure

Arise question regarding efficacy of RDN

Further read from intervention book
- *Sympathetic overactivity* occurs in
  - Early 1° HTN
    - Other forms of HTN (HTN associated with obesity, OSB early T2 DM, CKD, HF, immunosuppressive therapy with calcineurin inhibitors)
  - In all this situation
    Central symp outflow can result from deactivation of baroreceptors, activation of chemoreceptor, renal afferent or circulating angiotensin 2
  - In HTN baroreceptor at higher level of BP
  - Baroreceptor control of sinus node function is abnormal even in mild HTN
  - Baroreceptor control of SVR and BP is well preserved until late HTN DBP rise
  - Complete baroreceptor failure – leads to labile HTN (seen in throat CA patient who survive with local therapy)

  Partial baroreceptor dysfunction
  Common in elderly HTN trial of
  - Orthostatic hypotension
  - Supine hypertension
  - Symptomatic postprandial hypotension (due to splanchnic pooling)

- Obesity related HTN

    Weight gain
    ↓
    Excessive sympathetic stimulation to burn fat but at expense of sympathetic overactivity in target tissue
    ↓
    Hypertension

- OSA as a cause of HTN

    OSA
    ↓
    Markedly elevated pl and renal catecholamine levels (mimicking those seen in patient with pheocroma)
    ↓
    With repeated periods of arterial desaturation, carotid chemoreceptor are activated
    ↓
    Dramatic pressure fluctuations throughout night and reset chemoreceptor reflex
    ↓
    Daytime normoxia is interpreted as hypoxia and lead to sustained reflex SNS activation
    ↓
    Daytime HTN

C. Renal mechanism

Acquired/inherited abnormality of kidneys ability to excrete excessive sodium load imposed by a modern diet high in salt
↓
Retention of Na^+ and H_2O
↓
Plasma volume expansion
↓
Increase cardiac output
↓
Triggering autoregulatory response
↓
Increased SVR (HTN)

Resetting of pressure natriuresis

Normotensive subject	In all HTN patients pressure natriuresis curve is shifted to rt
↓	↓
BP increases	Resetting off pr natriuresis curve prevents return of BP to normal
↓	↓
Increased Na^+ excretion to shrink plasma volume and return of BP to normal	So fluid balance is maintained but at the cost of increased BP

This resetting can also lead to nocturia (bothersome feature in patients with uncontrolled HTN)

HTN patients excrete the same amount of given dietary load as normotensive patient but at higher BP

Low birth weight: LBW with reduced nephrogenic increased risk of development of adult salt dependent HTN

Genetic contribution
- APOL1 gene are found to be strongly associated with increased risk of ESRD and HTN
- As kidney fail BP become increasingly salt dependent

D. Vascular mechanism

- *Endothelial cell dysfunction*

    Endothelial lining - major defense against HTN
    Dysfunctional endothelium

Increased vasoconstrictor	Decreased vasorelaxants
Proinflammatory	NO
Prothrombin	Pal2
Growth factors	Endothelium derived hyperpolarizing factor

- No:
    - Formed by NO synthase in endothelium
    - Diffuse to adjacent vasc SMC and activate series of G kinase that culminate in vasodilatation
    - Endothelial dependent vasodilatation can be assessed by measuring increase in the large artery (forearm/coronary) diameter after intra-arterial infusion of acetylcholine or release of ischemia (arrested forearm circulation) or sudden elevation in BP (cold pressor test)
- Strong correlation between raised CRP and arterial stiffness and elevated PP
    - CRP is marker for new onset of HTN and accelerated progression of hypertensive target organ damage
- Oxidative stress (SO_2-) – also contribute to endothelial dysfunction in HTN
    SO_2 produced by
    - NADPH oxidase
    - NO synthase when imp cofactor (tetrahydrobiopterin) is deficit
    - Xanthine oxidase
    - Mitochondria
- *Vascular remodeling*
    - Endothelial dysfunction
    - Neurohormonal activation ⎤ over time vascular
    - Increased BP ⎦ → remodeling
        - *Hypertensive remodeling:* Increased media to lumen ratio (medial thickness) is hallmark of HTN in large arteries.

Increased size of SMC CSA
- Resultant large art stiffness is hallmark of ISH
- *Eutrophic remodeling:* Induced by vasospasm, smooth muscle cells rearrange themselves around a smaller lumen diameter
- Media to lumen ratio increases
- Medical cross sectional area unchanged
- By increasing lumen dia in peripheral circulation, inward eutrophic remodeling increases SVR (Hemodynamic hallmark of diastolic HTN)

E. Hormonal mechanism
- RAAS system

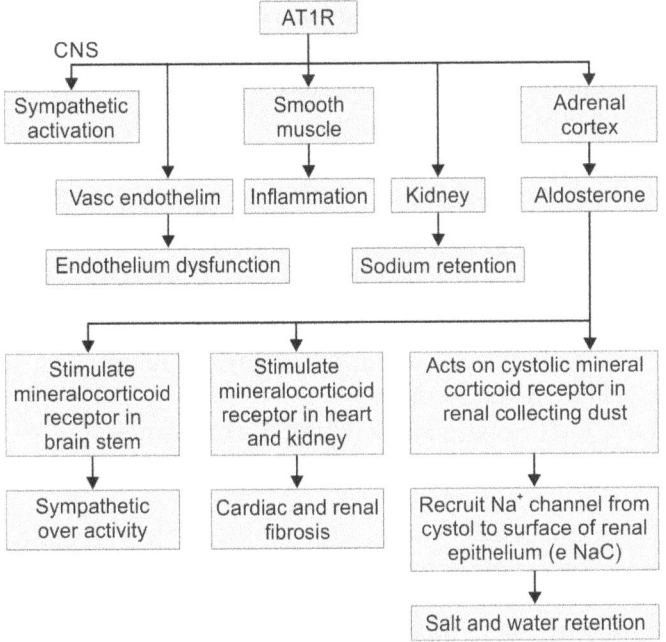

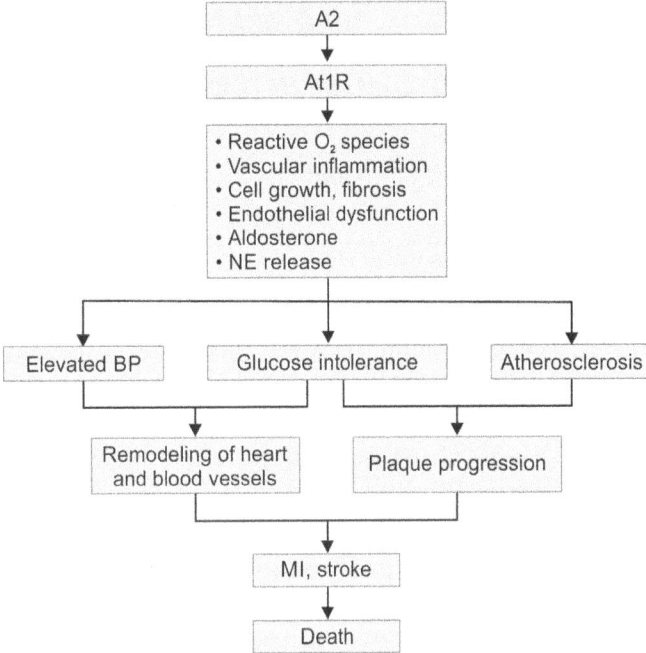

In modern fast food diet – Na⁺ is high – RAAS should be completely suppressed – low level of aldosterone – allow Na^+ and H_2O excretion
↓
If RAAS is activated even minimally
↓
Risk of developing HTN

Receptor mediated role of angiotensin

Receptor mediated role of renin and pro renin
- Kidney converts inactive pro renin to renin by enzymatic cleavage

Newly found Pro renin receptor
↓
When pro renin binds to pro renin receptor in heart and kidney – hinge is opened and this non enzymatic process fully activates prorenin
↓
Increased TGF beta receptor
↓
Collagen deposition and fibrosis
- AECI and ARBs trigger large release of pro renin and renin
- Reactive increases are even greater with direct renin inhibitors
(aliskiren)
↓
Counteract some cardioprotective action

9.10 MANAGEMENT OF HTN AND SPRINT TRIAL

*SPRINT: (SYSTOLIC BP INTERVENTION TRIAL)

Intensive vs standard BP control

WHAT GUIDELINES SAY?

ESC 2013

- SBP goal of <140 mm Hg is recommended in patients at low-moderate CV risk (class 1B) in patients with DM (class 1A) and should be considered in patients with prev stroke/TIA, CHD and in patients with diabetic/nondiabetic Ckd
- In elderly hypertensive <80 years old with SBP >160, there is strong evidence to support recommendation of reducing SBP to between 100-140 (class 1A)
- In fit alderfly <80 yrs SBP <140 mm Hg may be considered, where as in fragile elderly patient, SBP goal should be adjusted to the extent the individual tolerates (class 2 b C)
- DBP target of <90 mm Hg is always recommended except in patients with DM in when <85 mm Hg are recommended (class 1A)

ASH/ISH HTN Guidelines 2014

- Treatment goal for SBP <140 and DBP <90
- 80 or older, achieving SBP of <150 is associated with strong CV and stroke protection. EA hence target of <150/90 is recommended

ACC/AHA/ESH (2015)

- In patient with CAD, BP goal is <150/90 mm Hg
- For patients >80 years; and <140/90 mm Hg
- For patients of CAD, ACS and HF

Indian Guideline (2013)

BP < 140/90 in young and middle age HTN
    140/80 in diabetics
    130/85 in patients who survived stroke
    140-145/90 in elderly

SPRINT

- 9,361 patients
- Inclusion ≥50 years older; SBP 130-180; increased CV risk
- Exclusion DM and prior H/O stroke
- *Groups:* BP target <140 and BP target <120
- Stopped early after median follow up of 3-20 years - Intensive treatment showed significant benefit
- *Results:*
  Intensive BP lowering resulted in
  - 25% reduction in 1° composit outcome of CV disease and death
  - 27% reduction in all-cause mortality
  - Stroke no benefit
  - S/E -hypotension, syncope, electrolyte abnormality and ACEI - observed in high intensity group
- Office BP was recorded
- SPRINT result apply to SPRINT like population
  - Elderly
  - No H/O stroke
  - Increased CV risk
  - Numeral high adv effect with intensive treatment

Remember ACCORD Trial

- 4,744 patients with DM and High risk of CVD
- No significant diff between intensive control (avg 119) vs moderate control (avg 133) of BP
- Stroke was only prespecified 2° outcome which showed significant benefit with intensive treatment

9.11 PATHOGENESIS OF HYPERTENSIVE HEART DISEASE

PRESSURE OVERLOAD HYPERTROPHY

- Structural abnormality in hypertensive heart
  - Myocyte hypertrophy
  - Medial hypertrophy of intramyocardial coro art
  - Collagen deposition

↓

Leads to cardiac fibrosis (Hallmark of pathological LVH)

IMPAIRED CORONARY VASODILATATION RESERVE

Hypertensive heart

↓

Impaired vasodilatation reserve due to excessive myocyte mass

↓

Subendocardial ischemia and cardiac fibrosis

↓

Impaired diastolic relaxation

↓

Exertional dyspnea and HFPEF

HEART FAILURE

- HTN is most common cause of HFPEF
- HTN also indirectly leads to systolic HF as a major risk factor for MI

9.12 HTN AND ERECTILE DYSFUNCTION

INTRODUCTION
- 2/3rd of men with HTN have erectile dysfunction
- *TOMHS:* The only RCT on HTN to study erectile dysfunction
  - Most of erectile dysfunction precedes initiation of anti-HTN medications and w related to both age and baseline SBP
  - Chlorthalidone was the only drug that increases incident erectile dysfunction > placebo (J main anti-HTN meds studied)
  - PDE-5 inhibitor are safe and effective in treating erectile dysfunction (they should be avoided in patients taking nitrate or alpha-blocker)

RESISTANT HTN
Definition

High BP uncontrolled with three or controlled with at least 4 antihypertensive drugs (including a diuretic)
- Associated with higher prevalence of 2°HTN and worse CV and renal outcomes
  - >50% of this had "pseudoresistant HTN"
  - White coat reaction
  - Improper BP measurement
  - Medication nonadherence
  - Pressor substances (e.g., NSAIDs, excessive alcohol, psychiatric drugs)

Drugs that can TBD
- NSAIDs
- Steroid
- Anti depressant
- Cocaine
- Erythropoietin and analog
- OC pills
- Immunosuppressant

Causes of True Resistant HTN
1. Chronic kidney disease
2. 1° aldosteronism
3. Other 2° hypertension (COA, Cushing, OSA, pheochroma)
4. Difficult primary hypertension
- True drug resistant patients have
  - High risk of CV disease
  - Severe HTN along with target organ damage
- All true drug resistant cases
  - Should be screened for 2°HTN
    Esp. cKD, OSA, 1° aldosteronism and pheochroma

- In absence of an identifiable cause, mineralocorticoid receptor antagonist or vasodilating beta-blocker can serve as highly effective add-on therapies
- RDN is an option

Common Correctable Issues
- Clonidine rebound
- Inadequate diuretics
- Inappropriate use of loop diuretics in patient with normal renal function
- Infrequent dosing with short acting loop diuretic
- Low dose thiazide in patients with impaired renal function

Circumstances Req. Rapid Treatment
- Accelerated HTN with papilledema
- *Cerebrovascular disease:* HTN enceph, ICH, SAH, atheroembolic infarct
- *Cardiac:* AOD, Ac LVF, Ac MI, impending MI, S/P cABG
- *Renal:* Ac GN, renal crisis from collagen vasc disease
- Excessive circ catecholamine
  Pheochroma, food or drug interaction with MAO inhibitors, sympathomimetic drug (cocaine)
- Eclampsia
- Severe epistaxis
- *Postsurgical treatment:* Post op HTN, post op bleed from suture site

MANAGEMENT OF HYPERTENSIVE CRISIS
Definitions
- *Hypertensive crisis:* Heterogeneous group of disorder char by severe HTN and acute target organ damage to brain, heart, kidney retina or blood vessel
  - Typically BP is 220/130 mm Hg or higher
  - Require immediate reduction of BP
- *Hypertensive urgency:* Denotes severe uncontrolled HTN without evidence of target organ damage
  - Should be treated with short acting oral meds
- *Severe HTN:* Defined as BP of 180/110 mm Hg to 220/130 mm Hg without symptoms of acute target organ damage; almost always occurs in patient with chronic HTN- long acting oral medication can be restarted if it occurs because of patients noncompliance

IV drugs for hypertensive Emergency
1. *Labetalol:*
   - Onset – 5–10 min
   - $T_{½}$ – 3–6 hours

- *Dose* – 0.25–0.5 mg/kg; 2–4 mg/min until goal –BD is reached and there after 5–20 mg/hour
- *S/E:* 2°CHB, systolic HF, COPD, bradycardia

	Onset	t₁⁄₂	Dose	S/E
Nicardipine	5–15 mins	30–40 min	5–15 mg/h cont Infusion, starting Dose of 5 mg/h; Increase every 15-min with 2–5 mg Until 25 mg until Goal BP achieved	liver failure
Nitroprusside	Immediate	1–2 min	0.3–10 µg/kg/min Increase by 0.5 µg/kg/min every 5 min till goal BP achieved	liver/kidney failure, cyanide toxicity
Nitroglycerin	1–5 min	3–5 min	5–200 µg/min 5 µg/min increase Every 5 min	
Urapidil	Acts on central	Seronergic	Pathway (central sympatholytic)	
Esmolol				
Phentolamine	1–2 min	3–5 min	2.5 mg; repeat 5–15 mins until goal BP is reached	Tachycardia Angina pectoris
Other Fenoldopam Hydralazine Labetalol				

MANAGEMENT OF SPECIFIC HYPERTENSIVE CRISIS

- Hypertensive crisis with advanced retinopathy
  - BP ≥220/130 mm Hg + Gr 3–4 hypertensive retinopathy
  - Accompanied by – headache, visual disturbance, nausea/vomiting, heart failure, encephalopathy, LVH, renal impairment, microangiopathic hemolytic anemia
  - Drug of choice – any of above (table)
  - In patient with impaired cerebral autoregulation, labetalol causes small adverse fall in cerebral flow than nitroprusside, but its long acting – more systemic hypotension
  - Nicardipine produces more predictable and consistent reduction in PB
- *Hypertensive crisis with encephalopathy*
  - Hypertensive enceph char by decreased level of consciousness, delirium, agitation, stupor, seizure or cortical blindness in setting of acute severe high BP
  - FND are rare
  - Hypertensive enceph is a cause of reversible posterior leukoencephalopathy syndrome
  - CT/MRI – area of cerebral edema – confirms diagnosis (area of edema localize in posterior region because vertebral artery-per fusing posterior brain – have less sympathetic innervation – less dampening of BP oscillation in vertebral than in carotids)

Treatment
- Target MAP – decrease by 20–25%
- Immediate action required
- DOC = labetalol
- Enceph occur when BP exceeds upper limit of threshold of cerebral auto regulation (MAP 60–150)
- In normotensive patient; increase of MAP to >150 can lead to enceph
- In chronic HTN patient; cerebral auto regulatory curve shifted to rt so threshold has increased; But sudden decrease of BP to normotensive range can lead to cerebral hypotension
- *Rule of thumb:* Lower initially elevated pr by 10% in 1st half and additional 15% in next 12 hours to a BP no <160/110. BP can be reduced further during next 48 hours.
- *Acute ischemic stroke/hemorrhagic stroke*
  - BP should be lowered cautiously to avoid ischemic insult to salvageable ischemic penumbra
  - *2013 ACC/AHA*
    1. If stroke cannot be treated with thrombolytic therapy, BP should be treated if it remains higher than 220/120 mm Hg
    2. If stroke can be treated with thrombolytic, BP needs to be lowered to 185/110 mm Hg
  - *INTERACT-2:* With acute hemorrhagic stroke, lowering SBP to K 140 mm Hg showed improved functional outcome without more adv event

- *Treatment:* Ac ischemic stroke and BP >220/120 – labetalol
- Cerebral hemorrhage and SBP >180; or MAP – labetalol
- Ac ischemic stroke and lysis indicated – labetalol
- Avoid nitroprusside and hydralazine

- *Acute coro synd*
  - IV NTG after administering IV beta-blocker to prevent reflex tachycardia
  - Avoid nitroprusside (coronary steal)

- *Acute aortic dissection*
  - Immediate lowering of BP
  - SBP target < 110 mm Hg
  - DOC – nitroprusside + metoprolol
- *Acute pulm edema*
- *Acute HF*
- *Adrenergic crisis*
  - Pheochromocytoma crisis should be treated acutely with phentolamine followed by administration of beta-blocker
  - Nitroprusside and urapidil are effective alternatives

9.13 SECONDARY HTN

RENAL PARENCHYMAL DISEASE
- MC cause of 2° HTN
- Responsible for 2-5% cases
- DM and HTN most common risk factor for cKD
- *Markers for renal disease*
  - eGFR (Cockcroft-Gault equation) or (Modification of diet in renal disease)
  - Microalbuminuria
  - Cystatin C
  - Sr creat (Inadequate)
- Renal disease – loss of filtration surface – both glomerular and systemic HTN – more glomerular sclerosis – cycle of progressive disease
- *Precipitating/aggravating factors:*
  - Obst of urinary tract
  - Depletion of effective circulating vol
  - Nephrotoxic agent
  - Uncontrolled HTN

ACUTE RENAL DISEASE
Mech of HTN
- Markedly impair Na^+ and H_2O excretion
- Activation of RAAS (B/L ureteral obst)
- Reduce renal blood flow (sudden B/L renal ischemia due to chol. Emboli)
  - HTN can be presenting sign of vasculitis of kidney
  - NSAIDs and ACE/ARBS can precipitate acute kidney dying in patient with preexisting renal disease

CHRONIC RENAL DISEASE
- All cKD are associated with HTN
- HTN accelerates progression of disease
- Control of HTN slows progression
- Patients with cKD have nocturnal HTN
- Patients with cKD require 2 or more drug in addition to ACEI/ARB for control of HTN

HEMODIALYSIS PATIENT
- HTN is a risk factor for mortality
  - Excess fluid vol ⎤
  - Accumulation of endogenous inhibitor of NO synthase ⎬ Aggravates HTN
  - Sympathetic overactivity ⎦
- BP falls progressively after dialysis is complete – remain depressed during 24 hours and rise again during 2nd day due to fluid retention.

RENAL TRANSPLANT
- Successful transplant may cure HTN
- But 50% recipient becomes hypertensive within 1 year
  Reason:
  - Stenosis of renal art at anastomotic site
  - Rejection reaction
  - High dose of glucocorticoid and cyclosporine or Tacrolimus
  - Excess renin derived from retained diseased kidney
- HTN occurs more frequently if donor has F/H/O HTN or donor died of SAH with probable H/O HTN

RENOVASCULAR HTN
*Clinical clues to presence of renovasc HTN
- History
  - HTN before 30 years or after 50 years
  - Abrupt onset of HTN
  - Severe or resistant HTN
  - Symptoms of ath disease elsewhere
  - Neg. F/H of HTN
  - Smoker
  - Worsening renal function after renin angiotensin inhibition
  - Recurrent "flash" pulm edema
- *Examination:* Abd bruit; advanced fundal changes
- *Lab:*
  - Secondary aldosteronism
  - High pl renin level
  - Low sr potassium level
  - Low sr sodium level
  - Proteinuria
  - Elevated Sr. Cr. Level
  - Unilat small atrophic kidney (CNG)

*Classification
- Atherosclerotic disease
  - Affect mainly prox 1/3rd of main renal art
  - Mostly in older patients
  - Patients with atherosclerotic risk
- Fibromuscular disease
  - Mainly distal 2/3rd of renal art
  - MC in women between 20-60 years
  - Typically affects media
  - B/L carotid FMD can be present with renal FMD

*Other Causes of Renovasc HTN
- Cholesterol emboli renal art
- Eternal compression by tumor

*Most Renovasc HTN Develop from Partial Obstruction of 1 Main Renal Art

- If complete occlusion of renal art develops slowly – collaterals are adequate to maintain viability of kidney- such kidney may secrete renin and cause HTN
- B/L disease should be suspected in those with renal insufficiency, particularly if rapid prog renal failure develop without c/o obstructive uropathy and even more so if it develop after ACEI/ARB initiation

Mech

Decreased PP in Renal Art
↓
50% reduction in renal perfusion
↓
Activation of RAAS

Diagnosis

1. As mentioned clinical features
2. Renal duplex sonography –50% sensitivity
3. CT/MRI - better sensi and speci (gadolinium enhanced MRI is contraindicated in patients with advanced cKD to avoid nephrogenic systemic fibrosis)

Management

Outcome of revascularization is associated with use of resistance index to assess flow in renal artery

- High resistance index (>80) reflects marked intrarenal vasc disease
  - Poor outcome
- Low resistance index – good outcome
- Balloon angioplasty without stent: Choice for FMD
- For atherosclerotic HTN
  - Medical management (antihypertensive, statin, antiplatelet)
    Is cornerstone of treatment
  - ACEI/ARB – double edged sword
  - Balloon angioplasty 1 stent
    Only 2 indications
    1. Medically refractory HTN
    2. Prog decline in renal function
  [Further read from intervention]

RENIN SECRETING TUMOR

2° hyperaldosteronism manifested by hypokalemia

ADRENAL CAUSES

- *Includes:*
  - 1° hyperaldosteronism
  - 1° excess of cortisol and catecholamine
  - Excess deoxycorticosterone (cong. adrenal hyperplasia)
- *Compromise:* <1% of HTN in gen practice
- Adrenal incidentaloma found in 5% of CT scan obtained for non-adrenal purposes
- Most incedentaloma are nonfunctional

*Syndromes of mineralocorticoid excess

A. Adrenal origin
  1. Aldosterone excess (primary)
     - Aldosterone producing adenoma
     - B/L hyperplasia
     - 1° unilat adrenal hyperplasia
     - Adrenal CA
     - Extra adrenal tumor
     - Glucocorticoid remediable aldosteronism (familial hyper aldosteronism)
  2. Deoxycorticosterone excess
     - Deoxycorticosterone secreting tumor
     - Cong adrenal hyperplasia
     - l/B hydroxylase deficiency
     - 17 alpha-hydroxylase deficiency
  3. Cortisol excess
     - Cushing synd
     - Glucocorticoid receptor resistance

B. Renal origin
   - Activating mutation of mineralocorticoid receptor
   - Pseudohypo-aldosteronism type 2 (Gordon)
   - I/B hydroxysteroid dehydrogenase def

- 1° hypervaldosteronism
  - MC of mineralocorticoid excess
  - Spont or inherited K^+ channel mutation in approximately 1/3rd of aldosterone producing adenoma
  - MC cause = bilat adrenal hyperplasia

*Pathophysiology

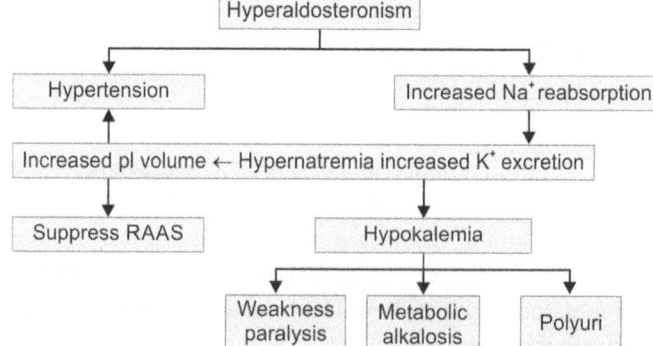

- Most of patients with 1° hyperaldosteronism are normokalemia

Diagnosis

Step 1: Screening: (for plasma renin and aldosterone lev)
- Elevated aldosterone + suppressed renin
- Recommended for patients with HTN who have high likelihood for aldosterone producing adenoma (unprovoked hypokalemia, excessive hypokalemia on diuretics, F/H/O aldosteronism, resistant HTN, adrenal incidentaloma)

Step 2: Oral salt leading suppression test (if abnormal)

Step 3: B/L renal vein sampling to differentiate U/L adenoma from B/L hyperplasia

*D/D Familial glucocorticoid remediable HTN mutation in:
- Aldosterone synthase gene
- L/B hydroxylase enzyme gene

Management
- Solitary adenoma (>4 cm) – surgical resection
- BAH – spironolactone/eplerenone
- Cushing syndrome
- Cong adrenal hyperplasia
- Pheochromocytoma
  - Rare catecholamine secreting tumor of adrenal chromaffin cells
  - Spells of pheochroma – (headache + seating + palpitation + pallor)

*Features suggestive of pheochroma
- HTN persistent/paroxysmal
  - Markedly variable BP (1 orthostatic hypotension)
  - Sudden paroxysm in response to
    - Stress-anesthesia, angio
    - Pharmacological provocation – histamine, nicotine, caffeine, beta-blocker
    - Manipulation of tumor – abd palpation
  - Unusual setting
    - Childhood, preg, familial
    - MEN-2, MEN 2B
    - Von Hippel–Lindau synd
    - Neurocutaneous lesion; neurofibromatosis
- Aso symptoms
  - Sudden spell
  - Pain in chest/abd
- Associated signs
  - Sweating, tachycardia, arrhythmia, pallor, weight loss

OTHER CAUSES

- Coarctation of aorta
- Hormonal disturbance
  - Acromegaly
  - Hypothyroidism
  - Hyperparathyroidism

SECTION 10

Infective Endocarditis

10.1 CARDIOVASCULAR IMPLANTABLE DEVICE INF

RISK FACTORS

- Device placement in older patients
- Those with more comorbid condition (especially renal failure)
- More number of leads
- Need for device replacement
- Complication of pocket site (e.g., hematoma, delayed or poor wound healing)
- C/F – MC – Erosion and/or inflammation at pocket site with/ without systemic manifestation of infection
- Pleuritic pain, lung infiltrate and lung abscess can develop

MICROBIOLOGY

- *Staph aureus* – 60–80%
- CONE 2nd common
- *Other:* Streptococci, enterococci
- Gm negative bacilli/fungi – uncommon

PATHOGENESIS

Bact and yeast can attach and accumulate on the surface of a device
    Bio film formation
    Evade normal host immune system and antimicrobial therapy

- Most occur due to contamination of device at time of placement
- Less freq. made of device contamination is lead infection by bloodstream infection

DIAGNOSIS

- *Straight forward:*
  - Device erosion at pocket present
  - Purulent discharge from pocket
  - Erythema/Pain/Swelling
- *Blood culture:* Should be obtained in all cases
- In patients with positive blood culture – TEE
- Ultimately, intra op findings and gm staining and culture of deep pocket tissue and device sample

MANAGEMENT

- Complete device removal (if infection cure is the goal)
- Antibiotic treatment for 6 weeks or longer (if valvular IE)
- Optimal timing of new device placement is undefined
- Some experts advocates that,
- New device can be implanted 72 hours after removal of infected device provided
  - Blood culture negative
  - No valvular IE
  - Control of infection at pocket site

PROPHYLAXIS

- Perioperative antibiotic
  Cefazolin 30–60 min before implant or vancomycin 2 hours before procedure
- No post op dosing required
- Secondary prophylaxis of patients with implanted device who undergo surgery is not required
  CIED = cardiac implantable electronic device

Infective Endocarditis

APPROACH

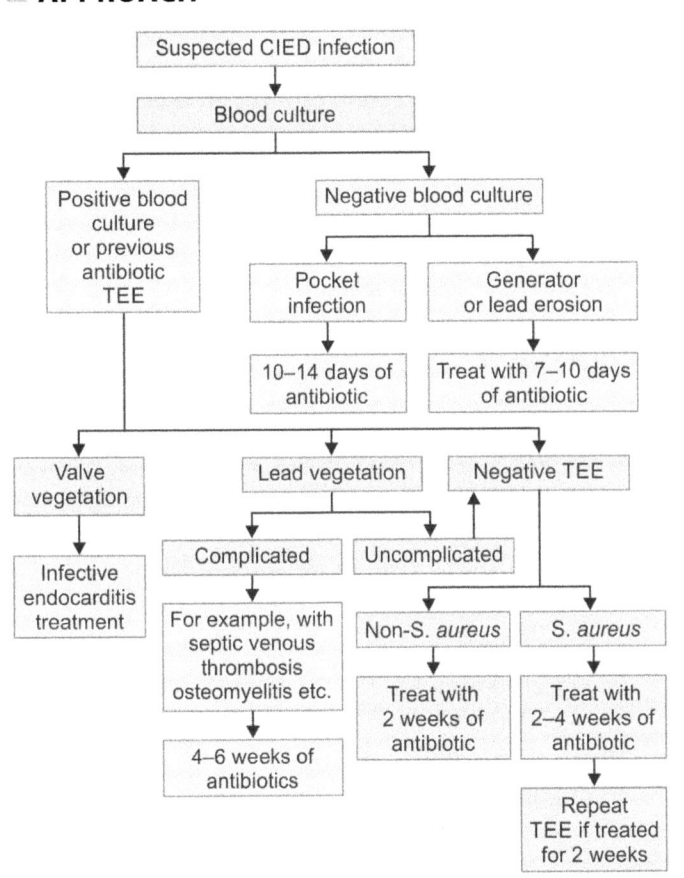

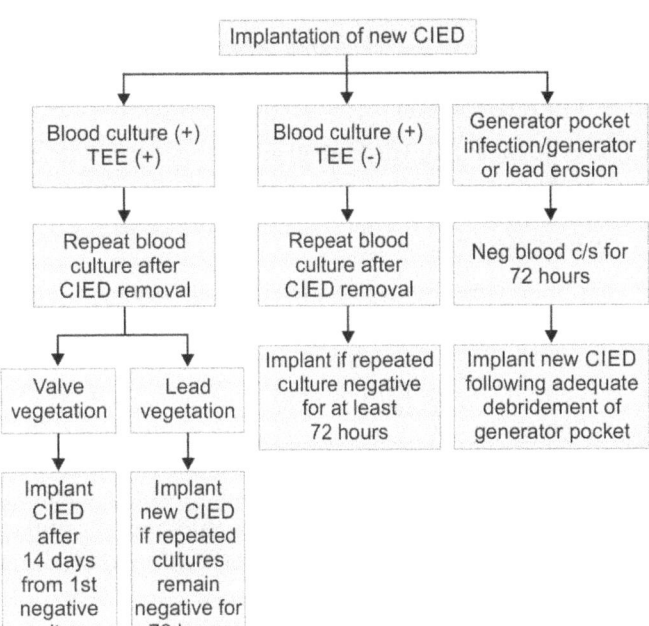

10.2 INFECTIVE ENDOCARDITIS PROPHYLAXIS

INTRODUCTION
*Should be considered for patient at highest risk for infective endocarditis.

CLASS 2A/C
- Patients with any prosthetic valve, including a transcatheter valve or those in whom any prosthetic material was used for cardiac valve repair
- Patients with prev episode of IE
- Patients with CHD
  - Any type of cyanotic CHD
  - Any type of CHD repaired with a prosthetic material, whether placed surgically or percutaneously – up to 6 months after procedure or lifelong if residual shunt or valvular regurgitation remains

CLASS 3
Not recommended in other forms of valvular or CHD.

WHICH PROCEDURE?
2a – Dental procedure requiring manipulation of gingival or peripheral region of teeth or perforation of oral mucosa.

3 – Not recommended for dental procedure with anesthetic injection in noninfected are, treatment of superficial caries, removal of suture, dental X-ray, placement or adjustment of removable orthodontic appliances or brace:
- Respi tract procedures
- GI or urogenital procedures
- Skin and soft tissue procedure

*Which Drug?
- No allergy to penicillin/ampicillin
  - Amoxicillin or ampicillin 2 gm oral/iv 30-60 min before procedure (child 50 mg/kg)
  - Alternative
    - Cephalexin 2 gm IV for adult or 50 mg/kg IV for children
    - Cefazolin
    - Ceftriaxone 1 gm IV for adults or 50 mg/kg IV for children
- Allergy to penicillin or ampicillin
  - Clindamycin 600 mg oral IV (child 20 mg/kg)

10.3 INFECTIVE ENDOCARDITIS

Q.1 Microbiology of IE, Pathogenesis of vegetation in IE Enumerate for surgery in native valve IE and prosthetic valve endocarditis (3+3+4)
Q.2 IE prophylaxis- newer guideline
Q.3 Gen principles, indi and regimens for IE prophylaxis (Dec 11) (June 12)
Q.4 Rt sided IE (Dec 07)
Q.5 Newer criteria for diagnosing IE
Q.6 Prosthetic valve IE
Q.7 Etiopathogenesis of bact IE (Dec 03)
Q.8 Diagnosis of IE (Dec 03)
Q.9 Treatment of culture neg. endocarditis (Aug 01)

DEFINITION

Microbial infection of endocardial surface of the heart or iatrogenic foreign body such as prosthetic valve
- IE usually involves valvular surface, but it can also involve septal defect, area with high turbulent jet flow and chordae tendineae.

FACTORS INFLUENCING RISK OF IE

Host factors
- Underlying anatomic cardiac condition
  - Valvular heart disease
  - Prosthetic heart valve
  - Septal defects
- Aging of population
  - Myxomatous degeneration with subsequent prolapsed and insufficiency
- Poor oral health in low SE class
- Gender (Previously M > F) But now M = F
- Health care exposure
  - Both nosocomial and non-nosocomial inf
- Injection drug abuse

TYPES

A. Left sided — Native valve
            — Prosthetic valve
   Right sided — Native valve
               — Prosthetic valve
               — Device related
B. Community acquired
   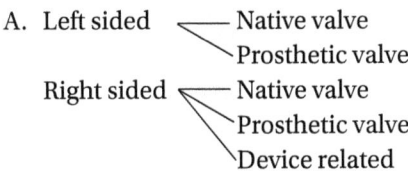
   IV drug abuser

C. Acute
   Subacute
   Recurrence — Relapse
              — Reinfection

MICROBIOLOGY

- Vast array of bacteria and fungi can cause IE
- Gram positive cocci predominates (*Streptococcus*, staphylococci, enterococci)
- Modified Duke Criteria consider only these 3 organisms as "typical microorganism"

1. *Streptococcal species*
- *Viridans group* – predominant organisms
  - Sub acute presentation
  - Weeks to months
  - Low-grade fever, night sweats, and fatigue
  - Normally found in oral flora
  - Causes indolent infection
  - Produce sustained bacteremia
  - Include several species
    - *Sanguis*
    - *Orilis (mitis)*
    - *Salivarius*
    - *Mutans*
    - *Intermedius* ⎤ *Streptococcus milleri* group
    - *Anginosus*   ⎬ - Abscess formation
    - *Constellatus* ⎦ - Metastatic inf foci
    - *Gemella*
    - *Abiotrophia*
    - *Granulicatella*

Viridans group
- Predominant cause of native valve endocarditis
- Predominantly community acquired NVE
- Common substrate = rheumatic valvular disease
- Have developed resistance to some antimicrobials
- *beta-hemolytic streptococci:* (<10% of all IE)
  - Injection drug user and elderly
  - Acute presentation
  - Complications are frequent
  - Often lead to valve destruction and distant site infection
  - Susceptible to penicillin
  - Surgery is often required
- *Streptococcus gallolyticus/Streptococcus Bovis (<10%)*
  - Found in GI tract
  - Common in patients with CA colon

- *S. pneumonia* (rare)
  - Related with bloodstream inf and pneumonia
  - Susceptible to penicillin
  - Acute presentation
  - Associated with valve destruction

2. *Staphylococcal species*
- *Staph. aureus*
  - Acute presentation
  - Associated with considerable syst toxicity
  - High morbidity and mortality (lt heart NVE)
  - Common cause for rt heart NVE (Injection drug abuser)
    - Low mortality and morbidity
      Higher cure rate
  - Resistance to oxacillin and methicillin is increasing
- *Coagulase neg. Staphylococcus (CONS)*
  - Subacute presentation
  - Freq. presentation for prosthetic valve IE
    - *S. epidermis*
      - Most common
      - Causes bacteremia and IE
    - *Staphylococcus lugdunensis*
      - Both native and PVE
      - More virulent than other species
  - CONS are more drug resistant than S aureus

3. *Enterococci*
- Subacute presentation
- Age is strongly associated factor
- Common in elderly (twice than young)
- Associated with health care exposure and central venous catheter use
- *Enterococcus faecalis:* Associated with genitourinary tract abnormalities
- Treatment penicillin + aminoglycoside (gentamicin)
- **VRE:** Vancomycin resistance enterococci is found

4. **HACEK organism:** Fastidious gram-negative bacilli
- *Haemophilus* species (other than *H. influenzae*)
- *Actinomycetemcomitans*
- *Aggregatibacter aphrophilus*
- *Cardiobacterium hominis*
- *Eikenella corrodens*
- *Kingella kingae*
- *Kingella denitrificans*
  - Colonize oropharynx and upper respi tract
  - Subacute presentation
  - Community acquired
  - Indolent clinical course
  - Large vegetation
  - Embolism common

5. *Aerobic Gm neg bacilli*
- Rare
- *E. coli, Klebsiella, Pseudomonas, Enterobacter*
- Acute presentation
- Associated with systemic toxicity

6. *Fungi*
- Extremely rare
- Difficult to identify (do not grow on routine culture media)
  E.g., *Candida* species
  - Usually health care associated (CVC)
  - Prosthetic valve endocarditis
  - Injection drug use is well-recognized risk factor
  - Surgery intervention is recommended

7. *Culture neg endocarditis*
Reason:
- Recent exposure to antimicrobials
- Organism does not grow in routine media
- Delayed growth of organism
  - Culture for 14 days
- Fungi, *Coxiella burnetii, Bartonella Brucella, Tropheryma whipplei, Legionella*

In Summary

- *Oral cavity - Strepto viridans*
  Skin – staphylococci
  Respi tract – HACEK group
  GI tract - *Streptococcus gallolyticus*
  Urinary tract – enterococci
- *Native valve – health care associated*
  - *Streptococcus viridans* (MC in India)
  - *Staphylococcus aureus* (MC worldwide)
  - CONS
  - Enterococci

  Prosthetic valve endocarditis (within 2 months)
  - S. aureus
  - CONS MRSA
  - Gm negative bacilli (*Pseudomonas*)
  - Fungal (*Candida*)

  PVE >12 months and NVE – community acquired
  - Streptococci –MC
  - HACEK group
- *Right-sided endocarditis*
  - *Staph aureus* (MRSA)
- *Nonbacterial thrombotic endocarditis*
  - Marantic – uninfected vegetation seen in patients with malignancy and chronic disease

PATHOGENESIS

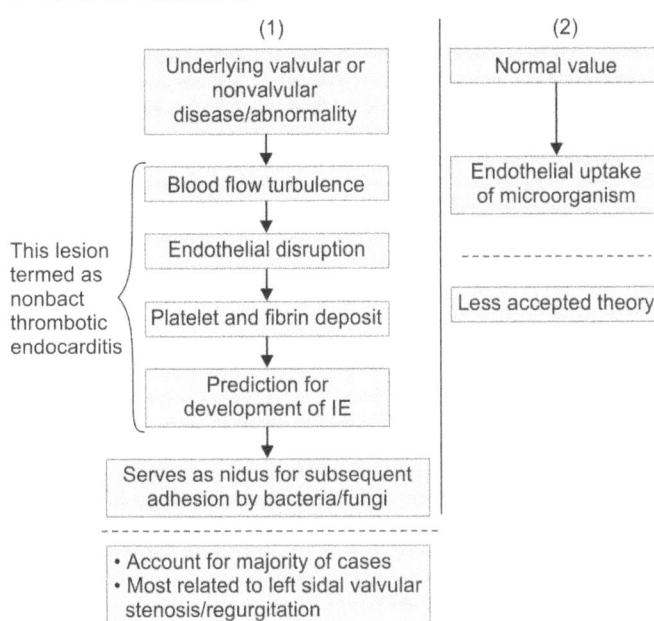

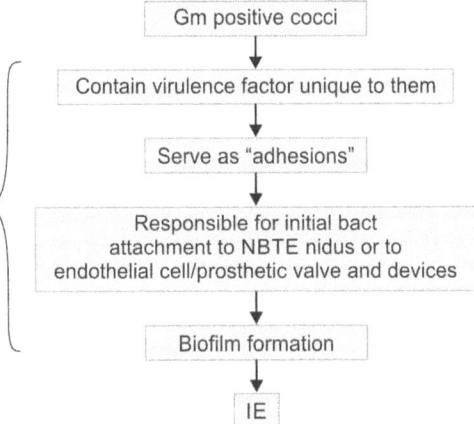

CLINICAL PRESENTATION

Types: (Data from ICE- PCS cohort – 278 patients)
1. NVE – 72%
   PVE = 21%
   Pacemaker/ICD = 7%
2. MV = 41%
   AV = 38%
   TV = 12%
   PV = 1%

(*) *Predisposing condition*
- Regurgitation lesion
  - More prone to IE than stenotic lesion

Regurgitation
↓
Venturi effect
↓
High velocity, low pressure eddy zone of regurgitant orifice on receiving chamber
↓
Localization of vegetation on upstream aspect of infected valve

- MR related with MVP (myxomatous degeneration thickened leaflet) – MC cause
- Aortic regurgitation – 2nd MC cause
- Function MR associated with LV remodeling
- BAV
  - Risk of IE is low as such
  - Associated with high incidence of periannular complication of IE
  - Strong independent factor predicting periannular extension of inf
- Non rheumatic as in elderly patients
- Rheumatic heart disease
- Congenital heart disease
  - Unrepaired VSD – MC
  - Ventricular outflow tract obst (2nd)
       E.g., TOF
  - Palliative shunt or conduits
  - Residual shunt after surgery
  - Low velocity flow turbulent lesions
       E.g., ASD
- Other predisposing conditions
  - Previous H/O IE
  - Chronic IV access
  - IV drug abuse
  - In dwelling endocavitary devices
  - DM
  - Renal failure/HD
  - Underlying malignancy
  - Chronic immunosuppressive therapy
  - Invasive dental procedure within 60 days

(*) *Symptoms*
Depends on
- Virulence of organism
- Persistence of bacteremia
- Extent of local tissue destruction and its HD sequence
- Peri valvular extension
- Septic embolization to systemic circulation or lung
- Consequences of circulating immune complexes and systemic immunopathological factors
  - Fever MC   –80–90%
  - Chills   ⎤
  - Weakness ⎦ 40–50%
  - Malaise   ⎤
  - Sweats
  - Anorexia
  - Headache ⎬ 20–40%
  - Dyspnea
  - Cough
  - Weight loss⎦

- Myalgia
- Arthralgia
- Stroke
- Confusion   } 0–20%
- Delirium
- Nausea/vomiting
- Edema
- Chest pain
- Abd pain   } 5–10%
- Hemoptysis
- Back pain

Absence of fever
- Elderly patient
- Immunocompromised patient
- Patients treated with prev empiric antibiotics
- Patients with infection of implantable devices

*Usually fever disappear in 5-7 days of treatment

Persistence of fever
- Prog. Inf with perivalvular extension
  E.g., abscess, septic embolization
- An extracardiac site of infection (native or prosthetic)
- Infected in dwelling catheters or device
- Inadequate antibiotic therapy
- Adverse reaction to antibiotic therapy

Dyspnea due to
- Severe HD lesion (e.g., left-sided valvular regurgitation)
- Onset of HF
- Septic emboli to lungs

Physical examination
- Heart murmur 80–90%
- New murmur
- Changing murmur
- Central neurologic abnormality/CVA
- Splenomegaly (2nd MC site of septic emboli; 1st brain)
- Petechial/conjunctival hemorrhage
- Splinter hemorrhage
  - Sublingual
  - Painless dark red lesion in prox
  - Nail bed
- Janeway lesion
  - Due to peripheral septic embolization
  - Painless hemorrhagic macule on soles or palms
- Osler nodes
  - Located in pads of fingers and toes
  - Painful erythematous nodular lesion
  - Due to immune complex deposit and focal vasculitis
- Retinal lesion/Roth spots – due to immune complex Mediates vasculitis
- Seizure, visual deficit, cranial nerve deficit, SAH, Toxic encephalopathy

INVESTIGATION
- Anemia
- Leukocytosis
- Microscopic hematoma
- Increased ESR
- Increased CRP
- Circulating immune complex
- Rheumatoid factor

DIAGNOSIS
D/D
- Acute rheumatic fever
- LA myxoma
- APLA syndrome
- NBTE/marantic endocarditis
- SLE, reactive arthritis, polymyalgia rheumatica and vasculitides

(*) *Duke criteria*
Sensitivity – 80%; specificity (90%)
Modified dukes criteria (2000)
  By Li and colleagues

A. *Major criteria*
- *Blood culture findings positive for IE:*
  - Typical microorganisms consistent with IE from 2 separate blood cultures (in absence of 1° focus)
    - *Strepto viridans, Streptococcus gallolyticus, Staphylococcus aureus,* HACEK, community acquired enterococci
  - Microorganism consistent with IE from persistently positive blood culture findings defined as
    - ≥2 positive culture of blood samples drawn >12 hours
      Apart (or)
    - 3 or most of ≥4 separate culture positively (with 1st and last sample drawn ≥1 hour apart)
  - Single positive culture for *Coxiella burnetii* or anti-phase IgE titv ≥1:800
- *Evidence of endocardial involvement:*
  - Echocardiographic findings positive for IE (TEE in patients with prosthetic valve or suspected paravalvular abscess and TTE in other patients) defines as
    - Oscillating intracardiac mass on valve or supporting structures, in the path of regurgitant jets or on implanted material (in absence of alternate anatomical explanation) or
    - Abscess or

- New partial dehiscence of prosthetic valve or
- New valvular regurgitation
Added in ESC 2015
↓
- Abnormal activity around the site of prosthetic valve implantation detected by 18 FOG PET CT or SPECT
- Definitive paravalvular lesion by cardiac CT

B. Minor criteria
- Predisposing heart condition or IV drug abuse - now?
- Fever; Temp >38°C/100°F
- *Vascular phenomena:* Major arterial emboli, septic pulm infarct, mycotic aneurysm, IC hemorrhage, conjunctival hemorrhage, Janeway lesions
- *Immunologic phenomena:* Glomerulonephritis, Osler nodes, Roth spots, Rheumatoid factor
- *Microbiologic evidence:* Positive blood culture findings does not meet a major criterion or serological evidence of active infection with organism consistent with IE

*DEFINITIVE ENDOCARDITIS
- *Pathologic criteria*
  - Microorg demonstrated by cultures for histopath examination of vegetation/a vegetation that has embolized/intracardiac abscess specimen or
  - Pathological lesion/vegetation or intracardiac abscess) confirmed by result of HP examination showing active endocarditis
- *Clinical criteria*
  - 2 major criteria
  - 1 major + 3 minor criteria or
  - 5 minor criteria

*POSSIBLE ENDOCARDITIS
1 major + 1 minor criteria or
3 minor criteria

*REJECTED DIAGNOSIS
- Firm alternative diagnosis or
- Resolution of IE syndrome with antibiotic therapy for ≤4 days
Or
- No evidence of IE at surgery or autopsy on antibiotic therapy ≤4 days or
- Does not meet criteria of possible IE

Other Laboratory Testing
- *Microbiology*
  - *Community acquired:* Strepto viridans - MC - S. aureus
  - *Health care associated:* S. aureus MC (esp. MRSA)
  - *IV drug abuser:* S. aureus (70%)
  - *Early PVE (<2 months):* S. aureus - CONS
  - *Late PVE:* Staph
  - Blood culture neg in 5-15%
- Other blood surgery
  - Normocytic normochromic anemia
  - Low serum iron and TIBC
  - Leukocytosis (left shift)
  - Thrombocytopenia (10%) - poor prognosis
  - Raised ESR
  - Elevated CRP
  - Elevated rheumatoid factor
  - Renal dysfunction (if in first 8 days - poor prognosis)
  - Microscopic hematuria and proteinuria
  - RBC cost if glomerulonephritis
  - Cardiac troponin and BNP may be elevated

D/D of mobile echodensity = Lamb's excrescence, endocardial fenestrations, ruptured or retracted chordate, acoustic artifact reflected by calcified tissue
- *ECG:*
  - Nonspecific findings
  - New AV block of any degree or BBB
- *ECHO:*
Modality of choice
Sensitivity 82-89%
Specificity 70-90%
  - TEE can diagnose vegetation with 2-3 mm size
    - Sensitivity 90-100%; specificity 90%
  - PVE with periannular infection and also compli
    - TTE sensitivity = 50%
    - TEE specificity = 80-90%
      Sensitivity = 80-95%
  - Vegetation of IE typically occurs on upstream low-pr side of regurgitant valve, multiple and lobulated, motion independent of valve structure

(*)ECHO features that suggest potential need for surgical Intervention:
- *Vegetation*:
  - Persistent vegetation after systemic embolization
  - AML vegetation, esp if it is highly mobile with size >10 mm
  - One or more embolic events during first 2 weeks of antimicrobial therapy
- *Valvular dysfunction:*
  - Ac AR/MR with signs of failure
  - HF unresponsive to medical management
  - Valve perforation or rupture
- *Perivalvular extension:*
  - Valvular dehiscence, rupture or fistula
  - New heart disease
  - Large abscess or extension of abscess despite appropriate medical management

Approach to ECHO Imaging

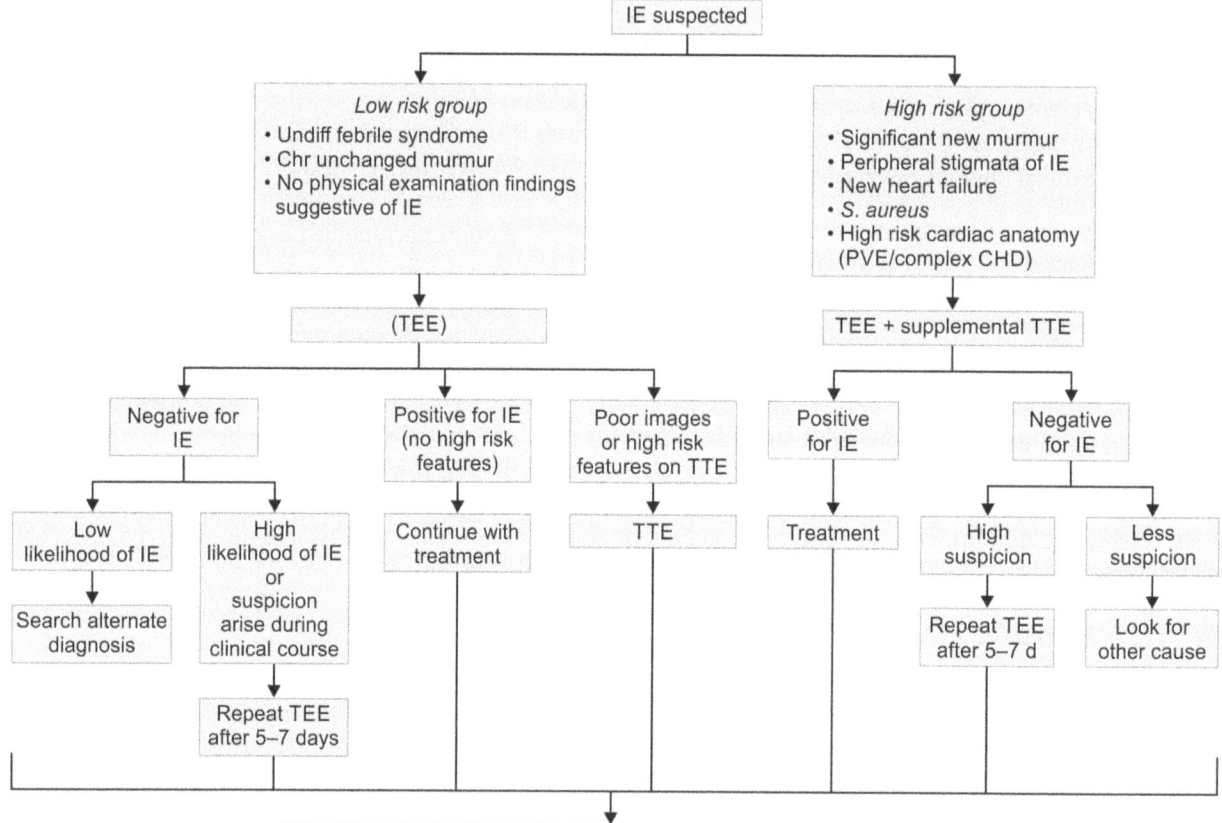

*When to do ECHO?

- *Early*
  - As soon as possible (<12 hours after initial evaluation)
  - TEE preferred; obtain TEE views of any abnormal findings for later comparison
  - TTE if TEE not available
- *Repeat ECHO*
  - TEE after TTE if high risk features
  - TEE 7-10 days after initial TEE is suspicion exists without diagnosis of IE or with Worison Clinical course during early treatment of IE
- *IntraOp*
  - Prepump (identification of vegetation, mechanism of regurgitation, abscess, fistulas and pseudoaneurysm)
  - Postpump (confirmation of successful repair)
- *Completion of treatment*
  - Establish new baseline for valve function and morphology and vent size and function
  - TTE is adequate

COMPLICATIONS

- *Local valvular destruction*
  - MC with left sided value regurgitant lesion
- Develop HF
  - 30-40% of patients with IE
  - 3 times more common in patients with NVE
  - 1° indication for surgery
  - NYHA 3-4 - in hospital mortality = 25-50%
  - MC with AV (30%) - MV (20%) - TV (<10%)
- New mod-severe regurgitation develop in up to 70% presenting with IE
- Mech for regurgitation
  1. Perforation
  2. Prolapse
  3. Flail leaflet
  4. Extensive vegetation impede valvular coaptation
- Saccular mycotic aneurysm situated on atrial side of MV may rupture - large defect in leaflet
- *Perivalvualr extension*
  - Periannular or intra myocardial abscess
  - Mycotic false aneurysm
  - Fistula
    - Incidence 10-30% for NVE
                30-50% for PVE
    - Predictor
      1. PVE
      2. AV IE

3. Staph inf
4. BAV - 50% patients develop periannular abscess
- 2nd MC indication for surgery
- TEE sensitivity 80-90%; specificity >90%
- AV IE - can extend to aortomitral continuity (MAIF)
  (MAIF = mitral Ao intervalvular fibrosa) - Least vascular
  Str of heart - prone to inf - mycotic false aneurysm or fistulas
  Communication into Ao/LA - compression of prox LCA/syst embolization/rupture into pericardium
- Prosthetic valve dehiscence is another complication of PVE
  Perivalvular extension
- TEE and CT is superior imaging

- Embolism
  - Incidence = 20-50%
  - Common in early course (even before antibiotic)
  - Stroke rate = 10-20%
    Other emboli = 15-25% / Silent = 15%
  - More common in younger patients (<65 years)
  - Sites of emboli
    - CNS (38%) - MC
    - Spleen (30%) - 2nd
    - Renal (13%)
    - Lung (10%)
    - Peripheral art (6%)
    - Mesenteric (2%)
    - Coronary (1%)
  - Risk factors
    - Vegetation >10 mm in greatest dimension
      Higher risk with dimension >15 mm
    - Pedunculated and highly mobile vegetation
    - MV vegetation esp AML in native valve IE
    - Equal risk in NVE and PVE
    - Staph aureus IE
  - Risk decrease dramatically within 1 week of antibiotic therapy
  - Rec emboli event or prog increase in vegetation size despite antibiotic treatment - indication for surgery
  - No antiplatelet or no anticoagulants

ANTIMICROBIAL TREATMENT

A. *Streptococci (viridans group and Streptococcus gallolyticus)*
- Native valve endocarditis
  Highly penicillin sensitive (MIC <0.12 μg/mL)
  - Penicillin G (12-18 MV cont inf/6 divided dose) × 4 weeks
    Or ceftriaxone (2 gm/24 hours) IV or IM × 4 weeks
    Or Amox (100-200 mg/kg/d in 4-6 divided dose)
  - Penicillin G (12-18 MV cont inf/6 divided dose) × 2 weeks
    Or ceftriaxone (2 gm/24 hours) IV or im × 2 weeks
    Or amox
      Plus
    Gentamycin (3 mg/kg/24 hours) IV/IM × 2 weeks
    Or netilmicin (4-5 mg/kg/d) in 1 dose
  - Vancomycin (30 mg/kg/24 hours iv in 2 doses)
    (max dose = 2 gm/24 hours) × 4 weeks

Note: 2 week regimen not for patients with
- Cardiac or extracardiac abscess
- Creat clearance <20 mL/min
- Impaired 8th CN function
- *Abiotrophia/Granulicatella/Gemella* spp)
- Gentamicin should be adjusted to achieve peak serum conc 3-4 μg/mL or through serum conc <1 ug/ml (when divided doses used)
- Vancomycin only for patients who are not able to tolerate penicillin or ceftriaxone

Relative penicillin resistance (MIC 0.12-0.5 μg/mL)

Class 2a
- Penicillin G (24 MV/24 hours - cont inf or 6 doses) × 4 weeks
  Or Ceftriaxone (2 gm/24 hours) IM/IV × 4 weeks
  Or Amoxicillin
    Plus
  Gentamicin (3 mg/kg/24 hours) IV/IM × 2 weeks

Class 2b
- Vancomycin (same as above) × 4 weeks

Penicillin resistance (MIC > 0.5)

Class 2a
- Ampicillin (12 gm/24 hours in 6 doses divided) × 4-6 weeks
  Or Penicillin G (18-30 MV cont or 6 divided) × 4-6 weeks
  Or Amoxicillin
    Plus
  Gentamycin (3 mg/kg/24 hours in 3 divided doses) × 4-6 weeks

Class 2a
- Ampicillin (12 gm/24 hours in 6 doses divided) × 4-6 weeks
    Plus
  Ceftriaxone (4 gm/24 hours in 2 doses) × 4-6 weeks

- **Class 2b** (Vanco only for patient unable to tolerate ampi/peni)
  - Vancomycin (30 mg/kg/24 hours in 2 doses) × 6 weeks
    Plus
    Gentamycin (3 mg/kg/24 hours in 3 doses) × 6 weeks

- Prosthetic valve endocarditis

Penicillin susceptible
- **Class 2a**
  - Penicillin G (24 MV/24 hours) × 6 weeks
    Ceftriaxone (2 gm/24 hours) × 6 weeks
    Plus
    Gentamycin (3 mg/kg/24 hours) in 1 dose × 6 week
- **Class 2a**
  - Vancomycin (30 mg/kg/24 hours) in 2 divided doses × 6 weeks

Penicillin-relatively or fully resistance
- **Class 2a**
  - Penicillin (24 MV/24 hours) × 6 weeks
    Or Ceftriaxone (2 gm/24 hours) × 6 weeks
    Plus
    Gentamycin (3 mg/kg/24 hours) in 1 dose × 6 week
- **Class 2b**
  - Vancomycin (30 mg/kg/24 hours) in 2 divided dose × 6 weeks

B. Nutritionally variant streptococci:
E.g., *Abiotrophia, Granulicatella, Gemella* spp
- Unusual metabolism – diminished activity of cell wall - active antibiotics to kill these organisms
- Treatment as per native valve endocarditis with strepto viridans

C. Beta hemolytic streptococci
- Acute onset with rapid valve destruction
- Often require surgery
- Treatment Group A: Penicillin G/Ceftriaxone × 4 weeks
  Group B, C, F, G: Add genta for first 2 weeks

D. Staphylococci
- *Native valve*

1. Oxacillin sensitive
- Nafcillin or oxacillin (12 gm/24 hours - 4-6 divided doses) × 6 weeks
  Or [Cotrimoxazole (4800 + 960/d) + Clindamycin 1800/d]
- For penicillin allergic patients (nonanaphylactoid type)
  - Cefazolin (6 gm/24 hours in 3 divided doses) × 6 weeks
- For penicillin allergic patients (anaphylactoid type)
  - Vancomycin (30 mg/kg/24 hours in 2 divided dose) × 6 weeks
  Or daptomycin or cotrimoxazole + clindamycin

2. Oxacillin - resistant
- Vancomycin (30 mg/kg/24 hours in 2 divided doses) × 6 weeks
- *Prosthetic valve*
  *) Oxacillin sensitive
  All 2a Class
  1. Nafcillin/Amoxicillin ≥ 6 weeks
     Plus Rifampin (900 mg/24 hours IV/PO in 3 divided dose) ≥ 6 weeks
     Plus Gentamycin (3 mg/kg/24 hours in 2-3 divided dose × 2 weeks
     - If resistance - Levoflox
  *) Oxacillin resistance
     Vancomycin ≥ 6 weeks
     Plus Rifampin ≥ 6 weeks
     Plus Gentamycin 2 weeks

E. Enterococci
- *Gentamicin susceptible*
  (same as penicillin resistant strepto)
- *Gentamycin resistant*
  - Substitute gentamycin with streptomycin
  - Streptomycin (15 mg/kg/24 hours IV or IM) in 2 equally divided doses × 6 weeks

F. HACEK org
- Ceftriaxone (2 gm/24 hours IV or IM one dose) × 4 weeks
- Or ampicillin (12 gm/24 hours in 4 divided doses) × 4 weeks
  Or Ciproflox (1000 mg/24 hours in 2 doses) × 4 weeks

G. Gram-negative Bacilli and fungi
- Combined medical and surgical approach
- For gm negative bacilli
  - Beta lactam with aminoglycoside
    Or beta lactam with fluoroquinolones
- For fungal
  - Amphotericin b
  - Echinocandins (caspofungin, micafungin, anidulafungin)
  - Long term oral suppressive treatment once initial induction therapy is completed
  - Fluconazole and voriconazole can be used

H. Culture negative endocarditis
- Clues of microorganism can be obtained from epidemiological data
- Regimen should be broad to cover
  - Streptococci

- Staphylococci
- Enterococci
- HACEK org

Epidemiological duo

	Common organism
1. Injection drug use or indwelling CV device	▪ S. aureus ▪ CONS ▪ Beta hemolytic streptococci ▪ Fungi ▪ Aerobic gm negative bacilli
2. Genitourinary inf	▪ Enterococci ▪ Gr B streptococci ▪ *Listeria/Neisseria* ▪ Aerobic gm negative bacilli
3. Chronic skin inf	▪ *Staph aureus* ▪ B - hemolytic streptococci
4. Poor dental hygiene	▪ *Streptococcus viridans* ▪ Nutritionally variant strepto ▪ HACEK
5. Early (≤1 year valve)	▪ CONS ▪ *Staph aureus* ▪ Aerobic gm negative bacilli ▪ Fungi ▪ *Corynebacterium* ▪ *Legionella*
6. Late (>1 year valve)	▪ CONS ▪ *Staphylococcus aureus strepto viridans* ▪ Enterococcus ▪ *Fungi/Corynebacterium*

7. HIV infection – *Salmonella/Streptococcus pneumoniae/ S. aureus*
8. Solid organ transplant – *Strepto, Aspergillus, Enterococcus, Candida*
   - Empirical treatment for acutely ill patients
     - Ampicillin + cloxacillin + genta/vanco + genta – community acquired NVE or late PVE (>12 months)
     - Vanco + genta + rifampin – for PVE <12 months
   - *Monitoring of treatment*
     - Serum and through conc of aminoglycoside and vancomycin
     - Renal/hepatic/hematological toxicity
     - Blood culture daily till negative
       *Usually blood culture becomes negative by
       - 4-6 weeks after therapy (max)
       - HACEK/viridans/enterococci - sterile in 2 days
       - MRSA - 7-9 days
       - S. aureus - 3-5 days
     - If fever persists >7 d of treatment with appropriate antibiotics

Check for paravalvular abscess, extracardiac abscess, embolic events

INDICATIONS FOR SURGERY

MC - ▪ Heart failure – acute AR/MR; intracardiac fistula
2nd - ▪ Partial dehiscence of prosthetic valve
      Sinus of Valsalva rupture
      Rupture into pericardial sac
      Septal perforation
      Perivalvular abscess/pseudoaneurysm/ fistulas
- Large (>10 min) hyper mobile vegetation Which increases risk of embolization
- Valve obstruction by vegetation
- Persistent fever in spite of antibiotic treatment
- Fungal endocarditis
- Beta hemolytic streptococci IE
- Gm negative bacilli
- Multi drug resistant org

Earlier surgery indicated in
- HF and uncontrolled inf
- After stroke - surgery should not be delayed in the absence of coma and once cerebral hemorrhage has been excluded by CT
- After TIA or a silent cerebral embolism, surgery is recommended without delay
- In case of surgery for PVE, general principle outlined for NVE should be followed
- All patients with stroke should have repeat CT brain immediately before surgery to rule out hemorrhagic transformation

} Stroke and IE management

Delay surgery
- ICH – Delay surgery for at least 1 month
- Presence of hematoma – cerebral angio to rule out mycotic aneurysm

RIGHT-SIDED VALVE IE

- Medical management is mainstay
- Surgery can be deferred in absence of
  - Diuretic resistant rt heart failure with severe TR
  - Fastidious organism resistant to antimicrobial treatment (fungemia or persistent bacteremia >7 d)

- Vegetation >20 mm diameter with multiple pulm emboli and possible rt heart failure

FOLLOW-UP

- *Before or at completion of therapy*
    - Obtain TTE
    - Drug rehabilitation for IV drug abuser
    - Educate regarding signs of endocarditis
    - Thorough dental evaluation and treatment
    - Prompt removal of CVC
- *Short-term follow-up*
    - Obtain at least 3 sets of blood culture from separate sites for any febrile illness and before initiation of antibiotic therapy
    - Physical examination for C/O CHF
    - Evaluate for toxicity (e.g., ototoxicity)
- *Long-term follow-up*
    - Evaluation of valvular and vent function
    - Oral hygiene and regular dental check up

SECTION 11

Interventions

11.1 CAROTID ARTERY STENTING

ANATOMY

Three types of Aortic Arch (based on relationship of innominate art to ao Arch)

Type 1: All 3 great vessels arise in horizontal plane of the outer curvature of Ao arch

Type 2: Innominate art arise between the horizontal planes of outer and inner curvatures of Ao arch

Type 3: Innominate art arise below horizontal plane formed by inner curvature of Ao arch

Type 2 and 3 Arch possess difficulty for carotid interventions

OTHER ANOMALIES

- Common origin of Innominate and left CCA (Bovine)
- Left CCA originates separately from Innominate (Bovine)
- Single brachiocephalic trunk–splits into B/L Subclavian and B/L carotids.

REVASC

Current guidelines: It is reasonable to consider revasc for patient with Asymptomatic stenosis >70% or symptomatic stenosis >50%; Provided risk of revasc <3% and 6% respectively.

PRESTENTING/REVASC ASSESSMENT (ON CAROTID CONGLO/CT)

- *Anatomic variations* (as described)
- *Lesions characteristics:*
  - Precise location with prox and distal extent
  - Lesion length
  - Complex lesion ulceration
  - Severity of stenosis
  - Severity of lesion calcification
  - Diameter of vessel prox and distal
- *ICA distal to lesion:*
  - Assess cervical portion of ICA for presence of disease and tortuosity
  - Diameter of cervical ICA
- Potency of ext carotid

ENDARTERECTOMY/STENTING

- *EVABS:* Risk of stroke is low and similar
- *SPACE 2:* Recurrent stenosis more common in stenting
- *SAPPHIRE:* Premature termination
- *Wall stent:* Prematurely terminated
- *CREST:* Risk of composite 1° end point of stroke, MI or death did not differ among symptomatic and asymptomatic patient between CEA and CAS
- *KSS:* No significant diff between 2 groups.

Procedure

Steps 1 = Vascular access
    2 = Guiding sheath placement
    3 = Angiographic assessment (including intracranial angio)
    4 = Crossing the stenosis with guidewire
    5 = Embolic protection device
    6 = Lesion predilatation
    7 = Stent development
    8 = Stent post dilatation
    9 = Removal of EPD
    10 = Final angio assessment
    11 = Removal of guidewire and sheath

EMBOLIC PROTECTION DEVICES

Three types
1. Prox protection with balloon occlusion
   Adv:
   - Transient reversal of flow in ICA
   - Operator can select guidewire of choice
   - Avoids embolization during initial passage of guidewire and throughout procedure

   Disadv:
   - More cumbersome—longer profile larger sheath
   - Arterial occlusion may be poorly tolerated

2. Distal protection with balloon occlusion
   Adv:
   - Easy
   - Compatible with all stents
   - Aspirate large and small particles
   - Reliably trap debris

   Disadv:
   - No antegrade flow
   - Balloon induced injury
   - Not as steerable as PTCA guidewire
   - Difficult to image during procedure
   - Loss of apportion during procedure

3. Distal protection with filter:
   Adv:
   - Presence antegrade flow
   - Imaging possible throughout procedure
   - Some device allow individual guidewire selection

   Disadv:
   - May not capture all debris
   - Difficult to evaluate retrieval of debris during procedure
   - Filters may clog
   - Delivery/retrieval catheters may cause embolization
   - Filter entrapment in stent

   Available filter devices:
   - Interceptor
   - Filterwire EZ
   - Embosheild NAV
   - Spider
   - Fiber net

Stents:
1. Wall stent- Stainless steel
2. Treatment Accelink / Vivexx / Precise — Open cell nitinol
3. Endotex—Nex stent / α act (Abbot) — Closed cell nitinol

COMPLICATIONS

1. Vasovagal
2. Vasodepressor reaction — CVS
3. MI

1. Dissection
2. Thrombosis
3. Perforation — Carotid
4. External carotid A stenosis/occlusion
5. Transient vasospasm
6. Restenosis

1. TIA/Stroke (2-3%)
2. ICH — Neuro
3. Hyper perf synd
4. Seizure

1. Access site injury
2. Blood Transfusion — Other
3. Contrast Nephropathy/reaction

Flowchart: Hemodynamic effect of carotid stenting

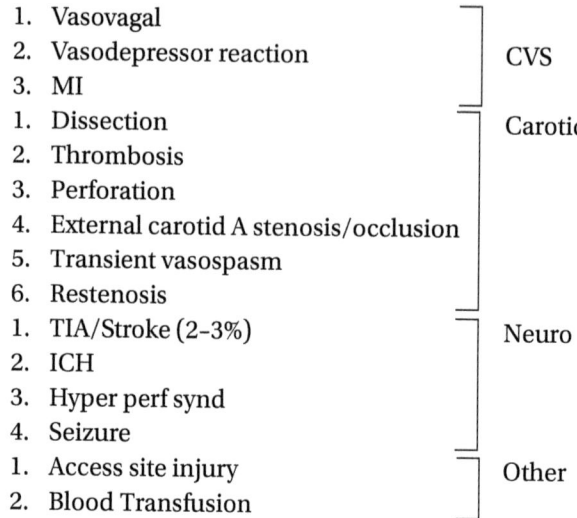

HYPER PERF SYND

- Rare (<1%)
- Life threatening
- Improve flow to chronically ischemic cerebral territory

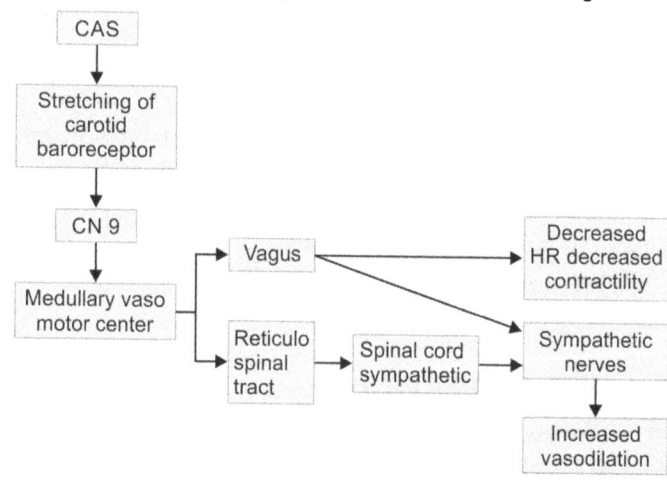

Most presents in 24-48 hours post procedure

C/F

Troubling I/L headache (on side of revasc)
- Nausea/vomiting
- Confusion

- Visual disturbance
- FND ⎤
- Seizure ⎦ Severe cases

Compli
ICH/SAH

Management
Prompt diagnosis and treatment
Diagnosis based on C/F
- Reduce Art BP (to decrease cerebral perfusion)
  - GTN, Nitroprusside, CCB, ACEI— Contraindicated
    - Because they increase CBR
  - Recommended agents
    - BB/Labetalol/and Clonidine
- After BP lowering

↓

CT/MRI

↓

Confirms ICH
Confirms edema
- Trans-cerebral Doppler ultrasound to demonstrate significant increase in flow velocity in I/L MCA confirms diagnosis

11.2 CORONARY PERFORATION

Q.1 Coronary perforation—classification and management (Dec 14)

DEF
Persistent extravascular loss and accumulation of contrast medium through the vessel wall

INCIDENCE
0.1–0.2%

CLASSIFICATION (EILIS)
Gr 1 Extra luminal crater without extravasation
Gr 2 Pericardial or myocardial blush without contrast extravasation in pericardium
   Limited extravasation producing a patch of blushing or staining within the myocardium or pericardium
Gr 3 Persistent extravasation with streaming or jet of contrast
   3A - Directed towards pericardium
   3B - Directed towards myocardium (cavity)

MECHANISM
- Guidewire penetration
- Vessel rupture
  - Balloon overdilatation (Balloon: Artery >1.2:1)
  - Stent mismatch (oversized)
- Extensive dissection; lack of vessel wall integrity; extensive calcification
- Athero-ablative devices

MANAGEMENT
Coronary perforation
↓
- Keep calm
- Immediate re occlusion of vessel with balloon inflation (Low pressure dilation 2-4 atm or for prolonged period) (Not >20 mins - may provoke myocardial ischemia)
- Reversal of anticoagulation
  - Heparin—Protamine
  - Bivalirudin - No antidote - Stop infusion
- Stop Gp 2b/3a infusion
  - Abciximab - Reversal with platelet
  - Eptifibatide ⎤ Cannot be reversed
  - Terofeban ⎦ with platelet
- Treat vagal reaction
  Restoration of hemodynamics
  - Atropine
  - Phenylephrine
  - Inotropes
  - IV fluids—IABP
- Urgent echocardiography (pericardiocentesis if cardiac tamponade)

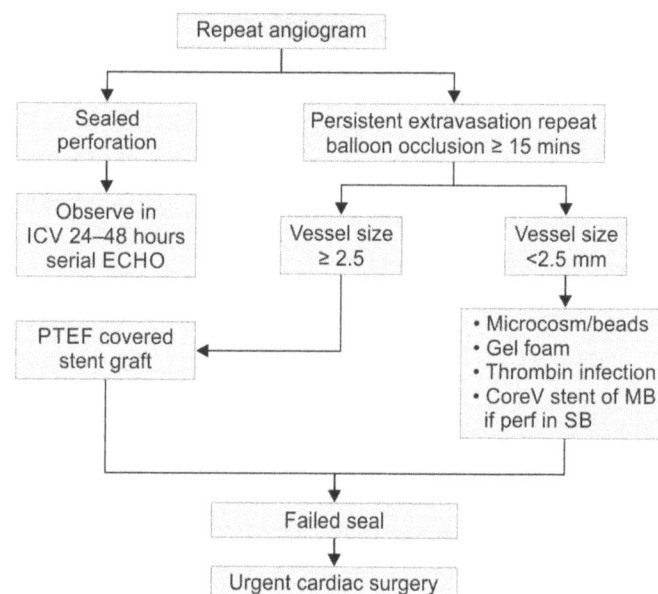

Drawbacks of Cover Stent
- Sub acute stent thrombosis 5-7%
- Angiographic restenosis rate 32%

RISK FACTORS FOR PERFORATION
- *Complex lesion:* Type B and C; calcification, tortuous vessel
- CTO
- Small vessel (<2-5 mm)
- Concomitant Gp 2b/3a inhibitor
- *Balloon dilation:* Compliant; cutting
- *Type of guidewires:*
  - Standard (nonhydrophilic)
  - High support (nonhydrophilic)
  - Hydrophilic
- Rotablation
- Female sex
- Old age

11.3 CTO INTERVENTION

WIRING TECHNIQUE (ANTEROGRADE)

Shaping wire

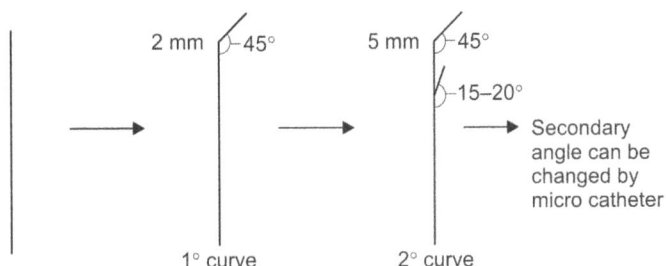

- Conventional techniques
  - Controlled drilling
  - Penetrating wire technique
  - Sliding wire through microchannel
  - Parallel wire technique
  - Antegrade intimal or subintimal tracking

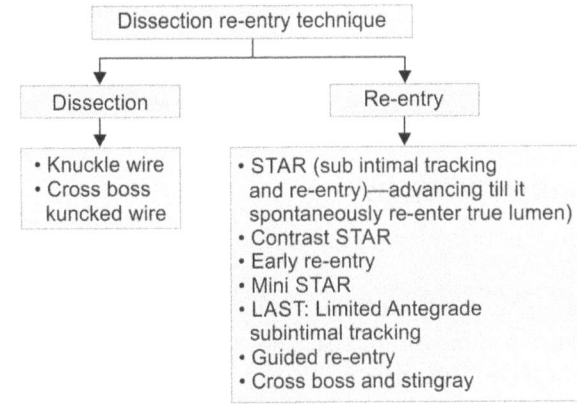

WIRING TECHNIQUE (RETROGRADE)

- Retrograde wire cross
- Kissing wire cross
- CART and reverse CART

1. CTO

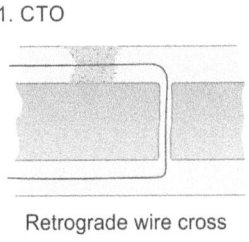

Retrograde wire cross

2.

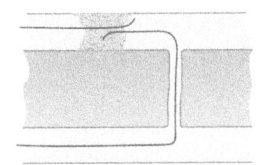

Kissing wire cross

3. Balloon on retrograde wire

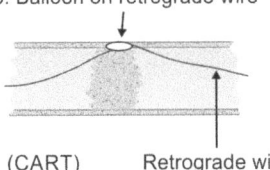

(CART)   Retrograde wire

4. Balloon on anterograde wire

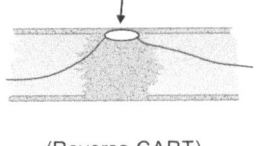

(Reverse CART)

Definition

CTO are described as obstruction of coronary arteries (1) ≥99% stenosis (2) of more than 3 months duration (3) with poor or no anterograde flow (TIMI 0-1)

Q1. Re-entry devices in CTO (June 15)
- Bridge point medical system
  - Over the wire catheter with 1 mm blunt tip rotated rapidly by operator to dissipate friction to facilitate CTO crossing
    If the crossing catheter traverses the CTO into distal true lumen
    Cross boss ↓
    Long PCI wire can be placed and the catheter is removed
    ↓
    Standard balloon dilatation and stenting
  - If the Catheter enters subintimal space
    ↓
    Advanced next to angiographically visible true lumen (distal to CTO - re-entry site)
    ↓
    Exchange wire is left in space
    Stingray ↓
    Re-entry balloon catheter advanced over guidewire to re-entry site
    ↓
    12 gm tapered tip angulated guidewire designed for re-entry is advanced through re-entry catheter
    ↓
    Exit through one of the exit port oriented towards true lumen
- SAFE CROSS system
  Method to optically access CTO using optical coherence reflectometry
  ↓
  OCR uses OCT along a single line of sight rather than producing a true image
  ↓
  RF energy used to penetrate lesion
  Device success rate = 50–60%

FAST-CTO TRIAL

Use of bridge point medical system in coronary CTO refractory to cross with standard technique was associated with higher success rate (77%)

11.4 DRUG-ELUTING BALLOONS

Q.1 DEB (June 15)
Q.2 DEB and their current status (June 12, 13)

DEB

Conventional semi compliant angioplasty balloon covered with antiproliferative drug ↓ which is released into the vessel wall during inflation of balloon.

Active substance on DEB is lipophilic with high absorption rate through vessel wall.

Paclitaxel

- Highly lipophilic
- Short incubation time (3 min)
- Paclitaxel completely inhibits vascular smc proliferation for
  12-14 days
- Concentration = 3 µg/mm^2
  (3 times higher than that of DEB)

First gen: Paclitaxel + IOPROMIDE carrier
Second gen: Paclitaxel + Hydrophilic Urea
  Paclitaxel + Hydrophilic resin "shellac"
  Paclitaxel + Butyryl trihexyl citrate (BTHC)
  (Panteralux)

INDICATIONS

- *Instant Restenosis:* BMS
  Trials: PACCOCATH ISR 1 and 2: DEB vs. POBA
  PEPCAD 2: DEB vs. PES
  RIBS 5: DEB vs. EES
- *Instant Restenosis:* DES
  Trials: PEPCAD DES: DEB vs. POBA
  ISAR DESIRE 3: DEB vs. PES vs. POBA
  RIBS 4: DEB vs. EES

Esc guidelines (2014):
DES for DES and BMS ISR (1A)
DEB for DES and BMS ISR (1A)

- *De-novo lesions small vessels:*
  PICOLETO Trial: DEB vs. PES
  BELLO Trial: DEB vs. PES
  DEDCAD—1
  Worldwide registry
- *Bifurcation lesions:*
  - Sequential DEB treatment of both branches followed by BMS in MB
  - MV stenting followed by DEB of SB
  Trials: PEPCAD 5
- *DENOVO lesions DEB + BMS*
  Trials DEB—AMI

Most Promising Indications

- ISR in BMS/DES
- De novo lesions in small vessel (<2-5 mm)
- Pt with contraindications to prolonged DAPT
- DEB in PAD

CURRENT STATUS

DEB has emerged as potential alternative to combat restenosis

DEB technology demonstrated safety and efficacy in preclinical and in randomized clinical trials for ISR

- *PACCOCATH 1 and 2*
  - Benchmark trials for DEB in ISR.
  - Showed superiority of DEB in treatment of BMS—ISR in comparison to POBA
  - *-6 month CAG:* Reduced in late lumen loss
- *PEPCAD 2:* Similar positive response
  DEB vs. PES

11.5 DEDICATED BIFURCATION STENT

INTRODUCTION
Dedicated bifurcation stents help to improve result of distal LM bifurcation and non-LM bifurcation
- Most data of dedicated bifurcation stents is from non-LM bifurcation

NEED FOR DEDICATED BIFURCATION STENT
- To maintain adequate patency of side branch throughout the procedure
- To provide ease of side branch rewiring
- To ascertain full coverage of SV ostium by stent scaffold

WHAT SHOULD AN IDEAL BIFURCATION STENT SYSTEM ACHIEVE?
- Improved short term and long term outcome
- It should be low profile and highly deliverable even in challenging anatomy
- Adequate coverage of carina
- Versatility—provisional stenting as well as 2—stent strategy compatibility

CATEGORIES
- *Bifurcation Y stent:* Implanted in both MB and SB simultaneously e.g., Medtronic bifurcation stent
- *Stent for provisional stenting:* Facilitates or maintain access to SB after MB stenting and do not require recrossing of MB struts
  For example: Petal, Boston scientific
  - Invatec twin rail
  - Antares
  - Y. Med sidekick
  - Nile Cro Co
  - Multi link frontier

  These stents allow placement of second stent in SV if needed
- Stents that require another stent Implanted in the bifurcation
  e.g., Side guard ⎫
        Tryton   ⎬ Treat SB First
        Biguard   ⎭
        Axxess plus → Implanted in proximal MB at level of carina. It may require additional 2 stents to completely treat some bifurcation lesions

FEW FREQUENTLY USED STENTS
Axxess

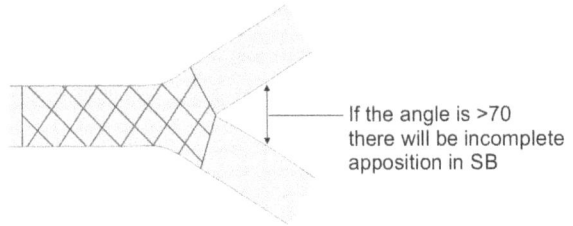

Trial: AXXENT- Good results in LM but not favorable in distal branches
  Advantage: Treat for 1-0-0 bifurcation lesion with narrow Bifurcation angle

Tryton SV Stent

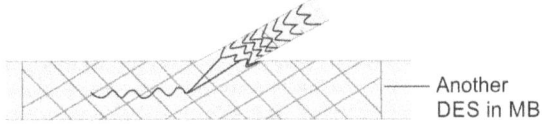

Trials: Triton with combination of DES in MB is feasible strategy to treat distal LM bifurcation

Advantages
- Compatible with natural anatomy of bifurcation in terms of diff between size of proximal MB and SD
- Reduce metal burden in proximal MB as compared to cullothe
- Suitable for wide variety of bifurcation angle

Disadvantages:
- Committed 2 stent strategy
- Only available in bare metal version—increased risk of repeat revascularization of SB

Stentys

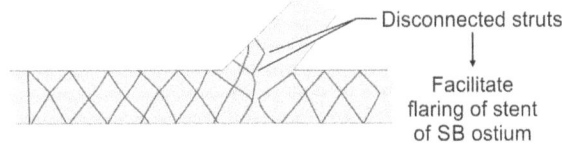

Advantages:
- Device will adjust itself to the natural step down phenomenon of bifurcation
- Less carina shift
- Potential to open stent by disconnecting the connecting struts (see **Figure**)

Disadv:
- When two proximal cell is crossed with a wire, not much advantage to be expected from strut disconnection

Nile Stent

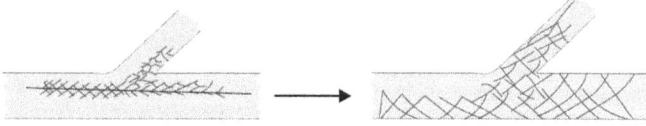

Advantages:
- Ensure access to MB and SB during procedure
- No tailing of wire or no need of recrossing

Disadv:
Straight stent—so prox malapposition is possible—POT is necessary

11.6 DEFERRED STENTING

Q.1 Deferred stenting (Dec 16)

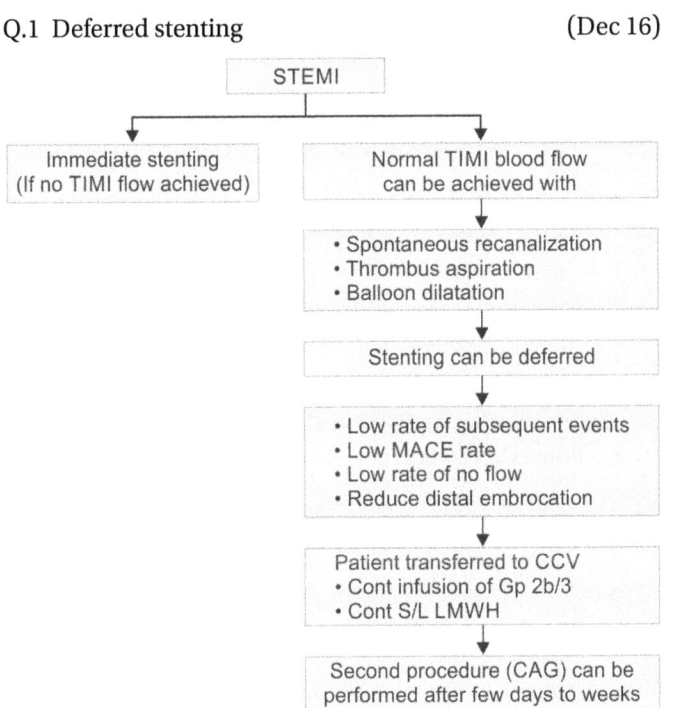

TRIALS SUPPORTING STRATEGY

- *DEFER STEM 1 (2013)*
  - Deferred completion of PCI reduced no reflow, distal embolization and intraprocedural thrombotic complication compared with conventional treatment of immediate stenting
  - Final coronary flow grade and MBG was better in deferred stenting group
  - Myocardial salvage measured with MRI was better in deferred group (after 6 months)
  - Approach to PCI at second procedure differ
    - Maximal stent diameter at second procedure was 0.5 mm greater
    - Vessel dimensions were greater due to attenuation of coronary artery tone with time from reperfusion
- *MIMI trial (2016)* (Comparison of immediate versus deferred stenting using minimalist immediate mechanical intervention approach in acute STEM)
  - This trial did not support deferred stenting and even suggested a deleterious effect of deferred stenting on microvascular obstruction size
- *DANAMI—3 DEFER (2016)*
  Routine defer stenting in STEMI pattern does not reduce occurrence of death, heart failure, MI, or repeat revascularization (compared with PCI)
- *INNOVATION Study*
  Routine defer stent did not significantly reduce infarct size and microvascular obstruction compared with immediate stenting
- *Meta analysis (2017)*
  Compared with immediate stenting, deferred stenting did not reduce occurrence of no—or slow—flow, death, MI, or repeat revascularization; But showed improved LV function at long term

Caution: Re—MI

11.7 DISTAL PROTECTION DEVICES

Q.1 Distal protection device (Dec 15)

EPD in catheter-based procedures:
- *TAVI/TAVR:*
  - To reduce number and volume of cerebral lesions in high-risk patients
  - *Trial:* Clean—TAVI (Claret Embolic Protection and TAVI)
- *SVG intervention*
  - To reduce MACE rate in patients undergoing SVG intervention
  - *Trial:* SAFER trial
  - ACC/AHA Guidelines (Class 1 indication)
- *Carotid artery stenting*
  - To reduce major adverse events i.e., stroke, death, or MI within 30 days
  - Retrospective analysis
- *For PAMI*
  - Multiple studies
  - No significant difference in angiographic and clinical outcome
- *Femoro—Popliteal intervention*
  - FDA has approved spider Fx filter and Proteus embolic capture balloon for embolic debris capture
  - No epidemiologic to illustrate its usefulness
  - No cost—effective data
  - Use of embolic protection device in fem—pop intervention should be reserved to lesions, procedure and patients who are at high risk.
- *Renal angioplasty*
  - Data suggested to reduce atheroembolic events
  - Prevention of deterioration of renal function
  - Larger studies awaited

Mechanism of embolic protection device
1. Distal occlusion
2. Distal filter
3. Proximal occlusion
4. Local plague trapping

1. Distal occlusion device
   For example: Guard wise temporary occlusion catheter connected to distal occlusion balloon
   - Low profile of balloon allows passage of balloon distal to lesion without embolizing
     ↓
     Balloon is inflated
     ↓
     Aspiration catheter used to remove collected thrombotic debris
   Adv:
   - Easy to cross lesion
   - Aspirates large and small particles
   - Reliability traps debris
   - Traps soluble substances that can cause vasospasm
   - Easy device retrieval
   Disadv:
   - No antegrade flow transiently can lead to ischemia
   - Balloon induced injury
   - Not as steerable as PTCA wires
   - Difficult to image during procedure

2. Distal filter device
   - Consist of angioplasty guidewire with expandable porous filter at distal tip
   - Pore size 100 mm
     Or
   - Distal aspiration system
   e.g., Filter wire (Boston scientific)
   Adv:
   - Preserve antegrade flow
   - Simple to use
   - Contrast imaging possible throughout the procedure
   Disadv:
   - Filters may clog
   - Delivery catheters may cause embolization before filter deployment
   - May not capture all debris and soluble substance
   - Difficult to evaluate retrieval of debris during procedure

3. Proximal occlusion device
   - Occlude inflow proximal to target lesion to suspend antegrade flow
     ↓
     Stagnant blood containing suspended debris and particles must be evacuated before restoring flow.
   e.g., Proxis system (St. Jude)
   Adv:
   - Protects myocardium during wire crashing
   - Use contrast suspension for lesion visualization
   - Large lumen catheter can aspirate large thrombus
   - No distal landing zone required
   Dis adv:
   - No antegrade flow ischemia
   - Cannot use with ostial disease

4. Local plague trapping device:
   - Stent covered with microporous PTFE (polytetrafluoroethylene) could also serve as a form of 'local filter' during SVG interventions
   - No clinical evidence
   - No FDA approval

11.8 ENDOMYOCARDIAL BIOPSY

INDICATIONS

- New onset HF<2 wk duration
  Associated with normal sized/dilated LV and HD compromise
- New onset HF 2 wk-3 mth associated with dilated LV and new vent arr, 2nd/3rd degree block or failure to respond to usual care within 1-2 week
- HF >3 month duration associated with dilated LV and new onset vent arr, 2nd/3rd degree block or failure to respond to usual care in 1-2 wks
- HF associated with DCM (any duration) associated with suspected allergic reaction and/or eosinophilia
- HF associated with suspected anthramycin CMpathy
- HF associated with unexplained RCMP
- Suspected cardiac tumors
- Unexplained empathy in children.

CONDITION IDENTIFIABLE WITH EMB

Treatable condition
- Cardiac allograft rejection
- Cardiac amyloidosis/Sarcoidosis
- Giant cell myocarditis
- Hypereosinophilic Synd
- Anthracycline toxicity
- Cardiac hemochromotons
- Lymc carditis
- Fabry's disease

Less treatable condition
- Myocarditis (Nongiant cell)
- ARVD
- Rheumatic carditis
- Glycogen storage disease
- Chagas disease

RELATIVE CI

- Patient not co-operative/No consent
- Profound H.D. compromise
- No surgical back up
- Coagulopathy (INR >1.5)
- Mechanical tricuspid prosthesis
- Significant root to it stunt(risk of air embolism)
- Thinning of myocardium after MI or in case of ARVD
- RA/RV thrombus

PROCEDURE

- Consent
- Patient education
- <1% chance of perforation
- Sedation seldom needed
- Cont HR, ECG, BP and SPO_2 monitoring
- IJV, Subclavian or femoral venous approach
- Fluoroscopic/ECHO guided
- Port procedure patient observed for couple of hours for pericardial diffusion

PROPERTIES

Two types:
1. *Stiff:* Does not require long sheath
   Rely on operator skill to maneuver safely into RV
2. *Flexible:* Require longer sheath advanced into RV for positioning.

IJV or Subclavian -50 cm long bioptome
   Femoral - upto 105 cm bioptome
- Usually 4 to 6 specimens obtained in different areas of the septum to reduce sampling error.
  RV Biopsy - from IJV/Subclavian/Femoral vein
  LV Biopsy - from femoral A.A
  → Digital inserted into LV.

COMPLICATION

In general EMB can be safely performed in transplanted heart because of scarred, thickened pericardium in transplanted heart

- Mortality (procedure related) <0.05%
- *Cardiac tamponade/perforation:* - 0.3-0.5%
  Can be minimized by obtaining samples from thicker IVS and by gentle catheter advancement
  S/E: Chest pain during or after procedure
    SOB
    Pericardial rub
    Altered H.D
- In patient with early port transplant, attend sutures are also at high risk of perforation
- *Thromboembolism:*
  - Chances of thromboembolism during LV Biopsy is higher as compared to RV biopsy
  - Right side thromboembolism are rarely clinically significant
- *Arrhythmia:*
  Mainly atrial arrhythmia—stopped by touching atrial or ventricular endocardium by bioptome
  - Rarely VT
  - Very rarely bradyarrhythmia or BBB
    → responds only to B1 agonist and not to atropine
- *Tricuspid valve dysfunction:*
  - Bioptome can damage cardiac/pap muscle and produce significant vascular dysfunction
- Damage to IVC, CS, hepatic vein, coro art ⎤
- *Local compli:* Hematoma, inf, injury to lung, nerve ⎟ Rare
  (recurrent laryngeal) ⎦
- *Pain* while bioptome touches heart or biopsy is taken

11.9 FFR

Q.1 Role of FFR in ostial intervention
Q.2 What is noninvasive FFR? How does it compare and contrast with invasive FFR? (June 14)
Q.3 Role of FFR in Coronary artery disease

FFR

Definition: Ratio of maximal blood flow in stenotic artery to normal maximal blood flow

Maximum flow = hyperemic flow

$$FFR = Q\ max\ S/Q\ max\ N$$

Now flow = pressure difference/resistance

$$Q = \Delta P/R$$

So,

$$FFR = \frac{Q\ max\ S}{Q\ max\ N} = \frac{(Pd - Pv)/Rmax\ S}{(Pa - Pv)/Rmax\ N}$$

Pd = pressure distal to stenosis
Pv = central venous pressure
Pa = aortic pressure

Now, during hyperemia resistance is minimal so it cancels out each other
So,

$$FFR = \frac{Pd - Pv}{Pa - Pv}$$

FFR myo = Pd - Pv/Pa - Pv = Pd/PV
FFR coro = Pd - Pw/Pa - Pw (Pw = wedge pressure)
FFR coll = FFR myo - FFR coro
PV is negligible most of time
So,

$$FFR = Pd/Pa$$

Technique

Guiding catheter is preferred (as diagnostic catheter's smaller lumen leads to higher level of friction)

Pressure wire
Sensor located 30 mm from tip at the junction of radio-opaque and radiolucent part 0.014 inch wire

Hyperemia
Maximal vasodilatation of both epicardial coronaries (conductance vessel) and microvasculature (resistance vessel)
1. Adenosine (t1/2 = 1-2 min) (intravenous): 140-180 ug/kg/min ⎤
2. Adenosine (t1/2 = 30-60 sec) (intracoronary): 50-150 ug bolus ⎬ Micro vascular dilatation
3. Nitroprusside (t1/2 = 1 min) 0.6 ug/kg intracoronary bolus
4. Papaverine (t1/2 = 2 min) (intracoronary): 16-20 mg for LCA 12-16 mg for LCA ⎦

5. Isosorbide dinitrate ≥ 200 ug intracoronary bolus wait for ≥ 30 seconds before first measurement ⎤ Epicardial dilatation
6. Dobutamine (iv) 10-40 ug/kg/min (t1/2 = 1 min) ⎦
   - Disadv of papaverine—can induce arrhythmia
   - Disorder of IC adenosine—does not allow pullback
   - Disadv of IV adenosine—unpleasant feeling in chest/throat

Defer study: Incidence of death and nonfatal MI 5 years was not significantly different between patients who were deferred on the basis of functionally nonsignificant lesion and patient undergoing PCI in spite of negative FFR

Application

A. *For intermediate lesion*
   - To determine functional relevance
   - FFR <0.75—physiological significant
   - FFR >0.80—physiologically insignificant
     - Stenting can be deferred
   - DEFER study

B. *Left main disease*
   - LMCA is generally short
   - Atherosclerosis is often diffusely distributed so normal segment is lacking
   ↓
   Underestimation of reference segment
   ↓
   Underestimation of stenosis by CAG as well as QCA
   ↓
   FFR is helpful

C. *Bifurcation lesions*
   Difficult to evaluate angiographically due to
   - Overlapping segments
   - Radiographic artifacts
   ↓
   FFR helps to delineate physiological significance of SB stenosis
   It also helps in case of provisional stenting
   - FFR <0.75 in SB (across stent strut) warrants treatment of SB ostium in terms of kissing balloon dilatation or stenting of SB

D. *Multivessel disease*
   FFR significantly reduces the rate of MACE, Death, MI, and repeat revascularization at 1 year (FAME study)
   FFR guided strategy
   - Reduce number of stents

- Do not prolong the procedure
- Reduce amount of contrast used
- Cost saving

E. Acute myocardial infarction

AMI
↓
Myocardium is replaced by scar tissue as time passes
↓
Reduces functional myocardium
↓
Reduces physiological significance of any stenosis with time
↓
So when viable myocardium mass supplied by stenotic IRA decreases
↓
Functional significance of stenosis decreases
↓
FFR increases (number)

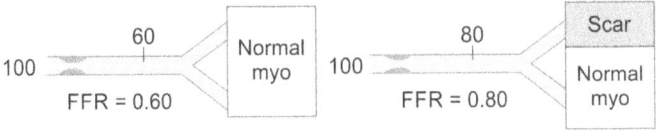

Physiological significance has decreased with formation of scar

FFR can identify viable myocardium that may recover following revascularization
↓
May be used as alternative to noninvasive viability tests

F. *CABG*
- Only 1 small study
- Cut-off value is 0.75

G. *Post stenting*
- Post stenting FFR is strongest independent of 6 months clinical outcome
- Post PCI FFR <0.9—unfavorable outcome

H. *Diffuse coronary artery disease*

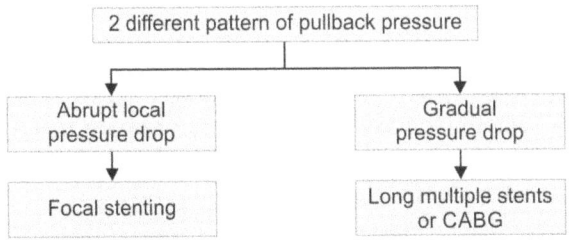

I. *Tandem lesions*
- Pullback FFR can be obtained like in diffuse diseases
- Another approach

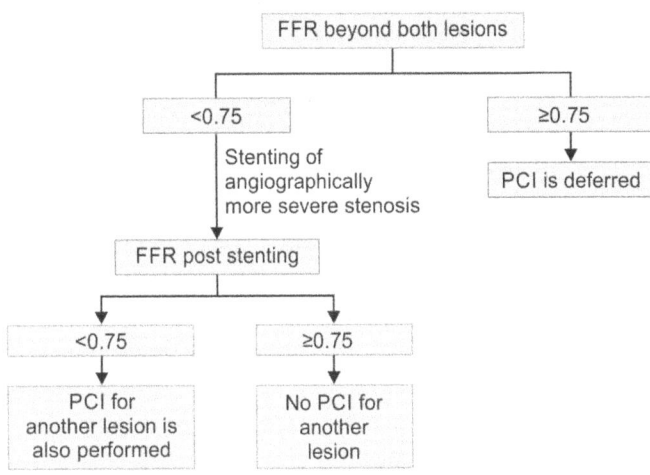

Trial: FAME; FAME 2
DEFER

Background

Two different approaches to evaluate functional relevance of CAD
1. Assessment of myocardial perfusion under stress
2. Measurement of fractional flow reserve

→ Depends on coronary flow reserve
↓
CFR is pressure gradient between epicardial coronary artery and microcirculation
↓
Reduced in case of
1. Collateral circulation
2. Microvascular disease
↓
Stress perfusion tests are not able to distinguish between these 2 entities
↓
FFR is preferred even in presence of collateral circulation

FFR
- Not influenced by systemic hemodynamic
- Takes into account contribution of collaterals
- Related to severity of stenosis and the mass of tissue to be perfused
- Per lesion accuracy rather than per myo territory
- High spatial resolution

Noninvasive FFR

CT coronary angio
 Sensitivity -99%
 Specificity 89–91%
 PPV 93–94%
 NPV 99–100%

Limitation

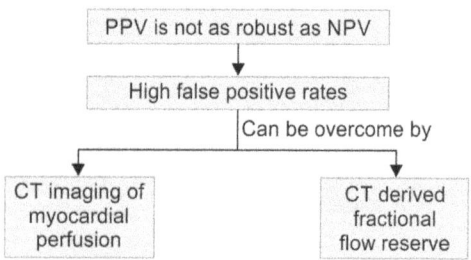

CT derived FFR (FFRCT) is novel diagnostic technique
- Allows derivation of FFR from raw data acquired during CT coronary angio

FFRCT can be derived from
- Typical CT coronary angio images
- No additional contrast
- No additional medication
- No additional radiation
- No additional imaging protocol

Procedure to Obtain FFRCT

Acquisition of CCTA images
↓
Upload CT images to "heart flow"
↓
Reconstruction of physiological model with ventricular myocardium (LV mass)
↓
Computation of blood flow on supercomputer (based on Newtonian fluid dynamics)
↓
FFRCT computation (including hyperemia)
↓
FFR can be calculated at any point
Approximate time required to calculate 5–6 hours/study

Trials

	Discover flow	DeFACTO	NXT
Year	2011	2012	2013
Patients	103	252	251
Design	Single center	Multi center	Multi center
	CT FFRCT	CT FFRCT	CT FFRCT
Sensitivity	94–93	84–90	94–86
Specificity	25–82	42–54	34–79
PPV	58–85	61–67	40–65
NPV	80–91	72–84	92–93

DISCOVER FLOW concluded
- FFRCT and FFR was well correlated
- Slight underestimation by FFRCT
- Diagnostic accuracy of FFRCT is superior and additive to CTCA stenosis for diagnosing ischemia—causing lesion

DeFACTO concluded
- Use of FFRCT + CCTA among stable patients with suspected or known CAD is associated with improved diagnostic accuracy
  - Specificity of FFRCT was low in DeFACTO because
    - They used early generation algorithms
    - Beta blockers not given as routinely—poor CT quality image
    - Nitroglycerin not used in all cases
      - Underestimation of maximum coronary artery diameter

NXT study concluded
- Good correlation of FFRCT with invasive FFR
- Slight underestimation by FFRCT (0.03)
- Reproducibility of FFRCT was high
- Accuracy of FFRCT in predicting lesion specific ischemia was superior to anatomic assessment by coronary CTA

Clinical Use of FFRCT

PLATFORM study
- Examined clinical effectiveness of FFRCT
- 584 patients
- Design

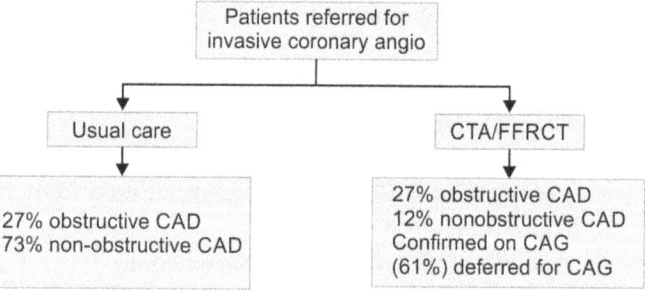

Conclusions

- No adverse clinical events among patients in whom CAG was deferred on basis of FFRCT
- No difference in clinical outcome between usual care and FFRCT guided groups at 90 days
- QOL score was higher in FFRCT group

PROMISE Trial (resent)
CREDENCE Trial (future trial)

Limitation of FFRCT
- Technical artifacts
  - Misregistration
  - Coronary motion
- Poor image quality
- Issue of poor-image can be minimized by administration of beta blockers
- Sending of image to 3rd party is required (rather than on site image analysis)
- FFRCT is only studied in stable CAD patients
  FFRCT in LVH, DM, previous PCF/CABG is not yet standardized
- No study comparing noninvasive functional testing modalities vs. FFRCT using invasive FFR as reference standard
- Long time required
- Long-term prognosis of management using FFRCT is yet unknown
- US FDA approval (2015)
  No guidelines recommend use of FFRCT
  ↓
  Recently NICE guidelines has approved FFRCT as cost effective solution for non-invasive evaluation

  No study comparing FFRCT with invasive FFR

iFR

Instantaneous wave free ratio
          Or
Instantaneous flow reserve

Introduced in TCT 2011

Principle

It is pressure derived, hyperemia free index for assessment of relevance of coronary stenosis

Technique

- Similar as FFR
- Same pressure wire is used
- Different software is used with special algorithms (By volcano corp)

Principle

         Flow = pressure difference/resistance
- When Coronary resistance is stable—pressure can be used as surrogate for flow to assess coronary stenosis
- If we can identify a period of naturally occurring stable resistance
  - Why we need to use adenosine for hyperemia

↓
Resistance remains stable during diastole (wave free period)
↓
Used to calculate iFR

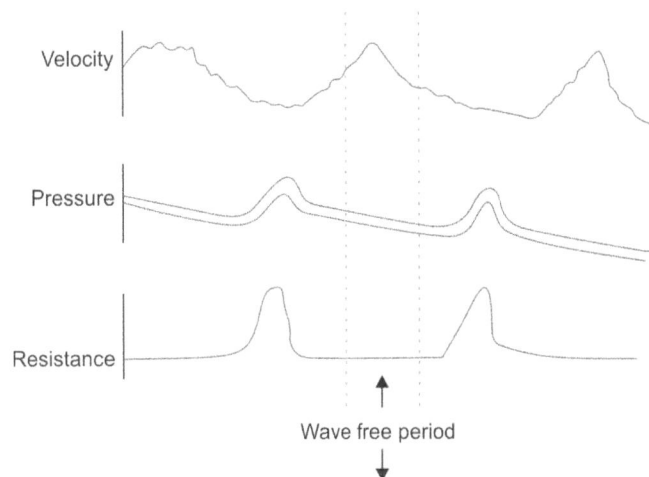

- Identified by fully automated algorithms
- Identification of naturally low resistance period
- Uses pressure only

Cut off value (0–90)

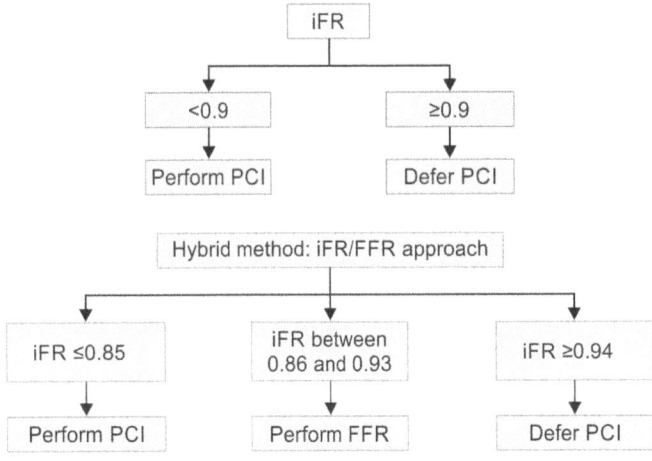

Advantages of iFR

- Simple, safe and cost effective
  - No adenosine (no side effect)
  - No doubt whether hyperemia is achieved or not
  - Few seconds to perform (5 beats)
  - Avoids serious complication related with adenosine (1%)
- iFR and FFR has similar ability to detect ischemia

Studies of iFR

- *ADVISE:* Adenosine vasodilatation independent stenosis evaluation

- Identified a wave free period in cardiac cycle when resistance is naturally stabilized and minimal
- iFR measured during wave free period gives an estimate of stenosis severity similar to FFR
- *ADVISE 2*
  - iFR is not replacement for FFR
  - Hybrid approach is possible with volcano system
- *CLARIFY study* (diagnostic classification of the instantaneous wave free ratio is equivalent to fractional flow reserve—and is not improved with adenosine administration)
  - iFR and FFR had equivalent agreement with classification of coronary stenosis severity
  - Adenosine did not improve diagnostic categorization
  - iFR can be used as adenosine free alternative to FFR
- *RESOLVE study*
  - Comparing iFR with FFR and nonhyperemic Pd/Pa with FFR

    ↓

    Overall accuracy of 80% for both
  - Clinical outcome studies are required
- *Johnson et al.*

  iFR does not equal mean hyperemic resistance
- *VERIFY study*

  iFR which is said to be independent of hyperemia, did changed markedly during adenosine induced hyperemia

  ↓

  Finding challenged underlying concept and clinical applicability of iFR
- *VERIFY 2*
  - Confirms result of VERIFY
  - Whether used as a part of binary or hybrid algorithm, resting index is not sufficiently accurate to be used as a guide to the need for revascularization
- *Outcome studies*
  - DEFINE-FLAIR
  - iFR-SWEDEHEART

11.10 FICK'S PRINCIPLE

Q.1 Fick's principle and cardiac output assessment
Q.2 What is Fick's principle? How do you determine cardiac output by Fick method? (Dec 11) (June 12)
Q.3 Values of different methods for measurement of cardiac output (Aug 97)
Q.4 Measurement of cardiac output (June 15)

CARDIAC OUTPUT

Quantity of blood delivered to the systemic circulation per unit time is termed cardiac output
    Expressed in liters per minute

Arterio venous difference: Extraction of a given nutrient by tissue from circulation is expressed as AV difference

Extraction Reserve: Factor by which the AV difference can increase at constant flow (due to change in metabolic demand) is termed extraction reserve

　　e.g., For O_2: 1L of blood can carry 200 mL O_2
　　Arterial O_2 sat = 95% = > so 95% of 200 mL = 190 ml/L
　　Venous O_2 sat = 75% = so 75% of 200 mL = 150 ml/L
　　　　　　　　↓
　　　　AV difference = 40 mL/L
　　　　　　　　↓
　　　Extraction reserve for O_2 = 3
　　　　　　　　↓
　So under extreme demand tissue can extract 40 × 3 = 120 mL/L of O_2
　　　　　　　　↓
　　Venous O_2 sat will be 190 – 120 = 70 mL (35%)

Lower Limit of CO

O_2 extraction reserve is 3
　　　　↓
　So CO can fall upto one-third without compromising oxygen delivery to tissue　↓
Any further fall will result in
- Tissue hypoxia
- Anaerobic metabolism
- Acidosis
- Circulatory collapse

Upper Limit of CO

- Largest increase achieved by trained athletes
- 600% of resting output
  =~ 5 × 6 = 30 L/min or =~ 3 × 6 = 18 L/min/m²

Normally Cardiac Output

- Varies with age
  4.5 L/min at 7 years
  2.5 L/min at 70 years
- Varies with posture
  Decrease by 10% when person rise from lying—sitting
  Decrease by 20% when person rise from lying—stand
- Body temp, anxiety, env heat, humidity also affects CO

FICK PRINCIPLE

- Described by Adolf Fick in 1870
- Never actually applied by Fick
- First used by O'Klein in Prague to measure cardiac output

Principle

Total uptake or release of any substance by an organ is the product of blood flow to the organ and arteriovenous concentration difference of the substance

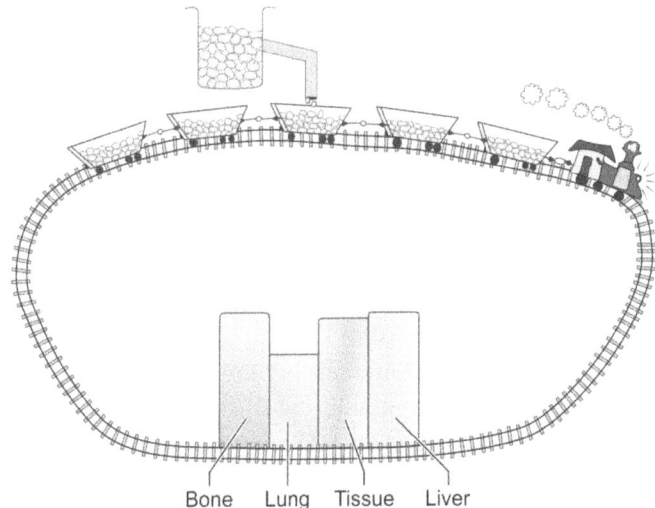

- Train represents circulation; Hopper represents lung; marble is O_2
- Say each box car contain 16 marbles before and 20 after passing under the Hopper
- Say speed of delivering marbles by hopper is 20/min
- So Train's speed = marble delivery rate/marbles delivered
　　= 20 marbles/min/4 marbles/box car
　　= 20/4 boxcar/min
　　= 5 box cars/min

Now if oxygen is 1L of blood and each marble is 10 mL of O_2
↓
We have an AV O_2 difference = 40 mL/L
And total O_2 consumption is 200 mL/min
↓
Cardiac output = $\dfrac{200\ \text{mL/min}}{40\ \text{mL/L}}$ = 5 L/min
↓

So to know cardiac output we must know
- Total uptake or release of substance by given tissue
- AV difference for that particular substance at given tissue level

Measurement of Cardiac Output

Fick's Oxygen Method

Pulm blood flow is determined by
- Pulmonary AV difference
- Rate of O_2 uptake

↓

If there is no shunt (intracardiac) and PBF = SBF
↓
CO can be measured

$CO = \dfrac{O_2\ \text{consumption}}{AV\ O_2\ \text{difference}}$

O_2 consumption calculation

A. In actual practice,

Equal at steady state
- Rate at which O_2 is taken up by blood is not calculated
- Uptake of O_2 from room air by lung is measured

↓
3 methods

1. *Douglas bag method (old)*
   - Collection of expired air for 3 mins in Douglas bag and measure its volume and O_2 content
2. *Metabolic rate meter (MRM) polarographic method*
   - Uses variable speed blower to maintain a unidirectional flow of air from room through hood and via connecting hose to polarographic sensing cells

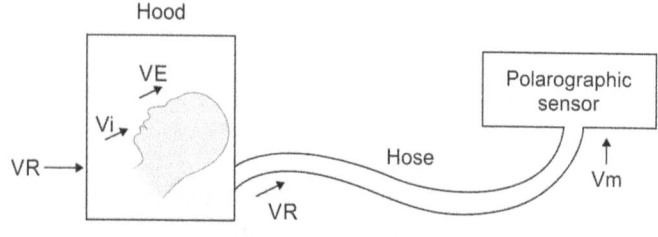

VR = room air enters hood at rate (mL/min)

Vm = Blower's discharge rate which determines VR
Vi = inhaled air
Vc = exhaled air

Patient's O_2 consumption,
$VO_2 = (FRO_2 \times VR) - (FMO_2 - Vm)$
FRO_2 = fractional O_2 in room air
FMO_2 = fractional O_2 in air flowing to polarographic light
↓
Now Vm = VR − Vi + Ve
So VR = Vm + Vi − Ve
So VO_2 = [FRO_2 (Vm + Vi−Ve)] − (FMO_2 − Vm)
   = FRO_2·Vm − FMO_2·Vm + FRO_2 Vi − FRO_2 Ve
   = Vm (FRO_2 − FMO_2) + FRO_2 (Vi − Ve)
↓
FRO_2 = @ room air = 0.209
↓
So VO_2 = Vm (0.209 − FMO_2) + 0.209 (Vi−Ve)
↓
At steady stage Vi and Ve are constant
In practice FMO_2 is kept at 0.199
↓
So VO_2 = Vm (0.209 − 0.199) + 0.209 (Vi − Ve)
VO_2 = 0.01 Vm + 0.209 (Vi−Ve)
Vi = Ve
So $\boxed{VO_2 = 0.01\ Vm}$

3. *Sensormedics deltatrac 2 (paramagnetic method)*
   (No longer available)
   - More sophisticated
   - Directly measure FO_2 and FCO_2 in expired air

B. *AV O_2 difference calculation*
- Blood collected by precisely positioned catheter simultaneously and as close to the midpoint of O_2 consumption determination process
↓
Three methods
1. Manometric technique of Van Slyke and Neil
   Disadv: 15–30 min required to run 1 sample
2. Lex-O_2-con fuel cell technique
   - No longer available
3. Co-oximeter
   - Uses hemolyzed blood (by ultrasonic or chemical method)
   - Simple and quick
   ↓
   How to calculate]
Ideally PV blood − 1. Saturation of arterial blood SaO_2 %

Ideally on PA blood
2. Saturation of mix venous blood SvO_2 %
   By above 3 methods
3. Blood's O_2 carrying capacity = Hb × 1.36 (O_2 carrying capacity of Hb) mL/gm × 10
   = mL/L
4. O_2 content of arterial blood = SaO_2 × O_2 carrying capacity
5. O_2 content of venous blood SvO_2 × O_2 carrying capacity
6. AV O2 difference
   Arterial O_2 content − venous O_2 content

$$CO = \frac{O_2 \text{ consumption}}{AV\ O_2 \text{ difference}}$$
↓
$$= \frac{VO_2}{(Hb \times 1.36 \times 10)(SaO_2) - (1.36 \times 10\ O_2\ Hb)(SvO_2)}$$
$$CO = \frac{VO_2}{Hb \times 1.36 \times 10 (SaO_2 - SvO_2)}$$

How CO is calculated by Fick's principle

Source of Error

- Fick's principle assumes that a steady state exists
  ↓
  Strict quiet, calm environment must be maintained in cath lab
- Errors in determining O_2 consumption
  - (Approx 6%)
  - Respi quotient is believed to be 1 in Fick's principle - actually it is 0-9—gives 1.6% error
  - If RQ is 0.8—error is 3.2%
- Errors in measuring AV O_2 difference
  - (Approx 5%)
  - Mixed venous blood taken from RA
  - Partial contamination of PA blood with pulm capillary blood (falsely high SPO_2)
  - Presence of air bubble in syringe
  - Presence of dye/contrast in circulation hamper with co-oximeters
  - SPO_2 determination hamper by presence of carboxyhemoglobin or other abnormal Hb
  - Oximetry is valid from SO_2 45-98 it is not reliable when $SO_2 < 40\%$
- Total error in CO calculation = ~10%
- Narrow AVO_2 difference is more prone to have errors
  ↓
  So in low CO State where AVO_2 difference is high
  ↓
  Fick's method is more reliable

- Some laboratory assumes O_2 consumption value to be 110–125 ml/m²
  ↓
  This further adds to error

Indicator Dilution Method

- Specific application of Fick's principle
- Two methods
  1. Continuous injection method
  2. Single injection method (widely used)

Principle
1. Nontoxic substance—mixes completely with blood
   - Concentration can be measured
   - Neither added to nor subtracted from blood during its passage between injection and sampling site
   - Most of indicator passes sampling site before recirculation starts
   - Indicator substance must pass through central circulation
2. *Indicators*
   1. Indocyanine green dye method
   2. Cold (Thermodilution method)

	Indocyanine green	Thermodilution
Dye injected	PA	vena cava/ RA
Sampling site	Radial/femoral	PA

$$Q = \frac{I}{\int_0^\alpha c(t)dt}$$

Q = flow
I = indicator
t = time
C = constant

Thermodilution method
- Cold dextrose used historically
- 2 thermistors were used
  1st at injection site
  2nd at sampling site

$$CO = \frac{V1\ (TB-T1)\ (S1.C1/SB.CB)\ 60}{\int_0^\alpha \Delta T(t)dt} \times 0.825$$

S1 and SB = specific gravity of injectate and blood
C1 and CB = specific heat of injectate and blood

CO is multiplied by 0.825 (correction factor for catheter warming)

Adv of Thermodilution method (over indocyanine dye)
- No withdrawal of blood
- No arterial puncture
- Inert and inexpensive Indicator
- Virtually no recirculation

Errors: (5-10%)
- Unreliable in presence of TR
- Temp in pulm art fluctuates acc to respiration and cardiac cycles
- In low flow, low output state cold indicator may get warm by myocardial walls—overestimate cardiac output
- Correction factor (0.815) (empiric) maybe inadequate
- Many labs use normal temp saline—can lead to variability in results

Continuous CO Monitoring

- Catheters based on thermodilution principle
- Uses warm Indicator rather than cold
- Prox thermal filament located in RA and distal thermistor in PA

$$\downarrow$$

Thermal filament warms the blood

$$\downarrow$$

Signals processed and interpreted by distal thermistor
- Used for continuous monitoring of CO in ICU
- More accurate measurement

11.11 HYBRID REVASCULARIZATION

Q.1 Current status of hybrid revascularization (Dec 16)
Q.2 Role, method and current status of hybrid revascularization (Dec 13)

INTRODUCTION

Concept introduced by Angelini and colleagues (1996)
- Minimally invasive thoracotomy LIMA – LAD and balloon angioplasty of non-LAD vessel

    LIMA patency is excellent in long term

    Sva to non-LAD patency is suboptimal
    50–70% at 10 years
    30% at 20 years
    ↓
    Hybrid revascularization is superior. (ACC/AHA 2011)

CANDIDATES FOR HCR

- Ostial, complex or occluded LAD lesion with simple lesion of other coronaries
- Elderly patients, LM disease with low SYNTAX score
- Overweight or diabetic patients
- Comorbidities making sternotomy high risk
- Younger patients, life expectancy >10 years and who are not complete PCI candidate
- Patients requiring redo revascularization for multivessel disease and LMA not used for LAD.

INDICATION

- Ungrafable non-LAD vessels
- Lack of conduits
- Reoperations
- Severe aortic atherosclerosis
- Severe calcification of mitral annulus
- Prior chest radiation
- High-risk patients
  - Recent MI
  - Prior stroke
  - ESRD on dialysis in whom less invasive approach may reduce operative time and ischemic time

CONTRAINDICATION

- LAD is nongraftable
- LAD is intramyocardial
- Inability to undergo off—pump beating heart revascularization
- Left SCA stenosis (unsuitable GMA)
- Dense adhesion in left chest (previous surgery/infection)
- Morbid obesity
- Severe lung disease

METHOD

- *MIDCAB:* (Minimally Invasive Direct Coronary Bypass)
  Via small anterior mini thoracotomy
  Via left 4th/5th ICS
- *EndoCAB:* (Endoscopic Atraumatic CAB)
  Thoracoscopic LIMA harvest with Lima-LAD Bypass
- *Robotic Assisted CAB*
  LIMA harvest through 3 endoscopic parts
- *Robotic TECAB* (Totally endoscopic CAB)

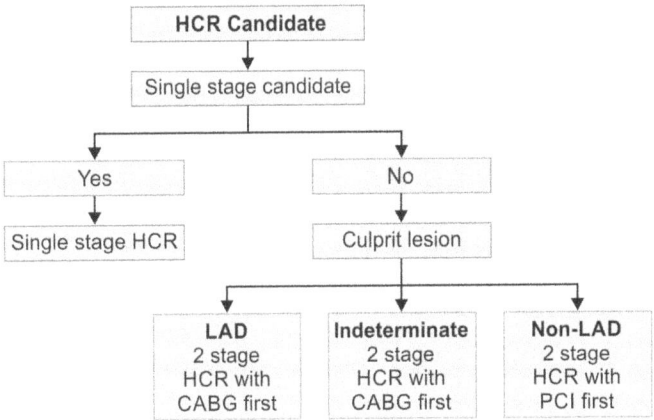

CABG First

Ideal timing of PCI not determined

Adv:
- Permits CABG to be performed without risk of antiplatelet agents
- Patency of LIMA can be determined during PCI
- Complex LM or LAD—Diag bifurcation can be attended under protection of LIMA

Caution: One must be sure about PCI of non-LAD lesion to avoid unfortunate situation of performing sternotomy to rescue a failed PCI

PCI First:
Adv:
- If PCI fails/suboptimal result → traditional CABG remains an option
- Addressing non-LAD lesion facilitate CABG by minimizing potential for ischemia

Disadv:
- Risk of Acute stent thrombosis

11.12 IABP

INDICATION

- *Cardiogenic shock*
  - Bridge to revascularization
    - Temporary HD stabilization in patients with cardiogenic shock caused by AMI
  - Bridge to tertiary care center
- *AMI treated with PCI*
  Uncertain benefit
- *High risk revascularization*
  - Unprotected LM
  - LVEF < 40%
  - Target vessel supplying > 40% myocardium
  - Severe CHF
- *Mechanical Compli of AMI:* (class 1 ACC/AHA)
  - Acute MR
  - VSD
- *Refractory angina*
  - Refractory angina in patients with STEM 1 (class 1)
  - Refractory angina in NSTEMI/UA (class 2 a)
  - Refractory pulm congestion in STEM 1 (class 2 b)
- *Weaning from CPB/post op pump failure*
  - Patient with severe LV dysfunction or those with prolonged CPB (are difficult to wean because of stunned myocardium from prolonged cardiac arrest)
- *End stage disease-bridge to transplant:*
  - IAB improve CO and decreased filling pr
    ↓
    Improves hemodynamics
- *Refractory vent arrhythmias*-class 2 a
  IAB improve HD, lesion ischemia and controlled vent arrhythmia
- *Support during non-cardiac surgery*

CONTRAINDICATION

- Aortic dissection
- Abdominal or thoracic aortic aneurysm
- Severe PVD
- Descending aortic and peripheral vascular grafts
- Coagulopathy or CI to heparin
- Mod-severe AR

HEMODYNAMICS

- *Decrease afterload*

As systole begins	After load reduction
↓	Occurs because of decreased LVEDP
IAB rapidly deflates	After load reduction leads to
↓	↓
Creates neg pr in aorta	Increases CO by 20% approx
	Decreased PCWP by 20% approx
↓	
Reduce after load and promote LV forward flow	

- *Decreases LV wall stress*
  By decreasing LVEDP and decreased afterload
  ↓
  Improve SV and CO
- *Augmented coronary perfusion*
  Balloon inflates during diastole
  ↓
  Displace blood to prox Ao
  ↓
  Augments Ao dia pr
  ↓
  Increases coronary perfusion pr

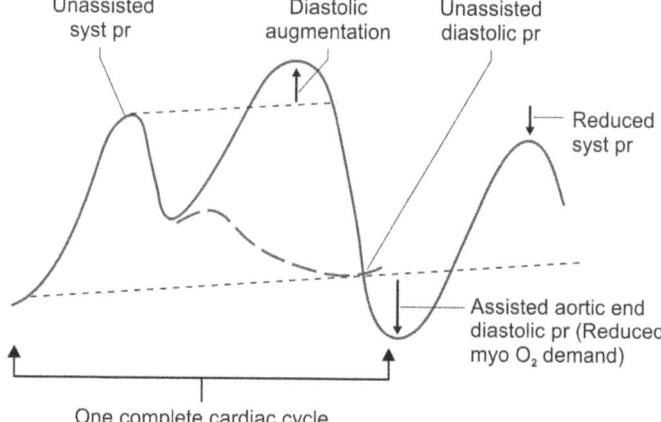

TIMINGS

- Ideally balloon pump should inflate on the down slope of systolic pr waveform before dicrotic notch
  ↓
  Deflate before onset of next systole

- *Early inflation*
  Inflation before Ao valve closure
  ↓
  Premature closure of aortic valve with increased afterload
  ↓
  Increased LV wall stress and increased MVO_2
- *Late inflation*
  Inflation well after closure of AV
  ↓
  Diminished diastolic pr augmentation and suboptimal coro perfusion
- *Early deflation*
  Deflation before isovolumic contraction
  ↓
  Suboptimal diastolic augmentation and coro perf as well as suboptimal afterload reduction
  ↓
  Increased myo O_2 demand
- *Late deflation*
  Deflation after onset of systole
  ↓
  Impaired LV emptying, increased afterload, increased preload, decreased SV and increased MVO_2

COMPLICATIONS

- *Vascular (5-20%)*
  - Hematoma around access site
  - Bleeding from access site
  - Limb ischemia
- *Infection*
- *Balloon rupture/leak (4.2%)*
  - Due to inflation against calcified plaque
  - Lead to helium gas embolism and balloon entrapment (when blood leaks into balloon, clots and prevents adequate deflation for removal)
- *Balloon entrapment*
  - Immediately carryout fluoroscopy to ascertain cause and position of entrapped catheter
- *RBC and platelet destruction*
  - Due to sheer force of balloon cath
  - Daily Hb and plt should be checked
  - Plt < 50,000 are unlikely to be caused by IABP-Find alternate cause
- *Other rare*
  - Renal failure by renal embolization
  - Mesenteric ischemia
  - Paraplegia from plaque embolization to spinal artery
  - Ao dissection
  - Ao perforation

11.13 IN-STENT RESTENOSIS

Q.1 Confronting neo atherosclerosis in BMS and DEC (Dec 16)
Q.2 Mechanism of ISR
Q.3 Risk factors of ISR
Q.4 ISR – definition, risk factor, diagnosis and management

DEFINITION

Clinically: The presentation of recurrent ischemia
Objective evidence of myo ischemia

Angiographically: >50% diameter stenosis in the stented segment or its edges (5 mm segments adjacent to the stent)

ETIOPATHOGENESIS

ISR is primarily a nonspecific inflammatory response to vessel wall injury due to the persistent insult by a foreign element such as stent strut

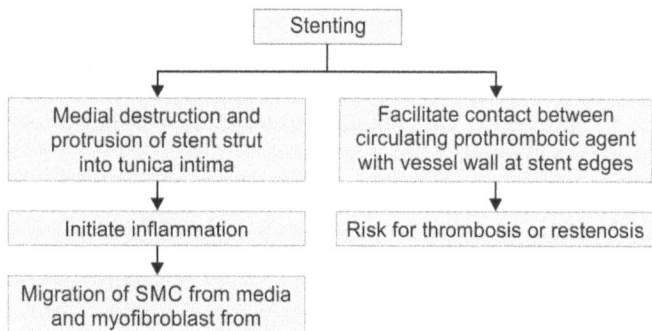

Additionally:
Mitogens released by
- Platelet
- Vascular SMC
- Endothelial cells
- Inflammatory cells
  ↓
  Hasten ISR
- Early (within days) with angioplasty
  - Elastic recoil
  - Relocation of axially transmitted plaque
  - Negative plaque remodeling
- Late (weeks to months)
  - Reorganization of thrombus
  - Neo intimal proliferation
    ◆ Vasc SMC proliferation
    ◆ Vasc SMC migration
    ◆ Vasc SMC matrix synthesis
  - Remodeling
  - Resolution of inflammation

Sirolimus: Stop proliferation at G1/S phase
Paclitaxel: Block proliferation at Go phase

RISK FACTORS

- *Patient related*
  - Age
  - Female gender ⎫ Interruption of
  - Diabetes mellitus ⎬ DAPT
  - Genetic factor ⎭
- *Lesion related*
  - Complex lesion (Type B2/C)
  - Ostial lesion and bifurcation
  - Small vessel
  - Multivessel CAD
- *Procedure related*
  - Number of stent and total length
  - Type of stent   • Plaque protrusion
  - Stent overlap   • Stent fracture
  - Stent under expansion/dissection
  - Minimal lumen diameter
  - Residual edge stenosis
  - Incomplete apposition/aneurysm

CLASSIFICATION

Mehran System

Type 1: Focal ISR (<10 mm)
  1A: Articulation or gap
  1B: Margin
  1C: Focal body
  1D: Multifocal
Type 2: Diffuse (>10 mm) intra stent
Type 3: Proliferative (>10 mm) extending beyond stent margin
Type 4: Total occlusion (TIMI grade 0)

Clinical Restenosis

- Req for ischemia driven repeat revascularization
- Diameter stenosis ≥ 50% and one of following
  - Positive h/o recurrent angina presumably related to target vessel
  - Objective signs of ischemia at rest (ECG) or during exercise related to target vessel
  - Abnormal test of avg functional diagnostic test (FFR < 0.8)
  - IVUS minimus CSA < 4 mm² (< 6 mm² for LM)
- TVR with stenosis of ≥ 70% even in absence of ischemic signs or symptoms

BMS vs. DES ISR

	BMS ISR	DES ISR
Angiographic OCT picture	Diffuse pattern common homogeneous, high signal band most common	Focal pattern common layered structure or heterogeneous most common
Time course	6–8 months	5 years
SMC cellularity proteoglycan mod content	Rich	Hypocellular high
Persistent fibrin and inflammation	Occasional	Frequent
Complete endothelization	3–6 months relatively in Freq late	Up to 48 months relatively Freq accelerated course
neoatherosclerosis		

TREATMENT

Options
0. Role of imaging (OCT > IVUS)
1. Conventional Balloon angioplasty
2. Cutting or scarring balloon
3. Drug eluting balloon
4. *Another stent:* Same DES/Another DES
5. Debulking
6. Vascular brachytherapy
7. Bypass surgery

1. *Balloon angioplasty*
   - For original stent under expansion
   - Larger high-pressure balloon (1:1)
   - Problem—slippage during inflation (watermelon seeding phenomena)
   - Early lumen loss

2. *Cutting or scoring balloon*
   - Avoid slippage during inflation
   - *Problem:* Difficult to deliver in distal areas through stented segment

     RESCUT
     ↓
     P.To
     ISAR-DESIRE-4
   - For scoring balloon
   Ongoing trial

3. *Another stent* (BMS or DES)
   DES: Result with DES for BMS restenosis superior
   - DES for DES restenosis is most popular
   - Better than cutting balloon
   - DES eluting a different drug might be better for drug resistance
   - Works better for Focal ISR (Focal ISR might not be due to drug resistance: diffuse ISR is more likely due to drug resistance)

   RIBS 2
   BAVS BMS for ISR
   Immediate result better in BMS
   Late lumen loss (MLD) equal in both group
   Sub gr: BMS superior for
   1. Large vessel > 3 min
   And
   2. Edge ISR
   Problem: Luminal loss
   Trial: ISAR-DESIRE Trial- DES is superior to BA

4. DEB (ESC 2014 1a)

   Adv Delivery of anti restenotic agent without adding a second metal layer
   - Effective for BMS as well as DES ISR
   - PEPCAD-DES—currently evaluating paclitaxel eluting DEB for treatment of DES ISR

   ISAR DESIRE-3 - non inferiority trial

RESCUT trial
Balloon slippage
Less freq with CB
↓
Less freq stent implantation to obtain satisfactory angiographic result

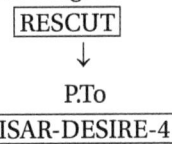

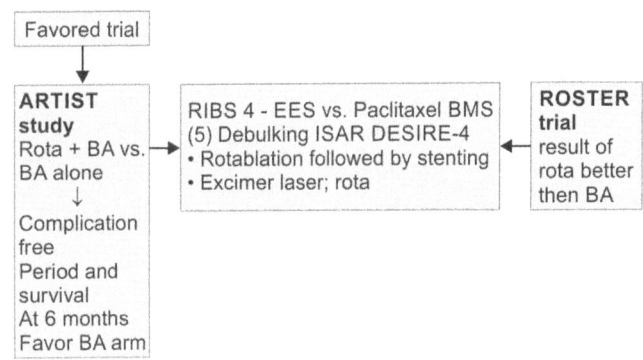

6. *CABG*
   For
   - Multi vessel DES + multi vessel ISR
   - Diffuse or even single vessel ISR at very critical location
   - Any complication or noncompliance issue

7. *Brachytherapy:* Anti proliferative technique
   Trials
   1. SISR (Brachytherapy with DES for BMS ISR Target vessel failure double at follow-up)
   2. TAXUS-V: (BMS ISR treatment with brachy or PES Target vessel revasc high in brachy)

   Problems
   Late catch-up phenomena with brachy — significant reduction of efficacy over time

APPROACH

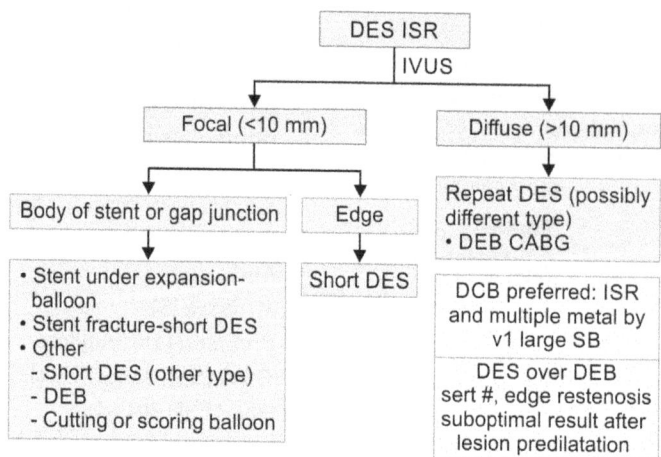

11.14 INTRAVASCULAR ULTRASOUND

Q.1 IVUS in angioplasty. Its limitation and usefulness (Aug 99) (June 03)
Q.2 Intravascular ultrasound (Aug 95) (Feb 97)
Q.3 Describe briefly the method of intravascular imaging. How do they help in imaging of complications after PCI? (Dec 11) (Dec 12)

PRINCIPLE

Intravascular ultrasound (IVUS) uses reflected sound waves to visualize the arterial wall in a two-dimensional tomographic format; analogous to a histological cross section

Used frequency of ultrasound: 20 to 60 MHz
Resolution: 100 to 200 μm

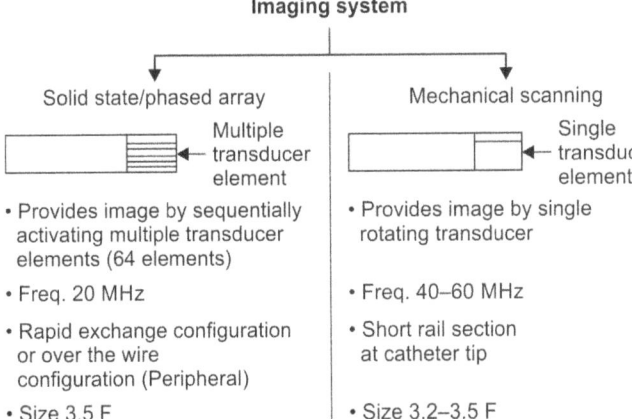

COMPARISON

Mechanical System

Adv:
- Better image quality (40–60 MHz)
- Excellent near field resolution
- No ring down artifact (outer sheath allows uniform movement of transducer in precise manner
- Distance between transducer and distal tip is less—allow its use for distal lesion and CTO lesions

Disadv:
- NURD (nonuniform rotational distortion) due to bending or friction of the drive cable—interferes with uniform rotation— causes wedge shaped smeared image

Solid State System

Adv:
- Rapid exchange desire allows better trackability
- No NURD artifact

Disadv:
- Ring down artifact
- Lower near field resolution—ring artifact

METHOD OF IMAGE ACQUISITION

100 iv/kg of heparin to be administered
↓
Maintain ACT > 250 seconds
↓
Engage LMCA/RCA as per area of interest
↓
0.014 inch PTCA guidewire passed across the lesion
IVUS catheter (outer sheath) thoroughly flushed with saline to remove air bubbles
↓
Catheter connected to pullback motor which is attached to monitor
↓
IVUS catheter passed over the guidewire into the guide catheter
↓
Extra step ["Masking process" is done in the aorta in case of solid state step catheter to avoid ring down artifact]
↓
100–200 ug of NTG given intracoronary to avoid vasospasm
↓
IVUS catheter passed at least 10 mm across the area of interest
↓
Manual/mechanical pullback
↓
Ideally scan from distal vessel upto entire proximal vessel—back to aorta

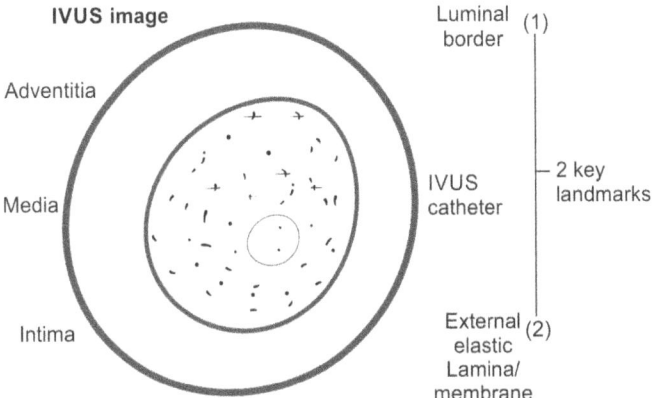

QUANTITATIVE ASSESSMENT

Various parameters obtained
- Lumen area (Intima-to-Intima)
- Total vessel area (EEM - to - EEM)
- Plaque area (difference between total vessel area and lumen area)
- Plaque burden (ratio of plaque area to total vessel area)
- Remodeling index (ratio of ECM CSA at lesion site versus reference site)
  - Positive remodeling index—>1.0 or 1.05
  - Negative remodeling index—<1.0 or 0.95
- Area stenosis = $\frac{RLA - MLA}{RLA} \times 100$

Reference segment: Most normal looking segment within 10 mm from the lesion with no intervening side branch

QUALITATIVE ASSESSMENT

- *Plaque characterization*
  - *Soft:* Echogenicity less than adventitia
  - *Fibrous:* Intermediate echogenicity between those of soft plaque and highly echogenic calcified plaque
  - *Calcified:* Echogenicity higher than that of adventitia with acoustic shadowing
  - *Mixed plaque:* More than one subtype contained in one
- *Plaque characterization by signal analysis technique* 3 different systems

Virtual histology (Volcano)	iMaP system (Boston scientific)	Integrated back scatter (YD corp)
• Fibrous (Dark green)	• Fibrotic (green)	• Fibrotic (green)
• Necrotic (red)	• Necrotic (pink)	• Dense fibrosis (yellow)
• Calcific (white)	• Calcific (light blue)	• Calcific (red)
• Fibro fatty (light green)	• Lipidic (yellow)	• Lipidic (blue)

Limitation
- Limited spatial resolution for detection of thin fibrous cap
- No classification for thrombus, blood or intimal hyperplasia
- Potential errors in plaque with extensive calcification
- *Abnormal lesion morphology*
  - *Thrombus:* Intra luminal mass with layered, lobulated or pedunculated appearance
    - *Fresh:* Relatively Echodense
    - *Old:* Darker ultrasound appearance

  D/D: slow flow; air bubble; stagnant contrast

- *Dissection:* Fissure or separation within intima or plaque
  - Severity can be quantified based on its depth and extent
- *Hematoma*
  - *Intramural:* Blood within medial space; displacing IEM inwards and EEM outwards
  - *Extramural:* Outside arterial wall

  Appear as homogenous, hyper echoic, crescent shaped area
- *Aneurysm*

  True Aneurysm: Intact vessel wall and maximum lumen area 50% larger than proximal reference

  Pseudo aneurysm: Loss of vessel wall integrity and damage to adventitia or perivascular tissue
- *Vulnerable plaque*
  - *Extensive positive remodeling:* Most consistent feature
  - Future events predicted by
    - Plaque burden >70%
    - Minimal lumen area <4 mm^2
    - VH—IVUS determined TGFA (>30% of the Necrotic core abutted the lumen in three or more consecutive frames)

INTERVENTIONAL APPLICATION

- Angiographically intermediate lesion (MLA cut off 3-4 mm^2)
- Calcified lesion
- High risk for distal embolization
  - Large plaque burden (noncalcium related) ⎫
  - Large low-echogenic region suggesting lipid rich plaque
  - Thrombus containing plaque ⎬ Indicators
  - Amount of lipid or Necrotic core on VH-IVUS ⎭
- Left main lesions
- Bifurcation lesions
- CTO lesions
- Restenotic lesion
- IVUS guided selection of device size and length
- IVUS for optimal stent expansion
- IVUS for acute and chronic stent problems

MUSIC = Multicenter ultrasound guided stent implantation in the coronaries.

*[IVUS in complications after PCI]

- *Acute stent problems*

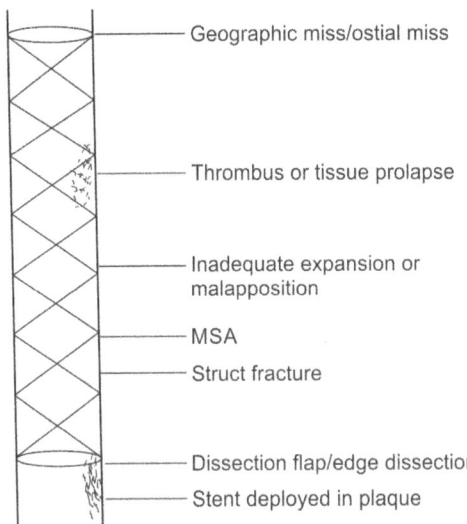

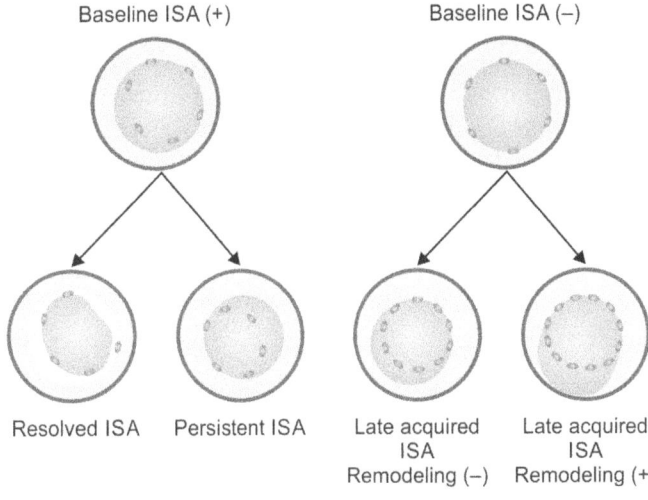

- **MSA: Minimal stent area**
  Optimal PCI results in >90% of mean reference lumen area without any malapposition or under expansion or edge dissection (MUSIC criteria)
- Stent landing in >50% plaque—prone for edge dissection/ restenosis
- Angiographic haziness in the stent
  - Thrombus prolapse—treated conservatively
  - Dissection flap can be treated by balloon
  - Tissue prolapse dilatation
- *Edge dissection*
  IVUS criteria for significant dissection
  - Flap length >0.6 mm
  - Extensive medial tears occupying >50% of vessel circumference (onion skin-like appearance)
  - Final lumen area < 4mm^2
  - Dissection angle >60°
  - Large, moving flap
  Free wall dissections (towards pericardium) are more prone to propagate as compared to dissection of mural wall
- *Under expansion*
  - When MSA <70% of balloon predilated maximal area
  - Stent expansion index (ratio between MSA to mean Proximal and distal reference area) <80%
- Malapposition or ISA (inadequate stent apposition)
  Part of stent structure is not fully in contact with vessel wall
  Acute / Chronic

- *Chronic stent problems*
  - *LISA* (late acquired incomplete stent apposition) due to
    - Thrombus resolution
    - Plaque regression
    - Positive vessel remodeling

Mechanism
- Mechanical vessel injury during stent implantation
- Biological vessel injury by biological agents or polymer
  - *Stent strut fracture*
    - *Def:*
      - Longitudinal strut discontinuity
    - *Char:*
      - Strut separation
      - Strut subluxation
      - Strut intussusceptions
    - *Types:* 1- with aneurysm; 2- without aneurysm
  - *In Stent restenosis:* Primary mechanism can be identified

LIMITATION OF IVUS
- Extensive calcification
- Severe angulations

RECENT ADVANCES
- Lipiscan (FDA approved): IVUS + NIRS
- FLIVUS (forward looking IVUS)
- Integration of RF ablation in FLIVUS (for CTO)
- OCT + IVUS

11.15 LA APPENDAGE AND CLOSURE

Q.1 Describe in brief the role of LA appendage in thromboembolism. Outline current status of LAA occluder device (Dec 12)
Q.2 Devices for LAA occlusion (June 16)
Q.3 Anatomy, imaging and flow pattern of LA appendage (Dec 12)

ANATOMY

- Derived from primordial LA, which is formed mainly by adsorption of primordial pulm vein and their branches
- Finger like projection from main body of LA
- Extends between ant and lat wall of LA and its tip is directed antero superiorly
- Overlaps the left border of RVOT or pulmonary trunk and main stem of LCc or Lcx

EXTERNAL APPEARANCE

- Slightly flattened
- One or more bends
- Pointed tip

Internally

- Orifice is usually oval
- Round, triangular and water drop shapes are observed less frequently
- Left lateral ridge separates the orifice of LPV from LAA
- Smooth muscular wall of LA vestibule separates the orifice from the mitral annulus

Various Shapes

- Chicken wing—MC—approx 50%
- Cactus
- Windsock
- Cauliflower

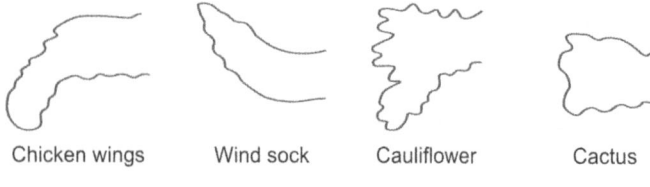

Chicken wings   Wind sock   Cauliflower   Cactus

IMAGING

- *Noninvasive*
  - *TTE and TEE*
    - Most widely used
    - Accurate assessment of morphology and flow pattern of LAA
  - Detection of LAA clot
    Sensitivity 92%
    Specificity 98%
    NPV—100%
    PPV—86%
  - Ultrasound contrast helps for enhanced visualization of LAA
  - Spontaneous echo contrast in LAA—18.2% risk of stroke (untreated)
  - Spont echo contrast ⎫
    Sludge   ⎬ Need anticoagulation
    Thrombus   ⎭
  - Pectinate muscles are part of LAA—no active Treatment (sometimes confused as thrombus)
- *Invasive*
  - Intracardiac Echo
    - Alternate imaging
    - Less sensile (compared to TEE) for detection of thrombus
    - Use is limited only during planned intracardiac procedure
      "Absence of visualizing LAA thrombus does not mean absence of LAA thrombus"
      ↓
      LAA Doppler helps to exclude LAA clot
      ↓
      Normally LAA contract: Biphasic
      Velocity: 50 + or - 60 cm/sec to 83 + or - 23 cm/s
      Highest velocity in NSR
      Intermediate in paroxysmal AF, AFL
      ↓
      Velocity <40 cm/s—highest risk of thrombus
      Velocity <20 cm/s—associated with identification of thrombus

Color Doppler with low Nyquist limit helps visualizing thrombus at tip of LAA
- *MDCT*
  - High spatial, low temporal resolution
  - NPV and sensitivity—100%
  - PPV range from 41–92%
  - Specificity—poor (high false positive rate)

Limitation
LAA mechanical function not routinely evaluated
Significantly low temporal resolution compared to TEE
- *CMRI*
  - Lower spatial resolution
  - Prolonged examination duration

- Dependence on breath holds
- Sensitivity 67%
- Specificity 44%

DEVICE THERAPY FOR LAA

Indication

- Alternative to 0 Acs in patients with nonvalvular AF and CHA2DS2 VAsc score >1
- Concomitant high stroke and bleeding risk
- Adjunct to OAC
  Inpatients developing thromboembolic event while on OAC despite therapeutic INR
- High stroke risk but intolerant to OAC
- Adjunct for patients with AF undergoing concomitant LA procedures such as AF ablation and MitraClip

Various Devices

- *PLATTO:* First device used for LAA closure
  Not available now
- WATCHMAN (Boston scientific)
  - Second generation device
  - Self expanding nitinol frame with PET (polyethylene terephthalate membrane)
  - PET covers 50% of outer frame
  - Blocks thrombus embolization
    - 5 different sizes available
    - 14 F compatible
    - *Study:* WATCHMAN trial

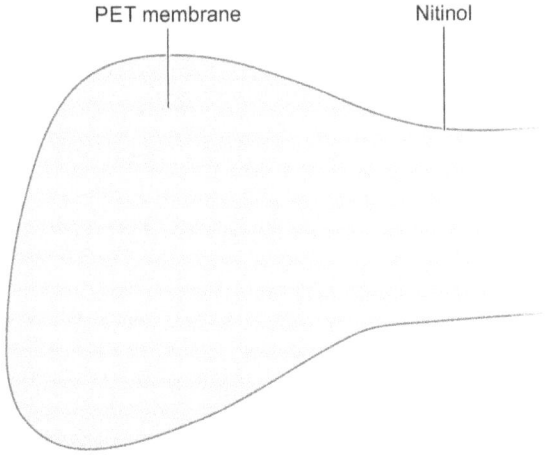

- AMPLATZER CARDIAC PLUG and AMULET (St. Jude)
  - Nitinol mesh and polyester patch
  - Developed on the basis of amplatzer double disk septal occluder
  - Consists of love and disc connected by central waist

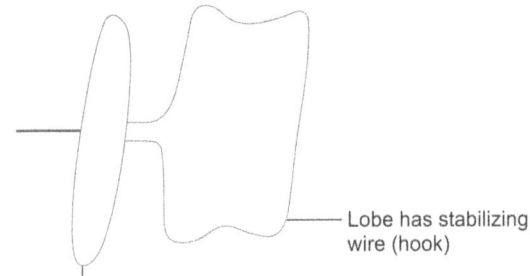

  - Available in 8 sizes
  - Appropriate size chosen to be 10-20% higher than narrowest diameter of LAA body (1-2 cm distal to orifice)
  Trial: AMULET
- *LARIAT Device* (sentreheart)
  (Percutaneous LAA suture ligation)
  Three components
  1. 15 mm compliant occlusion balloon catheter
  2. Magnet tipped guidewire (0.025 and 0.035)
  3. 12 F suture delivery device (LARIAT)
  Trial: PLACE 3

Contraindication

- Low risk for stroke (CHADS2VAsc = 0)
- Valvular heart disease (MS)
- Other indication for long term/lifelong OAC e.g., Mechanical valves, PE, DVT, Infracardiac clot
- Contraindication for Transseptal puncture
  1. LA clot/tumor
  2. Active infection
  3. Presence of ASD/PFO device
  4. Nonoperative patient

Current status
Trials: Protect AF
 Prevail
 CAP
 ASAP

Current Indi

- CHADS2 VAsc ≥ 2 but CI to OAC
- CHADS2 VAsc ≥ 2 and HAS-BLED ≥3
- Embolic events despite OAC
- CHADS2 VAsc ≥ 2 and ESRD
- CHADS2 VAsc ≥ 2 and triple anticoag treatment
- CHADS2 VAsc ≥ 2 and PV isolations
- Alt to OAC in patients with no Increased risk of bleeding

11.16 LEADLESS PACEMAKER

Q.1 What is a leadless pacemaker? Current status of needless permanent cardiac pacing device (June 12)
Q.2 Water leadless pacemaker discuss advantage and disadvantages (June 14)
Q.3 Leadless pacemaker (June 15)
Q.4 Leadless cardiac pacing and give a note on current follow up.

LEADLESS LV PACING

What is CRT with wireless LV endocardial pacing (4 + 4 + 2) (June 17)

Leadless Pacemaker

It is a small implantable device that send electrical impulse to the heart.

It is miniaturized single chamber pacemaker system that is delivered via catheter through femoral vein and directly implanted in RV eliminating need for pocket leads and subclavian access.

Advantages

- Less invasive
- Less procedure time (20–40 mins)
- Less recovery time
- No visible lump or scar

Eliminates complication reputed to transvenous leads
- No lead dislodgement/insulation break
- No lead fracture
- No infection
- No Venous obstruction

No hemothorax/pneumothorax
Maintain shoulder mobility
Less radiation
Better quality of life

Disadvantages

Pace only RV (no DDD pacing)
→*Pacemakers syndrome:* LV dysfunction
No defibrillation capability
No LV pacing
Small risk of procedure related cardiac tamponade
Unanswered question
- Long term follow-up
- Will the device be retractable?
- What is patience develop systemic infection
- Thrombogenic risk of device in long term

Contraindication

- Other implanted devices which uses electrical current (pacemaker, ICD, CRT, neurostimulator)
- Unstable angina/recent MI
- Implanted IVC filter
- Mechanical tricuspid valve
- LV assist device
- Limited or missing femoral venous access-intolerance to titanium or nitinol

Available Devices

Nanostim (St Jude)	Micra (Medtronic)
Released 2012	Released 2013
<10% of size of traditional pacemaker	<30% smaller than Nanostim
Battery life 8.5 to 12.5 years	Battery life 10 to 15 years
Screw in fix to RV	4 times anchor to RV
2 gram rate	2 gram weight
Introducer 18 F	Introducer 24 F

Implantation Procedure

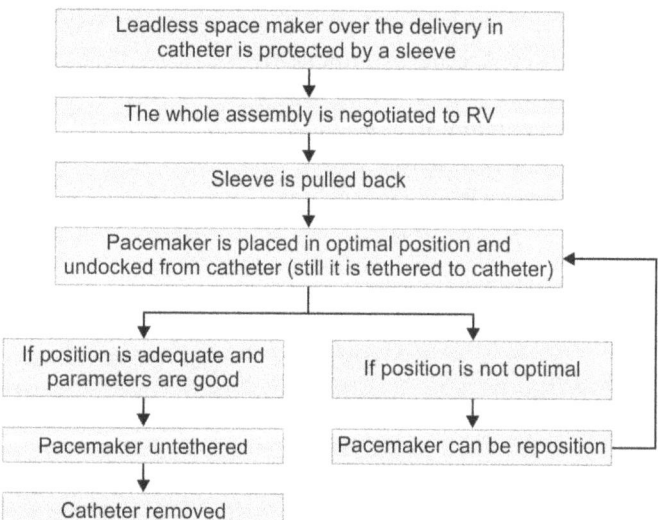

Current Status

- *Leadless trial* (2014)—33 patients
  - Done with Nanostim
  - Implant success rate 97%
  - 5 patients required >1 leadless pacemaker during implantation
  - 1 patient had RV perforation and Cardiac tamponade
  - *Result:* Leadless pacemaker is safe and feasible
- *1 year follow-up of lead less trial*
  - Very stable performance and reassuring safety results
  - Continued evaluation is needed to for the characterize the system

- No device related to adverse events between 3 to 12 months
- *Leadless 2 trial:* 300 patients (2015)
  - Implant success rate = 96%
  - Primary safety and point (freedom from serious adverse effect) achieved in 93%
  - Primary efficacy endpoint (pacing threshold 2V at 0.4 msec) achieved in 90%
  - Therapeutic acceptable sensing (R wave 5.0 MV) achieved in 90%
  - Cardiac perforations 4 patients (1.3%)
    - 2 require Intervention 2 conservative treatment
  - No device migration during implantation
  - Device dislodgement on follow-up = 5 (1.7%)

  Result: Trial met prespecified safety and efficacy endpoint Device is found to be retrievable in subgroup analysis (n = 7)

Leadless LV pacing

- WISE (wireless stimulation endocardially) CRT technology
- Novel, innovative approach
- Alternative to conventional epicardial LV pacing (through coronary veins)

Components

- Intracardiac receiver electrode which paces LV
  - Transmitter with synchronize with RV pacing impulse to transmit ultrasound energy to receiver electrode
- Battery powers the transmitter

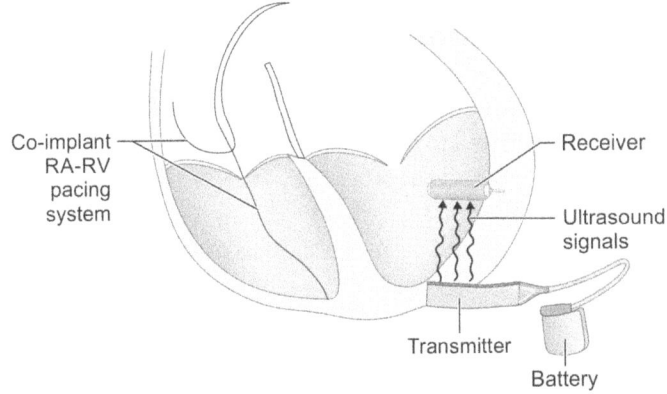

Procedure

- Battery is implanted into left axilla subcutaneous space
- Screening done to find appropriate intercostal space which allows acoustic window to posterior LV that is not impeded by lung—transmitter inserted in this intercostal space
- Implantation of receiver
  - via retrograde root through RFA
  - 12 F sheath

- 8 F electrode catheter inserted in delivery sheath and negotiated into LV
- Optimal position for device confirmed
  Long stimulus -LV timing
  Low threshold
  No latency
  Narrow QRS (adequate synchronization)
- Implant released
- Intracardiac ECG done to check viability of site

Transmitter now synchronizes with RV pacing impulse and activate receiver (LV) via ultrasound waves

Receiver converts ultrasound energy to electrical energy and paces LV

Current Status
- WISE-CRT study (WICS)
  - Total number = 17
  - Successful implantation in 13
  - 3 patients had pericardial effusion
    One patient—no sufficient pacing threshold achieved
  - BiV pacing documented in 83%
    Clinical efficacy in 92%
- SELECT LV study
  (Cardiac recolonization therapy with wireless LV endocardial pacing)
  - 34 patients
  - Successful implant in 33 patients
    - 28 (84.8%) had improvement in clinical composite score at 6 months
    - *Structural remodeling:* Absolute increase in LVEF by 7% and relative decrease in LV ESV by 15%
    - *Electrical Remodeling:* Of intrinsic U QRS by at least 20 minutes in 35% of patients

  Result WISE-CRT system is safe

Advantages
No complications related to subclavian lead
Can be done in cases of
  Failed CRT
  Difficult OS anatomy
  No optimal coronary vein for CRT
  Upgrading PPM/ICD
  High pacing threshold/phrenic nerve stimulus with CS lead
- More advantages anatomical pacing site with longer stimulus-LV time
- Better resynchronize
- Maintain physiological endo-epicardial activation
- No anticoagulation required

11.17 MITRACLIP AND PERCUTANEOUS MITRAL VALVE

Q.1 Outline Percutaneous Interventions to treat with mitral regurgitation. Discuss Indication and contraindication for MitraClip (June 14)
Q.2 Transcatheter treatment of MR (Dec 14)
Q.3 Development of transcatheter mitral valve repair. MV repair studies in heart failure (5+5) (June 17)

MITRACLIP

- MR found in 24% of adults with valvular heart disease
- Mod severe MR prevalence in elderly (>75 years) = 10%

Surgical therapies for MR
- Leaflet repair
- Indirect and direct annuloplasty
- Chordal replacement
- Left ventricular remodeling
- MVR

Transcatheter therapies for MR
- MitraClip
- Carillon mitral annuloplasty device
- Percutaneous MVR

Development

Experiments started by Fredrick SJ Goar in 1998 (based on surgical technique of edge to edge closure for MR creating double orifice)
↓
2003: First human implant by Jose candado in 48 years old lady having severe MR (patient remains asymptomatic and MR remains mild for 7 years)
↓
CE approval in 2008
FDA approval in 2013

Trials

- *EVEREST:* Only patient with DMR, preserved EF and low surgical risk
  Lowest success rates seen EVEREST
- EVEREST high risk ⎤ Function MR with high risk/elderly patients
- ACCESS-EU ⎦ • Good benefit with MitraClip
- TRAMI
- *PERMIT CARE:* Function MR; Ineligible for surgery - MitraClip reduced MR, improved function (LV) and improved function class
- EVEREST 2
- COAPT
- RESHAP-HF

MitraClip Procedure

Device: MRI compatible cobalt chromium device with 2 arms and 2 grippers covered by polypropylene
- Done under GA
- Fluoroscopy and TEE guidance (3D)
- Hemodynamic monitoring by Swan-Ganz catheter
- Trans-septal puncture through RFV route
- Trans-septal sheath exchanged by 24 F steerable guide catheter (22 F at septum)
- MitraClip device advanced through sheath and pushed into LV just below mitral Leaflets

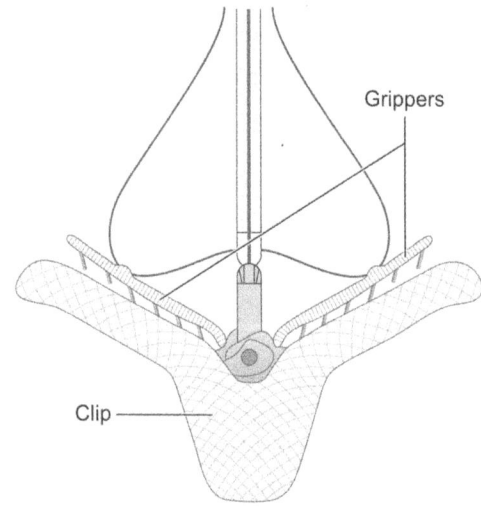

- 2 arms are opened and leaflets edges are allowed to fall into arms
  - Leaflets grasped with grippers
  - Arms are closed to grasp leaflet edges
  - If position satisfactory—device deployed otherwise—reposition
- Width of clip is 5 mm—so flail area >15 mm requires more than 1 clip
- Vena contracta width >10 mm and complex jet involving wide area usually require multiple clips
- Cut off for nock using additional clips are MVA ≤ 2.5 cm and mean PG ≥ 4 mm Hg
- Patient on OAC should continue it
- Rest all patients DAPT × 6 months

Indications

Indicated for percutaneous reduction of
- Significant symptomatic MR (MR ≥ 3t)
- Due to primary abnormality of mitral valve apparatus (degenerative MR) in

- Patients who are determined to be at prohibitive risk for SMVR by heart team and
- In whom existing Comorbidity would not preclude the expected benefit from reduction of MR

Patient Selection

- Prohibitive risk for CMVR by heart team (one or more of following)
  - 30 day STS predicted mortality
    - ≥8% for patients likely to undergo MV replacement
    - ≥6% for patients likely to undergo MV repair
  - Porcelain aorta/extensively calcified ascending aorta
  - Frailty
  - Hostile chest
  - Cirrhosis (MELD >12)
  - Severe PH
- Data regarding safety and efficacy not available for
  - RV dysfunction with severe TR
  - Degenerative MR with LVEF <20% or LVESD >60

TRANSCATHETER THERAPY FOR MR

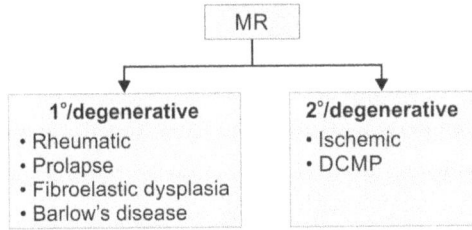

A. *Transcatheter therapy addressing MV annulus*
Principle: Clinching force by device into CS, reducing MV annular size

- Indirect annuloplasty
  - *Coronary sinus approach* (CS reshaping)
    - *MONARC*
      - Historical importance
      - 2 self expanding stents with connecting bridge
      - Late Lcx compression as complication
    - *Carillon mitral contour system*
      - 2 self expanding anchors
        1 in distal greater vein
        2 nd in CS
      - Can be retrieved if Lcx/RCA compress
      - Trials: Amadeus (distal anchor slippage)
        Titan (Prox ankle fracture)
        Titan 2 (improvement in design)
    - *VTGcor:* Delivery of 1-3 stiffening bars inside CS to exert tension on post annulus
      Problem: Dislodgement
    - *ARTO system:* Anchor placed in CS connected to interracial septal occluder
      - Under phase 1 trial
  - *Asymmetric approach:* NIH-cerclage
    - Only animal tested
    - Wires inside CS
    - Creates a near complete circumferential annuloplasty
- Direct annuloplasty
  - *Percutaneous mechanical cinching*
    - *Mitralign*
      - Emulate suture segmental annuloplasty
      - 2 sets of paired surgical pledgets are delivered percutaneously through post annulus and pulled together to plicate annulus
    - *Accucinch*
      - 15 anchor along ventricular surface of MV annulus
      - via LV approach
    - Millipede ring system
    - Ample PS3 system
  - *Percutaneous energy mediated cinching*
    1. *Quantum cor:* Uses RF energy at sub ablative temperature to produce contraction of MV annulus to reduce MR
    2. *Recor:* High freq ultrasound based MV annuloplasty
  - *Hybrid (needing surgery)*
    - *Adjustable annuloplasty ring:* Surgically implanted catheter that can be adjusted late
    - *Encor dynaplasty ring:* Surgically implanted annuloplasty can be adjusted post surgery under physiological condition
    - *Cardinal ring*
    - *Valtech cardioband*
    - *TASRA:* (Transapical segmented reduction annuloplasty): Transapical based approach to annuloplasty

B. *Transcatheter therapy addressing leaflet*
Principle: Based on surgical technique of suturing anteromedial and posterolateral leaflet to reduce MR

- Edge to edge leaflet plication
  - MitraClip (see later)
  - *Mitraflex* Designed for direct thoracoscopic approach through apex of o beating heart
  - *Mobius:* Used as suture to create double orifice MV
    Problem: Suture dehiscence
        Program was abandoned.
- Space occupier (leaflet coaptation)
  - *Percu-pro:* Using space occupying "buoy" anchored at the LV apex through trans-septal approach—fills the gap between 2 leaflets in systole

- Leaflet ablation
  - Thermocol irrigation ablation electrode RFA approach
    Catheter placed in contact with AML and RFA delivered—scarring and fibrosis and reduced leaflet motion

C. Transcatheter therapy addressing chordae
- Chordal implant
  Transapical—artificial cord
  - *Neochord:* Suffering of flail segment
  - *Miraflex:* Putting anchor on inner LV myocardium and another anchor on leaflet—connecting 2 will reduce MR

  Transapical—Transseptal cord
  - *Babic:* Device introduced trans apically and exteriorized through transseptal route. An elastic polymer tube is interposed between leaflet and free myocardial Wall and secured to the epicardial surface by adjustable knob

D. Transcatheter therapy addressing papillary muscle and LV
- *Myocor i-coapsys system:* 2 epicardial chords connected by a load bearing transventricular chords. All delivered through a post inserted in pericardium with percutaneous subxiphoid approach
- *Mardil BACE:* Wide band slipped around base of beating heart without CPB
- *Tendyne repair:* Self expanding transapical mitral valve implant with LV apical tether
- Parachute LV partitioning device

E. Transcutaneous MV replacement
- Right minithoracotomy—endovalve Hermann prosthesis (foldable mitral prosthesis)
- Transapical—Lutter prosthesis, TIARA, Fortis valve, Tendyne
  1. *TIARA:* Nitinol based valve
     Self expanding frame
     Covered by bovine pericardium
     Ventricular anchor fixed the valve onto fibrous trigone and post annulus
  2. *Tendyne:* Transapical
     Self expanding tri Leaflet porcine pericardium bioprosthesis with LV tether
  3. *Fortis valve:* Consists of central valve body and a cylinder; 3 pericardial leaflet and paddles
- Trans septal
  - *Cardia and prosthesis:* Unique frames suffer annular anchoring without radial force and preserve chords and uses native leaflets
- Transatrial Medtronic valve

MitraClip

Indications
- Candidates for MV surgery
  - Symptoms with >25% EF and LVEDV ≤ 55
  - Asymptomatic with one or more of
    LVEF 25–60%
    LVESD >40
    PAH
    AF
- Mod to severe (3t) or severe (4t) MR
  - Large and central color flow jet (>6 cm², or >30% of LA area)
  - Pulm vein flow may show systolic blunting or systolic flow reversal
  - Vena contracta width >5 cm (PLAX)
  - Regurgitant vol >45 mL/beat
  - Regurgitant fraction ≥ 40%
  - Regurgitant orifice area ≥ 0.3 cm²
- Sufficiently leaflet tissue for mech coaptation
- Nonrheumatic/endocarditis valve pathology
- Pathology in A2-P2 area
- Coaptation length >2 mm and width <11 mm
- Flail gap <10 mm
- Flail width <5 mm
- MV orifice >4 cm
- Mobile Leaflet length >1 cm

Contraindications
- Infective endocarditis
- Rheumatic MV disease
- Presence of LA clot and venous thrombosis
- Inability to tolerate antiplatelet and anticoagulation
- AMI within 12 wks
- Need for other cardiac surgery
- Renal insufficiency
- Anatomical exclusion
  - MVA <4 cm²
  - Leaflet flail width ≥ 15 mm and gap ≥ 10 mm
  - Leaflet tethering/coaptation depth >11 mm and length <2 mm
  - Short PML
  - Jet origin involvement in A1P1 or A3P3
  - Restricted PML + mobile AML
  - Calcification in grasping area
  - Severe annular calcification
  - MV cleft
  - Extensive immobilization of leaflet
  - Severe calcification in papillary muscle or chordae
- Systemic disease affecting MV apparatus

Complications

- *Allergic reaction:* (Anesthetic, contrast, heparin, nickel alloy, latex)
- Vascular site complication
- Arrhythmias (AF)
- Iatrogenic ASD requiring intervention
- Device embolization or partial clip detachment
- Leaflet tear
- Chordae entanglement/rupture
- Cardiac perforation/tamponade

Trials

- EVEREST 1
- EVEREST 2
- COAPT
- RESHAP-HF
- REALISM
- ACCESS-EV
- TRAMI
- Valki et al. systematic review

Topol-799

Causes of Mic:
1. Annular dilatation
2. Papillary muscle dysfunction
3. Chordal tethering
4. Loss of annular contraction
5. Spherical LV
6. Apical and post displacement of pap muscle

11.18 OPTICAL COHERENCE TOMOGRAPHY

Q.1 What is OCT? Discuss its utility and compare with IVUS (June 14)

Q.2 Role of OCT in predicting vulnerable plaques what are other modalities of intravascular imaging (6 + 4) (June 27)

Q.3 Principle and cardiovascular application of OCT (June 12)

INTRODUCTION

Principle: Back scattered reflections of infrared light
Resolution: High (10 times higher than OCT)
Infrared light 1300 nm wavelength

IMAGING SYSTEM

Components
- Computer processor and display console
- Fiber Optic catheter
- Catheter interface unit including motor drive
- Optical engine emitting and receiving infrared light

Optical Engine

- Includes super luminescent diode as a source of infrared light
- 2 generations of system
  First generation (TD-OCT)
  Second generation (FD-OCT)

1st gen (TD-OCT)	*2nd gen (FD-OCT)*
Time domain -OCT	Frequency domain OCT
↓	Fourier domain OCT
	↓
Obtain a line at low speed as frame rates are low (15–20 FPS)	Obtain a line at higher speed so achieves higher frame rates (100–160 FPS)
Axial resolution: 10–20 um	10–20 um
Lateral resolution: 25–30 um	25–30 um

Catheter

- Fiber optic care encapsulated in an optically transparent, imaging sheath
- *TD-OCT:* Fiber optic core within translucent sheath outer diameter 0.019 inch
  St. Jude; St. Paul
- *FD-OCT:* Imaging probes integrated in short monorail catheter outer dia = 2.6 to 3.2 F

Image Acquisition Process

Same as IVUS except
- Achieving blood free medium for OCT

Two methods
1. Occlusive technique with proximal balloon inflated at 0.3 to 0.5 atm pr (for TD-OCT)
2. Continuous flushing technique (for FD-OCT/TD-OCT)
   Flush with
   - Contrast
   - Low mol wt dextran
   - Ringer's lactate

Flushing speed (FD-OCT) = 3–6 mL/sec (Power injector)
Pull back speed = 20–40 mm/sec

For TD-OCT flushing can be done from distal part of balloon while its inflated @ rate of 0.5–1.0 mL/sec

Image Interpretation

Three layered vessel wall
1. *Intima:* Highly back scattering
2. *Media:* Low back scattering
3. *Adventitia:* Heterogeneous and highly back scattering

Periadventitial tissue presents as an appearance consistent with adipocyte (large clear structure resembling cells and/or vessels)

OCT can image through calcium with shadowing

ARTIFACTS

- Point artifact—due to guidewire
- NURD—wedge shaped smeared appearance in one or more image
- Seam line—appear as axial discontinuity due to cardiac motion or rapid pullback
- Tangential signal dropout when the optical beam is directed nearly parallel to tissue surface—appear like thin cap fibroatheroma
- High intensity area in imaging sheath (due to blood in sheath)
- Sunflower or merry-go round artifacts—appear as smeared stent strut towards OCT catheter seen when OCT catheter is off-centered within the artery
- *Saturation artifacts:* Linear streak of high intensity/low intensity. Due to strong refractors like guidewire or stent shut (high intensity backscatter)
- Reverberation appears at replica at a fixed distance from primary image of an object

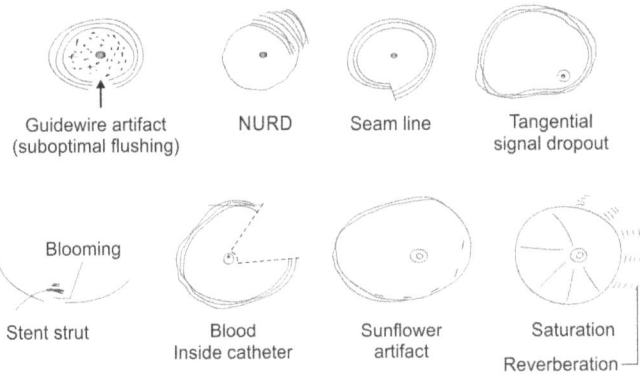

QUANTITATIVE ASSESSMENT

Same as IVUS except
- OCT is not suitable for study of plaque burden or vessel remodeling due to its limited signal penetration through the diseased arterial wall

QUALITATIVE ASSESSMENT

- Plaque characterization
  - *Fibrous:* Signal rich (high backscatters)
  - *Calcified:* Signal poor region with sharply defined borders
  - *Lipid rich:* Signal poor region with poorly defined, diffuse borders
  - Fibrotic cap—appears as signal rich band overlaying a lipid pool or Necrotic core
  - Macrophage in fibrous cap—signal rich distinct punctate regions that exceeds in the intensity Cholesterol crystal Thin linear region of high intensity
  - *Erythrocyte—rich (Red) thrombus:* High backscattering with high signal attenuation
  - *Platelet rich (white) thrombus:* Less back scattering with low signal attenuation and homogeneous appearance
- Vulnerable plaque
  OCT can identify
  - Lipid pool ⎤
  - Thin fibrous cap ⎥ OCT is suitable for identification of vulnerable plaque
  - Macrophage accumulation ⎥
  - Detailed surface morphology ⎦
    * Lightest resolution 10-20 um
    * Excellent sensitivity and specificity
    * The only imaging modality that can identify plaque with cap thickness of 65 μm or less
    * Gold standard to identify plaque neovascularization

THIN CAP FIBRO ATHEROMA (TCFA)

OCT definition: OCT delineated lipid or Necrotic core with an overlying fibrous cap, where minimum thickness of the fibrous cap is less than predetermined threshold

↓

Most commonly used threshold = 65 um
(based on histopathologic studies)

↓

Needs to be adjusted for in vivo analysis, to correct for tissue shrinkage (10-20%) that occur during histopathological processing

*Cap thickness alone is insufficient to identify lesion at risk of rupture

Additional parameters
- Lipid or Necrotic core should cover are of >90°
- Plaque comprises more than 1 quadrant of vessel circumference

CLINICAL APPLICATION OF OCT

- Peri Interventional plaque assessment
  - Plaque characterization
  - Red/white thrombus
  - TCFA
  - Plaque rupture/erosion
  - Luminal and EEM-EEM area
  - OCT can penetrate calcium - ability to assess thickness of superficial calcium
- Acute stent problems
  - *Stent geometry:* Apposition and expansion
  - Apposition can be measured (unlike IVUS) as distance between adluminal surface of strut and vessel wall
  - If strut vessel distance>strut thickness—malapposition
  - Thrombus/plaque protrusion
  - Dissection
  - Geographic miss/ostial miss
- Chronic stent problems
  - Stent apposition (types)
    * Apposed and covered
    * Apposed and uncovered
    * Nonapposed but covered
    * Nonapposed and uncovered
  - Discriminate between neo intimal coverage of stent vs. ISR (fibrin covering)
  - ISR
  - Assessment of BRS
    (preserved box; open box; dissolved bright box or dissolved black box)

FUTURE PERSPECTIVES

- OCT + IVUS
- OCT + rotational atherectomy catheter (approved in Europe for peripheral intervention)
- Spectroscope analysis of infrared light
  Color adding of OCT image (like VH-IVUS)
- Polarization analysis measuring degree of birefringence in the tissue—discriminate in plaque content
- OCT + elastography

	OCT	IVUS
Resolution	10–20 um	100–200 um
Penetration	2 mm	10 mm
Based on pull back	Infrared light 20–40 mm/sec	Sound waves 0.5–2 mm/sec
Blood less field	Required	Not required

Contd...

Contd...

	OCT	IVUS
Frame Rate	100 FPS	30 FPS
Application	Cardiac only	Cardiac + peripheral
Vessel border	Limited	Yes
Lesion length	Limited	Yes
Dissection, thrombus prolapse	Yes	Yes
Incomplete stent apposition	Yes	Yes
Stent strut coverage	Yes	Limited
Thin cap fibroatheroma	Yes	Limited
Ostial lesion evaluation	+	Better than OCT
Calcium	Can see beyond Calcium	Cannot

11.19 OTHER MODALITIES OF INTRAVASCULAR

OTHER MODALITIES OF INTRAVASCULAR IMAGING

Percutaneous Coronary Angioscopy

- Provides real-time fully colored images of luminal surface of coronary artery
- Visualize surface color and structure
- Visualize
  - Morphology of atherosclerotic plaque
  - Thrombus
  - Intimal flap
- Uses fiber-optic catheter for illumination and recording system
- High intensity white light is used for imaging
- Blood free field is required
  - Occlusion technique—SF compatible
  - Flushing technique—CF compatible
- Image interpretation based on surface color and endoluminal morphology
- Normal grayish white and smooth in contour
- *Atherosclerotic plaque:* Varying degree of yellowish color with or without visible irregularities on luminal surface
  ↓
  Yellowness increases as fibrous cap thins
- Dissection can be seen as crack/fissure
- Red/white thrombus based on color
- *Intramural hematoma:* Bulge with reddish surface

Spectroscopy (To Identify Components of Plague)

- Near infrared spectroscopy (NIRS)
- Raman spectroscopy
- Fluorescence Spectroscopy

Principle: When tissues are exposed to a light beam containing a broad mixture (spectrum) of wavelengths, wavelengths absorbed by illuminating surface will be absent from the spectrum.

NIRS: Analyze amount of these absorbance as a function of wavelengths within near infrared window.
↓
Tomographic 20 image with 'chemogram' current system is specifically designed to detect lipid (yellow color) Color scale from red to yellow indicates increasing probability of lipid component in vessel wall.

Intravascular Paleography/Elastography

- Thin fibrous layer, large lipid core and inflammatory cells can alter stress—strain relationship of coronary vessels.
- Elastography determine mechanical property of vascular wall
- Color coding of strain values are done and superimposed on IVUS image
- Color coding
   Purple: Hard and stiff part (low strain)
   Yellow: Soft and deformable (high strain)
- Highly sensitive and specific for vulnerable plague determination.

Intracoronary Thermography

- Atherosclerotic lemon with high levels of inflammation produces heat due to
- Leukocyte metabolic activity
- Ineffective metabolism
- Increased neoangiogenesis
  ↓
  Coronary temperature monitoring catheters are under investigations
  ↓
  Can detect temperature change of 0.05°C with spatial resolution of 0.5 mm

Disadvantage:
- Chances of vessel wall injury due to direct contact
- Multiple artifacts due to hemodynamic variations.

INTRAVASCULAR RADIATION DETECTOR

In early stage of development
- 18FDa—to detect metabolism
- 99mTc monocyte chemotactic peptide to detect receptor expression
- 99mTc annexin V—to detect apoptosis

Intravascular MRI (under investigation)

11.20 RADIATION HAZARDS

INTRODUCTION

- Unit of absorbed radiation = Gray
- Absorbed dose of radiation expressed as "Effective dose"
    Effective Dose expressed in sieverts (SV) units (SI unit) or REM (non-SI unit)
      1 SV = 100 REM
      1 Gray = 0.75 SV

LIMIT

- Occupational dose limit for adults = 5 REM/yr = 5,000 m REM = 50 SV
- Nonoccupational dose limit for adults = 0.1 rem/yr = 100 m REM
- Pregnant worker dose limit = 0.5 rem/0 month

Annual occupational dose limit (per year)
- Whole body—5,000 mrem
- Extremities—50,000 mrem
- Lens of eye—15,000 mrem
- Fetus—500 mrem
- Gen public—100 millirem

ASSESSMENT OF RADIATION EXPOSURE

- *Dosimeter:* Highly sensitive
  - Two types
    - Body dosimeter
    - Ring dosimeter
  - Protocol
    - Single badging
    - Double badging

  Estimated dose range for cath lab = 1 to 10 nsV
  Equivalent to 2-3 yrs of natural background radiation
  1 Diagnostic CAG = 7 MSV
  1 PCI = 15 MSV
  1 RFA = 15 MSV

- *Effective Dose Equivalent* (risk of doses from CA/hereditary defects) (HE = 1.5 HW + 0.04 HN)
    (W = waist and N = neck)

  It is recommended that occupational worker's cumulative effective dose equivalent should not exceed that person's age multiplied by 10

EFFECT OF RADIATION

- Deterministic effect—dose related
- Stochastic effect—related to probability and not proportional to dose
    ↓
  Both char by delay between effect and radiation
  Delay means hours to years

Symptoms of Ac Radiation

0–0.25 SV = None
0.25–1 SV = Nausea, loss of appetite, bone marrow, LN
1–3 SV = BM, LN, Spleen, severe Nausea
3–6 SV = Infection, Diarrhea, sterility, skin peeling
6–10 SV = above + CNS impairment
>20 SV = Death

- *Immediate effects:* Can damage esp fast growing cells
  - Brain = Fatigue, nausea
  - Hair follicle—Hair loss
  - Intestine—Diarrhea, malnutrition
  - Skin cells—sores, peeling
  - WBC and BM-Immune syst failure
- *Later effect*
  - DNA damage
  - Egg and sperm cells with damaged DNA
  - Body cells develop tuner/abnormal growth
  - Blood cell damage—leukemia
- *Stochastic effects:*
  - Neoplasm
  - Heritable genetic effects

CLINICAL PRESENTATION OF CV RADIATION

- Chronic skin injury
- Eye cataract (post surface)
- Vascular Aging
- Thyroid Disease
- Carcinogenesis—Brain, skin, thyroid
- Brain tumor—86% in (lt) side of brain

PROTECTION

- *Operator and team*
  - Use appropriate protective garments
  - Maximize distance of operator from X-ray source
  - Keep above—table and below table shield
  - Keep all body parts out of the field of view
  - Keep table height high
  - Keep exposure time to minimum
  - Minimum cine images
    - Less steep angles
    - Lower frame rate
    - Less magnified view
    - Use collimation
  - Real time dose tracking system
  - Nearer fluoroscopic techniques
  - Robotic assisted PCI

- *To patient:*
  - Plan procedure before hand
  - Keep table height high
  - Keep extremities-out of brain
  - Minimize cont exposure to any 1 area (try changing views)
  - Keep radiation close in check

ALARA
- As low as reasonably achievable
- Can be achieved by applying triad of
  - Increasing distance
  - Decreasing time
  - Use of shielding

11.21 RENAL STENTING AND DENERVATION

RENAL ARTERY STENOSIS

Q.1 Role of renal denervation in treatment of hypertension. (June 12)

INTRODUCTION
Renal artery stenosis is recognized cause of 2° HTN
- Flash pulm edema
- Renal dysfunction

CAUSES OF RAS
- Part of systemic atherosclerotic disease (90%)
- FMD
- Systemic vasculitis
- Post radiation
- Transplant graft scarring

Prevalence of RAS increases with
- Age
- DM
- PVD

CLINICAL CLUES FOR RENAL ART STENOSIS (RAS)
- Onset of HTN before 30 yrs
- Severe HTN after 55 yrs
- Accelerated, resistant or malignant HTN
- New azotemia or worsening renal function after administration of ACEI or ARBS
- Unexplained atrophic kidney (size discrepancy >15 cm between 2 kidneys)
- Sudden unexplained pulm edema
- Unexplained renal dysfunction
- Multi vessel CAD or PAD
- Unexplained CHF or refractory angina

DIAGNOSIS
- Conventional angio
  - Elevated trans-stenotic gradient >21 mm Hg
- CT angio
- MR angio
- Renal Doppler
  - Post stenotic dilatation
  - Elevated trans-stenotic velocity
  - Elevated trans-stenotic gradient
  - Blood flow turbulence

MEDICAL TREATMENT
- Control of dyslipidemia
- Antiplatelets
- *Control of HTN:* ACE/ARBS

Surgery
Reserved for
- Complex anatomy
- Need for concurrent aortic surgery
- Nephrectomy of an atrophic, nonfunctional kidney—improves BP

PTRA (Renal Angioplasty)
Indication
- Resistant or uncontrolled HTN and failure of 3 anti-hypertensive drug (including diuretic)
- HTN with intolerance to medication
- Ischemic nephropathy
- Post transplant RAS
- Cardiac destabilization syndrome (recurrent unexplained CHF or sudden unexplained pulm edema)

+ RAS >70% or 50–70% with significant gradient

Contraindication
- Advanced disease—creat > 3–4 mg/dL
- Kidney length <8 cm
- Limited life expectancy
- Generally poor surgical or PTCA candidate
- Bleeding diathesis
- Recent MI
- Pregnancy

Success Rate
Meta-analysis of 14 studies
- Angiographic success—98%
- Clinical response for HTN—70%
  - 20% Cured
  - 50% Improved
- Renal function improvement 30%
- Renal function stabilized 40%

Patient Selection
- Translesional gradient ≥ 20 mm Hg
- Translesional resting FFR (Pd/Pa) <0.90 (measurements should be done with 4 Fr catheter)

- Hyperemic gradient (paperesin, dopamine, Ach)

    Paparenin - 32 mg   - S/E: Hypotension
    Ach   - 100 ug - S/E: Hypotension, tachy arr
    Dopamine - 50 ug /kg - S/E: Tachyarrhythmia

    Cut off for FFR = 0.7–0.8
- Renal frame count: Total number of frames for contrast to reach visible distal artery RFC >30—predicts improvement post stenting

Recent trials
- *Recent RCT:* Renal revascularization does not confer significant benefit with respect to preservation of kidney function or prevention of adverse kidney and cardiovascular events

  ↓

  Possible due to selection bias
  High risk patients with clinically significant RAS were excluded
- *ASTRAL (2009):* Stent placement in patients with atherosclerotic renal artery stenosis and impaired renal function
  STAR (2009) angioplasty and stenting for renal artery lesion

  ↓

  Failed to detect any benefit regarding GFR decline, BP, kidney function, mortality CV events

  ↓

  Concluded, renal artery revascularization carries substantial procedure related risk without any clinical benefits
- 2014
  CORAL study: (cardiovascular outcomes in renal atherosclerotic lesion)
  Comparing OMT vs. renal stenting
  - Compared with OMT, lower SBP was observed in stented group but number of anti hypertensive did not differ

  ↓

  Conclusion: RAS does not have significant benefit for prevention of clinical events in atherosclerotic renal artery stenosis patients
  Limitation: Enrolment did not require true renovascular hypertension
  - Exclusion criteria precluded patients with recent episode of CHF (might have benefited from stenting)

From above studies:
- Medical management should be considered for patients with RAS
- Revascularization should be reserved for selected subgroups

- Cardiac disturbance syndrome (flesh pulmonary edema or ACS) with severe HTN
- Resistant HTN
- Ischemic nephropathy with CKD with CGFR <45 cc/min and global renal ischemia (unilateral significant RAS with solitary kidney or bilateral significant RAS)

FMD
- Balloon angioplasty only
- Rarely require stenting
- Procedural success 82–100%
- Restenosis <10%
- Cure of HTN 58–60%
- Improvement in HTN 35%

Nonspecific Aortoarteritis
- Balloon angioplasty treatment of choice
- Procedural success 80–90%
- Restenosis 13–26%
- Cutting balloon improve procedural success rate

Pediatric RAS

Takayasu and FMD are most common cause

  ↓   ↓
  India   Western data

RENAL DENERVATION

Q.1 Current status of renal sympathetic denervation
                                               (Dec 14)
Q.2 Renal denervation current role   (June 16)

Catheter based renal denervation using RF energy is an approach to disrupt renal sympathetic nerve activity—results in lowering BP in patients with resistant HTN

  ↓

- Underlying pathophysiologic concept is sound
- Historical observation shown that surgical sympathectomy can lead to significant reduction in BP and CV mortality

  ↓

  Latest SYMPLICITY HTN-3 trial

  ↓

  Brought renal denervation under question

MOA
Target of RON are both post ganglionic efferent nerves and renal stenosis (afferent nerves)

Overactivity of efferent nerves causes' renal vasoconstriction stimulates renin release and impairs Natriuretics

Overactivity of renal afferent nerve causes triggers reflex efferent symp nerve activation not only in kidney but also in heart, skeletal muscle and spleen

- SYMPLICITY HTN-3

  Conclusion: Catheter based RDN was safe but was not associated with significant reduction of office or ambulatory BP

  Criticism
  - Baseline office BP ≥180 mm Hg, aldosterone Antagonist use and nonuse of vasodilators were predictor of SBP change at 6 months follow up in RDN group patients
  - 22% patients had change in antihypertensive medication 2-6 weeks prior to screening

  Possible reasons for neg SYMPLICITY HTN 3 trial
  1. *Patients' selection:* All patients with resistant HTN will not have overactive symptoms
  2. *Incomplete denervation:* No procedure to verify completeness of RDN
  3. *Trial design issue:* Medication noncompliance may be confounding factor
     - Only 84% received complete ablation of 120s duration
     - 6% of all patients received 2 four quadrant ablation; 20% received 1 four quadrant ablation; 74%—no four quadrant ablation
     - Non-African American receiving renal denervation had a significantly greater change in office BP

- PRAGUE-15
  - Studied efficacy and safety of catheter based RDN
  - Used medtronic's SYMPLICITY DEVICE vs. OMT
    - Patients with OMT group received significantly more drugs after 6 months
    - RDN significantly lower 24 hr and office BP. OMT does also
    - In OMT group S. CR increased and in group difference it borderline favored RDN in decreasing creat

- RAPID study
  - One shot renal denervation system used
  - Suggests effective ablation of renal symp nerves lowers office and ambulatory BP in patients with uncontrolled HTN

- Reduced HTN study
  - RDN with balloon based multi electrode bipolar RF system provides clinically meaningful BP reduction and favors safety profile for patients with resistant HTN

Present scenario

- Currently available evidences strongly suggest that RDN lowers BP in hypertensive patients
- However, SYMPLICITY-3 questioned effectiveness (superiority) of RDN over OMT

↓

Much more scientific evidences are needed before any conclusion is drawn

↓

Time has come to turn the page on RDN for HTN, but by all means let's not close the book

11.22 ROTATIONAL ATHERECTOMY

MECHANISM OF ACTION

Rota excavates tissue and reduces lesion rigidity by attacking calcified atherosclerotic plaque by drill
↓
Based on theory of differential cutting, rotablation pulverizes rigid atherosclerotic plaque which is not able to deflect and still preserve the integrity of flexible artery wall
↓
Hard plaque abraded into small particles (average size <5 μm)

EQUIPMENT

- Rotalink burr and advancing device that contain turbine and drive shaft
- Consol to regulate motion of burr
- Dynaglide foot padel
- Rotawire
  - 0.009 inch
  - Flexible distal platinum part (20 mm)

Burr:
- Nickel coated
- 2000-3000 microscopic diamond crystals on leading surface
- Diamonds are 20 um size and protrude only 5 um beyond surface
- Various size = 1.25-2.5 mm
- 140-190 RPM (lower speed associated with lower platelet activation and aggregation)
- Runs 15-20 second

TRIALS

- ROSTER (1996)
- COBRA (1996)
- DART (1998)
- ERBAC (1998)
- SPORT (1999)
- STRATAS (2000)
- CARAT (2000)
- ARTIST (2002)
- ROSTER (2002)
- ROTAXUS (2013) (1° endpoint was late lumen loss)

1. *STRATA:* Study to determine transluminal rotational emulator and transluminal angioplasty strategy
   - Compared aggressive debulking with mod debulking
     - *Aggressive:* Burr size: artery ratio = 0.7-0.9
     - *Moderate:* Size art less than 0.7
     ↓
   - Clinical success similar
   - Higher MI and restenosis with aggressive rota
2. *CARAT:* Coronary angioplasty and rotablator atherectomy
   Compared large burr (>0.7 ratio) with small burr (<0.7 ratio)
   ↓
   Large burr caused more angiographic complication
   These two trials recommended single burr for each procedure with size based on ratio of 0.5-0.6
3. *Multiple trials*
   Angiographic restenosis and 30 days MACE rate higher than conventional PTCA

LESION SELECTION

- Rigid lesion
  - Unable to cross balloon
  - Undilatable at >20 atm prq
- Long calcified lesion—small burr recommended

PRECAUTION

- Angulated lesion (>60%) relative C/I
- Band
- Lesion in band of >90% stenosis strong C/I
- Rotating burr not allowed to go beyond the point of contact with spring tip of rota wire
- Burr not allowed to stop at one location
- Gental retraction and readvancement
- Never pull back rotating burr in guiding cath
- Avoid rota in dissected segment lesion with visible thrombus

ORBITAL ATHERECTOMY

MOA: Based on principle of elliptical burr movement, in which rotational speed determines the effective burr size

It uses eccentrically mounted diamond coated crown

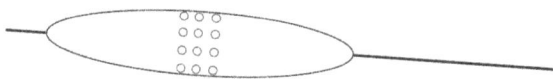

- Speed 80,000-120,000 rpm
- Repeated passes of crown across calcified lesion "sands" away rigid plaque but allow elastic wall to flex away from the crown

Equipment: Diamond back 360° orbital atherectomy system (burr size up to 2 mm)

Procedure is same as except
- Leading tip never advanced within 5 mm of distal opaque portion of viper wire
- Ablation runs limited to 30 seconds

Note: Allows blood to flow across the elliptical burr
↓
So micro particles smaller than rota and blood allow its clearing easily

Trials: Based on Oct (15 mm Ca^{++}) and IVOS (270° of Ca^{++} arc) ORBIT-1 and Orbit 2

Cutting Balloon

3–4 sharp metal microtome blade mounted on noncomplaint balloon
↓
Incise and score coronary atheroma

MOA: Reduce risk of uncontrolled tear (longitudinal) in vessel wall which can be caused by conventional balloon
↓
CBM makes controlled micro incision in atheromatous plaque in controlled fashion
↓
Lesion can be dilated at lower pressure as compared to conventional balloon

Equipments:
- Flextome cutting balloon or
- Cutting balloon ultra 2 (monorail)

Flexstome: Contain flex point every 5 mm along the length for greater flexibility and deliverability
- Length = 6, 10, 15 mm
- Bounded to pad mounted on balloon
- Number of blades (atherotomes)
    3 on 2 mm and 3.25 mm 4 on 3.5 mm balloon
    4 on 3.5 mm and 4 mm balloon

Lesion Selection
- Bifurcated lesion
- Ostial lesion
- ISR

Complication
Risk of coronary perforation slightly higher than conventional RTCA

Trials
- CAPAS (1997)
- CUBA (1997)
- GRT (1997)
- CBASS (1999)
- BETACUT (2002)—ISR
- RESCUT (2002)—ISR
- REDUCE-2 (2002)—ISR
- REDUCE-3 (2003)—Stenting

GRT: Reported no difference in CAG restenosis between CBA and balloon PTCA

RESCUT: (Restenosis cutting balloon trial)

Reported no difference in restenosis between CBA and balloon PTCA

REDUCE 2: Reported slightly higher restenosis rates after CBA than PTCA

REDUCE 3: Reported lower restenosis rate with CBA (11.8%) vs. PTCA (19.6%)

11.23 STENT THROMBOSIS

Q.1 What is stent thrombosis? Discuss its etiopathogenesis and diagnostic criteria (June 12)

INTRODUCTION

Stent thrombosis	ISR
Freq presents as MI Time frame from Original implantation—short Angio picture—thrombus is soft	• Presents as MI rarely • Long time Neo intimal Hyperplasia reliably seen and measured on CAG Neointimal tissue is hard and associated with balloon slippage

DEFINITION (ARC—ACADEMIC RESEARCH CONSORTIUM)

- *Definite stent thrombosis*
  Angiographic confirmation
  - Occlusive or non—occlusive thrombus within or 5 mm proximal or distal to stent
  - And at least 1 of following (within part 48 hours)
    1. Acute ischemic symptoms at rest
    2. New ischemic ECG changes
    3. Positive cardiac bio marker
  - Or pathological confirmation
- *Probable stent thrombosis*
  - Unexplained death within 30 days after stent implantation
  - Any MI in the territory of implanted stent without angiographic confirmation and in the absence of any other obvious cause
- *Possible stent thrombosis*
  Any unexplained death > 30 days after stent implantation

CLASSIFICATION

- *Early* 0–30 days
  - *Acute:* 0–24 hours
  - *Sub acute:* >24 hours–30 days
- *Late:* 3 days to 1 year
- *Very late:* > 1 year
  INTRA PROCEDURE THROMBIC EVENTS are not considered as stent thrombosis

MECHANISM

- *Patient related factors:*
  - Diabetes
  - Smoker
  - CKD
  - AES presentation
  - Thrombocytosis
  - High post treatment platelet relativity
  - Prematured discontinuation of DAPT
  - Surgical procedure (unrelated to PCI)
- *Lesion related factors:*
  - Diffuse CAD with long stented segment
  - Small vessel disease
  - Bifurcation disease
  - Thrombus containing lesions
  - Significant inflow or outflow lesions proximal or distal to stented segment
- *Stent related factors:*
  - Poor stent expansion
  - Edge dissection limiting inflow/outflow
  - Delayed or absent endothelialization
  - Thicker stent struct
  - Hypersensitivity/inflammatory or thrombotic reaction to stent polymer
  - Struct fracture
  - Late malapposition/aneurysm formation
  - Development of neoatherosclerosis within stent struct with new plaque rupture

TREATMENT

- Urgent Reperfusion
  - Emergent PCI (preferred)
  - Mechanical/aspiration thrombectomy
  - Balloon angiography
    +
    More potent antiplatelet
  - Avoid additional stent
  - IVUS/OCT guidance
- In the absence of mechanical cause search for hematological cause
  - Hypercoagulable state, resistance to antiplatelet, thrombocytosis
- Escalation of antiplatelet therapy

PREVENTION OF STENT THROMBOSIS

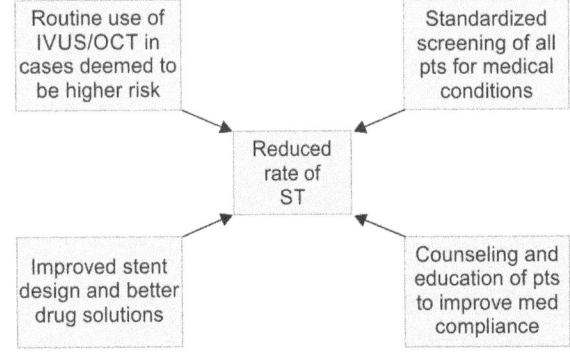

11.24 SUBCUTANEOUS IMPLANTABLE CARDIOVERTER-DEFIBRILLATOR

INTRODUCTION

- Entirely Subcutaneous implantable cardioverter-defibrillator (S-ICD)
- Developed initially for special group of patients in whom implantation of transvenous ICD was not practical

  Example: Pediatric population where congenital heart disease preclude placement of transvenous ICDs

  or

  In whom venous access is obstructed due to any reason

DESIGN

Four components
1. Pulse generator
   - So J Biphasic shock
   - 5.1 yr longevity
   - 30 seconds post shock pacing
2. Subcutaneous electrode
3. Guide electrode insertion tool
4. TECH programmer

IMPLEMENTATION OF S-ICD

- Three subcutaneous incision
- Components implanted below the skin

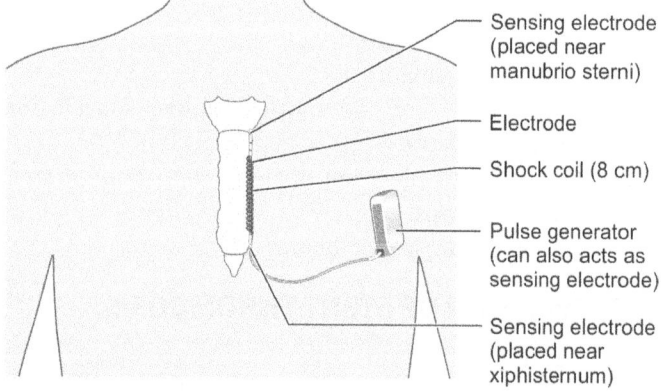

- Implantation process guided by anatomical landmarks with the option of Fluoroscopy to confirm *optimal shock vector* crossing the heart silhouette

  Three shock vectors
  1. *B-CAN:* Primary
  2. *A-CAN:* Secondary
  3. *A-B:* Alternate

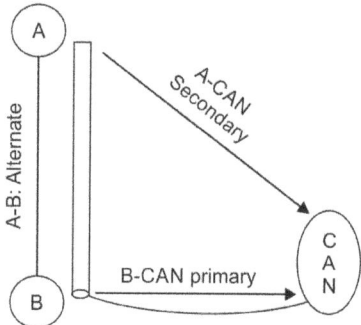

- (A), (B), and (CAN) also work as surface electrode—Helps in arrhythmia detection
- START study (Subcutaneous VS Transvenous Arrhythmia Recognition Testing): Sensitivity for detection of ventricular Arrhythmias were excellent
- Conditions/factors that can hamper arrhythmia detection
  1. Myopotentials sensing
  2. Double counting
  3. Suboptimal sensing vector selection

ARRHYTHMIA DETECTION

Different algorithm applied to all 3 vectors
↓
S. ICD choose appropriate vector to avoid Double sensing/sensing of T waves
↓
H.R calculated as avg of art 4 RR interval
↓
Arrhythmia discriminated based on H.R and morphology of P-QRS.

Advantages

- No risk of vascular injury
- Very low risk of systemic infection
- Reduce risk associated with lead extraction (as in case of TV ICD failure)
- Cosmetic advantage (Battery placed in lateral axilla)
- Shock energy is more evenly distributed throughout myocardium—relatively low voltage gradient—Avoids transient myocardial stunning and myocyte damage (useful especially in patients with poor LV function)
- Less invasive procedure
- Less procedure time
- Can be done on OPD basis

LIMITATIONS

1. No backup pacing ability for brady arrhythmia (except 30 sec pacing post shock)
2. No Antitachycardia pacing (ATP) mode
3. Cannot upgrade to CRT-D

4. Large pulse generator
5. Large amount of shock (higher joules) is required to terminate arrhythmia
   ↓
   Less battery life (approximately 5 years)
6. No long term data/follow-up

PATIENT SELECTION

Favorable factors	Relative contraindications
• Young and active	• Recurrent MMVT
• CHD that limits lead placement	• Brady arrhythmia requiring pacing
• Indwelling catheters	• Indications for CRT
• Immunocompromised (High risk of systematic infection)	• High risk for VT (sarcoidosis; ARVD)
• Inherited channelopathies	• Preference for remote monitoring

Available devices
- *First generation:* SQ-Rx 1000
- *Second generation:* Emblem (Boston)

TRAILS SUPPORTING
- CE Trails
- UK cohort
- Dutch cohort
- German 1 and 2 cohort
- EFFORTLESS S-ICD Registry (5 years follow-up)

11.25 TRANSCATHETER AORTIC VALVE IMPLANTATION

Q.1 Discuss indication for transcatheter aortic valve implantation (TAVI). How does balloon expandable valve differ from self expandable in technique of implantation (June 14)
Q.2 Advances in TAVR/TAVI technology (June 16)
Q.3 Valve-in-valve TAVR. Enumerate various valves used in TAVR. Recent clinical trials in TAVR (2 + 3 + 5) (June 17)
Q.4 Discuss concept, design, and initial results of percutaneous aortic valve replacement (Dec 11)
Q.5 Percutaneous erotic valve replacement (June 15)
Q.6 Discuss catheter erotic valve implantation what are the current indication and complications (June 13)

NATURAL HISTORY OF AS

Progression of mod As
- Mean velocity increase by 0.3 m/s/yr
- Mean gradient increase by 7 mm Hg/yr
- AVA decrease by 0.1 cm^2/yr

Event free survival= 30-50% @ 2 yrs
Mortality for symptomatic severe As = 50% at 2 yr
Prevalence of severe As among
- 50-60 yr = 0.2%
- 60-70 yr = 1.3%
- 70-80 yr = 3-9%
- \>80 yr = 9-8%

With each decade risk of incident As doubles

CT before TAVR
- *Ao annulus* (3D CT) - In systole
  - Long and short axis dia
  - Planimetry area
- *Valvular landing zone Ca^{++} burden*
  - Symmetric/asymmetric
  - Predictor of para valve leak
- *Ao Root*
  - Ht of coro ostia
  - SOV to annular plane ⎤
  - Leaflet length   ⎥ Predict coro occlusion
  - Width of SOV   ⎦
  - Sinotubular junction
  - LVOT
  - Asc Ao
- CT based prediction of angiographic projection angles for TAVR
- Access route assessment
  - Atheroma or bulky calcium in Ao arch
- Concomitant cardiac disease
  - First TAVR coas performed by Cribier et al., in 2002
  - TAVR is minimally invasive available treatment option for patients with severe As who are too sick or too old for an open heart surgery

- In this procedure a stent like scaphoid with metallic frame containing bio prosthetic valve is deployed with the help of a catheter delivery system

WORK UP
- Pre-anesthetic work up
- Cardio thoracic evaluation
  - Access
  - AVR
  - Risk assessment
- Imaging
  - As Severity; morphology; calcification
  - 3D-CT
  - 3D MR
  - 3D TEE
  - Preferred
    - Annulus size and shape (preferred systolic-max)
    - Aortic root size
    - Atheroma burden
    - Sub aortic obstruction
    - LV function; other valvular disease
    - Vascular anatomy from access site to annulus
    - Cerebrovascular imaging

FACTORS TO CONSIDER
- Landing zone
- Access site
- Aortic valve type
- Coronaries
- LV
- Cond. Syst
- Cerebral prot
- Renal prot
- Management and anticipated Compli

PROCEDURE
- LA + conscious sedation/GA
  - Maintain hemodynamic stability
    - SBP~120 mm Hg; MAP >75 mm Hg
- *Vascular access*
  - Sites
    - Transfemoral (14-24 Fr)
    - Transapical (18-26 Fr)
      - Left anterior thoracotomy
      - More direct, short catheter
      - Ascendra 2, sapien valve
    - Transaortic
      - Upper partial sternotomy
      - Mini sternotomy ⅔ RICS
      - Aorta 5 cm above valve

- Manipulation of ascending aorta
- Subclavian
- Pacing leads
  - Transvenous
  - Epicardial
- *Anticoagulation*
  - Heparin
  - Maintain ACT > 300 sec
- Intra op TEE for
  - Guidewire placement
  - Valve placement
    - Stable position
    - No coronary obstruction
    - No interference with mitral valve function
    - No conduction system impingement
    - No overhanging native aortic root complications (rupture and dissection)
  - Port deployment assessment (MR, AR)
- *Balloon aortic valvotomy*

  C/L femoral artery punctured
  ↓
  6 F sheath and pigtail catheter
  ↓
  Iliofemoral angio of opposite site
  ↓
  Site of punctured marked
  ↓
  Arterial access: 14 F long (24 cm) sheath (percutaneous/surgical)
  Venous access for right heart cath and pacing
  ↓

  Valve crossing
  - AL-1/JR with 0.035 guidewire
    Advanced into aorta up to valve
  - Wire exchanged to straight tip
  - AV crossed and guiding cath advanced to LV
  - Wire exchanged with amplatz extra stiff guidewire (260 cm)
  ↓

  Balloon valvuloplasty
  - 20/30 mm or 23 × 30 mm
  - Appropriate angio projection LAO 20°; Cran 20°
  - Rapid LV pacing
  - Rapid inflation-deflation cycle
  - Stop pacing
- *TAVI procedure*

  Expandable sheath with advancer negotiated up to aortic root
  ↓
  Valve with assemble is advanced to aortic root and valve placed across the aortic valve
  ↓
  Valve position checked on aortogram with catheter from C/L grain and on TEE
  ↓
  Rapid LV pacing
  ↓
  Valve is inflated
  ↓
  Stop pacing

POST OP CARE AND MONITORING

- Immediate or early extubation
- Early mobilization
- Adequate analgesia
- Control of post op hypertension
- Monitor vital parameters; fluid balance; renal status; AV conduction system
- Pre discharge TTE
- DAPT

COMPLICATION/PROBLEMS

- *Vascular complications*
  Major
  - Thoracic aortic dissection
  - Access site related vascular injury (dissection, perforation, Rupture, arterio venous fistula, pseudo aneurysm, hematoma, nerve injury, compartment syndrome, visceral ischemia due to hypogastric artery occlusion; paraparesis due to spinal artery occlusion)
  - Distal embolization

  Minor
  - Failure of percutaneous site closure resulting in interventional or surgical correction
- *Conduction disturbances*
  - *LBBB* due to mechanical compression on AV conduction tissue
  - *AV block:* (14-44%) after core valve 12% after Edwards's sapien

  PPM implantation
  - 18-49% for core valve
  - 0-12% for SAPIEN

  AF
- *Paravalvular leak*
  - Even mid paravalvular leak is associated with significant mortality
  - First generation valves were more prone to have paravalvular leak
- *Stroke and CVA*
  - Low stroke risk (2-9%)
  - No difference between stroke rate and type of valves
  - Acute (within 24 hrs) related with procedure
  - Early (within 30 days)

- Late (1-2 months) related with disease factor
- Cerebral protection by
  - Filtration (EMBOL-X; Edwards and Claret montage device)
  - Diversion (Embrella embolic deflector: Edwards and Triguard cerebral protection device)
- *Coronary occlusion*
  - Low coro (<8 mm)
  - Small SOV
  - Long leaflet
  - Bulky calcification
    - Very rare
    - Mortality as high as 50%
    - Require immediate coronary intervention
    - More common during valve-in-valve procedure
- *Annular Rupture/LVOT Rupture/ periaortic hematoma*
  - Very rare
  - 1.1%
  - *Predictor:* LVOT calcification
        Over sizing of prosthesis
  - Very high mortality
  - Surgery is almost always required
- *Hypotension after TAVI*
  - Vascular Rupture; ventricular rupture
  - Acute valve dysfunction; coronary obstruction
  - Multiple rapid pacing in patients with poor LV
  - *Suicidal LV:* In severe LVH; after removing LV obstruction LV decompress to such an extent that the subvalvular hypertrophy obstructs outflow (treatment fluid; W/H diuretics)
- *Patients prosthetic mismatch:* Defined as 1° EPA ≤0.65 cm²/m²
  Associated with mortality

CORE VALVE SYSTEM (MEDTRONIC)

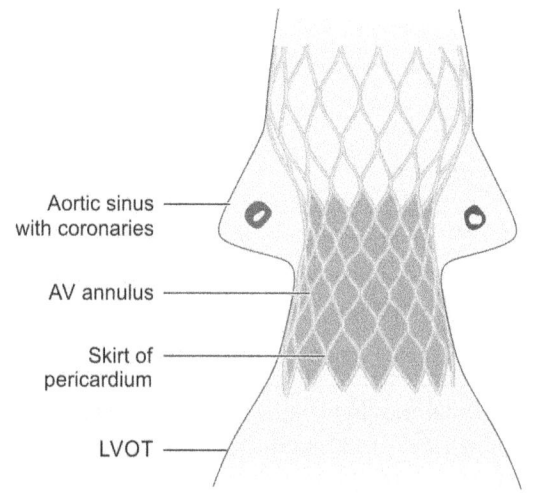

- Upper one third low radial force—sits in ascending aorta—orient valve into Ao root
- Middle one third—high strength—valve attaches here
- Lower one third—high radial strength—sits in LVOT. Has a skirt of pericardium that seals the system

Second generation valves:

Bovine - 1. Medtronic evolut
Porcine - 2. SAPIEN-3 (Edward life science)—Sapien XT
Bovine - 3. Lotus medical (Boston scientific)
          4. Direct flow medical valve
Porcine - 5. Symetis acurate
Bovine - 6. Portieo (St. Jude)
Bovine - 7. Centera (Edwards's life science)
Bovine - 8. Engager (Medtronic) transapical valve
Porcine - 9. Transapical jenavalve

Sapien-3
- Presence of skirt around distal part of stent frame to prevent paravalvular leaks
- Balloon expandable valve

New1: Tissue engineered valve
- Implanted bone marrow mononuclear cells →Self repair

	SAPIEN	SAPIEN-XT	SAPIEN-3
Delivery	Retroflex 3	Novaflex	Commander
Sizes	23/26	20/23/26/29	23/26/29
Vessel size	≥ 7 mm	6/6/6.5/7	5.5/5.5/6
Sheath	22/24	16/16/18/20	14/14/16
Sheath model	Retroflex	Esheath	Esheath
Expanded length	16 mm	17.2 mm	20 mm

Balloon expandable	Self

Edward sapien THV
   XT
   S3
• Myval
• Direct flow
• Brail inovare
• Colibri
	• Core valve
	• Core valve evolut R
	• Core valve evolut pro
	• Portico
	• Lotus
	• Jenavalve
	• Edward Centera
	• Accurate neo
	• Optimum TAV
	• Trinity
	• Vita flow
	• Allegra
	• Perc
	• Triskele

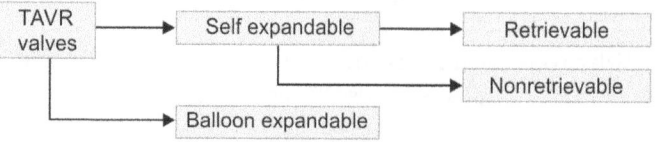

	Edwards SAPIEN (smaller)	Medtronic core valve
Structure	Porcine pericardium	Bovine pericardium
Delivery	Balloon mounted	Self expandable
Vascular access	16–18 F (XT) 22 (SAPIEN)	18 F
LV apical approach	Possible	Not possible
Implantation	Require asystole induction (rapid pacing)	Can be delivered in beating heart
Staged deployment (Partial retrieval)	Not possible	Reposition possible (only minor adjustment)
Main force fixing the valve	Aortic elasticity dependent	Radial force also involved
Ascending aortic support	Nil	Yes
Coronary ostium flow	Unrelated	Can be related to strut
Potential AV block	Less	High unique feature of confirming the shape of native annulus

CHOICE Trial (2014) balloon expandable valve resulted in greater rate of device success than self expandable valve

Pragmatic: No difference between Medtronic core valve vs. Edward sapien

CURRENT STATUS

- TAVR for high surgical risk population is well backed by robust data from various registries and trials

PARTNER cohort B: Showed 20% reduction in all cause mortality at 1 year follow up

PARTNER cohort A: Compared TAVR and SAVR in high risk but operable patients showing similar mortality in 2 arms (TAVR 24.2% SAVR 26.8%) and at 2 years (TAVR 33.9% SAVR 35%)

↓

TAVR is considered effective alternative modality of treatment for high surgical risk cases and is the choice of treatment for inoperable patients

PARTNER 2 Trial: In intermediate risk patients, SAPIEN-3 TAVR resulted in low 1 year mortality by all cause (7.4%), all stroke (4.6%) and moderate or severe As (1.5%) SAVR vs. SAPIEN-3 TAVR
- Noninferiority for 1° end points
- Superiority of SAVR for AR ≥ mod

SURTAVI
- TAVR with self expanding core valve is noninferior to SAVR for all cause mortality or disabling stroke at 24 months
- TAVR has significantly less 30 day stroke AKI, AF and transfusion use
- TAVR related with superior quality of life
- SAVR had less residual AR, major vascular complications and fewer new pacemaker
- Need for new pacemaker after TAVR was not related with increased mortality

2014 ACC/AHA

- SAVR in patients who meet an indication for AVR with low or intermediate risk `1A`
- For patients undergoing TAVR or high risk SAVR, heart valve team approach should be used `1A`
- TAVR is recommended in patients who meet indication for AVR for As who have a high prohibitive surgical risk and predicted post TAVR survival>12 months `1B`
- TAVR is reasonable alternate to SAVR in patients who meet an indication for AVR and who have high surgical risk `2a/b`
- TAVR is not recommended in patients in whom existing Comorbidities would preclude the expected benefit from correction of As `3`

FRAILTY

- ≥ 2/6 activity of daily living impairment   ⎫
- S. Albumin ≤ 3.5   ⎬ Each score 0–3 is most frail
- Grip strength<30 kg male and <18 kg female   ⎪
- 15 feet walk test ≥ 7 sec   ⎭

Frailty score >5
- Poor outcome with TAVR

PATIENT SELECTION

TAVR acceptable only in patients with
1. Life expectancy >1 yr
2. Those with chance of "survival with benefit" >25% at 2 years follow-up
3. Favorable anatomy

- Patient and prosthetic selection are crucial
- Heart team approach; cardiologist; CVTS surgeon; cardiac anesthetic; cardio-radiologist; electrocardiographer
- *Patient selection*
  - STS score >10% + modified euroscore

Euroscore logistic >20%
Severe risk factor not covered by high risk score
- *Frailty:* Decline in function status post TAVR
- *Comorbid conditions:* CAD, COPD, CKD, cirrhosis, stroke/TIA, malignancy, immunodeficiency
- *Patient benefit*
  - *Females:* PARTNER A found that high risk females who underwent TAVI had better survival compared to SAVR
  - *Diabetes:* In PARTNER trial, diabetics had significant benefit
  - *Renal dysfunction:* Poor outcome with SAVR
  - O_2 *dependent COPD:* Better with TAVR
  - *Mod severe MR:* Increased 2 yr mortality with SAVR not with TAVR

LIMITATION

- *Durability*
  - Matter of concern and risk for its use in younger patients
  - UCL TAV is a device with polymeric leaflet
  - Vanguard 2 valve
  - Expected to have an increased durability as it allows in vivo replacement of its leaflets when these begins to fail

DEVICE SUCCESS

- Successful vascular access, delivery and deployment of device and successful retrieval of system
- Correct position of device in proper anatomical position
- Intended performance of prosthetic valve (Ao area > 1.2 cm^2; mean AVA gr < 20 mm Hg or peak velocity<3 m/s, without moderate or severe prosthetic valve AR)
- Only 1 valve implanted in proper anatomical position

TAVR IN BAV

- Problem of malposition
- Optimum TAV is dedicated for BAV (still in trial phase)
- BAV was contraindication for TAVR in PARTNER and core valve US pivotal trials
- Difficulties
  - Asymmetric ensp size
  - Asymmetric distribution of calcium
  - Raphe may prevent complete apposition
  - Elliptical annulus maker circular expansion of valve difficult
  - Large annulus require large sized valve

TAVR for AR

(Reg et al. JACC 2013)
- 43 patients
- Pure severe AR
- TAVI done in 42 patients
- 8 patients required second valve during index procedure for residual AR
- Post procedure AR Gr1 or low - 34 patients
- 30 day stroke
- 30 day all cause mortality 9.3%
- 12 months all cause mortality 24%

Future

- Nanotechnology based valve
- Autologous tissue engineered valve

Valve-in-valve TAVI

For
- Bioprosthetic valve failure
- Post TAVI failure

Reoperation mortality =15–23% (depending on comorbidities)

Challenges

- Identify bioprosthesis suitability
- Evaluate role of balloon predilatation
- Creat new sizing
- Positioning and deployment

11.26 TIMI-MBG-NO FLOW

Q.1 Role of PPCI in AMI. Discuss mechanism of slow flow and treatment of slow flow (Dec 11)
Q.2 Coronary slow flow and no reflow (June 15)
Q.3 TIMI flow and TMP grading. Methodology and significance (June 04)
Q.4 TIMI flow and MBG grade and its utility clinically (Dec 15)

TIMI GRADING

Grade 0: No anterograde flow beyond point of occlusion

Grade 1: Contrast media able to pass beyond the area of obstruction but fails to opacify the distal coronary bed

Grade 2: Contrast is able to pass through the area of occlusion and fills the distal coronary bed; however it is perceptually slower than other coronary vessels unaffected by coronary occlusion

Grade 3: Antegrade flow into distal coronary bed of obstructed artery is as prompt as flow in uninvolved artery

TIMI MYOCARDIAL BLUSH GRADE

Grade 0: Minimal or no ground glass appearance (blush) of the myocardium

Grade 1: Dye slowly enters but fail to exit microvasculature Blush fails to clear and dye staining present on the next injection (approx 30 seconds between injections)

Grade 2: Delayed entry and into exit of dye from microvasculature. Blush strongly persists at the end of washout phase (after 3 cardiac cycle dye does not or only minimally diminish in intensity

Grade 3: Normal entry and exit of dye from microvasculature. Blush clears normally present at the end of washout phase (3 cardiac cycle)
    Similar to that in uninvolved artery

Mortality	TMP grade
6.2%	<- 0
5.1%	<- 1
4.4%	<- 2
2.0%	<- 3

TYPES OF CORONARY LESION

Type-A	Type-B	Type-C
Discrete (<10 mm)	Tubular (10–20 mm)	Diffuse (>20 mm)
Concentric	Eccentric	
Readily accessive	Mod tortuosity of prox	Ext tortuosity of prox
Nonangulated <45°	Mod angulated 45–90	Extreme angulation >90
Smooth contour	Irregular contour	
Little/No calcification	Mod-heavy calcification	
Less than total occlusion	Total occlusion <3 mth	Total occlusion >3 mth
Nonostial lesion	Ostial lesion	
Nonbifurcation	Bifurcation lesion	Inability to predict major
Absence of thrombus	Some thrombus	Degen vein graft with friable lesion

NO REFLOW

Inability to perfuse myocardium after opening of a previously occluded or stenosed epicardial coronary artery

MECHANISM

- Suspected to result from combination of endothelial damage, platelet and fibrin embolization, vasospasm and tissue edema that overwhelms the coronary microcirculation
- Reperfusion—infiltration of microcirculation with neutrophils and platelets—contribute to no reflow state

INCIDENCE—0.6–2%

- More frequent when using atherectomy
- PCI in SVG—high incidence

RISK FACTORS

- Angiographic presence of thrombus
- Cardiogenic shock
- Increased reperfusion time
- Hyperglycemia
- Leukocytosis

PREVENTION

- *Pre-treatment*
  - IC calcium channel blocker for SVG
  - Abciximab prior to PAMI (ADMIRAL Trial)
  - IC abciximab did not significantly improve TIMI/MBG score as compared to IV abciximab
  - Go 2b/3a Inhibitor treatment
- Use of distal protection device for SVG intervention (SAFER Trial)
  (No flow reduced from 9.7-4.8%)
- Routine use of nitroglycerin, verapamil and heparin in combination with flush solution while doing rotational atherectomy
- Minimize balloon inflation and consider direct stenting in patients with bulky atheroma/SVG graft
- Thrombus aspiration during STEM 1 (TAPAS trial)

TREATMENT

*First Line

- Adenosine (10-20 ug)
- Nitroprusside (50-200 ug; upto total 1,000 ug)
- Verapamil (100-200 ug bolus; upto 1,000 ug total with TPM standby)

**Evidence Less Strong

- Rapid, moderately forceful injection of saline or blood (to unplug microvasculature)
- Papaverine
- Nicorandil (200 ug)
- Nicardipine (2 ug)
- Epinephrine (50-200 ug)

**Never Shown to be Effective

- Intracoronary NTG
- CABG (contraindicated)
- Stent placement; If original stenotic site is widely patent
- Thrombolytics
  - Distal contrast injection through micro catheter can be made to exclude dissection
  - Vasodilator through microcatheter
  - IABP for patients with cardiogenic shock

11.27 VALVE AREA CALCULATION

Q.1 How will you calculate aortic valve area in cardiac cath lab (Dec 10)

Q.2 Pressure gradient measurement during cardiac cath flow to calculate stenotic valve area in cath lab (June 14)

Q.3 Gorlin's equation for MV and AV

INTRODUCTION

Dr Richard Gorlin and his father developed a formula for calculation of area of stenotic valve based upon flow and pressure gradient area

GORLIN'S FORMULA

Based on Torricelli's law
"Flow across a round orifice F = AVCc"
F = flow rate
A = orifice area
V = velocity of flow
Cc = coefficient of orifice contraction

$$\text{So } A = \frac{F}{VCc}$$

Cc compensate for physical phenomena:
"Except for a perfect orifice, the area of a stream flowing through an orifice will be less than the true area of the orifice"
Second principle used for Gorlin's equation
↓

Pressure gradient and velocity of flow according to Torricelli's law
$$V^2 = (C_V)^2 \cdot 2gh$$
$$\text{So } V = (C_V) \cdot \sqrt{2gh}$$

V = velocity of flow
CV = coefficient of velocity
g = gravitational constant = 980 cm/s²
h = Pr. Gradient in cmH$_2$O

CV corrects for the energy loss as pressure energy is converted to kinetic or velocity energy

$$\text{So area} = \frac{F}{\sqrt{Cc}}$$
$$= \frac{F}{Cv \cdot \sqrt{2gh} \cdot Cc}$$
$$= \frac{F}{Cv \cdot Cc \cdot \sqrt{2 \times 980 \times h}}$$
$$= \frac{F}{C \cdot 44.3 \sqrt{h}}$$

C is empirical constant accounting for Cc and Cv, and the expression of h in mm Hg, and correcting calculated valve area to actual valve area

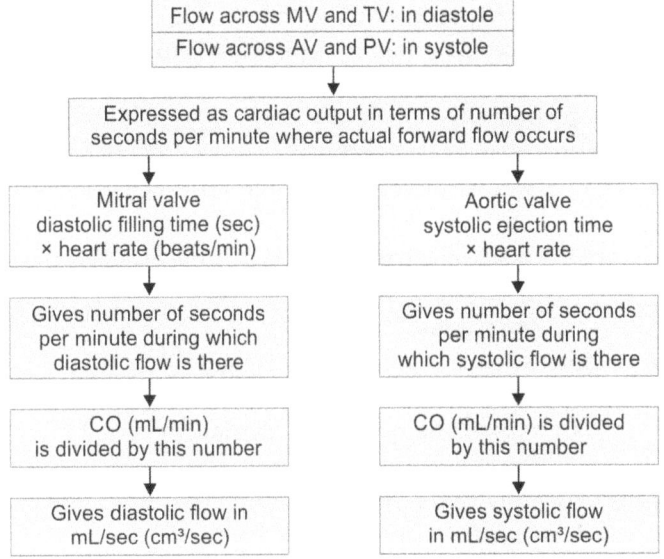

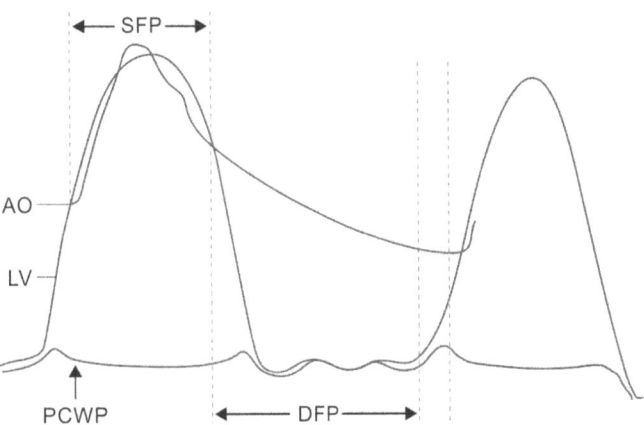

So final equation
$$\text{Area} = \frac{CO/(PFP \text{ or } SEP) \times HR}{C \cdot 44.3 \sqrt{\Delta P}}$$

C = 0.7 (now 0.85) was empirical constant derived from autopsy study
↓

When c is taken as 0.7 – calculated MVA deviates from actual MVA by 0.2 only

No such constant derived for AV, TV and PV
It is considered to be 1

MVA CALCULATION

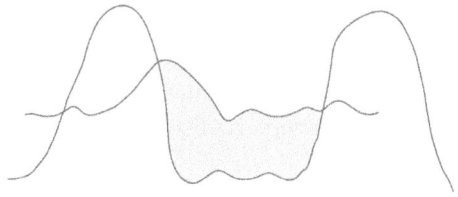

$$\text{Area} = \frac{\text{CO}/(\text{DFP}) \times \text{HR}}{0.7 \times 44.3 \times \sqrt{\Delta P}}$$

- Heart rate = beat/min
- Cardiac output (as per Fick's principle): mL/min (or indicator dilution)
- C = 0.7 (or 0.85)
- New to calculate DFP and ΔP
- DIP (or average diastolic filling period) of such 5 beats
  ↓
  Avg DIP = avg length (of such 5 beats)/paper speed
  = mm/mm/sec
  = Seconds
- Gradient = Area of gradient / Length
  (calculated by / of
  planimetry of / diastolic
  area between / period
  LV and PCWP)

Such avg gradient calculated for 5 beats
↓
Mean gradient = avg gradient × scale factor
(mm)   (mm Hg/mm)
= mm Hg
↓
Putting all in the above formula gives MVA (cm²)
↓
Indexed for BSA
Indexed MVA = valve area/BSA
(cm²/m²)

Pitfalls

- If PCWP is not obtained properly it deviates from LAP by 3–5 mm Hg
  ↓   PCWP error
  LAP is overestimated
  ↓
  Reduce area between LV and PCWP
  ↓
  Gradient is underestimated
  ↓
  Valve area is overestimated

■ PROPER PCWP IS

1. Mean wedge pressure is lower than mean pulmonary artery pressure
2. Blood withdrawn from wedge catheter has sat ≥95%
- PCW and LV pressure alignment does not match LA and LV pressure alignment (because LA pressure takes time to transmit back to pulm capillaries)
  ↓   Figment error

- Mismatch is very small if measured in distal PA with Cournand or Goodale-lubin catheter
- Mismatch is large if measured with balloon tipped catheter in proximal pulmonary tree
  ↓
  Ideally PCWP should be aligned with LV by shifting it leftwards 50–70 msec (ideally V wave peak should not be bisected by down stroke of LV pressure)
- If both transducer are not zeroed properly   Calibration error
  ↓
  Can underestimate/overestimate the gradient
  ↓
  To check; both transducers are exchanged
  ↓
  If pressure gradients remain same
  ↓
  Everything is fine
- If MR is present with MS
  ↓
  Fallacies in calculating cardiac output
- *Early diastasis*
  Even when LA and LV pressure Equalize (diastasis) before end of diastole
  ↓
  Flow across MV persists
  ↓
  DFP used in calculating valve area should include all of such diastasis period

AVA calculation

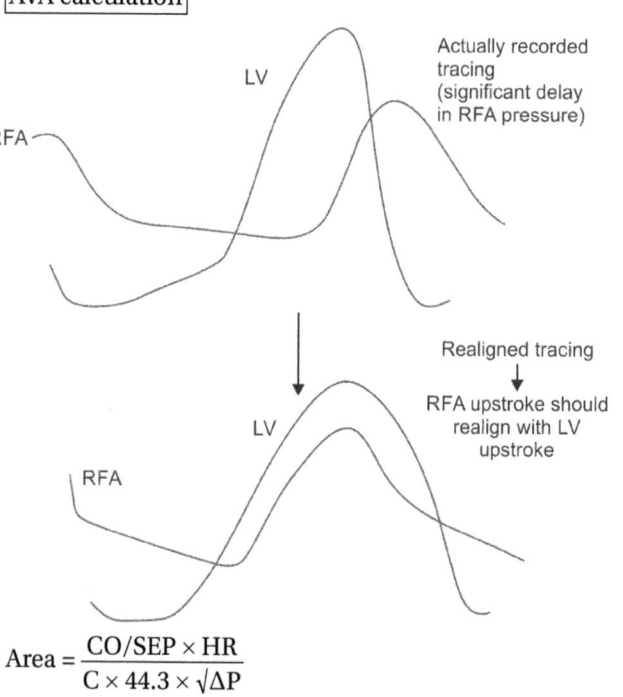

$$\text{Area} = \frac{\text{CO}/\text{SEP} \times \text{HR}}{C \times 44.3 \times \sqrt{\Delta P}}$$

- CO obtained from Fick's principle or indicate dilution say 5,000 cm³/min
- SEP = mean ejection period = average/length/paper speed say 0.33 seconds/beat
- HR = heart rate (say 74 BPM)
- C = 1 (Constant)
- Δp = mean avg pr Gr
    = Avg Gradient × scale factor
    = Area of Gradient × length of systolic period × scale factor
    = Say 40 mm Hg

So area = $\dfrac{5000/0.33 \times 74}{44.3 \sqrt{40}} = 0.7$ cm²

Pitfalls

1. *LV and femoral artery pressure*
    a. Peripheral artery pressure curve is delayed—needs to realign
    ↓
    If not, it will overestimate gradient and underestimate AVA
    b. Systolic amplification and spreading out of pressure waveform in peripheral artery
    ↓
    Peak systolic pressure is high
    ↓
    Planimetered Gradient is underestimated
    ↓
    AVA overestimated
2. a. Misplaced catheter tip, If tip placed in LVOT (rather than LV body)
    ↓
    Underestimate LV-Ao gradient by 30 mm Hg
    b. Ideally aortic catheter should be placed in ascending aorta
    ↓
    Farther the catheter tip; it will underestimate gradient (due to pressure recovery phenomena) in spite of alignment
    ↓
    Overestimate valve area
    To overcome this
    - Difference between peak central aortic pressure and peak peripheral artery pressure is added to planimetered gradient
    - Mean LV gradient during A and mean aortic gradient during B is calculated

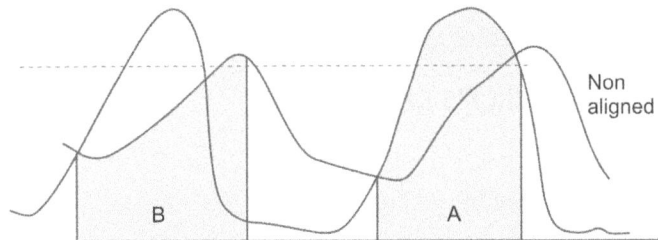

The diff between A and B found to be nearly equal as LV-As Ao gradient
- Use 2 separate catheters (1° in LV and 2nd in Asc. Ao) or double lumen catheter (Langston catheter)
↓
Ideal and accurate
3. Improperly calibrated/zeroed catheters
4. *Pullback hemodynamics*
    a. In severe As—6F catheter can reduce effective orifice area significantly - hamper simultaneous aortic gradient recording
    b. If arterial pressure increases by >5 mm Hg after pullback—stenosis is severe

ACC/AHA guidelines
If severity of As is known accurately from noninvasive tests
↓
Class 3 recommendation for crossing the aortic valve invasively

ALTERNATE TO GORLIN'S FORMULA

Proposed by Hakki et al.

Valve area = $\dfrac{CO}{\sqrt{\Delta P}}$

(It is observed that product of heart rate, SEP or DIP and Gorlin's formula constant was same for all patients and it is close to 1.0)

Low flow low gradient As
- Gorlin's formula is flow dependent
- If flow is low—AVA calculated low
↓
To overcome this
1. Increase flow across the valve
2. Remove inaccuracy in Gorlin's formula
   (Constant C to be assured as 1.0; that's improper)

METHODS

1. Infusion of nitroprusside or dobutamine increases forward flow

Caution: In patients with As, nitroprusside can decrease gradient and lead to hypotension
- Dobutamine can precipitate ischemia in patients with known CAD

11.28 MEASUREMENT OF VASCULAR RESISTANCE

POISEUILLE'S LAW

$$Q = \frac{\pi (P_i - P_o) r^4}{8nl}$$

Q = volume of blood
$P_i - P_o$ = Inflow – outflow pressure
r = radius of tube
l = length of tube
n = viscosity of blood

Applies in a steady state laminar flow of homogenous fluids through a rigid tube
Now, OHM's law states that
Resistance is defined as ratio of mean pressure drop to flow

$$R = \frac{(P_i - P_o)}{Q} = \frac{8nl}{\pi r^4}$$

- Resistance depends mainly on dimension of tube and viscosity of blood
- Resistance is markedly sensitive to change in radius of the tube

Pitfalls

- Blood flow is pulsatile
- Blood is not homogeneous   ⎫ Ambiguity in
- Vascular bed is nonlinear elastic ⎬ calculating
  and frequency dependent   ⎭ resistance
  ↓

To assess blood vessel elasticity and caliber, concept of vascular impedance is developed.
"Vascular impedance is defined as instantaneous ratio of pulsatile pressure to pulsatile flow"

Estimating Resistance in Clinical Scenario

$$\text{Systemic resistance} = \frac{Ao - RA}{Qs}$$

Ao = mean system pressure
RA = mean RA pressure

$$\text{Pulmonary Resistance} = \frac{PA - LA}{QP}$$

PA = Mean Pa pr
LA = Mean LA pr
↓

Mean PCWP can be taken as mean LA pr
(flow measured as L/min and pressure measured as mm Hg)
So Resistance unit = $\boxed{mm\ Hg/L/min}$
Known as
- Hybrid Resistance unit (HRU)
- Woods unit

Conversion to metric unit

$$\text{Resistance} = \frac{\Delta P\ (mm\ Hg) \times 1{,}332\ dynes/cm^2/mm\ Hg}{Q\ (L/min) \times 100\ mL/L \div 60\ sec/min}$$

$$= \frac{\Delta P}{Q} \times 80\ dynes - sec - cm^{-5}$$

Pediatric Cardiology

Resistance expressed as resistance index

$$\text{Resistance index} = \frac{\Delta P}{C.I} \times 80$$
↓

Blood flow index substitute for blood flow
SVR = 1170 +/– 270 dynes – sec – cm^{-5}
PVR = 67 +/– 30 dynes – sec – cm^{-5}

Clinical Application

- Resistance can change by
  - Change in length of vessel—Unusual after growth
  - Change in viscosity
  - Change in dimension of vessel
- SVR/PVR is dominated by arterioles, but other components do contribute
  Arterioles = 60%
  Capillaries = 15%
  Small veins = 15%
  Arterial system prox to arterioles = 10%
- Hypotension or decreased C.O.   ⎤ Blunted in CCF
  ↓   │ due to tissue
  Stimulate baroreceptors   │ hypoperfusion
  α Adrenergic neural pathway   │ ↓
  ↓   │ Hypoxia and
  Release of vasoconstrictors   │ acidosis
  ↓   │ ↓
  Increased SVR   │ Blunting of Baro
                                    ⎦ receptor reflex
- SVR falls in response to dynamic exercise but PVR remains unchanged
  ↓
  Transient elevation in SVR can be provoked by infusion of vasopressor drugs to evaluate LV response to increase in after load.
- PVR may be elevated by hypoxia, hypercapnia, increased sympathetic tone, polycythemia, local release of serotonin, mechanical obstruction pre capillary pulm edema or lung compression (pl effusion, artificial respirator)
- PVR decrease by O_2, adenosine, isoproterenol, α antagonists (phentolamine, tolazoline) inhaled NO, prostacyclin, nitroprusside and high dose of COB.

11.29 WEARABLE IMPLANTABLE CARDIOVERTER-DEFIBRILLATOR

Q.1 Wearable implantable cardioverter-defibrillator (ICD) – design and Indication (Dec 16)

DILEMMAS WITH ICD

- Recent MI with arrhythmias
  - Standard guidelines do not recommend the implantation of ICD
  - Patient still at risk of demise due to life threatening arrhythmia
- Infected ICD
- Newly diagnosed nonischemic cardiomyopathy who is at risk of arrhythmias and who is recently started on GDMT
  ↓

WCD is an option

1998: Preliminary data published by Auricchio and associates

2002: US FDA approval for patient who is at risk of SCD but not immediate candidate for ICD therapy

Model: Life west 3100 (old) ⎤ by 2011, USA
Life west 4000 (new)   ⎦

DESIGN

- Wearable garment with elastic belt and 2 shoulder strap
- 4 Dry nonadhesive sensing electrode
- 3 defibrillation electrodes (2 large posterior and one apical)—with self gelling capsule

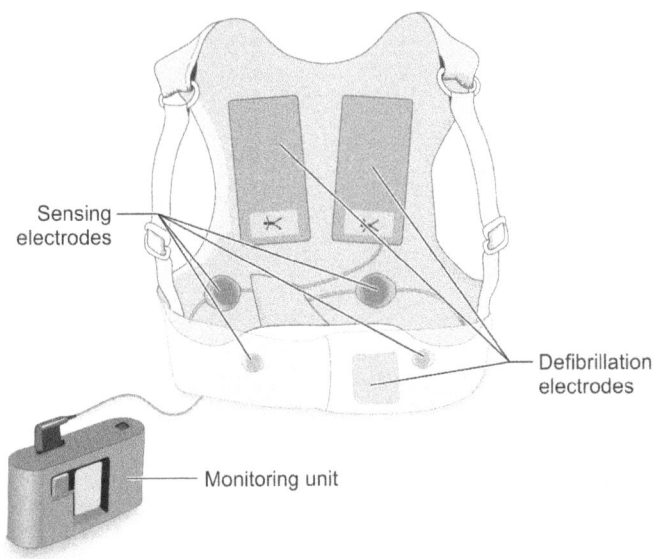

- Monitor unit (500 gm)
  - Battery
  - Digital signal processor of ECG analysis
- LCD display
- Patient response button
  ↓

Arrhythmia detection by 2 nonstandard channels
1. Front—back
2. Side—side

WORKING PATTERN

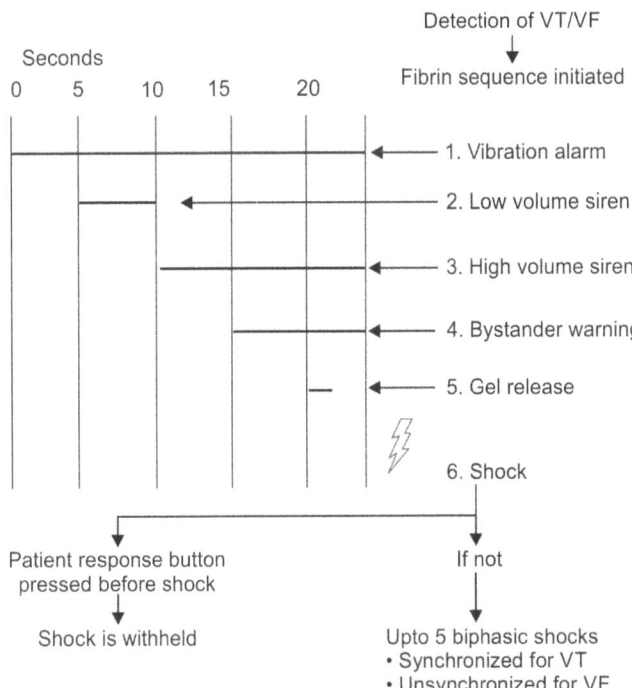

ECG can be stored
30 seconds prior to arrhythmia and 15 seconds after alarm stops

STUDIES

- *Auricchio et al.:* Proposed role of WCD as a bridge to subsequent ICD
- WEARIT and BiROD
  - First outpatient trial
  - 289 patients
  - Advanced heart failure (NYHA 3-4)
  LVEF <30% or at high risk of arrhythmia post MI or CABG
- WEARIT - 2
  - Prospective registry
  - 2,000 patients
  - Inappropriate stock rate = 0.5%
  - No death related to unsuccessful termination of VT/VF

- ICD implantation deferred in 41% due to improvement in EF at follow up
- *Ongoing trial:* VEST, WED-HED

ADVANTAGES
- Noninvasive
- Cost effective
- Inappropriate shock can be prevented in conscious patient (pressure response button)
- Long term use can aid in arrhythmic risk stratification and definitive intervention
- Allows adequate time for myocardial recovery (immediate post MI period)

DISADVANTAGES
- No anti-tachycardia pacing
- No backup pacing for bradyarrhythmia
- External electromagnetic influence can potentially affect WCD more than ICD
- Need to wear throughout the day
  - Hamper quality of life

COMPLICATIONS
- Unsuccessful defibrillation
  - Failure to detect arrhythmias
  - Electrode misplacement
- Inappropriate shock (0.5–3%)
  - False detection and patient fail to respond
  - *False detection due to:* Artifact rapid SVT, loss of signal; double counting; NSVT
  - *Failure to respond:* Sleep inadequate training, mental or physical inability
- VF can be induced by inappropriate unsynchronized shock
- Poor compliance due to discomfort

INDICATIONS
- When there is clear indication for implanted device accompanied by a transient contraindication or interruption in ICD care such as infection 2a/c
- As a bridge to more definitive therapy (e.g., Cardiac transplant) 2a/c
- Heightened risk of SCD that may resolve over time with treatment 2b/c
  - IHD with recent revascularization
  - Newly diagnosed nonischemic DCM
  - Secondary cardiomyopathies (Tachycardiomyopathy, thyroid mediated)
- Bridging therapy in situations associated with increased risk of death and ICD has been shown to reduce SCD but not overall survival 2b/c
  - Immediate post MI period
- Nonarrhythmic risk > arrhythmic risk 3
  Life expectancy <6 months

SECTION 12

Ischemic Heart Diseases

12.1 STEMI: PATHOLOGY, PATHOPHYSIOLOGY, AND CLINICAL FEATURES

UNIVERSAL DEFINITION OF MI

Criteria for Acute MI

- The term acute MI should be used when there is evidence of myocardial necrosis in a clinical setting consistent with AM ischemia
- Any one of the following criteria meet diagnosis of AMI
  - Defection of rise and/or fall in cardiac biomarker value (preferably CTN) with at least is value above 99th percentile of URL and with at least one of the following:
    - Symptoms of ischemia
    - New or presumed new significant ST segment T wave changes or new LBBB
    - Development of pathologic Q waves on ECG
    - Imaging evidence of new RWMA or new loss of viable myocardium
    - Identification of an intracoronary thrombus by CAG or autopsy
  - Cardiac death with symptoms suggestive of Myo. Ischemia and presumed new changes on the changes on the ECG or new LBBB

    Death occurred before cardiac biomarker value were determined or before cardiac biomarker value would be increased
  - *PCI related MI:* Arbitrarily defined by elevation of CTN value (to >5 times the 99th percentile of URL) in patient with normal baseline value, or a rise in CTN value > 20% if baseline values were elevated and were stable or falling. In addition, either
    - Symptoms of myo ischemia

    or
    - New ischemic changes on ECG

    or
    - Imaging demonstration of new loss of viable myocardium or new RWMA

    or
    - Angiographic finding consistent with procedural compt
  - *Stent thrombosis:* Associated with MI when detected by coro angio or autopsy in sitting of myo ischemia and with a rise and/or fall in cardiac biomarker value at least 1 value higher than 99th percentile of URL
  - *CABG mediated MI:* Defined by value of cardiac biomarker (>10 times the 99th percentile of URL) in patient with normal baseline CTN Value. In addition
    - New pathological Q wave or new LBBB
    - Imaging c/o new RWMA or new visible myo. loss
    - CAG documented new graft or new coro art occlusion

Criteria for Prev. MI

Any of following criteria
- Pathological Q waves with or without symptoms in absence of non-ischemic cause
- Pathological findings of prev MI
- Imaging c/o regional loss of viable myocardium that is thinned and fails to contract in absence of non-ischemic cause

UNIVERSAL MI CLASSIFICATION

Type 1: Spontaneous MI—Related to ath plague rupture, ulceration, following erosion or dissection with resulting intraluminal thrombus in one or more arteries that lead to decreased myocardial blood flow or distal platelet emboli with ensuring myocardial neurosis.

Type 2: Myocardial Infarction to Ischemic imbalance e.g., coro endothelial dysfunction, coro art spasm, coro embolism, tachy/bradyarrhythmias, anemia, respiration failure, hypotension.

Type 3: MI resulting in death when biomarkers are unavailable.

Type 4a: MI related to PCI.

Type 4b: MI related to stent thrombosis.

Type 5: MI related to CABG.

12.2 APPROACH TO PATIENTS WITH CHEST PAIN

*COMMON CAUSES OF AC CHEST PAIN

- *Cardiac*
  - Angina
  - Rest or unstable angina
  - AMI
  - Pericarditis
- Vascular
  - Aortic dissection
  - Pulm embolism
  - Pulm HTN
- Pulmonary
  - Pleuritis/pneumonia
  - Tracheobronchitis
  - Spont pneumothorax
- Gastrointestinal
  - Esophageal rupture
  - Peptic ulcer
  - Esophageal reflux
  - Gall stone
  - Pancreatitis
- Musculoskeletal
  - Costochondritis
  - Cervical disc disease
  - Trauma/strain
- Infection
  - Herpes zoster
- Psychological
  - Panic disorder

SHORT-TERM RISK FOR DEATH/NONFATAL MI IN PATIENTS WITH UA

- High risk
  - Accelerating tempo of ischemic symptoms in prior 48 hours
  - Prolonged ongoing (>20 min) pain at rest
  - Pulm edema
  - New onset or worsening of MR murmur
  - S3 or new onset or worsening rates
  - Hypotension/bradycardia/tachycardia
  - Age >75 years
  - Angina at rest with transient ST changes (>0.05 mv)
  - BBB, new or presumably new
  - Elevated cTnI, cTnT or ckMB.

INDICATION AND CONTRAINDICATION FOR EXERCISE ECG IN EO

Requirement for Performing Exercise Testing

- Two sets of cardiac enzymes at 4 hrs inter should be normal
- ECG at time of arrival and pre-exercise 12-lead show no significant abnormality
- Absence of rest ECG abnormality that will preclude accurate assessment of exercise ECG
- From adm to 2nd enzyme patient is asymptomatic, lessening chest pain, persistent atypical symptoms
- Absence of ischemic chest pain at time of exercise testing.

Contraindication

- New or evolving abnormality on rest testing
- Abnormal cardiac enzyme levels
- Inability to perform exercise
- Worsening or persistent ischemic chest pain symptoms from adm to the time of ex
- Clinical risk profiling indicate need for CAG.

12.3 CARDIOGENIC SHOCK

INTRODUCTION

- Most severe clinical manifestations of LVF
- *Char by:* Increased LV filling pr, decreased CO, syst Hypotension, e/o vital organ hypoperfusion
- Incidence 5–8%
- Less of >40% myocardium
- *Patho:* Piecemeal necrosis—prog myocardial necrosis from marginal extension of the infarct into ischemic zone bordering on infarct
  - Associated with persistent elevation of cord biomarkers.

DEFINITION

Marked and persistent (>30 min) hypotension with systolic BP <90 mm Hg and reduction in CI (<2.2 L/min/m^2) in presence of elevated LV filling pr (PCWP > 18).

MANAGEMENT

- Inotropic and vasopressor (lowest possible dose)
- Dopa and dobu
- Ca^{++} sensitizing agent—levosimendan (shown little increment value in RCT)
- Mechanical support
  - IABP (1) Support of circulation
    - (2) Cardiogenic shock
    - (3) Refractory ischemia
  - LVAD
- Revascularization
  SHOCK study—benefit from early revascularization.

RVMI

C/F

- Mild RV dysfunction to cardiogenic shock
- Approx one third of IWMI
- Rt sided filling pr (CVP, RAP, RVEDP) increased
- LV filling pr normal or slightly increased
- CO markedly decreased.

Diagnosis

- Elevated JVP
- Steep of descent
- Square root sign (early diastolic drop and plateau)
- Kussmaul sign (↑ in JVP with inspiration)
- Pulsus paradoxus (fall in SBP >10 mm Hg with inspi)
- ST elevation in rt sided leads
- ECHO.

Treatment

Avoid nitrate and diuretics
Expansion of pl vol to increased RV preload
Arterial vasodilator if associated with LV failure
(further expansion may lead to pulm edema)
↓
PAP catheter for HD monitoring
↓
Arterial vasodilator to empty LV
↓
Decreased impedance to RV emptying.

MECHANICAL CAUSES OF HF

	Vent septal rupture	**Fee wall rupture**	**Pap mu rupture**
Incidence	• 1–3% without reperf • 0.2–0.34% with reperf	• 0.8–6.2% fibrinolysis does not reduce • PCI may reduce risk	1% CPM (more Freq than AL)
Time course	*Bimodal peak:* within 24 hr and 3–5 d: range 1–14 d	Same	Same
C/F	Chest pain, dyspnea Hypotension	Pleuritic/pericardial, syncope, hypotension, arrhythmia, Nausea, restlessness SCD	Abrupt onset SOB pulm edema, hypotension
O/E	Harsh syst murmur Thrill+, S3, accentuated 2nd HD, pulm edema, RV and LV failure, shock	JVP increased, pulsus paradoxus, electro mechanical dissociation cardiogenic shock	Soft ESM, no thrill, variable sign of RV overload severe pulm edema cardiogenic shock
ECHO	VSD, lt to rt shunt, RV overload	• >5 mm pericardial fluid high acoustic echo in Pericardium (blood clot) • Direct visualization of tear	Hypercontractile LV, ruptured pap mu or chordae, severe MR
Rt heart cath	Increase in O$_2$ sat from RA-RV, large V waves	Classic signs of tamponade not always present. Rt heart Cath insensitive	No increase in O$_2$ sat from RA - RV large V waves (PCWP) very high PCWP

Rupture of IVS

- With AWMI—Apical in location
- With IWMI—basal septum—worse prognosis

Increased risk with

- HTN
- DM
- Chr angina
- Prev MI
- Lack of collaterals
- Advanced age
- Female sex
- CKD
  - High 30 d mortality
  - Prompt surgical repair is necessary.

Free Wall Rupture

- More common in LV (Ant or Lat wall)
- Usually preceded by large infarct
- Risk factors
  - Old age
  - Female sex
  - HTN
  - Absence of collat circ
  - First MI.

Pseudoaneurysm

- Incomplete rupture of heart
- Organizing thrombus and hematoma together with pericardium seals Rupture of LV and prevent development of hemopericardium
- Pseudoaneurysm maintain communication with cavity
- Can become quite large (as equal as vent cavity)
- Have marrow neck
- Have significant quantity of old and recent thrombi—can cause arterial emboli
- *Management:* Prompt surgical treatment.

Papillary Muscle Rupture

- *Complete rupture:* Incompatible with life—sudden massive MR cannot be tolerated
- *Partial rupture:* Head or tip—severe MR—very high mortality
- *IWMI:* Post med pap mu rupture
- *AWMI:* Ant—lat pap mu rupture
- *RVMI:* Rupture of RV pap mu—severe TR.

Management

- Invasive monitoring
- PAP and PCWP guide fluid therapy or use of diuretics
- Measure of CO and MAP/SVR—direct vasodilator treatment
- For AC MR and VSD—NTG/Nitroprusside (unless SBP <90)
- Inotropes to maintain CD
- IABP
- Operative intervention
- In patients with stable HD surgery can be postponed up to 2-4 weeks to allow some healing of myocard.

Dynamic LVOT Obstruction after AMI

- Rare
- Thought to occur due to distorted LV geometry and hypercontractility of preserved LV segments
- Usually with AWMI. Caused by mid LAD lesion
  - LV apical akinesia and hyperkinesia of basal segments → increased LVOT gradient.

Management

- LV filling with fluid (with caution)
- BB to decrease contractility
- Inotropes, IABP and vasodilators avoided (because they decrease afterload and worsen LVOT obst).

12.4 CORONARY BLOOD FLOW AND MANAGEMENT ISCHEMIA

CONTROL OF CORONARY BLOOD FLOW

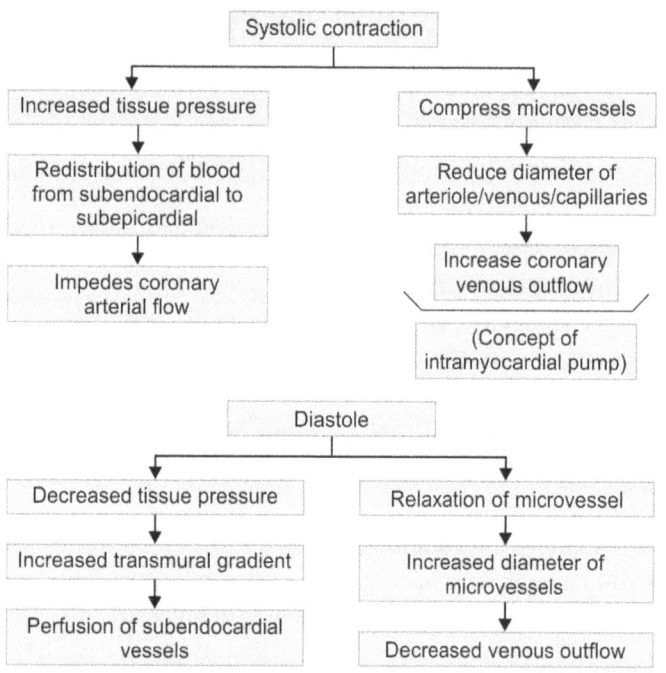

Determinants of Myocardial Consumption

- Myocardial O_2 extraction is near maximal at rest (~60–80%)
- Ability to increase O_2 extraction is limited
- Coronary venous O_2 (PVO_2) can only decrease from 25 mm Hg to 15 mm Hg

↓

Because of high resting O_2 extraction increase in myocardial O_2 consumption primarily depend on Increase in [Coronary flow] and [O_2 delivery] depends on 1. HR 2. SV

Depends on
1. Hemoglobin
2. Arterial O_2 content (CaO_2)
3. O_2 dissolved in plasma

1. Anemia results in proportional reduction in O_2 delivery
2. Hypoxia results in relatively small reduction due to non-linear O_2 dissociation curve. Once PO_2 falls to approx 50 mm Hg (steep portion of O_2 dissociation curve)— Fasten reduction in O_2 delivery

So, major determinants of myocardial O_2 delivery are
1. Heart rate ⎤
2. Systolic pressure (myocardial stress) ⎬ Double product
3. LV contractility ⎦

Note: The basal myocardial O_2 requirement to maintain critical membrane function are low (approx 15% of resting O_2 consumption)

And

Cost of electrical activity is trivial

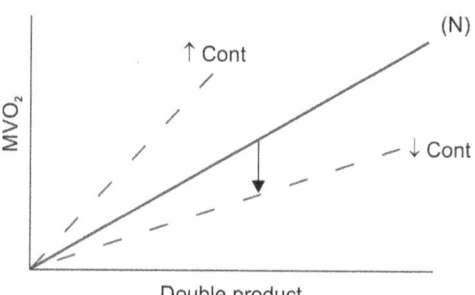

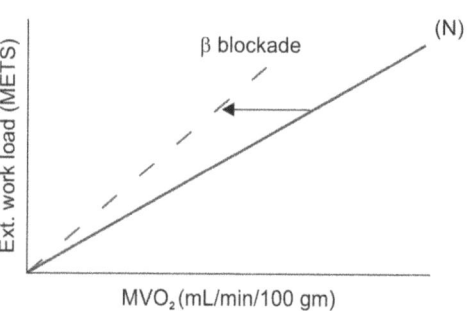

Auto Regulation

Definition

- Regional CBF remains constant as coro art pr is reduced below aortic pressure over a wide range when the determinants of myo O_2 consumption are kept constant. This phenomenon is termed autoregulation

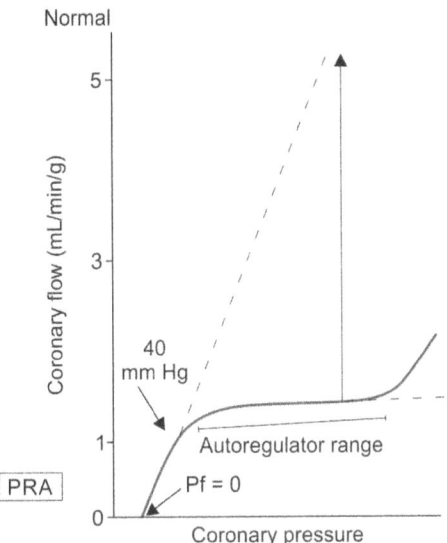
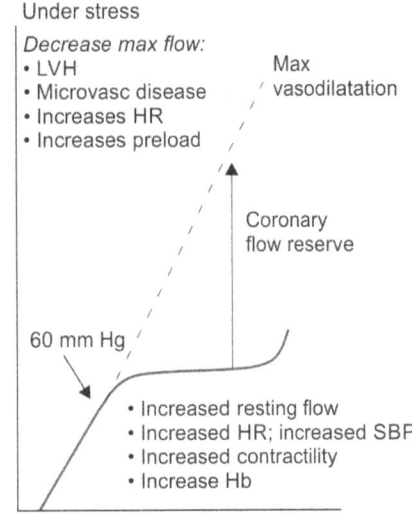

Under basal condition: Normal heart maintains CBF constant as regional coro pr is varied over a wide range when global determinants of O_2 consumption are kept constant. Below lower autoregulatory pr limit (40 mm Hg) subendocardial vessels are maximally dilated and myo ischemia develops. Coro flow ceases at a pr higher than RA pr (PRA) called zero flow pr (Pf = 0), which is effective back pr to flow in absence of coro collaterals

Under stress: Tachy—increased compressive force—increased coronary and decreased diastolic time
Resistance:
- Decreased Max vasodilatory flow
- LVH and microvasc disease also reduce max coro flow
- Increased O_2 demand and decreased PaO_2 - increased resting flow

When pressure falls to the lower limit of autoregulatory pr (~40 mm Hg)
↓
Resistance vessels are maximally dilated
↓
Flow becomes pressure dependent
↓
Onset of subendocardial ischemia

Resting flow under normal circumstances is 0–7 mL/min/gm can increase between 4–5 fold during vasodilatation

Coronary Flow Reserve

Ability to increase coronary flow in response to pharmacological vasodilatation is termed "coronary flow reserve"
- Determinants of CFR (8 maximal perfusion)
  - *Heart rate:* CFR decreases when the diastolic time availability for subendocardial perfusion is decreased
  - *Increased preload:* Increased compressive determinant of diastolic perfusion—CFR decreases

- Increased resting flow
  - Increased O_2 consumption (SBP, increased HR, increased contractility)
  - Decreased O_2 supply (Anemia, hypoxia)
  ↓

These circumstances can produce subendocardial ischemia even in presence of normal coronaries.

Subendocardium vs. Subepicardium

- Subendocardial flow occurs primarily in diastole and begins to decrease below a mean coro pressure of 40 mm Hg. By contrast subepicardial flow occurs throughout cardiac cycle and is maintained until coro pr falls below 25

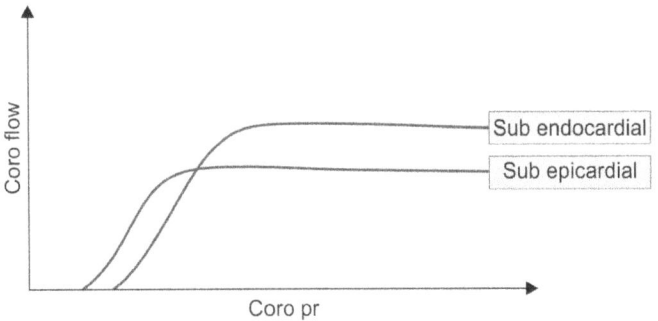

Difference occurs due to
1. Increased O_2 consumption in subendocardium
   ↓
   Requires a higher resting flow
2. More pronounced effect of systolic contraction on subendocardial vasodilator reserve
   ↓
3. Subendocardial vessels become maximally vasodilated before those in subepicardium as coro art pr falls (Autoregulatory lower limit for subendo = 40 and sub epi = 25)

↓
This transmural pr diff in autoregulatory limit makes the subendocardium vulnerable to ischemia in presence of stenosis.

Role of Endothelium in Coronary Tone Regulation

- Conductance vessel as well as resistance vessels exhibit Endothelial modulation of diameter
- Major endothelium dependent biochemical pathways involved in regulating coronary epicardial and resistance artery diameter are as follows
  - *Nitrate oxide*
    - Produced in endothelial cells
    - By NO synthase (conversion of L-arginin—citrullin)
    - No diffuse albuminally into vasc SMC

    ↓
    Binds to guanylyl cyclase
    ↓
    Increased cGMP production
    ↓
    Decreased intracellular calcium
    ↓
    SMC relaxation
    ↓
    Vasodilatation

    - No mediated vasodilatation enhanced by
      - Cyclic or pulsatile change in coro shear stress
      - Chronic upregulation of NOS in response to episode increase in CBF (e.g., exercise training)
    - *No mediated vasodilatation impaired by*
      - *Oxidative stress*—superoxide anion—inactivate NOS (e.g., Atherosclerosis, HTN, DM)
      - *Endothelium dependent hyperpolarizing factors*
        - For selected agonists (e.g., Bradykinin)
        - Shear stress induced vasodilatation
    - Produced by endothelium
    - Opens Ca^+; activated K^+ channel—hyperpolarize VSMC—vasodilatation
  - *Prostacyclin*
    - Produced during metabolism of arachidonic acid via cyclooxygenase
    - Produces coronary vasodilatation when administered exogenously
  - *Endothelin*
    - ET-1, ET-2 – ET-3
    - Peptide endothelium dependent constricting factors
    - *ET-1:* Potent constrictor derived from enzymatic cleavage of a large precursor molecule (pre-pro endothelin)
    - Constriction to endothelium is prolonged
    - Mainly mediated through transcriptional control—produce long-term changes
    - ET A and ET B receptor

ET A	ET B
Activation of protein kinase C in VSMC ↓ Vasoconstriction	ETB mediated constriction is less pronounced and it is counterbalanced by ETB mediated endothelium dependent NO production and vasodilatation

12.5 CORONARY COLLATERAL CIRCULATION

INTRODUCTION

Total coronary occlusion
↓
Native coronary collateral channels open with development of intracoronary pr gradient between source and recipient vessel.

ADVANTAGES

- Maintain resting perfusion normal.
- Prevent stress induced ischemia at submaximal workload.
  - Ischemia does not develop during balloon PCI when FFR is > 0.25

PATHOPHYSIOLOGY

- Arteriogenesis and Angiogenesis
  - Respective stress induced ischemia ⎤
    +
  - Transient development of interarterial pressure gradient between source and recipient vessel ⎬ Arteriogenesis
    ↓
Proliferation of collateral vessel ⎦
Resting distal coro pr gradually falls with increasing severity of stenosis beyond 70%
↓
Creat intraarterial pr—gradient
↓
Increasing shear stress in preexisting collaterals of <200 mm
↓
Flow mediated no dependent dilation and release of VEGF
↓
Collateral formation

Note: Patient with impaired endothelial no mediated vasodilatation will have impaired collateral circulation.
- Arteriogenesis in existing epicardial anatomosis can reach up to 1–2 mm in diameter.
- *Angiogenesis* Do novo vessel growth
  - Sprouting of smaller, capillary like structure from pre-existing blood vessel.

Function: 1. Provide nutritive collateral flow when they develop in border between ischemic and nonischemic regions
2. Can reduce intercapillary distance for O_2 exchange.

Note: As capillary resistance is small component in coronary vas resistance—increasing density of capillaries will not significantly affect coronary flow reserve.

INTERVENTION

For example: Record growth factors, gene transfer
- No intervention has resulted in measurable increase in maximum vasodilated myocardial perfusion or CFR indices.

REGULATION OF COLLATERAL RESISTANCE

- Collateral resistance is major determinant of perfusion
- Coro pr distal to CTO is always near the lower auto-regulatory pr limit
↓
Subendocardial perfusion is critically dependent on mean aerotic pr and preload (Ischemia easily provoked by syst hypotension, increase LVEDP, tachycardia)
- Collaterals constrict when no synthase is blocked
- Collaterals are under tonic dilation from prostaglandins and blocking Cox with aspirin exacerbates ischemia (animals)—rate of PG in human collat is unknown.

12.6 CORONARY FLOW RESERVE

INTRODUCTION
- Concept proposed by Gould
- *Definition:* Ability to increase coronary blood flow in response to maximal vasodilatation
- Can be measured by
  - *Invasive:* CAG + FFR
  - *Noninvasive:* CT FFR; PET; SPECT; CMR

(*See* "autoregulation")

TYPES
Three indices to quantify coro flow reserve
1. Absolute CFR
2. Relative CFR
3. Fractional flow reserve.

Absolute Coronary Flow Reserve

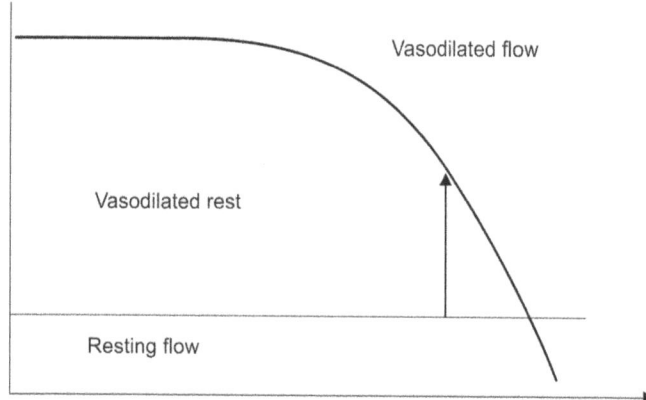

- *Concept:* Assessing relative increase in flow after ischemic vasodilatation or pharmacological vasodilatation (Adenosine, papaverine, dipyridamole)
- Using intracoronary Doppler or Thermodilution method or quantitative approach based on CMR/PET
- Expressed as maximally vasodilated flow and resting flow
- Quantifies ability of flow to increase above resting value
- Absolute flow reserve depends on
  - Decrease in maximal coro flow
  - Increase in resting flow (anemia, hypoxia, increased SBP × HR

Limitation
Importance of epicardial stenosis cannot be dissociated from changes close to function abnormality in microcirculation which are common in patients (e.g., LVH, impaired endothelial dependent vasodilatation).

Relative Flow Reserve

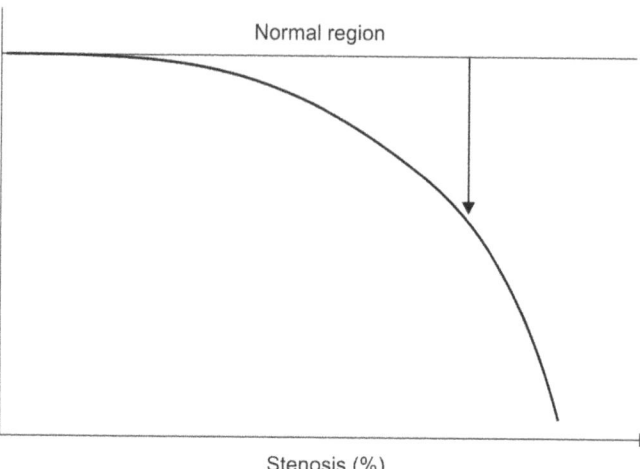

Concept: Relative differences in regional perfusion are assessed during maximal vasodilatation and expressed as a fraction of flow to normal region of heart.

Used mainly in nuclear perfusion imaging.

Limitation
- Requirement of relative normal segment of LV—Relative flow reserve cannot determine exact severity when diffuse abnormality is present either due to multivessel CAD or impaired micro circulation vasodilatation
- Large differences in maximal vasodilated flow are required to detect SPECT perfusion difference.

Fractional Flow Reserve

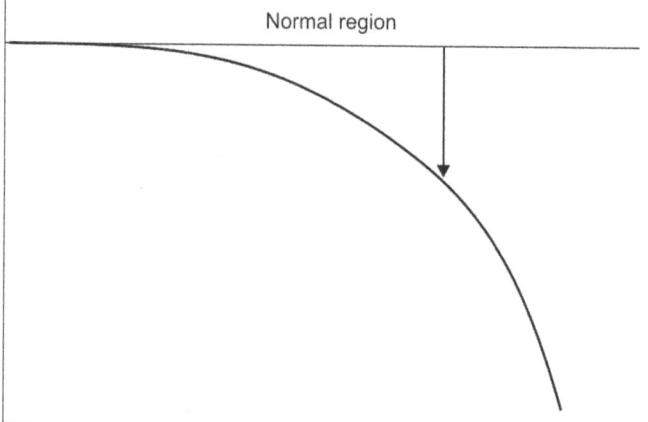

- Pioneered by pryls and colleague
- *Principle:* Distal coronary pr measured during vasodilatation is directly proportional to maximum vasodilated perfusion

- FFR is indirect index
- Determined by measuring during pr for microcirculatory flow distal to stenosis relative to coronary driving pressure available in absence of stenosis
- FFR assumes
  - Linearly of vasodilated pr flow relationship (which is actually curvilinear)
  - Coro venous pr is zero

  $$FFR = Pd/Pao$$
- Conceptually similar to CFR

Limitation

1. FFR can only assess function significance of epicardial art stenosis and cannot assess limitation in Myocardial perfusion (that arises from abnormality in microcirculatory flow reserve)
2. Critically dependent on achieving max vasodilatation
3. Assuming the back pr (venous pr) to zero and ignoring curvilinearity of pressure flow relationship—FFR may underestimate physiological significance

Adv

Physiological assessment of coro stenosis and deferred stenting.

Disadv:

- *Major assumption to all 3 measures:* Administered pharmacological vasodilator achieve maximum vasodilatation of resistance vessel in normal subject as well as in atherosclerotic vessel also
  - Str abnormality in microvessel (regional hypertrophy) or function abnormality in microvessel (altered endothelium dependent vasodilatation)—fallacies in reality
- Currently available approaches can measure only CFR averaged across the entire wall of the heart. They have insufficient spatial resolution to assess transmural variations (this is now possible with CMR).

Pathophysiologic State Affecting Microcirculatory CFR

- LV hypertrophy
  - Flow needs to be considered in mL/min/g
  - Acquired hypertrophy—resting flow per gram of myocardium remains constant (But increase in LV mass require increase in absolute CBF) mL/min
  - Maximal flow (mL/min) during vasodilatation also remain unchanged, but increase in LV mass reduces the max perfusion per gram of myo

  ↓

  Net effect CFR at any given coronary arterial pressure is reduced in a manner that is inversely related to change in LV mass

  Clinical
  1. LVH 2° to systemic HTN has higher coronary flow reserve than LVH of AS
  2. LVH 2° to systemic HTN with increased pulse pr can reduce CBF reserve as coro filling depends on diastolic pr (reduced in increased PP situation)
  3. Some degree of LVH is present in all patients with CAD

- *Coro microvascular disease and dysfunction*
  - Similar to that in LVH
  - Differ in terms of effect on max CBF
  - Max flow pr gm of LV remains normal at rest and reduced during pharmacological vasodilatation
  - *Absolute flow:* Normal at rest and decrease at vasodilatation

	LVH	Microvasc disease
Max flow/gm		
• Resting	Normal	Normal
• Vasodilatation	↓	↓
Absolute flow mL/min		
• Resting	↑	↓
• Vasodilatation	Normal	Normal

  - Because absolute flow across stenosis during vasodilatation is major determinant of pr drop; a similar stenosis will have smaller pr gradient and higher distal pr in patient with microvasc disease than in patients with LVH
- Impaired endothelium dependent vasodilatation
  - Associated with risk of CAD esp hypercholesterolemia
  - Resting BP is not altered
    - Marked increase in coro pr at which intrinsic auto regulatory adjustment becomes exhausted

    ↓

    Flow beginning to decrease at distal coro pr of 60 (rather than 40-45)
    - Excess resistance in penetrating art (which depends on shear stress dependent NO release)—subendocardial infarct

    CFR is markedly reduced in endothelial dysfunction even in absence of coro stenosis (e.g., familial hypercholesterolemia)

    ↓

    Improving endothelial function leads to increased CFR (treatment with statin)

- *Impact of microcirculatory abnormality on physiological measure of stenosis severity*
  - No microcirculatory dysfunction

    ↓

    Absolute FR, Relative FR and fractional FR all will be similar
  - Microvasc dysfunction in presence of normal coronary artery attenuate coronary flow reserve
  - For any given stenosis, FFR measured in presence of microvasc dysfunction will be higher

    ↓

    So when maximal vasodilatation not achieved FFR will underestimate Severity of stenosis

New Availability of high fidelity pr and flow measure on a single wire—facilitated development of approaches to assess stenosis pr flow relation as well as abnormality in microcirculatory reserve by determining FFR and absolute flow reserve simultaneously

↓

Identify circumstances in which mixed abnormality from stenosis and abnormal microvasc contribute to functional impact of a lesion.

12.7 HEART MUSCLE AND CAUSES OF MYOCARDIAL INJURY

HEART MUSCLE

- Cellular effect of ischemia begins within seconds of onset of hypoxia with loss of ATP
- Irreversible cell injury begins within 20 min
- Necrosis usually completes within 6 hours (until and unless reperfusion occurs or extensive collaterals are present)

Gross Findings

- *Two types:* (1) Transmural and (2) Subendocardial

Histologic and Ultrastructured Findings

- Gross alterations are difficult to find until 6–12 hours
- Some histochemical stains can identify zone of necrosis within only 2–3 hours

Microscopic Findings

- Earliest ultrastructural change (within 20 min)
  - Decrease in size and no. of glycogen granules
  - Intracellular edema and swelling
  - Distortion of transverse tubule, SR and mitochondrial this early changes are reversible
- After 60 mins of occlusion
  - Myocyte swelling
  - Internal disruption of mitochondria
  - Development of amorphous, flocculent aggregation
  - Margination of nuclear chromatin
  - Relaxation of myofibrils

Patterns of Myocardial Necrosis

- *Coagulation necrosis*
  - Severe ischemia
  - In central region of infarct
  - Causes arrest of mu cell in related state and passive stretching of ischemic muscle cell
- *Necrosis with contraction band/coagulative myocytolyis*
  - Severe ischemia followed by reflow
  - Hyper contracted myofibrite with contraction band
  - Caused by increased influx of Ca^{++} into dying cell, which causes current in contracted state in periphery of large infarct
  - In nontransmural rather than transmural
- *Myocytolysis:* Severe prolonged ischemia can lead to myocyte vacuolization, termed myocytolysis
- Apoptosis

Cellular Events During MI and Healing

First day: Accumulation of granulocyte
After first day: Mononuclear phagocyte
Finally: Granulation tissue

Now

Day 1–3: Proinflammatory subset of monocyte (high proteolytic and phagocytic capacity and elaboration of inflammatory cytokines)

Day 3–7: Less inflammatory monocyte predominates and produce angiogenic mediator VEGF and fibrogenic growth factor (TGF-beta)

Temporal Sequence

EM: Glycogen depletion: Sarcolemma disruption
     Mitochondrial swelling → Mitochondrial amorphous
     Relaxation of myofibrils   densities

LM: Waviness of fibers at border
↓
Beginning of coagulation necrosis
↓
Continuous coag necrosis
↓
Coag necrosis with loss of nuclei and striations
↓
Disintegration of myofibers and phagocytosis in macrophage

Modification by Reperfusion

- If within 15–20 minutes—prevent necrosis
- Beyond that, salvageable myo tissue depends on
  - Length of time of total occlusion
  - Level of myo O_2 consumption
  - Collateral flow

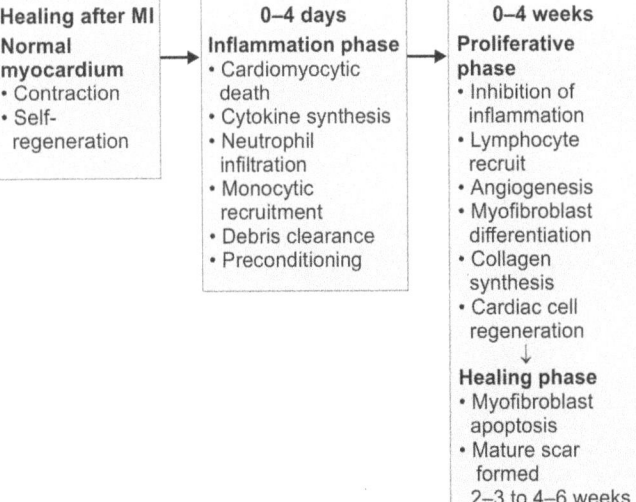

| Healing after MI
Normal myocardium
• Contraction
• Self-regeneration | 0–4 days
Inflammation phase
• Cardiomyocytic death
• Cytokine synthesis
• Neutrophil infiltration
• Monocytic recruitment
• Debris clearance
• Preconditioning | 0–4 weeks
Proliferative phase
• Inhibition of inflammation
• Lymphocyte recruit
• Angiogenesis
• Myofibroblast differentiation
• Collagen synthesis
• Cardiac cell regeneration
↓
Healing phase
• Myofibroblast apoptosis
• Mature scar formed
2–3 to 4–6 weeks |

CAUSES OF MYOCARDIAL INJURY

- *Related to 1° myocardial ischemia*
  - Plague rupture
  - Intraluminal coro art thrombus formation
- *Related to supply demand imbalance*
  - Tachy/bradyarrhythmias
  - Aortic dissection/severe aortic valve disease
  - HCM
  - Cardiogenic, hypovolemic, septic shock
  - Severe anemia
  - Severe respi failure
  - HTN with/without LVH
  - Coro spasm
  - Embolism or vasculitis
  - Coro endothelial dysfunction
- *Injury not related to myocardial ischemia*
  - Cardiac contusion, surgery, ablation, pacing, defibrillation shock
  - Rhabdomyolysis with cardiac involvement
  - Myocarditis
  - Cardiotoxic agents (anthracycline, transtuzumab)
- *Multifunctional/indeterminate myo injury*
  - Heart failure
  - Stress cardiomyopathy
  - Severe PHTN/pulm embolism
  - Sepsis and critically ill patient
  - Renal failure
  - Severe Ac neurological disease (stroke, SAH)
  - Infiltrative disease (amyloidosis, sarcoidosis)
  - Strenuous exercise

12.8 LVF IN STEMI

INTRODUCTION
- Predictor of mortality
- Normal wedge pressure and hyperfusion benefit from infusion of fluids (because peak SV is not reached until LV filling pressure reaches 18-24)
- Low level of LV filling for
  - Relative hypovolemia
  - Concurrent RV MI

AIM
- Reduce preload
- If possible, lower after load
- Meat arrhythmia

TREATMENT

Hypoxemia
- Caused by
  - Pulm vase engorgement
  - Decreased vertical capacity.
  - Respi depression from narcotic analytics
- Hypoxia can impair function of ischemiad to do at margin of infarct
- *Treatment*
  - O_2 via facemask/NP
  - Invasive ventilation
  - Noninvasive venti
- PEEP may diminish syst venous return and reduce effective LV filling pressure—this may require reducing amount of PEEP, infusion of NS to maintain LV filling pressure

Diuretics
- Furosemide
- Decreasing pulm cap pressure—decrease dyspraxia
- Decrease LVEDV decrease LV wall tension—decrease myo O_2 requirement
  - Improve contractility and increase EF, SV, and CO
- Reduction in LV filling pressure—also enhance myo O_2 delivery by diminishing impedance to coro flow
- Decreased pulm congestion—increase salts
- Diuretic reduce pulm vasc congestion and PVP within 15 mins before renal exertion of Na and water has occurred

After Load Reduction
(AECI Long-acting Nitrates)
- IV vasodilation in pt with ocmy with
  - HF—unresponsive to diuretics
  - HTN
  - MR
  - VSD
- Vasodilator to decrease after load—increase SV and decrease myo O_2 demand

Lessen ischemia

Target: 3 simultaneous effects required to improve LV function
1. Reduction of LV after load
2. Avoidance of excessive syst hypotension to maintain effective coro perfusion
3. Avoidance of excessive reduction of LV filling pressure

- In general DCWP should be maintained at 18 and art pr >90/60
- In MR/VSD—vasodilation alone or in combination with IABP

NTG: 10-15 mg/mm infusion—increase 10 mg/mm every 5 mins until improvement of HD relief of ischemic pain is achieved or SBP cyo or SBP fall >15 mm Hg

Diagnosis
- Normally digitalis increase contraction and O_2 consumption
- In HF
  - It decrease heart size and wall tension
  - Decrease myo O_2 requirement

Use: Should be reversed in management of AF/AFL in setting of poor LV function and HF precipitating despite treatment with diuretics and vasodilations

Beta-agonist
- When LVF is severe (CI <2.2 and PCWP >18)
- Dopamine
  - Adrenergic action low only at high dose
  - Vasodilating effect on splanchnic and renal vessel and its positive inotropic action improve HD and renal function
  - Start 2 mg/kg/min—increase up to 20 mg/kg/min
  - *Target:* Decrease in PLWP <18 and CI >2

- Dobutamine
  - Positive inotropic similar to dopamine
  - Slightly less positive chronotropic dopa
  - Less vasoconstriction than dopa
  - Dose 2–30 mg/kg/min
- NE
  - Increase myo O_2 consumption because of its peripheral vasoconstriction effect
  - However trial of NE versus dopamine drowned efficiency similar to or better than dopa

Isomotereral potent cardiac stimulant should be avoided in STEMI patient

Other Positive Inotropic Agents

Milrinone: Noncatecholamine, nonglycoside, phosphodiesterase inhibitor with inotropic and vasodilating agent

- Useful in pt in whom HF persists despite diuretic, who are not hypotensive and who are likely to benefit from both enhancement contractility and after load reduction

Dose: Loading 0.5 mg/kg/min over 10 mins between infusion 0.375 to 0.75 mg/kg/min

12.9 DETERMINANTS OF CORONARY VASCULAR RESISTANCE

COMPONENTS

Three major components

1. *R1: Epicardial coro art resistance*
   - Normal circumstance—No measurable pr drop in epicardial coronaries
   - Stenosis >50%—epicardial artery begins to contribute to coro resistance
   - When stenosis >90%—may reduce resting coro flow
2. *R2: Microcirculatory resistance* (artery and arterioles)
   - Secondary to metabolic and autoregulatory adjustment
   - Distributed throughout myocardium
   - Change in response to physical factor. (Intraluminal pressure and shear stress) as well as metabolic need
   - (Normally—little resistance pr contributed by capillaries and venules and it remains fairly constant during change in vasomotor tone)
   - Minimal coronary vasc resistance of microcirculator is primarily determined by the size and Density of arterial resistance vessels and results in substantial coronary flow reserved in normal heart.
3. *R3: Intravascular compressive resistance:*
   - Varies with time throughout cardiac cycle
   - Related to cardiac contraction and system pressure development
   - HF—increase filling pr—increase extravascular tissue pr during diastole—passive compressor of microcirculatory vessels—impede filling

   (*See* systole and diastole changes)
   (Normal heart - R2> R3 >> R1) and (severe epi stenosis - R1 > R3 > R2)

Phasic systolic cork blood flow determined by
- Intra-myocardial capacitance
- Compressive changes in effective coronary back pressure
- Increase in systolic coro resistance
- Time varying driving pressure

CONCEPT OF DIASTOLIC DRIVING PRESSURE

Effective back pressure to flow in positive heart is higher than right atrial pressure. This has been termed zero flow pressure (Pf = 0)

↓

Its minimum value is approx 10 mm Hg in maximally vasodilated heart

↓

When preload increases; this value increase to 20 mm Hg (close to LV diastolic filling pressure)

↓

Reduce coronary arriving pressure

↓

Reduce subendocardial perfusion

(Important when coronary pressure is reduced by coronary stenosis as well as in failing heart)

CONCEPT OF TRANSMURAL VARIABILITY

Subendocardial vulnerability due to compressive determinants of vascular resistance

↓

Can be partially compensated by reducing minimal resistance

↓

Can be achieved by increasing arteriolar and cap density

STRUCTURE AND FUNCTION OF CORONARY MICROCIRCULATION

- *Conduct artery* (> 400 um in dia)
  - Epicardial coronaries
  - Flow sensitive
  - Dia primarily regulated by shear stress
  - Contribute little pressure drop (<5%)

- Resistance vessels
  Small arteries (100-400 um)
  - Pressure sensitive
  - Reduce their tone in response to shear stress and luminal pressure change

  Arterioles (<100 um)
  - Metabolic sensitive
  - Directly control perfusion of low resistance capillary bed
  - Under resting conditions, most of pressure drop in microcirculation arise in resistance artery (50-200 mm) with little pressure drop across capillaries and vessels
  - After pharmacological vasodilation—resistance art vasodilators—attenuate precapillary pressure drops in arterial resistance vessel to increase pressure drop and redistribution of resistance to venules
  - *Heterogeneity in microvascular dilatation*

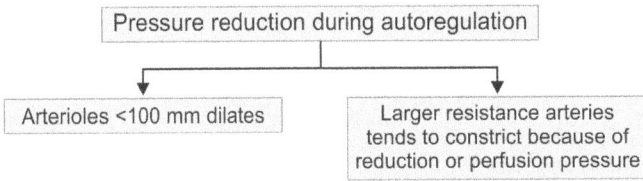

  - By contrast metabolic vasodilation results from more uniform vasodilatation of resistance vessels of all sizes.

12.10 METABOLIC MANAGEMENT IN CAD

INTRODUCTION

- *Drugs that reduce/inhibit FA oxidation:*
  1. Carnitine palmitoyltransferase 1 (CPTI) inhi
     - Etomoxir, Oxfenicine, Perhexiline
  2. 3-Ketoacyl CO A thiolase inhibitor; trimetazidine
  3. Late inward Na^+ channel blocked; ranolazine
- *Activator of Glucose oxidation:*
  - L-Carnitine
  - CO. - Q
  - Lipolic Acid
  - Ribose
  - Dichloroacetate

METABOLIC ALTERATION IN CAD

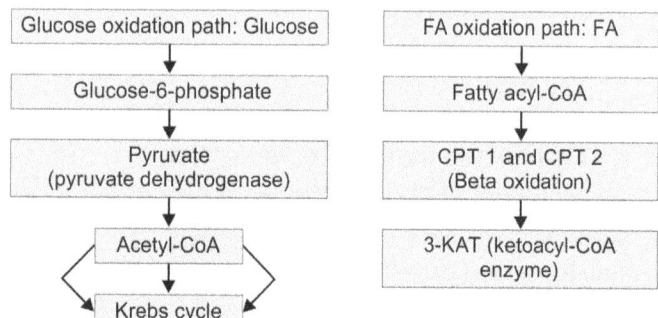

METABOLIC MANAGEMENT IN CAD

- GIK (Glucose, Insulin, and K^+) infusion
  ↓
  - During cardiac ischemia
    ↓
    Metabolism of cardio myocyte shifts from glucose to FA
    ↓
    Generate free radicals—VT/VF
                        Not used
                        Hepatotoxic

- *CPT 1:* Inhibitor (Etomoxir, Perhexiline, Oxfenicine)
  - Inhibit key enzyme in FA oxidation ⎤
  - Improve angina |
  - Increased ex tolerance |
  - Increased LVEF   ⎬ Perhexiline
  - MVO_2 improves |
  - Improve symptoms |
  - Improves resting and peak myofunction|
  - Improves skeletal muscle energetics ⎦

S/E: Cardiac hypertrophy
  Oxidative stress
  Hepatotoxicity (Etomoxir)
  ↓
  Use decreased because of S/E

- *3-KAT inhibitor* (Trimetazidine)
  - Enzyme involved in FA beta oxidation
  - No inotropic/vasodilator
  - No effect on CBF/BP/HR
  - Stimulate membrane phospholipid turnover during ischemia and reperfusion.
    ↓
    Redirect FA toward phospholipid
    ↓
    Improves cell tolerability towards reperfusion injury
  Dose: 35 mg BD
  CI–CKD
      Allergy
      PD/Restless leg syndrome/movement disorder
  TRIMPOL I study: Improve total duration of ex
                    Improvement takes work (mets)
                    Improves time of onset of angina
  TRIMPOL 2: Trimeta + Metoprolol - Addictive
  METRO and VASCO - Improves Angina

- *Ranolazine:*
  - Piperazine derivative

MOA
- Inhibit late Na^+ current ⎤
  In diseased state: |
  Enhanced late NCx (?) |
  ↓ |
  Increased Cytosolic Ca^{++} level ⎬ Inhibited by ranolazine
  ↓ |
  Increased LV relaxation and |
  increased LV EDP; DAD |
  ↓   ⎦
  Compromise blood flow
- Inhibit Ikr—Prolongs APD—QT increases
- Reduced HbA1C
$t_{1/2}$ = 7 hrs
Meta—Cyst P450
Exc—Renal
S/E: Dizziness, nausea, asthenia, constipation, dose dependent QTc

TRIALS

MARISA: Increased ex duration
    Dose dependent adv effect
    CARISA
    ERICA
    TERESA

RIVER PCI—Did not show benefit in chr stable angina incomplete PCI
MARLIN- TIMI—No benefit in NSTEMI

- *Activation of Glucose oxidation:*
  L Carnitine ⎤
  CO Q   ⎬ Limited use due to lack of evidence
  Dichloroacetic Acid ⎦

12.11 METABOLIC AND FUNCTIONAL CONSEQUENCES OF ISCHEMIA

INTRODUCTION

Thrombotic coro occlusion
↓
Sudden cessation of blood flow
↓
Cessation of aerobic metabolism
↓
Onset of anaerobic glycolysis
↓
Accumulation of tissue lactate, reduction in tissue ATP level and accumulation of catabolites
↓
Development of tissue acidosis and efflux of K^+ in extracellular space
↓
Once ATP level falls below threshold that is necessary for critical memb function
↓
Onset of myocyte injury

Irreversible Injury and Death

- Begins after 20 mins of total occlusion
- Subendocardium to subepicardium
- Factors that increase myo O_2 consumption and worsens ischemia
  - Tachycardia
  - Anemia/hypotension
- Repetitive reversible ischemia/angina before an occlusion—can reduce irreversible injury through ischemic preconditioning
- When collat flow is approx 30% of resting flow values, it prevents infarction after ischemia for >1 hour
- Moderate subendocardial ischemia from subtotal occlusion (flow reduction ≤50%)—can persist for at least 5 hours without irreversible damage

Reversible Injury and Perfusion Contraction Mismatch

- *Supply induced ischemia*
  - Transient coronary occlusion from vasospasm → Increased LV compliance
  - Transient thrombosis in critically stenosed artery
  ↓
  Both can produce transmural ischemia
- Demand induced ischemia
  - Inability to increase flow in response to increased myocardial O_2 demand → Decreased LV compliance
  - Predominantly affect subendocardium

Coronary occlusion
↓
Decreased coronary venous O_2 saturation
↓
Decreased ATP production
↓
Decline in regional contraction within several beats—reaching dyskinesia within a minute
↓

- Reduction in global LV contractility (dp/dt)
- Progressive rise in LVEDP
- Fall in SV and SBP
- Significant OCG change within 2 mins as effect of K^+ into extracellular space reaches critical level
- Chest pain is variable and last to appear in events of ischemia
- If perfusion restored, chest pain disappear first followed by HD abnormalities
↓
Regional contraction can remain impaired (Stunned myocardium)

Acute Perfusion Contraction Matching During Subendocardial Ischemia

- Linear relation between relative reduction in subendocardial flow vs myocardial regional wall thickness (at rest, tachy and during ex induced dysfunction)
- This forms basis for using Myocardial regional wall thickness and function as an index for severity of subendocardial ischemia during stress imaging

CONSEQUENCES OF ACUTE ISCHEMIA

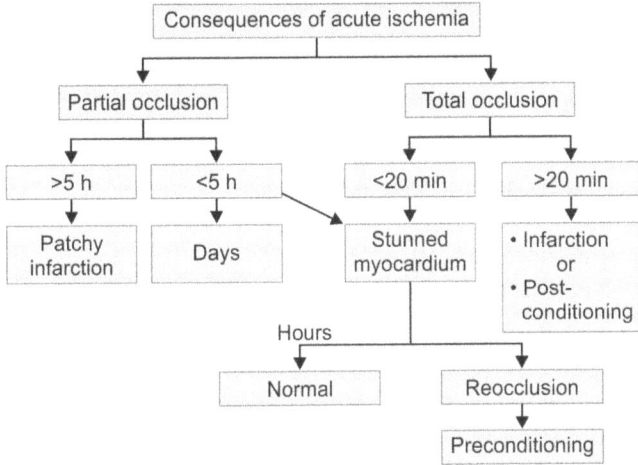

CONSEQUENCES OF CHRONIC REPETITIVE ISCHEMIA

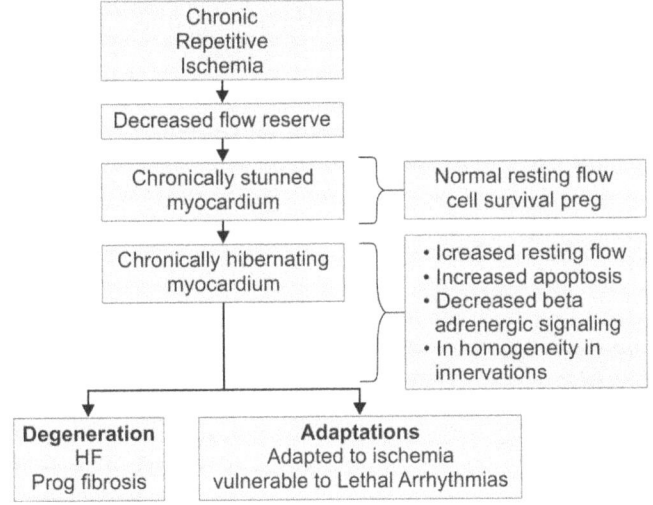

ISCHEMIC PRECONDITIONING AND POSTCONDITIONING

Preconditioning: Brief episodes of reversible ischemia preceding—prolonged coronary occlusion reduce irreversible myocyte necrosis. This phenomenon termed as preconditioning

- It reduces myocardial infarct size and protects heart from ischemia induced stunning
- Preconditioning can also develop on a chronic basis (delayed preconditioning)
- Once induced it persists up to 4 days
- Mech of chronic preconditioning are:
  - Up regulation of inducible form of NO (iNO)
  - Up regulation of Crx-2
  - Opening up of mitochondrial k ATP channels
- Can be induced pharmacologically by
  - Adenosine A1 receptor stimulation
  - Pharmacological agonist that stimulates protein kinase C or
  - Opening of kATP channel
  - During coronary angioplasty with successive coronary occlusion (with balloon)

Postconditioning: Ability to cause cardiac protection by producing intermittent ischemia or administer pharmacological agonist at the time of reperfusion

- Can be induced after myocardial ischemia is established rather than pretreatment
- Protection occurs principally through reperfusion injury salvage kinase pathways—thereby limiting opening of the mitochondrial permeability transition pore

12.12 PHYSIOLOGICAL ASSESSMENT OF CORO ART STENOSIS

STENOSIS PRESSURE FLOW RELATIONSHIP

- Normally coro art accommodate large amt of coronary blood flow without any significant pressure drop (conduit function)
- In CAD, fixed stenosis limits maximal myocardial perfusion (because epicardial artery resistance increase with increasing severity)
- Pressure drop across stenosis can be predicted by Bernoulli's equation
- Pressure drop depends on
  - Viscous losses
  - Separation losses
  - Turbulence (minimal)
  - Single most imp determinant of stenosis resistance if minimal luminal CSA

ΔP = vicious loss + separation loss
 = $S1\, Q° + S2\, Q°$ F1 = vicious coefficient
            S2 = separation coefficient

$$S1 = \frac{8\pi uL}{As^2}; \quad S2 = \frac{P}{2}\left[\frac{1}{As} - \frac{1}{An}\right]^2$$

Flow separation

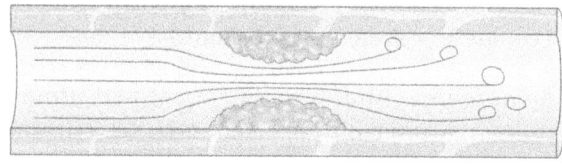

L = Length of stenosis
As = Area of stenosis
An = Area of normal segment
uP = Blood viscosity
P = Blood density

- So resistance is
  Inversional proportional to square of CSA
  ↓
  Small change in CSA by thrombi/vasospasm leads to major change in stenosis pr flow relationship

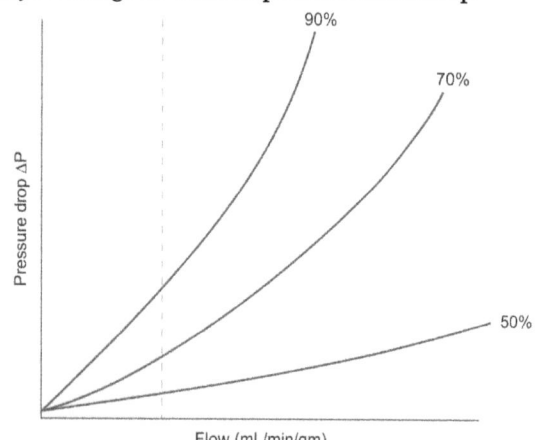

(epicardial art stenosis pr flow relationship)

- Separation losses determine curvilinearity or steepness of pr flow relationship
  ↓
  Becomes increasingly important as stenosis severity and/or flow rate increases
  ↓
  Pressure drop is also flow dependent and varies with square of flow or flow velocity
  ↓
  Small reduction in luminal area results in large reduction in post stenotic pressure
  ↓
  Limits maximal coro perfusion of distal microcirculation

INTERPRETATION OF DISTAL CORO PR FLOW AND STENOSIS SEVERITY

- Max myocardial perf is determined by coro pr distal to a stenosis
  ↓
  Effect of stenosis on resting and vasodilated flow is summarized in this figure

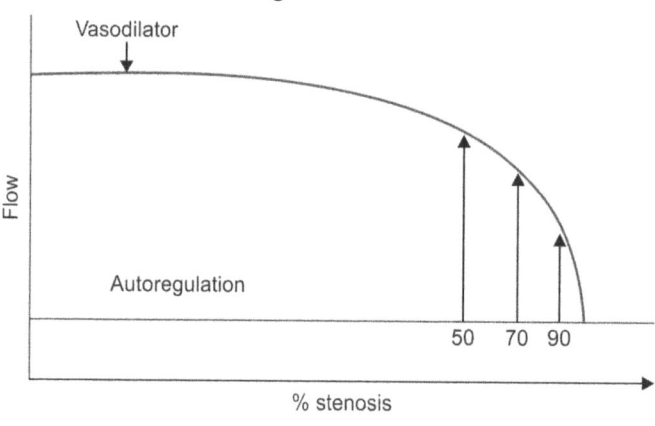

  ↓
- Autoregulatory flow remains constant even if stenosis severity increases
- Vasodilator pr flow relationship is more important to detect physiological significant stenosis
- No significant pr drop occur until stenosis Severity increases >50% diameter reduction (75% CSA reduction)
  ↓
  As stenosis severity crosses 50%; pr flow relationship steepens
  - Stenosis resistance increases
  - ΔP across stenosis also increases
- Critical stenosis is one in which subendocardial flow reserve is completely exhausted at rest (usually >90%)

12.13 NSTE-ACS

DEFINITION

Patients without persistent ST segment elevation in 2 or more contiguous leads but with biomarker evidence of myocardial necrosis are classified as having NSTEMI.

In patient without such evidence of Myocardial necrosis are classified as UA.

Features that differentiate from stable angina (vs ACS)
- Onset of symptoms are rest (or with minimal exertion) and lasting longer than 10 min
- Severe compressive pressure or chest discomfort
- Accelerating pattern of symptoms that develop more frequently, with greater intensity or awaken the patient from sleep

PATHOPHYSIOLOGY

Four processes
1. Rupture of unstable atheromatous plaque
2. Coronary artery vasoconstriction
3. Imbalance between supply and demand
4. Gradual Intraluminal narrowing of an epicardial artery because of progressive atherosclerosis or post restenosis

- Leads to formation of superimposed thrombus, typically non occlusive in NSTE-ACS—impaired myocardial perfusion—myocardial necrosis
- Can result from vasospasm (Prinzmetal angina), vasoconstrictor released by platelets, endothelial dysfunction or adrenergic stimuli (fight-or-flight response), cold, cocaine or amphetamines

Plaque rupture/erosion
↓
Vascular injury or endothelial dysfunction
↓
Adhesion of platelet to arterial wall via platelets Gp1b to subendothelial von Willebrand factor
↓
Exposure of platelets to subendothelial collagen and/or circulating thrombin causes plt activation
↓
Degranulation of platelet with release of ADP and TxA2
↓
Further platelet activation and expression of Gp2b/3a
│
Platelet aggregation—platelet fibrin thrombus
↓
Fibrinogen → fibrin
↑
Thrombin (factor 2a)
↑
Activated factor 10 (10a)
↑
Complex of tissue factor and 7a and 5a
↑
Activates coagulation cascade
↑
Tissue factor expressed within the lipid rich core of atherosclerotic plaque exposed to circulating blood

MARKERS OF MYOCYTE DAMAGE

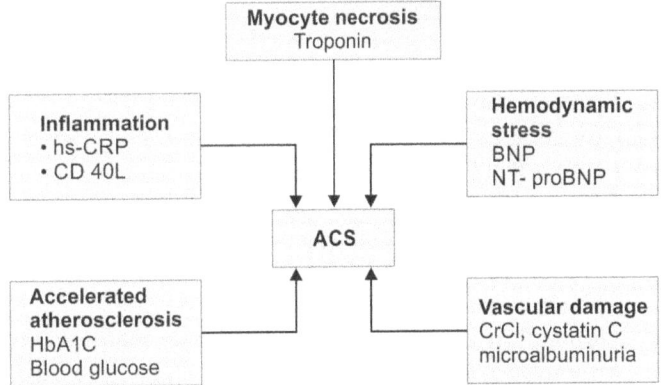

MECHANISM OF TROPONIN RELEASE

- Myocyte necrosis (ischemia, infarction, Inflammation, trauma)
- Apoptosis
- Normal myocyte turnover (low grade annual turnover of myocyte)
- Cellular release of proteolytic troponin degradation products (creation of small fragments that pass through the intact myocyte membrane without cell death)
- Increased cellular wall permeability (reversible injury to myocyte membranes resulting in altered permeability
- Formation and release of memb blebs (active secretion of vesicles or membrane expression with shedding).

EMERGING BIOMARKERS OF ACS

A. *Markers that can predict death/ischemic events*
   - *Growth differentiation factor 15:* Memb of TGF-B superfamily. Release from cardiomyocyte
   - *Heart type FA binding prot:* Cytoplasmic protein involved in intracellular uptake and buffering of FFD in myocardium
   - *Myeloperoxidase* released during degranulation of neutrophils and monocytes

- Preg associated pl protein A—expressed abundantly in eroded and ruptured plaque
- *Placental growth factor:* Strongly upregulated in ath lesions
- *Secretory phospholipase A2:* Hydrolyzes phospholipid to generate lysophospholipids and FA
- Interleukin-6
- Chemokine ligand 5 and 18

B. *Markers that predict HF*
- *Mid regional pro adrenomedullin:* Peptide fray of vasodilatory peptide adrenomedullin
- *Neopterin*—marker of monocyte activation
- *Osteoprotegerin* modulator of immune function and inflammation

MANAGEMENT

General
- Transport rapidly to ED
- Directed history and examination and ECG within 10 mins of arrival
- CTn assay should be obtained
- CBC, electrolyte, creatinine, glucose
- Bed rest, O_2 supplement if SPO_2 <90% and in patients with HF or basal rates
- Ambulation as tolerated is permitted if patient stable without recurrent chest discomfort or changes on ECG for at least 12–24 hrs
- *2nd Tn assay:* 3 hours if hs TN
  6–9 hrs if 4th gen CTN

Nitrates
- Endothelium independent vasodilator
- *MOA:*
  1. Increased Myocardial blood flow by coro vasodilatation
  2. Decreased myo O_2 demand by lowering preload through venodilation
  3. Decreased cardiac afterload by inducing arterial dilatation and thereby decreased vent wall stress
- *Dose:*
  S/C NTG (0.3 to 0.6 mg up to 3 times at 5 mm internal)
  If ischemia symptoms persists and patient is hypotensive (iv NTG ≥70 ug/min with dose gradually increase to 200 ug/min as needed)
  Topical or long-acting nitrate if patient pain free >12–24 hrs
- *Tolerance:*
  - Within 12–24 hrs
  - Can be ameliorated by nitrate free period
  - If symptoms do not allow nitrate free period-increasing dose may help

C/I
- Hypotension
- PPE-5 inhibitors within prev 24–48 hours
  ↓
  Decreased breakdown of cGMP and causes exaggeration and prolongation of vasodilatory effect of nitrate
- Caution in severe As, HCM, RV Infarction or HD significant PE

Beta-blockers
Adv: Reduce infarction ⎤
   Vent fibrillation ⎬ Reduce
   Death ⎦
   Also reduce risk for Progression to MI

Indi: Should be initiated in 24 hrs with follow exception
  1. S/O decompensated heart failure
  2. e/o low CO state
  3. Increased risk for cardiogenic shock
  4. AV block, asthma or reactive airway disease

Can be administered in patients with HF once their condition has stabilized

Morphine
- In patients with persistent pain despite nitrate and BB
- *Dose:* IV 2–5 mg every 10 mins × 3 times
- Monitor BP, respi and mental status
- *MOA:* Analgesic, anxiolytic, venodilator
- *S/E:*
  - Hypotension
  - Respi dep—naloxone 0.4 to 2 mg

CCB
- Vasodilator effect—decreased arterial pr
- Verapamil and diltiazem also slows HR, decreased myo O_2 demand
- Effective in decreasing ischemia in patients with NSTE-ACS and persistent ischemia despite treatment with full dose nitrate and BB (also in patients with CI to BB)
- *Nifedipine:*
  - Short acting
  - Can increase HR—harm in patients with ACS if not co-admin with BB

Ranolazine
- Novel antianginal agent
- No alteration in HR/BP
- *MOA:* Inhibition of late sodium current in myocardial cells—reduce some of deleterious effects attributed to overload of intracellular sodium and Ca^{++} during ischemia

- *Adv:* Reduces ischemic episodes and need for NTG in patients with chr stable angina both as monotherapy and in combi with CCB/BB
- In trial population, ranolazine did not reduce 1° composite outcome of CV death, MI, or recurrent ischemia but did decrease incidence of recurrent ischemia
- 1° outcome, however was reduced significantly in sub groups of patients with elevated natriuretic peptide and in those with prev angina

DECISION MAKING

Urgent Invasive (<120 min)

- Refractory angina
- Recurrent angina despite intense antianginal treatment associated with ST dep (≥2 mm) or deep neg T inv
- Clinical symptoms of HF or HD instability
- Life threatening arrhythmias (VF/VT)

Early Invasive (<72 hours)

- Elevated troponins
- Dynamic ST-T changes
- DM
- Reduced renal function (eGFR <60)
- Decreased LVEF (<40%)
- Early post-MI angina
- PCI within 6 months
- Prior CABG
- Intermediate to high risk acc to risk score

Conservative

- No recurrence of pain
- No high of HF
- No abnormality on initial ECG or 2nd ECG (6-12 hrs)
- No elevation of troponin (arrival and 6-12 hrs)

ANTIPLATELETS

Aspirin

MOA:

Acetylation of cor-1 (irreversible Inhibition)
↓
Blocks synthesis and release of TxA2 (G. plt activator)
↓
Decreased platelet aggregation and arterial thrombus formation
↓
Anti plt action lasts for life tire for plt (7-10 d)

Aspirin:
- Decreased adv cardiac events early in course
- Decreased Freq of ischemic event in 2° prev

CURRENT OASIS 7:
- High dose (300-325) vs. low dose (75-100)
- No diff in the risk for CV death, MI or stroke between two doses, but at bleeding increase with higher dose

PLATO: Another reason to favor low dose ASA

C/I: Documented allergy (e.g., ASA induced asthma)

	Treatment
Nasal polyp	
Active bleeding	Desensitization
Known platelet disorder	Substitute
	Anti-platelet

Resistance (2-8% of patients)
Reason:
- Poor compliance (pseudo resistance)
- Decreased absorption (interaction with ibuprofen)
- Over expression of COX 2 MRNA
- Enteric—coated dosage forms
- Rarely genetic or other intrinsic reason

Recommendation: Aspirin should be given to all patients without CI at initial loading dose of 150-300 and maintenance of 75-100 regardless of treatment strategy

P2Y12 Inhibitors

- *Thienopyridine:* Ticlopidine, clopidogrel and Prasugrel
- Cyclopentyl—triazolopyrimidine: ticagrelor
  Acts directly as reversible Inhibitors of P2Y12 rec
  Irreversible blocking binding of ADP to plt surface P2 1/12 rec
  ↓
  Interfering with both plt activation and aggregation
- They are prodrugs—require oxidation by hepatic cytochrome P450
- Also reduce fibrinogen, blood viscosity and erythrocytes deformability and aggregability (mechanism that appears to be independent of ADP)

Clopidogrel

- Avoids neutropenia and TTP (associated with Ticlopidine)
- 85% hydrolyzed by circulating esterase and render inactive
- Remaining oxidized by CYT -P- 450—active metabolite
- *Trials*
  1. CURE: Addition of clopidogrel to ASA Reduced CV death, MI or stroke by 20% in both low and high risk patients with NSTE-ACS regardless of treatment strategy. Benefit seen as early as 24 hrs with Kaplan meter beginning to diverge after just 2 hrs. Benefit continued throughout trials 1 yr period

2. *CURRENT-OASIS 7:* High dose clopidogrel (600 mg loading: 150 for 7 d and then 75 mg) did not reduce CV death, MI or stroke in NSTE-ACS
- Analysis of subgroup of patients who underwent PCI showed reduced CV events following PCI with 600 mg when compared with 300 mg

Recommend

- P2Y12 Inhibitors should be added to Aspirin ASAP and maintain over a period of 12 months unless there is CI - class 1
- PPI (omeprazole) in combination with DAPT is recommended in patients with H/O CI hemorrhage or peptic ulcer and (Cl-I) patient with other risk factors (*H. Pylori*, ≥ 65 yr)
- Prolonged/permanent withdrawal of P2Y12 Inhibitors within 12 month after index event is discouraged until clinically indicated (1)
- Clopidogrel 1300 mg loading, 75 mg/d is recommended for patients who cannot receive ticagrelor/Prasugrel (1)
- 600 mg loading recommended for patients scheduled LV invasive strategy (C1)
- Higher maintenance dose 1150 mg/d should be considered for 1st 7 d in patients with PCI without Increased risk of bleeding (2a)

Hyporesponder to Clopidogrel

5–30%
DM
Obesity   ⎫ More common
Adv age
Genetic polymorphism ⎭

- *Reason* Several polymorphism of gene encoding for CYP2C19 enzyme
  *production of active metabolite
  Reduced function* C2 allele – up to 50% of Asian
- *Trial:* Patients with UA undergoing PCI, maintenance dose of 225 mg or more is necessary in heterozygous carries a CYP2C19*2 allele to achieve same effect on 75 mg

PPI modestly decreases effect of clopidogrel because of competition for metabolism by CYP3A4 (esp Omeprazole)
↓
However RCT of ticagrelor vs clopidogrel showed that significant interaction between clopidogrel and PPI is unlikely.

Prasugrel

- Prodrug like clopidogrel
- Active metabolite is irreversible inhibitor of P2Y12 rec
- Oxidized rapidly in 1 step to its active metabolite
- Become active within 30 mins of ingestion
- Generation of active metabolite is 10 times greater than clopidogrel—so 10 times potent
  (60-10, 300-75)

Trial

1. *TRITON TIMI 38* Prasugrel vs. Clopidogrel
   - CV death, mortality and stroke—decreases by 19% with Prasugrel 30% in patients with DM
   - Prasugrel decrease stent thrombosis by 50%
2. Wiviott and coauthors—60 mg loading of Prasugrel resulted in higher plt Inhibition than 600 mg clopidogrel

C/I

1. High bleeding risk (TRITON TIMI 38)
   esp • Patient ≥75 yrs   ⎤ Avoid prasugrel
       • Body weight <60 kg ⎦ except in high-risk patients
                                ↓
                             Can be used at 5 mg maintenance dose
2. H/O stroke /TIA

TRILOGY ACS (Prasugrel vs Clopidogrel for OMT)
- No diff between 1° composite end patients of LV death, MI, stroke
- No diff in severe bleeding

Recommend

- For P2Y12 Inhibitors naive patients (esp diabetics) in whom the coronary anatomy is known and who are proceeding to PCI unless there is high risk of bleeding
- Patient undergoing non emergency surgery, postponing surgery for 5 d after cessation of ticagrelor/Clopidogrel 7d after cestabo or Prasugrel

Ticagrelor

- Reversible blockade of P2Y12
- Act directly on plt
- $t_{1/2}$ - 12 hrs
- It too has active metabolite (potency of which is similar to parent drug)
- Both excreted in bile
- Inhibit P2Y12 mediated aggregation completely

Trial (1) PLATO (Clopidogrel vs Ticagrelor)

- 1° end patient (composite CV death, MI and stroke) decreased by 16%
- MI reduced by 16%

- CV death by 21%
- Relative risk reduction of total mortality by 22%
- Significant reduction of stent thrombosis
- No benefit of ticagrelor in patients who had received high dose of aspirin

↓

FOA recommended ASA dose to be 75-100 when used with ticagrelor
- Plato also showed
  -0.7% absolute higher incidence of non-CABG-related major bleeding with Ticagrelor
- Moderate—minor dyspnea ⎤ Occurred more
- Vent pauses >5 seconds ⎦ frequently with Ticagrelor
- As Ticagrelor is reversible inhibitor—can be started at the time of arrival to ER and can be continued for 1 yr in medically managed patient or those undergoing PCI
- Should be discontinued 5 day before surgery

Protease-activated Receptor-1 (PAR 1) Antagonist
Vorapaxar
- Investigational drug
- Inhibit thrombin mediated platelet activation
- TRA-2P TIMI 50 Addition of vorapaxar to std therapy reduced ischemic events while increasing bleeding compared with placebo
- 2 weeks to 1 year after MI received vorapaxar and showed 20% decrease in CV death, MI and stroke

↓

It may be used as 2° preventive measure
No role in early after ACS

Gp 2b/3a Inhibitors
MOA: Block final common pathway of plt aggregation, fibrinogen mediated cross linkage of plt caused by variety of stimuli (thrombin, ADP, collagen, serotonin)

Three Agents
1. Abciximab
   - Major surgery deferred until 24 hours
   - Cannot be reversed rapidly
   - Prolonged action (~12 hrs)
   - Approved only in patient undergoing PCI
2. Tirofiban ⎤ Reversible
3. Eptifibatide ⎦ short $t_{1/2}$ (2 hrs)
   - Restoration of plt function in hours
   - Discontinued 2-4 hr before surgery

Trials
1. Tirofiban + heparin and Aspirin significantly reduce the rate of death, MI or Refractory ischemia at 7 d when compared with Heparin + ASA
2. Eptifibatide also significantly decrease MI at 30 d
3. No benefit and higher mortality found in patients with abciximab in NSTE-ACS in whom an early conservative strategy was planned
4. Benefit appears to be greater in patients with ST segment changes and/or elevated troponin or diabetes (This subgroups have more thrombosis at CAG and have high risk of microvasc embolization
5. *Major bleeding:* Significantly high severe Thrombocytopenia slightly high
   - Daily platelet monitoring is required
6. *Two large trials:* When to initiate?
   - Routine early administration vs delayed provisional use before PCI

↓

- No diff in 1° efficacy
- Bleeding more in patients with early admin

Recommend
- Routine administration of Gp2b/3a inhibitor to patients with NSTE-ACS who receive DAPT is not recommended
- Selective use [in patients with high risk of ischemia (DM, CAG evidence of thrombus) and at low risk of bleeding who are to undergo PCI] is more prudent

ANTICOAGULANTS
Heparin:
MOA
- Blocks thrombin (factor 2a) and factor 10a
- Also binds to circulating plasma protein, acute phase reactant and Endothelial cells

↓

Unpredictable anticoagulant effect
- Short $t_{1/2}$—cont infusion needed
- 33% reduction in death or MI with UFH + aspirin vs. aspirin alone
- Variability in effect due to
  - Heterogeneity in MOA
  - Neutralization by plasma factor and protein released by platelet

Guideline (ACC/AHA):
- Weight adjusted dose 60 u/kg bolus - 12 u/kg/hr infusion
- APTT every 6 hourly till target range achieved and then 12-24 hours thereafter

Ischemic Heart Diseases

Heparin reversal
- Protamine sulfate
- Binds heparin to form a stable salt
- 1 mg of protamine = 100 U of UFH
- Because of $t_{1/2}$ of heparin is 1-15 hrs, total dose of protamine needed to be administered is based on UFH administered in prev 2-3 hours
- Slow iv to avoid hypotension and Brady
- S/E:
  - Hypotension
  - Brady
  - Flushing
  - Feeling warmth
  - Dyspnea

Note: Protamine Neutralize approx 60% of anticoag activity of heparin, but does not affect its anti alpha a activity

LMWH

Advantages
- Greater anti alpha a activity—inhibit thrombin generation more effectively
- Greater release of tissue factor pathway Inhibitors than UFH does—not neutralized by PF4
- LMWH less freq causes H/T
- High and consistent bioavailability—s/c dose
- Monitoring not req
- Bind less avidly to patient prot—more consistent anticoag effect

Note:
1. Renal dysfunction affect LMWH more
   - Dose reduction is required

Dose
- 1 mg/kg s/c × 12 hourly
- Once a day for patient with CrCl <30 ml/min
- Upto 80 days (until hospital discharge)

UFH should not be administered in cath lab
- If LMWH given in prev 10 hours
- LMWH effect can be reversed with protamine
- Less effectively than UFH

Direct Thrombin Inhibitor

Adv:
- Do not require anti-thrombin and can inhibit clot bound thrombin
- Do not interact with plasma protein
- Provide very stable level of anticoagulation
- Do not cause Thrombocytopenia (choice for H/T)

Bivalirudin
- Binds Reversibly to thrombin
- $t_{1/2}$ approx 25 mins

ACUITY trial: Patients with NSTE-ACS
Three groups
1. UFH or Enoxaparin with/without Gp2b/3a
2. Bivalirudin with Gp2b/3a
3. Bivalirudin alone

   Biva alone reduced bleeding
   No diff between all 3 arms in terms of ischemic events
   ↓
   Bivalirudin monotherapy is now considered an acceptable alternative in patients with NSTE-ACS managed with early invasive strategy and may be preferred in patients with increased risk of bleeding who undergo PCI

Dose: 0.1 mg/kg bolus –0.25 mg/kg/hr
If started during procedure
0.75 mg/kg bolus –1.75 mg/kg/hr
↓
Discontinue shortly after PCI

Renal dysfunction
- CrCl <30; not on HD: 1 mg/kg/hr
- Patient on HD: 0.25 mg/kg/hr

Factor 10a Inhibitors: Fondaparinux
- Indirect factor 10a inhibitor
  - Require presence of antithrombin for its action
- *OASIS 5 trial*
  Daily s/c fondaparinux vs. Enoxaparin

  - No diff found in 1° ischemic composite through 9 days
  - Fondaparinux did reduce major bleeding by nearly half and mortality at 30 days tended to be lower with fondaparinux
  - In patients undergoing PCI—fondaparinux was related with 3 fold increased risk of catheter related thrombi
- So, fondaparinux is an alternative for patient being managed noninvasively and esp. for patients at high risk of bleeding.

Otamixaban
- Direct Factor 10 a inhibitor (investigational)
- Phase 3 trial is underway

Oral Anticoagulation
- *ASA + warf:* More effective than ASA alone very high risk of serious bleeding

- Another indication for warf + ASA are patients without cons stents but with another indication such as chr AF, severe LV dysfunction, high risk for systemic embolization
- *Triple therapy* ASA + P2Y12 inhibitor + warf
  Sometimes required in NSTE-ACS post stenting who have AF or another strong Indi for warf
  > High risk of bleeding
  > No large RCT
- Low dose aspirin + warf (INR 2-2.5) + clopidogrel for short time can be used
  > BMS is recommended (they can reduce duration of P2Y12 Inhibitor)
- 2010 ESC—short cause of triple therapy followed by long-term single anti platelet + warf
  - *ATLAS ACS 2 TIMI 51:* Low dose rivaroxaban (5 BD) and very low dose (2.5 BD)
    - Both decreased primary composite end point of death, MI or stroke by 16%
    - Rivaroxaban substantially decreases overall mortality and stent thrombosis
    - Higher rate of IC bleed
    - 2.5 mg BD has favorable profile
  - *APPRAISE 2:* Apixaban 5 mg BD
    Stopped prematurely due to excessive major bleed

Bleeding Risk

Steps to Reduce Chances of Bleeding

- Weight adjusted dose of anticoagulant
- Modified dosing of antithrombosis in patients with renal dysfunction
- Selection of anticoagulants with low-risk bleeding profile (e.g., Fondaparinux, Bivalirudin)
- Low dose aspirin after initial loading
- GI protective agents
- Avoid Concomitant treatment with NSAIDS/steroid
- Radial access, smaller sheath size and timely removal of sheath
- BMS, which permit short course of DAPT

Crusade Bleeding Risk Score

- Baseline hematocrit
- Cr clearance
- HR
- Gender
- Sign of CHF at initial evaluation
- Prev vasc disease (PAD/stroke)
- DM
- Syst BP

Score <20—very low risk
  21-30—low risk
  31-40—intermediate risk
  41-50—high
  >50—very high

Lipid-lowering Therapy

- *LIPID trial:* Pravastatin leads to 26% reduction in mortality
- *PROVE-IT-TIMI 22*
  Intestine lipid lowering (Atorva-80/prava-40)
  - 16% reduction in 1° end point (CV death + MI + stroke + revascularization or UA leading to hospitalization)
  - 25% reduction in death, MI or urgent revasc
- *NCEP recommended*
  - Optional therapeutic LDL goal <70 in high-risk patients with CAD
- *Meta-analysis*
  - No adv effect of ultra low LDL (<40-50) and statin dose should not be routinely titrated downward in asymptomatic patient.

12.14 CAUSES OF MI WITHOUT CORONARY ATHEROSCLEROSIS

- *Coronary arterial disease other than atherosclerosis*
  - *Arteritis*
    - Syphilitic
    - Granulomatous (Takayasu)
    - PAN
    - Kawasaki disease
    - SLE/RA/AS
  - *Trauma to coronaries*
    - Laceration
    - Iatrogenic
    - Radiation therapy
  - *Coronary mural thickening with metabolic disease or intimal proliferative disease*
    - Mucopolysaccharidosis (Hurler)
    - Homocystinuria
    - Fabry disease
    - Amyloidosis
    - Pseudoxanthoma elasticum
    - Intimal hypertrophy associated with contraceptive steroid or post-partum period
  - *Luminal narrowing by other causes*
    - Spasm (Prinzmetal)
    - Spasm after NTG withdrawal
    - Dissection of aorta
    - Dissection of coro art
- *Emboli to coro art*
  - IE
  - Non-bact thrombotic
  - MV prolapse
  - Mural thrombi (LA, LV)
  - Prosthetic valve thrombi
  - Cardiac myxoma
  - Associated with CAG and CABG
  - Paradoxical emboli
  - Papillary fibroelastosis
  - Thrombi from intracardiac catheters
- *Cong coro anomalies*
  - ALCAPA
  - LCA from ant sinus
  - Coronary AV fistula
  - Coronary cameral fistula
  - Coro art aneurysm
- *Myo O_2 demand-supply*
  - AS/AI
  - CO poisoning
  - Thyrotoxicosis
  - Prolonged hypotension
  - Takotsubo
- *Hematological*
  - Polycythemia vera
  - Thrombocytosis
  - DIC/TTP
  - Hypercoagulability
- *Miscellaneous*
  - Cocaine abuse, myocardial contusion
  - MI with normal coronaries; compli of cardiac cath

12.15 CORONARY VASOSPASM

INTRODUCTION

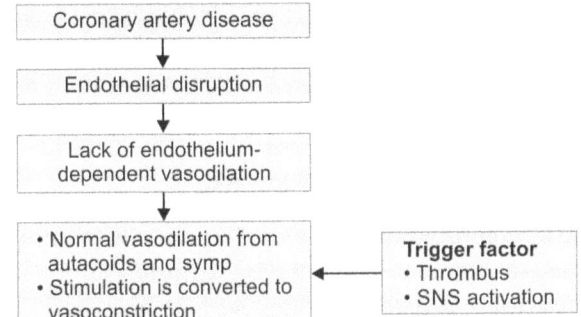

PHARMACOLOGICAL VASODILATION

- Direct action on vasc AMC
- Secondary adjustment in resistance art—tons
  - *NTG:* Dilates epicardial conduct arteries and small resistance arteries but does not increase CBF in normal heart (because transient arterials dilatation is counter acted by autoregulatory escape which brings resistance to control levels

Beneficial effect of NTG
- It dilates epicardial art—improve subendocardial perfusion
- Reduce LVEDP via systemic vasodilation in HF—improve subendocardial perfusion
- Coro collar vessels dilate—improve regional flow
- *CCB:*
  - Induce VSMC relaxation
  - Also pharmacological vasodilation
  - Effective in preventing coro vasospasm
  - Nifedipine is potent
  - Can lead to coronary steal phenomena
- *A2 receptor agonists:*
  - Regadenoson
- *Dipyridamole:*
  - Vasodilation by inhibiting myocyte uptake of adenosine released from cardiac myocyte
- *Papaverine:*
  - Short acting coro vasodilator

12.16 PATHOPHYSIOLOGY OF STEMI

INTRODUCTION

- *Left vent function*
- *Systolic function*

Four abnormal contraction patterns
1. *Dyssynchrony:* Dissociation of the time course of contraction with adjacent segment
2. *Hypokinesia:* Reduction in extent of shortening
3. *Akinesis:* Cessation of shortening
4. *Dyskinesis:* Paradoxical expansion and syst bulging
- *Hyperkinesia of remaining normal myocardium initially* accompanies dysfunction of the infarct
  - Due to increased activity of SNS and Frank Starling mechanism
  - Portion of hyperkinesis is ineffective because contraction of noninfarcted segment causes dyskinesia of infarct zone
  - Increased hyperkinesia subsides within 2 weeks
- Sometimes *reduced myo contractile function in non-infarct zone* — Ischemia at a distance
  - Result from prev obst of coro supplying non infarct region and loss of collaterals from freshly occluded IRA
- Preservation of systolic function may occur due to collaterals

↓

If sufficient portion of myocardium undergo ischemia

↓

LV pump failure

↓

CO decreases, SV decreases, BP decreases, peak dp/dt decreases

ESV increases
↘ Powerful predictor of mortality
- In some patients,
  Vicious cycle (Dilatation begetting further dilatation)
- With time
  - Increased stiffness of infarcted myocardium — Edema, Fibrosis
  ↓
  Slightly improve LV function because it prevents dyskinesia
- Earliest abnormality vent stiffness in diastole
- When infarcted segment is >15% - LVEF falls and LVEDV + LVEDP increases

Abnormally contracting segment
- >25% - clinical HF
- >40% - cardiogenic shock

DIASTOLIC FUNCTION

- Decreased peak rate of decline in LV pr (dp/dt)
- Increase in time constant of fall in LV pr
- Rise in LVEDP—after few week—LVEDV tends to increase and LVEDP comes to normal

CIRCULATORY REGULATION

- If the infarct is of sufficient size, overall LV function falls—lowers aortic pr and coro perfusion pr—intensify myocardial ischemia—vicious cycle—cardiogenic shock
- Systemic inflammation 2° to MI leads to release of cytokines that contribute to vasodilatation and decreased SVR
- Inability of LV to empty normally—increased preload— increased SV but at expense of low EF
- Dilatation of LV—increased afterload (Laplace law)
  - Decreased LV stroke volume and also elevate myo O_2 consumption—intensity MI

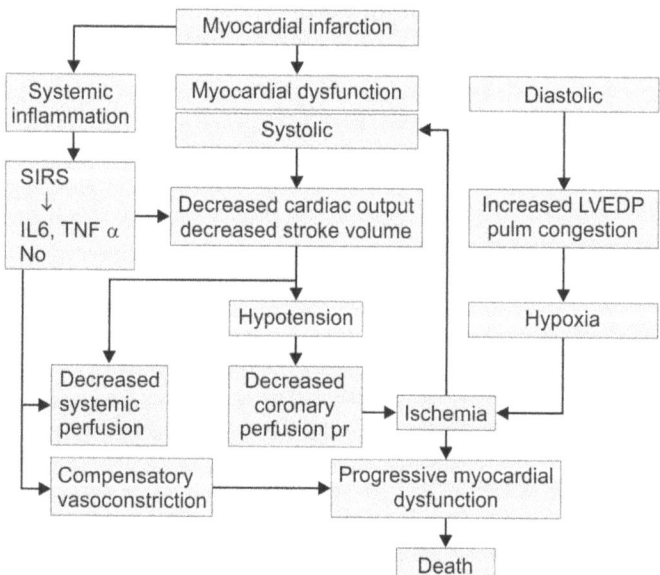

VENT REMODELING

STEMI
↓
Change in LV size, shape and thickness involving both infarcted and noninfarcted segment
↓
Collectively referred as LV remodeling
(Changes in LV dilatation combined with hypertrophy of residual noninfarcted myocardium causes remodeling)
↓

Depends on
- Infarct size
- Patency of IRA
- Vent volume
- Loading condition

INFARCT EXPANSION

Definition
Acute dilatation and thinning of the area of the infarction not explained by additional myocardial necrosis

Causes
- Slippage between muscle bundles—reduce no of myocyte across infarct wall
- Disruption of normal myocardial cells
- Destruction of ESM within Necrotic zone

Degree of infarct expansion depends on
- Pre infarct wall thickness
- Hypertrophy possibly protect against it
- Intensity of inflammatory response to Necrotic cells—it's suppression limits infarct size
(Apex the thinnest portion—prone to infarct expansion)

STEMI - Infarct - Infarct expansion - final scar

Complication (of infarct expansion)
- Higher mortality
- Higher incidence of nonfatal complication
- Higher HF and vent Arrhythmia

Investigation
Best recognized as elongation of non contractile region of ventricle on ECHO/CMR

Vent Dilatation
- Remodeling is also caused by dilatation of viable portion of vent which commences immediately after STEMI and progress for months—years
- Shift of pr vol curve of LV to rt will result in large LV volume at any given diastolic procedure
- Dilatation of noninfarcted zone can be viewed as compensatory mechanism that maintains stroke volume in presence of large infarct

Effects of Treatment
- Reperfusion—limits infarct size
- Glucocorticoid and NSAIDS—causes scar thinning and greater infarct expansion
- RAAS inhibitor—decreased vent enlargement
- Aldosterone inhibitor—decreased fibrosis and decreased vent arrhythmia

Pathophysiology of Other Organs

- *Pulmonary function*

If STEMI + hypoxia
↓
Increased pulm capillary hydrostatic or
↓
Interstitial edema
↓
Arteriolar and bronchiolar compression
↓
VQ mismatch
↓
Further hypoxia
↓
Hyperventilation
↓
Hypocapnia + respi alkalosis

- Decrease in airway conductance
- Decreased Pulmonary compliance
- Decreased FEV
- Decreased mid exp flow rates
- Increased closing volume

Due to widespread closure of small dependent airways during first 3 days after MI

- Ultimately,
  Severe increase in extravasc volume of water
  ↓
  Leads to pulm edema

- *Reduction of affinity of HB for O_2*
  - Affinity of HB for O_2 falls due to increased 23 DPG (diphosphoglycerate)

- *Endocrine function*
  - *Pancreas*
    - Absolute conc of insulin is normal
    - But it's relatively low level
    - Insulin resistance

    → Marked hyperglycemia

Reason
- Decreased pancreatic blood flow 2° to splanchnic vasoconstriction
- Increased activity of SNS will augment circulatory catecholamines—inhibit insulin secretion and glycogenolysis

- Glucose can generate energy (ATP) via anaerobic metabolism—this uptake of glucose require insulin
  ↓
  Insulin deficiency hamper glucose uptake and can lead to decreased ATP generation in myo
  - *Adrenal medulla*
    - Plasma and urinary catecholamine levels peak during first 24 hours
    - High level correlate with occurrence of arrhythmia and increased myocardial O_2 demand
    - Circulating catecholamine enhance plt aggregation—release TxA2—vasoconstriction—Impair cardiac perfusion
  - *Activation of RAAS*
    - A2—promote TGF-Beta and PDGF—compensatory hypertrophy
    - A2—release of endothelin, PAI-1, aldosterone—vasoconstriction, impaired fibrinolysis and increased Na^+ retention (respectively)
  - *Natriuretic peptide*
    - Risk in BNP and NT pro BNP correlate with infarct size and RWMA
  - *Arterial cortex*
    - Plasma and urinary 17-hydroxycorticosteroids and ketosteroid as well as aldosterone rise markedly in STEMI patients
    - Correlate with peak level of ck, infarct size and mortality
    - Glucocorticoid also contribute to impaired glucose metabolism
  - *Renal function* impaired
- *Hematological alteration*
  - *Platelet:* Increased propensity to aggregate
  - *Hemostatic marker:* Increased FDP
    Increased fibrinopeptide A, TAT, F1.2—associated with increased risk for mortality
  - *Leukocyte:* Accompanies necrotic process, elevated glucocorticoid level and possibly inflammation
    - Associated with mortality

12.17 PRINZMETAL ANGINA

INTRODUCTION
- Ischemic pain that occurs at rest and accompanied by ST segment elevation
- May be associated with AMI, VT/VI and SCD
- Diagnostic Hallmark: Spasm of prox coro art with resultant transmural ischemia and abnormality in LV function.
- Mechanism of spasm—not established
  - Decreased NO production
  - Imbalance between endothelium—derived relaxing and contracting factors
  - Inflammation (increasing hs-CRP)
  - Polymorphic of alpha-2 presynaptic and beta-2 postsynaptic receptor

CLINICAL PROFILE
- Younger
- No classical coro risk factor
- Heavy cigarette smokers
- Severe anginal pain may be accompanied by syncope
- Tend to Chester between midnight and 5am
- One third patient also exhibit fixed coro obst and may have combination of exertion induced angina with ST seg dep and episode of angina at rest with ST elevation
- Rarely, generalized vasospastic disorder associated with migraine and/or Raynaud's phenomenon
- Can also develops in associated with aspirin induced asthma
- Ergot derivative used to treat migraine can precipitate PVA

DIAGNOSIS
Key to diagnosis—C/o episodic ST elevation with severe chest pain

Provocative test
- Hyper ventilation
- Coro acetylcholine
- IC ergonovine—not available
- Performed only in patient without obstructive CAD and in whom PVA is suspected

MANAGEMENT
- Discontinue smoking
- Calcium channel blocker—DOC
    (alone or in combination with long-acting nitrate)
- S/L or iv NTG often abolishes attack of PVA promptly
    Long-acting nitrates useful to prevent attacks
- Response to BB is variable
- Revasc—CI in pt with only spasm
  - May help in pt with prox obst lesion in combination with spasm
- ICD for pt who cont to have vent arrhythmic inspite of OMT

NATURAL HISTORY
- Many patients with PVA pass through acute, active phase with freq episodes of angina and cardiac events occurring during first 6 months
- Remission occur more freq in patient without significant fixed stenosis and in those who have discontinued smoking

PROGNO
- Excellent (if no CAD underlying)
- *CASPAR:* No MI or cardiac death noted

12.18 REPERFUSION INJURY

INTRODUCTION

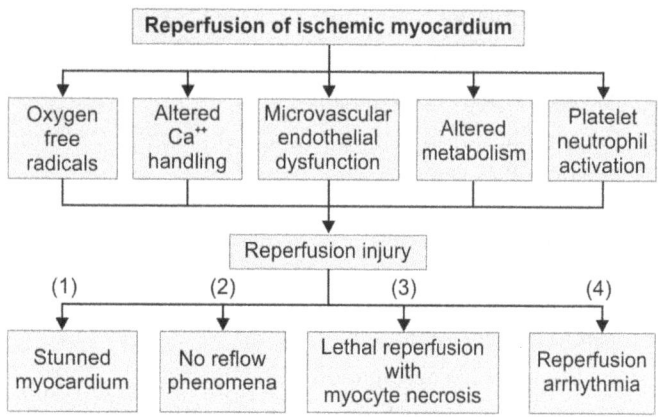

MEDIATORS OF REPERFUSION INJURY

- *Oxygen paradox:* Reperf—sudden restoration of O_2 level - oxidative stress—Myo injury
- *Calcium paradox:* Abrupt increase in intracellular Ca^{++} due to sarcolemnal memb damage and oxidative stress induced dysfunction of SR—excess of Ca^{++} induce cardiac myocyte death of hypercontracture of heart cells and increasing mitochondrial permeability
- *Ph paradox*
- *Endothelial dysfunction and microvasc injury*
- *Metabolic modulation*

STRATEGIES TO INCREASE REPERFUSION INJURY

- Inotropic stimulation of perfused stunned heart
- *Ischemic postconditioning:* 3–30 sec cycle of ischemia-reperfusion
- Therapeutic Hypothermia
- Mg^{++} therapy
- Treatment for no-flow phenomena
- Metabolic stimulation with insulin
- *Antioxidants:* Vit E
- Sodium hydrogen anti post inhibition
- Stimulating endogenous cardioprotectants
- Targeting risk pathway
- Targeting mitochondrial PTP

12.19 STEMI: MANAGEMENT

CONTRAINDICATION TO FIBRINOLYSIS
- Absolute
  - Any prev IC blood
  - Known structural cerebral vasc lesion (AV malformation)
  - Known malignant IC neoplasm (1°/mets)
  - Ischemic stroke within 3 month except acute ischemic stroke within 4.5 hrs
  - Suspected aortic disease
  - Active bleeding/bleeding diathesis (except menses)
  - Significant closed head or facial trauma in 3 months
  - Intracranial or spinal surgery within 2 months
  - Severe uncontrolled HTN (unresponsive to emergency treatment)
  - For STk, previous treatment within 6 months
- Relative
  - H/O chronic, severe, poorly controlled HTN
  - Significant HTN at initial evaluation (SBP>185; DBP>110)
  - H/O prev ischemic stroke > 3 months
  - Dementia
  - Known I/C pathology not covered in absolute CI
  - Traumatic/prolonged CPR (>10 min)
  - Major surgery < 3 weeks
  - Recent internal bleeding (2-4 wks)
  - Noncompressible vasc puncture
  - Pregnancy
  - Active peptic ulcer
  - Oral anticoagulant

Beta-blocker
Adv:
- Limit infarct size
- Relief of ischemic pain
- Reduce need for analgesics
- Reduce life-threatening arrhythmias

Routine use of IV beta-blocker is not recommended because-risk of precipitating cardiogenic shock

Practical Approach
- Exclude patient with hypotension, heart failure, Bradycardia or significant AV block
- Administer Metoprolol 5 mg × 3 iv boluses
- Observe patient for 2-5 min after each bolus
  - If HR<60 or SBP < 100—no further dose
- If HD stability continues 15 min after last iv dose—begin oral Metoprolol (25-50 mg every 6 hourly for 2-3 days and then step up to 100 mg BD)

Esmolol: Short acting IV beta-blocker
- Can be used in patient with relative CI to administration of beta-blocker and in whom slowing HR is necessary

LIMITATION OF INFARCT SIZE
- Important prognostic factor
- Large infarct size—late impairment of vent function
Long-term mortality is higher
- Approach to limit infarct size
  - Early reperfusion
  - Reduction of myo energy demand
  - Manipulation of energy production source
  - Prevention of reperfusion injury
  - Ischemic preconditioning

> Spontaneous recanalization of IRA occurs in up to *one-third of patient* beginning at *12-24 hours*
>
> Enhance LV function and limits infarct size

- Relief of coro spasm
- Prevention of damage to microvasculature
- Improved systemic hemodynamics (augmentation of coro perf and reduced LVEDP)
- Collateral circulation

Measures
- Timely reperfusion
- Myocardial O_2 consumption minimized by
  - Maintaining patient at rest both physically and emotionally
  - Mild sedation
  - Quiet atmosphere
- Avoid adrenergic agonists
- Prompt treatment of tachy arrhythmias
- Treatment of HF to minimize SNS activation and hypoxia
- Correction of anemia (by caution)
- Associated condition esp Infection—Tachy, fever and elevated O_2 needs—required management

REPERFUSION THERAPY

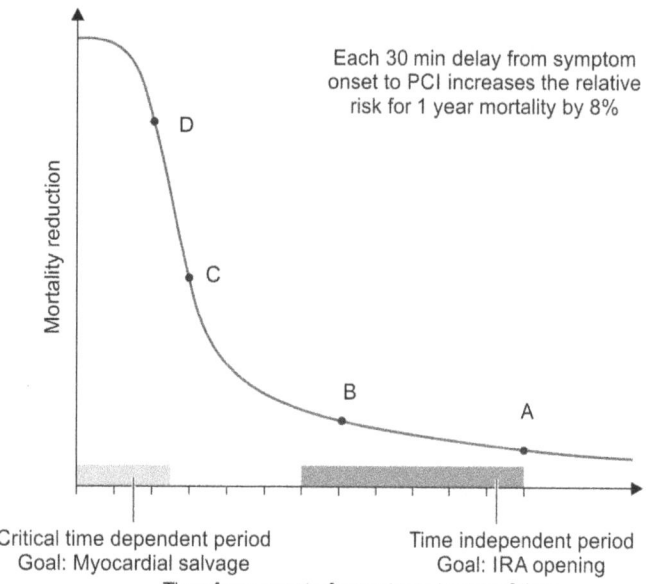

Each 30 min delay from symptom onset to PCI increases the relative risk for 1 year mortality by 8%

Critical time dependent period
Goal: Myocardial salvage

Time independent period
Goal: IRA opening

Time from onset of symptoms to reperf time

- Even after successful reperfusion and despite the absence of irreversible myocardial damage, a period of post ischemic contractile dysfunction can occur a phenomenon referred to as *"Myocardial stunning"*

REPERFUSION INJURY

- Process of reperfusion might be accompanied by adverse sequelae described by the terms *reperfusion injury*

Types

1. Lethal reperfusion injury—reperfusion related cell death
2. Vascular reperfusion injury—progressive damage to microvasculature—expanding area of no-reflow and loss of coronary vasodilatory reserve
3. Stunned myocardium—salvaged myocytes display a prolonged period of contractile dysfunction because of abnormality in intracellular metabolism leading to reduced energy production
4. Reperfusion arrhythmias
   - 2., 3., 4. can occur in STEMI
   - 1. Concept of lethal reperfusion injury is controversial
     - Microvascular injury in reperfused myocardium can lead to hemorrhagic infarct
       (More likely with fibrinolytic than catheter)

*Protection Against Reperfusion Injury

- Preservation of microvasc integrity by using
  - Anti platelets ⎤ To minimize embolization of
  - Antithrombin ⎦ atheroembolic debris
- Prevention of inflammatory damage
- Metabolic support of ischemic myocardium

- *Remote conditioning:* Phenomenon of induction of transient ischemic in other vascular bed has been associated with reduction in reperf injury
- *Post conditioning:* Introducing brief episodes of ischemia alternating with reperfusion—activates cellular mechanism centering around prosurvival kinases

*Reperf Arrhythmias

- Transient Brady and Hypotension in patient with IWMI at time of acute reperfusion—due to bezold—Jarisch reflex
- PVC, AIVR, NSVT—also types of reperf arrhythmias
  - IC beed with fibrinolytics: <1%

*Assessment of Reperfusion

- TIMI flow grade
- TMP grading
- TIMI frame count
    TIMI frame count can also be used to quantitative CBF
    CBF = 21 ÷ (observed TIMI frame count) × 1.7
- *ECG:* Persistence of ST elevation—higher risk for LV dysfunction and mortality (because of microvascular damage)
- Noninvasive testing
  - CECT
  - CMR
- Invasive assessment
  - Doppler flow wire studies
  - TMP grading

*Effect of Fibrinolytic Therapy on Mortality

- *Fibrinolytic therapy trialists* (FTT)
  18% reduction in short-term mortality
  25% reduction in mortality in patients with STEMI
- *LATE and EMERAS*
  Reduction in mortality may still be observed in patients treated with thrombolytic agents between 6 and 13 hours after onset of ischemic symptoms
  ↓
  All 3 trials are basis of extending window of fibrinolysis up to 12 hrs
- Bedside risk scoring system for predicting 30 day mortality at initial evaluation of fibrinolytic eligible patient
- Developed by Morrow
- In time 2 trial

Myocardial Salvage Index

Difference between initial perfusion defect (e.g., by sestamibi scintigraphy) and final perfusion defect

Useful means for comparing the effectiveness of reperfusion therapy
- Characterization of LV volumes concurrently with extent of scar as revealed by myocardial delayed enhancement as well as ischemia with adenosine stress perfusion and cardiac MRI, provide prognostic information. It is emerging strategy for risk stratification after MI

TIMI risk for STEMI	(Predicting 30 d mortality)
Age 65–74/≥75	2/3 patient
SBP<100	3 patient
Killip I 4	2 patients
HR>100	2 patients
Anterior STE/LBBB	1 patient
DM, H/O HTN, H/O angina	1 patient
Wt < 67 kg	1 patient
Time to treatment> 4 m	1 patient

ANTICOAGULANT THERAPY FOR STEMI

A. Heparin
RCT in pre fibrinolytic era—Heparin to STEMI patients lower risk of reinfarction, pulm embolism and stroke

↓

ISIS-2 trial—substantial reduction in most with aspirin alone confusing data regarding risk benefit ratio of hex used as adjunct to aspirin or in combine with aspirin and fibrinolytic agent

Other effects of heparin:
- Mortality benefit and amelioration of LV after STEMI indicates that use of heparin for at least 48 hours after fibrinolysis
- Major A/E occurs more frequently iv patient with low body weights advanced age, marked prolongation of APTT performance of invasive procedure

Potential disadv of UFH
1. Dependency on anti thrombin 3 for inhibition of thrombin activity
2. Sensitivity to platelet factor 4
3. Inability to inhibit clot bound thrombus
4. Marked inter patient variability
5. Freq. monitoring of APTT

↓

To circumvent these disadvantages

↓

B. Newer anticoagulants
- *Hirudin and Bivalirudin*
  - Direct thrombin inhibitor
  - Bivalirudin decreases incidence of rec MI by 25-30%
  - Higher rates of major bleeding

HORIZONS-AMI: Biva vs. heparin + Gp2b/3a inhi
- Reduced 30 d major bleed or major adv CV events, including death, reinfarction, TVR for ischemia and stroke
- Significant 40% reduction in major bleeding
- Biva significantly decreased mortality at 30 days and 1 year

- *LMWH: Adv* (1) Stable reliable anticoagulant effect (2) High bioavailability (3) High anti f alpha 1 to anti 2 a ratio producing blockade of coagulation cascade in upstream location
  - Compared with heparin,
    - Rate of early (60-90 mins) reperfusion of IRA is not enhanced
    - Rate of reocclusion of IRA, reinfarction or Recurrent ischemic events however appears to be reduced with LMWH
  - Trials demonstrating superiority of LMWH against UFH
    - *ASSENT 3 trial:* Enoxaparin 30 mg IV followed by S/C 1 mg/kg ever 13 hr—decreased 30 d mortality, in-hospital reinfarction or in-hospital refractory ischemia. Rate of IC bled—similar
    - *EXTRACT AMI 25:* Enoxaparin
      - Decreased death/ rec non-fatal MI by 17%
      - 33% in reinfarction
      - Nonsignificant favorable trend on overall mortality
      - Improvement of rec MI was balanced against increased major bleeding
    - *Meta-analysis:* LMWH clearly reduced recurrent MI but with a pattern of increased bleeding
- *Parenteral anti f α a*
  - *OASIS-6* fondaparinux reduced composite end point of death or reinfarction in patients where UFH was not indicated "but not in patients where UFH was indicated"
    - Superior to placebo but not to UFH

Recommendations
- IV UFH bolus of 60 unit/kg (max 4000 U) followed by initial infusion at 12 u/kg/hr (max 1000 u/hr) for 48 hrs (maintain APTT 1.5–2 times)
- Alternative anticoagulation regimens are preferred if administered for longer than 48 hrs (because of risk of HIT)
- *EXTRACT TIMI 25* and *OASIS-6*—patients managed with pharmacological reperfusion should receive anticoagulation therapy for minimum 48 hrs and preferably for duration of hospitalization after STEMI (upto 8d)

- *Enoxaparin/fondaparinux preferred* when >48 hr and anticoagulation is planned
  Enoxaparin: iv—s/c after 15 mins
  Fondaparinux iv—s/c after 24 hrs
  When PCI done in patient receiving fondaparinux, additional agent with anti factor 2 ~ activity (Heparin) is required
- For patients with HIT—Bivalirudin is option
- For patients undergoing CABG-UFH preferred
- Fondaparinux not recommended as sole agent when PPCI is contemplated

ANTIPLATELETS

- *ISIS-2* study single strong piece of evidence that aspirin reduces mortality in such patients
  - Aspirin within 4 hr—25% reduction
    - Within 5-12 hr—21% reduction
    - 13-24 hr—21% reduction
    - Aspirin + STK—42% reduction
    - Aspirin + STK (within 6 hours)—13% reduction
- *CLARITY TIMI (28)* (clopidogrel)
  Addition of clopidogrel to background treatment with Aspirin in patients with STEMI<75 years and received fibrinolytic therapy reduce risk for clinical events (death, reinfarction, stroke) and reocclusion of a successful reperfused IRR
  STRES (ST resolution) - substudy from CLARITY TIMI 28
  - Treatment with clopidogrel resulted in greater benefit in those with c/o STRes and greater odds of having an open artery at late angiography in patients with partial/complete STRes
  - Significant reduction in in-hospital death or MI who achieved partial or complete STRes
    ↓
    Clopidogrel did not increase the rate of complete opening of occluded artery when fibrinolysis uses administered, but was highly effective in preventing reocclusion of IRA
  COMMIT: (Clopidogrel and Metoprolol in MI)
  - Clopidogrel reduced death, reinfarction and stroke

C. Combination of Gp2b/3a inhib + fibrinolytic
- Large outcome trials revealed no significant effect on survival and reduction of reinfarction bleeding risk increases
  ↓
  Combination not recommended

D. Antiplatelet therapy for PCI
- All patients with STEMI should receive Aspirin—ASAD
- *CLARITY TIMI 28* Pretreatment with clopidogrel significantly reduced CV death, MI, or stroke following PCI and decreased MI or stroke before PCI
- *PCI + CLARITY + PCI - CURF + CREDD* (meta analysis) Pretreatment with clopidogrel significantly reduce risk for 30 d CV death or MI
- *CURRENT OASIS 7:* Doubling the std dose of clopidogrel (loading 600 and daily 150) for first 7 d did not improve outcome in overall ACS population referred, but there was benefit in ACS who underwent PCI
- *TRITON TIMI-38:* Prasugrel reduced definite or probable stent thrombosis by 42% when compared with clopidogrel
- *PLATO* Ticagrelor in STEMI reduce primary end points of CV death, recurrent MI or stroke

Recommendations

- *Aspirin:* ASAP 162–325 mg chewable
  Maintenance phase 75–162 mg/d
- *Clopidogrel* (COMMIT & CLARITY TIMI-28)
  - 75 mg/d for all patients with STEMI regardless of whether they receive fibrinolytic therapy, undergo PPCI or do not receive reperfusion therapy
  - Loading dose of 300 for patient 75 year and undergoing fibrinolysis
  - Insufficient data to recommend loading for >75 years
  - Loading dose of 600 for patient undergoing PPCI
- *Prasugrel* (Triton TIMI 38)
  Loading-60
  Daily-10
- *Ticagrelor* (PLATO)
  Loading—180
  Daily 90-BD

BETA-BLOCKERS

- Both immediate effect and long-term (2°) prevention
- MOA
  - Decreased HR
    Decreased SBP
    Decreased cardiac index
    ↓
    Decreased myocardial O_2 consumption
    ↓
    Reduce chest pain
  - Antagonize lipolytic effect of catecholamine
    ↓
    Diminish circulating level of FFA
    ↓
    [FFP can diminish myo O_2 demand] - this is prevented by beta-blocker
    ↓
    Benefit to ischemic heart
  - Prevent vent Arrhythmias

Data

A. *Pre fibrinolytic CrG:* BB decreases mortality, re infarct and cardiac arrest
B. *Reperf ECG:* BB to fibrinolytic patients did not reduce mortality.
   But helped reduce rate of recurrent ischemic events
   Concern: Risk of provoking cardiogenic shock

COMMIT Trial: BB iv (5-15)—followed by - 200 mg/d oral
- Composite end point (death, reinfarction, or cardiac arrest) did not differ from placebo
- Significant reduction in reinfarction and episodes of VF in Metoprolol group
- Risk of cardiogenic shock was greatest in patients with mod-severe LV dysfunction

Recommendations

- All patients without contraindication (irrespective of fibrinolytic therapy/PCI) should receive oral beta-blocker within first 24 hrs
- Prompt iv BB is reasonable if a Tachyarrhythmia or Hypotension is present in absence of HF/low output state/high risk of development of shock/any other contraindication
- Cont BB during and after hospitalization (of no CI)

*C/I to BB

- Signs of HF/c/o low output state
- Increased risk for cardiogenic shock
  - Age >70
  - SBP <120
  - Sinus tachy >110 or HR <80
  - Increased time since onset of symptoms
- Other contraindication
  - PR prolongation>240
  - 2nd - 3rd degree heart block
  - Active asthma/reactive airway disease

Choice of BB

- Metoprolol, atenolol, carvedilol, bisoprolol
- BB with intrinsic sympathomimetic activity (Pindolol, oxprenolol)—unfavorable evidence—should be avoided
- *CAPRICORN:* (carvedilol vs. placebo)
  All cause mortality decreased (23%) at 30 days and 1-3 year

- When clinician wish to give BB to patients with mild HF, tachycardia, mild asthma, 1° CHB—trial of esmolol ($t_{½}$ = 9 min—effect disappear in <30 min)

RAPS INHIBITORS

Adv:
- Favorable effect on vent remodeling
- Improvement in HD
- Decrease incidence of CHF
- Decreased mortality from STEMI

Trials (ACEI)

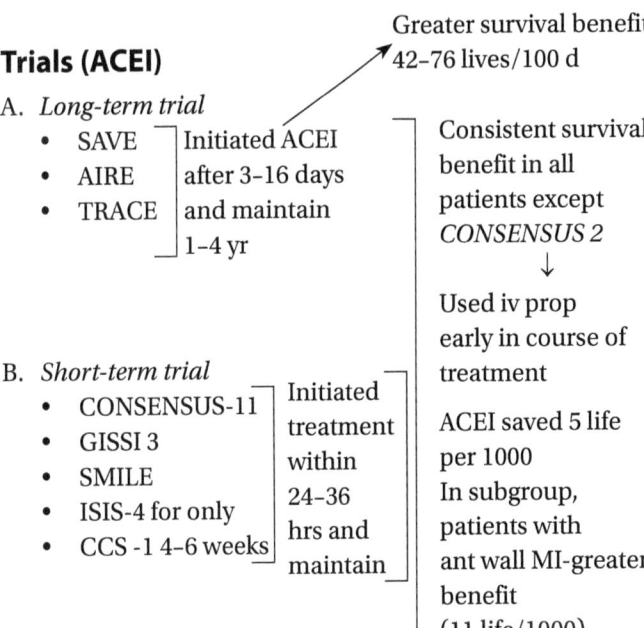

A. *Long-term trial*
- SAVE
- AIRE
- TRACE

Initiated ACEI after 3-16 days and maintain 1-4 yr

Greater survival benefit 42-76 lives/100 d

Consistent survival benefit in all patients except CONSENSUS 2
↓
Used iv prop early in course of treatment

ACEI saved 5 life per 1000
In subgroup, patients with ant wall MI-greater benefit (11 life/1000)

B. *Short-term trial*
- CONSENSUS-11
- GISSI 3
- SMILE
- ISIS-4 for only
- CCS -1 4-6 weeks

Initiated treatment within 24-36 hrs and maintain

- Chronic administration of ACEI decreased incidence of ischemic events, Recurrent Infarction, need for coro revascularization, significant reduction in HF
- Mortality benefit was additive to those achieved with Aspirin + BB

C/F

- Hypotension in setting of adequate preload
- Known hypersensitivity
- Preg

S/E: Hypotension, intolerable cough, angioedema

Trials (ARBS)

- *VALIANT:* (valsartan vs. valsartan + captopril vs. captopril)
  - Similar mortality in all 3 groups
- *EPHESUS:* (eplerenone vs. placebo)
  - 15% Decrease in RR for mortality in eplerenone
  - Also decrease CV mortality or hospitalization

Recommendations

1. All patients with STEMI should be considered for RAAs blockade
2. High-risk patient (elderly, AMI, prev Infarction, killip class ≥2, c/o depressed global vent function) should receive lifelong ACEI
3. Choice between ACEI and ARB should be based upon physician experience
4. Long-term aldosterone Antagonist flow high risk patient (EF<40%, HI, DM) who are already receiving ACEI + BB

NITRATE

MOA

- Decreased LV filling pr, wall tension and cardiac work
- Improvement in CBF in ischemic zone
- Decreased PCWP and SBP, LV chamber vol, Infarct size, incidence of mechanical Compli

Note: Routine administration of nitrates do not alter survival in patients with STEMI

Trials

- Trials in pre reperf era did not show any benefit with nitrate
- GISSI-3 and ISIS-4—no independent effect of nitrate on short-term mortality

S/E of iv Nitrate

- Reflex tachy
- Systemic hypotension
- Catastrophic in IWMI/RVMI
- Clinically significant methemoglobinemia
  (When large dose used) → Impair O_2 carrying capacity of blood
- Lethargy
- Headache

Recommendations

- NTG indicated for relief of persistent pain and as a vasodilators in patients with MI associated with LVEF or HTN
- In absence of recurrent angina or HF NTG not recommended

HEMODYNAMIC ASSESSMENT

Indication

- Management of complicated AMI
  - Hypovolemia vs cardiogenic shock
  - VSD vs. AMR
  - Severe LV failure
  - RV failure
- Refractory VT
- Difficult to differentiate severe pulm disease from LVF
- Assessment of card tamponade
- Assessment of therapy
  - After load reduction in patients with LVF
  - Inotropic agent
  - BB agent
  - Temporary pacing
  - IABP
  - Mech—ventilation
  - Uncomplicated STEMI do not require invasive HD monitoring

Hemodynamics Classification/Subset

	Clinical exam	Invasive monitoring
Normal syst perf and without pulm congestion	Rates and S3 Absent CI >2.2	Normal HD PCWP <18
Normal syst perf and with pulm congestion	Pelles + S3+; ↑JVP	PCWP >18 CI>2.2
Decreased perfusion and without pulm congestion	Frank pulm edema	Peri hypoperf PCWP<18; CI<2.2
Decreased perf and pulm congestion	Shock	PCWP>18, CI<2.2

PROPHYLACTIC ANTIARRHYTHMICS

- Routine use of antiarrhythmics (except BB) does not improve outcome (in fact some of them may cause harm)
  CAST: Encainide, flecainide or moncozine
- Slipped prematurely because of increased mortality in treatment group
  SWORD: Similarly stopped
  CAMIAT: Amiodarone reduced Freq. of VPC in patients with recent MI—related with reduction of arrhythmic death or resuscitation from VF
- However 42% discontinued amio because of intolerable S/E
  EMIAT: (Amiodarone) reduction in arrhythmic death after MI in patients with decreased LVEF, but total mortality and other CV related mortality did not decrease

Routine use of antiarrhythmic is not recommended
ICD in first few weeks after MI has not shown benefit

ANTICOAGULANTS POST-MI

- *ATLAS-ACS-TIMI 51*
  - Tested rivaroxaban 25 and 5 mg BD
  - Both significantly reduced CV death, MI or stroke in comparison to placebo
  - Both also decrease stent thrombosis
  - 2–5 mg showed significant decrease in CV mortality (not seen with 5 mg)
  - Increased major bleeding (2.1% vs. 0.6%) (without significant increase in fatal bleeding)
- ATLAS-ACS TIMI 46 (Phase 2 study)
  Similar findings
- APPRAISE - similar findings with apixaban
- APPRAISE 2 (phase 3)
  - Terminated early because of increased major bleeding without significant improvement in efficacy

12.20 *RISK STRATIFICATION POST-STEMI

SEVERAL STAGES

- Initial Findings
  1. Age >65 year ⎫
  2. H/O Dm   ⎪
  3. Prev Angina Pectoris ⎬ Worse prognosis
  4. Prev MI   ⎪
  5. 12 Lead ECG   ⎭

  DM—40% increase in risk for death by 30 days

  DM—More complicated post MI course due to extensive atherosclerosis and higher risk for thrombosis and HF associated with DM

  AWMI>IWMI

  RWMI—More risk

  Higher sum of ST segment elevation—High risk

  Persistent adv HB (2nd degree type 2 or 3 degrees) and bifasicular/trifasicular block—high risk

  Persistent non or downsloping ST dep, Q wave in multiple lead, ST dep in ant leads in art infarction and atrial arrhythmia—High risk clinical sign of HF (tachy, Hypotension)—more risk

- Hospital course:
  - Depend on severity of LV function
  - Physical findings, infarct size and invasive HD parameters
  - HD significant MR ⎫
  - LVH after MI   ⎬ Poor prognosis
  - Recurrent infarction ⎪
  - New stroke   ⎭

- Assessment of hospital discharge:
  Factors: 1. Resting LV function
  Most imp 2. Residual potentially ischemic myocardium
  3. Susceptibility to serious vent arrhythmia

Assessment of LV Function

- LVEF
- Cant differentiate stunned/ hibernating myo (ECHO)
- Exercise and pharmacological stress ECHO, stress radionuclide angio, perfusion imaging with pharmacological stress, PET and CMR—can differentiate
- <5% Myocardium is infarcted—Best prognosis

Assessment of Myo Ischemia

- Exercise testing/pharmacological stress
- Helps risk stratification
- Boost patient's self confidence
- Submaximal protocol
- Exercise until symptom of angina appears, ECG evidence of ischemia of target workload (SMETS) achieved
- Magnitude of ST seg depression, development of angina, exercise capacity and SBP response - predict future course

Assessment of Electrical Instability

- QT dispersion, vent arrhythmia on Holter, invasive EP testing, signal averaged ECG, HR variability, barrow reflex sensitivity
  ↓
- None of these have proved to be useful for routine practice

12.21 STABLE ISCHEMIC HEART DISEASE

Q.1 Clinical manifestation of stable AP. List positive D/D of chest pain. Indi of PCI in stable IHD. (2+2+2+4)
(June 17)

STABLE ANGINA PECTORIS

Clinical Manifestation

AP: Discomfort in chest or adjacent areas caused by myocardial ischemia
- Associated with disturbance in myocardial function
- Precipitated by exertion
  - Heberden's initial discussion of angina
    Sense of strangling and anxiety
  - Other adjectives used for AP
    - Constricting
    - Heavy
    - Suffocation
    - Squeezing
    - Crushing
  - In some patient
    - Mild pressure like discomfort, tightness, uncomfortable numbers or burning sensation
  - *Site:*
    - Usually retro sternal
    - Radiation is common outer surface of lt arm, right arm and outer surface of both arms
    - Epigastric discomfort
- AP discomfort above mandible and below epigastrium - rare
- Angina equivalent Dyspnea Fatigue
  Faintness Eructations
  Abnormal exertional dyspnea
- Nocturnal angina may be manifestation of IHD (UA)
- Postprandial angina may be marker of CAD
- *Typical episode of angina:* Begins gradually, reaches its max intensity over a period of minutes, dissipates
- Unusual for AP to reach max intensity within seconds
- Patient prefers to rest, sit or stop walking

Features Against AP

- Pleuritic pain
- Pain localized with 1 finger
- Pain reproduced by movt or palpitation and chest wall
- Constant pain lasting many hours
- Very brief episode of pain lasting seconds

Effect

- Typical AP is relieved within mins by rest or NTG
- Delay of >5-10 min
  - AP either not caused by ischemia
  - Or caused by severe ischemia

Warm up phenomena: Angina develop with exertion—continue subsequently at same or even greater level of exertion without symptoms after intervening period of rest (due to ischemic preconditioning)

Gradings

- NYHA functional score
- CSS angina grading
- Specific activity scale by Goldman and association
- Angina score by Galiff and colleagues
  - Integrates C/F and tempo of angina together with ST-T changes

Mechanism

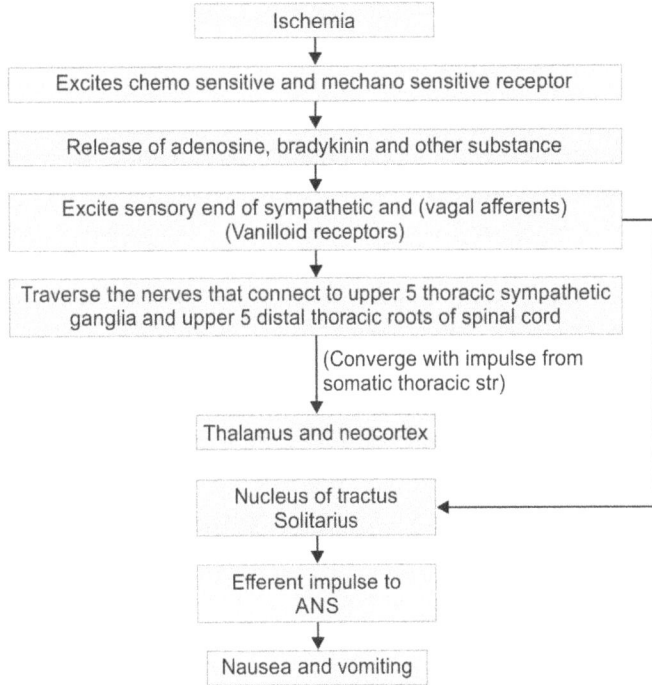

D/D of Chest Pain

- Esophageal disease
  - GI reflux
  - Diffuse spasm
  - Nutcracker eso
- Esophageal motility disorder
- Biliary colic
- Costo chondrites—Tietz syndrome
- Other musculoskeletal disease
  - Cervical radiculitis
  - Compression of brachial plexus by cervical ribs

- *Other*
  - Severe PHTN
  - Pulm embolism
  - Ac pericarditis
  - Ao dissection

Pathophysiology

- AP results from myo ischemia caused by
- Imbalance between O_2 req and myo O_2 supply

  Depends on   CBF
  - HR O_2 content
  - LV wall stress Ao LVEDP gradient
  - Contractility

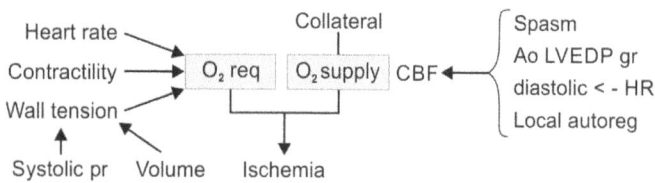

Demand Angina

- From release of NE by adrenergic nerve endings in heart and vascular beds
- Physiologic response to exertion, emotion, mental stress
- Mental and emotional stress
- Physical exertion and emotional association in sexual activity
- Anger—may constrict coro arteries
- Heavy meal and excessive metabolic demand imposed by chills, fever, thyrotoxicosis, tachycardia exposure to cold and hyperglycemia

Supply Angina

- Coro vasoconstriction (by vasoconstrictor substances such as serotonin and TxA2)
- Endothelial dysfunction—decreased release of vasodilators
- Circadian variation in angina (more common) in morning
- Precipitated by cold, emotion and mental stress

■ EVALUATION

Biochemical Tests

- Hypercholesterolemia and dyslipidemia
- Carbo intolerance and insulin resistance
- Lipid profile + Lp(a) + lp asso phospholipase Az
  ↓
  Associated with high risk of CAD (inhibitor of Lp-PLA2 decreased investigation)
- Homocysteine
- Inflammatory biomarker
  - hs-CRP
    - Increased risk of CV events
    - Prognostic value
  - Il-6,
  - MPO,
  - Growth factors
  - Metalloproteinases Genetic testing decreases investigation (Peri: blood gene expression score)

High hs-CRP in LDL 130 mg/d was associated with increased CV risk

Biomarkers of myo injury ischemia and HD stress Differentiate patient with AMI from those with S1HD
- BNP increases in spont or provoked ischemia
- Novel biomarker
  - Mid regional pro adrenomedullin
  - Mid regional pro ANP
- Growth differentiation factor 15, ST 2 and galctin 3—may reflect myocardial ischemia or its consequences

Resting ECG

- Normal in 50% patients
- MC abnormality—nonspecific ST-T changes without Q wave especially if obtained during ischemia
- Normal resting ECG—favorable prognosis
- LBBB, LAFB may occur—associated with LV dysfunction and relatively poor prognosis
- VPBs—low sensitivity and specificity
- Hypertrophy (LVH)—poor prognosis
- During AP—50% patient shows abnormal finding After pain subsides—pseudo normal ECG

Noninvasive Stress Test

- Based on Bayes principle
- Depends on NPV/PPV (lens/specs) as well as pretest sport test probability

Exercise ECG

sens = 68 spec = 77

- Provide degree of function limitation
- Diagnosis of CAD
- Influence of antianginal treatment: long-acting BB should be stopped 2-3 d before testing short acting BB, nitrate and CCB. Should be stopped the day before testing

Nuclear Testing

- *Stress MPI*

sens = 88 spec = 78

  - Exercise MPI with simultaneous ECG
  - Superior than stress test
  - Exercise SPECT
  - Should not be used as screening

- *MPI with pharmacological vasodilators*
  - For patient who are unable to exercise
- *Stress ECHO*   sens = 88 spec = 80
  - Exercise/pharmacological stress
  - Allow detection of regional ischemia
  - Accuracy similar to stress MPI
  - Superior to stress ECG
- Stress MRI and CT

CT Angio

- Highly sensitive for coro classification
- *Provides:*
  - Coro arterial tree anatomy
  - Assessment of myo perfusion
  - Quantification of vent function
  - Myocardial viability
- Low specificity (50%)
- Not recommended as routine approach
- Also used to characterize plaque composition and PET-CT provide info about coro anatomy + perfusion + metabolism
- CMC char arterial atheroma
- Vulnerability to rupture
- Predict function recovery
- Discriminate between ischemic and non ischemic dysfunction
- CAE
- Definitive diagnosis
- 25% each have SVD, DVD or TVD
- 5-10% have LM
- 15-30% have critical obstruction
- Role of IVUS, OCT

Findings
- Coro ectasia and aneurysm
- Collateral vessels
- Myocardial bridging
- LV function
- Myo metabolism—ant and venous lactate measurements (lactate produced by anaerobic metabolism)—its appearance in CS at rest or after stress determine myo ischemia

RISK STRATIFICATION

Based on Noninvasive Testing

- *High risk:* >3% risk of death/MI annually
  - Severe resting LV dysfunction (LVEF <35%) not explained by non coronary causes
  - Resting perfusion abnormality involving >10% myocardium
  - High risk stress finding
    - ≥2 mm ST seg depression at low workload or persisting into recovery
    - Exercise induced ST elevation
    - Exercise induced VT/VF
  - Severe stress induced LV dysfunction (peak <45% or drop in WEF with stress ≥10%
  - Stress induced perfusion abnormality ≥10% of myocardium or stress segmental scores indicating multiple territories with abnormality
  - Stress induced LV dilatation
  - Inducible WMA (involving >2 segment or 2 coro beds)
  - Wall motion abnormality developing at low dose of dobutamine (≤10% mg/kg/min) or at a low heart rate (<120 beats/min)
  - CAC score > 400 AV
  - Multi vessel CAD (≥70% stenosis) or LM stenosis (≥50% stenosis) on CCTA
- *Intermediate risk* (1-3%)
  - LVEF 35-49%
  - Resting perf abnormality 5-9.9%
  - *Stress test:* ≥1 mm ST dep with exertional symptoms
  - Stress induced perf abnormality 5-9.9% or stress segmental score indicating 1 vascular territory
  - No LV dilatation
  - Small WMA involving 1.2 seg and only 1 coro bed
  - CAC 100-399
  - 1 vessel CAD (≥90%) or mod CAD (50-70%) in ≥2 art on CCTA
- *Low risk* <1%
  - Low risk TMT score (>15): No new ST seg changes or ex induced chest pain
  - Normal or small myo perf defect at rest or with stress (<5%)
  - NO stress WMA
  - CAC score <100
  - No coro stenosis >50% on CCTA

MEDICAL MANAGEMENT

Five components

Treatment of Associated Diseases

- This may increase O_2 demand or decrease O_2 delivery
- Anemia
- Marked wt gain
- Occult thyrotoxicosis
- Cocaine abuse
- Heart failure/MR/Tachyarrhythmias
- Fever
- Infection
- Tachycardia

Reduction of Risk Factors

- *HTN*
  - 40-70 yrs of age—risk of IHD doubles for each 20 mm Hg increase in SBP across range of 115-185 mm Hg
  - HTN predispose to vasc injury, accelerate dev of atherosclerotic plaque, increased O_2 demand, intensity ischemia predisposes to AF
  - LVH is strong predictor of MI and CAD death
  - Goal BP < 140/90
  - *ACCORD-BP* - did not reveal any additional benefit of lowering SBP <120
- *Cigarette smoking*
  - Increased 5 yr mortality, MI and SCD
  - Increased myo O_2 demand and reduce coro blood flow by alpha adrenergic mediated coro spasm
- *Dyslipidemia:* Statin significantly improves endothelial mediated response in positive coronary and syst arteries of patients with dyslipidemia or known atherosclerosis
  - *Statin:* Reduce circulating level of hs-CRP
    Decreased thrombogenicity
    Favorably alter collagen and inflammatory comp
    Antiatherothrombotic property of statin
    Plaque stabilization
    Improvement in blood flow
    Reduction of inducible myo ischemia
    Decreased coro events
  - High intensity statin therapy in all patients with established IHD who are less than 75 years in absence of CI with less emphasize or LDL target goal

  Low HDL: Diet + exercise
  - LDL reduction
  - VA—HIT—gemfibrozil
  - Extended release niacin (heart protection study 2)—no significant reduction
  - Torcetrapib (CETP inhibitor)—did not decrease progression of ath and was associated with increased ischemic events
  - Dalcetrapib Trials stopped early because of reported lack of clinically meaningful efficacy
- *DM:* Weight management exercise BP control and lipid management
- *Obesity and exercise:* Less info is available on benefit of exercise in patients with SIHD. Small RCT showed improved in effort tolerance, O_2 consumption and QOL and decreased evidence of ischemia on MPI
- *Inflammation*
  - Lower level of hs-CRP associated with statin in patients with SIHD are associated with better long term outcome

Secondary Prevention

- *Pharmacological measures*
  - *Aspirin*
    75-182 mg daily
  - *Clopidogrel*
    - May be substituted for aspirin
    - *CAPRIE trial:* Clopidogrel resulted in modest 87% reduction in risk of vasc death, ischemic stroke or MI
    - CHARISMA No overall benefit of adding clopidogrel to aspirin
    - Vorapaxar significant risk reduction
  - *BB:* Sensible to use when angina and/or HTN is present in patients with SIHD
  - *ACEI/ARBS*
    - Decreased LVH
    - Decreased vasc hypertrophy
    - Decreased prog of atherosclerosis
    - Decreased pl rupture
    - Decreased thrombosis
    - Favorable influence on myo O_2 supply-demand relationship
    - Favorable effect on cardiac hemodynamics
    - Decreased symp overactivity
    - Improve endothelial vasomotor function
    - Decreased inflammation
    - *HOPE:* Ramipril significantly decrease risk for major vasc events
    - *EUROPA:* Similar result
    - *PEACE:* Trandolapril showed no effect
      ↓
    - ACEI recommended for all patients with LV dysfunction and CAD esp. For those with HTN, DM or CKD
    - Optional use in all other patients with SIHD, normal LVEF and well controlled CV risk factors
    - ARB equivalent to ACEI
  - *Antioxidants*
    - High dietary intake of antioxidant vitamin (A, C and B-carotene) and flavonoids naturally present in fruit, vegetables, tea and wine is associated with decreased CAD events
    - Supplements including vit C, vit E, B-carotene, folic acid, vit B6 and B12 - did not reduce major CV effect in RCTS
- *Nonpharmacological*
  - *Counseling and change in lifestyle*
    - Dietary habits, goal for physical activity
    - Isometric activity such as weightlifting

- Most angina have lower threshold shortly after arising in morning
- Morning activities should be done at slower pace (showering, shaving etc)
  Prophylactic nitrate can be used

Pharmacological Management

Beta-blockers

- Anti-ischemic property
- Effective anti hypertensive
- Antiarrhythmic
- Reduce mortality in patients with HF
  - It reduces freq of anginal episodes and increases threshold for angina
  - Can be given alone or in combination

MOA:

- Competitive inhibition of effect on neuronally released and circulating catecholamines on beta receptors
- Decreased myocardial O_2 requirements by slowing HR
- Decreased HR—increased diastolic period—increased CBF
- Decreased exercise induced increase in BP and limit induced increase in Contractility—decreased myo O_2 demand during exercise
- Beta (nonselective blocker) unopposed alpha activation decreased blood supply to other organs—decreased blood supply to patients with PVD—decreased max exercise capacity
- Beta-blocker may increase LV volume and thereby increase O_2 demand in patients with pre-existing LV dysfunction

Action of Beta receptors:

- SA node Beta-1—increased HR
- Atria Beta-1—increased contractility and cond velocity
- AV node Beta-1—increased cond velocity
- His Purkinje Beta-1—increased cond velocity
- Vent Beta-1—increased automaticity, Contractility and cond velocity
- Peripheral, coro, carotid art—Beta-2—dilatation
- Other (Beta-2)—increased insulin release; increased liver and muscle glycogenolysis
- Lung Beta-2—dilate bronchi/uterus (Beta-1)—5M relaxation

Characteristics of Beta blocking agents

- Selectivity
  Beta-1
  - Predominate in heart
  - Stimulation increase HR, AV conduction and contractility
  - Release of renin from JG apparatus and lipolysis in adipocyte

  Beta-2
  - Bronchodilatation
  - Vasodilatation
  - Glycogenolysis

  Cardioselective Beta-blocker: (Acebutolol, Betaxolol, Atenolol, Bisoprolol, Esmolol, Metoprolol, Nebivolol)—Blocks Beta-1 receptors—decreases myo O_2 demand

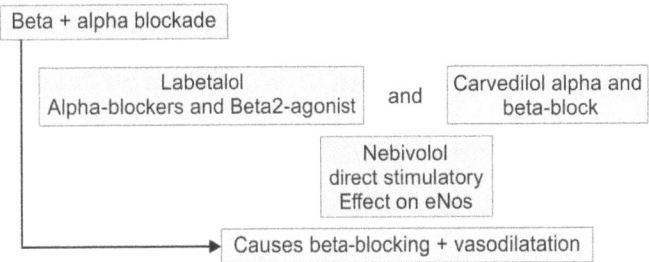

- *Antiarrhythmic action*
- *Intrinsic sympathomimetic activity*
  - Acebutolol, bucindolol, celiprolol, pindolol
  - Partially stimulate beta receptors
  - May not be as effective as those without these property
- *Potency:* Timolol and pindolol are most potent
  Acebutolol and labetalol are least
- *Lipid solubility:* Metoprolol, propranolol and pindolol are readily absorbed from GIT
- *Genetic polymorphism*
  - Metabolism of metoprolol, carvedilol and propranolol might be affected (metabolized by liver) - (cyt P450)
  - Poor hydroxylators have significant prolongation of $t_{1/2}$
  - Angina might be controlled by single dose in patients with poor metabolizer
- *Effect on lipid profile*
  No change in LDL
  Increased TG and HDL

S/E and CI

- Severe sinus brady, AV block, sinus arrest, decreased LV contractility
- Bronchospasm
- Fatigue
- Sexual dysfunction
- Intensification of insulin induced hypoglycemia
- Cutaneous reaction
- Lethargy, weakness, fatigue (due to decreased CO) (or direct CNS effect)
- HF may be intensified
- Enhance vasoconstriction (unopposed alpha action)
  Noncord selective beta-blocker—Ppt Raynaud

- *Abrupt withdrawal:* Increased total ischemic activity in patients with chr stable angina

Candidate selection
- Ideal candidate
  1. Prominent reaction of physical activity with angina
  2. Coexisting HTN
  3. H/O SVT/VT
  4. Prev MI
  5. LV syst dysfunction
  6. Mild to mod HF
  7. Prominent anxiety
- Poor candidate
  1. Asthma or reversible airway component in patients with 6OLD
  2. Severe LV dysfunction with HF symptoms (class 4)
  3. H/O severe depression
  4. Raynaud
  5. Symptomatic PVD
  6. Severe brady
  7. Brittle DM

CCB

MOA
- Noncompetitive blockade of voltage sensitive L-type calcium channel
- Phenylalkylamines (verapamil-diltiazem) impair channel recovery—depressant effect on conduction system
- Dihydroxy Riding (Nifedipine)—no effect on conduction system
- Negative inotropic action ← protect against this
- Relaxing VSMC—peri vasodilatation
- SNS activation in response to drug induced hypotension
- Decreased myocardial O_2 demand ⎤ Relieves
- Increased O_2 supply ⎦ ischemia
- Especially imp in prinzmetal angina

Metabolism
- By liver
- $t_{1/2}$ between 3-12 hrs
  (except amlodipine and felodipine)

Antiatherogenic action
Amlodipine may improve endothelial function and reduce progression and coro atherosclerosis

Nifedipine:
- Dihydropyridine
- Dilator of VSMC
- More potent than dilzem and vera

- Decreased myo O_2 req (due to after load reduction) Increased O_2 supply (vasodilatation)
  S/E:
  - Due to vasodilation—headache, dizziness, palpitation, flushing, hypotension, leg edema
  - In patients with severe CAD—Nifedipine can aggravate angina by (1) lowering arterial pressure excessively and (2) reflex tachy
  - Worsen HF in patients with preexisting severe HF
  - CI in patients who have hypotensive or have severe As

Verapamil
- Dilate syst and coro resistance vessel as well as large conductance vessels
- INVEST Combining sust release verapamil + trandolapril vs atenolol
- Equal outcomes with respect to death, MI or stroke
- In patients with cardiac dysfunction
  Vesa car:
  1. Decreases CO
  2. Increases LV filling pr
  3. Causes clinical HF
- Not to use iv beta-blocker
  S/E Gingival hyperplasia (rare)
  After 1-9 months

Diltiazem:
- Intermediate between vara and nifedipine
- Vasodil effects are less profound than Nifi and cardiac depressant on action on conduction system less profound than verapamil
- Infrequent side effects

>2nd gen CCB:
- Amlodipine
  - Slow, smooth onset and ultralong duration of action ($t_{1/2}$ = 36 hours)
  - Esp useful in patients with chr angina and LV dysfunction
  - Significant changes in BP seen after 2-3 days of initiation of treatment
- Nicardipine $t_{1/2}$ similar to nifedipine
  - Great vasc selectivity
- Felodipine and Isradipine
  - Approved for HTN but not for angina

Nitrates

MOA:
- Relax VSMC
- Systemic (including coro) artery and vein
- Effect on veins predominates

- Decreased vent preload—decreased wall tension and O_2 requirement
- Decreased heart's mechanical activity, vol and O_2 consumption—increased exercise capacity in patients with IHD
- Nitrate + CCB ⎤
- Nitrate + BB ⎦ Improved antianginal effect

Effect on coro circ
1. Dilatation of epicardial stenosis
2. Prevent vasoconstriction and vasospasm caused by endothelial dysfunction of resistant vessel
3. Redistribution of blood flow by increasing collat flow increased blood flow to decreased LVEDP ischemic areas (esp subendocardial)
4. *Antithrombotic effect:* Stimulation of guanylyl cyclase by nitric oxide (NO) result in inhibition action on plt in addition to vasodilatation
5. *Cellular MOA:* Nitrate—enter VSMC—converted to reactive NO—activate intracellular guanylate cyclase—produce cGMP—trigger SMC relaxation and anti plt aggregator effect
   - Arterial vasodilator effect depends on endothelial Ca^{++} activated K^+ channels

S/E:
- Headache, fatigue, flushing, hypotension
- Nitrate induced hypotension is associated with paradoxical bradycardia consistent with vasovagal or vasodepressor effect
- Methemoglobinemia (rare)

Preparation
- Short acting NTG (SL tablet and spray)
- Isosorbide dinitrate
- Isosorbide mononitrate
- Topical nitroglycerin

Nitrate tolerance
- Demonstrated with all prep which leads to continuous stable blood level of nitrate
  Mech Hypothesis that increased gen of vasc superoxide anion is central to process of tolerance
- Multiple possible contributors
  1. Effect of NTG or eNOS uncoupling
  2. Counter regulatory neurohormonal activation
     ↓
     Increased superoxide anion
     ↓
- Plasma vol expansion and neurohormonal activation
- Impaired bio transformation of nitrate—NO
- Decreased end organ responsiveness to NO

Management
- Provide nitrate free interval
- Optimal interval—unknown
- Recommend—12 hours

Ranolazine
- Piperazine derivative
- Anti ischemic effect achieved without clinically significant change in BP or HR—unique activation

MOA
- Shown to shift myocardial substrate uptake from FA—glucose (potential myocardial metabolic modulator)
- Decreased Ca^{++} overload in ischemic myocyte via inhibition of late inward Na^+ current
- Preserve tissue level of ATP
  - Improve myocardial contractile function
  - Decreased extent of myo injury (irreversible)
  - Decreased pre procedural management in patients undergoing elective PCI

RCT
- Improved exercise performance
- Increased time to ischemia during exercise
- Decreased angina freq
- Decreased incidence of worsening angina
- Decreased incidence of recurrent ischemia
- In patients with angina and ischemia without CAD Reduced symptoms with elo improved myo perfusion reserve index
- $t_{1/2}$ = 7 hr
- Steady state achieved in 3 d
- Metabolized primarily through cyt P450 pathway conc increase with cyp P-450 inhibitors
  - Verapamil increase absorption by inhibition of pylycoprot

Dose: 500 BD—max 1000 BD

S/E: Nausea, Gen weakness, constipation, dizziness, minor QR prolongation

Ep effect: Inhibition of delayed rectifier current and inhibition of INa
↓
Shorten AP duration and suppress EAD
↓
Effect on vent and atrial arrhythmias

CI
1. In patients with long QT or receiving other QT prolonging drug
2. Hepatic impairment

Ivabradine

MOA
Specific and selective inhibitor of If
↓
Reduce spont firing rate of sinoatrial pacemaker cells and thus slows HR through meth that is not associated with negative inotropic effect
- Approved in Europe for AP and chr HF
- Can be used in adult who cannot tolerate BB

Selection of therapy
- Long term admin of BB has shown prolong life in patients after ac MI—It is reasonable to consider BB over CCB as agent of choice
- Sinus brady—CCB preferred
- Sinus tachy—BB preferred
- SVT—BB preferred (verapamil also)
- AV block—CCB preferred
- Rapid AT—BB/vesa
- VT—BB
- LV dysfunction—BB
- SHTN—BB/CCB
- Severe pre-existing headache—BB
- COPD with bronchospasm/asthma—CCB
- Hyperthyroid—BB
- Claudication—CCB
- Sev depression, sleep disturb, sexual dysfunction—CCB
- Variant angina—CCB
- Sympt PAD—CCB

EECP
- 7 weeks—35 sitting—each 1 hr
- Decreased freq of angina and use of NTG
- Improve ex tolerance and QOL
- Response lasts for upto 2 years
- MOA:
  1. HD changes—decreased myo O_2 demand
  2. Increased transmyo pr to open collatuab—increased O_2 supply
  3. Elaborate various substances which improve endothelial function and vasc remodeling

Spinal cord stimulation
- For refractory angina
- Based on gate theory

Revascularization

Patient selection
1. *Presence and severity of symptoms*
   Revasc should be considered if ischemic symptoms persists despite OMT
2. *Significance of coro lesion*
   - >70% dia stenosis—anatomically significant
   - IVUS
   - OCT
   - FFR
3. *Extent of ischemia and presence of LV dysfunction*
   - Extent of ischemia
   - No of vessels involved
   - LV function of risk   4 major determinant of risk
   - Electrical substrate
4. Risk associated with procedure and comorbid condition

In general
- For most patients with chr angina—OMT is first choice followed by revascularization
- When improvement in survival is not a relevant consideration, severity of angina or impairment in health status should play significant role in determining whether revasc is appropriate or not
- Patients prey 2 SE status should be considered
- Symptoms that are atypical or nondiagnostic of obst CAD—does not improve with revasc

PCI
- Imp treatment modality in patients with SIHD esp chronic angina who remain symptomatic despite optimal GDMT

PCI vs. OMT
- No randomized trial or meta-analysis has shown reduction in death/MI with PCI vs. OMT
- *COURAGE (1998-3004):* PCI did not reduce death, MI or other major CV events when added to OMT
  - Patient treated with PCI has less angina at least 1-3 years but not at 5 years
- *Subgroup of COURAGE*
  - No diff between PCI + OMT vs. OMT in patients with multivessel CAD, for low LVEF, CCS class 2 or 3 and DM

FFR strategy
- FAME-2 trial terminated prematurely
  Highly significant reduction in the composite 1° end point of death, MI or urgent Revascularization
  Both trials
  ↓
  1. PCI reduce ischemia symptoms and need for Revascularization
  2. None of above trial showed reduction in rate of death/MI with PCI vs. GDMT

Meta-analysis
- Mortality, MI, severity and extent of ischemia and long-term angina to not differ between PCI and OMT

- *ISCHEMIA:* Ongoing trial to evaluate long-term GDMT + PCI vs. long-term GDMT

SUMMARY

- It appears reasonable to pursue a strategy of initial GDMT for most patients with SIHD and CCS class 1 or 2 symptoms ←──── Indication
- Reserve revascularization for those with persistent and/or more severe symptoms despite GDMT or those with high risk criterion on non invasive testing

Pt selection for PCI
- Likelihood of success based on angiographic char of lesion
- Risk and potential failure of PCI (which are related to coro anatomy), the percentage of viable myocardium at risk, presence of HF and underlying LV function should be considered
3. Likelihood of restenosis with clinical (DM, prev restenosis) and angio factors (small vessel, long lesion, total occlusion and SVG)
4. Need for complete revasc based on extent of CAD and vol of myocardium and severity of ischemia in distribution of artery

CABG
- First used in 1964. IMA used in 1967-1970
- Documented to prolong survival, relieve angina and improve QOL in specific subgroup of patients
- Excellent short and intermediate term results in patients with SIHD
- Long-term results affected by occlusion of venous grafts

Minimally invasive CABG
1. *Post access CABG:* Through limited incisions with femoro-femoral CPB and cardioplegic arrest
2. Totally endoscopic robotically assisted CABG
3. Off pump CABG standard median sternotomy with small skin incisions
4. Minimally invasive direct CAB (MIDCAB) through left art thoracotomy without CPB

Adv:
- Decreased post op discomfort
- Minimize risk for wound inf
- Short recovery time
- No CPB decreased risk of bleeding, systemic thrombo embolism, renal insufficiency, myo stunning and stroke

Patient selection
Indi:
- Need for improvement in quality and duration of life
- CABG vs PCI—coro anatomy, LV function, comorbidities; patient pref
- CABG indicated regardless of symptoms for patients with CAD in whom survival is likely to be prolonged and for those with multivessel CAD with high risk noninvasive testing

Operative mortality
Risk factors
- Preoperative factors related to CAD
  - Recent acute MI, hemodynamic instability, LV dysfunction, extensive CAD, presence of LM CAD; severe or unstable angina
- Preoperative factors related to aggressiveness
  - Associated carotid artery disease/PAD
- Preop biological factors
  - DM, other comorbid conditions, pulm and renal disease, female sex
- Intraoperative factors
  - Intraoperative ischemia damage and failure to use IMA grafts
- Environmental or institutional factors
  - Specific surgeon and treatment protocol used

*Most potent predictor of mortality
- Age
- Urgency of surgery
- Prev cardiac surgery
- LV function
- Stenosis of LMCA
- No of epicardial vessel with significant disease

*Periop complications:
- *Myocardial infarction*
  - 0% to >10%
  - *Definition:* 10 times increase in cardiac enzymes (cTn/ckMB)
- *Cerebrovasc complications*
  - Emboli from atherosclerotic aorta
  - Emboli from CPB
  - Intra op hypotension
  - Peri op silent injury in 25-50% on MRI
- *Atrial fibrillation*
  - Upto 40% patients, within 2-3 d
  - 2-3 fold increase in post op stroke
  - Old age, HTN, prev AF, HF-associated with high risk for dev of AI
  - Prev statin therapy may be accompanied by less freq post op
  - Management
    - Prophylactic BB
    - Amiodarone

- Upto 80% spontaneously revert to NSR within 24 hrs
- Off-pump associated less freq with AF
- **Renal dysfunction**
  - Incidence = low 0.5 to 1.0%
  - Decline in renal function defined as post op Sr—cr higher than 2 or an increase of >0.7 mg/dl
  - *Risk:* adv age, DM, pre existing renal dysfunction, HF
  - High risk criteria that identify patients who are likely to sustain more substantial survival benefit:
    - LM CAD
    - Single or double vessel disease with prox LAD disease
    - LV syst dysfunction
    - Composite evaluation that indicates high risk (including severity of symptoms, high risk ex tolerance test, H/O prev MI, presence of ST dep on ECG)

Guidelines for CAG

Class 1
- SIHD who have survival SCD or life threatening vent arrhythmias
- SIHD in whom symptoms and signs of HF develops
- For patients with SIHD whose clinical characteristics and result of noninvasive testing indicate high likelihood of severe IHD (Benefit>risk)

Class 2a
- Further risk assessment in patients with depressed LV function (LVEF <50%) and moderate risk criteria on non-invasive testing
- Further assess risk in SIHD and inconclusive prognostic info after noninvasive testing or in patients for whom noninvasive testing is contraindicated or inadequate
- For patients with SIHD who have unsatisfactory QOL because of angina have preserved LV function (EF>50%) have intermediate risk criterion on noninvasive test

Class 3
- Not recommended for patients who elect not to undergo revascularization or who are not candidate for revascularization because of comorbidity
- For patients who have preserve LV function and low risk on noninvasive
- Patients who are at low risk acc to clinical criteria and who have not undergone non invasive testing
- For asymptomatic patients who do not have e/o ischemia on noninvasive testing

Guidelines for Revascularization
1. ≥1 significant stenosis amenable to Revascularization and unacceptable angina despite GDMT
1a. ≥1 significant stenosis and unacceptable angina in whom GDMT cannot be implemented because of medication contraindications, asv effects or patients pref
   - Prev CABG with ≥1 significant stenosis associated with ischemia and unacceptable angina despite GDMT
     - PCI 2a
     - CABG 2b

   Complex TVD (SYNTAX score ≥22)—CABG preferred over PCI

2b. Viable ischemic myocardium that is preferred by coro arteries that are not amenable to grafting—TMR (transmyocardial revasc) as adjunct to CABG

Patient specific consideration for PCI
A. Extent of jeopardized myocardium
   - Role of anatomical vs physiological stenosis
   - FFR and FAME
B. Baseline lesion morphology
   - CTO
   - SVG graft
   - Bifurcation lesion
   - Lesion classification
   - Thrombus
   - LMCA
C. Underlying cardiac function
   10% decrease in LVEF—mortality increases twice
   IABP support may help
D. Renal insufficiency
   - Mild renal dysfunction—20% higher risk for death at 1 year following PCI
   - CIN
E. Associated comorbid conditions
   - Bleeding diathesis
   For resistant angina
   1. TMR—trans myocardial laser revasc
   2. CVBG
   3. Temp cardiac sympathectomy
   4. Spinal cord stimulation
   5. Cell based treatment for therapeutic angiogenesis
   6. Cardiac transplant

12.22 REGULATION OF CORONARY MICROCIRCULATION

TRANSMURAL PENETRATING ARTERIES

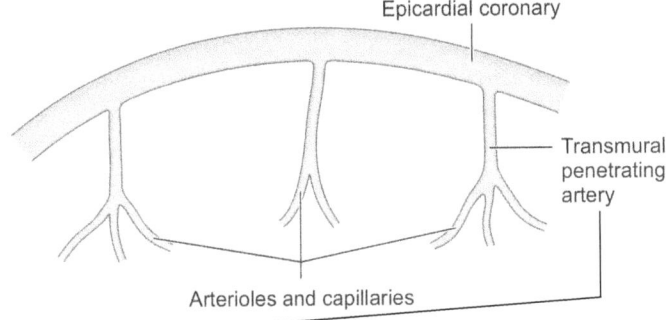

- Less sensitive to metabolic signals
- Removed from metabolic signals that develop when ischemia is confined to subendocardium
  ↓
- Shear stress and myogenic response to local pressure change becomes utmost importance in these vessels
  ↓
- Even during max vasodilatation, this vessels create resistance channel that must be crossed before reacting microcirculation
  ↓
- And because of these channel, microcirc pr in subendocardial coronary arteries are lower than in subepi vessels

*REGULATION OF CORONARY MICROCIRCULATION

Intraluminal Pressure Force

- Myogenic regulation—ability of VSMC to oppose changes in coronary artery diameter
  - Distending pr decrease—vessel relax
  - Distending pr increase—vessel constrict
- Property of VSMC
- Dependent on VSMC Ca^{++} entry through L-type Ca^{++} channels
- Myogenic response primarily occurs in arterioles smaller than um - 400 um
- Important component of coro art autoregulation

Flow Mediated Control

- At level of small arteries and arterioles
- In response to local shear stress
- Flow induced dilatation is dependent on endothelium dependent NO release and vasodilatation
- Can also be mediated by EDHF (endothelium derived hyperpolarizing factors)

Metabolically Mediated

- Vasodilatation—adenosine, PO_2 and PH + autacoids
  - *Adenosine:* Released from cardiac myocyte when rate of ATP hydrolysis exceeds its synthesis (e.g., Ischemia)
    - Extremely short $t_{1/2}$
    - Rapidly deactivated by adenosine deaminase
    - Binds to A2 receptor on VSMC—increased cAMP—opens Ca^{++} activated K+ channels
    - No effect on conduit arteries and larger resistance vessels
    - Vasodilating effects on vessels <100 um
    - As arteriolar resistance falls—flow across those vessels increase—local shear stress related vasodilatation of these vessels too
  - *ATP—sensitive K^+ channels*
    Many candidates for metabolic flow regulation (e.g., NO, adenosine, Beta 2 receptor, Prostacyclin) acts through this channels of VSMC
  - *O_2 sensing/hypoxia*
    - CFR increases in response to reduction in PO_2 or anemia
    - *Mech:* Activation of release of NO and ATP
      ↓
      Vasodilatation
  - *Acidosis:* Potent vasodilator independent of hypoxia

Neural Control

- *Cholinergic innervation*
  - Resistance vessels—dilate in response to Ach
  - Conduit vessels—mild vasodilatation
  - Ach action on VSMC—contraction of SMC
  - Net effect
    Direct muscarinic
    Constriction of VSMC—counterbalanced by
    ↓
    - Direct stimulation of NOS which leads to endothelium dependent vasodilatation
    - Flow mediated vasodilatation in resistance vessels
  - In atherosclerosis
    - Resistance vessel of dilatation to Ach is reduced
    - Flow mediated NO production reduced
      ↓
    Epicardial conduit vessel vasoconstriction esp. stenotic segment
- *Sympathetic innervation*
  - *Basal condition:* NO resting sympathetic tone

- During symp activation—NE released

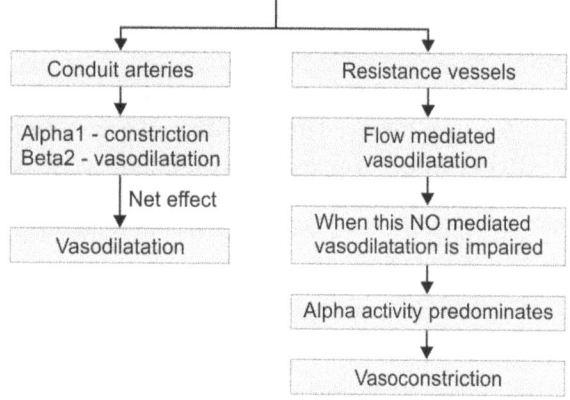

- Overall action of SNS on myo perfusion depend on
  - Beta-1 mediated increase in myo O_2 consumption
  - Beta-2 mediated vasodilatation
  - Alpha-1 mediated vasoconstriction
- Under normal condition Beta-2 mediated vasodilatation predominate
- After nonselective Beta-blockade—Alpha-1 mediates vasoconstrict (but this is counterbalanced by increasing O_2 extraction and reduced in coro venous PO_2 at similar level of cardiac workload)

Paracrine Vasoactive Mediators

- Released from epicardial artery thrombi after activation of thrombotic cascade initiated by plaque rupture
- They can modulate tone in eccentric ulcerated plaque which are still responsible to stimuli
  ↓
  Leads to dynamic change in physiological significance of a stenosis
  They can also have effect on downstream vessels
  - *Serotonin:* Released from activated platelets
    - Causes vasoconstriction in normal and atherosclerotic conduit arteries
    - Dilates coronary arterioles
    - Increased flow through endothelium dependent NO
    - In atherosclerosis NO release is impaired with net effect of serotonin is vasoconstriction
  - *Thromboxane—A2:* Potent vasoconstrictor
    - Conduit art as well as resistance vessel
    - Can accentuate AMI
  - *Adenosine diphosphate*
    - Platelet derived vasodilator (NO mediated)
    - Both conduit and resistance vessel
    - Abolished by removing endothelium
  - *Thrombin*
    - Release prostacyclin and NO—vasodilate resistance vessels
    - Also release TxA2 → vasoconstriction of epicardial stenosis (in which endothelium dependent dilatation is impaired)

12.23 STUNNED MYOCARDIUM

INTRODUCTION

- Myocardial function normalizes rapidly after a brief episode of ischemia lasting <2 min
- When ischemia increases in duration and/or severity
  ↓
  Delay in recovery of function occurs despite normal blood flow established ⎤
  ↓   ⎥ STUNNING
  Regional myocardial function remains depressed for upto 6 hours after resolution of ischemia lasting for 15 mins, in absence of any tissue necrosis ⎦
  - Function remains depressed while resting myocardial perfusion is normal—defining feature of stunning
  - Association between subendocardial flow and function
  - Stunning can also develop after demand induced ischemia
  - Stunning can also develop after CABG
    ↓
    Responsible for post-op pump dysfunction
  - Stunned myocardium can also coexist with irreversibly injured myocardium—contributes to time dependent partial recovery of myocardial function after MI
  - *Cellular mechanism:* Probably involves free radical mediated myocardial injury and reduced myofilament calcium sensitivity.
  - Important to recognize stunning because contractile function normalizes during stimulation and various inotropic agent (e.g., Beta-agonist)

HIBERNATING MYOCARDIUM

Short-term Hibernation

Definition: In steady state ischemia, close matching between perfusion and contraction leads to reduced regional O_2 consumption and energy utilization. A phenomenon termed as short-term hibernation.
↓
Re-establish balance between supply and demand
↓
Reflected by restoration and creatinine phosphate and ATP with resolution and lactate production despite of persistent hypoperfusion
↓

Any short-term increase in O_2 demand can precipitate ischemia and leads to rapid deterioration in function and metabolism
↓
Irreversible injury frequently occur after a period of 12–24 hrs

Chronic Hibernating Myocardium

- Chronic segmental dysfunction arises from repetitive episodes of ischemia
  ↓
1. When resting flow (relative to a normal remote region) is normal in dysfunctional myocardium, the region is called chronically stunned.
2. When relative resting flow is reduced in absence of signs and symptoms of ischemia, hibernating myocardium is present.

Both entities exist in patients and represent extreme in spectrum of adaptive and maladaptive response.

Viability studies are required to distinguish infarction from hibernating myocardium because the myocardium is always viable when resting flow is normal.

Experimental studies have shown that:

Delayed subendocardial infarction is rare in chronically hibernating myocardium; when moderate flow reduction is maintained for >24 hrs
↓
Many patients with hibernating myocardium present with LV dysfunction rather than ischemia symptoms
(Relative decreased resting flow is rather consequences and not the cause)

Studies have shown that chronic stunning (normal resting flow) proceeds chronic hibernation (decreased resting flow for approximately 1 week—3 months)
↓
Cause for progression from chr stunned—chr hibernation
1. Significance of chronic stenosis
2. Repetitive supply or demand induced ischemia
   As progression from stunned—Hibernation occurs
   Myocyte takes on regional characteristics similar to those from an heart with advanced HF

Some of the major cellular responses are:

- *Apoptosis, myocyte, and myofibrillar loss*
  - Prominent during transition from chronically stunned to hibernating myocardium
  - Results in compensatory regional myocyte hypertrophy to maintain normal wall thickness

- *Cell survival and antiapoptotic program in response to repetitive ischemia:*
  - Upregulation of cardioprotective mechanisms
  - Downregulation of glycogen synthase kinase 3 Beta which can ameliorate cell death
  - Physiological significance of a stenosis has been demonstrated to be a major determinant of intrinsic myocardial adaptation to ischemia
- *Metabolism and energies in hibernating myocardium*
  - Glycogen content increased
  - Max rates of glucose uptake during insulin stimulation not allowed
  - Down regulation of energy utilization and energy consumption—slows ATP utilization and maintain cell viability during superimposed acute ischemia
- *Inhomogeneous symp innervation* (Beta adrenergic) response with SCD
  - Contractile reserve of hibernating myo is blunted and partially related to regional down regulation in beta adrenergic adenylyl cyclase coupling (similar to adv HF)—maybe be related to local NE overflow—make myocardium vulnerable for HF and vent arrhythmia
- *Successful adaptation v/s Degeneration:*
  - Some investigator believes that hibernating myocardium is destined to undergo fibrosis degeneration.
- At other extreme there are incidences where fibrosis is not prominent and myocardium can maintain for long period without degeneration.

VIABLE DYSFUNCTIONAL MYOCARDIUM

It is defined as myocardium region in which contractile function improves after coronary revascularization

Three categories:

	Contractile reserve	Resting flow	Time course for recovery
A. Transient reversible ischemia:			
• Post ischemic stunning	Present	Normal	<24 h
• Short-term hibernation	Present	Normal	< 7d
B. Chronic receptive ischemia:			
• Chronic stunning	Present	Normal	Day-week up to 12 months
• Chronic hibernating mgo	Variable	Decreased	
C. Structural remodeling:			
• Subendocardial infarction	Variable	Decreased	Weeks
• Remodeling heart	Present	Normal	Months

SECTION 13: Lipid Disorders

13.1 PHARMACOLOGICAL MANAGEMENT

Q.1 Current guidelines for treatment of dyslipidemia (June 16)
Q.2 Statin and their role in pl regression
Q.3 Role of statin in management of dyslipidemia
Q.4 Lipid lowering strategies

PHARMACOLOGICAL MANAGEMENT

Bile Acid Binding Resins

- Interrupt enterohepatic circulation of bile acid by inhibiting their reabsorption in Intestine
- *Use:* Adjunctive therapy in patients with severe hypercholesterolemia 2° to increase LDL-C
- Not absorbed systemically
  Remain in intestine } Safe in children
  Excreted in stool
- E.g., Cholestyramine-4 g unit dose } Always taken
  colestipol -5 gm unit dose   with mod
- *S/E:* Constipation, sensation of fullness, GI discomfort decreased absorption of other meds (should be given 1 hour before or 4 hours after bile acid binding resins)
- *Colesevelam*: Bioengineered bile acid binding resin
  - Twice capacity then cholestyramine
  - Useful as 3rd line therapy (who do not achieve target LDL-C or statin side effect)
  - Also decrease HbA1C levels
    (Useful for patients with dyslipidemia + DM)

Statin

MOA:
- HMG-COA reductase inhibitor
  Rate limiting step of sterol synthesis
  ↓

To maintain cellular chol homeostasis, expression of LDL-R increases and rate of cholesteryl ester formation declines

↓

Increased clearance of LDL from plasma and decreased hepatic production of LDL and VLDL

- Also interfere with synthesis of lipid intermediate

  Intermediate of chol synthesis pathway produce geranylgeranyl and farnesyl
  ↓
  Participate in protein prenylation
  ↓
  Mech by which lipid attaches to prot
  ↓
  Anchoring into cell membrane and enhance its biological activity

Statin increase HDL level by preventing geranylgeranylation of Rho A and PPAR—alpha

- Anti-inflammatory property statin
  - Decreased CRP level
  - Augment collagen content of plaque
  - Alter inflammatory component of plaque
  - Alter endothelial function.

Pharmacology

Drugs that interface with metabolism of statin by inhibiting cy + P450 3 A4 and 2C9 system can increase pl conc of statin, e.g., Antibiotics, antifungal, antiviral, grapefruit, cyclosporine, amiodarone, etc.

S/E

- Diffuse myalgia (normal ck level) to myositis (defined as diffuse muscle pain with e/o muscle inflammation and elevated ck level)
- Rarely rhabdomyolysis (life threatening)
  - Precipitating factors (advanced age, frailty, renal failure, shock, concomitant, antifungal, antibiotic, and hypothyroidism)
- Reversible elevation of transaminases
- Statin are generally well tolerated
- Myalgia seen in 10%
- Discontinuation required in 1%

Clinical Trials

- Total 27 trials
- A t02
- PROVE IT (Pravastatin or Atorva)
- TNT
- IDEAL
- SEARCH

Showed that more intensive reduction of LDL-C in patients at high or very high risk for CAD events further reduce risk

Reversal

(Reversal of atherosclerosis with Lipitor) used IVUS to examine effect of degree of lipid lowering on plaque
↓
More aggressive lipid lowering regimen reduced lesion volume

ASTEROID

Showed that rosuvastatin at a dose of 40 mg promotes regression of coro ath

SATURN

Rosuvas 40 vs. Atorva 80
Both proved equivalent in decreasing lesion progression

Use of statin in particular population

- *DM:* Patients with DM should receive statin
  Statin markedly decreased risk of CV disease
- *Older patients:* No reason to withdraw statins from older patients if clinically indicated
- *Women:* Meta-analysis showed that significant reduction in AMI, stroke, CVD related death, arterial revascularization and hospitalization for UA in favor of statin
- *Advance HF:* CORONA and CUSSI-HF Trial
  - Statin (rosuvas) did not reduce CVD related morbidity or mortality in patients with advanced HF

- Renal failure
  SHARP:
  - Statin reduced all-cause mortality, CV mortality and CV events in person not receiving dialysis
  - Statin has little or no benefit among person undergoing hemodialysis

Risk Associated with Low LDL Level

Evidence against this concern

- Most animals have no or low LDL level and they produce only when dietary consumption of chol and saturated fats increases
- Most cell type have machinery to produce cholesterol endogenously
- HDL transport system via SR-B1 receptor appears to be able to deliver chol from Hepatic source to organs
- LDL deficiency state in human (1) Hypobeta-lipoproteinemia (mutation in APO B genes and (2) loss of function mutation in PCSK9—associated with normal health and marked reduction in lifelong CV events
  - CTT meta-analysis
  - JUPITER Trial

  Did not show increase in CA, renal/hepatic disease or hemorrhagic stroke despite low LDL levels

Statin and Risk of DM

- Small risk of developing DM
- Overwhelming benefit of statin use in subjects at high risk for in 2° prev of CVD exceeds the small risk for dev of DM

Cholesterol Absorption Inhibitor

Ezetimibe: Interfere with NPCIL—limit selective uptake of cholesterol and other sterol by intestinal epithelium

- Lower LDL-C by 15%
- Adds to effect of statin
- Prevent absorption of sitosterol (DOC for sitosterolemia)
- Dose 10 mg/day
- *SHARP:* Suggest that Ezetimibe combined with simvastatin can decrease CV events in patients with impaired renal function (but no arm to compare with statin alone).

Fibrates

For example, Gemfibrozil -600 mg BD
Fenofibrate 200 mg/d
C/O Fibrate
Bezafibrate

Indicated for hypertriglyceridemia and 2° prev of CVD in patients with low HDL-C level

MOA

Interaction with nuclear transcription factor PPAR-Alpha
↓
PPAR-Alpha regulates transcription of LDL, apo C2 and A1

S/E

- Cutaneous manifestation
- GI effect (Abd distention, increased bile lithogenicity)
- Erectile dysfunction
- Elevated transaminases level
- Interaction with oral anticoagulants
- Elevated pl homocysteine
- Elevated LDL level (Fibrate increase LDL activity).

Gemfibrozil + Statin

Gemfibrozil inhibit glucuronidation of statin and retard its elimination—increased risk of myotoxicity—such combi is contraindicated

Clinical Usefulness

- FIELD ⎤
- ACCORD ⎦ Failed to show benefit
- Small subgroup of patients with baseline raised TG—showed benefit
  ↓
  - Fibrate might be indicated in high risk subjects with residual CV risk char by elevated TG, reduced HDL-C and elevated non HDL-C who are on statin therapy
  - For prevention of pancreatitis in patients with severe hypertriglyceridemia.

Nicotine Acid

- Niacin increased HDL-C
  - Lowers TG
  - Modest effect on LDL
- Dose = 2000–3000 mg/d
  (Escalating dose schedule)
- Niaspan (slow release from of niacin)—decreased S/E profile

MOA

Decreased hepatic secretion of VLDL and decreased FFA mobilization in periphery

S/E

Flushing, hyperuricemia, hyperglycemia, hepatotoxicity, acanthosis nigricans, and gastritis.

Clinical Use

- Raise HDL-C level in combination with low dose statin
- Retard angiographic progression of CAD and decreased Freq of adverse cardiac events

AIM High

Testing the hypothesis that patients with CAD optimally treated with statin and still have residual risk of developing CAD owing to low HDL and high TG level would benefit from niacin
↓
Trial stopped after 3 years because of lack of beneficial effect

HPS2-THRIVE

Niacin did not produce clinically meaningful reductions in CV events

Cholesteryl Ester Transfer Protein Inhibitor

Torcetrapib: Proved toxic and increased mortality
Dalcetrapib: Use stopped because of lack of effect in clinical trials
Anacetrapib ⎤
Evacetrapib ⎦ Under evaluation

Fish Oils

- Rich in PVFA (eicosapentaenoic acid and docosahexaenoic acid)
- Lower plasma triglyceride level and have antithrombotic property
- Reserved for patients with severe hyperglyceridemia resistant to therapy
- Response to fish oil depends on dose
  (With a daily intake of 10 gm of EPA/DHA)
- Lack of clinical trials.

Phytosterols

- Derivatives of cholesterol from plants and trees
- Interfere with micelles formation in Intestine and prevent intestinal absorption of chol
- Available as nutraceuticals
- Current guidelines include them as part of lifestyle modification

Novel Agents

- Inhibition of MTP with small molecule lomitapide reduces LDL-C by approximately 50% (FH)

- Inhibit Apo B MRNA with phosphorothionate linked antisense oligonucleotide: MIPOMERSEN—First such approved compound for FH—20–30% LDL reduction.

TARGET LEVELS

- NCEP ATP 3 recommendations
  - Patient with CAD/Ath of other vasc bed (carotid)
  - Adult with DM
  - Estimated 10 year risk >20%

  } High risk

  ↓

  Aggressive treatment
  Medication along with lifestyle modification, exercise and diet

  ↓

  Achieve 1° target of LDL-C<100 mg/dL

- In subjects with TG>200

  ↓

  2° target of non HDL-C<130 mg/dL

- LDL-C target for patients with ACS <80

Whom to treat (2013 guidelines)

TNT, ideal PROVE-IT	
Group 1 Clinical ASCVD (CAD, stoke, PAD)	*Group 2* LDL-C ≥190 mg/dL (No trials)
Group 3 DM +age -40–75 +LDL-C 70–190 TNT, HPS	*Group 4* ASCVD risk ≥7.5% No DM +Age 40–75 ASCOT-LLA HPS, JUPITER

13.2 NUTRITION AND CV METABOLIC DISEASE

FATS AND CV DISORDER

- Early ecological studies suggested that higher fat intake might increase cardiometabolic risk
- Percentage of total fat in foods or diets has little influence on weight loss, weight gain or overweight/obesity
- When total fat is reduced, carbohydrate intake typically increase, which can induce adverse effect if carbo are more refined and of lower quality
- Quality of fat (specific type of fat and fatty acid consumed) has major effect on health
- Classification of dietary fat
  - Based on numbers (saturated, unsaturated, mono-unsaturated, polyunsaturated) of double bond
  - Based on position (omega 3; omega 6) of double bond.

SATURATED FATTY ACID

- Meat, dairy product, tropical oil (palm, coconut)
- SFA increases risk of CVD
- 12-,14- and 16- carbon SFA raised LDL, lower TG, raise HDL-C and increased apo A1 level
- When compared with carbohydrate total/HDL-C ratio:
  - Not altered by 14-0 or 16-0 SFA
  - Non-significantly decreased by 18-0 SFA
  - Significantly decreased by 12-0 SFA
- Overall, SFA intake minimally affect risk
- Replacing SFA with PUFA decrease risk of CVD
- Replacing SFA with isocaloric carbo: little effect on risk (Indeed carbo has high GI—associated with high risk)
- Replacing SFA with MUFA—uncertain effects
- SFA from meat—higher risk for CVD
- SFA from dairy—lower risk for CVD.

MUFA

- Animal fat and vegetable oil (olive, canola)
- Largely oleic acid
- Oleic acid favorably influence blood chol conc yet increase ath risk—due to alteration in LDL-C composition
- Overall incidence does not strongly support increasing intake of MUFA per se to reduce CVD.

PUFA

- n-6 PUFA (linoleic acid)—from vegetable oil
- n-3 PUFA (alpha linoleic acid)—from plants (flaxseed, canola, walnuts, soybeans)
- EPA and DHA—from seafood
  - Linoleic acid
    - Accounts for >90% of dietary PUFA
    - Compared with carbo, LA decrease LDL-C and TG raises HDL-C and improve total /HDL-C ratio
    - Greater PUFA intake in place of SFA was associated with lower incidence of CAD
    - Greater PUFA intake in place of carbo
      - Similar effects
    - *Conclu:* PUFA recommended in place of either SFA or carbohydrate
  - *EPA/DHA:*
    - Benefit on HR, BP, TG level, cardiac function, possibly inflammation reaction, endothelial function and autonomic tone
    - Short-term use (6-12 months) does not appear to have substantial antiarrhythmic benefit in patients with established recurrent arrhythmias
    - Peri op use doesn't reduce post op AI
    - Long term use decreases mortality in HF
    - For reducing CHD death, modest dietary intake ($\cong$250 mg/d CPA plus DHA) is advisable (~1-2 savings 1 week of oily fish).

TRANSFATTY ACID/UNSATURATED FA

- 20–50% of FA in partially hydrogenated oils, which are used in baked goods, deep fried foods, packaged snacks
- Associated with higher risk of CAD and SCD
- Increased LDL-C, TG and Lp(a); lower HDL-C
- Increased total/HDL-C and increased apoB/A1 ratio
- Promote inflammation, endothelial vasodilator dysfunction, insulin resistance, visceral adiposity and arrhythmias.

DIETARY CHOL

- Raises both LDL-C and HDL-C
- Small net effect on total/HDL-C ratio
- Major sources are egg, shellfish
- Higher dietary chol associated with higher risk for CAD and DM.

13.3 STATIN INTOLERANCE

DEFINITION

Occurs when a patient is unable to tolerate statin either because of the development of side effects or because of evidence on a blood test (liver enzyme or marker of muscle injury) are abnormal
- *Complete:* All statin at any dose
- *Partial:* Some statin at a particular dose

C/F

- Muscle aches, pain, weakness, cramps
- Occurs in up to 15% of treated patients
- *Clinical trials:* 5-10% of patients are intolerant
- Reversible shortly after discontinuation of statin
- Some of muscles are due to
  - Effect of statin on muscle metabolism or
  - Attributable to reduced level of co-enzyme.

S/E OF STATIN

Adv Effect with Good Supp. Evidence

- Myopathy (myositis, myalgia, rhabdomyolysis)
- Increased liver enzymes
- New-onset DM

Adv Effects with Little or No Supp. Evidence

- Cancer
- Hemorrhagic stroke
- Cognitive disorder (Alzheimer)
- Lung disease
- Erectile dysfunction
- Fatigue, headache, dizziness
- Cataract
- Permanent liver/kidney damage.

FACTORS ASSOCIATED WITH INCREASING RISK OF STATIN INTOLERANCE

- H/o muscular symptom with other drug
- H/o unexplained muscular symptoms
- H/o unexplained ck elevation
- F/H/o muscular symptoms with lipid lowering therapy
- Strenuous exercise
- Hypothyroidism
- Vit D deficiency
- Advance age
- Female gender
- Low BMI
- Alcohol abuse

(HOW TO IDENTIFY?) DIAGNOSIS

- Statin induced ck elevation >10 times ULN
- Statin induced hepatic transaminases elevation >3 times ULN

PRIMO TRIAL

- Found statin induced muscle symptom frequency 10.5% (more than reported in RCTs)
- Fluvastatin lowest (5%)
- Simvastatin highest (18%)
- Median time of onset—1 month after initiation or titration to higher dose.

STOMP STUDY

- High dose of Atorva (80 mg) significant increased frequency of myalgia (9-4%)
- CK level also increased in asymptomatic patients (<10 ULN)
  - Suggesting that high dose statin may induce low grade muscle injury

MANAGEMENT OF STATIN INTOLERANCE

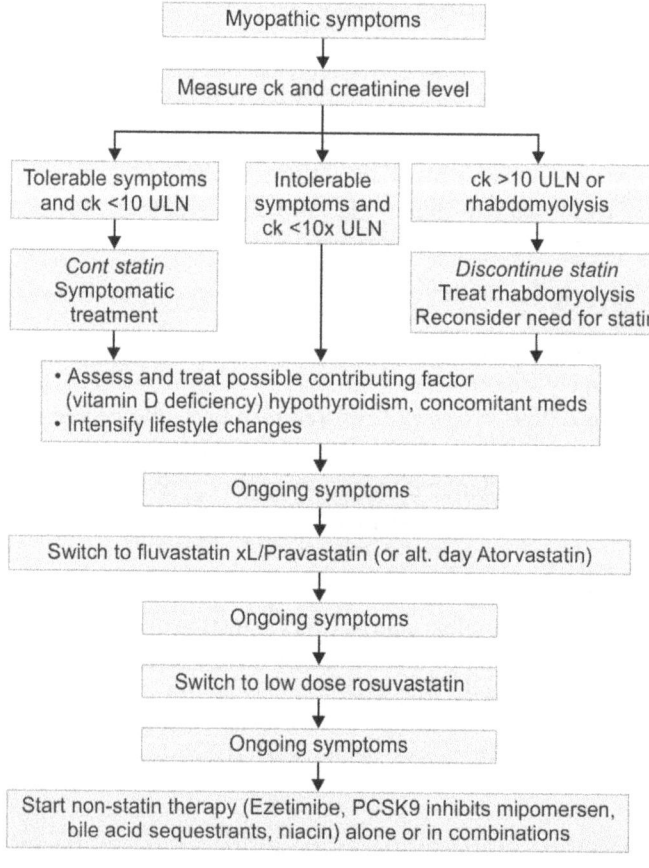

SPECIFIC PHARMACOTHERAPY
- Many studies have reported significant improvement in S/E if COQ given as co-therapy with statin
  - Q10 (200 mg/d) with statin reduced incidence of muscle related S/E
- Vitamin D supplementation have shown ameliorative effects in statin induced myopathy
  (*Recent trial:* 92% patient become symptom free after 3 month of vitamin D supplementation)
- Nutraceuticals may help.

13.4 SECONDARY CAUSES OF HYPERLIPIDEMIA

Q.1 2°causes of hyperlipidemia ways to treat it (June 14)

METABOLIC
- DM
- Lipodystrophy
- Glycogen storage disease

RENAL
- CRF
- Glomerulonephritis with nephritic synd
- Port losing enteropathy

HEPATIC
- Cirrhosis
- Biliary obst
- Porphyria
- 1° Biliary cirrhosis (With 2° LCAD def).

HORMONAL
- Estrogen
- Progesterone
- GH
- Hypothyroidism
- Corticosteroid.

LIFESTYLE
- Physical inactivity
- Obesity
- Diet rich in fats
- Alcohol intake
- Smoking

MEDICATION
- Retinoic and derivatives
- Glucocorticoids
- Exogenous estrogen
- Thiazide diuretics
- Selective BB
- Testosterone and other anabolic steroids
- Immunosuppressive meds
- Antiviral
- Antischizophrenic.

13.5 2013 ACC/AHA GUIDELINES (MANAGEMENT AND LIPIDS)

CLINICAL BENEFIT GROUP

- Clinical atherosclerotic CVD - 2° prevention
- LDLC ≥ 190 mg/dL without 2° cause
- 1° prevention with DM
  Age 40-75 years; LDL 70-190 mg/dL
- 1° prevention without DM
  Age 40-75 years; LDL 70-190 mg/dL estimated CVD risk using new pooled cohort algorithm ≥ 7.5%.

CATEGORIES OF INTENSIVE STATIN THERAPY

A. *High intensity statin therapy*
   - Daily dose lower LDL—C by approximate 50% on average
     E.g., Atorva 40-50; Rosuvas 20-40
B. *Moderate intensity statin therapy*
   - Daily dose lower LDL—C by approximate 30-50%
     E.g., Rosuvas 5-10; Atorva 10-20; Simvastatin 20-40; Pravastatin 40-50, Lovastatin 40, Fluvastatin 40 BD
C. *Low intensity statin therapy*
   - Daily dose lowers LDL - C by < 30%
     E.g., Simva 10, Rosuva 10-20, Lova 20

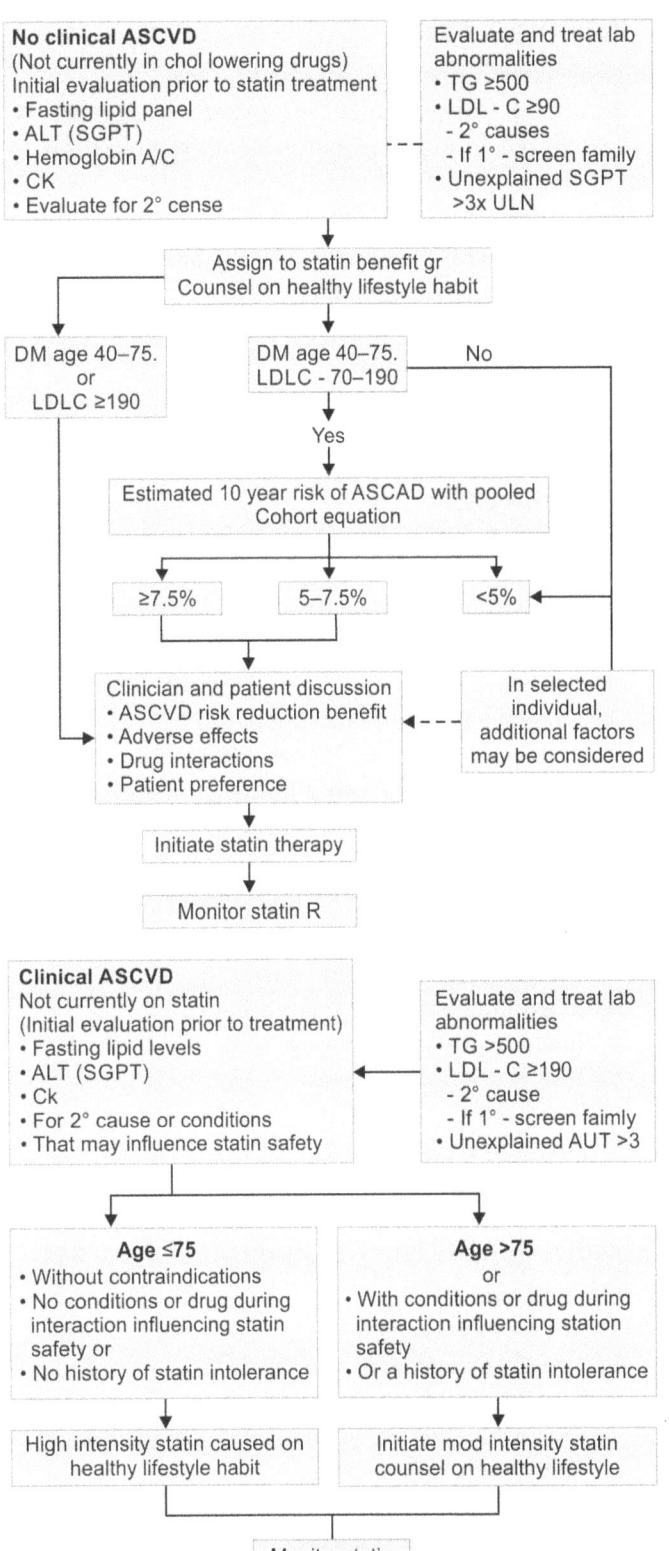

13.6 LIPOPROTEIN DISORDERS

INTRODUCTION

Original classification Frederickson, Lees and Levy.

Based on measurement of plasma chol and TG and analyzed lipoprotein patterns after separation by electrophoresis

Type 1 : Elevated chylomicrons
- 4 : Elevated VLD2 or pre Beta lipoprotein
- 2 : Elevated Beta lipoprotein (LDL)
- 5 : Elevated both chylomicron and LDL
- 3 : Broad beta disease
- 2b : Combined elevation of pre beta (VLD2) and beta (LDL Lipoprotein)

DRAWBACKS

- Does not include HDL-C
- Does not diff severe monogenic lipoprotein disorder from more common polygenic disorders
- WHO, European Ath society and more recently NCEP (Natural chol education program) classified lipoprotein disorder on basis of arbitrary cut points
- Practical approach describes lipoprotein disorder by absolute plasma level of lipids (chol and TG) and Lipoprotein chol level (LDL and HDL)

GENETIC LIPOPROTEIN DISORDER

- Monogenic lipoprotein disorders are rare
  - Familial hypercholesterolemia
- Most lipoprotein disorders results from
  - Interaction of increasing age with
  - Lack of physical exercise
  - Weight gain
  - Suboptimal diet
  - Individual genetic makeup

Classification of Genetic Lipoprotein Disorder

A. *LDL particles*
  1. AD hypercholesterolemia
  2. Familial hypercholesterolemia
  3. Familial defective apo blood
  4. Gain of function mutation of PCSK of mutation
  5. AR hypercholesterolemia
  6. Abetalipoproteinemia
  7. Hypo Beta lipoproteinemia
  8. Familial sitosterolemia
  9. Familial Lp(a) hyperlipoproteinemia

B. *Remnant Lipoprotein*
  1. Dysbetalipoproteinemia type 3
  2. Lipoprotein lipase def
  3. Hepatic lipase def
  4. Apo AV def
  5. Apo C 2 def; Apo A1 def
  6. Familial hypertriglyceridemia
  7. Familial combined hyperlipidemia
  8. HDL particles
  9. Tangler disease/familial HDL def
  10. Familial LCAT def
  11. CETP def
  12. Niemann–Pick disease type A and B
  13. Niemann–Pick disease type G

A. *LDL Lipoprotein (type 2 hyperlipidemia)*
  1. *AD hypercholesterolemia* (Familial hypercholesterolemia) (FH)

(1), (2), (3), (4) included in familial hypercholesterolemia
- Most thoroughly studied
- Elevated LDL-C level
- Defective LDL-C receptor gene
- *C/E:* Corneal, arcus, tendinous xanthoma over exterior tendons (MCP joints, patellar, tricuspid, and Achilles tendons) xanthelasma
- Autosomal co dominant
- High risk of CAD by 3rd–4th decade in men and 8–10 years late in female
- *Diagnosis:* Based upon increasing plasma LDL-C, F/H/O premature CAD, presence of xanthoma

DIAGNOSTIC CRITERIA (ESC)

a. 2 mutant allele at LDL-R, apoB, PCSK 9 or LDL-RAD-1 gene locus
b. Untreated LDL-C (500 mg/dL) or treated LDL-C (300 mg/dL)
c. Cutaneous/tendon xanthoma before 10 years of age
d. Untreated raised LDL-C level as per criteria in both parents

For diagnosis
- (a)/(b) + (c)
- (d) alone

	Heterozygous	homozygous
C/F	• Tendon xanthoma • CAD > 25 year • LDL 5–12 mmol/L	• -Same- • Cutaneous xanthoma • CAD <25 year • LDL >12
Genetic disorder	• LDL receptor – 1 allele • ApoB – 1 or 2 allele • NARC – 1 – 1 allele	• LDL-R both allele • AR hyperchol • Phytosterolemia

DUTCH LIPID CLINICAL NETWORK CRITERIA

A. *F/H*
- 1° relative with premat atheroscleotic (<55 in male and <60 in female) (CAD/PAD)
  Or
  1° relative with known LDL-C >95th percentile } (1)
- 1° relative with tendinous xanthoma and/or circus cornealis
  Or
  Child <18 year with LDL-C >95th percentile } (2)

B. *Clinical history*
- Patients with premat CAD (2)
- Patients with premat PAD (1)

C. *Examination*
- Tendinous xanthoma (6)
- Arcus cornealis <45 years (4)

D. *Chol level*
- LDL-C 155–190 (1)
- 190–250 (2)
- 250–325 (5)
- ≥325 (8)

E. *DNA analysis* (class 1 recommended)
  Function mutation in LDL-R, PCSK 9 gene or ApoB
  ↓
- >8 = Definitive FH
- 6–8 = Probable FH
- 3–5 = Possible FH

Patients on statin require correction of LDL with correction factor
e.g., Atorva 40 = correction factor = 2-0
      Rosuvas 20 = correction factor = 2-1

TREATMENT

Goal
To decrease risk of ASCVD
1. Lifestyle modification
   - Dietary change
   - Exercise
   - Behavior therapy
2. Statin (Targets: child <135 LDL
            Adult <100
            Adult with CAD /DM <70)
3. *CETP Inhibitor:* Ezetimibe (+statin) (Trial IMPROVE IT)
4. Bile acid sequestrant
   - Cholestyramine, colestipol, colesevelam
5. *New:* PCSK9 inhib mipomersen, lomitapide
6. LP apheresis
7. Gene therapy

Treatment Goal
LDL<100
LDL<70 (if CVD risk)

2. *Familial defective apolipoprotein B*:
   - Mutation in APO B gene
   - AD form of hypercholesterolemia
   - Clinically indistinguishable from FH
   - Defective APO B has decreased affinity for LDL-R
   - Defective APO B pl $t_{½}$ is 3-4 fold greater than normal LDL
   - LDL can undergo more oxidative modification
   - LDL-C elevated up to 400 mg/dL
   - Prevalence similar to FH (1 in 500)

3. *PCSK 9 gene (proprotein convertase subtilisin/kexin)*
   - AD
   - Chr/p34.1
   - Mutation in PCSK 9 gene
   - PCSK 9 codes for proprotein convertase belong to subtilase family of convertase
   - PCSK required for cleavage of SREBP
   - Gain of function mutation—decreased surface availability of LDL-R—accumulation of LDL-C in pl
   - Loss of function mutation—markedly lower LDL-C than do subject without mutation
   - Therapeutic target
   - Parenteral administration of injectable, humanical, monoclonal antibody directed against PCSK9 markedly reduce LDL-C in human

4. *AR hypercholesterolemia*
   Mutation in gene coding for LDL-R (LDL-RAP-1)

5. *Hypobetalipoproteinemia and abetalipoproteinemia*
   - Mutation in APOB gene—truncation of mature APO-B100 peptide

6. Gene therapy—cascade screening (family screening)—class 1
   - Synd char by reduced LDL-C and decreased VLDL-C
   - Little or no clinical manifestation } Hypobeta
   - No known CVD risk } lipoproteinemia
   - APO B truncated near its amino terminal loses the ability to bind lipids—syndrome similar to abetalipoproteinemia
   - *Mental retardation*
   - Growth abnormality
   - Resulting lack of Apo-B containing lipoproteins causes marked def of fat soluble vitamin (A,D,E,K)

7. *Sitosterolemia*
   - Rare condition
   - Increased intestinal absorption of plant sterol and decrease it's excretion
   - Can mimic severe FH
   - Extensive xanthoma
   - Premature atherosclerosis
   - *Diagnosis:* Specialized analysis of plant sterol
   - Pl chol level normal and TG decreased
   - Mutation in ABCG 5 and ABCG 8

B. *Triglyceride rich lipoproteins*
   Severe elevation of pl TG
   - Genetic disorder
   - Poorly controlled DM
     ◆ *Familial hypertriglyceridemia*
       - Not associated with clinical signs of FH
       - TG, VDL-C and VLDL-TG are moderately to marked elevated
       - LDL-C and HDL C low
       - TC normal or elevated
       - Fasting TG 200–500; PPTG: >1000
       - Calorie intake/carbohydrate—intake/alcohol intake potently stimulate hypertriglyceridemia
       - Weaker relation with CVD
       - 1 in 1000 to 1 in 50
       - Several genes and strong env influences
       - Hepatic over production of VLD2–familial hypertriglyceridemia
       - Excess TG load, esp ath fatty meal, may lead to impaired processing of VLDL particles
         - *Treatment:* Lifestyle modification, limit alcohol, limit caloric intake and increased exercise
     ◆ *Familial hyperchylomicronemia (Type 1 hyperlipidemia)*
       - Increased fasting pl triglyceride>1000 mg/dL
       - Recurrent boils of pancreatitis, eruptive xanthoma, xerostomia, xerophthalmia, behavioral abnormality
       - Due to markedly reduced or absent LDL activity (rarely absence of its activator APO C2)
       - Lack of hydrolysis of chylomicron and VLDL - Accu in plasma (esp after meals)
       - *Diagnosis:* plasma is milky white
         Clear band of chylomicron can be seen on top of pl after it stand overnight in refrigerator
       - *Treatment:* Treatment of pancreatitis
         Avoidance of alcohol and dietary fat
         Addition of short chain FA can increase palatability of diet
     ◆ *Type 3 hyperlipoproteinemia*
       (Broad beta disease/dysbetalipoproteinemia)
       - Accumulation of remnant lipoprotein particle in plasma
       - Electrophoresis show broad band between pre beta VLDL and beta LDL Lipoprotein
       - *C/F:* Pathognomonic tuberous xanthomas and palmar striated xanthomas
       - *Diagnosis:* Increased chol and TG level
         Decreased VLDL-C
       - Due to abnormality APO-E gene - does not bind to hepatic receptor
       - Ratio of VLDL chol to TG (normally <0.7) is elevated
   - *Familial combined hyperlipidemia*
     - MC lipoprotein disorder
     - Char by presence of elevated total chol and/or TG levels
     - *C/F: Corneal arcus, xanthoma xanthelasma* Infrequent
     - *Diagnosis:* (Increased TC, LDL-C and/or increased TG)
       Often in correlation with low HDL-C and elevated apoB level
       - *Mech:* Hepatic over production of apo B containing lipoproteins, delayed PP clearance of this and increased flux of FFA to liver (Increased FFA delay to liver also occur in insulin resistance and visceral obesity—increased hepatic apo B secretion)
     - Complex genetics
     - Considered to be AD tract
     - *Modifying factors:* Sex, age at onset and comorbid state

C. *High density lipoprotein*
   - Decreased HDL–CV risk
   - Most case of decreased HDL-C result from increased pl TG or apo B level
   - *Plasma TG and HDL levels vary inversely:* Reasons
     ◆ Decreased lipolysis of TRL decreased availability of substrate for HDL maturation
     ◆ HDL enriched with TG gas increased catabolic rate and hence decrease pl conc
     ◆ Augmented pool of TDL saps chol from HDL compartment of LETP mediated exchange
   - Genetic disorder of HDL result from
     ◆ Decreased production
     ◆ Abnormal maturation/increased catabolism
   - Familial hyperchylomicronemia ⎤
   - Familial hypertriglyceridemia   ⎬ Associated with decreased HDL-C
   - Familial combined hyperlipidemia ⎦
     ◆ *Apo A 1 gene defect*
       - Affecting production of HDL
         - *C/F:* Vary from extensive atypical xanthomatosis and corneal infiltration to no manifestation at all
     ◆ *Tangier disease (Familial HDL deficiency)*
       - Rare disorder of HDL deficiency
       - *Defect:* Reduced cellular chol efflux in skin fibroblasts and macrophytes from affected subjects
       - Mutation in ABCA-1 gene
       - Increased risk of CVD (counterbalanced by their very low levels of LDL-C)

- *Niemann-Pick type C disease*
  - Disorder of lysosomal cholesterol transport
  - Mental retardation and neurologic manifestation
  - Cellular defect appears to be proximal to the transport of chol to pl memb
  - Gene 189 21
- *Disorder of HDL processing enzyme*
  - *Lecithin cholesterol acetyltransferase* (LCAT def)
    - LCAT catalyze formation of cholesteryl ester in plasma
    - LCAT def – corneal infiltration (fish eye disease) Hematological abnormality due to abnormal RBC memb
    - No Increased risk for CAD
  - *CETP def (cholesteryl ester transfer prot def)*
    - Very high level of LDL-C
    - CETP facilitates transfer of HDL cholesteryl ester into TRLs
    - Def of CETP - accumulation of cholesteryl enter in HDL particle
    - Not associated with premat CAD Neither protect against CAD
    - CETP Inhibitors–negative trials
  - *Niemann-Pick disease Type A and B*
    - Mutation in sphingomyelin phosphodiesterase 1 gene
    - Associated with low HDL level
    - Appears to be due to decrease in LCAT reaction because of abnormal HDL constituents.

13.7 NON-HDL CHOLESTEROL

IDEAL TRIAL

- Elevated non-HDL-C and Apo B were best predictors after Acs of adv. CV outcome
- LDL-C was not associated with poor outcomes once non-HDL-C or apo – B was controlled

REASON FOR USEFULNESS OF NON-HDL-C

- Non-HDL-C measure cholesterol content of all atherogenic lipoprotein (including CDL)
- Easily calculated from lipid profile (no additional information required)
- Increased non-HDL-C and normal LDLC identify a subset of patient with increased "LDL particle "and" increased App B core"

↓

Measuring apo B and LDL particle core separately adds expense to positive patient and it is not standardized

↓

Non-HDL-C can identify this subset without any extra cost

- In patient with met syndrome LDL not sensitive marker
  - Non-HDL-C, LDL particle and apo- B has good predictive capacity
  - Elevated levels of non-HDL-C are treatable with currently available lipid lowering agents
  - Non-HDL-C correlate more closely with apo B level than LDLC → Better indicator of the total burden of atherogenic particles

Risk Cat	Criteria	LDL/Non-HDL-C	
		Treatment goal	Consider treatment
Low	• 0-1 major ASCVD risk factor	<130	≥190
	• Consider other risk indicators If known	<100	≥160
Mod	• Consider quantitative risk scarring	<130	≥160
	• Consider other risk indicator	<100	≥130

Contd...

Contd...

Risk Cat	Criteria	LDL/Non-HDL-C	
		Treatment goal	Consider treatment
High	• ≥3 major ASCVD RI	<130	>-130
	• DM (Type 1 or 2) – 0-1 other major ASCVD RF and – No e/o end organ damage	<100	≥100
	• CKD (3rd or 4th stage) • LDLC ≥190 (severe hyper chol)		
Very high	• ASCVD	<100	≥100
	• DM – ≥2 major ASCVD RF or – e/o end organ damage	<70	≥70

LIPID METABOLISM AND SITE OF DRUG ACTION

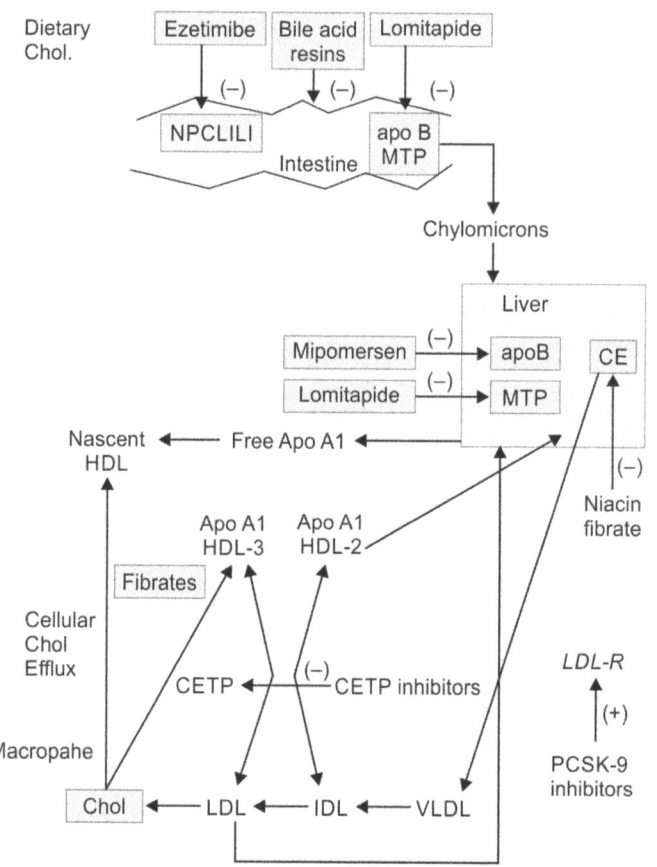

13.8 LA(A) AND SGLT2

LIPOPROT(A)

- Apo B100 containing protein
- LDL like particles containing apo B covalently linked to apolipoprot (a)
- Apo (a)-gene-Chr 1
  - Extensive variation in size
  - >40 diff isoform
  - >40 diff size
- Synthesized exclusively in liver
- During assembly apcas docks onto LDL
  ↓
Formation of disulfide bond between apo B and apo (a)
  ↓
Apo (a) binds near LDL-R binding site
  ↓
Reduce clearance of apo cas by LDL-R

METABOLISM UNDER

- Statin don't reduce LP(a)
- PCSK 9 inhi can decrease LP(a)

Patho

- Proinflammatory
- Proatherogenic
- Prothrombotic

Lp(a): Level determined by gene (LPA) on Chr-6
Very little effect of diet and exercise
  ↓
Level measured only once and no further testing required
More harmful than LDL
  ↓
Contain B100: As LDL ⎤
Apo(a) in addition   ⎦ More harmful
  ↓
So even in patient with LDL <70
  ↓
Apo(a)/ LP(a) continues to have risk of CVD.

Treatment

No approved treatment
   (AIM HIGH)
- Niacin and PCSK9 inhi have some effect
- CETP inhi (Anacetrapib) also
     (AIM HIGH)
  ↳ But no clinical benefit shown
- Apheresis decreased Lp(a) by >50% with some clinical benefit

New: Mipomersen (Antisense Oligonucleotide)

- Target apo B MRNA

SGLT 2 INHIBITOR

- Novel class of anti-DM agent
- Facilitate excretion of glucose through urine + metabolic modulators
  ↓
Improve preload, after load and cardiac efficiency

Normally: Filtered glucose is completely absorbed in prox tubule by
SGLT (Sodium glucose co-transporter)
   (Mainly SGLT-2)
  ↓
   Up regulated in DM
(SGLT-1 present in body in gut, skeletal muscle and myocardium)
  ↓
So selective SGLT-2 inhibition increasing average urine glucose excretion by 60–80 gm/d
  ↓
Higher glycemia level – more glucose excretion
  ↓
Associated with 400–500 mL of fluid loss for initial few weeks
Transient natriuresis also observed

DO NOT increase pl renin activity or Aldosterone
ASSO improve tubuloglomerular feedback in T2DM

H D. Effects and Meta Effect

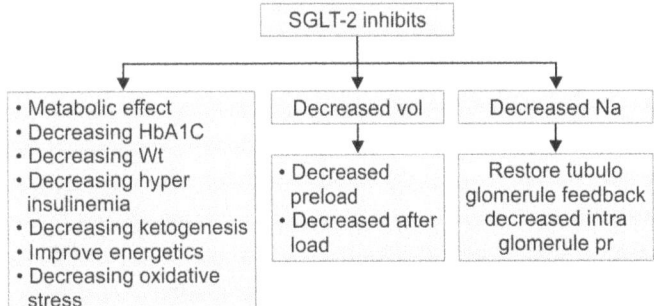

Clinical Effect

- Improve Art stiffness
- SBP and DBP reduction
- Presentation of renal function
- Improve LV function
- Metabolic efficiency

TRIALS

Lowest non-specific tissue distribution → *Empagliflozin:* EMPA REG outcome—benefit—increase bone #

Higher → *Canagliflozin:* Canvas—no benefit—increased amputation

Intermediate → *Dapagliflozin:* Declare TIMI 58—ongoing—increased bladder CA

S/E: Genital target inf (mild)/increased Cr level (mild)

CAUTION: NOT A SUBSTITUTE OF INSULIN

- Small increase in LDL-C and HDL-C (ratio unaltered)
- Don't use with other nephrotoxic drugs
- Maintain adequate hydration
- Avoid in frail patients
- Avoid fasting
- Stop 2-3 days prior to surgery

CI: KNOWN HYPERSENSITIVITY

- CKD (eGFR<45)
- Severe stress (medical illness, surgery, trauma, fasting, catabolic state).

OTHER ANTIDIABETICS

Liraglutide (LEADER Trial)

- Decreased MACE
- Decreased CV death
- Decreased all cause death
- No signi decrease in hospitalization for HF.

Semaglutide

- Decreased 3P-MACE
- NS decrease in CV death/all cause death.

13.9 EMERGING THERAPIES FOR DYSLIPIDEMIA TREATMENT

REDUCTION OF LDL-C
Cholesterol Absorption Inhibition
Ezetimibe

MOA: Inhibit chol absorption at the level of brush border of intestine
Interact with Niemann-Pick-C1 like prot
↓
Decrease amt of cholesterol delivered to liver
↓
Liver reacts by increasing LDL receptors expression
↓
Increased clearance of LDL-C from blood

Clinical Use
- Ezetimibe reduce LDL-C by 15–22%
- Ezetimibe + statin—increased LDL reduction by 15–20% more
- *Improve it trial:* Ezetimibe was added to simvastatin. No harm caused by further reduction of LDL-C. Support the proposal that Ezetimibe should be used as 2nd line therapy in association with statin
  - Recommendation endorsed in 2013 ACC/AHA and 2016 ESC guideline

Dose: 10 mg/d (No adjustments for mild hepatic: mid-mod renal dysfunction)
S/E: No major adv events
Most Freq: Mild elevation of liver enzymes and myalgia

LDL binds to LDL receptor and internalized
↓
PCSK9 controls whether LDL-R is recycled or catabolized
↓
Circulating PCSK9 binds to LDL-R and directs it to lysosome for degradation
↓
So inhibition of PCSK9
↓
Promote recycling of LDL-R
↓
Increased LDL uptake in hepatocyte
↓
Increased LDL-C level

PCSK9 Inhibitors
- Alirocumab and evolocumab—approved
  - Bococizumab, SIRNA, Adnectin—decreased phase 3,2,1 trial respectively

- *MOA:* Interaction of PCSK9 + LDL-R trigger intracellular degradation of LDL-R
↓
Inhibition of PCSK9 leads to over expression of LDL-R
↓
Decreased circulating LDL levels

Strategies to Inhibit PCSK9
- Development of R antisense oligonucleotide against PCSK9—stopped due to safety outcomes
- SIRNA Inhibitor of PCSK9—40% reduction of LDL level in phase 1 trial
- Inhibition by Adnectins—phase 1 trial
- Peptide based anti PCSK9 are approved alirocumab and evolocumab (bococizumab in clinical trials)

Efficacy
- In combination with statin or as monotherapy decreased LDL-C by 45–70%; decreased non HDL-C, decreased apolipoprotein B and Lp(a)
- *S/C:* Injection every 2–4 weeks
  - ODYSSEY long term (alirocumab) will provide
  - FOURIER (evolocumab) info about
  - SPIRE 1 and 2 (bococizumab) long term safety
- Efficacy has been demonstrated in
- Familial hypercholesterolemia
- High risk patient not controlled by max tolerance statin dose
- In combination with statin in patients with high LDL-C
- As monotherapy
- Who can't tolerate statin

Trials
1. ODYSSEY LONG TERM (alirocumab) ⎤ Shown to reduce
2. OSLER (evolocumab) ⎦ CV events

Dose: 150 mg s/c every 2 weekly
S/E: well tolerated

PROFICTO with evolocumab decreased progress SPIRE with bococizumab	- Rarely injection site reaction - Neurocognitive events reported with both - *EBBINGHAUS* trial—currently evaluating the possibility of neurocognitive disorder - *DESCARTES* Provided long term safety info

3. *Mipomersen*

Antisense oligonucleotide against Apo-B	MOA Antisense oligonucleotide ↓ Blocks in RNA translation into Apo B containing lipoprotein (LDL, VLDL)

Dose: 200 mg s/c once a week ($t_{1/2}$ = 1–2 months)
Action: Decreased LDL Apo B and Lp(a) by 25–35% in patients with severe hypercholesterolemia including FH (HeFH and HoFH)

Major safety concern is increased accumulation of TG in liver	*S/E*: Frequent: (injection site related reaction, flu like symptoms, hepatic fat accumulation and transaminases elevation)

Approved by FDA with box warning only for homozygous FH (2013 approved)

PROFICIO (evolocumab) ⎫
ODYSSEY (alirocumab)   ⎬ PCSK9 shown to reduce CV events
OSLER (evolocumab)   ⎪
SPIRE (bococizumab)   ⎭

PROFICIO PCSK9 inhi well tolerated and no diff in adv events
    Compared to placebo
DESCARTES-Long term safety (Evolo)
    S/E: Nasopharyngitis, URT 1, Influenza
MENDEL 2 (Evolo)—monotherapy
    Decreased LDL by 55–57%
RUTHERFORD 2 (Evolo) well tolerated
    OSLER (Evolo) decreased LDL-C by 60%
No published trial of bococizumab

4. *Lomitapide*

Microsomal TG Transfer Inhibitor	*MOA*: Inhibit MTP (microsomal TG transfer protein) ↓ Hamper assembly of VLDL in liver and chylomicron in Intestine ↓ Inhibit secretion of both

Approved for homozygous FH
Dose: Start at 5 mg/d and titrated 4 weeks interval to max 60 mg daily
Action: Decreased LDL-C by 50–40%
S/E: Poor tolerability
    GI intolerability, elevation in hepatic enzymes, increased hepatic steatosis

5. *Bempedoic acid*: (phase 2 trial)
   - Oral agent
   - Novel dual MOA
     1. *Inhibit ATP citrate lyase—decreased LDL-C*
     2. *Activate AMP kinase*—beneficial effect on glucose, lipids, inflammation and weight gain

6. *Gemcabene* (phase 2 trial)
   - Oral drug
   - *MOA:* Acetyl CO-A carboxylase and enhancement of VLDL clearance by decreasing apo C 3

INCREASED HDL-C

- 10% increase by lifestyle changes
- No clear evidence that increasing HDL-C and CV events

ILLUMINATE (torcetrapib)   ⎫
Dalcetrapib OUTCOMES   ⎪
ACCELERATE (evacetrapib)   ⎬ Failed to show such events
HPS 2 THRIVE (Nicotinic acid)   ⎪
AIM-HIGH (Nicotinic acid)   ⎭

REVEAL ongoing study with CETP will provide more info
- CETP inhibition
  - Can induce increase in HDL-C by ≥100%
  - Torcetrapib-withdrawn because of excess mortality in ILLUMINATE Trial (due to off target toxicity related to RAAS activation)
  - Dalcetrapib
  - Anacetrapib
  - Evacetrapib -ACCELERATE trial terminated due to futility
  - Dual outcome trial did not show any benefit
  - REVEAL trial ongoing

- Infusion of reconstituted HDL (phase 2 trial)
- Apo AI upregulators (phase 2 trial)

REDUCTION OF TG

- New omega 3 FA preparation
  - Vascepa (EPA)   ⎫ Approved
  - Epanova (EPA, DHA) ⎭
  Clinical: Decreased TG by 30% at 4 gm daily dose
  Trial: REDUCE-IT for Vascepa
        STRENGTH for Epanova
- PPAR-alpha—agonists
  - Decreased TG and Apo C3 levels
  New 1 pemafibrate (PROMINENT Trial ongoing) saroglitazar first approved dual action PPAR agonist for diabetic dyslipidemia uncontrolled on statin
- Lipoprotein lipase gene therapy
- Angio protein like protein Inhibitor

FOR TARGETING LP(A)

- PCSK9 Inhibitors
- Mipomersen
- Lomitapide
- Antisense therapy targeting Lp(a)
  (ESC guideline recommend TG <1.7 mmol/L)

13.10 LIPOPROTEIN DISORDERS AND CV DISEASE

Q.1 LP transport system and role of HDL in CAD
Q.2 Lipoproteins

LIPOPROTEIN DISORDERS AND CV DISEASE

Lipids

- 70% of dry weight of body
- 50% of circulating lipids are sterols

Others: Glycerophospholipids, glycerolipids

Dyslipidemia/Dyslipoproteinemia

- Disorder of the lipid transport pathway associated with arterial disease
- Better term than hyperlipidemia.

LIPOPROTEIN TRANSPORT SYSTEM

Biochemistry of Lipids

- Water insoluble
- Biologic lipid refers to broad group of naturally occurring molecules—fatty acid, waxes, eicosanoid, monoglyceride, diglyceride, phospholipids, sphingo lipids, sterols, terpenes, prenols, fat-soluble vitamins (A, D, E and K)
- Major biological function of lipid
  - Contributions to biological membranes
  - Energy storage
  - Backbone or modifiers of many signaling molecule
- *Metabolism of cholesterol and FA*
  - FA undergoes oxidation and can generate substances highly toxic to cells
  - Sterol nucleus resists enzymatic degradation
  - Chol must therefore be modified into bile acids or hormones or be shed with the skin to be eliminated
- Most of the cholesterol in plasma circulate in the form of cholesteryl esters in core of lipoprotein particles
- *Enzyme LCAT* (Lecithin-chol Acyl transferase) forms cholesteryl ester by transferring a fatty acid chain from phosphatidylcholine to cholesterol
- *Glycerolipid* = 3 carbon glycerol backbone covalently linked to 3 FA chain
  Aka triglyceride
  - Nonpolar and hydrophobic
  - Transported in core of lipoprotein
- *Glycerophospholipid:* Constituent of all cell memb and consists of glycerol molecule lined to 2 FA (designated R1 and R2)
  - Third carbon of glycerol moiety carries a phosphate group, to which one of 4 molecules is linked
    1. Choline—phosphatidylcholine (Lecithin)
    2. Ethanolamine—phosphatidylethanolamine
    3. Serine—phosphatidylserine
    4. Inositol—phosphatidyl inositol
- *Complex phospholipid*
  Cardiolipin = fusion of 2 phosphatidyl glycerol sphingomyelin

Lipoprotein, Apolipoprotein: Receptor and Processing Enzyme

Lipoprotein

Complex macromolecule structure composed of envelop phospholipids and free cholesterol, core of cholesteryl esters and triglyceride

- Classification of Lipoprotein refers their density in plasma
- TG rich lipoproteins = chylomicrons, chylomicron remnants, and VLDL
  ↓
- Density <1.006 gm/mL (pl. Density = 1.006)
- Rest consists of LDL, HDL, Lp(a)

Apolipoprotein

Four major roles
1. Assembly and secretion of the lipoprotein (apoA1, B100, B48)
2. Structural integrity of Lipoprotein (apo B, E, A1 and A2)
3. Coactivator or inhibition of enzymes
4. Binding or docking to specific receptors and proteins for cellular uptake of the entire particle or selective uptake of a lipid component

Lipoprotein	Engin	Major Apo
Chylomicron	Intestine	B48
Chy remnant	metabolism of chylo	B48 (E)
VLDL	Liver	B100
IDL	VLDL	B100 (E)
LDL	IDL	B100
HDL	Liver, Intestine	A1, A2
Lp(a)	Liver	B100(a)

LDL-R: Regulates entry of chol into cells and tight control of its expression in cell depending upon its need

Note: Macrophage express receptor (scavenger Lipoprotein Receptor) that mediate uptake of oxidatively modified LDL—This scavenger receptors not inhibited by intracellular LDL receptors not inhibited by intracellular LDL conc (unlike LDL-C receptor)—accumulate large amt of LDL—foam cell—atherosclerosis.

Receptors for HDL

- Scavenger receptor chess B
- ATP binding cassette transporters A1
- ATP binding cassette transporters G1

LIPOPROTEIN METABOLISM AND TRANSPORT

Two major role
1. Efficient transport of TG from Intestine and liver to site of utilization
2. Transport of cholesterol to peripheral tissue for membrane synthesis and steroid hormone production or to liver for bile acid synthesis

1. *Intestinal pathway*
   Essential fatty acids
   Linoleic acid – arachidonic acid
   Linoleic acid – eicosapentaenoic acid

- Chylomicron remnants
   Particles, delivered from LDL action on chylomicron are transported to liver for degradation and utilization of their constituents

2. *Hepatic pathway*

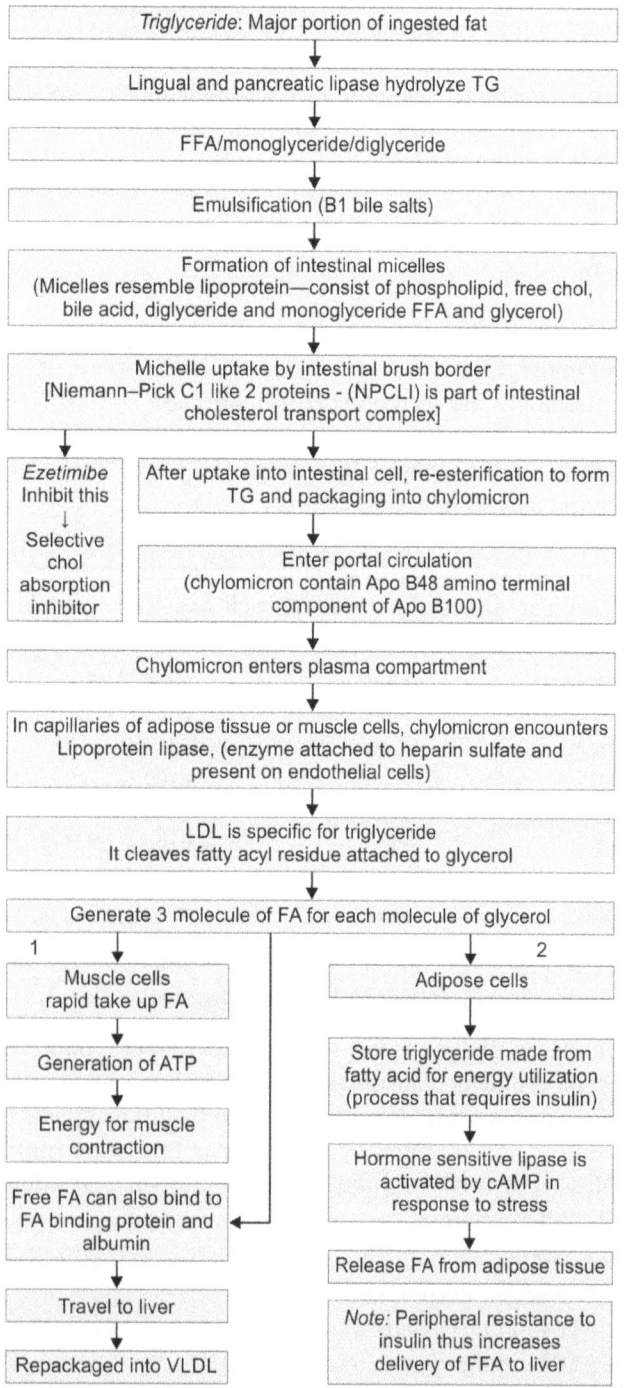

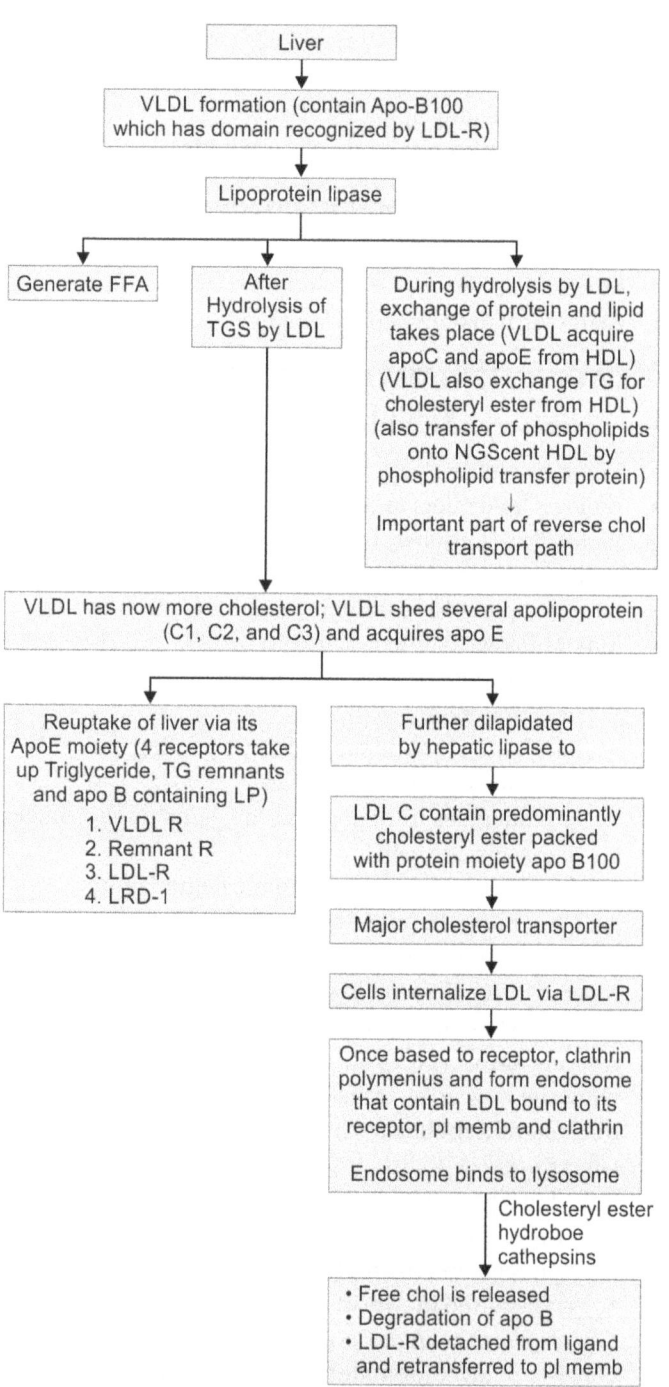

Cells can either make cholesterol form Acyl coenzyme A through enzymatic reaction or obtain it as cholesteryl ester form HDL and LDL

↓

SREBP2 regulates these 2 pathways at gene transcription level

Cells tightly regulate their chol by
1. Synthesis of chol in smooth ER (via rate limiting step HMG Co A reductase)
2. Receptor mediated endocytosis of LDL (via SREBP 2—steroid responsive element binding protein 2)
3. Efflux of chol from pl memb to cholesterol acceptor particles like HDL
4. Intracellular cholesterol esterification via ACAT (Acetyl COA acetyltransferase)

Depends on ABCA 1 pathway

Regulate chol content in membrane

- Cleavage of SREBP depends on Proprotein convertase subtilisin/kexin (PCSK)
- Another member of convertase superfamily

PCSK 9: Regulate internalization and cellular processing of LDL-R
  → Gain of function mutation → AD hypercholesterolemia
  → Loss of function mutation → Increased LDL-R and LDL-C significantly

3. *HDL and reverse chol transport*
   HDL: Promote reverse chol transport
   - Prevent Lp oxidation
   - Exert anti-inflammatory action
   - Promote cell proliferation and survival
   - Promote production of NO (in vitro)

80% HDL originate from liver/20% from intestine (Both organ synthesize Apo A1, main prot of HDL)
↓

Lipid free Apo A1 acquire phospholipid from cell membrane and from phospholipids shed during hydrolysis of triglyceride by phospholipid transfer protein
↓
Lipid free Apo A1 binds to ABCA-1 and promotes its phosphorylation via cAMP
↓
Perceive phospholipid and cholesterol onto Apo A1 to form nascent HDL
↓
On reaching a cell membrane, the nascent HDL particles capture memb associated chol and promote efflux of free chol onto other HDL particles

Two steps:
1. Binding of HDL Apo A1 to ABCA-1 and generation of specific memb microdomain that allows subsequent lipidation of Apo A1
2. Plasma enzyme LCAT, activated by Apo A1—esterify free chol—transferred to HDL particle (known as selective uptake of cholesterol)—cholesteryl ester is hydrophobic-moves to nuclears—HDL forms
↓
With further increase in cholesterol esterification HDL particle increase in size to form HDL2

- Inhibition of CETP ↑ blood HDL level TRL to HDL
- Cholesterol within HDL particle can be exchanged with triglyceride via CETP equimotor most of chol from HDL–TDL and movement of TG from
- Cholesterol on HDL particle is taken up by liver

13.11 HOPE 3 TRIAL: IMPLICATION IN INDIA

HOPE-3 (HEART OUTCOME PREVENTION EVALUATION-3)

- Initiated in 2007
- To evaluate effect of low dose potent statin to lower LDL-C, low dose fixed combination of ARB +D and their combination to prevent major CV events in patients who are at intermediate risk and no previous CAD.
- 12,705 Participants
- Inclusion criteria:
  - Elevated WHR
  - HPL children < 3g ♂; < 50 ♀
  - Current or recent smoking
  - Prediabetes/diet controlled DM
  - Premat CAD in 1st degree relative
  - Early renal days function

  } At least one of this as inclusion criteria

- Randomly assigned to 4 groups
  1. Rosuvas 10 mg + combi pill (candesartan 16 mg and HCTZ 12.5 mg)
  2. Rosuvas 10 + placebo
  3. Placebo + combipill
  4. 2 placebo pill
- Median follow-up 5-6 years

FINDINGS

- Compared with placebo, rosuvastatin decrease mean LDL-C level by 35 mg/dL and antihypertensive drugs lower mean SBP/DBP by 6/3 mm Hg
- 1st co-primary outcome (CV death, nonfatal stroke or nonfatal MI) occurred significantly less frequently with rosuvas than with placebo.

  Absolute reduction were   0.3% – CV related death
                                          0.4% – MI
                                          0.5% – stroke

- Overall candesartan HCTZ did not significantly lower incidence of 1st co-primary end point. However it lowered incidence in subgroup with highest baseline SBP (> 143)
- Overall outcome with rosuvas + candesartan + HCTZ was not better than outcome with rosuvas alone
- All-cause mortality was not lowered by active Tx compared with placebo
- Neither treatment increased risk for DM.
- Significantly differ from JUPITER trial

SECTION 14

Miscellaneous

14.1 CV MANIFESTATION OF AUTONOMIC DISORDERS

NEURAL CIRCULATORY CONTROL

- Sympathetic
- Parasympathetic
- Enteric

A. *Baroreceptor:*
- Autonomic response ⎫
- Capillary shift mechanism ⎬ All interact to maintain control of BP
- Hormonal response ⎪
- Kidney and fluid balance ⎭
- Most rapid response system
  ↓
  Acts via—increased contractility of heart or vasoconstriction of arterial/venous circulation in response to baroreceptor stimulation (Known as baroreflex)

- *Arterial Baroreceptors* (aka high pr receptors)
  - Location: Carotid sinus ← inverted by CN 9
    Aortic arch ← innervated by CN 10
    Origin of subclavian art
  - Baroreceptor stretch receptor sense change in pr
  - Baroreceptor are tonically active decreases normal circumstances at MAP higher than 70 mm Hg (Baroreceptor set point)
  - MAP<70 → Baroreceptors are silent
  - In chronic HTN, set point is increased
    Normal circumstance
    ↓
    Baroreceptor tonically active
    ↓
    Sense impulse to NTS
    ↓
    Inhibitory signal to vasomotor center (Sympathetic center)

    Excitatory signal to vagal nuclei (parasymp center)
    MAP falls below set point
    ↓
    Baroreceptor become silent
    ↓
    Inactive NTS
    ↓
    ⎡Induce sympathetic activation
    ⎣Inhibit parasymp activation
    Increased cardiac contractility
    Increased HR
    Art vasoconstriction
    Veno constriction
    ↓
    Increased CO and SVR
    ↓
    Increased BP

- *Cardio pulm baroreceptor:* (low pr receptor)
  - Location:
    - In heart
    - In vena cava
  - Less strong than baroreceptor (arteria)
  - Respond primarily to change in volume and occasionally to chemical stimuli
    - Activation (high volume state)
      ↓
      Vagal afferents to NTS and spinal symp afferent to spinal cord
      ↓
      Vasodilatation and inhibition of vasopressin release
    - High volume state
      ↓
      Stretch stimulus
      ↓

Depress renal sympathetic nerve
↓
Modulate renin release
↓
Diuresis and natriuresis
↓
Regulate where body vol to maintain BP homeostasis

B. Heart rate modulation
- *During rest:* Little sympathetic efferent input and low conc catecholamines
- *During any activity:* Sympathetic activity increases and parasympathetic activity decreases

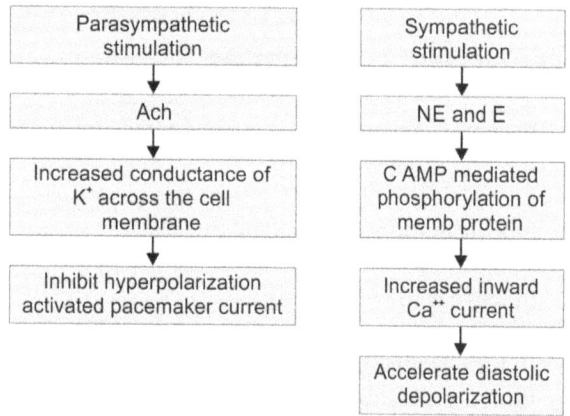

C. Breathing and chemoreflex

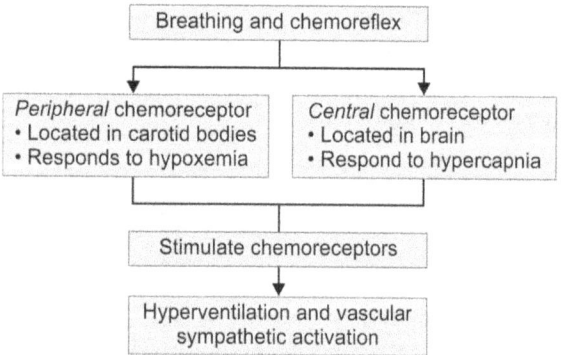

Role of chemoreceptor
- OSA: Symp vasoconstrictor response to hypoxia is potentiated because of elimination of inhibitory influence of chemoreceptor by stretch of pulm afferents
- Early HTN: Ventilatory response to early hypoxemia is increased in addition to increase in symp tone due to impaired baroreflex sensitivity and increased chemoreflex drive
  ↓
  - 100% O_2 can reduce tonic chemoreflex drive in OSA-reduce HR, BP
  - 100% O_2 to early hypertensive patients also reduce vasoconstrictor tone

D. Diving reflex
Prolonged apnea
↓
Diving reflex
↓
Increased parasymp drive to heart ⎤
Increased symp drive to vasculature ⎦ Unique
Prolonged apnea
↓
Hypoxia
↓
Body seek increase ventilation and blood flow to end organs
↓
To maintain O_2 supply to vital organs (Brain and heart)
↓
- Sympathetic vasoconstriction—decreased O_2 delivery to much of rest of body
- Parasympathetic to heart—Brady—decreased O_2 demand
  ↓

So it is possible for individual to survive for prolonged period of up to 5 min or more under anoxic condition (exceptional cases).

AUTONOMIC TESTING
- *Orthostatics*
  - Orthostatics hypotension defined as decrease of >20 mm Hg in SBP or decrease of >10 mm Hg in DBP after rising from supine to standing. BP and HR measured after symptoms develop or 3 mins have passed.
  - If not able to stand can be done in sitting position (with leg dangling) from supine
  - OH means inability to maintain sufficient BP and adequate cerebral perfusion against gravity.

    Significant drop in BP 'Without rise in HR' suggest autonomic dysfunction and underlying neuropathy, chronotropic incompetence or drug therapy (BB) that blunts HR response
- *Valsalva*
  - Patient blows continuously in closed system for 12 seconds at 40 mm Hg
  - Note fastest HR during maneuver and divide it by slowest HR immediately afterward
    ↓
    <1.4—autonomic dysfunction
    ↓
  - Nonspecific test
    BP response also provide useful info
    Phase 1: Increased BP with onset of Valsalva
    Phase 2: Normalization during sustained Valsalva

Phase 3: Dip after Valsalva
Phase 4: Overshoot several seconds later
↓

- Sympathetic index—derived from change in BP at baseline and phase 2 has been suggested as useful sign of OH and sympathetic failure
- Prompt fall in SBP during phase 2 suggested normal PCWP; Sustained elevation suggests left sided congestion] Provide non-invasive Basis of Mech of PHTN
- Can also provide effectiveness of septal ablation for HCM by calculating gradient across LVOT during Valsalva

- *Baroreceptor sensitivity*
  - Measured reflex increase in RR interval in response to BP increase (In short decrease in HR with increase in BP)
  - Injection of Phenylephrine
    ↓
    20-30 mm Hg increase in BP
    ↓
    Increased RR interval is linear to increase BP
    ↓
    Slope is used to quantify sensitivity of baroreflex
    - Steep—healthy individual
    - Decreased slope—with advancing age
    - Flatten more—with severe CV disease—HTN/HF
  - Baroreceptor sensitivity decreases with symp dominance (steep slope)
  - Relation between beat to beat RR interval and change in BP is being studied as possible alternative to Phenylephrine Infusion

- *Heart rate variability*
  - Commonly used but difficult to interpret
  - Phenomena being measured are
    - Oscillation in intervals between consecutive beats
    - Variance in heart rate
  - *Methods*
    - Time domain method—calculation of std-deviation of beat to beat interval
    - Freq domain method—graph shows how much of signal lies within given Freq bands over a range of frequencies
  - Reduce HR variability associated with
    - Higher risk of post infarction mortality
    - HTN
    - Hemorrhagic stroke
    - Septic shock
  - Impaired HRV and baroreflex dysfunction
    ↓
    May help identify patients with ESRD at greatest cardiac risk

- *Heart rate recovery*
  - During exercise—HR increases due to symp activity
  - After exercise—parasymp activation occurs again and reduce symp activation—to recover
  ↓
  Rate at which HR returns to baseline measured over 1st min post exercise is termed HR recovery
  ↓
  Delayed recovery is marker of decreased vagal activity and risk factor for SCD
  Impaired HRR also seen in patients with HFPEF

- *Tilt table testing*
  - Indication—unexplained syncope
  - Aim—to diagnose possible dysautonomia
    - *Positive:* If patient experience syncope associated with drop in BP or arrhythmia

    Cardio inhibitory syncope = syncope associated with decreased HR

    Vasodepressor syncope = syncope associated with decreased BP

- *Orthostatic hypotension*
  Nonneurogenic or neurogenic
  - Hypovolemia
  - Cardiac dysfunction
  - Medications
  - Prolonged bed rest

  OH increased risk of stroke, MI, mortality
  Treatment: Compression of venous capacitance bed
  Use of physical counter maneuvers
  Intermittent fluid boluses

DYSAUTONOMIA/AUTONOMIC DYSREGULATION

- Most common dysautonomias are those affecting sympathetic symptoms
- Due to disordered release/function/reuptake of NE
- Two groups: 1. Associated with decreased function (orthostatic often occurs)
  2. Associated with increased outflow (HTN and/or tachy)

A. *Primary chronic autonomic failure:*
- Orthostatic intolerance is key manifestation
- Most OH occurs from blood loss, vol depletion or prolonged bed rest
- Rarely it occurs from autonomic failure
  Chronic autonomic failure
  - Progressive nature
  - Poor prognosis

  Chr autonomic failure
  - Primary
  - Secondary

  Primary Chr autonomic failure divided into three

1. *Pure autonomic failure*
   - OH in absence of central neurodegeneration
   - Dysfunction at peripheral neurons in CNS
   - Basic error—low NE level in supine minimally rise in standing

   ↓

   Oh and inadequate chronotropy

2. *Multisystem atrophy*
   - Autonomic failure + s/s of neurodegeneration
   - Three types:
     1. *Parkinsonia*
     2. *Cerebellar*
     3. *Mixed*
   - Symptoms in 6th – 7th decade
   - Symp + parasymp dysfunction
     - C/F: OH, loss of sweating, impotence, Reduced IOP, urinary incontinence, alveolar hypoventilation, and central sleep apnea
   - OH is striking (as much as 100 mm Hg fall in SBP and minimal rise in HR)

3. *Parkinson disease with autonomic failure*
   Clinically appears to MSA + PD features

Investigation

- D/D is pure autonomic failure vs. MSA and PD is early
  - MRI shows neurodegeneration in MSA and PD
- D/D between MSA and PD
  - MSA - NE transport is preserved
    GH response to clonidine is impaired
  - PD - NE uptake is impaired
    GH response to clonidine is preserved
  - Neuroimaging technique
  - Autonomic dysfunction more striking in MSA
  - Progression is rapid in MSA

Treatment

- Change lifestyle
- Meal before bedtime—avoids night time supine hypotension
- Caffeine ingestion—attenuate HD response to food
- Water intake—can help increase BP
- Compression of lower limbs
- Fludrocortisone
- Adding sodium to diet
- Midodrine (alpha adrenoceptor agonist)
- L-threo 3-4 dihydroxyphenylserine (NE precursor)
- Ma Huang and yohimbine—sympathomimetic amine/alpha 2 receptor

B. *Secondary autonomic failure*
- Diabetes-MC cause
- Amyloidosis
- Renal failure
- Paraneoplastic syndrome
- Vitamin B_{12} deficiency
- HIV

C. *Congenital autonomic failure*
- Due to Dopamine Beta-hydroxylase def
- Dopamine Beta-hydroxylase convert—DOPA → NE

↓

So NE deficiency ensues

↓

Poor vasoconstrictor response to upright posture

↓

OH

ORTHOSTATIC INTOLERANCE

- Entity distinct from OH
- Seen in young women
  - C/F: Visual change, poor conc while standing, fatigue WITH Standing, tremor, and syncope

1. Postural tachycardia syndrome (POTS)
   Char by Orthostatic symptoms, tachycardia and absence of significant hypotension (within 5 min of standing)

   Diagnostic criteria
   - >30 beats/min Orthostatic tachycardia usually ≥120 BPM
   - Transient decrease in SBP >20 mm Hg with recovery within 1st min of tilt
   - Standing plasma NE level >600 pg/mL
   - Severe Orthostatic symptoms
   - Absence of signi BP charge within 5 min of standing or upright tilt

   C/F: F>M = 5:1
         Between 20–40 years age
         Symptoms due to brain hypoperfusion/symp overdrive

   Mech
   1. Denervation   ⎫ Exacerbated
   2. (Neuropathic POTS)   ⎬ by
   3. Deconditioning   ⎪ hypovolemia
   4. Hyperadrenergic state ⎭

   - Excessive tachy is a physiological response to maintain arterial pr during venous pooling
   - Patient with POTS also demonstrate excessive tachy during exercise
   - Orthostatic function is intact in POTS

   ↓

Marked tachy is due to small heart coupled with reduced blood volume-attributable to cardiac atrophy and hypovolemia

Treatment:
- Exercise training—improve/relieve POTS
- Increased intravasc vol with salt and fluid
- Compression garments
- Low dose BB—propranolol
- Low dose vasoconstrictor—midodrine
- Fludrocortisone

2. *Neurally mediated syncope/neurocardiogenic syncope*
- Periodic syncopal episode with normal autonomic function between episodes — 2 components
  1. Vasodepressor
  2. Cardioinhibitory
  3. Mixed
- Vasovagal like fainting
- *Mech:*
  - Controversial
  - Presumed to be 2° to decreased volume return to heart due to increased peripheral venous pooling—decreased venous return—decreased CO—increased SNS activity → cardiac hypercontractility (Vigorous contraction increase cardiac mechanoreceptor stimulation - stimulate vagus)
  - Possible nitrate mediated dilatation suggest vascular sensitivity to nitrates

Paradox stimulation of vagus and withdrawal and peri symp tone

Cardiac hypercontractility
↓
Activates cardiac mechanoreceptor
↓
Paradoxical reflex Bradycardia and decreased SVR (despite already decreased venous return)
↓
Elicit presyncopal symptoms
(Weakness, lightheadedness, feeling of warmth, brief loss of consciousness)
↓
Reflex Brady and hypotension are similar to those evoked by Bezold-Jarisch reflex

Diagnosis: Exclude—cardiac causes
- Situated syncope
- Phobia
- Other organic disorder

Tilt table testing
Implantable loop recorder

Treatment
- Education—Determine potential, predisposing factors and recognize prodromal symptoms
- Increased fluid and salt intake
- BB—Inhibition of mechanoreceptor
- Fludrocortisone—expand central fluid volume via sodium retention
- Vasoconstrictor / modulate SNS
- SSRI
- Cardiac pacing—compensate for Brady but not for vasodepressor component

3. *Chronic Fatigue syndrome*
Def: New unexplained fatigue that lasts for at least 6 months, unrelieved by rest and has no clear cause
- Dysautonomia is common
- Some data implicate role of impairment in skeletal muscle and cardiac muscle metabolism and bioenergetics
- *Tilt table test:* >60% shows abnormal BP or HR
- Syncope related to decreased symp outflow in absence of vent ← D/D with neuro cardiogenic hypovolemia or hypercontractility syncope

Treatment: Midodrine/BB
- No benefit from fludrocortisone/high risk salt intake

4. *Baroreflex failure*
Cause:
- Surgery, radiation therapy, CVA
- Damage to afferent (vagas and glossopharyngeal) or damage to brainstem nuclei or interneurons

C/F: (like pheochromocytoma crisis)
Palpitation, diaphoresis, headache
- Post Intervention/trauma/surgery
- BP is labile and may rise to extreme level
- Severe hypotension and Brady occurs during sleep
- Concomitant change in HR and BP
- No OH initially—may appear later

Diagnosis:
- Clinical
- Right carotid baroreceptor are more effective usually → suggests diff in clinical outcome depending on which carotid is affected
- Pl and urine NE >1000 pg/mL

Treatment: Initial treatment (first 72 hours)
        Nitroprusside
        Clonidine
- Max require long term treatment
- Chronically patients may have tachy + HTN with alternating Brady + hypo
  → Treat with clonidine and methyldopa
- During period of stress and anxiety (excess cortical stimulation)—low dose BZD and clonidine may help

5. *Carotid sinus hypersensitivity*
Def: Vent pause >3 seconds and/or fall in SBP of >50 mm Hg with carotid sinus massage

Carotid sinus synd: CS hypersensitivity + spont syncope
Treatment: Pacing may help
6. Norepinephrine transporter deficiency
7. Addison's disease

VARIANTS OF NEUROCARDIOGENIC SYNCOPE

- Aortic stenosis
- Renal failure and HD
- Right coronary thrombolysis
- IWMI
- HOCM
- Blood phobias

DISORDERS OF INCREASED SYMPATHETIC OUTFLOW

- Occur in number of diseases either as
  - Primary event or
  - Secondary to underlying disease
- Sympathetic outflow increases with age (even in absence of any disease)—contribute to increased risk of HTN

1. *Neurogenic essential HTN*
   High symp outflow may be 2° to
   - Impaired baroreceptor reflex
   - Increased chemoreflex
   - Insulin resistance
   - Genetic factors

   Treatment options
   - Renal denervation
   - Baroreceptor stimulation
2. *Panic disorder*
3. *Coronary art disease*
4. *Congestive heart failure*
   - Failing heart becomes partly sympathetically denervated
   - HF also exhibits baroreflex and chemoreflex dysfunction and disrupted HR variability and ventilatory control
   - Presence of sleep apnea may worsen cardiac sympathetic activation

   ↓

   All associated with poor long term outcome
5. *OSA*
6. *Pheochromocytoma*
7. *Stroke*
8. *Sleep associated disorders*

DISORDER OF INCREASED PARASYMP TONE

Associated with number of pathological and physiological condition

- *Physiological*
  - During sleep (esp REM)
  - Trained athletes
- *Pathological*
  - Weight loss
  - Spinal cord trauma

14.2 COCAINE AND HEART

COCAINE
*Pharmacology and MOA
- Two forms
1. *Cocaine Hydrochloride*
   - Water soluble
   - Can be taken orally, IV or Intranasally
   - High absorption through all mucosa
2. *Free base*
   - Heat stable
   - Can be smoked
   - Known as "crack"
   - Most potent and addictive
   - Effect starts within seconds and short lived

Cocaine
↓
Metabolized by liver cholinesterase
↓
Water soluble metabolic
↓
Excreted in urine

- $t_{1/2}$ = 45–90 mins
- Detectable in blood and urine only for few hours
- Metabolites persist for 24–36 hrs.
- *Applied locally*
  - Acts as anesthetic agent (due to its inhibition of membrane permeability to sodium—Block transmission of electrical impulse)
- *Given systematically*
  - Blocks presynaptic reuptake of Dopamine and NE- powerful sympathomimetic action

Cardiovascular Complications + Cocaine
- Myocardial Ischemia/Infarction
- Angina pectoris
- Arrhythmia
- Sudden death
- Pulm edema
- Endocarditis
- Myocarditis
- Ao dissection

COCAINE RELATED MI
Mechanism
Cocaine is patent sympathomimetic agent
- Myocardial O_2 demand with limited O_2 supply due to- increased HR
  - Increased myocardial contractility
  - Increased LV wall tension
  - Increased SBP
- Vasospasm/vasoconstriction due to
  - Increased alpha-adrenergic stimulation
  - Increased endothelin production
  - Decreased NO production
- Accelerated atherosclerosis and thrombosis due to
  - Increased plasminogen activator Inhibition
  - Increased platelet aggregation and activation
  - Increased endothelial permeability
- *Char of patient with cocaine induced MI*
  - *Dose:* Variable
  - *Freq. of use:* Variable
  - *Route of administration:* with all route → 75% after inhibitional use
  - *Age:* mean 34
  - *Gender:* M>>F (80–90% male)
  - *Timing:* Within minutes of cocaine use
  - 50% patient with cocaine induced MI have no c/o obstructive CAD
  - Death in <2%
  - Most common presenting features = chest pain
  - Risk greatly increased with concomitant smoking
- *Cocaine induced myocardial dysfunction*
  - LVH
  - Systolic/Diastolic dysfunction
  - May also cause Takotsubo cardiomyopathy
  - *Mech:*
    - Cocaine induces myo ischemia
    - Repetitive symp. Stimulation—cardiomyopathy and char Subendocardial cont bond neurosis
    - Concomitant adulterants or infectious agent- myocarditis
    - Increased production of ROS, altered cytokine production—change composition of myocardial collagen—myocyte apoptosis
- *Arrhythmias*
  - S. Tasty, S Brads, SVT, BBB, CHB, AIVR, VT, VE, Asystole, Tdp, Brugada
  - *Mech:*
    - Sympathomimetic property-increased ventricular irritability and lower threshold for fibrillation
    - Na^+ and K^+ channel blocking property
      - Inhibit AP generation and conduction
      - BBB/Brugada/TdP

- Cocaine increased intracellular Ca^{++} core EAD and triggered vent Arrhythmias
 - Reduces vagal activity—Potentiate its symptomatic effect
- *Endocarditis*
 - Reason unknown
  Probably due to
  - Drugs immunosuppressive effect
  - Direct effect of adulterant
- Ao dissection
 - Due to cocaine induced increase SBP

Cocaethylene

Cocaine + Alcohol $\xrightarrow[\text{Meta}]{\text{Hepatic}}$ cocaethylone

- More lethal than cocaine
- Synergistic effect

14.3 CARDIORENAL SYNDROME

Q.1 CRS, diagnosis, pathophysio and management (Dec 13)
Q.2 CRS: C/F types and management

DEFINITION

Disorder of heart and kidney where acute or chronic dysfunction in one organ may induce acute or chronic dysfunction in other organ

TYPES

CRS Type 1: Acute Cardiorenal Syndrome

Acute worsening of cardiac function leading to acute kidney injury

CRS Type 2: Chronic Cardiorenal Syndrome

Chronic abnormality in cardiac function leads to progressive and permanent chronic kidney disease

CRS Type 3: Acute Renocardiac Syndrome

Abrupt worsening of renal function leads to acute cardiac disorder

CRS Type 4: Chronic Renocardiac Syndrome

Chronic kidney disease contributing to decreased cardiac function, cardiac hypertrophy and/or increased risk of adverse CV events

CRS Type 5: Secondary Cardio Renal Syndrome

Systemic condition (e.g., DM, sepsis) causing both cardiac and renal dysfunction

PATHOPHYSIOLOGY

- Role of RAAS

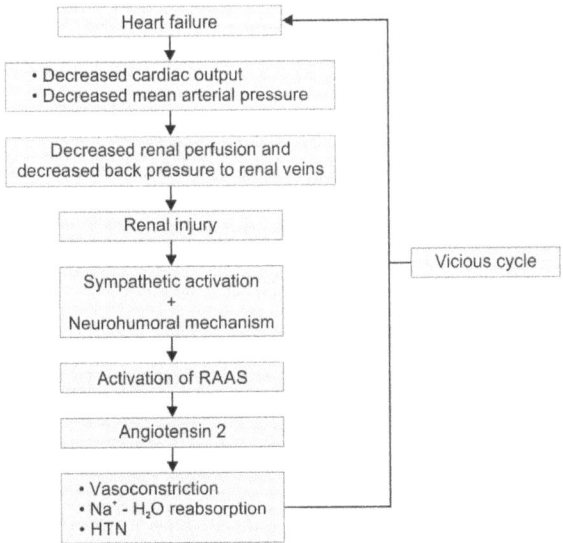

- *Role of endothelium*
  It releases endothelin
  ↓
  Vasoconstriction and
  Hypertrophy of cardiac myocyte
  ↓
  Damage to heart

- *Role of vasopressin*

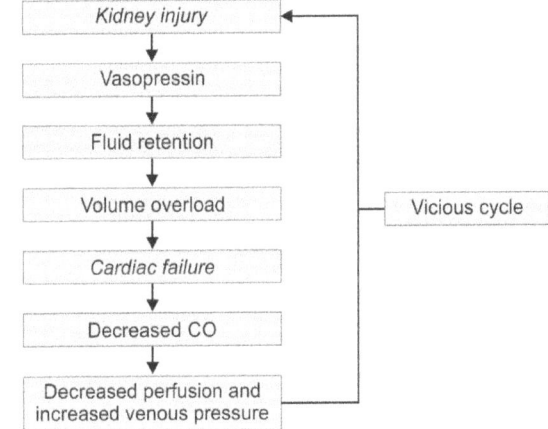

- *Role of BNP:*
  - Inhibit RAAS
  - Inhibit endothelin 1   } Beneficial
  - Promote Diuretics
  - Promote natriuresis

- *Role of NO and ROS*
  Decrease in NO   } Damage to both heart and kidney
  Increase in ROS

- *Role of sympathetic nervous system overactivity*

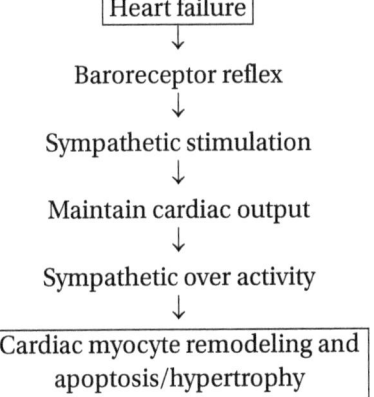

Type Specific Pathogenesis

Type 1: Acute cardio renal syndrome
Due to
- Cardiogenic shock
- Acutely decompensated chr HF

- Predominant RV Failure
- Hypertensive pulm edema

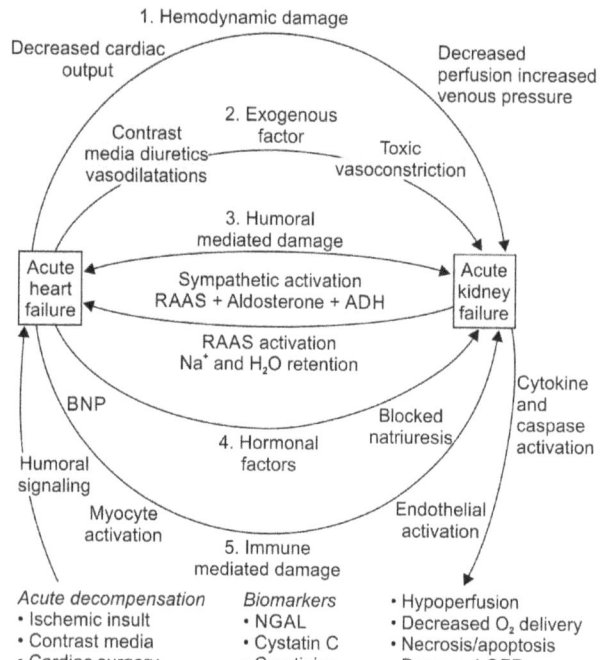

Type 2: Chronic cardiorenal synd

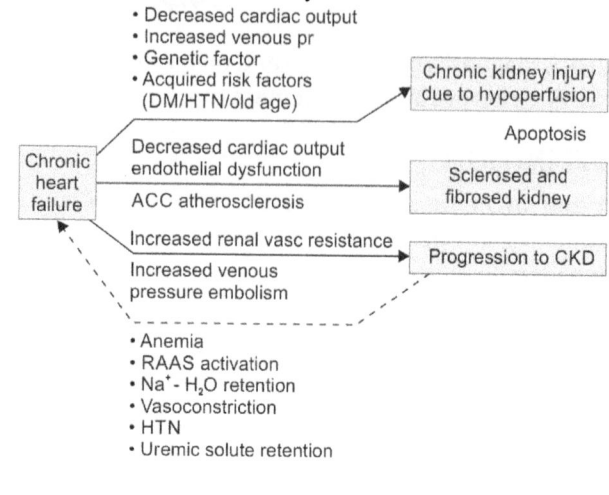

Type 3: Acute renocardial CRS

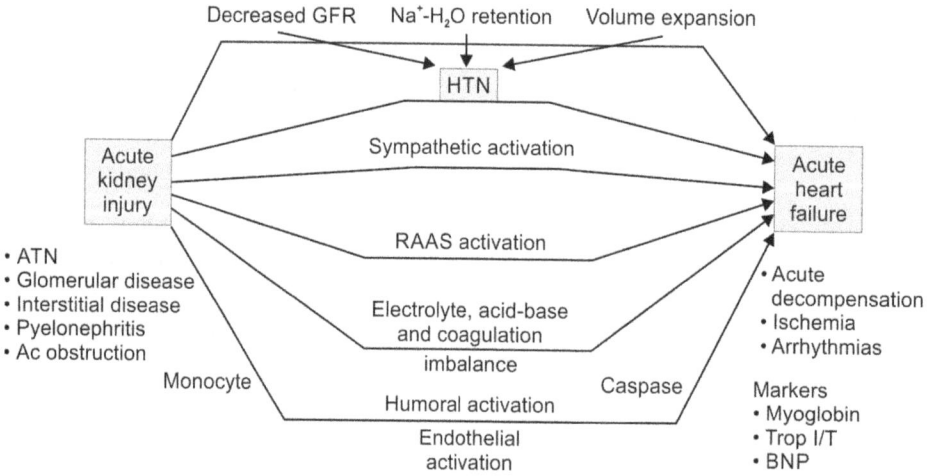

Type 4: Chronic Reno-cardiac syndrome:

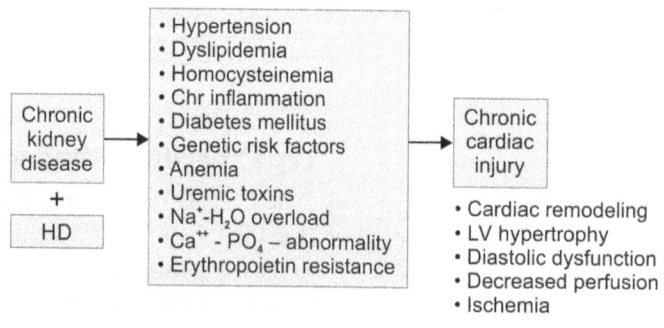

Type 5: Secondary CRS

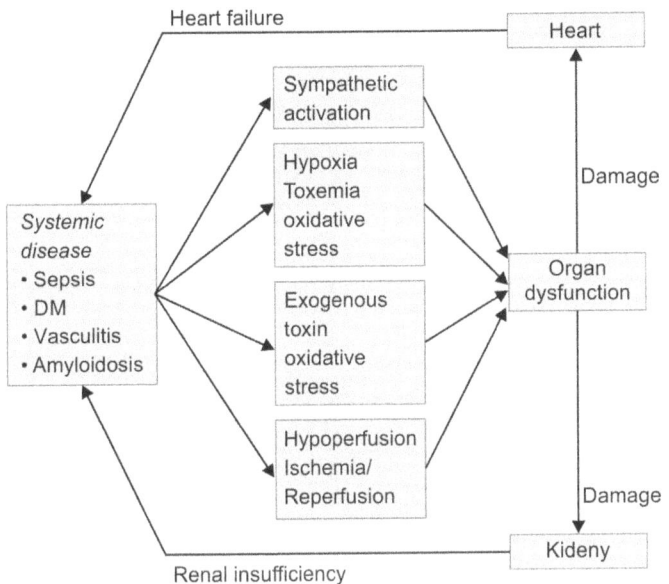

MANAGEMENT

- Regular monitoring of renal function by S. Creat /S. K$^+$ and other electrolyte
- Regular monitoring of cardiac function
- Regular monitoring of volume status
  - CVP monitoring
  - Art pr monitoring
  - Renal perfusion pr
- Body weight monitoring
  A. *Role of diuretics*
     - First line of treatment
     - Loop diuretics first choice
     - If diuretic resistance (not responding to >240 mg of furosemide daily)
       ↓
     - Consider thiazide/K$^+$ sparing diuretic/metolazone
  B. *Rise of dopamine*
     - Low dose of dopamine in conjunction with diuretics
  C. *Inotropes*
     - If CRS is mainly due to low cardiac output
       ↓
     Inotropes like dopamine will be helpful
  D. *Role of ultrafiltration*
     - Helpful in type 2 or 4 CRS patients who are in renal compromise in spite of optimal diuretic therapy and who are severely edematous
  E. *Role of RAAS Inhibitor*
     - Should be used cautiously in patients with renal insufficiency/Hyperkalemia
     - To reduce incidence of renal dysfunction (CRS 1 and 2) ACE inhibitor can be started in low dose
  F. *Newer modalities*
     - AVP receptor antagonist (Tolvaptan)
     - Adenosine A1 receptor antagonist
     - Hypertonic saline with diuresis
     - Nesiritide

PRECAUTION

- Patients with stable renal function should be monitored for S. K$^+$ and creatinine if combination therapy used
- If Sr. Cr is increasing—sought for reversible causes such as NSAIDS/Hypotension/urinary tract obstruction/hypovolemia
- Oliguria patient who is stable—daily review dose of diuretics/ARBS

14.4 RENAL DISEASE AND CV ILLNESS: CONTRAST INDUCED NEPHROPATHY

DEFINITION
(By Acute kidney injury network criteria)
Increase in serum creatinine conc of >0.5 mg/dL or 25% above baseline within 48-72 hours after contrast administration (in absence of alt expansion)

INCIDENCE
- 13% in nondiabetics
- 20% in diabetes
  CI-AVI leading to dialysis is rare (0.5 to 2.0%)

PROGNOSIS
- 36% in-hospital mortality rate
- 2 year survival—only 19%

PATHOPHYSIOLOGY
Mode of Injury
- Direct toxicity of iodinated contrast material to nephron (tubule)
- Microshower of atheroemboli to kidney
- Contrast material and atheroemboli induced internal vasoconstriction of Vasa recta
  - Direct toxicity depends on ionicity and osmolality of contrast material

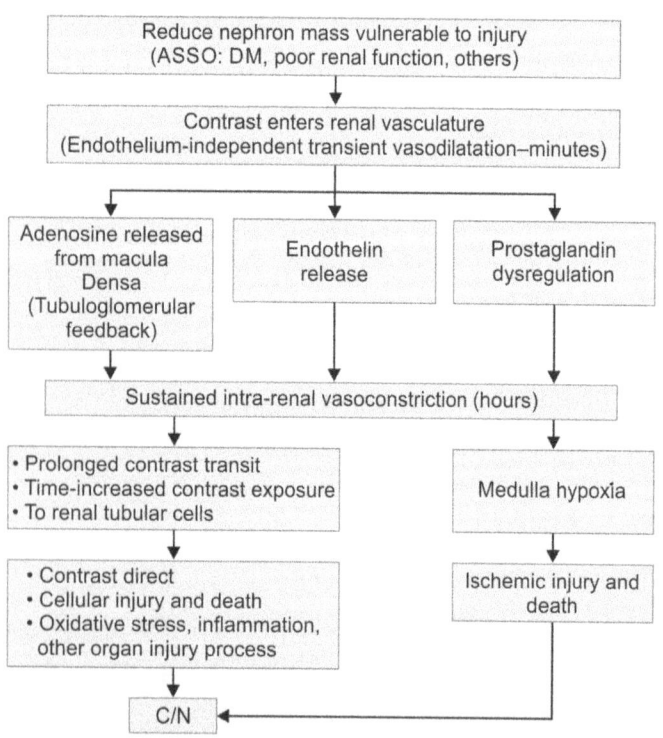

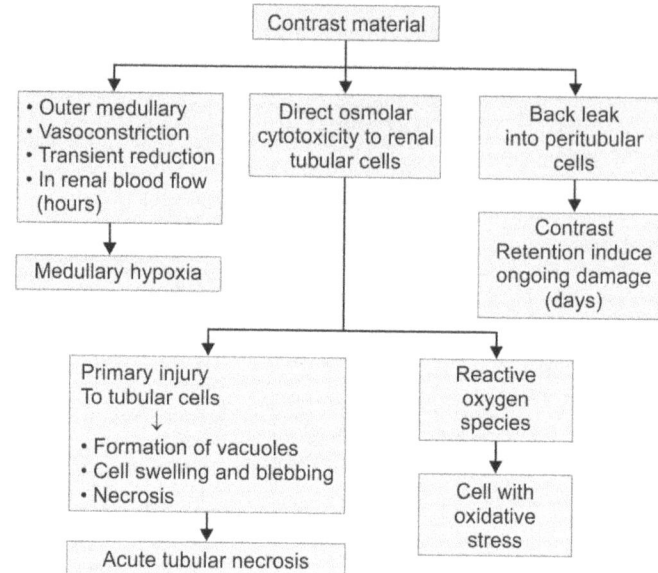

PRESENTATION
- Rise in S. Creat starts at 1-2 days post procedure peaks between 3-5 days
  Returns to baseline 7-10 days
- *Risk factors*
  A. *Patient related*
     - Renal insufficiency
     - Diabetic nephropathy
     - Advanced age (>75 years)
     - Effective volume depletion
       - Dehydration, CHF, CLD, hypotension, nephrotic syndrome
     - Concomitant exposure to nephrotoxins
     - Male
     - HTN
     - Hyperuricemia
     - Proteinuria
  B. *Procedure related*
     - Type of contrast (HOCM>LOCM/IOCM)
     - Dose of contrast used
     - Repeated exposure within 72 hours
     - Mode of administration (IA>IV)
     - 1° coro intervention for AMI

Risk Scores
A. *Mehran risk score*
   Includes: Age, hypotension, CHF, anemia, IABP, DM, vol of contrast media, S. creat/eGFR
   Risk of C/N and risk of dialysis calculated by scoring system

B. *ACFE score* $\dfrac{Age + 1 \text{ (if S. creat >2)}}{EF\,(\%)}$
- Age
- Creat
- Ejection fraction
- Predict C/N in patients with AMI undergoing PCI
- If score <1.48—NPV is 100%
- For each 1 point increase in ACFE value—5 fold increase risk of CTN

Ionic
High osmolar = Diatrizoate
                 Iothalamate
                 Ioxithalamate
Low osmolar = Ioxaglate

Nonionic
Low osmolar = Iopamidol
                 Iohexol
                 Iopromide
                 Ioversol
Iso osmolar = iodixanol
                 Iotrolan

C. *AGEF score:* (Age, GFR, EF)
$\dfrac{Age + 1 \text{ (if eGFR <60)}}{EF(\%)}$
- Better sensitivity and neg predictive value

PREVENTION

A. *Minimize contrast volume*
- Total vol of contrast should not exceed MACD
- MACD = max acceptable contrast dose
    Cigarroa's formula = 5 × body weight/S. Creat
    Laskey's formula = 3.7 × eGFR

Contrast vol/MACD <50%—low risk   C/N 2.5%
Contrast vol/MACD 50-100%—intermediate C/N 5%
Contrast vol/MACD >100%—high risk   C/N 15%
Target volume should be 30 mL for diagnostic
                           100 mL for interventional
- Nonionic contrast are better
- Use DOCM/LOCM whenever possible

B. *Minimize risk by*
- Discontinue concomitant nephrotoxic meds (e.g., NSAIDS) whenever possible >3 days
- Hydration and vol expansion (allow oral as well as iv hydration)
- Pre, intra and post procedure end-organ protection with pharmacotherapy
- Post procedure management and monitoring

Hydration
- Most efficient method
- Regimes
  - IV crystalloid 1 mg/kg/h beginning 12 hours before procedure and continue up to 24 hours after procedure (if no contraindication)
  - In patients with EF<40%—0.5 mL/kg/h
- 0.45 saline or 0.9 saline both can be used   [Isotonic salin better than 0.45] [Can also use renal guard system]
- *Mech*:
  - Both increased delivery of Na^+ to distal nephron—reduce activation of RAAS
  - Both increase free water clearance—dilution of contrast agent within tubule lumen
- Maintain vo 150 mL/h
- Post op volume expansion is more imp than pre-op volume
- IV hydration better than oral
- Soda bicarbonate
  - Mech. Alkaline renal tubular fluid and prevent free radical injury through Haber-Weiss reaction   [Sodium bicarbonate better than sodium chloride]
  - *Dose:* Regimes
    - 3 mL/kg/h infusion 1 hour before and 1 mL/kg/h 6 hours after
    - 1 mg/kg/h 6 hours before to 10 hours after
    Trials have shown ambiguous results
  - *N-acetyl cysteine*
    Dose: Regime
    - Oral 600 mg BD—1 day before cont procedure—cont 48 hours post procedure
    - IV 150 mg/kg in 500 mL NS over 30 min immediately before contrast exposure and then 50 mg/kg in 500 mL NS over 48 hours

Current status (ACT trial) (NAC does not reduce risk of C/N)

- Loop diuretic ⎤
- Mannitol   ⎦ Can worsen C/N if hydration is poor
- Low dose dopa ⎤
- Fenoldopam   ⎬ Not useful
- Adenosine receptor antagonist ⎦
- Statin   ⎤ Unclear benefits
- Hemofiltration ⎦

STRATEGY

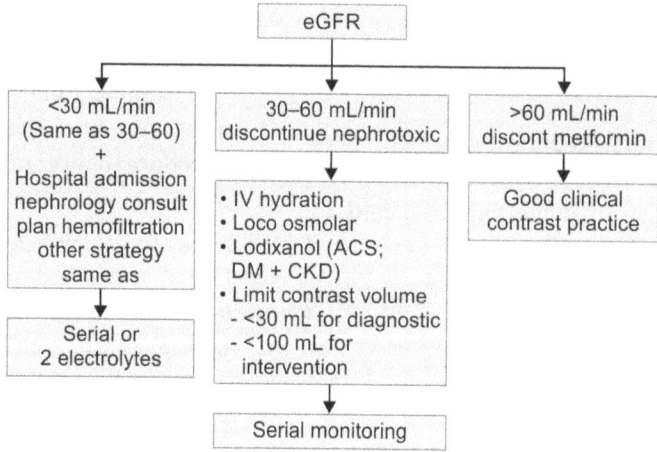

NOVEL BIOMARKERS, PROGRESSION OF KIDNEY DAMAGE AND RELATIONSHIP TO COMPLICATION

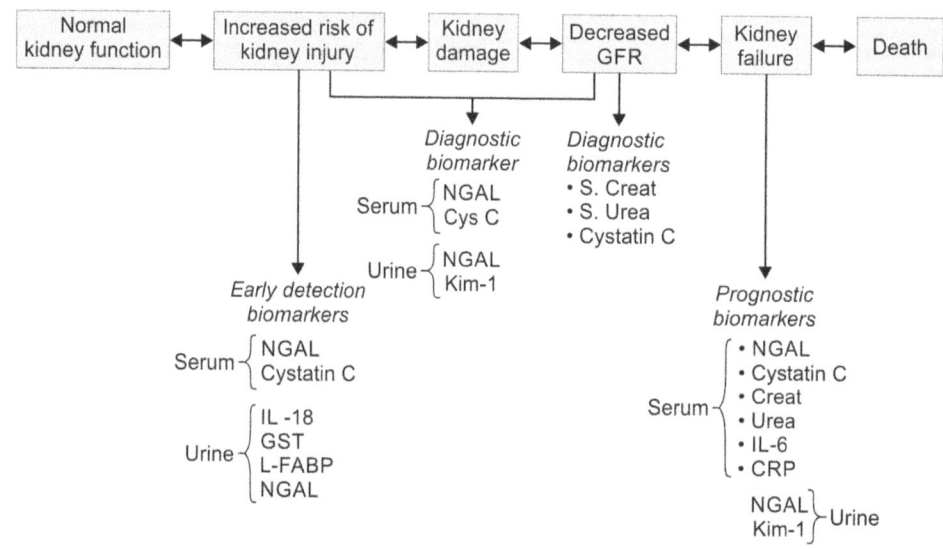

AkI
- Defined as increase in S. Cr by ≥ 0.3 mg/dl within 48 hours or increase in S. Cr to ≥1.5 times baseline (within last 7d) Urine vol <0.5 mL/kg/h for 6 hours

Stage:	S. Cr	Urine output
1	1.5–1.9 times baseline or ≥0.3 mg/dL increase	<0.5 mL/kg 1 hour × 6–12 hours
2	2–2.9 times baseline	<0.5 mL/kg/h ≥12 hours
3	≥3 times baseline or ≥4.0 S. creat increase or <eGFR <35	<0.3 mL/kg/h ≥24 hours or amine ≥12 hours

14.5 RHEUMATIC FACTOR

Q.1 Management and prevention of acute rheumatic fever
Q.2 Rheumatic fever vaccine prophylaxis

EPIDEMIOLOGY

- Four changing patterns over post 150 years
  1. Pre-antibiotic fall in incidence of rheumatic fever (typical of industrialized countries)
     Due to improved SE status, less over crowded housing and improved access to medical care
  2. Persistently high incidence in developing region who do not have comprehensive national prog (Africa, middle East, Asia, eastern Europe and south America)
  3. Some developing countries, falling incidence of RF following implementation of comprehensive public health prog for 1° and 2° prevention of RF
  4. Incidence of RF in central Asia fell in middle 1970s but rare sharply in post-soviet period

  Kyrgyzstan have highest incidence

India

- 25–50% of global burden of RHD (2002 WHO)
- 0.2–0.75/1000/year
- Around one third develop RHD
- Recent ICMR registry—0.0007–0.2/1000 in urban population

PATHOGENESIS

Multifactorial disease
- *The host:* Susceptible individual
- *The agent:* Group A beta hemolytic streptococci pharyngeal infection
- *Environment:* Deprived SE condition

A. The agent:
- Group A Beta hemolytic streptococci (GAS)
- GAS: GM positive cocci
  Chains or pairs
  Usually capsulated
  Nonmobile

Cross reactivity
- Autoantibodies that target the dominant GAS epilope of group A carbohydrate N-acetyl-beta-D glucosamine
  ↕
  Cross react with laminin and laminar BM in heart valve endothelium
- T cells cross react between M-protein
  ↕
  Cardiac myocyte myosin
- Autoantibodies against collagen (not cross reactive) forms due to release of collagen from heart valves

Two-hit hypothesis
Attack of valve endothelium by antibody
↓
Facilitates extravasation of T cell through activated epithelium into valve tissue
↓
Formation of granulomatous nodule called "Aschoff bodies" (Char by rheumatic myocarditis)
↓
Area of central necrosis is surrounded by ring of plump histiocytes called antichlor cells

> Discovered index pendantly by
> 1. Ludwig Aschoff and
> 2. Paul Giepel
> ↓
> Occasionally called as Aschoff Geipel bodies

Sydenham chorea
- Auto antibodies cross react between GLCNAC and ganglioside and dopamine receptor on surface of neuronal cells in brain
  ↓
  Activate calcium-calmodulin dependent Protein kinase-2

Streptococcal pharyngitis
- ~15–20% of pharyngitis in children 5–15 years
- Most common with Gr A streptococci (60%)
- Infection defined as rising trend in Ab titers
- Sudden onset, severe odynophagia, fever, vomiting, headache, Abd pain

RF following GAS pharyngitis
- Latent period 1–5 weeks
- Incidence 0.3–3%
- Rheumatogenic M serotype = 1, 3, 5, 6, 14, 18, 19, 24, 27, 29

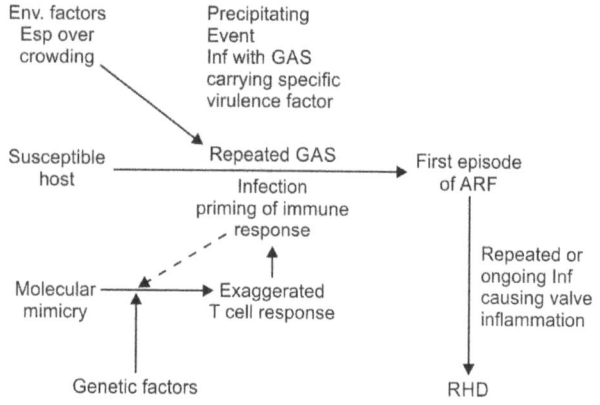

*Streptococcal skin infection
- Not thought to cause HF
- Reports of RF following streptococcal wound infection
- High prevalence of pyoderma in Aboriginal communities of Australia with high incidence of RF has raised question about link between skin inf and RF

B. The host
1. Role of hereditary factors
   - Lifetime cumulative incidence of RF in population exposed to GAS is constant 3-6% regardless of geography/ethnicity—suggest role of hereditary factors
   - Familial aggregation of rheumatic fever
2. Genetic susceptibility factors
   - Several genes controlling adaptive immunity (HLA class2 allele and cytotoxic T cell lymphocytes antigen 4), innate immune response (ficolin 2, mannose binding lectin 2, Ig4 and toll like receptor 2), cytokine gene (TNF Alpha, TGF-Beta, IL1 and IL10) and B cell alloantigen has been implicated in development of disease.
   At present it is not possible to predict individuals risk for development of RF following episode of untreated streptococcal pharyngitis.

C. Environment
- Low socioeconomic status
- Overcrowding
- Less access to 1° health care

CLINICAL FEATURE

- RF follows an episode of streptococcal pharyngitis: Latent period = 2-3 weeks
  ↓
  - No clinical/lab evidence
- One third patients who develop RF, develops it after an asymptomatic GAS infection

1. *Polyarthritis*
- More common (almost 100%)
- More severe in young adults
- Migratory-inflammation resolving in one joint and beginning in another
- Sometimes jt involvement is additive rather than migratory
- If untreated no of joints involved vary from 6 to 16
- Affected jt inflamed for few days to week
- Resolves completely
- If jt swelling persist > 4 weeks → consider other condition (e.g., Juvenile idiopathic arthritis or SLE)
- Joint involvement is asymmetric
- LL involved early than UL
- Monoarthritis reported in 17-25%
- Large joints (knee, ankle, elbow, wrist are involved more frequently)
- Hip, shoulder and small joints affected less frequently
- *Analysis of synovial fluid:* Sterile Inflammatory fluid
- Reduction in complement component C19, C3 and C4 - suggesting consumption by immune complex

*Jaccoud arthritis/chronic post RF arthropathy
- Rare
- Char by deformities of finger and toes
- Occur after repeated attack of RF
- Result from inflammation of fibrous articular capsule
- Ulnar deviation of finger
  Flexion of MCP joint
  Hyperextension of proximal TP jt
- Hand is usually painless without any sign of inflammation
- Generally correctable deformity
- No erosive lesion
- RA factor usually negative

(D/D) Post Streptococcal Reactive Arthritis
- Short talent period
- Not typical of rheumatic fever
- Respond less well to anti-inflammatories

2. *Carditis*
- Most serious
- In some carditis may be asymptomatic
- Incidence of carditis during the initial attack = 40-91%
- Clinical diagnosis based on
  - Detection of organic murmur that was not previously present (to indicate endocarditis)
  - Presence of pericardial friction rub or signs of pericardial effusion (to indicate pericarditis)
  - Presence of cardiomegaly/CHF (to indicate myocarditis)

- Myocarditis in absence of valvulitis is unlikely to be rheumatic in origin
- Cardiac tamponade is rare and constrictive pericarditis do not occur
- MC valvular lesion = MR
  AR occur less frequently
  Stenotic lesions are less common in early stage

3. Sydenham chorea
- Max be the only manifestation of RF
- F>M
- Latent period= 6-8 weeks
- Involuntary, purposeless, jerky movement of hands, arms, shoulders, feet, leg and trunk, along with hypotonia and weakness. Interfere with voluntary activity and disappear during sleep
- *Jack in box tongue:* Involuntary withdrawal of tongue when attempting to protrude it for 30 seconds
- *Milking sign:* repetitive irregular squeezing
- Chorea lasts for 8 weeks—15 weeks
- When chorea occurs alone; ESR, CRP and streptococcal anthoag may be normal
- Chorea does not appear simultaneously with arthritis but may coexist with carditis
  - *PANDAS:* (Pediatrics autoimmune neuro-psychiatric disorder with streptococcal inf)
    - Tic/OCD triggered by GAS
    - No association cardiac valve damage

4. Subcutaneous nodule: (only 1.5%)
- Nodule around elbow tend to occur on olecranon (while RA nodule occur more distally along extensor aspect of upper part of forearm)
- Firm, painless and freely movable
- 0.5-2 cm
- Occur in crops
- May persist for few weeks

5. Erythema marginatum: Less common
- Occur on upper part of arm/trunk (not on face)
- Extends centrifugally whereas the skin at the center returns to normal
- Irregular serpiginous border
- More after hot water bath

INVESTIGATION
Recommended for all cases
- WBC
- ESR/CRP
- Throat swab for GAS culture (before antibiotics)
- Blood culture if febrile
- Antistreptococcal serology (ASLO, Anti DNAs B)
- ECG
- CXR
- ECHO

Diagnostic criteria

A. Original Jones criteria 1944

Major manifestation	Minor manifestation
1. Carditis	1. Fever
2. Arthralgia	2. Abd pain
3. Chorea	3. Precordial pain
4. Subcutaneous nodule	4. Rashes (erythema maginature)
5. H/O prev definitive RF or RHD	5. Epistaxis
	6. Pulm findings
	7. Lab findings
	– ECG
	– Microcytic anemia
	– Elevated TLC
	– Raised ESR

B. Modified Jones 1956

Major manifestation	Minor manifestation
1. Carditis	1. Fever
2. Polyarthritis	2. Arthralgia
3. Chorea	3. Prev H/O RF or RHD
4. Subcut nodule	4. Prolonged PR interval
5. Erythema marginatum	5. Increased ESR, increased CRP, leukocytosis
	6. E/o preceding B-hemolytic streptococcal infection

C. Revised Jones criteria 1965

Major manifestation	Minor manifestation
Same as above	1 to 5 same as above

Essential criteria +
Supporting evidence of preceding streptococcal inf
- Positive throat c/s for GAS
- Increased ASO titer
- H/O recent scarlet fever

D. Jones criteria update—1992

Major criteria	Minor manifestation
Same as above	(1), (2), (3), (4) and (5)
+	
Supporting evidence (same)	

E. WHO manifestation (2003)

Major manifestation	Minor manifestation
1. Carditis	1. *Clinical:* Fever, polyarthralgia
2. Polyarthritis	2. *ECG:* Prolonged PR
3. Chorea	3. *Lab:* increased acute phase reactant (ESR/CRP) or leukocytosis
4. Erythema marginatum	
5. Subcut nodule	

Supporting evidence of preceding streptococcal infection within 45 days
1. Elevated or rising ASO or other streptococcal antibody
2. Rapid antigen test for GAS/Positive throat culture
3. Resent scarlet fever

Diagnostic Categories

1. *1° episode of RF* = 2 major or + evidence of
   1 major and preceding
   2 minor GAS infection
2. *Recurrent attack in patients without established RHD*
   As for 1° episode of RF
3. *Recurrent attack in* 2 minor manifestation
   Patients with established RHD + e/o GAS infection
4. *Rheumatic chorea*
   Other major manifestation or E/o GAS infection not required
5. Chr valve lesion of RHD (i.e., patients seen first time with pure MS or mixed MV disease with or without AOV disease) ≥ Do not require any other criteria for diagnosing RHD

F. 2015 Jones criteria

	Low risk population	High risk population
	ARF incidence ≤2 per 100,000 school aged children Or All age RHD prev ≤1 per 1,000 population year	
Major criteria		
1. Carditis	Clinical and/or subclinical (seen only on ECHO without auscultatory finding)	Clinical and/or subclinical
2. Arthritis	Polyarthritis	Monoarthritis Polyarthritis and/or Polyarthralgia
3. Chorea	Chorea	Chorea
4. Erythema marginatum	Erythema marginatum	Erythema marginatum
5.	Subcutaneous nodule	Subcutaneous nodule
Minor criteria		
Carditis Arthralgia Fever Markers of inflammation	• Prolonged PR int polyarthralgia ≥38.5°C • Peak ESR ≥60 mm in 1 hour and/or CRP ≥3.0 mg/dL	• Prolonged PR int monoarthralgia ≥38°C • Peak ESR ≥30 min in 1 hour and/or CRP ≥3.0 mg/dL

A.

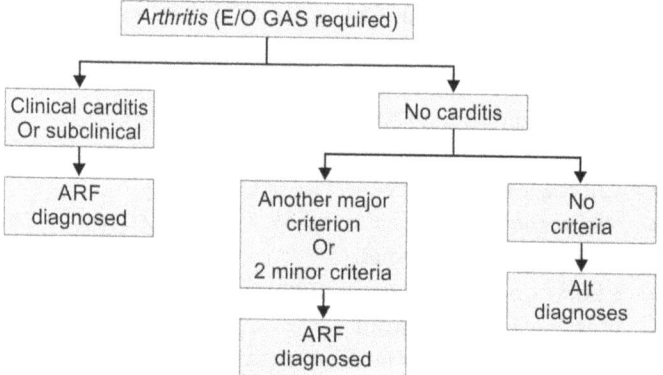

B.

C.

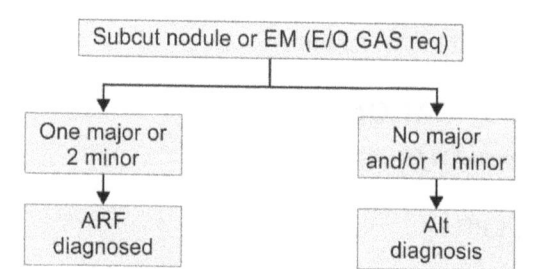

Contd...

D.

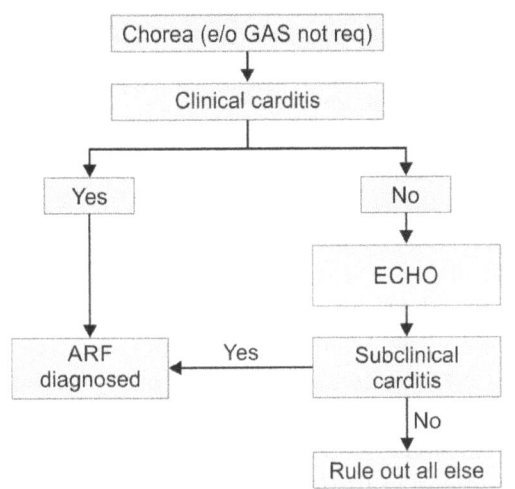

For all group of patients with e/o preceding GAS inf
A. Initial ARF diagnosed if
   1. 2 major
   2. 1 major + 2 minor
B. Recurrent ARF diagnosed if
   1. 2 major
   2. 1 major and 2 minor
   3. 3 minor

D/D OF

Arthritis	Carditis	Chorea
Septic arthritis	Physiological MR	Drug intoxication
CTD such as Juvenile idiopathic arthritis	MVP	Wilson disease
	Myxomatous MV	TiC disorder
	Congenital MV disease	Choreoathetoid cerebral poly
Viral arthropathy	Fibroelastoma	Encephalitis
Reactive arthropathy	Congenital AoV disease	Familial cholera
Lyme disease	IE	Intracranial tumor
Sickle cell anemia	Cardiomyopathy	Lyme disease
IE	Viral/idiopathic	Hormonal
Leukemia/Lymphoma	Myocarditis	APLA
Gout/pseudogout	Kawasaki disease	Sarcoid
HSP		Hyperthyroid
Post streptococcal reactive arthritis		

ECHO

Should be done in all cases of confirmed and suspected ARF (class 1 indi)

A. *Doppler findings in rheumatic valvulitis*

Pathological MR (all 4)	Pathological AR (all 4)
1. Seen in at least 2 views	1. Same
2. Jet length ≥2 cm in at least 1 view	2. ≥1 cm
3. Peak velocity >3 m/s	3. Same
4. *Pansystolic* jet in at least 1 envelope	4. *Pandiastolic* jet in at least 1 envelope

B. *Morphological findings on ECHO in rheumatic valvulitis*
   1. *Acute MV changes*
      * Annular dilatation
      * Chordal elongation
      * Chordal Rupture resulting in flail leaflet with severe MR
      * AML tip prolapse (less commonly PMC)
      * Beading/nodularity of Leaflet tips
   2. *Chronic MV changes (not seen in Ac carditis)*
      * Leaflet thickening
      * Chordal thickening and fusion
      * Restrict Leaflet motion
      * Calcification
   3. *Ao valve changes in acute/chronic carditis*
      * Irregular or focal leaflet thickening
      * Coaptation defect
      * Restricted leaflet motion
      * Leaflet prolapse

TREATMENT

Aims

- To suppress inflammatory response
- Minimizing effect of Inflammation on joint and heart
- Eradicate GAS organism from pharynx
- Symptomatic relief
- 2° prophylaxis

A. *Bed rest*
   * Mainly to relieve joint pain
   * Ambulation to be decided on individual bases
   * In general
      * *No carditis*—bed rest for 2 weeks and gradual ambulation over 2 weeks
      * Carditis with no cardiac enlargement: bed rest × 4 weeks and gradual ambulation over next 4 weeks
      * Carditis with cardiac enlargement: bed rest × 6 weeks and gradual ambulation over next 6 weeks
      * Carditis with HF strict bed rest as long as HF present, gradual ambulation over next 3 months
B. *Treatment of GAS*
   * Oral penicillin 500 mg BD × 10 d
   * Benzathine penicillin 12 L units IM
   * Erythromycin 250 QD × 10 d

C. *Treatment of carditis*
- *No CHF*—aspirin only—100 mg/kg/d in 4-5 divided doses × 1 month
- *CHF*—steroids at a dose 2 mg/kg × 8 weeks—12 weeks to be overlapped with aspirin when it is tapered
- *Antifailure:* Diuretics, ACEI, BB, Digoxin

D. *Treatment of arthritis*
- Aspirin—100 mg/kg/d in 4-5 divided doses × 2 weeks and gradually toper to 60-80 mg/kg for another 4 weeks
- Naproxen—alternative

E. *Skin lesion:* No specific treatment

F. *Chorea*
- Reassurance and sedation (if required)
- Haloperidol
- Carbamazepine and valproate—for refractory cases
- No benefit of aspirin/steroid

G. *Surgery:*
- Patients with refractory carditis
- Ideal after acute inflammation settles
- Valve replacement better

H. *Secondary and primary prevention*

PREVENTION

A. *Primordial prevention*
- Improvement in S-E status
- Prevention of overcrowding
- Improving nutritional status
- Availability of prompt medical care
- Public education
- Vaccine

B. *Primary prevention*
- Antibiotic treatment of proven or presumed GAS pharyngitis is effective in reducing RF by 70%
  - Benzathine penicillin 1.2 MV single IM injection (50% dose if <30 kg)
  - Oral penicillin v 250-500 mg TDS × 10 d
    <30 kg >30 kg
  - Amoxicillin 50 mg/kg OD oral × 10 d
- *For penicillin allergy*
  - Erythromycin × 10 days
  - Clindamycin
  - Azithromycin another alternatives
  - Clarithromycin

Post-treatment throat culture 2-7 days after completion of treatment are indicated
- If patient remain symptomatic
- Whose symptoms recurs
- Patients who have had RF and are at high risk of recurrence

C. *Secondary prevention*
- Benzathine penicillin: IM every 3-4 weeks
  6 L unit for <30 kg
  12 L unit for >30 kg
  (Every 2 weeks injectanly strongly reduces recurrence by 50% as compared to 4 weeks. But WHO still recommend 3-4 weeks)
- Penicillin v—250 mg BD
- Erythromycin 250 mg BD
- Sulfadiazine 1 gm daily for weight >30 kg
  500 mg daily for weight <30 kg

Duration

- Patients without carditis—5 year after last attack or 1 year age (whichever is longer)
- Patients with carditis—10 year after last attack or 25 year age (mild MR/healed) (whichever longer)
- More severe valvular disease—life long
- After valve surgery—life-long

Recurrence after
- Benzathine penicillin 0.4% 1 year
- Oral penicillin 5.5%
- Sulfadiazine 2-8%

VACCINES

*Components of GAS used in vaccine development
- M protein
- GAS C5a peptidase—a major surface virulence factor
- Fibronectin binding protein sfb 1
- Chimeric peptide 58 from conserved region of M protein
  - M protein vaccine less likely to succeed because
  - Heterogeneous distribution of strain varies from place to place and keeps changing even in a closed community in short period
  - On the basis of emm typing of M protein, >250 strain of GAS can cause infection and provide only strain specific immunity
  - GAS has strong tendency for mutation

14.6 CARDIOVASCULAR ABNORMALITIES IN HIV

Q1. Discuss cardiovascular involvement in HIV disease
(June 13)

*CV Complications of HIV Infection
- Tends to occur late in disease
- Esp in those with AIDS or Prolonged viral infection

1. Accelerated atherosclerosis
- Can occur in HIV infected young adult/children
- AMI is frequently 1st manifestation
- Patient is often young and have single vessel disease
- Plaque rupture is cause of MI
- Features suggestive of both coronary atherosclerosis and transplant related vasculopathy

Mech and Cause
- Endothelial dysfunction
- Increased oppression of adhesion molecule ICAM-1, VCAM, E-selection, TNF alpha, IL 6
- Dyslipidemia and insulin resistance (2° to protease inhibitor)
- NRTI (didanosine and abacavir) also increases risk NNRTI (efavirenz, nevirapine) does not increase risk
- Atherogenesis with viral infected macrophage
- Chronic inflammation
- Glucose intolerance
- Dyslipidemia—lipodystrophy

Treatment
- Low fat diet, aerobic exercise - improve both atherogenesis and lipodystrophy
- Smoking cessation
- BP control
- Statin use
- PCI/CABG

2. LV systolic dysfunction - (up to 25% autopsy cases)
Causes
- *Drug induced:* Zidovudine, cocaine, interferon
- *Infectious*: HIV, toxoplasma, Coxsackie virus, CMV, Adenovirus
- *Metabolic/Endocrine:* Anemia, or carnitine deficiency, hypocalcemia, hyponatremia, hypokalemia, hypoalbuminemia, hypothyroidism, hormone deficiency, adrenal insufficiency
- *Cytokines:* TNT alpha, TGF beta, IL-6, endothelin
- *Immunodef:* CP4 count<100
- *Autoimmune*

*HIV persists in reservoir cells in myocardium even after antiretroviral treatment—causes progressive tissue damage by Chronic release of cytotoxic cytokines
  *Prog LV dilatation is common

Treatment
- Standard treatment for non-ischemic LV dysfunction
- HAART
- Treatment of infection
- Nutritional supplement
- IvIg for SIRS

3. LV diastolic dysfunction (37% asymptomatic patient)
Cause:
- HTN
- Chronic viral inf
- TNF-alpha, IL-6

4. DCMP
Cause: Coro art disease

5. Primary pulm HTN: (0.5%)
- *Cause:* Plexogenic pulm arteriopathy
  - Char by remodeling of pulm vasculature by intimal fibrosis and replacement of normal endothelium
  - Poor prognosis

Treatment: Anticoagulant; PDE-5 inhibitor, endothelin antagonist, prostacyclin

6. Pericardial disease (pericardial effusion and pericarditis)
- Approximately 11%/year decrease with HAART

Causes: Bact: *Staph, Strepto, Proteus, Klebsiella, Enterococcus,* and *Mycobacterium*
Viral: HSV, HIV, CMV, Adenovirus
Other- Cryptococci, *Histoplasma, Toxoplasma*
Malignancy: Kaposi sarcoma, Lymphoma
Hypothyroidism
Immunodeficiency
Uremia
Treatment: Treat cause

7. Infective endocarditis
Causes: Autoimmune
Bacterial: Staph, salmonella, others
Fungal: *Candida, Aspergillus,* and *Cryptococcus*

8. Nonbacterial Thrombotic endocarditis
Cause: Valvular damage
Vitamin C deficiency
Malnutrition
Wasting
Hypercoagulable state/MC

9. *Malignancy*
   - Kaposi sarcoma (related with HHV 8)
   - NHL/lymphoma - 1° cardiac malignancy associated with HIV
   - Leiomyosarcoma
   - Kaposi sarcoma involving heart rarely causes any symptoms, can cause mild pericardial effusion (serosanguinous)

NHL/Lymphoma
   - Dyspnea, rt heart failure, BiV Failure, chest pain, arrhythmia
   - SVC syndrome
   - Pericardial effusion (contain malignant cells)
   - Intracardiac mass associated with poor prognosis

10. *Other*
   - *Right ventricular disease*
     Due to recurrent pulm inf
       Pulm arteritis
       Microvasc pulm emboli
   - *Vasculitis*
     Due to—drug therapy
   - Autonomic dysfunction
     Due to
     - Drug therapy
     - Malnutrition
     - Prolonged immunodeficiency
     - Sedentary lifestyle
   - *Arrhythmia/SCD*
   - *Lipodystrophy*

Complication of Drug Therapy

- *NRIT:* (zidovudine, stavudine, abacavir, lamivudine, etc.)
  - Rare CV side effects
    Lactic acidosis, hypotension myocarditis
- *NNRTI:* (Efavirenz, delavirdine, and nevirapine)
  - Arrhythmia
- *Protease inhibitor* (darunavir, indinavir, saquinavir, ritonavir, etc.)
  - Premature atherosclerosis, dyslipidemia, DM, insulin resistance, increased risk for MI
- Integrase Inhibitor (elvitegravir, raltegravir) ⎤
- CCR5 antagonist—maraviroc   ⎬ No reported S/E
- Fusion Inhibitor—enfuvirtide   ⎦

14.7 NONCARDIAC SURGERY IN CARDIAC PATIENTS

ASSESSMENT OF RISK

1. *Revised cardiac risk index* (RCRI)
   Six independent predictors
   1. High risk type of surgery
   2. H/O IHD
   3. H/O CHF
   4. H/O cerebrovascular disease
   5. Pre op treatment with insulin
   6. Pre op treatment creat ≥2.0

0 Risk factor	→ low CV risk
1-2 risk factors	→ intermediate CV risk
3 or more risk factor	→ high CV risk

2. Another risk index developed by American college of surgeons:
   Five predictors of periop MI/cardiac arrest
   1. Type of surgery
   2. Abnormal creat level
   3. Functional status
   4. American SOC of anesthesiologist class
   5. Increasing age

NONCARDIAC SURGERY AND CV DISEASE

A. *IHD:* (stress related to surgery—increased HR—worsen ischemia)
   ACC/AHA task force suggested that
   - Highest risk patients are those within 30 days of MI during which time plaque and myocardial healing occurs
   - After this period risk stratification is based on features of the disease (i.e. those with active ischemia are at higher risk)
   - Mortality remains elevated for at least 60 days after MI
   - Increased incidence of reinfarction after non-cardiac surgery if prev MI had occurred within 6 months of operation
   - *Stable angina*
     ♦ Patients with angina only after strenuous exercise often do not LV dysfunction and can generally tolerate surgery well and stabilized with adequate aspirin, BB and statin
     ♦ Patients with dyspnea on mild exertion are at high risk for development of periop MI. Such patients have high probability of having extensive CAD. They need additional testing depending on surgical procedure

B. *HTN*
   - Poorly controlled HTN associated with untoward HD response
   - Antihypertensive should be continued perioperatively
     ♦ *Hypertensive crisis:* DBP >120 mm Hg and clinical evidence of impending or actual end-organ damage (Papilledema, MI or renal failure)
       – Risk for MI and CVA
       – *Recipients:* Preeclampsia/eclampsia
           Pheochromocytoma
           Abrupt withdrawal from clonidine treatment
           Inadvertent discontinuation of anti-HTN meds
     ♦ *Chronic HTN:* Predispose to periop MI
       – *Severe HTN:* (DBP>110)—potential benefit of delaying surgery to optimize anti-HTN meds should be weighed against risk of delaying surgery

C. *Heart failure*
   - Associated with peri op mortality
   - S3/signs of HF—highest risk
   - Ischemic cardiomyopathy is of great concern

D. *HOCM*
   - Previously considered high risk condition
   - Now considered low risk
   - Spinal anesthesia contraindicated because LV function depends on preload

E. *Valvular heart disease*
   - Critical as associated with highest risk
   - MV disease associated with lower risk than AoV disease
     Can lead to severe HF in patients with tachycardia and/or volume loading
   - Patients with prosthetic valve who undergo procedure that can cause transient bacteremia should receive prophylaxis
   - Patients with prosthetic valve, risk of bleeding vs embolism should be weighted appropriately
   - *Commonly*, anticoag stopped 3-4 days before surgery and allow INR to fall <1.5 times normal. OAC can be resumed on POD-1
   - *Alternatively*, in patients with high risk of thrombo-embolism, conversion to heparin in peri op period— discontinue 4-6 hours before surgery and resume shortly after surgery

- High risk patient defined as (ACC/AHA)
  - Mechanical mitral/ tricuspid valve or mechanical AoV
  - AF
  - Prev thromboembolic episode
  - Hypercoagulable condition
  - EF <30%
  - >1 mech valve
F. *Arrhythmias:* common in peri op period
  Predisposing factors
  1. Prev arrhythmia
  2. Underlying heart disease
  3. HTN
  4. Periop pain
  5. Severe anxiety
  6. Heightened adrenergic tone

Periop AF
- Six fold increase in CV death, MI, UA and stroke in first 30 d
- 4 fold increased risk over next 12 months
- Arrhythmias in periop setting should provoke search for underlying CV disease, ongoing myocardial ischemia, drug toxicity or electrolyte—metabolic derangements
- IVCD even in presence of LBBB/RBBB rarely progress to CHB perioperatively

*CARDIAC CONDITIONS FOR WHICH PATIENTS SHOULD UNDERGO EVALUATION OF TREATMENT BEFORE NON-CARDIAC SURGERY

- *Unstable coronary syndromes*
  - Unstable or severe angina/recent MI
- *Decompensated HF*
- *Significant arrhythmias*
  - High grade AV block
  - Mobitz 2 AV block
  - 3° AV block
  - Symptomatic bradycardia
  - Symptomatic vent arrhythmias
  - Supravent arrhythmias (including AF)
  - Newly recognized VT
- *Severe valvular disease*
  - Severe As
  - Severe MS

Example of Procedures

1. *High risk:* (Reported cardiac risk >5%)
   - Aortic and other major vascular surgery
   - Peripheral vasc surgery
2. *Intermediate risk:* (reported risk 1.5%)
   - Intraperitoneal and intrathoracic surgery
   - Carotid endarterectomy
   - Head and neck surgery
   - Prostate surgery, orthopedic surgery
3. Low risk (Reported cardiac risk <1%)
   - Endoscopic procedure
   - Superficial procedure
   - Cataract surgery
   - Breast Surgery
   - Ambulatory surgery

Step Wise Approach

Patients scheduled for surgery with known risk factors for CAD

Step 1: Emergency —— Yes → • Clinical risk stratification perioperative surveillance
  No ↓
  • Proceed to surgery
  • Risk factor management

Step 2: Active/unstable cardiac—yes ——→ Evaluate
conditions   and treat
(UA/Recent MI/overt HF/   acc to GDMT
Severe Arrhythmias/severe VHD)

No ↓

Step 3: Estimate perioperative risk for MACE based on combined
  Clinical/surgical risk
  ↓   ↓
Elevated risk   Low risk (<1%) - Proceed with surgery
                                       No further testing

Step 4: Assess functional capacity

1 met = Take care of own self
        Eat, dress, use toilet
        Walk indoor around house
        Walk on level ground @ 3–5 km/h

4 met = Light work around house (dusting/dish washing)
        Climb a flight of stair/walk uphill
        Walk on level ground >6 km/h
        Run a short distance
        Heavy work around house-lifting or moving heavy objects
        Recreational activities dancing, bowling, golf

>10 mets: Strenuous activity: swimming, skiing, football, tennis
                            ↓
- Excellent (≥10 mets) ——→ Proceed to surgery
                            No further testing

- Moderate/good (≥4–10 METS) - Proceed to surgery No further testing
- Low/not known ——→ Will further testing impact decision making or perioperative core?

2a Step 5: pharmacological stress testing

Yes → Abnormal / Normal
No → Proceed to surgery acc to GDMT or alternate strategies
Normal → (Noninvasive treatment, palliation)

1 Coronary Revascularization ——→ Step 6

TIMING OF NON-CARDIAC SURGERY IN PATIENTS WITH POOR MI/PCI

(ACC/AHA 2014)

Class 1: Elective surgery should be delayed
- 14 days after balloon angioplasty
- 30 days after BMS
- 365 days after DES

Class 2: Elective surgery after DES
- Can be considered after 180 days if risk of further delay is greater than expected risk of ischemia and Stent thrombosis

Class 3: Elective surgery should not be performed
- Within 14 days of angioplasty
- Within 30 days of BMS
- Within 365 days of DCS where extended DAPT is req

PERIOP BETA-BLOCKER

Class 1: Continue BB in patients with undergoing surgery who have been on BB chemically

Class 2a: Patients with Intermediate to high risk M Ischemia noted in pre-op risk stratification, it may be reasonable to begin pre-op BB

Class 2b: In patients with 3 or more RCRT risk factors, it may be reasonable to begin BB preop

Class 3: BB should not be started on day of surgery

PERIOP ANTIPLATELET

Class 1

1. Patient undergoing urgent surgery during 4–6 weeks after BMS/DES, DAPT should be continued unless bleeding risk outweighs benefit of preventing stent thrombosis
2. If it is mandatory to stop P2Y12 Inhibitor, it is recommended to cont aspirin if possible and P2Y12 Inhibitor should be started ASAP after surgery

Class 2b:

1. Nonurgent surgery in patients who have not had prev stenting—it may be reasonable to cont aspirin when risk of potential increased cardiac event outweighs risk of increased bleeding

Class 3:

Initiation of aspirin in patients undergoing non-cardiac surgery is not beneficial

14.8 VASCULAR HEART DISEASE

Q.1 Epidemiology and pathophysiology in cong BAV. Clinical course of BAV-Non-inv evaluation in a case of BAV. Enumerate expected compli.

BICUSPID AORTIC VALVE

Epidemiology

- Cong BAV present in 1-2% population
- More prevalent in men (70-80% cases)
- Autosomal dominant inheritance
- Mutation in NOTCH-1 gene described
- Familial = Tumor - 30% have BAV
- Associate with other congenital malformation coarctation of AO/HLHS

Pathophysio

1. Most common: 2 cusp with right left systolic opening

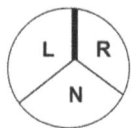
Fusion of RCC-LCC 70-80%

2. 2nd common: Antero posterior orientation

Fusion of RCC-NCC 20-30%

3. Least common: Fusion of LCC-NCC (rare)

- Prominent ridge of tissue/raphe present in the larger of two cusps
  ↓
  Closed valve may mimic a tri leaflet valve
  ↓
  Systolic leaflet opening shows only 2 aortic commissures

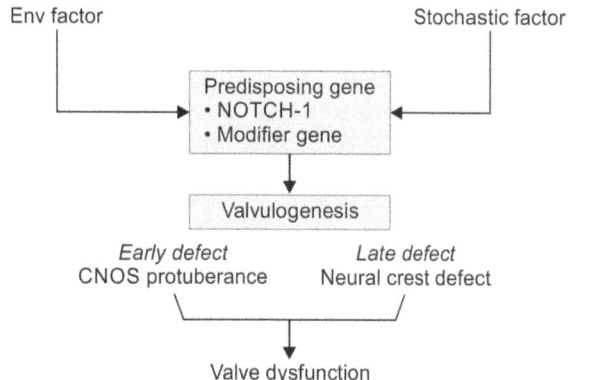

Aortopathy: (increased MMP—Loss of integrity in ECM)
- BAV associated with aortopathy
- Dilation of ascending aorta due to accelerated degeneration of aortic media
- Presence, location and severity of aortic dilation is not related to severity of valve dysfunction per se
- Risk of AOD is 5-9 times higher than gen population

MC *Type 1:* Dilation of tubular asc Ao along convexity with Mild - mod root dilation
   Type 2: Isolated tubular Asc Ao dilation which may extend into arch with relative sparing of root
   Type 3: Isolated root dilation

Diagnosis

TTE—92% Sensitivity; 96% specificity
Andy's—Raphe; Eccentric closure, 2 commissures

Clinical Cause

- Most bicuspid valve function normally until late In life
- Overall survival is not diff from gen population
- Risk factors for cardiac events
  1. Age >30 years
  2. Mod—severe AR (in 20% patient)- 10-40 years of age
  3. Mod—severe AS (more common than AR)
- BAV patient are at increased risk of endocarditis
- Most patient with BAV develop calcific As later in life
  - Presenting around 50 years or later age
  - Turbulent flow and increased leaflet stress caused by abnormal architecture are postulated to result in accelerated valve changes—Explanation for earlier avg age at presentation in BAV
- Portopathy associated with BAV often results in Ao dilation and carries an increased risk of AOD

Management

- No effective medical treatment to prevent progressive valve deterioration
- Follow-up for valve dysfunction
- Evaluation for Asc Ao with CT/MRI
- AVR + root replacement (if max Ao dia >45)
- Even in absence of Aortic valve replacement not replacement required when Ao diameter >55 mm
  - Even considered early (Ao dia >50 mm) in Patient with positive family history or evidence of rapid progression

14.9 ETHANOL AND HEART

ETHANOL

- Effect of ethanol on cardiac myocyte—str and function mechanism of ethanol induced myocardial injury
  - *Direct toxic effect:*
    - Uncoupling of excitation/contraction system
    - Reduce Ca^{++} sequestration in SR
    - Inhibit sarcolemal ATP dependent $Na^+ - K^+$ pump
    - Reduction in mitochondrial respiratory ratio
    - Altered substrate uptake
    - Increased interstitial/extracellular protein synthesis
  - *Toxic effect of metabolites:*
    - Acetaldehyde
    - Ethyl esters
  - *Nutritional or trace metal deficiencies*
    - Thiamine
    - Selenium
  - *Electrolyte disturbance:*
    - Hypokalemia
    - Hypomagnesemia
    - Hypophosphatemia
  - *Toxic additives*
    - Cobalt
    - Lead
    - Arsenic

Sustained exposure

- *Myofibritor* degeneration and replacement fibrosis
- Increased accumulation of collagen in ECM

- *Effect of ethanol on organ function:*
  - *Diastolic dysfunction*:
    - Due to interstitial fibrosis
    - 50% of asymptomatic chronic alcoholics have ECHO evidence of LVH with DP
    - LV relaxation time prolonged
      Peak early diastolic velocity is reduced (E decreasing)
      Acceleration of early diastolic flow slowed
    - Even small amount of alcohol can lead to diastolic dysfunction
  - *Asymptomatic systolic dysfunction*:
    - 30% of asymptomatic chronic alcoholics
    - Can occur even in social drinker
    - With continued ethanol ingestion—HF symptom usually develop due to DCM
  - *Nonischemic DCM*
    - Ethanol is leading cause
    - > 80 gm of ethanol for at least 5 years (daily)
      - (1 liter of wine, 8 standard size beer or half pint of hard liquor)
    - Women are more susceptible
  - *Protective effect*
    - 5-25 g/day of ethanol consumption have lower incidence of CHF than do those who don't drink at all
  - Patient who stop alcohol or substantially decreased alcohol ingestion—substantial improvement in LV systolic function within 6 months
- *Ethanol and syst HTN:*
  - Casual factor in up to 11% of men with HTN
  - > 1.5-2 drinks/day increase likely had of HTN
  - > 5 drinks/day (30 gm ethanol)—double risk
  - Mech:
    - Poorly understood
    - Ethanol increases pl level of catecholamines, renin, cortisol and aldosterone
  - Abstinence normalize SBP
- *Ethanol and lipid metabolism:*

  Ethanol
  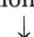
  Inhibit oxidation of FFA by liver

  Stimulate hepatic TG synthesis and VLDL secretion
  ↓
  Heavy ingestion also increase LDL level
  - Regular mild—mode consumption increases HDL level
- *Ethanol and CAD*
  - Heavy ethanol ingestion—increase CAD due to
    - Increase system HTN
    - Increase LV muscle mars
    - Syst and diastolic dysfunction
    - Hypertriglyceridemia
  - Mild—mod consumption decreases risk of CAD
  - Some authors suggested cardio protective effect only with wine
- *Arrhythmias:*
  - Atrial fibrillation—MC
  - APC/VPC
  - SVT
  - Atrial flutter
  - Vent tachycardia
  - Vent fibrillation
    - Ethanol responsible for ⅓ rd—⅔ rd cases of AF

- - Most episode after binge drinking (Holding Heart)
  - Mechanism:
    - AC ethanol indigestion—Diuresis—Urinary loss of Na$^+$, K$^+$, MG^{++}—arrhythmia
    - Ethanol (chronic)—interstitial fibrosis, vent hypertrophy, cardiomyopathy and autonomic dysfunction—arrhythmia
    - Ethanol—prolong QT, decreased HR variability, decreased vagal modulation and decreased baroreflex sensitivity—arrhythmia
    - Associated HTN, sleep apnea, metabolic abnormality and cigarette smoking—arrhythmia
- *Sudden death:*
  - Daily ethanol ≥ 80 gm - 3 fold increased mortality
  - Binge drinking also increases mortality

PROTECTIVE EFFECT

- Light to mod ethanol ingestion (>2 drink/day)
- Maximum benefit with wine
- Increase in HDL, decrease in CAD, decreased CHF, decrease in inflammation, decreased stroke and decrease in SCD

MECHANISM

- Increase of serum conc of HDL, apo-A1, adiponectin
- Inhibition of platelet aggregation
- Decrease of SR fibrinogen concentration
- Increase of antioxidant activity (phenolic compound and flavonoid in red wine)
- Anti-inflammatory effect
- Improve fibrinolytic (due to increased concentration of endogenous tissue plasminogen activator and concomitant decrease in PAI activity)
- Improve insulin sensitivity
  - Cardio protective effect of ethanol is greater for middle aged and old (than young person)

14.10 TRAUMATIC HEART DISEASE

CAUSES

- *Blunt injury*
  - Motor vehicle injury (seat belt, air bag, steering)
  - Vehicular—pedestrian accident
  - Fall from height
  - Crushing (industrial)
  - Blast
  - Assault
  - Sternal or rib
  - Recreational sports (e.g., baseball)
- *Penetrating*
  - Stab wound
  - Projectile wound-handgun, rifle
  - Shotgun wound
- *Iatrogenic:*
  - Catheter induced
  - Pericardiocentesis-induced
  - Percutaneous
- *Metabolic*
  - Traumatic response to injury
  - Stunning
  - SIRS
- *Other*
  - Burn
  - Electrical shock
  - Factitious—needles, foreign body
  - Embolic—missiles

BLUNT INJURY

- Septal rupture, free wall rupture, Coro art thrombosis, cardiac failure, complex and simple dysrhythmias and/or rupture of chordae tendinae or papillary muscle
- Fatal cardiac dysrhythmia can occur when sternum struck by a ball
- A form of commotio cordis

Mech

- Direct transmission of intrathoracic pr
- Hydraulic effect of pr transmitted to abdominal vein—RA
- Decelerating force
- Direct confusion causing myonecrosis and delayed rupture
- Penetration from broken rib
  - Blunt rupture of IVS occur near apex
  - Blunt trauma followed by rupture of vent involve LV more commonly
  - Patient arriving alive at ER, RV disruption is more common
  - Heart can be displaced into pleural cavity or even abd
  - Clue to cardiac reposition—sudden ion of pulse when patient is repositioned

EEG: 8-Tachy (MC)

14.11 RHEUMATIC DISEASE AND CV SYSTEM

CORONARY ARTERY INVOLVEMENT IN RHEUMATIC RISE

A. *Premature atherosclerosis*
- SLE
- RA
- Ankylosing spondylitis
- Gout
- Giant cell arthritis
- Takayasu's arteritis

B. *Coronary arthritis*
- SLE
- Takayasu's arteritis
- Kawasaki disease
- Churg-Strauss syndrome
- PAN
- Granulomatous polyangiitis
- RA

GIANT CELL ARTRITIS

- Large and medium sized arteries
- >50 years of age
- Typically affect extracranial branches of Aorta, temporal arteries, subclavian art, axillary art, thoracic aorta and occasionally femoral and iliac art.

CV Complication

- Rare
- Thoracic and abd aneurysm, limb ischemia, pericarditis, coronary arthritis, IHD, MI

TAKAYASU'S ARTERITIS

- Granulomatous Pan arthritis
- Affect aorta and major branches
- Age < 40 years
- Predominantly female
- F:M = 10 : 1

C/F

- Initial symptoms—Nonspecific
  - Fever, night sweat, arthralgia, malaise, profound tiredness, lethargy
- May be accompanied by Raynaud phenomena or upper extremity claudication and carotidynia
- (MC) Affect subclavian and common carotids
- Stenotic/occlusive arterial lesion found in >90%
- Aneurysms noted in approximately 25%
- Pulm art involved in up to 50%

Red Flag Sign

In patient younger than 40 years following indicates TA
- Unexplained acute phase response (increased ESR/CRP)
- Carotidynia
- HTN
- Discrepancy between BP in norms (>10 mm Hg)
- Absent/weak peripheral pulse
- Limb claudication
- Arterial burst
- Angina

Diagnosis

- Above C/F and red flag sign
- No specific autoantibody or serology
- FOG—PET, may reveal e/o active arthritis and leads to early detection

Involved art	Presentation
Subclavian	Arm claudication, Raynaud's, subclavian steal syndrome
Carotids	CVA, TIA, syncope, visual changes
Abd Ao	abd pain, nausea, vomiting
Renal	HTN, renal failure
Ao arch/root	Aortic insufficiency, CHF
Vertebral	Visual changes, CVA
Celiac axis	Abd pain/Nausea/Vomiting
Iliac	Leg claudication
Pulm	Atypical chest pain, dyspnea
Coronary	MI; Arthritis and aneurysm

CV complications:
  Aortic valve insufficiency
  Accelerated atherosclerosis
  Cardiac ischemia
  MI
  Heart failure
  Coronary artery lesion typically involving Ostia and prox segment (LMCA MC)—in 30% patients TA

Treatment

- Glucocorticoids
- Methotrexate
  Cyclophosphamide
- Anti TNF-alpha
- Medical treatment to control inflammation
  or PTCA
  or CABG

KAWASAKI DISEASE

- Predominantly children <5 years
- Peak incidence 6-24 months of age
- Affect medium and Small vessel
- Self-limited illness—resolve in 1-2 months

C/F

- Fever of 5 days duration or longer
- B/L conjunctivitis
- Mucocutaneous lesions—red fissured lips and strawberry tongue
- Prominent cervical lymphadenopathy
- Erythema affecting pulms and soles
- Polymorphous Xanthoma

Pathogenesis

- Unknown cause
- Infection may trigger the disease
    - Streptococci, staphylococci, and *Propionibacterium* acne
- No definitive e/o infectious disease
- Infiltration of arterial wall by neutrophil, T-cell and macrophage is associated with dev of arterial stenosis/aneurysm

Diagnosis

- Clinical features
- Neutrophilia, thrombocytosis: 2 increase ESR/CRP acutely
- ECHO can detect coronary involvement in 2nd week of illness
- CAG not performed actually because of risk of precipitating MI—can be done after 6 months
- ECG (50% patients)—Tachycardia, ST depression, T inversion, AV block, vent arrhythmia

CV Compilations

- Coro aneurysm develop in 20-25% patients
- MI, myocarditis, pericarditis, cardiac failure, vascular dysfunction
- Sudden death can occur due to a cute coro thrombosis or aneurysm rupture

TREATMENT

- Aspirin 80-100 mg/kg/d in divided doses along with IvIg
  $\downarrow$
  Reduce development of coro aneurysm to 5% significant effect on mortality
- Good outcome over all
  In up to 20% of those with coro aneurysm, stenosis eventually develops and may require follow-up.

14.12 VITAMIN D AND HEART DISEASE

RISK FACTORS FOR VITAMIN D DEFICIENCY

- Inadequate exposure to sunlight
- Malabsorption
- Liver or renal disease
- *Medications:* Glucocorticoids, phenytoin, phenobarbital
- Physical inactivity
- Obesity

CV RISK

Vitamin D deficiency increases risk of
- CAD
- PVD
- HTN
- HF
- Arrhythmias

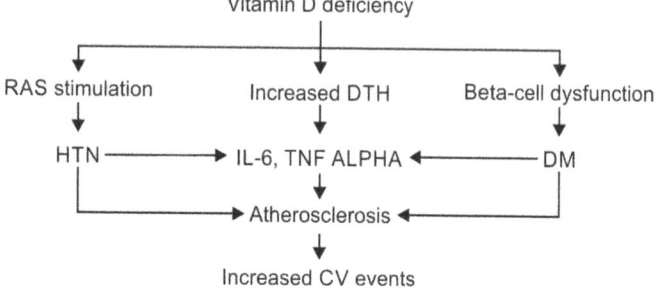

14.13 VENTRICULOARTERIAL IMPEDANCE (ZVA)

DEFINITION

In aortic stenosis Zva represents the cost in mm Hg for each ml of blood indexed for body size pumped by LV during systole.

It provides estimate of the global LV hemodynamic load that results from the summation of valvular load vascular load

$$Zva = \text{Valvular load} + \text{Vascular load}$$

DEPENDS ON

- Stenosis severity
- Volume flow rate across AV
- Body size
- Systemic vascular resistance

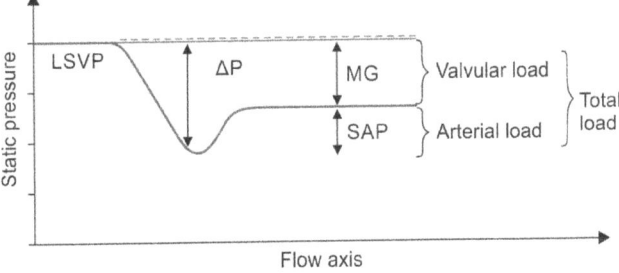

So,

$$Zva = \frac{LVSP}{Svi} = \frac{MG + SAP}{Svi}$$

\>3.5—moderate
\> 4.5—severe

CLINICAL SIGNIFICANCE

- Symptoms of As develop at lower degree of stenosis severity in hypertensive patients; probably because of the additional overload due to hypertension
- LV dysfunction is common in patients with increased Zva
  - Especially in the subgroup with low flow As
- High Zva is associated with poor mid and long term outcome even in asymptomatic patients
- High Zva in As patients is an accurate marker of advanced stage of disease
- High Zva is associated with reduced maximal exercise capacity
- Patients with severe symptomatic As and high Zva— follow-up should be shorter

14.14 EXERCISE CARDIOLOGY

INTRODUCTION

Aerobic exercise: Exercise requiring primarily an increase in O_2 transport (e.g., treadmill)

Resistance exercise: Exercise primarily stressing skeletal muscular system (e.g., Weight lifts)

CV RESPONSE TO EXERCISE

*Basic Principle of Exercise Physiology

A. *Maximal O_2 uptake*
- Aerobic and resistance exercise increase body's O_2 requirement to supply energy to exercising muscle
- Amount of energy used indirectly measured as amt of O_2 consumed-referred as "Ventilatory O_2 consumption" (VO_2)
- Fick Equation: C.O. = VO_2/Art-ven O_2 diff
  So,
  VO_2 = C.O. × ΔA - VO_2

So, VO_2 can be increased by
1. Increased C.O. (product of HR and S.V)
2. Increased ΔA-VO_2 =Increased by
   1. Redistribution of blood from nonexercising tissue (e.g., Kidney and splanchnic bed)
   2. Increased O_2 extraction in exercising muscle and
   3. Hemoconcentration as a result of plasma fluid loss into intestinal space of exercising muscle
- Maximal exercise capacity measured as VO_2 max., i.e., and max amt. of O_2 that an individual can transport during exercise before being fatigued.
- Maximum increase in A.VO_2 Δ is fixed, So VO_2 max depends on CO or SV

B. *Myocardial O_2 uptake:*
- Myocardial O_2 demand (MO_2)—estimated as product of HR and SBP (Double product)
- Increase in HR and SBP are determined by the exercise VO_2 requirement as a percentage of VO_2 max
- So for an individual with larger VO_2 max, he uses less maximal capacity for a given level of exercise and has lower HR and SBP response to exercise
- So, MO_2 is not determined by external exercise work rate, but by exercise work rate relative to maximal exercise capacity.

C. *Ventilatory threshold*:
- Expired CO_2 (VCO_2) also increase as exercise work rate increase
- VO_2 and VCO_2 are parallel during early exercise
- As exercise work rate increases = CO_2 expiration increases more.
  So, VO_2 and VCO_2 diverge = This point is termed respiratory/ventilatory threshold
- Divergence occurs due to increase blood lactic—acid, buffering of lactic acid H^+ ion by bicarbonate and subsequent exhalation of additional CO_2
- Also known as aerobic threshold
- VT occurs at approx. 50% of VO_2 mam.in non-trained individual. But at higher level in exercise trained

CV EFFECT OF AEROBIC EXERCISE TRAINING

- Increase maximal exercise capacity
- Increase VO_2 max. (Max. CO and max ΔAVO_2)
  ↓
  Max H.R. is determined by age and largely immutable.
So, C.O. determined by max SV.
- Increase in S.V. means performing same exercise which requires same VO_2 can be performed at a slower HR and lower MO_2 (internal work)
- Reduction in HR and thereby reducing MO_2 contributes to increase in exercise capacity in patients with Angina pectoris after exercise training.
- Ex. training also increase endurance capacity (ability to perform submaximal) effort for a prolonged period.

*Athlete's Heart

- Intense and prolonged aerobic ex. training produce CV adaptation termed as athlete's Heart
  - Increase resting SV
  - Decrease resting SV
- May be produced by increase resting vagal tone or decrease resting sympathetic tone
- Associated with
  - Resting brady
  - Marked sinus arrhythmia
  - 1° AV block
  - Mobitz I 2° HB
  - Even 3° AV block
  - WPCD (because AV cords reduced)
  - Early repolarization (due to increase vagal time)
- Regression of eccentric LVH can occur in highly trained athletes after 12–13 weeks of abstinence from exercise

Endurance/aerobic training ↓	Strength training ↓
Eccentric LVH and pr dilatation	Conc LVH but no RV remodeling
Biatrial Enlargement	Normal to mildly enlarged LA
Normal to slightly reduced LVEF	Normal to hyperdynamic LVEF
Normal or enlarged early LV diastolic function	Normal or slightly reduced early LV diastolic function
Normal or enhanced LV twisting/untwisting	increase in late LV diastolic function

DECREASE EXERCISE CAPACITY

Due to
- Inappropriate fast HR at low levels of exercise due to hyperthyroidism
- Ex. Induced asthma
- Disease of skeletal muscle
- Reduced O_2 carrying capacity from anemia
- AF or freq premature beats during exercise
- Occult CAD
- LV diastolic dysfunction
- Borderline HTN
- Psychological factors

SECTION 15

Pericardial Diseases

15.1 ACUTE PERICARDITIS

DEF

Acute pericarditis defined as symptoms and/or signs of pericardial inflammation of no more than 1–2 weeks duration
- Upto 5% of patients with nonischemic chest pain.

ETIOLOGY

A. *Idiopathic*
B. *Infection*
   - *Viral:* Echovirus, Coxsackie, adenovirus, CMV, EBV, HIV, Help B
   - *Bact:* Pneumococcus, Staph, *Strepto*, *Mycoplasma*, Lyme disease, M. Influenza, Neisseria
   - *Myobact:* (M-TB, *M. avium intracellulare*)
   - *Fungal:* (Histoplasma, coccidioidomycosis) Protozoal
C. *Inflammatory*
   - Connective tissue disorder (SLE, RA, scleroderma, Siogen)
   - Drug induced (procainamide, hydralazine, isoniazid, cyclosporine)
   - Arteritis (PAN, temporal arteritis)
   - IBD
   - After cardiotomy/thoracotomy
   - After cardiac injury
   - Genetic immune system disorder
   - Miscellaneous—sarcoidosis, Churg-Strauss IgG4 related disease
D. *After MI*
   - Early
   - Late (Dressler syndrome)
E. *Malignancy*
   - Primary
     2' – breast and lung CA, lymphoma, Kaposi sarcoma
F. *Radiation induced*
G. *Hemopericardium*
   - Trauma
   - Post MI free wall rupture
   - Device and procedure related PCI, ICD, PPI, RFA, closure of ASD, valve repair/replacement
   - Dissecting Ao aneurysm
H. *Misc*
   - Chr renal failure, HD associated
   - Cholesterol—Gold paint pericarditis
   - Hypo/hyperthyroidism
   - Amyloidosis
   - Pneumo/chylopericardium.

C/F

- Chest pain (always)
  - Severe
  - Always pleuritic
  - No compressive or oppressive feature
  - Relatively rapid onset
  - Substernal
  - No radiation to lt arm
  - Trapezius ridge—most characteristic and highly specific
  - Relieved by leaning forward and worsen by lying supines
- *Associated:* Dyspnea, cough, biscups
- *H/O* fever with chills
  Viral illness
  Rash
  Weight loss
  Malignancy

D/D

Pneumonia, pulm embolism/Infarction, costochondritis, GI reflux, Ao dissection, intraabdominal processes, pneumothorax.

EXAMINATION

- Uncomfortable and anxious
- Low grade fever
- S. Tachy
- Pericardial friction rub
  - Three components: (1) vent systole, (2) early diastolic, and (3) filling and atrial contraction
  - Resembles sound made when walking on crunchy snow
  - Loudest at lower left sternal border
  - Best heard with patients leaning forward.

INVESTIGATION

ECG

- Diffuse ST elevation
- ST vector points leftward, anterior and inferior with ST elevation in all leads except V1 and aVR
- Coved upward ST segment
- Some uses ST elevation resembles early reply
- ECG changes can be dynamic
- PE depression
  - Can occur without ST elevation
- Some ECG reverts to normal over a period of days or weeks. In other elevated ST passes through isoelectric point and progress to ST segment depression and T inversion.

D/D

- AV block indicates lyme disease
- Pathological Q—Myocardial ischemia
- Alternans and low voltage—effusion

CBC

- Modestly elevated WBC with lymphocytosis
- Anemia and high WBC—search for other cause

Biomarkers

- S. Troponin increase by 15% hs-CRP in 75%
- Serial hs-CRP useful for monitoring
- Most cases hs-CRP normalize in 1 week and almost all cases by 4 week

CXR Usually Normal

Can show sign of pneumonia/Kochs.

ECHO

- Normal in patients with AC pericarditis
- Normal LV function (except myopericarditis)
- Mod-severe effusion-other than idiopathic Ac. Pericarditis
  (ANA) consider if patient is young female.

MANAGEMENT

Initial Management

- Focused on screening for specific cause
- Detection of effusion and other ECHO abnormality
- Symptomatic relief and appropriate treatment if specific case is discovered.

Investigation

- ECG, hemogram, CXR, Trop I, hs-CRP, ECHO
- In young women—ANA (SZE)—esp recurrent idiopathic pericarditis.

Treatment

- Ac idiopathic pericarditis—self-limiting (70-90%) without complication/or recurrence
  - *Symptomatic treatment:* NSAIDs + colchicine
    - Ibuprofen (600-800 mg TDS)
      ASA (2-4 gm/d in divided doses)
      Gastric protection (PPI)

    - Many patients respond to 1st and 2nd dose
    - Fully respond after 10-14 d and no additional treatment required
    - hs-CRP normalization as a guide to treatment

      Those who do not respond/have large effusion/cause other than idiopathic pericarditis—hospitalize for further investigation and management
  - *Colchicine*
    - Now used as a part of initial treatment
    - Prev used to treat pericarditis that did not respond to NSAIDs or Recurrent pericarditis
    - It improves initial response in conjunction with NSAIDs
      - Reduces dance of recurrence
    - Anti-inflammatory effect by blocking microtubule assembly in WBC
    - *Dose:*
      < 70 kg—0.5 mg/d
      > 70 kg—0.5 mg BD
      Dose reduction in renal impaired
    - *S/E*: GI side effect
    - *Duration:* 3 months of colchicine after initial episode

- *Narcotic analgesia*
  - For those who respond slowly to NSAIDs + colchicine
- *Corticosteroid + colchicine*
  - Those who respond poorly to NSAIDs + Colchicine
  - Their use appears to promote recurrence
  - Lower initial dose with gradual taper is preferable with respect to both recurrence and S/E

Dose: Prednisone 0.2-0.5 mg/kg/d
Tapering every 2-4 weeks
Tapering guided by symptoms and hs-CRP.

COMPLICATION

- Effusion
- Tamponade—3.1%
- Constriction—1.5%

15.2 CONSTRICTIVE PERICARDITIS

INTRODUCTION
CP is end stage of an inflammatory process involving the pericardium.

ETIOLOGY
- Idiopathic—(MC)
- Irradiation
- Related to surgery
- Infection—Koch's (MC)
- Neoplastic
- Autoimmune
- Uremia
- Related to trauma
- Sarcoid
- Methysergide therapy
- ICD patches.

PATHOPHYSIOLOGY
- Inflammation - fibrosis + calcification + adhesion of parietal and visceral pericardium
  ↓
  Markedly restricted filling of heart
  ↓
  Elevated and equal filling pr in all chambers and systemic and pulm veins
  - *Early diastole:* Vent fills very rapidly because of marked elevated Atrial pr and early diastolic vent suction (due to small ESV)
  - *Early mid diastole:* Vent filling abruptly stops when intracardiac volume reaches the limit set by stiff pericardium (total cardiac vol fixed)
    ↓
    So atmost all filling occur in early diastole
    - Systemic venous congestion
    - Hepatic congestion
    - Peripheral edema
    - Ascites
    - Anasarca
    - Cardiac cirrhosis
    - In pure constrictive pericarditis—contractile function is preserved, although EF can be reduced because of low preload
- Failure of transmission of changes in intrathoracic respiratory pr to chamber (pr continues to transmitted to pulmonary circulation)
  ↓
  Inspiration: Drop in intrathoracic pr transmitted to pulm veins but not to left side of heart
  ↓
  Pulm vein to LA gradient decreases
  ↓
  Transmitted Inflow decreases
  ↓
  Decreased LV filling
  ↓
  Allow more RV filling and shift of IVS to left
  ↓
  Exaggerated respi variation/vent interdependence in transmitral and transtricuspid inflow, LV and RV systolic and diastolic pr and volume

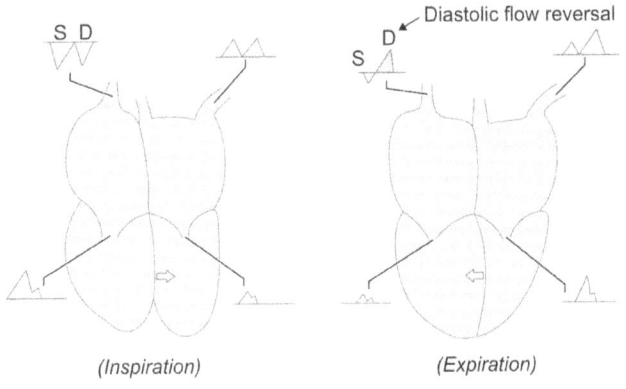

(Inspiration)   (Expiration)

C/F
- Sign and symptoms of rt heart failure
  - Passive hepatic congestion and discomfort LL edema
  - Ascites, anasarca and jaundice/2° to cirrhosis
- Sign and symptoms of left HF also appear
  - Dyspnea, orthopnea, PND, cough
- AF
- *End stage:* Low output state (chronically low CO)
  - Fatigue, muscle wasting, cachexia
- *Other:* Recurrent pleural eff and syncope.

EXAMINATION
- Markedly elevated JVP
- Prominent Y descent (with normal X descent)
  - Result in M or W shaped JVP contour
- In patients with AF
  - X descent lost
  - Only Y descent present
- *Kussmaul sign:* Inspiratory increase in venous pr (due to loss of normal increase in venous return to rt side of heart on inspiration, even though tricuspid flow increases)
- Paradoxical pulse in 1/3rd (esp with effusive-constrictive)
- With extensive calcification and adhesion
  - Cardiac impulse does not change with position
  - *Pericardial knock:* Most notable finding

- Early diastolic sound best heard at left sternal border and/or cardiac apex. High freq than S3
- Widening of S2 splitting
- Secondary TR with murmur
- *Other:*
  - Jaundice
  - Hepatic enlargement
  - Spider angioma
  - Palmar erythema
  - LL edema
  - *End stage:* Muscle wasting, cachexia, massive ascites and anasarca.

LABORATORY INVESTIGATION

ECG
- No specific findings
- Reduce voltage, non-specific T wave changes, left atrial abnormality
- AF common

CXR
- Cardiac silhouette—normal
- Cardiac silhouette enlarged if effusion +
- Pericardial calcification can be seen (suggest tuberculosis)
- Pl effusion—common (can be initial sign)
- Pulm vasc congestion may be present.

ECHO
- Pericardial Thickening
- Abrupt displacement of IVS, during early diastole (septal bounce)
- Signs of syst venous congestion such as dilatation of hepatic vein and distention of IVS with blunted respi fluctuation
- Exaggerated septal shifting during respiration
- Exaggerated respi variation in mitral and tricuspid Inflow
- Patient with constriction demonstrates 25% or greater increase in mitral E velocity during expiration than during inspi
  And
  Increased diastolic flow reversal in hepatic vein with expiration
  - Good sensitivity and specificity
  - Helps distinguishing restrictive cardiomyopathy from constriction
- 20% patients do not exhibit typical respi changes due to
  - Marked increase in LA pr
  - Mixed constrictive-restrictive pattern due to myocardial involvement
- In patients without typical respi variation
  ↓
  Maneuvers that decrease preload (head up tilt, sitting) can unmask char respi pattern
  Tissue Doppler increase E' velocity: Septal bounce
- As sensitive as mitral tricuspid Inflow pattern.

D/D
Similar Pattern of MV Inflow velocity can be observed in normal RV infarct, pulm embolism and pl effusion
↓
SVC flow velocity can differentiate these conditions

TEE
- Superior to TTE for pericardial thickness.

Cardiac Cath
- Provides evaluation of HD
- Diff between constrictive and restrictive CM pathy.

Findings:
- RA, RV diastolic, PCWP and LV diastolic pr all increased and equal (=~20 mm Hg)
- Diff of >3-5 mm between lt and rt heart filling pr is rare
- *RAP tracing:* Preserved X descent and prominent Y descent; roughly equal w and v wave (M or W pattern)
- RV and LV pr—Early marked diastolic dip followed by a plateau (dip and plateau or square root sign)
- Exaggerated vent interdependence—increased repi variation in LV and RV syst and dia pr
  ↓
  Quantified by using "systolic area index" (ratio of RV to LV systolic pressure × area in inspiration vs expiration)
  ↓
  Ratio >1.1 suggest constriction (strongly)
- PAP and RVSP modestly increased (35–45 mm Hg) (PAP >45 is not a feature of CP)
  - Hypovolemia caused by diuretic can mask hemodynamic findings
  - Rapid infusion of 1L NS over 6–8 mins can revert typical findings

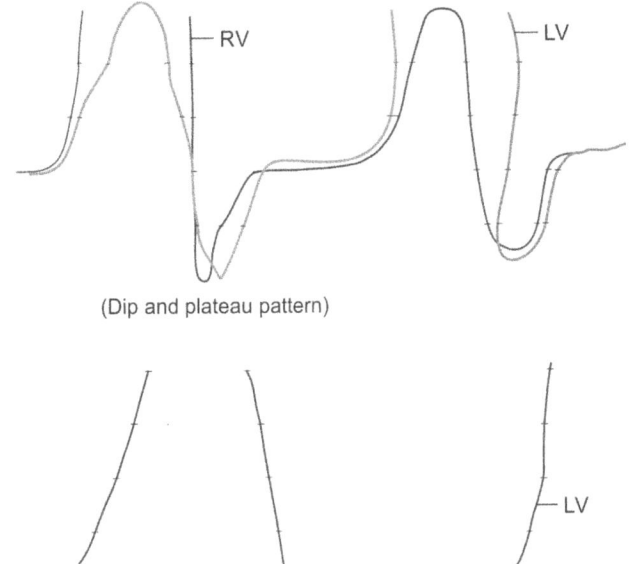
(Dip and plateau pattern)

Prom Y descent

CT and MRI

- Helpful in detecting even minute amt of calcification
- Thickness of normal pericardium =~2 mm (CT)
  3-4 mm (MRI)
- Thickened pericardium—Ac/chr pericarditis
- LGE on MRI—specific for active Inflammation
- Absence of thickening does not rule out CP.

MANAGEMENT

- CP—progressive but variable course
- Definitive treatment—pericardiectomy
  - Radiation induce disease is relative CI

For Very Mild CP

- Diuretic and salt restriction to avoid fluid overload
- Avoid BB and CCB as they cause Bradycardia with further decrease CO
- For patients with AF—digoxin to control rat
  - Can give BB/CCB
  - Rate maintained ~80-90/min
- Anti-inflammatory drugs for patients with increased LGE and pericardium >3 mm
  - *Pericardium*
    - Should not be delayed once diagnosis is confirmed
    - Median sternotomy/is 5th Ie thoracotomy
    - Radical excision of as much as pan ertor endocardium
    - Visceral pericardium is inspected and resected if involved
  - Ultrasonic/laser debridement is adjunct to conventional pericardium (for patients with extensive involvement)
  - "Waffle procedure" making multiple transverse and longitudinal incisions in epicardial layer is another alternative.

Postop

- H1D and symptomatic recovery in some patients achieved immediately
- In others it may take weeks to months
- LV diastolic function returns to normal in 40% early and in up to 60% late after surgery
- Persistence of abnormality filling is associated with post op symptoms
- Delayed response due to
  - Long standing disease with myocardial atrophy or fibrosis
  - Incomplete resection
  - Recurrent cardiac compression by mediastinal Fibrosis and inflammation
- 5-15% peri-op mortality
- Early mortality due to
  - Low CO often is debilitated patients with Prolonged CPB
  - Difficult dissection
  - Sepsis
  - Uncontrolled hemorrhage
  - Renal and respi insufficiency
- Highest mortality in patients with class 3/4 symptoms.

Transient CP

- MC cause is early after surgery
- Either resolve spontaneously or respond to NSAIDs.

EFFUSIVE-CONSTRICTIVE PERICARDITIS

- Combined element of effusion—tamponade and constriction
- Subacute
- Inflammatory effusion dominates early with constriction being prominent later
- Often identified when HD fails to normalize post pericardiocentesis
  ↓
  "Defined as failure of RAP to decline by at least 50% to a level below 10 mm Hg when pericardial pr reduced to at most 0"
- Incidence = 4-5% of all effusion
- Missed if HD not measured post trapping
- *Cause:* Idiopathic, malignancy, radiation, TB, pericardiotomy, connective tissue disease.

15.3 CONSTRICTIVE VERSUS RESTRICTIVE

INTRODUCTION

RCMP is relatively rare and caused mainly by amyloidosis. But it is becoming more common with increasing obesity and metabolic synd

	Constrictive pericarditis	Restrictive cardiomegaly
H/O	TB, radiation, Sx, CTD, pericardiocentesis	Geographic area, metabolic disease
Clinical examination	Pericardial knock	S3
CXR	Calcified pericardium	
ECG		Low voltage and biatrial enlargement – amyloidosis
Pulse	Paradoxical pulse in 1/3	NO
JVP	• Kussmaul sign usually present: Freidrich's sign • M or W pattern, prominent Y and X descent	• Kussmaul usually absent • NO/variable
Sympt	Abd distention, pedal edema, PND absent	Dyspnea, PND, and RV fail
ECHO 2D-image	• Septal bounce • Pericardium is thickened (apparent on TEE) • Normal vent wall thickness	• Thick walled vent due to infiltrate CM pathy • Marked biatrial enlargement
Doppler flow measurement	• RV and LV inflow show • Prominent E due to rapidly early diastolic filling • Short deceleration time of E • Small A wave • E/A >2 • DT<160 • IVRT<60	Early disease E<A late disease E>A constant IVRT
Respiratory variation	• Enhanced respi variation in mitral inflow velocity • >25% increase in insp velocity	Velocity varies <10%
Tissue Doppler	• (Contraction and relaxation property of myocardium preserved) so E' is normal or increased because lateral enlargement	

Contd...

	Constrictive pericarditis	Restrictive cardiomegaly
	is decreased due to fibrotic pericardium Peak E' ≥8 cm/s • Normal lat E' velocity>med E' in CP - medial E' >lateral E' (annular reversus) because of tethering of Lat annulus to fibrotic pericardium	E' decrease as severity increase Peak E' <8 cm/sec
Pulm venous Doppler	Not observed in constriction	Pulm venous systolic flow blunted and diastolic flow increases
Hepatic vein reversal	Enhanced expiratory flow reversal	Enhanced inspiratory flow
Speckle tracking	• Normal longitudinal restoration • Impaired circumferential/rotational mechanics	• Impaired longitudinal strain • Preserved rotational strain
Hemodynamic/ cardiac cath	• RV and syst pr markedly increase • LV and RV diastolic pr track closely and differ only by 3–5 mm Hg • PASP rarely exceed >45 mm Hg (or RVSP) • RV filling PR rarely >25 mm Hg • LV-RV discordance LV-RV discordance	• Same • LV syst pr >RV systole by >5 mm Hg • Significant PAH (>55 mm Hg) • Extreme high filling Pr (>25 mm Hg) is common
Rt heart catheterization	• M or W wave • Inspiratory rise in RA pressure (Kussmaul's sign)	• M or W wave • Normal respiratory variation
Square root sign	Present	Variable
CT/MRI	Provide detail of pericardium thickness and inflammation process (LGE)	Can detect infiltration
BNP	Normal	Elevated
EMB	Differentiate between CP and RCMP	

Contd...

15.4 PERICARDIAL EFFUSION AND TAMPONADE

Q.1 HD of tamponade (Dec 16)
Q.2 Management of cardiac tamponade (June 94)
Q.3 Pathophysiology of cardiac tamponade (June 89)

ETIOLOGY
Some as acute pericarditis.

PATHOPHYSIOLOGY AND HEMODYNAMICS

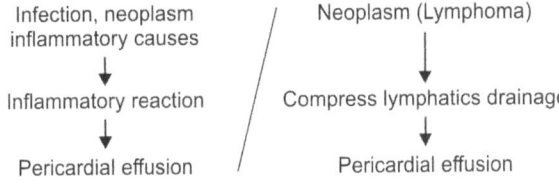

DETERMINANTS OF HD CONSEQUENCES
1. Amt of fluid in pericardium
2. Pressure in the pericardial sac
3. Pressure volume relationship
4. Ability of heart to compensate

- Relatively small amt (150-200 mL) rapidly accumulating fluid can have major effect of cardiac function
- Slowly accumulating large amt of fluid can be well tolerated
- *Compensatory response* to pericardial effusion/tamponade
  - Increased adrenergic stimulation
  - Decreased parasympathetic activity
    ↓
  Tachycardia and increased contractility to maintain CO
    ↓
  Eventually CO and BP declines
    ↓
  In terminal tamponade, depressive reflex with paradoxical Brady may supervene
- *Hemodynamics consequences*
  Accumulation of pericardial fluid
    ↓
  Increased pericardial sac pressure
    ↓
  Impaired filling of rt side of heart
    ↓
  Immediate drop in pulm sv (aortic SV remain unchanged for time being)
    ↓
  This transient inequality results in transfer of blood out of pulm circ [Explains decrease in pulmonary vascularity in patients with tamponade]
    ↓
  Effect on left side of heart due to underfilling eventually develop
    ↓
  LV SV also decline
    ↓
  New steady state develop with both RV SV and LV SV are low

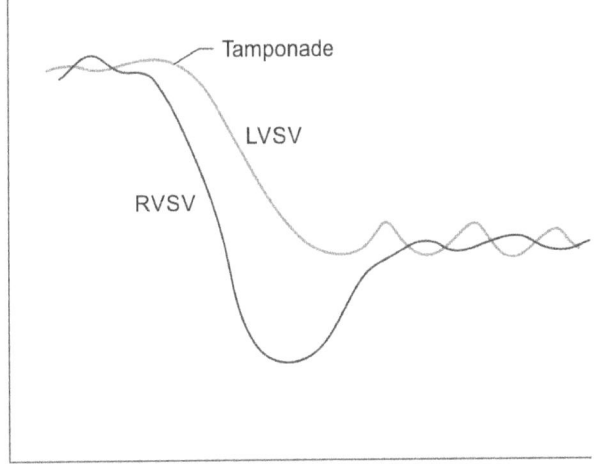

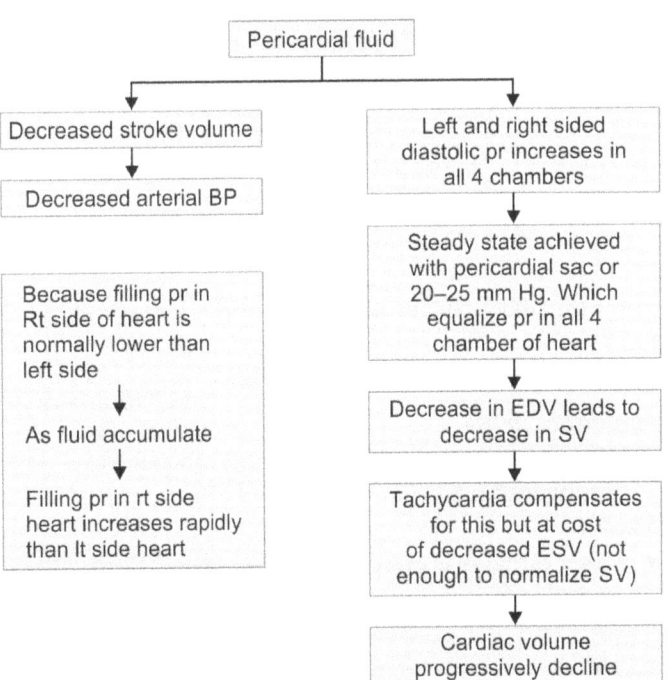

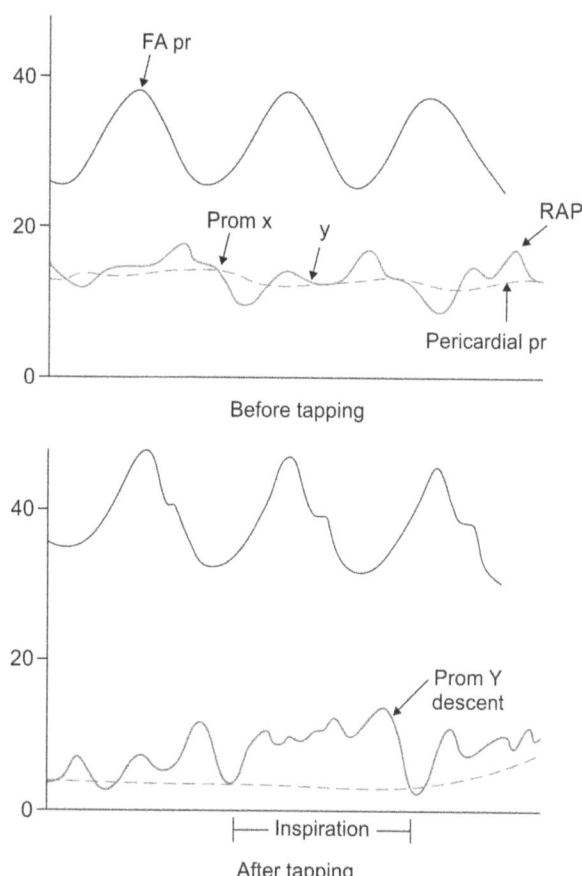

(Figure shows both RA and pericardial pr are at new steady state level (15 mm Hg) during tamponade. Absence of Y descent before pericardiocentesis.
Pericardiocentesis—marked Y descent, marked increase in FA pr and decrease in RA pr)

Loss of Y descent

Tamponade
↓
Increased pericardial sac or
↓
Total cardiac volume is decreased and fixed
↓
Sn inflow can't be increased and descent is lost
↓
Loss of Y descent

Paradoxical pulse
- Abnormally large decline in SBP during inspiration (>10 mm Hg)

Mech:
- Respi variation is present in tamponade
  ↓
- During inspi rt heart filling increases
  ↓

In CP respiratory variation is abolished
↓
No inspiratory increase in syst venous return
↓
No decrease in syst venous pr
↓
Kussmaul sign

In situation of fixed total cardiac volume this lead to IVS shift to left side which is already underfilled
↓
Paradoxical drop in BP

- Increased afterload by transmission of negative intrathoracic pr to aorta
- Traction of pericardium caused by descent of diaphragm

Low pr tamponade
Tamponade can occur at low filling pr too (<20-25 mm Hg)

Mech:
- When blood volume decrease in setting of pre-existing effusion
  ↓
  Modestly elevated pericardial pr can lower transmural filling pr (because venous pr is only modestly elevated or even normal, the diagnosis may not be suspected)
- During hemodialysis
- Blood loss and volume depletion
- Diuretics administered to patients with effusion.

C/F
- Less often critically ill
- Signs of tamponade were less prominent

Investigation
- ECHO findings similar to those with high pr tamponade
- Regional tamponade should be considered when hypotension develop in setting of loculated effusion

	Tamponade	Constriction
Paradoxical pulse	Present	1/3rd cases
Equal lt and rt filling pr	Present	Present
Syst venous wave	Absent Y descent	Prominent Y descent (M or W shaped)
Inspiratory change syst venous pr	Decrease	Increase (Kussmaul or no charge)
Square root sign In vent pr	Absent	Present

C/F
- Asymptomatic large chronic effusion
- Associated pain because of pericarditis
- Effusion themselves so not cause any symptoms if no tamponade

Tamponade

- Dyspnea (uncertain mechanism)
- Comfortable sitting forward
- Symptoms due to decreased CO and increased BP
- Pericardial pain and/or nonspecific discomfort

O/E

- Difficult in palpate cardiac impulse
- Tubular BS in axilla (due to compression of bronchus)
- Hypotension
  - Muffled HS ⎫ Beck's trial
  - Increased JVP ⎭
- *Decreased CO* - shock, tachycardia, tachypnea, diaphoresis, cool extremity, dusky cyanosis, altered sensorium
- Paradoxical pulse (better in bronchial art)
- Tachycardia is rule
- Bradycardia—Preterminal depressive stage
- Absent Y descent in JVP.

INVESTIGATION

- *ECG:*
  - Decreased voltage
  - Electrical alternance (due to ant-post-swing)
- *CXR:*
  - Round flask like cardiomegaly with large effusion
  - *Lat CXR:* Fat pad sign linear translucency between sternum and ant surface of heart
  - Lungs appear oligemic
- *ECHO:*
  - Investigation of choice
  - Small effusion are first evident on posterior basal part of LV.

  ↓

  As fluid increases it spread anteriorly and laterally and then behind LA where its limit is demarcated by visceral pericardium
  - *Grading:* Small <10 mm ⎫
              Mod 10-20 mm ⎬ Circumferential effusion
              Large >20 mm ⎭
  - Frond-like-staggy appearing str in pericardium
    - Suggest clots, chronic inflammation or neoplastic process
  - *Finding suggest severity of tamponade*
    - Early diastolic collapse of RV ⎫
    - Late diastolic collapse or   ⎬ Sensitive and specific
      indentation of RA   ⎭
    - Exaggerated variation in RV v and LV chamber size
    - IVS shifting during inspiration.

Other Signs of Tamponade

- Small cavity sizes
- Distention of caval vessel which does not collapse during inspi
- Doppler velocity recordings demonstrate exaggerated respi variation in rt and lt sided venous and valvular flow, with inspiratory T on rt side and decrease on lt side ⎱ More sensitive for tamponade
- Caval Inflow occur largely during vent systole (because Y descent is absent)
- *Fluoroscopy:* Useful in cath lab for detecting procedure related effusion
- *CT and MRI:*
  - Complimentary
  - Not advised/required routinely
  - When
    - ECHO is inadequate
    - HD are atypical
    - Presence and Severity of tamponade are uncertain
  - *Additional info*
    - Pericardial thickness
    - Identify inflammation (CMR)
    - Transudative (attenuation similar to water), malignant, bloody, purulent (more than water) chylous (less than water).

MANAGEMENT

Initial approach
1. Determine whether tamponade is present or threatened —based on history, C/F and ECHO
2. If no tamponade
   - No apparent case—consider work up for Ac pericarditis
   - Large effusiong—NSAIDs + colchicine (+- steroids) and if no response—closed pericardiocentesis
3. If tamponade/threatened
   - Urgent or emergency closed pericardiocentesis
   - Close monitoring if medical management attempted

In patient without actual or imminent tamponade, pericardiocentesis may be undertaken for diagnostic purpose (but not usually required)

↓

Because:
- Diagnosis will be evident from initial investigation mostly (investigation for AC pericarditis, TB, malignancy, thyroid disorder, etc.)
- Pericardial fluid alone has low yield in providing specific diagnosis

Large pericardial fluid without effusion
- Can progress to tamponade unexpectedly (20-30%)

- NSAIDs + colchicine should be considered
- If reference after pericardiocentesis
  - Pericardiectomy
- *Patient with impending tamponade*
  - *Most:* Pericardiocentesis to prevent
  - *Few:*
    - Acute apparently idiopathic pericarditis with mild tamponade
    - Connective tissue and some other inflammatory disease
      ↓
    - Possible bact infection with small pericardial fluid
      ↓
      NSAIDs + colchicine can be tried under HD monitoring

- *Patient with tamponade: (medical emergency)*
  - IV hydration + or- positive inotropes
  - Urgent pericardiocentesis
  - Cholesterol rich (gold paint) effusion in severe hypothyroidism
- *Hemopericardium*
  Closed pericardiocentesis increase chance of bleeding due to sudden decrease in intrapericardial sac or without approaching site of bleeding
  ↓
  Should be avoided esp in trauma or rupture of LV wall (post MI)
  ↓
  If bleeding is slower (coronary perforation, puncture of cardiac chamber)
  ↓
  Closed pericardiocentesis is appropriate.

15.5 PERICARDIAL DISEASES

Q.1 Anatomy of pericardium, physiology of pericardium. Passive role of normal pericardium in heart disease. Usefulness of base area of pericardium (3+2+3+2) (June 17)

ANATOMY AND PHYSIOLOGY

- Two layers of pericardium
  1. *Visceral layer:* Monolayer of mesothelial cells and collagen and elastin fibers
     - Adherent to epicardial surface
  2. *Panetal layer:* Fibrous
     2 mm thick
     Surrounds most of the heart
     Largely acellular and contain collagen and elastin fibers
     ↓
     Major structural component.
- Visceral pericardium reflects back near the origins of great vessel and is continues with and form the inner layer of parietal pericardium
- Pericardial space is contained within these 2 layers and has 50 mL of serous fluid normally.
- Visceral pericardium reflects a few cm proximal to junction of the canal vessels with RA—portion of which lie within pericardial sac
- Posterior to LA the reflection occurs at the oblique sinus of the pericardium
- LA is largely extra pericardial
- Parietal pericardium has fibrous ligamentous attachment with diaphragm, sternum and other str—fix heart
- Only non CV str dissociated with pericardium are phrenic nerve (enveloped by panetal pericardium).

Function

- Maintain the position of heart relatively constant
- Provide lubrication
- Provide barrier to infection
- Participate in reflex arising from pericardium and/or epicardium (Bezold-Jarisch reflex)
- Transmission of pericardial pain (pericardium wall innervated with mechanoreceptors, chemoreceptors and phrenic afferent receptors)
- Secrete prostaglandin and related substance that modulate neural traffic and Cora tone
- Restraining effect on cardiac volume.

Physiology

- Parietal pericardium has tensile strength
  - At low stress it is very elastic
  - As stretch increases—tissue abruptly boom stiff and resistant to further stretch
- *Pressure—volume relationship*
  - PVR of parietal sac parallels property of isolated parietal pericardial tissue
  - The sac has relatively small reserve volume

  ↓

  When exceeded

  ↓

  The pressure within the sac operating on the surface of heart increases rapidly and is transmitted to the inside of cardiac chamber

  ↓

  Once a critical level of effusion is reached, relatively small amount of additional fluid cause large increase in intra pericardial pressure and have marked effect on cardiac function
  - Because of such PVR

  ↓

  Pericardium also restrain cardiac volume i.e., the force that it exerts on the surface of heart can limit filling with a component of intracavitary pressure
- This pericardiac contact pressure can be measured by
  1. Balloon to measure surface contact pressure
  2. Quantifying changes in rt and it heart diastolic PVR before and after pericardiotomy
  - In patient with normal cardiac volume undergoing pericardiotomy—mild post op increase in cardiac mass and volume develop (due to relief of underlying normal restrain to filling in pericardium)
  - Pericardium also contribute to diastolic interaction defined as transmission of intracavitary filling pressure to adjoining chamber

  ↓

  As cardiac volume increases above physiologic range, pericardium contribute increasingly to intracavitary—filling pressure
  - Directly because of external contact pressure
  - Indirectly because of increased diastolic interaction.

Q. Role of pericardium in Heart disease. (Dec 15)

PASSIVE ROLE OF PERICARDIUM IN HEART DISEASE

When cardiac chamber dilutes rapidly
↓
Restraining effect of pericardium and its contribution to diastolic interaction become augmented
↓
H-D features suggestive of both
1. Cardiac tamponade and
2. Constructive pericarditis
For example: RVMI: RV dilates rapidly
↓
Total heart volume exceeds pericardial reserve volume
↓
Increase of pericardial constrain and diastolic interaction
↓

- Lt and rt sided filling or equilibrate at elevated level and
- Paradoxical pulse and
- Kussmaul sign (paradoxical increase in inspiratory systolic venous pressure observed)

Chronic cardiac dilatation (e.g., DCMP and VHD)—Cardiac volume in excess of pericardial reserve volume—But exaggerated restraining effect not observed.

Because pericardium adepts to accommodate chronic increase in cardiac volume

- PVR shifts to right and its slope decreases.

15.6 RELAPSING AND RECURRENT PERICARDITIS

INTRODUCTION
- Incidence 15-35% of Idiopathic acute Pericarditis
- *High risk:* Women
- Who do not respond to initial treatment?
- Steroid treatment

INVESTIGATION
- Repeated evaluation to look for specific cause
- Hemogram, ANA, hs-CRP
- Rarely pericardial biopsy (in patients with no effusion)
- Genetic disorder of immune system
- TRAPS (Turner Necrosis Factor receptor-associated periodic syndrome)
  (Mutation of TNFRSFIA gene)
  (Periodic fever, rash, Abdomen pain, periorbital edema, polyserositis with pericarditis)
  (Treatment respond to steroid not to colchicine)

PROG
- Cured long term prognosis
- Very few complications
- Low rate of constriction

MANAGEMENT: EMPIRIC TREATMENT
For initial relapse
- Repeat course of NSAIDs (with hs-CRP monitoring)
- Colchicine effective for both treatment and prophylaxis
  - Cont. for 6-12 months
- Prednisone (for patient not responding)
- *Immunosuppression*, azathioprine, cyclosporine, cyclophosphamide, or alternative
- *Pericardiectomy* reserved for those whose quality of life is severely affected, failure of medical treatment who desire this option despite the fact that remission may occur.

15.7 SPECIFIC CAUSES OF PERICARDIAL DISEASE

*VIRAL PERICARDITIS
- Most common pericardial effusion
- (MC) Echovirus and *Coxsackievirus*
- CMV has predilection for immunocompromised
- (Investigation) viral DNA detection by PCR or in situ hybridization.

*BACT PERICARDITIS
Cause
- Direct extension from pneumonia/empyema
- Hematogenous spread
- Contagious spread after thoracic surgery or trauma *(MC)*: Staph, strepto, Pneumococci
- MRSA after surgery
- *Other:* Meningococci, *Neisseria*

Char by purulent fluid
- *Neisseria:* Sterile effusion accompanied by systemic reaction (arthritis, pleuritic, and opthalmist).

C/F
- High grade fever with chills
- Dyspnea, chest pain
- Friction rub
- *Fulminant course:* Rapid dev of tamponade
- Leukocytosis
- *Pericardial fluid:* Leukocytosis, low glucose, high protein, elevated LDH
- Gas producing bact may cause air-fluid interphase.

Management
- Medical emergency
- Prompt closed pericardiocentesis/Sx drainage
- 3-4 days of cont drainage
- Broad spectrum antibiotic—followed by modification acc to culture report
- Purulent pericardial effusion likely to recover
- Sx drainage with construction of window
- Intrapericardial fibrinolysis in some
- Extensive pericardiectomy in patients with dense adhesion, thick and purulent effusions.

HIV AND PERICARDIAL DISEASE
- Pericardial disease is MC cardiac manifestation of HIV
- Most Freq—pericardial effusion (constriction rare)
- Mostly small and asymptomatic
- Effusion may be due to "capillary leak syndrome"
- CHF, Kaposi syndrome, TB and other pulm inf associated with peri eff
- TB is MC cause.

TUBERCULOSIS
- 2% of patient with PTB
- Now rare cause of constrictive pericarditis
- Pericardial involve is 2° to retrograde spread from nearby LN or hematogenous spread
- Rarely contagious spread.

C/F
- Subacute to chronic
- Fever, malaise, dyspnea
- Cough, night sweats, orthopnea, weight loss, leg edema
- CXR-cardiomegaly
- Pericardial rub, fever, tachycardia
- Cardiac tamponade common
- Effusive-constrictive syndrome
- Definitive diagnosis by isolating org from fluid or pericardial Bx specimen
    1. ADA - 40 u/L in pericardial fluid has sensitivity of 85% and specificity of 83%
    2. Increased interferon 8 is additional marker
    3. PCR to detect M-TB

Treatment
Multidrug AkT 6 months

HIV + TB
- Anti TB in patients with CD4 >350 by ART
- CD4 100–350: ART after 2 months of AkT
- CD4 <100: Both together.

Renal Disease
- Physiology not fully understood
- Associated with BUN and creat level
- Incidence decreased with HD
- Char by shaggy, hemorrhagic, fibrinous exudate on both pericardial and visceral surface
- HD associated pericardial disease is now more common than uremic pericarditis.

C/F
- Ac pericarditis—chest pain, fever
- Small asymptomatic eff common
- Patients can have low pr tamponade
- Extremely large asymptomatic effusion are typical of uremic pericarditis.

Treatment
- Treat empirically
- Pericardiocentesis.

POST MI PERICARDITIS AND DRESSLER
- Early post MI pericarditis-1-3 day
  - No more than a week
- Due to transmural necrosis with Inflammation of adjacent visceral and parietal pericardium
- Early revasc has reduced its incidence
- Only 4% patients
- *Dressler:*
  - Late pericarditis
  - Polyserositis with pericardial and/or pleural eff
  - As early as 1 week to few months post MI
  - 3-4% of patients with MI - now 0.1%
  - Believed to be autoimmune cause
  - Antimyocardial antibodies noted.

C/F
- Early post MI pericarditis—asymptomatic
- Diagnosed by aug cultation
- Rarely large enough to cause tamponade
- Impl to distinguish pericardial pain from rec ischemia
- Typical change of pericarditis is rare on ECG post MI
- Pericardial inflammation is localized in infarcted area - can lead to subtle re ST elevation
  - *Dressler:*
    - Fever and pleuritic chest pain
    - Pleural and/or pericardial sub
    - Typical ECG changes +
  - *Treatment:*
    - Augmentation of post MI ASA dose (650 3-4 times a d)
    - Acetaminophen
- Avoid Corticosteroid—they interfere with conversion of MI into scar—wall thinning and high incidence of post MI rupture
- Ror Dressler: self-limited: NSAIDs + Colchicine is effective

Q. Causes, presentation and management of neoplastic pericardial effusion   (Dec 13)

PERICARDIAL DISEASE AND CANCER
Cause
- Pericardial tumor implants are usual cause various
- Infectious causes
- Radiation induced
- Obstruction of lymphatic drainage mediastinal LN

(Most common) lung CA (40% of malignant effusion)
- Breast CA
- Lymphoma –40%
- GI CA
- Melanomas
- Sarcoma
- Kaposi Sarcoma.

C/F
- Prominent feature in effusion
- Effusive-constrictive pattern common
- Most patient have symptomatic effusion and tamponade
- Asymptomatic incidentally discovered effusion can be a sign of malignancy.

ECG
- Non-specific T wave change and low QRS voltage
- ST elevation unusual

CT, CMR and PET helps in diagnosis.

Investigation
Pericardial tapping/BX to conf meds

Management
- Treatment of underlying cause
- Pericardiocentesis
- Generally it's recurrent so intrapericardial installation of drugs is necessary

Sclerosing agent:
E.g., tetracycline
   Chemotherapeutic agent
   Cisplatin (30 mg/mL)
   Bleomycin for nonsmall cell CA lung thiotepa

- External beam radiation is less effective preferred in patient with enlarged mediastinal LN
- Window/complete surgery pericardiectomy should be considered in patients with resistant and recurrent effusion with good Prognosis and life expectancy.

Patient with poor life expectancy and bad Prognosis-Coral of life care.

CONNECTIVE TISSUE DISEASE
- Pericardial involvement common in RA
- *Fluid:* Low glucose, neutrophilic, leukocytosis, elevated RA factor, low C3 level is rarely high cholesterol level.
- Constriction can occur after long standing inflammation

- Respond well to standard treatment
- ANA +ve.

CONGENITAL ANOMALIES AND PERICARDIUM

- *Pericardial cyst:* Rare benign, cong malformation, fluid filled, located at right costophrenic angle confirmed by echo, conservative management.
  Rarely can occur in patient with AOPKD.

- *Congenital absence of pericardium:* Very rare part of all of LV pericardium is absent associated with other anomalies like ASD, BAV, pulm malformation. Often symptomatic allow herniation of heart through defect or torsion of great vessels life threatening MRI diagnostic.

SECTION 16

Peripheral Artery Disease

16.1 ACUTE LIMB ISCHEMIA

DEFINITION
Acute limb ischemia occurs when an arterial occlusion suddenly decreases blood flow to arm or leg.

C/F
Depends on
- Severity of ischemia
- Location of arterial occlusion
- Resulting decrease in blood flow
- Disability claudication/pain at rest
- Sensory loss and no/or dysfunction
- *O/E:* Cool skin, pallor, delayed capillary return and venous filling, diminished or absent sensory perception, muscle weakness/paralysis
- *C.P:* Pain, paresthesia, paralysis, Pallor, pulselessness, poikilothermia.

PROGNOSIS
- Poor long term outcome
- 1 Year survived rate = 15-20%
- Risk of limb loss depends on
  - Severity of ischemia
  - Time elapsed between revasc.

CLINICAL CATEGORIES
- *Viable:* Not immediately threatened
  No sensory loss/no muscle weakness
  Doppler signal at arteries and vein-audible
- *Threatened:* Marginally (salvageable if treated promptly)
  Immediately: (salvageable with immediate revasc)
- *Irreversible:* major tissue loss/permanent nerve damage inevitable.

PATHOGENESIS
Causes
- Arterial embolism
- Thrombosis in situ
- Dissection
- Trauma.

Arterial Embolism
- From thrombotic source in heart MC
  - AT/CHF/CAD/HTN
- Rheumatic/prosthetic valve
- Vent thrombosis
- Paradoxical embolus.

Thrombus in Situs
- Occur in atherosclerotic peri art, influ inguinal bypass graft, peri art aneurysm normal art of patient with hypercoagulable state
- May complicate plague rupture
- Thrombosis complication pop art aney is common (10% of Ac limb ischemia)
- One of common cause-thrombosis occurs of infra-inguinal bypass graft
- *Thrombophilic disorder:* APLA, HIT, DIC, myeloproliferative disorder, protein C and S def, factor V Leiden mutation.

DIAGNOSTIC TESTS
Test could not delay urgent decade
- Doppler USG
- Duplex some
- CT
- MRI

TREATMENT

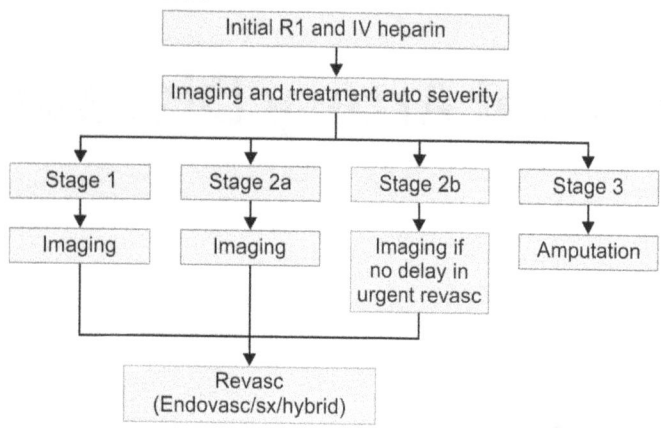

A. *Medical management*
   - Analgesic medication
   - Feet lower than chest level
   - Decreased pressure on heel, bone prominence and between toes
   - Keep room warm to prevent cold induced vasoconstriction
B. *Drugs*
   Heparin infusion

C. *Definitive decade*
   - Intraarterial thrombolysis
   - Prevent mechanical thrombectomy
   - Sx revasc
- Catheter directed intraarterial thrombolysis + thrombectomy is initial treatment for patient with either category 1 and 2 if there are no contraindication
  - rtPA, alteplase, reteplase, and tenecteplase
  - Cont flow 24-48 hours to achieve optimal benefit
  - Adjunent Gp 2b/3a shorten thrombolysis times but does not improve outcome
- Thrombic removal by aspiration, rheolysis, fragmentation or high energy ultrasound
- *Sx:* thromboembolectomy + bypass
- Hybrid

Summary: Cath based thrombolysis is an appropriate initial option in patient with viable or marginally threatened limb and when the ischemia of less than 14 d duration
- Treatment more appropriate in those with immediately threatened limb and in those whose symptoms have lasted for > 14 d
- Patient with irreversible injury amputation.

16.2 PERIPHERAL ART DISEASE

Q.1 ABI and classify PAD
Q.2 Evaluate and manage a case of LL PAD

RISK FACTORS OF PAD

- Cigarette smoking
- DM
- HTN
- CkD
- Hypercholesterolemia
- Hyperhomocysteinemia
- Insulin resistance
- CRP.

Cigarette
2-4 fold increase in PAD incidence.

DM
- Femoral and popliteal involvement is same as in nondiabetes
  But
- Tibial and peroneal involvement is more common 2-4 fold increase in PAD
- Increased risk of critical limb ischemia and amputation.

HTN
1.3-2.2 fold increased risk of PAD.

Bilirubin
Endogenous antioxidant with anti-inflammation property—associated with reduced incidence of PAD

PATHOPHYSIOLOGY

- *Factors regulating blood supply to limb*
  - Flow limiting lesion (stenosis severity, inadequate collaterals)
  - Impaired vasodilatation (decreased NO and reduced responsiveness to vasodilatations)
  - Accentuated vasoconstriction (TX A2, Serotonin, angiotensin 2, endothelin, NE)
  - Abnormal rheology (decreased RBC deformability, increase leukocyte adhesiveness, platelet aggregation, microthrombosis, increased fibrinogen)
- *Altered skeletal muscle str and function*
  - Axonal denervation of skeletal muscle
  - Loss of type 2, Glucolyte fast-twitch fibers
  - Impaired mitochondrial enzymatic activity
  - Stenosis reduce flow through an artery

Poiseuille equation:

$$Q = \frac{\Delta P \pi r^4}{8 n l}$$

ΔP = Pr Gradient
n = blood viscosity
l = length of vessel affected by stenosis

- As stenosis increased—flow progressively decrease
- Pr Gradient across the lesion increase in nonlinear manner

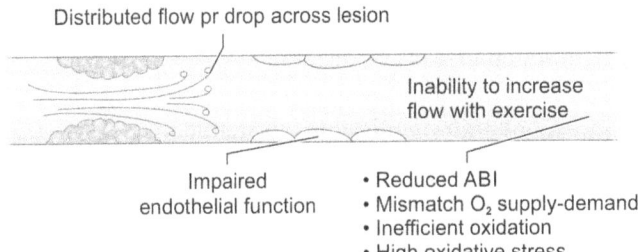

- Reduced ABI
- Mismatch O_2 supply-demand
- Inefficient oxidation
- High oxidative stress

Stenosis high resistance

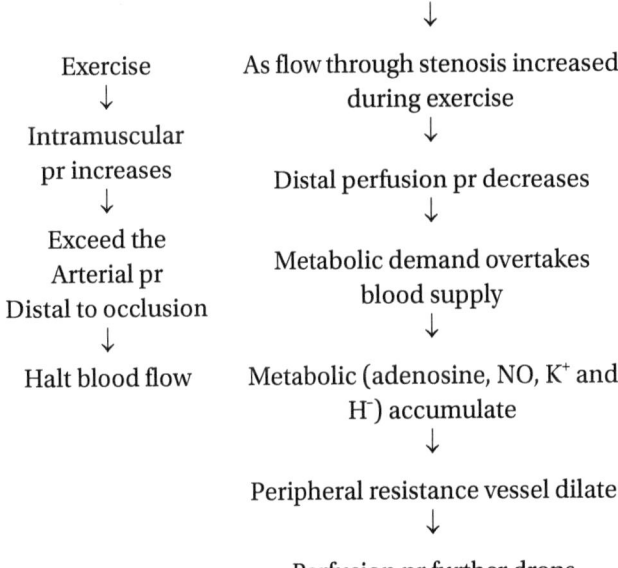

*Flow through collateral—can meet resting metabolic need of skeletal muscle tissue at rest but does not suffice during exercise.

*Patients with peri atherosclerosis have reduced vasodilator capacity of both conductance and resistance vessels.

In skeletal muscle distal to PAD, shift to anaerobic metabolism occurs earlier during exercise and persists longer after exercise.

C/F

Cardinal Symptoms

1. *Intermittent claudication/pain at rest*
   Pain, acute, sense of fatigue or other discomfort that occurs in the affected muscle group with exercise and resolve with rest
   - Buttock, hip, thigh claudication—Ao/iliac art
   - Calf claudication—femoral/popliteal art
   - Ankle/foot claudication—tibial/peroneal
   - Shoulder/biceps/forearm—subclavian/ax/brachial
   - Symptoms resolve several mins after rest
   - Nocturnal calf and thigh pain which occur at rest—not a part of PAD
2. Patient with CAD walks slowly and have less walking endurance than do patients without PAD
3. Questionnaires of claudication
   - Ross questionnaire
   - Edinburgh claudication questionnaire
   - San Diego claudication questionnaire
   - Walking impairment questionnaire
4. *Critical limb ischemia*
   - Pain occur at rest
   - Worsen on leg elevation and improves with leg dependency
   - Skin is very sensitive—even weight of bedsheet can cause pain.

D/D OF EXERTIONAL LEG PAIN

Vascular Causes

- Atherosclerosis
- Thrombosis
- Embolism
- Vasculitis
  - TAD
  - TA
  - GCA
- FMD
- Irradiation
- Endofibrosis of ext iliac art
- Extravascular compression
- Arterial entrapment
- Adventitial cysts

Nonvascular causes (neurogenic pseudoclaudication)
- Lumbosacral radiculopathy
  - Degen arthritis
  - Spinal Stenosis
  - Herniated discs
- Arthritis
  - Hips/knee
- Venous insufficiency
- Myositis
- Glycogen storage disease (McArdle syndrome)

O/E

- Palpation of all peripheral pulses and auscultate for bruit
- Absence of any pulse—gives insight into site of occlusion
- *Bruit:* Sign of accelerated blood flow velocity and flow disturbance at stenosis
- *Pallor:* On soles of PAD patients by performing a maneuver in which feet are elevated where level of heart and calf muscle are exercised by repeated dorsiflexion and plantar flexion—legs are then placed in dependent position and tire until the onset of hyperemia and venous distention is measured
- Muscle atrophy
- Signs of chronic low grade limb ischemia
  - Hair loss
  - Thickened and brittle toenail
  - Smooth and shiny skin
  - Atrophy of subcut fat of digital pad
- With severe ischemia
  - Cool skin
  - Petechiae
  - Persistent cyanosis
  - Pallar
  - Dependent rubor
  - Pedal edema
  - Skin fissure
  - Ulceration
  - Gangrene
- Uller (arterial)—pale base with irregular borders, involve sip of toes or the heel, vary in size and may be small as 3–5 cm

CLASSIFICATION

A. *Fontaine classification*
   Stage 1 - asymptomatic
       2 - Intermittent claudication
           2a - pain free, claudication > 200 m
           2b - pain free, claudication < 200 m
       3- Rest and nocturnal pain
       4- Necrosis, gangrene

B. *Modified Rutherford classification of chronic limb ischemia*

Grade	Category	Clinical
I	0	• Asymptomatic
	1	• Mild claudication
	2	• Mod claudication
	3	• Severe claudication
II	4	• Ischemic rest pain
	5	• Minor tissue loss; non-healing ulcer, focal gangrene with diffuse pedal ulcer
III	6	• Major tissue loss extending above the transmetatarsal level, functional foot no longer salvageable

TESTING FOR PAD

- *Segmental pressure measurement*
  - Pneumatic caffs placed on upper and lower thigh, on the calf, above ankle and are the metatarsal area of food
  - U: Over the biceps, over forearm and at wrist

  ↓

  SBP measured at each level by increased pr to suprasystemic and then gradual fall in pr to determine flow across the site

  ↓

  Flow determined by Doppler
  - BP gradient >20 mm Hg, b/w successive cuffs is generally used as evidence of arterial stenosis (LL)
  - For UL gradient > 10 mm Hg = stenosis with exercise SVR decrease—so ABP increase
- *Ankle brachial index*
  - Ratio of SBP measured at ankle to SBP measured at brachial artery
  - Normal ABI = 1.00–1.40
  - 0.91–0.99—borderline
  - <0.9—abnormal
  - 0.5–0.8—leg claudication
  - <0.5—critical limb ischemia
  - >1.4—indicate noncompressible artery

  In patients with skin ulceration—ankle pr <55 mm Hg - poor ulcer healing
- *Treadmill exercise test*

  Claudication onset time: Time at which symptoms of claudication first develops

  Peak walking time when a patient is no longer able to continue walking because of severe leg discomfort

  ↓
  - Quantitative measurement
  - Reproducible
  - Can be used to judge efficacy of treatment

  Ankle and brachial >BP measured at rest and 1 min after exercise

  ↓

  Normal = increase in BP should be same in both UL and LL

  Normal = ABI ≥1

  PAD = ABI decrease because increase in ankle SBP I'd not proportional to increase in branchial SBP
- *Pulse volume recording*
  - Plethysmographic measurement
  - Illustrate volumetric change in segment of the limb that occur with each pulse
  - Normal pulse volume contour depends on both local Arterial pr and vascular wall distensibility and resembles BP waveform

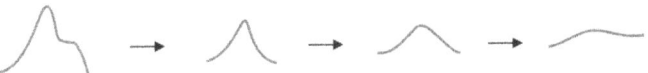

Normal Severe

Segmental analysis of pulse wave may indicate the location of art stenosis
- *Doppler ultrasound*
  - CWD and PWD
  - Normal Doppler waveform has 3 components
    1. Rapid forward flow—during systole
    2. Transient flow reversal—during early diastole
    3. Slow anterograde flow—during late diastole

Deceleration of systolic flow ⎤
Loss of early diastolic reversal ⎬ Characterize PAD
Diminished peak Freq ⎦ (distal to stenosis)

- *Duplex ultrasound imaging*
  - Assess both anatomic char of peripheral arteries and functional significance of stenosis
  - Blood flow velocity can be calculated with Doppler
  - Normal arteries have laminar flow with highest velocity at center of artery
  - In presence of stenosis, blood flow velocity increase through narrowed lumen—As velocity increases there is prog desaturation of color display and flow disturbance distal to stenosis causes changes in here and color
  - ≥2 fold increase in syst velocity at site of stenosis = 50% or greater stenosis
  - ≥3 fold increased velocity - ≥75% stenosis

  specificity 89–99%

  Sensitivity 80–98%
- Management angiography
- CT angio
- Contrast enhanced angio.

PROGNOSIS

- Patients with PVD—increased risk for CAD, limb loss, impaired QOL
- Abnormal ABT—2 rognosis 4 fold more likely than those with normal ABI to have a H/O MI, angina, CHF, CVA
- CAD occurs in 60–80% of patients with PAD
- Coro art stenosis in 15–25% of patients
- PAD also increases risk for mortality.

MANAGEMENT

Aims

- Decreased CV morbidity and mortality
- Improve QOL by increasing symptoms of claudication
- Eliminating rest pain
- Preserving limb viability

A. *Risk factor modification*
  1. *Lipid lowering therapy* (diet and drug)
     - *ACC/AHA and ESC guideline:* Target LDL ≤100
     - *TREADMILL Trial:* Atova (80) increase pain free walking distance by >60%
     - *FIELD trial:* Fenofibrate decreased risk of minor amputation
  2. Smoking cessation (behavioral + pharmacological)
     - Nonsmoker have lower rate of MI and mortality than do those who smoke
     - Patients who discontinue smoking-twice 5 years survival rate
  3. *Treatment of DM*
     - *Meta-analysis of 5 RCT:* Intensive glycemic control resulted in 17 reduction in CAD
     - No significant stroke/total mortality
     - *ACCORD:* Intensive glycemic control did not reduce 1° composite end point of non-fatal MI, nonfatal stroke or CV death
     - *ADVANCE:* Intensive glycemic control did not reduce microvasc complication
     - *VADT:* Intensive glycemic control did not affect 1° composite point (MI, stroke, CV death, CHI, revasc and amputation)
     - *PROactive:* No significant benefit of pioglitazone
     - *UkDDS:* 15% decrease in MI but not in PAD with intensive control
  4 *Control of BP*
     - Decreased risk for stroke, CAD and vascular death
     - Intensive BP control decrease CV death in diabetic patient with PAD
     - *ACCORD:* NS differ (<140 vs. <120)
     - *ADVANCE:* Decreased micro and macro vasc events
     - *HOPE:* Decreased vasc death, MI, stroke by 22%
     - *ONTARGET:* Decreased CV death, MI, stroke, or hospitalization
     - Treatment of HTN decreases perfusion pr to extremities already compromised by peri art stenosing
     - BB symptoms of claudication or critical limb ischemia
  5 *Antiplatelet*
     - To reduce adverse CV events
     - *POPADAD Trial:* Aspirin did not decrease risk
     - *CAPRICE:* Clopidogrel decrease advv CV events by 23%
     - *CHARISMA:* DAPT NS difference over aspirin alone
     - *CASPAR:* DAPT NS difference
     - *TRAZP-TIMI 50:* Varapaxar significantly decrease risk of MI, stroke, CV death by 12%
     - *WAVE:* Combined antiplt + anticoag vs. antiplt NS diff
     - Current recommendation—patients with symptomatic PAD treated with antiplatelet drug such as aspirin or clopidogrel to decrease CV events oral anticoagulants with warf is not recommended

B. *Pharmacological*
  - Two drugs approved
    1. *Pentoxifylline*
       - Xanthine derivative
       - MOA:
         - Hemorheologic property
         - Ability to decrease blood viscosity
         - Improve erythrocyte flexibility
         - Anti-inflammatory effect
         - Antiproliferative effect
       - Marginal efficacy
       - Increased max walking distance by 14%
    2. *Cilostazol*
       - Quinolinone derivative
       - MOA: Inhibit PDE-3—decreased degradation of cAMP and increase its conc in plt and Blood vessel—inhibit plt aggregation and vasodilatation
       - Improves absolute claudication distance by 40–50%
       - CI: In patients with CHF: PDE inhibition decreases survival in these patients
    ACC/AHA guidelines recommend cilostazol to improve symptoms and walking distance
  - *Other class of drugs*
    - Statin
    - ACEI
    - Serotonin inhibitor   ⎫
    - Alpha adrenergic antagonist ⎬ Under investigation
    - L arginine ornithine derivatives
    - Vasodilator prostaglandins
    - Androgenic growth factor   ⎭
    - Several trials have found statin to improve walking distance
    - 1 study - Ramipril improves walking distance
      - *Serotonin Inhibitor:* Naftidrofuryl improved symptoms of claudication in some trial
      - Buflomedil (alpha adrenergic antagonist) decrease risk for critical CV events angiogenic growth factor have shown promising result in primary evaluation

C. *Exercise rehabilitation*
   - 30 mins session, at least 3 times a week for 6 months
   - Walking is mode of exercise
   - Leg strength improves walking time
   - Treadmill is better
   - Arm ergometer too Increases walking time
   - *Mech:* Formation of collateral
     Improve endothelial function
     Sensitive vessel to endo dependent vasodilation
     Improve hemotheology, muscle str and metabolism
   - Current guidelines
   - Patient with int claudication undergo exercise rehab as initial therapy
   - 30–60 min session at least 3 times per week for min 12 weeks
D. *Percutaneous transluminal angioplasty and stents*
   For patients with critical limb ischemia and anatomy amenable to catheter-based treatment
E. *Peripheral artery surges*
   - Aortofemoral bypass
   - Extranomical surgery reconstructive procedure
     - Axillobifemoral bypass
     - Iliofemoral bypass
     - Femorofemoral bypass
   - Femoropopliteal, femorotibial, and femoral-peroneal artery bypass

MANAGEMENT ALGORITHM

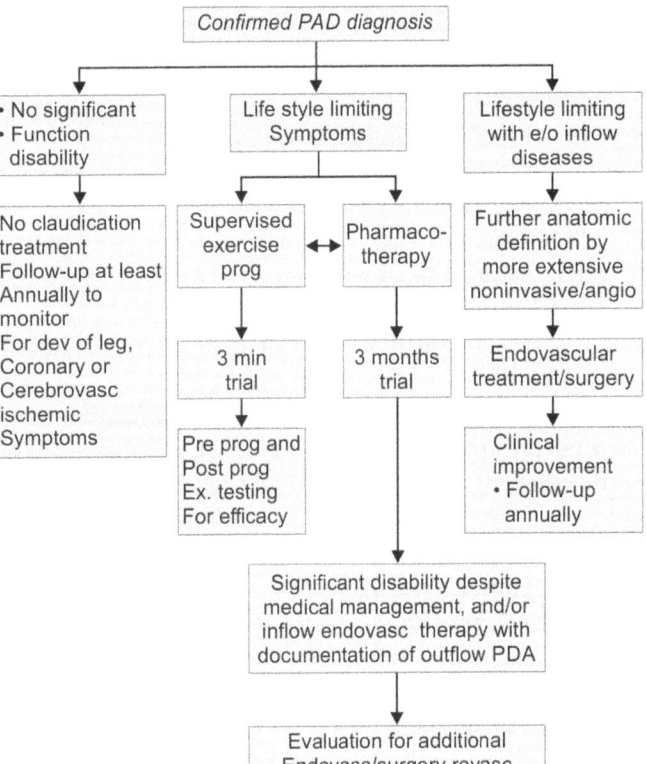

16.3 THROMBOANGIITIS OBLITERANS

INTRODUCTION
- Segmental vasculitis that involving distal arteries, veins and nerves of UL, LL
- Typically affect young person who smoke

PATHOPHYSIOLOGY
- TAD affects medium and small vessel of arms (radial, ulnar, Palma, digital arteries) and counterparts in legs (Tibrol, peroneal, planter and digital art)
- Cerebral, coroner, renal, aortoiliac, and pulm candidiasis
  ↓
- *Patho*: Occlusive, highly cellular thrombus that incorporates PMN leukocytes, microabscess and occasionally multinucleated giant cells
  ↓
  Inflammatory process can also affect vasc wall but int elastic lamina remain intact
  Decreased endo dependent vasodilatation

ECHO
- Precise cause—unknown
- Tobacco and smoking present in all patients
- Hypercoagulability, immunologic meln and endothelial dysfunction may contribute to progression of TAD

C/F
- 13 per 100,000 populations
- Most patients <45 years
- 70–90% men
- Claudication
- Pain at rest ⎤
- Ulceration (>1 extremity) ⎦ Most patients
- Raynaud phenomenon—45% of patients
- Superficial thrombophlebitis (may be migratory)—40%
- Amputation within 5 year—25%

O/E: Pulselessness
- Abnormal Allen test
- Pallar
- Discrete, tender, erythematous subcut
- Chords—indicates superficial thrombophlebitis

DIAGNOSIS
- No specific lab test
- Biopsy is Diagnostic
- Need to exclude
  - SLE, scleroderma, hypercoagulable, statin, DM, Embolism
- Normal ESR and CRP
- ANA as DNA, ANCA—Neg
- *Arteriography*: Segmental occlusion of small and medium sized arteries, absence of atherosclerosis and corkscrew collateral vessels circumventing occlusion
- Conclusive: Biopsy (rarely done)
- Prob: Biopsy site fail to heal due to ischemia
- So Δ depends on—age of onset <45 years, H/O tobacco use, physical examination showing distal limb ischemia, exclusion of other disease and if necessary angiography

TREATMENT
- Tobacco cessation
- Patient without gangrene who stop smoking rarely require amputation
- No definitive drug treatment
- Surgery is not ideal because of segmentary affection
- Saphenous venous bypass graft can be used if target vessel for distal anastomosis is available

FMD
- Medium and large arteries, typically renal and carotid
- May involve iliac and less so femoral
- Most common in young women
- Fibroplasia most commonly affect media but can involve intima/adventitia also
- *Angio*: Beaded appearance
  (Medial and perimedial fibroplasia and focal stenosis)

Treatment: Balloon angioplasty/PTRA

SECTION 17

Pulmonary Diseases

17.1 SLEEP APNEA AND HEART DISEASE

Q.1 Define OSA. Discuss physiology and association with CV disease (Dec 11)

Q.2 What is OSA? Discuss its diagnosis, management and effect on CV system (Dec 13)

AHI (Apnea Hypopnea Index):
Average no of apnea–hypopnea events per hour of sleep
AHI ≥ 5 - OSA
AHI ≥ 30 - severe OSA
Clinically important CV events are associated with an AHI as low as 5

INTRODUCTION

REM
- 25% of night sleep
- Tonic state punctuated by periods of phasic activity
- Autonomic and cardiac functions are erratic
- Sympathetic drive, HR and
- BP increases

NREM
- 75% of night sleep
- Autonomic and cardiac regulation is stable
- Sympathetic drive decreases, parasymp tone dominates, decrease baroreceptor set point, decreased BP, decrease in HR, decrease of CO and decrease of SVR

Marked sinus Brady
Marked sinus arrhythmia
Sinus pulse
1° and type 1 2° H.B.
} Possible during sleep

OBSTRUCTIVE SLEEP APNEA

Definition

Obstructive Apnea

Absence of air flow for at least 10 seconds in presence of active ventilatory efforts as reflected by abdomino thoracic movt.

Obstructive hypopnea

Decrease of more than 50% in throraco-abd movt for at least 10 seconds associated with decrease of > 4% in O_2 saturation

Mechanism

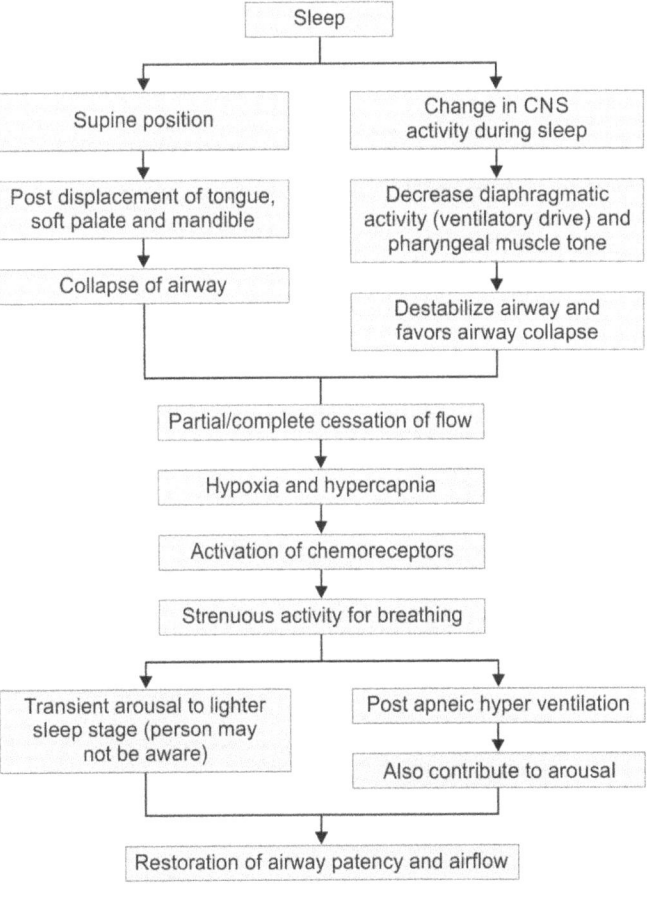

Pathophysiology "Linking OSA to CV Disease"

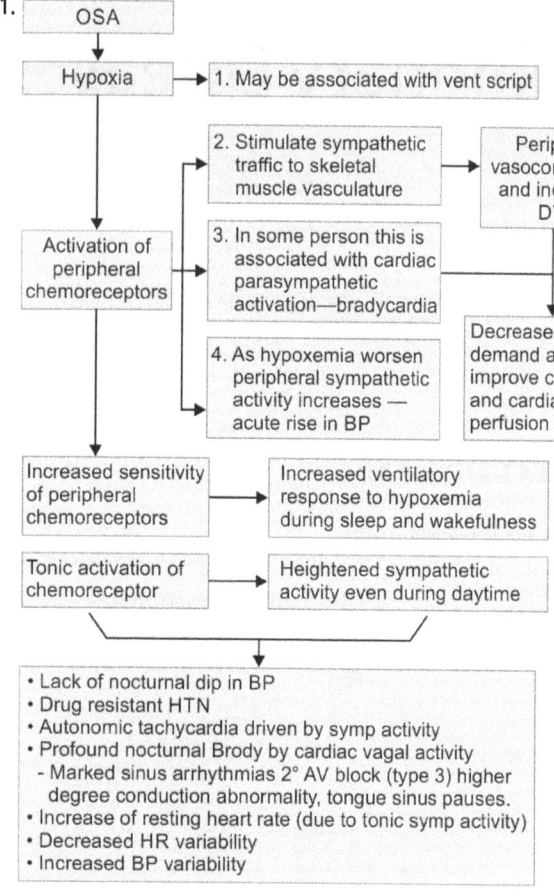

3. Intrathoracic pressure change + oscitation of symp parasympathetic activity
   ↓
   Atrial fibrillation
4. OSA also associated with
   - Endothelial dysfunction—increased endothelin—vasoconstriction
   - Syst and vasc inflammation—progression of atherosclerosis
   - Insulin resistance—increases risk of metabolic syndrome
   - Increased leptin level—associated with CV events
   - Hypercoagulability
   - Oxidative stress
5. OSA also associated with
   - Abdominal obesity
   - Diabetes
   - Dyslipidemia
   - Metabolic syndrome

OSA CV Disease and Outcomes

OSA associated with
- HTN
- CAD
- MI
- ACS
- HF with syst dysfunction
- Acute stroke
- AF requiring cardioversion
- Lone AI
  - Severity of nocturnal O_2 desaturation was associated with AF, obesity, HTN, HF
  - CPAP reduces BP, TG, HbA1C, total chol and LDL, metabolic synd, HTN and AF
  - Nocturnal desat of 4% or more–associated with CV disease increase all-cause mortality and CAD.

Summary

Pathophysiologic Consequence of OSA

- Hypoxemia
- Hypercapnia
- Intrathoracic pr fluctuations
- Reoxygenation
- Arousals.

Possible Intermediate CV Disease Mechanism

- Sympathetic activation
- Vasoconstriction
- Acute tachycardia

- Acute BP elevation
- Decreased CV variability
- Increased LV wall stress
- Increased after load
- Ac diastolic dysfunction
- LA stretch
- LAE
- Insulin resistance
- Hyperleptinemia
- Hypercoagulability
- Syst inflammation
- Oxidative strech
- Endothelial dysfunction.

CV Disease Associations and Risk
- HTN
- Syst dysfunction
- Diastolic dysfunction
- Sinus pause/arrest
- AV block
- AF
- Vent ectopy
- Nect angina
- CAD
- CV disease
- SCD.

Screening and Diagnosis

History and Clinical Examination
- Snoring
- Excessive day time sleepiness
  Excessive day time somnolence may be less common in patient with OSA and CV disease like HF/AF
- Tiredness on waking from sleep
- Witnessed nocturnal apnea noted by partner
- Nighty gasping/choking sensation
- Night time or morning headaches
- Morning dry mouth/sore throat
- Nocturia
- Cognitive and memory difficulties
- Psychological and behavioral changes
- History from partner is important.

On examination:
- Usually normal
  - Overweight or abdominal obesity
  - Increased neck circumference - > 17 inches
    More sensitive than BMI
  - Low soft palate, narrow oropharynx, large uvula, micrognathia, retrognathia.

Screening Trials
- Diagnosis based on history and physical examination = 50%
- Multiple prediction model and questionnaires
  - Epworth sleepiness score/modified Berlin questionnaire
    Response to
    - Sitting and reading
    - Watching TV
    - Sitting in active in public place
    - Sitting in car for an hour
    - Car at signal
    - Lying down to rest in afternoon

    Give 1-3 score
- ≥ 11 score = require further diagnostic procedure.

Polysomnography
- Gold standard test
- Performed during full night and if required, repeated on another night to apply and titrate CPAP therapy
- Gives information about
  - Sleep architecture
  - Sleep efficiency
  - Disordered breathing events
  - Oscillation in O_2 saturations
  - Cardia Arrhythmias
  - Neurophysiological signal
  - Muscle electromyogram.

Management
*Whom to treat?
- Symptomatic patients
*Asymptomatic patients with apnea/hypnea do not benefit
  A. *Gen measures*
     - Lifestyle modification
       - Weight loss
       - Exercise
     - Alcohol reduction
     - Smoking cessation
     - Avoid sedatives
     - For patients with positioned OSA (supine)- wearing well-fitting shirt with tennis ball sewn tightly to midback–maintain non-supine position.
  B. *CPAP*
     - *Indications*
       - AHI ≥ 15 or
       - AHI ≥ 5 in patients with symptoms (e.g., excessive day time sleepiness, impaired cognition, mood disorders, insomnia), HTN, IHD or H/O stroke

- *Mech*
  - PAP effectively splints airway open and prevents As collapse
- *Diff models*
  - Naso-oral mask
  - Nasal mask
  - Nasal pillow
- *Draw back*
  - Claustrophobia
  - Rhinitis or nasal congestion
  - Nosebleed
  - Abrasions of bridge of the nose
  - Drying of upper airway
- *CV benefits*
  - Decreased BP during sleep and daytime
  - Symptomatic relief
  - Relieve nocturnal ischemia/angina
  - Improve LV syst function
  - Decrease risk of major adv cardiac event, MI, coro revascularization, stroke and death
  - TG, LDL level decrease
  - Decreased HbA1C
C. *Mandibular repositioning splint*
   Holding tongue and lower jaw protruded
D. *Surgery*
   - Jaw advancement surgery
   - Uvulo-palato-pharyngoplasty
   - Tonsillectomy
   - Bariatric surgery
   - Rarely tracheostomy
E. *Medical management*
   Modafinil mofetil marginally improve OST.

CENTRAL SLEEP APNEA: (CHEYNE STOKES RESPI)

Definition
Form of periodic breathing in which ventilation waxes and wanes and gradually alternate between hyperpnea and tachypnea

- Common among infants and people travelling to high altitudes
- Associated with HF

Pathophysiology
- Principle defect is instability in Ventilatory control
  ↓
Oscillation in $PaCO_2$ above and below apneic threshold
  ↓
Periodic hyperpnea and apnea

HF
- Patients with HF have CSA due to
  - Heightened chemosensitivity to $PaCO_2$ (high loop gain) and long circulation tire (phase delay)—decreased apneic threshold
- Stimulation of pulm irritant mechanoreceptor by increased LV filling pr and pulm edema causes hyperventilation—drop in $PaCO_2$ below apneic threshold—apnea
- Prolonged lung to periphery time exacerbate apneic intervals

Diff between OSA and CSA
OSA- Respi efforts present
CSA- No respi efforts

CSA and CV Disease
Similar as OSA and CV disease

Management
A. *PAP therapy*
   Based not on treatment of CSA per se
   Based on treatment of HF

   PAP- decreased sympathetic activity
       Decreased vent afterload
       Increased LV EF
B. *Other:*
   - Low flow O_2 supplementation
   - Theophylline

17.2 PULMONARY EMBOLISM AND DEEP VEIN THROMBOSIS

Q.1 How do you classify acute pulmonary embolism (PE)? What is the classification of deep vein thrombosis (DVT)? List the major risk factor for VTE that is not readily modifiable (3+3+4) (June 17)?
Q.2 Catheter intervention in Ac PE (Dec 16).
Q.3 Management of submassive PE (June 15).
Q.4 Ac massive PE Dx and MX (June 04).
Q.5 Pathological consequences of PE (Jan 2000).

MOLECULAR PATHOPHYSIOLOGY

- VTE is now regarded as Pan cardiovascular syndrome that includes
  - Coro art disease
  - Peri art disease
  - Cerebrovascular disease

Inflammation hypercoagulability and endothelial injury activates pathophysiological cascade leading to VTE

Infection, transfusion or erythropoiesis stimulating factor
↓
Inflammation
↓
Recruit platelet
↓
Activated platelet releases phosphorylate, procoagulant microparticles and pro inflammatory mediator

It also binds neutrophil and stimulates them to release their nuclear material and form weblike extracellular network
↓
This web is called neutrophil extracellular traps
↓
NET is procoagulant
↓
Stimulate platelet aggregation and platelet dependent thrombin generation
↓
Thrombin flourish in an env of stasis, low O_2 tension, oxidative stress, if expression of proinflammatory product
↓
Impair endothelial cell regulatory capacity
↓
This venous thrombosis can persist as a subclinical, perhaps chronic inflammatory that becomes clinically apparent intermittently

ARIL study: Conc of hsCRP above 98th percentile was associated with increased risk of VTE
JUPITER: 43% reduction in symptomatic VTE in patient treated with Rosuvastatin for asymptomatic elevation of hsCRP

CARDIOPULMONARY DYNAMICS

PE
↓
- Increased pulm vasc persistence due to
  - Vascular obstruction
  - Neurohormonal agent
  - Pulm art baroreceptors
- Impaired Gas exchange due to
  - Increased alveolar dead space by vasc obst
  - Hypoxia from alveolar hypoventilation
  - Rt to lt shunting
- Alveolar hyperventilation due to
  - Reflex stimulation of irritant receptors
- Increased airway resistance due to
  - Bronchoconstriction
- Decreased pulm compliance due to
  - Long edema, lung hemorrhage and loss of surfactant

RV dysfunction determined by
- Extent of pulm vasc obstruction
- Presence of underlying cardio-pulm disease
- Neurohormonal response
- Vasoconstrictor compounds such as serotonin, reflex pulm art constriction, hypoxemia

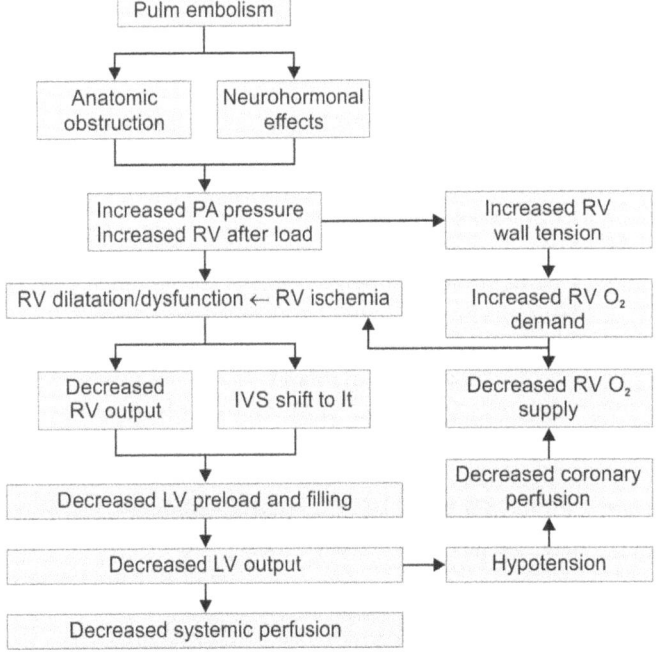

CLASSIFICATION OF PULMONARY EMBOLISM

- *Massive PE:* 5-10% of cases
  - Thrombosis is widespread, affecting at least half of pulm art vasculature
  - *Presentation:*
    - SBP <90 mm Hg/poor tissue perfusion or multi-system organ failure
    - Plus extensive thrombosis such as "saddle PE" or B/L pulm art involvement
    - Dyspnea is MC presentation
    - Transient cyanosis is common
    - Renal and Hepatic dysfunction and altered mentation are common
  - *Treatment:*
    - Anticoagulants (starting with iv UFH)
    - Systemic thrombolysis
    - Catheter directed intervention
    - Surgical embolectomy
    - IVC filter
- *Submassive PE:* 20-25% of cases
- Thrombosis involve 1/3rd or more of pulm vasculature
  - Presentation:
    - HD stable
    - Mod-severe RV dysfunction dilatation
    - Biomarkers elevation indicative of RV micro-infarction and/or RV pr overload
    - At risk of recurrent PE
  - *Treatment:*
    - Anticoagulation (starting with UFH) + or - advanced therapy (based on risk of circulatory collapse vs risk of hemorrhagic stroke)
    - For patients with low bleeding risk and severe RV dysfunction—consider advanced therapy same as massive PE
- *Low risk PE/small-mid PE* (70% of cases)
  Presentation: Normal hemodynamics and normal RV size and function
  Treatment: Parenteral anticoagulation followed by oral warf/oral rivaroxaban
- *Pulm infarction*
  - Char by pleuritic chest pain
  - Occ accompanied by hemoptysis
  - Due to embolus lodging in peripheral PA near pleura
  - Usually after 3-7 days of embolism
  - S/s: Fever, leukocytosis, increased
  - ESR, CXR evidence of infarct
- *Paradoxical embolus:* DVT that embolize to syst circulation through PFO/ASD
- *Non-thrombotic PE*
  - Source of embolism other than thrombus
    e.g., Arr, fat, tumor, and amniotic fluid Peripartum period
    After blunt trauma/# of leg bone
    During placement/removal of CVC; ICD/PPI

IV drug abuse—self inject hair, talc and cotton as contaminants.

CLASSIFICATION OF DEEP VEIN THROMBOSIS

- *Lower extremity DVT*
  - 10 times more common than UL DVT
  - More proximal thrombus—more likely to embolize
- *Upper extremity DVT*
  - Becoming increasingly important clinical entity
  - Can occur due to PPI/ICD/indwelling cath
  - At risk of PE, SVC syndrome and loss of vascular access
- *Superficial vein thrombosis*
  - 6-fold increased risk of DVT
  - 4-fold increased risk of PE
  - Short term use of fondaparinux is useful
- *Chronic venous insufficiency/post thrombotic syndrome*
  - DVT- dysfunction of valves of deep venous system
  - DVT- decrease output form veins—increased venous pressure with muscle contraction
  ↓
  This increases pressure in large veins of leg are transmitted to microchannels
  ↓
  Venous microangiopathy

O/E: Varicose vein, abnormal pigmentation of medial malleolus and skin ulceration
  - Chronic venous disease is associated with reduced QOL, due to chronic pain, decreased physical function and decreased mobility
  - DVT stockings (30-40 mm Hg) is mainstay of treatment.

Nonmodifiable Risk Factors

- Advancing age
- Arterial disease (carotid and coronary disease)
- Personal or F/H/O VTE
- Recent surgery, trauma or immobility
- Congestive heart failure
- COPD
- Acute infection
- Blood transfusion
- Erythropoietin stimulating factor
- Chronic inflammation
- cKD
- Air pollution
- Preg, OC pill or post menopause HRT
- PPI/ICD or indwelling catheters
- Hypercoagulable states
  - Protein C def
  - Protein S def

- Factor V Leiden mutation-3 times increased risk—prot C resistance
- Prothrombin gene mutation 20210—2 times increased risk
- MC acquired—APLA syndrome
- Antithrombin deficiency
- CA—adino CA of pancreas, stomach, esophagus, lung, prostate and colon/myeloproliferative—lymphoma leukemia.

Modifiable Risk Factors

- Obesity
- Cigarette smoking
- Diabetes mellitus
- HTN
- Hypercholesterolemia
- Persistent stress/depression/loneliness
- Long haul travel—18% increase in risk every 24 hours.

Clinical Presentation

- Clinical suspicion is of utmost importance
- MC symptoms
- Unexplained Dyspnea (MC)
- Chest pain—pleuritic/atypical
- Anxiety
- Cough

  → Severe pleuritic chest pain suggests that PE is small and located in distal PA system

Signs

- Tachypnea (MC)
- Tachycardia
- Low grade fever
- Hypotension
- ↑ JVP
- TR murmur
- Accentuated P2
- Hemoptysis
- Leg edema, erythema, tenderness

PE should be suspected in hypotensive patients with
1. E/O venous thrombosis/predisposing VTE risk
2. Acute RV failure (cor pulmonale)
3. ECG manifestation of RV dysfunction or ECHO findings of RV dilatation and hypokinesia.

Investigation

- *D-dimer*
  - Most patients of PE have ongoing endogenous fibrinolysis
  - Breakdown some of fibrin lot to D-dimer
  - Sensitive but not specific
  - High NPV
- ECG
  - Sinus tachy—MC
  - Slight ST-T abnormality
  - S1Q3T3
- CXR
  - Near normal CXR in severe respi compromise is highly suggestive of PE
  - Watermark sign focal oligemia due to massive central embolic occlusion
  - Hampton hump peripheral wedge-shaped opacity above diaphragm (due to pulm infarction)
  - Palla sign Enlargement of des RPA
- *VQ scanning*
  - For patients who can't tolerate contrast/preg
  - Vent scan with xenon/Krypton
  - Perf scan with radiolabeled albumin—r rays
  - ≥ 2 segment perf detect in presence of normal ventilation is highly diagnostic
  - High NPV
- *CT:*
  - Initial imaging test in patients with suspected PE
  - Can image thrombus up to 6th order vessel
  - Can also detect other pul disease
  - Signs of RV dysfunction
    - RV-LV diameter ratio >0.9
    - RV-LV volume ratio >1.2
    - IVS blowing
    - Reflux of contrast into IVC
      Any sign of RV dysfunction—poor prognosis
- *ECHO:*
  - Normal in 50%
  - RV overload
  - Mod-severe RV hypokinesia ⎤
    Persistent PH   ⎥ associated with
    RFO   ⎥ high risk of death
    Free floating thrombus in RV/RA ⎦
  - *McConnell's sign:* Hypokinesia of RV free wall with normal motion of RV apex.
- *USG:*
  - 50% patients with PE have no DVT
  - Signs of DVT
    1. Lack of vein compressibility (vein do not wink)
    2. Direct visualization of thrombus
    3. Abnormal flow dynamics—flow blunted with cold compression
- *MRI:* Less sensitive than CT
  Limited sensitivity for distal PE
  Can't be used as standalone test to exclude PE

- *Pulm angio:*
  - Rarely done
  - Replaced by CT angio
  - Used only when catheter-based interventions are required
- *Contrast venography:*
  - Rarely done
  - 1st step for patients with large femoral or iliofemoral DVT who are undergoing pharmacochemical catheter directed treatment.

Diagnostic Scoring System

- *For DVT*
  - Active CA   +1
  - Paralysis/paresis/cast recently   +1
  - Bedridden >3d; major surgery <12 weeks   +1
  - Entire leg swelling   +1
  - Unilat calf swelling >3 cm   +1
  - Pitting edema   +1
  - Collateral superficial veins   +1
  - Tenderness along vein distribution   +1
  - Alternative diagnosis as likely as DVT   -2
    ≤0 - low likelihood
    1-2 - moderate likelihood
    ≥3 - high likelihood
- *For PE (well's criteria)*
  - Sign/symptoms of DVT   +3
  - Alt diagnosis less likely   +3
  - HR >100/min   +1.5
  - Prior PE/DVT   +1.5
  - Immobilization/surgery within 4 weeks   +1.5
  - Hemoptysis   +1
  - CA treated within 6 months/mets   +1
    ≥4 - high likelihood

Diagnostic Approach

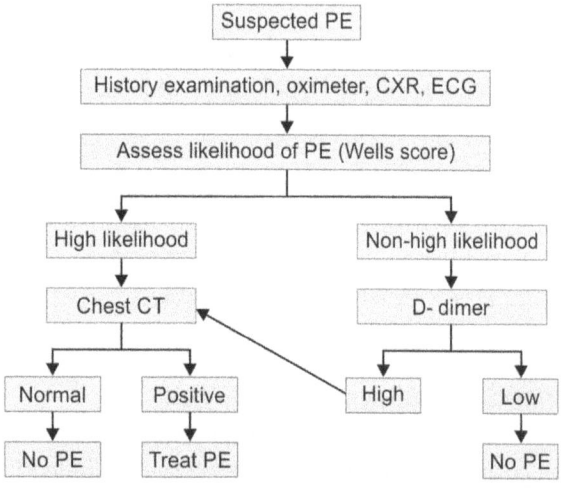

Risk Stratification

PESI (Pulm Embolism Severity Index) Criteria

Age > 80
Male sex
H/O CA
H/O MI
H/O Chronic lung disease
HR > 110
SBP < 100
RR ≥ 30
Terp < 36
Altered mental status
Arterial O_2 < 90%

Simplified PESI criteria

Age > 80 years	+1
H/O cancer	+1
H/O HF or COPD	+1
HR >= 110	+1
SBP < 100	+1
Art O_2 sat < 90%	+1

Score 0 = low risk
>=1 = high risk

- Low risk patients—excellent prognosis with intensive Anticoagulation
- High risk patients—require intensive HD and respi support

Components of Risk Stratification

1. Clinical evaluation—simplified PESI score
2. Assessment of RV size and function (Examination, ECG, ECHO)
3. Analysis of elevated CV biomarkers.

Massive PE with Hypotension

A.

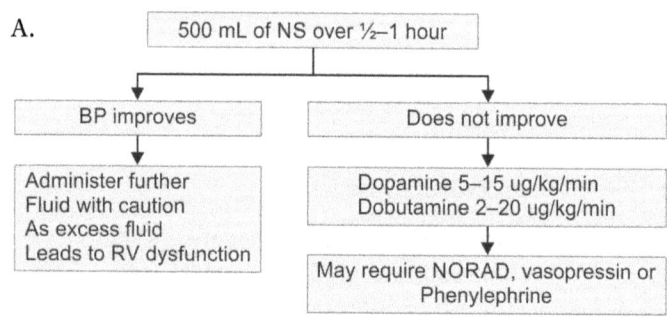

B. Once patients with stabilized hemodynamically
   ↓
   Attempt fibrinolysis

- *Alteplase:* 100 mg as a cont infusion over 2 hours without concomitant heparin
- *Streptokinase:* IV bolus 2,50,000 U over 30 mins followed by infusion of 100,000 units/hour for 12-24 hours

- Urokinase 4,400 unit 1 kg bolus followed by 4400 units 1 kg/hour for 12-24 hours
  - Thrombolysis reverses rt sided heart failure
  - Hallmark of successful therapy
    - Reduction of RV for overload
    - Prevention of continued release of serotonin and other neurohormonal factors that exacerbate PHTN
    - Dissolution of thrombus in pelvic and deep vein—prevent occurrence of PE
    - Improve pulm capillary blood flow and reduce likelihood of developing chronic thromboembolic pulm HTN
  - Time window of lysis = up to 14 days or new symptoms/signs
  - For patients with high risk submassive PE, PEITHO trial significant reduction in all-cause mortality or HD collapse within 7 d of initiation of therapy
  - But significant increase in major bleeding risk

C. *Catheter directed therapy*

Goals
1. Rapidly reducing PAP, RV strain and PVR
2. Increasing systemic perfusion
3. Facilitating RV recovery

Indi
- When thrombolysis is absolutely contraindicated or has failed
- When emergency Surgical embolectomy is unavailable or contraindicated

Tech
A. *Aspiration thrombectomy*
   - Uses sustained suction applied to catheter tip to secure and remove thrombus
   - Greenfield suction embolectomy catheter
B. *Thrombus fragmentation*
   - Performed with balloon angioplasty, pigtail rotation catheter or more advanced fragmentation device, amplatz catheter
C. *Rheolytic thrombectomy*
   - Angiojet, hydrolyzed and oasis cath
   - Use high velocity saline jet to fragment adjacent thrombus by creating Venturi effect
D. Low intensity ultrasound-facilitated fibrinolysis
E. Pharmachemical-low dose rtPA (25 mg)

Recommendation (ACC/AHA 2012)

Class 2a: Reasonable for patients with massive PE and CI to fibrinolysis or patients who remain unstable after fibrinolysis

Class 2b: May be considered for submassive PE judged with clinical evidence of adverse prognosis (new HD instability, worsening, respi failure, severe RV dysfunction or major myocardial necrosis)

Class 3: Not recommended for small and low risk PE

D. *Surgical embolectomy*

For patients with
- CI to lysis
- Acute PE who requires surgical excision of RA/RV thrombus
- Patients who require closure of PTO
- Failed lysis

E. *IVC filter*

For patients with
- Contraindications to anticoagulants
- Recurrent PE despite optimal anticoag
- Very poor cardiopulm reserve (including patients with massive PE)

Trials: PREPIC Trial

F. *Anticoagulants*
- Unfractionated heparin
  Acts by binding to antithrombin

  Promotes a confrontational change in antithrombin that accelerate its activity 100-1000 times

  Prevent additional thrombus formation and permits endogenous fibrinolytic mechanism to lyse some amt of clot

  Dose: 80 u/kg IV bolus followed by 18 u/kg/hour
  - Maintain aPTT 1.5-2.5 times
- LMWH:
  - Greater bioavailability (less binding to plasma protein and endothelial cells)
  - Long half life
  - More predictable effect

  Dose: 1 u/kg s/c daily (OD or divided)
  Decreased dose in patients with renal failure
- *Fondaparinux*
  - FDA approved
  - Inhibit activated factor X
  - Fixed dose, once a day s/c
  - Dose modification in patients with renal dysfunction
- Heparin-induced thrombocytopenia
  - Immune mediated complication
  - Serious complication
  - More with UFH than LMWH
  - Manifest as bilat DVT, PE, MI, stroke and unusual arterial thrombosis
  - IgG antibodies binds to Heparin—platelet factor 4 complex

Activate platelets
↓
Release of prothrombotic microparticles
↓
Promote excessive thrombin generation
↓
Paradoxical thrombosis despite thrombocytopenia

- Semiquantitative clinical screening test (4-T point score)
  - Thrombocytopenia
  - Timing of decrease in platelet count
  - Thrombosis or other sequelae (e.g., skin Necrosis)
  - Absence of other explanation
- Suspected when plt < to 100,000 or less than 50% of baseline
- Occurs after 5-7 days of heparin exposure
- ELISA quantification of anti PF4/Heparin antibody level (may be false positive)
- Gold std = Serotonin release assab
  Treatment
  - Stop Heparin/LMWH immediately
  - No plt transfusion
  - Asymptomatic—fondaparinux
  - Thrombosis—Biva, argatroban lepirudin
- *Warfarin*
  - Vit K antagonist
  - Prevent r-carboxylation of coag factor 2,7,9,10
  - Full effect evident after 5-7 days (because factor 2 has half life of 5 d approx)
  - Target INR = 2-3
  - Warfarin monotherapy—decreased level of protein e and s—increased thrombogenic potential
  ↓
  So need to overlap for at least 5 d
  S/E:
  - Hemorrhage
  - Hair loss
  - Increased coronary calcification
  - Drug and food interaction
  Warf pharmacogenetics
  - GYP2C9 variant alleles
    Impair hydroxylation of s-warfarin
    Extremely low dose requirements
  - VKORCI (variant in gene encoding vit K epoxide reductase complex 1)
    Variability in INR response to warf is strongly associated with VKORCI
    Genetic testing is not necessary or marginally useful as shown by multiple trials

Novel oral anticoagulants
- Fixed dose
- Rapid onset of action
- No lab monitoring
- Minimal drug-drug or drug food interaction
- Dabigatran noninferior to warfarin (RE cover; RE-MEDY; RECOVER 2)
- Rivaroxaban non-inferior to warfarin (EINSTEIN E, EINSTEIN -PE)
- Apixaban—Non-inferior (AMPLIFY)
- Edoxaban (Non-inferior) (HOKUSAI-VTE)

OPTIMAL DURATION OF ANTICOAG

- VTE-high risk of recurrence
- Factors that increase chance of recurrence
  - Male sex
  - PE symptoms at initial presentation
  - Magnitude of D-dimer elevation
  - Immobilization
  - Cancer
  - COPD
  - Overweight
  - Low HDL
  - Family history
  - Thrombophilia
  - Failure to recanalize leg vein after anticoagulation

"Persistent thrombus on CT does not predict recurrence. 50% patients have persistent thrombus 6 months after initial event"

Q. Chronic thromboembolic PHTN (Dec 14)
Provoked VTE—3 Months of Anticoagulation
Unprovoked with low-mod bleeding risk—extended anticoag

Patients with CA—extended anticoag

Role of aspirin
- Therapeutic benefit for patients who do not wish to restrict their lifestyle with burdens of indefinite duration anticoagulants
- It is for more effective than placebo

Chronic thromboembolic PHTN
- 2-4% of patients with PE
- 1° treatment = thromboendarterectomy
- Other
  - Sildenafil
  - Bosentan
  - Percute PA balloon dilatation

17.3 PULMONARY HYPERTENSION

Q.1 Drug therapy in PHTN (Dec 16).
Q.2 Management of PPH (June 16).
Q.3 Newer drugs for PAH (June 15).
Q.4 Pulm hypertensive crisis.
Q.5 Define idiopathic PHTN. Its etiopatho and treatment (June 13).
Q.6 Describe invasive and non-invasive evaluation of PHTN. How to assess reversibility (June 12)?
Q.7 Discuss clinical recognition, investigation, and management of PHTN crisis (Dec 10, 11).

DEFINITION

An "abnormal" elevation in pulm art pr, may be result of left heart failure, pulmonary parenchymal or vascular disease, thromboembolism or combination of these factors.

For group 1 or pulm art HTN also require that left sided filling pr (PCWP), LVEDP or LAP ≤15 mm Hg and calculated PVR ≥3 w.u.

By definition PH means mPAP >25 mm Hg (at rest)
>30 mm Hg (exercise)
Normal mPAP = 12–16 mm Hg (at sea level)
Mean PAP = (0.61 × systolic PAP) + 2
↳ Measured on ECHO

ANATOMY

- Each PA accompanies appropriate generation bronchus and divides with it down to the level of respi bronchiole
- PA are other elastic or muscular
- As the arteries decrease in size, no of elastic lamina decreases and smooth muscle increases
- Eventually in vessel between 100 and 500 mm^3, elastic tissue is lost from the media and arteries becomes muscular
- Intima of PA consists of a single layer of endothelial cells and their basement memb.

PATHOLOGY

- *In PAH:* Lesion mainly involve distal PA (<500 μm) char features
  - Medial hypertrophy
  - Intimal proliferation and fibrotic changes (concentric or eccentric)
  - Adventitial thickening
  - Perivascular inflammation
  - Complex lesions (plexiform, dilated lesion) and thrombotic lesion
- *In PVOD* (pulm veno-occlusive disease)
  - Septal vein and paraseptal venules affected
- Char by
  - Venous muscularization
  - Occlusive fibrotic lesions
  - Patchy capillary proliferation
  - Occult alveolar hemorrhage
  - Lymphatic dilatation
  - Pulm edema
- *In patients with PH due to lt sided heart disease*
  - Enlarged and thickened PV
  - Pulm capillary dilatation
  - Interstitial edema
  - Alveolar hemorrhage
  - Lymphatic vessel and UN Enlargement
- *PH caused by lung disease and/or hypoxia*
  - Medial hypertrophy
  - Intimal obstructive proliferation
- *CTEPH*
  - Organized thrombi tightly attached to PA metal layer and replace normal intima
  - May completely occlude positive lumen or form diff grade of stenosis, webs and bunds.

PATHOPHYSIOLOGY

Multifactorial - 1. Imbalance in vasoconstriction and relaxation
2. Cell proliferation and remodeling.

Pulm vascular remodeling involves intima, media and adventitia of small PA (<500 um) and it involves all cell type (Endothelial smooth muscle and fibroblast as well as inflammatory cells and platelets

Various pathological process involved

- Inhibition of voltage gated K$^+$ channel—vasoconstriction
- Endothelial dysfunction—impaired production of vasodilator (NO, prostacyclin) and overexpression of vasoconstrictor (endothelin-1)
- Mutation in bone-morphogenetic protein receptor 2
- Increased serotonin uptake in SM cells
- Excessive thrombin deposition related to procoagulant state
- Increased angiopoietin expression in SMC
- Abnormal proteolysis of ECM, autoimmunity, and inflammation.

GENETICS

- *Idiopathic PAH:* Without any family history of PAH or known triggering factor
- Many cases of familial PAH has been described
  - Autosomal dominant trait

- With incomplete penetrance
- Possible genetic anticipation phenomena (Age at onset disease significantly lower in each succeeding gen)
- BMP receptor type 2 was identified as first PAH-predisposing gene
  - BMPR2 is involved in regulation of growth, differentiation and apoptosis of PA endothelium and smooth muscle cells
- Other genes involved
  - Activin A receptor type 2 like kinase (ALK-1)
  - Endoglin
  - SMAD-9
  - CAV-1
  - KCN-3 gene—channelopathy
- Like IDAH, familial PH affect F>M
- BMPR2 mutation
  - Younger at time of diagnosis
  - More severe HD compromise
  - More likely to die sooner or to undergo transplantation than IDAH
- ECHO every 1-3 year or when sign/symptoms of PH develop in carrier or 1st degree relatives

HEMODYNAMICS

- Normal mPAP at rest = 14.0 + or - 3.3 mm Hg
  Independent of sex and ethnicity
  Slightly influenced by age
  Rarely exceeds 20
- Pulm circ is high flow, low pr and low resistance
- Normal PAP rarely exceeds 20
  By definition PH ≥25 mm Hg (mPAP)
  More work up required for mPAP 21-24
- PH can be precapillary (PCWP ≤1.5) or post capillary (PCWP>15)
  Some patients have mixed picture with elevated mPAP and PAWP with transpulm gradient (mPAP-PAWP) >12
- Exercise PAP depends on
  - Level of exercise
  - Age

  Data: Upper limit of normal mPAP flow relationship is 3 mm Hg/L/min with resistive vessel distensibility or the order of 1-2% change in diameter/mm Hg pr and that higher or is associated with decreased exercise capacity
- PVR can be calculated as
  1. $PVR = \dfrac{mPAP - PAWP}{CO}$
  2. TPR (total pulm resistance) = $\dfrac{mPAP}{CO}$

This can be multiplied by 80 to express result in dyne-sec.cm^{-5}
Or
Expressed in woods unit (mm Hg/L/min)
Normal = 1 wood unit (67 + or - dyne-sec.cm^{-5})

CLASSIFICATION

- *Pulm art HTN*
  - Idiopathic PAH
  - Heritable PAH
    - BMPR2
    - ALK-1, endoglin, SMAD-9, CAV 1, KCNK-3
    - Unknown
  - Drug and toxin Induced
  - Associated with
    - Connective tissue disease
    - HIV
    - Portal HTN
    - Cong heart disease
    - Schistosomiasis

  1a: Pulm veno-occlusive disease and/or pulm capillary
  1b: Persistent pulm HTN of newborn
- *Pulm HTN caused by lt sided heart disease*
  - LV syst dysfunction
  - LV diastolic dysfunction
  - Valvular heart disease
  - Cong/acquired lt sided heart inflow/ outflow tract obstruction
- *Pulm HTN caused by lung disease and/or hypoxia*
  - COPD
  - IHD
  - Mixed Restrictive and obst disease
  - Sleep related disordered breathing
  - Alveolar hypoventilation
  - Chr exposure to high altitude
  - Development of lung disease
    - Cong dia hernia
    - Broncho pulm dysplasia
- *Chronic thromboembolic pulm HTN*
- *Pulm HTN with unclear mechanism |multifactorial|*
  - Hematological disease—chr hemolytic anemia, myeloproliferative disorders, splenectomy
  - *Syst disorders:* Sarcoidosis, pulm Langerhans cell histiocytosis, vasculitis, neurofibromatosis
  - Metabolic-glycogen storage disease, Gaucher disease, thyroid disease
  - *Other:* Segmental PAH, tumoral obst, fibrosing mediastinitis, CRF.

GROUP 1: PULMONARY ARTERIAL HTN

- *Idiopathic PAH*
  - Formerly known as primary pulm HTN
  - MC type of group-1
  - Rare
  - Unknown cause
  - Female preponderance (2:1 to 4:1)
  - Mean age at diagnosis = 37–50 (4th–5th decade)
  - *Untreated:* 2–3 years survival after diagnosis
  - Survival depends on functional class (NYHA)
  - *Cause of death:*
    - RV failure
    - Hypoxemia
    - Tachycardia
    - Hypotension
    - Edema
- *Heritable PAH*
  - 6–10% of patients with PAH
- *Drug and toxin induced*
  - Anorexigen (serotonin reuptake Inhibitors)
  - Fenfluramine, dexfenfluramine
  - Rapeseed oil
  - Tryptophan
  - Illicit drugs (methamphetamines)
- *Associated with CTD:*
  - MC CREST syndrome — DLCO decreased first
  - 2nd scleroderma — Prominent hypoxemia
  - SLE, RA, Sjogren polymyositis

Investigation: PFT + ECHO

- *PAH associated with HIV* -rare
- *PAH associated with portal HTN*
  - Unknown Mechanism
  - Neither severity of liver disease nor degree of portal HTN predict presence of porto pulm HTN
  - Can increase mortality post liver transplant
- *PHTN associated with cong heart disease*
  - Eisenmenger syndrome
- *PAH with schistosomiasis*

Group 1': Pulm veno-occlusive disease: and pulm capillary hemangiomatosis

- Rare
- In addition to pathological change of PAH, this entity also exhibits findings of pulm venous HTN (pulm hemosiderosis, interstitial edema, lymphatic dilatation)
- May have crackles on examination and low DLco and SO_2
- Rapid development of pulm edema after administration of PAH specific therapy is first due to appropriate diagnosis
  ↓
  It can be life threatening
- Survival—poor
- Lung transplant is treatment of choice

Signs and Symptoms of Pulm Art HTN

- Develops insidiously over years
- MC = exertional dyspnea

Symptoms: Exertional dyspnea
   Fatigue
   Angina pectoris (RV ischemia)
   Syncope
   Near syncope
   Peripheral edema
   Orthopnea ⎤ If associated pulm venous HTN
   DND   ⎦

Examination: Gen: Raised JVP, decreased carotid pulse
   Peripheral cyanosis ⎤ later stage
   Peripheral edema   ⎦

CVS: Loud S2 (P2)
   Palpable RV impulse ⎤
   RV S4   ⎬ signs of RV dysfunction
   TR   ⎦

Signs that reflect severity of PH

- Accentuated S2 (P2); audible at apex
- Early systolic click
- Midsystolic ejection murmur
- Left parasternal lift
- RV S4
- Increased jugular a wave

Signs that suggest mod-severe PH

Mod-severe PH
- Holo systolic TR murmur
- Increased JVP V wave
- Pulsatile liver
- Diastolic murmur
- HJR

Advanced PH with RV fail
- RVS3
- distension of jug veins -Hepatomegaly
- Ascites
- Peripheral edema
- Low BP, low PP and cool extremities

Evaluation

- *ECG:* Neither sensitive nor specific
   RV hypertrophy + RAD (often with strain)
- *CXR:* Enlarged main and hilar PA with pruning of peripheral vasculature
   RV Enlargement on lat view
- *ECHO:* RAE, RV Enlargement, RV dysfunction
   Small underfilled left chambers
   IVS flattening
   TR
   Decreased TAPSE
  - Also helpful in assessment of Gr2 (LV dysfunction) and cong heart disease
  - Prognostic indicators 1. RV dysfunction severity
     2. Presence of pericardial eff

- *Vent perf scan:*
  - To rule out CTEPH
  - (*Note:* Diffuse defect of non-segmental nature can be often seen in PAH without thromboembolism)
- *Pulm function test:*
  - To check and rule out obstructive and restrictive disease
  - Gr 1 PAH usually have modest Restrictive defect
- *HCRT:* To rule out CTEPH and obstructive-restrictive disease
- *CMRI:*
  - Excellent assessment of RV function
  - Helpful in assessing CHD
  - RVEF <35% on CMR—poor prognosis
- *Overnight oximetry*
  - Detect OSA
  - Significant PAH (≥35 mm Hg) can rarely be due to sleep disordered breathing
  - However, untreated OSA will limit effectiveness of other treatment approach
- *Lab investigation*
  To screen for
  - Connective tissue disorder
  - HIV
  - Liver disease
  - Thyroid function test
- *Functional tests:* (6 min walk test/cardiopulm Ex)
  - To quantify exercise ability
  - Useful prognostic factor
  - Helps in monitoring during follow-up
- *Rt heart catheterization:*
  - To look for intracardiac shunt
  - To measure exact PAP and PCWP (Measured at end expiration)
  - To measure hemodynamics
  - To measure for reversibility with vasodilators
    Inhaled NO
    IV Adenosine
    IV Epoprostenol
    (Ac response defined as decrease in MPAP by at least 10 mm Hg to an absolute mPAP <40 mm Hg in setting of unchanged or Increased CD)
- *BNP:* Used to decide disease progression
  - Work up protocol

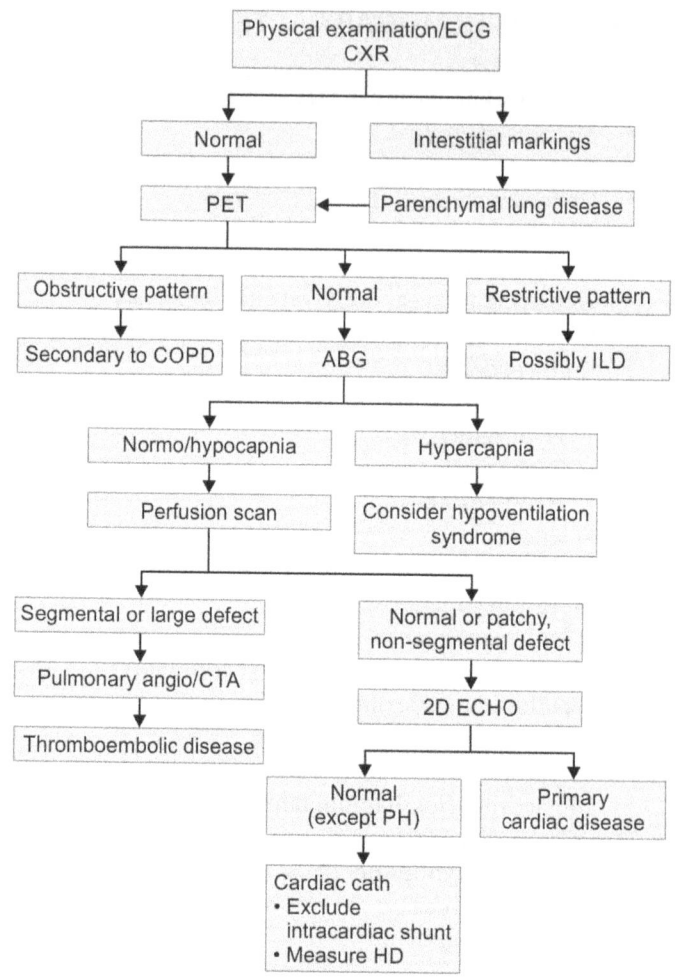

Management

Goal:
- Improve symptoms
- Improve RV function
- Improve exercise tolerance
- Improve hemodynamics

General measures
- Basic counseling and education + psychological support
- Low grade aerobic exercise (e.g., Walking)
- Avoid strenuous physical activity
- Avoid pregnancy (maternal mortality upto 50%)
- Influenza and pneumococcal vaccine
- O_2: Maintain SPO_2 >92%
- Salt restricted diet esp in patient with RV failure
- Diuretics
- Anticoagulants

Pulmonary Diseases

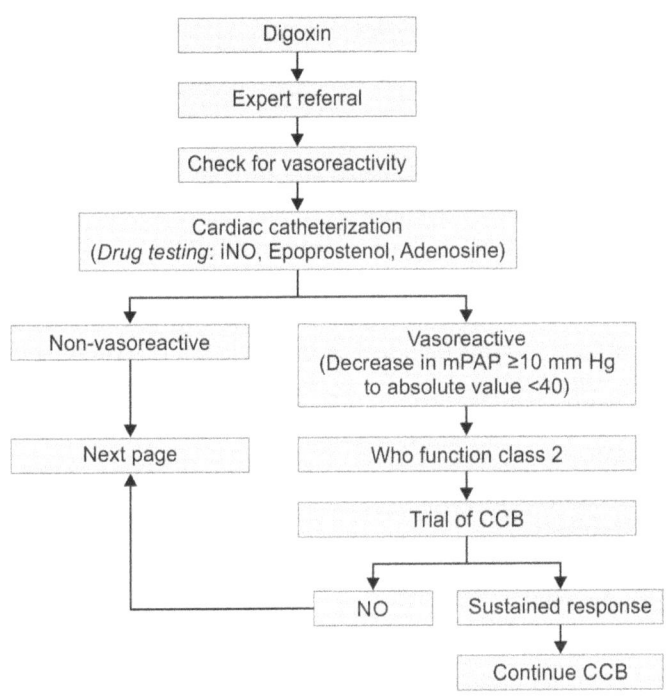

Medical Management (Drugs)

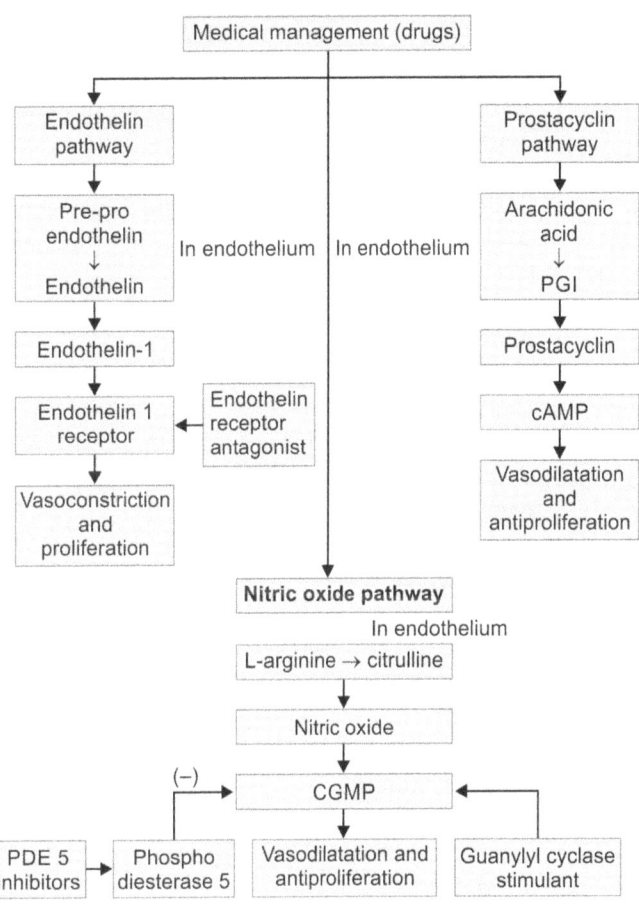

Initiate Treatment with PAH Approved Drugs

Class of recommendation	WHO FC 2	WHO FC 3	WHO FC 4
(1)	Sildenafil Tadalafil Bosentan Ambrisentan Macitentan Riociguat	Sildenafil Tadalafil Bosentan Ambrisentan Macitentan Riociguat Epoprostenol (IV) Treprostinil (SC/ inhal)	Epoprostenol IV
(2a)		Iloprost (iv) Treprostinil (iN)	All except epoprostenol (IV)
(2b)		Beraprost	

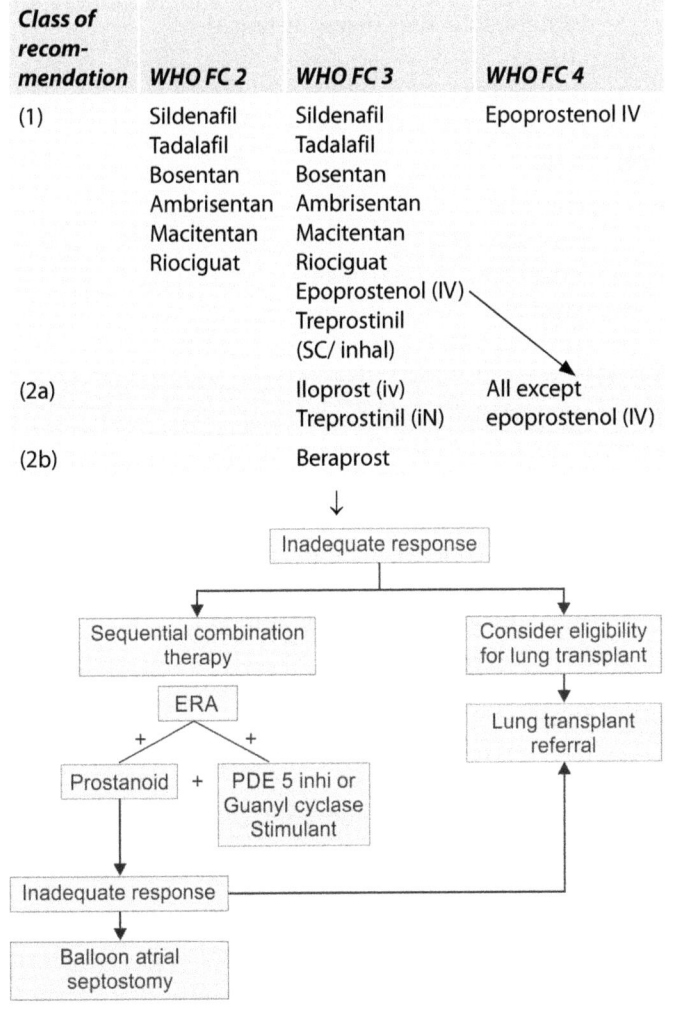

CCB

- Very effective for few patients with robust response to acute vasodilatation testing
- Very few patients do well over long term
- Not approved by USFDA
  - Nifedipine 240 mg/d
  - Amlodipine 20 mg/d
- If patient is non responder on cardiac cath, CCB should not be given as it may lead to given as it may lead to hypotension, reflex, achy, hypoxemia and RV failure.

Prostanoids

- Approved
- Improve symptoms and exercise tolerance
  - *Inhalational Iloprost*
    - 2.5–5 µg per inhalation
    - *S/E:* Cough, headache, Flushing, saw pain
    - Very short t ½ (<30 min)
    - Freq closing (every 2 hours)
    - *Adv:* Fewer systemic S/E
      Delivery limited to well-ventilated areas so reduce ventilation—perfusion mismatch

- *Intravenous—epoprostenol*
  - Was 1st therapy approved by US-FDA
  - Need cont IV infusion (LVC + ambulatory Infusion pump)
  - Stored in hospital at 2 mg/kg/min and titrated up optimal dose = 25–40 ng/kg/min
  - *S/E:* Diarrhea, Flushing, saw pain, rash
  - Positive Inotropic effect—long term high—output state have detrimental effect on cardiac function
- *IV/S/C: Treprostinil*
  - Stable prostacyclin analogue
  - Action similar to epoprostenol
  - Longer t ½ (4 hours)
  - Cont s/c or cont IV infusion
  - *Dose:* 75–150 ng/kg/min
  - *S/E:* Local pain at infusion site, headache, diarrhea, nausea, rash
  - Also approved for inhalation route
  - Oral treprostinil is not approved.

Endothelin Receptor Antagonist

- Bosentan, ambrisentan, macitentan
- Bosentan
- 62.5 mg BD × 1 month
- 125 mg BD to continue
- Require monthly LFT
- Improve symptoms and exercise capacity
- *Trial:* BREATH1
- *S/E:* Headache and LL edema, anemia
- Ambrisentan 5–10 mg daily
- No monthly LFT required
- *S/E:* Headache, LL edema
- Macitentan
- *S/E:* Headache, nasopharyngitis, anemia
- Edema and LFT derangement similar as compared to placebo.

PDE 5 Inhibitor

- Approved
- Improve symptoms and ex tolerance
- Sildenafil—20 mg TDS
- Tadalafil—40 mg OD
- *S/E:* Headache, Flushing, dyspepsia, myalgia, Epistaxis
- Rare episode of sudden loss of vision.

Soluble Guanylyl Cyclase Stimulator

- Riociguat
- Improve 6 mw distance and HD
- *S/E:* Headache, peripheral edema, Hypotension
- *Caution:* Not to be used concurrently with PDE 5 inhibitors.

Investigational Therapies

- Selexipag—oral, selective, prostacyclin, receptor antagonist
- Imatinib—tyrosine kinase inhibitor
  IMPRESS trial: Improved 6 mw distance and HD
  But serious adv events were more
- *Escitalopram:* Serotonin transport inhibitor
- Beraprost oral prostacyclin analog
- Inhaled NO and sodium nitrate

(Wait for 2 months for effect of any drug before switching to other therapy).

Surgery

- Balloon atrial septostomy
- Transplant

Prognosis

- 1, 2 and 3 year survival rate = 85.7%, 70% and 55%
- *Predictor of survival*
  - Male worse Prognosis
  - Functional class
  - Exercise tolerance (6 mw distance)
  - HD
  - RAP and CO.

Follow-up

- Patients who achieve
  - Function class 1 or 2
  - 6 mw distance >400 meters
  - Normal RV function
  - Normal cardiac cath RAP and CO/CI

Follow up every 3–6 months
- Functional class assessment every visit
- 6 MWT—every visit
- ECHO—yearly
- Rt heart cath if clinical deterioration
- BNP—center dependent
- If patient does not fulfill above criteria
- Follow-up every 1–3 months.

CTEPH

Definition

Based on findings described after at least 3 months of effective anticoagulation

Such findings include precapillary PH and at least one segmental perfusion defect detected by CT angio, lung scan and/or pulm angio.

Cause
Chronic obstruction of PA following PE.

Incidence
0.1 to 9.1% within 2 years after symptomatic events.

Pathophysiology
- H/O acute VTE observed in 75% patients
  - Inadequate anticoagulation ⎤
  - Large thrombus mass   ⎬ Risk factors
  - Residual thrombus   ⎪
  - Recurrence   ⎦
- Lupus anticoagulant/APLA ⎤ Found to be associated
  And coagulation factor 8 ⎦
- Pulm edema

↓

Pulm vascular remodeling process

↓

Modified by infection, immune phenomena, inflammation, malignancy, thyroid hormone replacement

↓

Hypercoagulation (sticky RBC, high plt count, uncleavable fibrinogen)

↓

Major vessel obliteration in CTEPH

- Other risk factors
  - Splenectomy
  - Ventriculo-atrial shunt for hydrocephalus
  - IBD
- CTEPH is small pulm vessel disease
  (Pulm arteriopathy)
  Caused by high flow or high pr state in prev unaffected artery or driven by hypoxia, infection and inflammation associated condition.

C/F: M = F
- Mean age = 63 years
- All age groups
- Almost normal on physical examination
- Late stage—non-specific signs of RV fail

- Symptoms similar to IPAH
- Edema and hemoptysis more common.

Investigation
- VQ scan is imaging of choice (initially)
- RHC will show precapillary PH
- CECT—PA webs and bands, wall irregularities, stenoses, aneurysms and complete vascular obstruction as well as bronchial collaterals
- Pulm angio confirms diagnosis.

Treatment
Surgery is treatment of choice: pulm endarterectomy

Operability criteria:
- NYHA 2, 3, or 4
- Pre op PVR >300 dysborsa cm^{-5}
- Surgery accessible thrombi
- HD severity
- Absence of severe comorbid disease

Four anatomical subtypes:

Type 1 (=~25%): Involve main and lobar PA with fresh red thrombus superimposed on white obstructions

Type 2 (40%): Intimal thickening and fibrosis of proximal to segmental arteries

Type 3 (30%): Fibrosis and intimal thickening confined to distal segmental and subsegmental arteries

Type 4 (<5%): Distal arteriolar vasculopathy

Not operable

Post OP
- Most patients exhibit almost normal HD and substantial release from symptoms
- 3-year survival 90%.

Medical Management
Anticoagulation
Diuretic
Chr O_2 supplement
Riociguat for inoperable CTEPH is under review by AHA

SECTION 18: Pregnancy and Heart

18.1 PREGNANCY AND HEART DISEASE

Q.1 Cardiovascular (CV) adjustment during normal preg (June 03, 04)

INTRODUCTION

- Symptoms and signs of normal pregnancy may mimic
  - Lightheadedness
  - Dizziness
  - Shortness of breath
  - Peripheral edema
  - Syncope

*Worrisome predictors of maternal cardiac events
- Prior cardiac events (e.g., HF, TIA, stroke) Arrhythmias
- Baseline NYHA class ≥2 or cyanosis
- L sided heart obstruction (MVA <2 cm^2, AVA <1.5 cm^2 or peak LVOT gr >30)
- LVEF <40%
- Mechanical valve prosthesis.

HEMODYNAMIC CHANGES

During Pregnancy

Profound and begin early in first trimester
- *Plasma volume:* Begins to increase in 6th week
  - By 2nd trimester—reaches 50% above baseline
  - Then plateaus until delivery
- Red cell mass increases—relative amenia of preg
- HR increases to 20% above baseline
- Uterine blood flow increases
- Fall in PVR—slight fall in BP
- Venous pr in LL increase—pedal edema (80% of healthy preg)
- Increased cardiac output = 30–50% above baseline by end of 2nd trimester.

Summary

Peripheral resistance decreases ⎫
Uterine blood flow increases   ⎬ Increased cardiac
Blood/pl volume increase 40-50% ⎬ output (30%)
Heart rate increases 10-20%   ⎬
Blood pr decreases slightly   ⎭
PVR decreases
Venous pr in LL increases = pedal edema (80% of normal preg).

Changes and CV Disease

- Increase in plasma volume is poorly tolerated by patients with low cardiac output status and impaired vent function with limited reserve
- Stenotic lesions are poorly tolerated because decrease in PVR increases gradient across AOV
- Tachycardia of preg decrease diastolic filling time
- So transmitral gradient increase in patients with ms leading to increased LA filling pr
- For MR—decrease in PVR improves cardiac output.

During Labor and Delivery

- With each uterine contraction 500 mL blood released into circulation

  ↓

  Rapid increase in CO and BP
  (CO increases 50% above baseline during 2nd stage labor and even higher during delivery)

  ↓

  During delivery: 400 mL blood lost during FTND
  800 mL blood lost during CS

  ↓

  Significant HD changes

- After delivery
  - Abrupt increase in venous return (because there is no IVC compression by fetus)
  - Autotransfusion of blood continues in 24 to 72 hours after delivery

  ↓

  Pulm of edema may develop
- For most patients with CV disease, vaginal delivery is feasible
- *Except:*
  - Patients on Anticoagulation—baby is also anti-coagulated—increased chances of ICH in vaginal delivery
  - Dilated unstable aorta (marfan synd)
  - Severe PH
  - Severe obstructive lesion (e.g., As)

  ↓

  If vaginal delivery is elected
  - Should be done in center with expertise
  - Left lat position, to avoid compensation on IVC
  - 2nd stage of labor should be assisted
  - Blood and vol loss should be replaced promptly
  - Swan-Ganz catheter and monitoring of HD should be done throughout labor and 24 hours after delivery (when pulm edema commonly occurs)
  - Antibiotics prophylaxis remains optional for patients most vulnerable to deleterious effect of endocarditis, i.e., with cyanotic heart disease and prosthetic valve.

Physical Examination in Normal Pregnancy

- Heart rate increases
- Pulse volume bounding
- JVP may be elevated with brisk descent (due to vol overload and decreased PVR)
- Apical impulse more prominent

D/D ASD
- S1 - loud, S2 - loud
- ESM at left sternal edge (not >3/6) due to increased flow through LVOT or RVOT
- S3 - common
- No diastolic murmur

- Cont murmur—cervical venous hum/mammary souffle
- Peripheral edema

Lab Investigation

- Women with heart disease have high BNP levels throughout pregnancy
  - BNP <100 pg/mL have a good NPV for predicting MACE.

2D-ECHO

- Cornerstone of evaluation
- Flow across left and right sided valve increases
- Careful comparison of 2D—anatomy will help differentiating this from true outflow abnormality
- Valve area calculation may be more helpful.

Fatal ECHO

- Can be achieved by 20th week of gestation.

Q.1 Management of aortic disease in preg (Dec 16)

Q.2 Management of patients with bileaflet valve in Ao position and preg

HIGH RISK PREG

- Pulm HTN (SPAP 60-70% higher than baseline SPAP)
- DCMP (EF <40%)
- Symptomatic obstructive lesions
  - As/ms/PS
- Coarctation of aorta
- Marfan syndrome with Ao root >40 mm
- Cyanotic lesions
- Mechanical valves.

CHD IN PREG

- *ASD:*
  - Usually tolerate preg, well without complication unless concomitant PHTN/AF
  - Elective closure is preferable before preg is contemplated
- *VSD:*
  - Usually tolerate preg
  - Large VSD with PHTN should be counseled not to undergo preg
- *PDA:* Tolerated well (except PDA with PH)
- *Cong As Usually 2° to bicuspid Ao valve*
  - Careful examination of entire Thoracic Ao for associated aortopathy, Ao dilatation, aneurysm
  - Preg CI of Ao diameter >4.5 cm
  - Mild As usually well tolerated
  - Mod As maybe well tolerated
    - (in absence of symptoms, normal result on exercise testing without ST-T changes)
  - Severe As (AVA <1 cm^2 or MG >50)—coursed not to have preg
  - Decrease in peri resistance exaggerate across AV
  - Patient respond well to bed rest and BB
  - Early delivery may be required
  - *Delivery*
    - Should be considered early CS

- Spiral block should be avoided (Hypotension)
- Central venous pressure monitoring
- Monitor for abrupt fall in afterload following delivery
- Monitor for blood loss
• Preg in women with severe As is char by increasing incidence of HF preterm labor and shorter preg duration
• BAV during 2nd trimester is possible with lead screening of mothers abd and pelvis
- *Coarctation of aorta*
  • May present first time during pregnancy with HTN
  • CoA impair flow to both uterus and fetus
    - Small for dates babies and fetal loss
  • *Treatment:* Control of BP (avoid Hypotension)
    - Percut stenting of Ao
    - Surgery
  • *Aortopathy:* Aorta is vulnerable to dilatation, Aneurysm and dissection
  • However, most women will have successful preg with core
- *PS:* Usually well tolerated
- *Cyanotic heart disease*
  • Risk for both mother and fetus
  • Pregnancy-decreased PVR—exacerbate right to left shunt-cyanosis
  • Pregnancy venous thrombosis—risk of paradoxical emboli
  • Degree of maternal cyanosis—impact on fetal growth with maternal oxygen less than 85%—poor fetal outcome
  • *problems:* HF
    Bact endocarditis
    Thrombotic complication (pulm and cerebral)
  • RV dysfunction-poor outcome
  • Controlled Anomalies (AD) - 22q11 deletion –50% chances of inheritance
- *Ebstein's anomaly*
  • Safety depends on RV function, degree of TR
  • If patient cyanotic at rest-risk increases
  • Atrial communication-risk for Paradoxical emboli
- *CCTGA:*
  • Usually successful preg if syst vein EF preserved
- *TOF:*
  • Most will have repaired surgery
  • Occasional adult without prev surgery or in whom palliation achieved with BT shunt
    - Pregnancy risk depend on cyanosis and RV function, residual PR, atrial Arrhythmias
  • Good surgical repair, good exercise capacity and minimal residual-preg well tolerated
- *TGA:*
  • Prognosis depends on
    1. Function of systemic ventricle
    2. Degree of syst AV valve regurgitation
    3. Degree of bare Obstruction
    4. Residual ASD
    5. Presence or absence of atrial Arrhythmias
- *Univent heart and Fontan*
  • High risk
  • Vulnerable to develop thrombosis in fontan circuit because of low flow and prothrombotic state of preg.

PULMONARY HTN

- High mortality
- Causes (ASD, VSD, PDA)
- When pulm HTN exceeds approx 60% of systemic level - freq is more likely to be associated with complications
- Maternal mortality ~ 50% in Eisenmenger
- *Problems:*
  • Volume load of preg—RV Failure
  • Fall in PVR—rt to lt shunt cyanosis
  • Hypovolemia at delivery—hypoxia, syncope and sudden death
  • Pulm embolism or pulm infarct
- Highest mortality during labor and peripar
- Even termination of preg. Pose a risk
- If NVD contemplated,
  • ICD delivery with monitoring
  • Epidermal analgesic (caution to prevent Hypotension)
  • Assisted 2nd stage of labor
  • Anti-DVT compression pump
- *If CS:* Cardiac anesthesia
- Post delivery, in hospital monitoring × 2 weeks
- Inhaled NO/sildenafil/epoprostenol useful
- *Post delivery:*
  • Appropriate advise for contraception
  • Estrogen containing contraceptives are contra-indicated.

VALVULAR HEART DISEASE

(MS)

- MC = bicuspid As and
- Worsen during preg due to increased pl volume, increased CO and decreased PVR
- Increased HR
  • Shorten diastole filling time
  • Exaggerate MV gradient

Management

- Cornerstone of therapy is BB
  - It slows HR—increased diastolic filling time and results in marked clinical improvement with control of symptoms
- Bed rest slow HR and clinical improvement
- Diuretics—only if pulm edema
- Anticoagulant
  - For AF
  - For patient with bed rest
- Balloon valvuloplasty (if favorable valve anatomy)
- *Surgical valvotomy:* For patient refractory to medical management and in whom BMV not possible

(MS/AR) well tolerated

PROSTHETIC VALVES

- *Tissue valves:* Less thrombogenic
  Do not req warfarin
- Mitral prosthesis degenerates faster than aortic prosthesis
- Use of homograft pose similar problem
- Mortality for 2nd valve replace surgery is as high as 6%-if death occurs after successful preg, child left without a mother
- *Mechanical prosthesis*
  - High thrombogenicity during preg
    - Significant increase in valve thrombogenicity and thromboembolism
  - Tilting disk in mitral position is most problematic
  - Anticoagulants increase risk of
    - Placental bleeding
    - Miscarriage
    - Fetal death
  - Addition of low dose aspirin confer additional benefits (but scant data)
- UFH does not cross placenta and is safe
  - Should be started as soon as preg detected
  - Cont until 13-14 week (fetal embryogenesis is completed)
  - Switch to warf
  - Studies show that valve thrombosis risk doubles on heparin (9 to 39%)
  - 33% increased risk in valve thrombosis if Heparin used throughout preg
- LMWH—does not cross placenta
  - Alternative to UFH
  - Recommended optimization of Anticoagulation based on monitoring anti Xa levels
  - Dose req changes dramatically throughout preg
  - Optimal data is limited regarding optimal anti Xa level, timing of measurement and Freq of testing
  - Valve thrombosis is still a problem
  - Recommends
    1. 12 hourly dosing
    2. Testing anti-alpha a level 4 hr post imaging
    3. Once weekly testing
    4. Maintain Anti alpha a level 1-1.2 u/mL
  - Switch to UFH at delivery
- *Warf:* 1st trimester: CI
  - Leads to fetal embryopathy
    Mild: Chondrodysplasia punctata
    Severe: Nasal hypoplasia, optic atrophy, and mental retardation
- *ESC:* Recommend use of warf in 2nd and 3rd trimester (until 36th week) with strict monitoring (class 1/c)
  - Because of fetal risk in 1st trimester is dose related, ESC recommends cont oral anticoag if warf dose is <5 mg/d (class 2a/c)
- No data on DTI or anti alpha a drugs.

ARRHYTHMIAS

- *Contributing factors*
  - Increase in preload causing Myocardial irritability
  - Increased HR may affect refractory period
  - Fluid and electrolyte shift
  - Changes in catecholamine levels
- Difficult to distinguish as symptoms of normal preg may mimic arrhythmias
- *Work-up*
  - Careful history
  - Look for precipitating cause
  - Concomitant medical problem (thyroid disease)
  - CBC
  - Electrolyte
  - ECHO
- *Management:*
  - In absence of underlying cardiac disease, pharmacological treatment (if patient is symptomatic or if Arrhythmia poses risk to mother/baby)
  - APC, VPC—no treatment required

- With underlying cardiac disease—treat cause as well as Arrhythmias
- Atrial Arrhythmias—treat conventionally
- SVT-vagal maneuver—adenosine
- Use lowest possible dose of any drug
- If medical management fails
  - Electrocardioversion with fetal monitoring is safe
- Catheter ablation should be considered only if unavoidable (high radiation exposure).

Antiarrhythmics
- Amiodarone—IUGR, Goiler, hypo and hyperthyroidism
- Beta-blocker—safe: can cause neonates Brady and hypoglycemia
- CCB—safe; concern during uterine tone during delivery
- Digoxin—safe; No S/E
- Flecainide—relatively safe
- Lidocaine—safe; High dose can cause neonatal CNS depression
- Adenosine—safe
- Atenolol and Amiodarone—contraindicated.

SECTION 19

Clinical Examination

19.1 DYNAMIC AUSCULTATION

Q.1 Dynamic auscultation: Its role in diagnosis of various heart disease (2003).
Q.2 Dynamic cardiac auscultation: Principle and clinical utility (June 16).

It is the technique of altering circulatory dynamics by variety of physical maneuvers and determining effect of these maneuvers on heart sound and murmur.

TYPES OF MANEUVERS

A. *Physical:* Respiration, position change, isometric hard grip, valsalva and Müller maneuver
B. *Non-deliberate:* Change in cardiac cycle length due to VPC, AF or heart blocks
C. *Pharmacological:* Vasoactive agents such as amyl nitrate, methoxamine and phenylephrine

Normal Respiration

- *Effect on heart sound:*
    - Inspiration—normal split of S2 ⎤
      Expiration—S2 heard as single sound ⎦ S2
    - S3, S4, and OS
        - RV S3 and S4 increase in intensity with inspiration
        - LV S3, S4 and MV OS increase in intensity with expiration (due to increased LV SV)
    - *Aortic ejection sound:*
        - Aortic valvular ES does not vary
        - Aortic vascular ES may increase with expiration
        - ES variable in large Bivent Truncus arteriosus and TOF with PA
    - *Pulm ejection sound:*
        - Best heard during expiration—intensity increased during inspiration
        - Inspiratory increase of venous return and RV SV leads to increased RVEDP beyond PADP—premature opening of PV in diastole itself—less upward motion of PV—decreased intensity of ES
        - Pulm vascular ES may increase with inspiration
- *Effect on murmur:*
    - All rt sided murmur increased during inspiration
    - All left sided murmur are best heard during expiration

Valsalva

- Effect on HS
    - During phase 2: S3 and S4 decrease; S4 split narrows
    - During phase 3: Due to sudden increase in SV return rt sided S3 and S4 augmented and S2 split widens
    - During phase 4: Left sided S3 and S4 increases
- *Effect on murmur:*
    - During phase 2: SV and SAP decreases—following murmur decreases
        - Syst murmur AS, PS, MR and TR
        - Diast murmur of AR, PR, MS and TS
    - During phase 2: Reduction in LV vol and size
        - Increased LVOTO with increased pr gr—increased syst murmur of HCM
        - Increased degree of valve prolapse in patients with MVP
            - Loud and early mid systolic click and murmur
    - *During phase 3:* Sudden increase in syst venous return result in increased rt sided murmur
    - During phase 4: Left sided murmur return to normal level and may transiently increases.

Müller Maneuver

- Exaggerates Inspiratory effort
- S2 split is widened
- RV S3 and S4 increases
- All rt sided murmur increases

Postural Changes

- *Sudden lying down from sitting/leg rising (passive)*
  - Increased syst venous return
  - Increased RV stroke vol initially
  - Increased LV stroke vol after several cardiac cycle
    ↓
  - Widening of S2 split in both phase of respi
  - Initially RV S3 and S4 increases; after several cardiac cycles LVS3 and S4 increases
  - Systolic murmur augmented AS, PS, MR, TR, VSD
  - Due to increased LVEDV and LV size
    ↓
  - SM of HOCM decreases
  - Click and murmur of MVP are delayed and decreases
- *Sudden standing from supine or squatting*
  - Reverse effects
- *Squatting from standing*
  - Increased venous return and SV
  - Increased SVR
  - Increased ABP with transient Brady
  - S3 and S4 accentuated
  - SM of PS and AS increases; DM of TS and MS increases
  - Decreased HOCM murmur and MVP murmur
  - Due to increased aortic reflux = inaudible murmur of AR becomes audible

Isometric Exercise (Hand Grip)

Increased SVR, Art pr, HR and CO and LV filling pr and size
↓

- LV S3 and S4
- DM of MS louder (due to increased CO)
- Increased DM of AR
- Increased SM of MR and VSD   (due to increased SVR)
- SM of HOCM decreases
- Click and SM of MVP is late and decreases

Change Cardiac Cycle Length Due to VPC/AF

VPC: Increase in vent filling pr and size
Increased contractility of next beat and transient elevation of SAP
↓

- Varying intensity of S1 (AF)
- SM of AS and PS increases
- DM of AR increases (due to increase in Art pr)
- SM of HOCM augmented due to increased LVOTO as a result of increased contractility—result in decreased vol of pulse (Brockenbrough Braunwald sign)
- Click and SM of MVP delayed because of decreasing prolapse due to increase in vent filling and size.

Pharmacological Agents

- *Amyl Nitrate:* During early relative hypotension after amyl nitrate inhalation, murmurs of MR, VSD and AR decrease whereas murmur of AS increases, during later phase of tachycardia, murmur of MS and rt sided lesion also becomes louder
- Help distinguished Austin-Flint from MS

Transient Arterial Occlusion

Compression of both brachial arteries by cuff inflation >20 mm Hg of SBP
↓

Augment murmur of AR, VSD, MR

DIASTOLIC MURMUR

MDM

Are diastolic murmur that begin at a clear interval after S2 in rapid vent filling phase

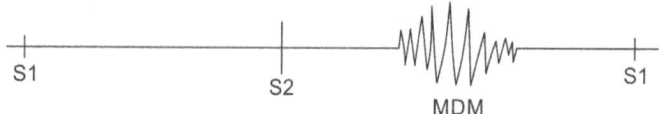

- Caused by forward flow across AV valves when atrial pr exceeds vent pr
- Low pitch and rumbling in character (because velocity of flow is relatively low)

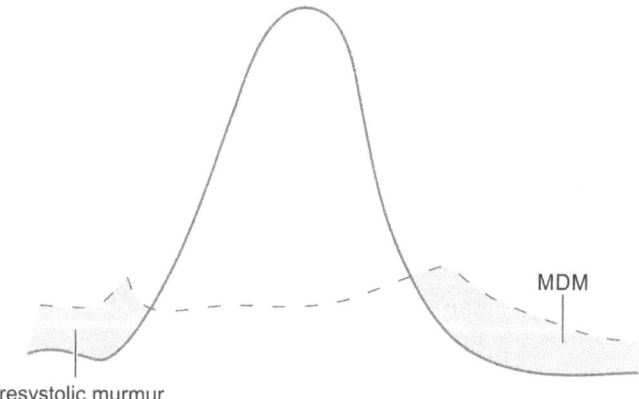

Etiologies

A. *LV inflow obstruction*
  - MS
  - LA myxoma
  - Cor triatriatum
  - Constriction around AV groove

B. *RV inflow obstruction*
  - TS
  - RA myxoma
  - Caranoid
  - Ebstein's anomaly

C. *Mitral diastolic flow murmur*
   - Severe MR
   - VSD
   - PDA
   - AP window
   - RSOV into RV
D. *Tricuspid diastolic flow murmur*
   - Severe TR
   - ASD
   - RSOV into RA
   - DAPVC
   - TAPVC
   - Single atrium

E. *MV opening interference*
   - Severe AR
   - Acute rheumatic carditis (Carey coombs)
F. *PR with No PH*
   - Organic PK.

PRESYSTOLIC MURMUR

- Occur in rapid vent filling phase which coincides with atrial systole
  Etio: MS
  TS
  CHB

19.2 HANGOUT INTERVAL

Q.1 What is hangout interval? Describe its mechanism and effect on Auscultation (June 13).

Q.2 Hangout interval mechanism and significance (Dec 15).

HANGOUT INTERVAL

- Semilunar valves are expected to close at the point of cross—over of the pressure, i.e., the point where vent pressure falls lower than the arterial pressure

  ↓

  However in reality, these valves close slightly latter (at incisura of aorta and pulm array)

  ↓

  This time interval from cross-over of pressure to actual closure (occurrences of A2 and P2) is called hangout interval

- Hangout interval depends on
  - Pressure in the arteries
  - Vascular resistance
  - Distensibility/compliance
  - Recoil of arterial system

Due to higher pressure and less compliance (distensibility) hangout interval on aortic side is less than that on pulmonary side.

- Hangout interval measured between incisura of aorta and LV pressure at same level on left side

  And

  Between incisura of PA and RV pressure at same level on right side

- Vent mechanical systole is sum of (IVCT + EP) = Hangout interval

On left side

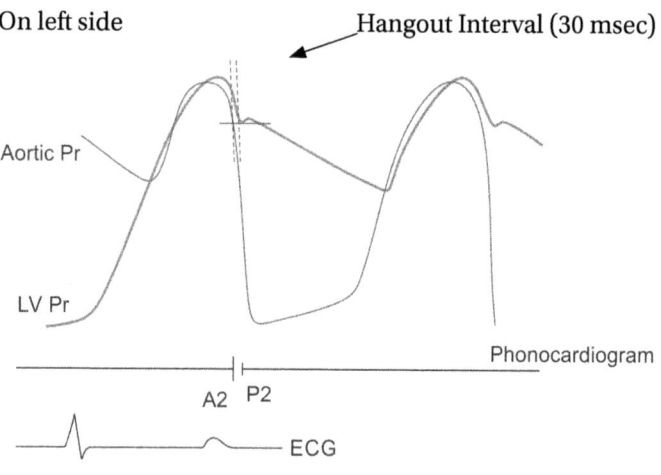

On right side

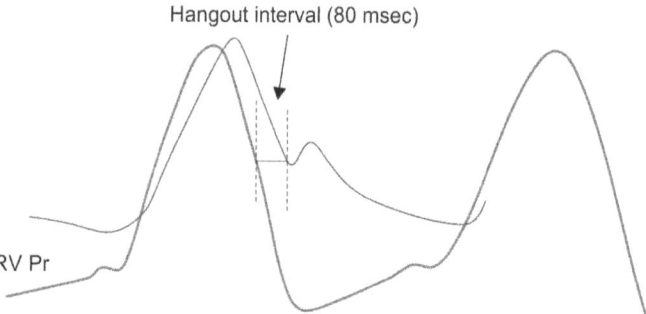

19.3 SECOND HEART SOUND

Q.1 Physiologic and hemodynamic basis of S2 in health and disease (Dec 12)
Q.2 Physiology and etiology of paradoxical split of S2 (June 2002)

INTRODUCTION

- S2 signals the onset of ventricular diastole
- Two component A2 (First component)
  P2 (Second component)
- Produced by sudden deceleration of retrograde flow of blood column in the aorta and pulm artery, which initiates the vibrations of hemocardiac structure coinciding with the closure of aortic and pulm leaflets.

CHARACTERISTICS OF S2

- High frequency
- 110 msec duration
- Incisura of aortic pr coincides with A2
- Incisura of pulm pr coincides with P2
- A2-P2 interval during inspi <30 msec
  Expiration 40-50 msec
- A2 is earlier than P2
- A2 is louder than P2 (even at pulm area)
- A2 well heard at aortic, pulm area and apex
- P2 well heard only at pulm area
- S2 is high pitch and Freq than S1 because
  1. Low elasticity of arterial trunk and SLV as compared to AV valve and ventricles
  2. Less blood volume in arteries than ventricle—so low inertia of vibrating mass—produce higher Freq of vibrations
  3. S2 is snappier and shorter than S2 because high freq. fibration damp out earlier and more rapidly.
- A2 early and loud than P2 because
  1. Louder due to high pr in Ao than PA
  2. Earlier than P2 due to
     - RV ejection begins early, lasts longer than LV ejection and ends after LV ejection resulting in delayed P2
     - Hang out interval on Ao side (30 ms) is less than that on pulm side (80 ms).

NORMAL PHYSIOLOGICAL SPLIT OF S2

- During expiration A2 and P2 separated by <30 ms, so heard as single sound
- While during inspiration A2-P2 separated by 40-50 ms
- Splitting best heard at 2nd or 3rd Lies

Mech of Normal Split

- Delayed P2 accounting for 73%
- Early A2 accounting for 27%

Abnormal Splitting of S2

Wide splitting	Reverse splitting
1. ASD	1. *LVOTO:* As
2. Significant MR	2. Complete LBBB
3. VSD	3. RV ectopic beats
4. Complete RBBB	4. RV pacing
5. VPC	5. PDA
6. LV pacing	6. WPW (type B)
7. Mod-severe PS with IVS	7. Chronic IHD
8. Acute PE	8. Hypotensive heart disease
9. PHTN with RV failure	9. Post stenotic dilatation of Ao 2° to AS and AR
10. Idiopathic dilatation of PA	

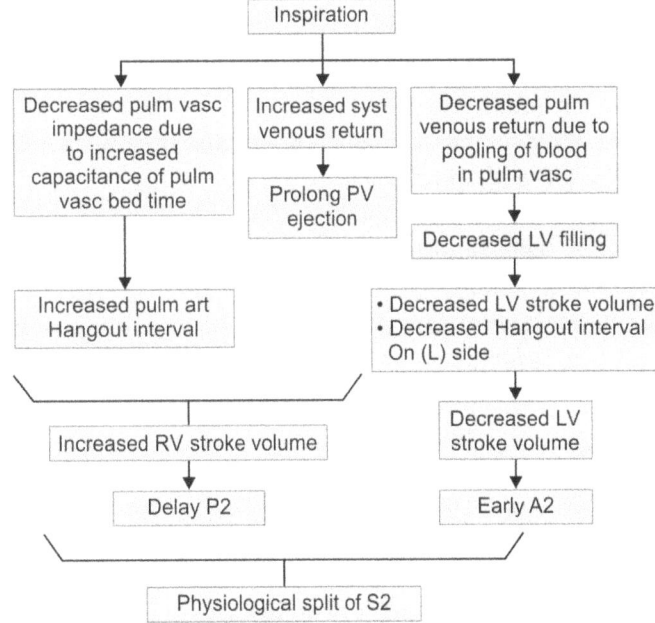

ABNORMAL SPLIT

- Defined as audible expiratory split both in supine and upright posture
  - Persistent physiological splitting
  - Wide splitting
  - Reverse or Paradoxical split
  - Single S2

A. *Wide physiological split:*
   - Due to delayed P2
     - *Delayed electrical activation of RV*
       - Complete RBBB
       - LV ectopic beat
       - LV pacing
     - *Prolonged RV mechanical systole*
       - Mod-severe PS with IVS
       - PH with RV failure
       - Ac PE
     - *Increased hangout interval*
       - Mild PS
       - Idiopathic dilatation of PA
       - Post op ASD
   - Early A2
     - *Shortened LV mechanical systole*
       - Significant MR
       - VSD
   - Other benign cause mimicking wide split
     - Pectus excavatum
     - Straight back syndrome
     - Occasionally in normal child
B. *Wide fixed split*
   - Wide because of increased pulm hangout interval (interval between crossing over of pr between RV and PA and closure of PV)
   - Fixed because LA and RA pr equalize because of ASD
   - ASD with variable split
     - ASD with AF
     - Sinus venosus type of ASD
C. *Reverse splitting*
   - See table on prev page
     - *Delayed Aortic closure A2*
       - *Delayed electrical activation of LV*
         - Complete RBBB
         - RV pacing
         - RV ectopic beats
       - *Prolonged LV mechanical systole*
         - LVOTO (As)
         - Hypertensive heart disease
         - Arteriosclerotic heart disease—chronic IHD
       - *Decreased impedance of SV bed (increased hangout interval)*
         - Post stenotic dilatation of AO
         - PDA
   - Due to early P2:
     - Early electrical activation of RV in WPW type 2
     - Rarely due to shortened LV filling as in RA myxoma or TR

D. *Single S2*

P2 absent/undetectable	A2 absent/undetectable
1. >60 years	1. Severe As
2. Obesity/thick wall/emphysema	2. Severe PS
3. Severe As	3. Severe PH
4. TOF	4. Aortic atresia
5. PA	5. Eisenmenger VSD
6. TA	6. Single vent
7. DORV with PS	
8. TGA	
9. Eisenmenger VSD	
10. Single vent	

S2 IN PATHOLOGICAL CONDITION

- *Valvular heart disease*
  - Mitral stenosis
    - *Mild-mod MS without PH:* Normal S2 and Normal O_2
    - *Severe MS with severe PH:* Narrow split with loud P2
    - Intensity of P2 correlate with PH severity
    - S2 - OS mistaken as wide split
      - S2-OS – S2 is louder (first component)
      - Split S2 – P2 is louder (second component)
  - Mitral regurgitation
    - *Mild-mod MR:* S2 split normal; P2 accentuated if PH
    - *Severe MR:* S2 split wide and variable
    - S2 split wide and fixed when complicated with HF; associated ASD; Associated AVCD
    - Reverse splitting of S2 in MR = Due to HDCM/CAD
  - Aortic stenosis
    - Single S2 due to masking effect of P2 or absent A2
    - Reverse splitting
  - Aortic regurgitation
    - Usually normal split of S2
    - A2 loud in aortic root cause of AR
    - A2 soft in valvular causes of AR
    - A2 may be loud when associated with VSD/ TOT
- *Congenital heart disease*
  - ASD:
    - Wide and fixed split S2 with loud P2 (even in absence of PH)
    - Eisenmenger—S2 split remain wide with loud P2
  - VSD:
    - Small VSD—Normal split with Normal P2
    - Mod VSD—Normal S2 split with moderate accentuation of P2
    - Large VSD—Narrow split with loud P2
    - *Eisenmenger:* Single loud P2
    - VSD with PS—single loud A2

- *PDA:*
  - *Small:* Normal S2 split and normal intensity P2
  - *Large:* Normal S2 split with accentuated P2
  - Eisenmenger PDA—closely split S2 with loud P2
- *PS:*
  - *Mild PS:* Normal S2 split with Normal intensity P2
  - *Mod severe PS:* Wide variable split with diminished P2
  - Dysplastic PV; Absent P2
- *BAV:* In absence of AS/AR—S2 normal with accentuated A2
- *COA:* Normal splitting of S2 with accentuated A2 due to HTN

- *Cyanotic heart disease*
  - *Single S2*
    - Single loud A2 in TOF (due to absent P2 and Ant-dextroposed aorta)
    - Single loud A2 in TGA, DORV, single vent: P2 inaudible due to post placed pulm trunk
    - Single loud A2 in TA due to absent P2
    - Single loud S2 in truncus arteries
  - *Wide splitting*
    - TAPVC
    - Eisenmenger ASD
    - Ebstein anomaly
    - Single atrium
    - PS with IVS

19.4 HISTORY TAKING AND PHYSICAL EXAMINATION

FUNCTIONAL CLASS

- *NYHA functional class*
  - Patient with cardiac disease without any limitation of physical activity—ordinary physical activity does not cause undue fatigue, palpitation, dyspnea or anginal pain
  - Patient with cardiac disease with slight limitation of physical activity—comfortable at rest. Ordinary physical activity results in fatigue, palpitation, dyspnea or anginal pain
  - Patient with cardiac disease with marked limitation of physical activity. Comfortable at rest less than ordinary activity results in fatigue, palpitation, dyspnea or anginal pain
  - Patient with cardiac disease with inability to carry any physical activity without discomfort. Symptoms of cardiac insufficiency or anginal syndrome may be present even at rest. If any physical activity is carried—discomfort is increased.
- *CCS functional class*
  - Ordinary physical activity (such as walking and climbing stairs) does not cause angina. Angina occurs with strenuous or rapid or prolonged exertion at work or recreation
  - Slight limitation of ordinary activity
  - Walking or climbing stairs rapidly, walking uphill, walking or stair climbing after meal, in cold, in wind or when under emotional stress or only during few hours after awakening
  - Walking >2 blocks on the level and climbing >1 flight of ordinary stairs at a normal pace and in normal condition
  - Marked limitation of ordinary physical activity. Walking 1-2 blocks on the level and climbing more than one flight of ordinary stairs in normal condition
  - Inability to carry on any physical activity without discomfort
- *Specific activity scale:*
  - Patient can perform to carry completion any activity req >7 mets
  - Patient can perform to carry completion any activity req >5 mets
  - Patient can perform to carry completion any activity req >2 mets
  - Patient cannot perform to completion activities requires ≥2 mets.

SECTION 20

ECG and Stress Test

20.1 ELECTROCARDIOGRAPHY

MEASURE OF VENT RECOVERY

- QT interval
- QT dispersion
  - In normal individual QT interval vary by up to 65 msec—referred as QT dispersion
  - Longest in lead V2 and V3
  - Increase in max range of intervals have been related to electrical instability and arrhythmogenesis
- QRST angle
  - Angle can be visualized in 3D space between the vector representing mean QRS force and vector representing ST-T force
    ↓
  - Known as QRST angle
    ↓
  - Angle between 2 vectors in horizontal plane is simplification and normally is <60°
  - Abnormal QRST angle reflect Abnormal relationship between properties of activation and recovery.
- *Vent gradient:* If the 2 vectors representing mean activation and mean recovery gradient are added—third gradient known as vent gradient is created. This vector represents the net area under QRST complex.

LA ABNORMALITY

- Prolonged P duration >120 msec on lead 2
- Prominent notching of P in lead 2, interval between notches of > 4 msec (P mitrale)
- Ratio between the duration of P wave in lead 2 and duration of PR seg >1.6
- Increased duration and depth of terminal negative position of P wave in lead V1 so that area subtended by it >0.04 mm-sec
- Leftward shift of mean P axis between −30 and −45.

RA ABNORMALITY

- Peaked P wave with amplitude in lead 2 to >0.25 MV (P pulmonale)
- Prominent initial positivity in lead V1 or V2 >0.15 MV
- Increased area under initial positive portion of P wave in lead V1 to >0.06 mm-sec
- Rightward shift in mean P axis (>+75).

LVH CRITERIA

- Sokolow-Lyon voltage: SV1 + R VS >3.5 mv
                              RaVL >1.1 mv
- Romhilt-Estes point score system
  - Any limb lead R wave or S wave >2.0 mv   (3 pt)
    - or SV1 or SV2 >3 mv   (3 pt)
    - or RV5 or RV6 >3 mv   (3 pt)
  - ST-T wave abnormality; NO digitalis therapy   (3 pt)
  - ST-T wave abnormality; digitalis therapy   (1 pt)
  - LA abnormality   (3 pt)
  - LAD ≥−30°   (2 pt)
  - QRSe ≥90 msec   (1 pt)
  - Intrinsicoid deflection in V5 or V6 ≥50 msec   (1 pt)
- Cornell voltage criteria
  SV3 + RaVL ≥2.8 mv (men)
                   ≥2.0 mv (women)
- *Cornell regression equation:* Risk of LVH = 1/lte^-exp
- Cornell voltage duration measurement
  QRSD × Cornell voltage >2,436 mm-sec^3
  QRSD × sum of voltage in all leads >1,742 mm-sec

RVH CRITERIA

- R in V1 ≥0.7 mv
- S in V5 ≥0.7 mv
- Rls in V1 >1 with R >0.5 mv
- R/s in V5 <1
- QR in V1
- RAD (>90 degrees)
- S1 Q3 pattern
- S1S2S3 pattern
- P pulmonale.

D/D OF Q WAVES

- Myocardial Infarction
- Physiological or positional
  - Normal variant septal Q waves
  - Normal variant Q waves in V1-V2, 3 and avE
  - Left pneumothorax/dextrocardia
- Myocardial injury/infiltration
  - Acute process—Myocardial ischemia without infarction, myocarditis, hypokalemia
  - Chronic process—Idiopathic cardiomyopathies, myocarditis, amyloid, tumor, sarcoid
- Vent hypertrophy/enlargement
  - LVH (slow and progression)
  - RVH (reversed R prog or poor R prog, esp with COPD)
  - HCM
- Conduction abnormality
  - LBBB
  - WPW

D/D OF AT ELEVATION

- Myocardial ischemia l infarction
  - Acute MI
  - Post MI
  - Non-infarction transmural ischemia (e.g., Prinzmetal angina, Takotsubo)
- Acute pericarditis
- Normal variants (early repolarization)
- LVH, LBBB (V1-V2, V2 only)
- Other
  - Acute PE
  - Brugada pattern
  - Class 1c antiarrhythmics
  - DC cardioversion
  - Hypercalcemia
  - Hyperkalemia
  - Hypothermia
  - ICH
  - Myo injury (trauma)
  - Myocarditis
  - Tumor invading LV.

20.2 EXERCISE TESTING

Q.1 Effect of exercise on myocardial O_2 demand and supply relationship. Diagnostic value of ex ECG for identification of coro art disease. Progno value of exercise ECG (4+4+2) (June 17).

PHYSIOLOGY OF EXERCISE TESTING

- Total body O_2 uptake

  Exercise
  ↓
  Exercise muscle require energy
  ↓
  Energy derived from O_2 metabolism to generate ATP
  ↓
  Can be estimated by measurement of total body oxygen uptake (VO_2)

  $VO_2 = CO \times \Delta A\text{-}VO_2$—Fick equation

  - VO_2 can be expressed in multiple of nesting O_2 requirements (metabolic equivalent)
  - 1 MET = 3.5 mL/kg/min
  - 5 META means energy required is 5 times than energy required at rest
  - VO_2 max is (maximum) peak O_2 uptake achieved during highest level of dynamic exercise
  - VO_2 max beyond certain level can't be achieved despite increase in work rate
  - CO can increase as much as 4–5 times ⎤
  - SV plateaus at 50% to 60% of VO_2 max   ⎬ Reason
  - O_2 extraction at periphery can increase as much as 3 fold and max A-VO_2 diff has a physiologic limit of 15–17 mL/100 mL blood ⎦

  During stress testing patients are prompted to exercise not until they attain VO_2 max but rather to the VO_2 that is obtained during symptom limited, maximum tolerated exercise
  - This is termed the VO_2 peak.

- *Effect on myocardial O_2 demand and supply:*
  Exercise testing enables clinician to
  - To assess for development of myocardial ischemia
  - Also evaluate at what level of myocardial O_2 demand and physical activity myocardial ischemia occurs

  Myocardial O_2 demand
  - Depends on HR, BP, LV contractility and LV wall stress
  - LV wall stress is related to these affects myocardial O_2 demand
    ↓
    Change in any of these affects myocardial O_2 demand

Rate pressure procedure (HR × BP) is a reliable index of O_2 demand

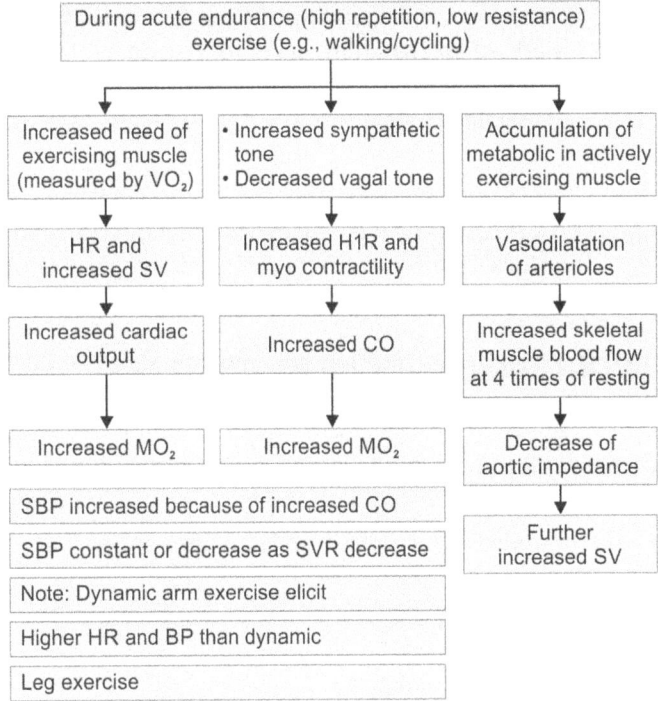

- *Resistance* (low repetition/high load) exercise (weight lifting)
  - Not generally used during exercise testing
  - Generate increased symp response—increased HR
  - However venous return may decrease during strain
    ↓
    So rise in CO is relatively small
  - Muscle contraction during strength training compress capillaries—increased SVR—increased both SBP and DBP
    (SBP increase because of increased CO)
    (DBP increase because of increased SVR)

Both endurance Ex and resistance Ex increase MO_2 because of:
1. Increased HR
2. Increased BP
3. Increased LV contractility
4. Increased wall stress

- Myocardial O_2 supply:
  - Coro blood flow increases during exercise in response to neurohormonal stimulation (primarily beta receptor stimulation—sympathetic) and as a result of release of endothelial substance (including NO)

↓
So in normal individual
Coro art dilates and CBF increases

In patient with atherosclerotic plaque

CBF decreases (depending on degree of obstruction, length of obstruction, no and size of collateral vessels, magnitude of muscle mass supplied and autoregulatory capacity)
↓
Exercise stimulates local change in vasomotor tone as a result of neuro modulation, endothelial dysfunction and local factors—can factor influence supply of O_2 to myocardium.

CONTRAINDICATIONS TO STRESS TEST

Absolute

- Acute MI within 2 days
- High risk UA
- Uncontrolled arrhythmias with HD compromise
- Active endocarditis
- Symptomatic severe As
- Decompensated HF
- Acute PE or pulm infarction
- Ac myocarditis/pericarditis
- Physical disability.

Relative

- Known LMCA disease
- Mod As with uncertain relation to symptoms
- Tachyarrhythmias with uncontrolled VR
- Acquired CHB
- HCM with severe resting gradient.

INDICATION FOR TERMINATING TMT

Absolute

- ST elevation >1 min (in leads without 2 because of prev MI)
  - Other than aVR, aVL, V1
- Drop in SBP >10 mm Hg when accompanied by any other evidence of ischemia
- Mod to severe angina
- Signs of poor perfusion (cyanosis, pallor)
- Sustained VT
- CNS symptoms (dizziness, near syncope)
- Technical difficulties monitoring ECG or BP
- Patients request to stop.

Relative

- Marked ST displacement (>2 mm horizontal or downsloping) in patients with suspected ischemia
- Drop in SBP >10 mm Hg without any other evidence of ischemia
- Increasing chest pain
- Arrhythmias other than sust VT (multiple actopy, vent triplet, NSVT, SVT, Bradyarrhythmias)
- Exaggerated hypertensive response (SBP >250 mm Hg and/or DBP ≥115 mm Hg)
- Fatigue, SOB, wheezing, leg cramps/claudication
- Development of BBB that can't be distinguished from VT.

EXERCISE TESTING IN PATIENTS WITH CAD

- Clinical response
  - Ex induced angina is imp clinical predictor of presence and severity of CAD
- Exercise capacity
  - Strong predictor of mortality and nonfetal CV outcomes with or without CAD
  - Most accurately measured by CPAX
  - Predicted METS
    Men: 18−(0.15 × age)
    Women: 14.7−(0.13 × age)
  - Reported METS can be expressed as percentage of expected METS
  - Multiple scores available for Ex capacity
    - Duke treadmill score
    - Cleveland Cline score
- *Hemodynamic response:* Maximum HR
  [HRmax = 220 − age]
  New equation has been proposed
  Men: HRmax = 208−(0.7 × age)
  Women: HRmax = 206−(0.88 × age)
  CAD with BB: HRmax = 164−(0.7 × age)
- Chronotropic incompetence
  Definition: Inability of heart to increase its rate to meet the demand placed on it
  - Independent predictor of cardiac or all-cause mortality
  Submaximal study: When peak HR achieved predefined goal, i.e., 80–85% of predicted MHR
  Inadequate study: Failure to achieve predefined goal, i.e., 80–85% of predicted MR

  Chronotropic incompetence incorporates
  - Baseline resting HR
  - Peak HR
  - Age adjusted HR

Chronotropic index = [(HR peak – HR rest) × 100]/[(220 – age) – HR rest]
- Failure to achieve chronotropic index >80% defined presence of chronotropic incompetence
- For patient on BB; index <62%—chronotropic incompetence

Before labeling chronotropic incompetence

Consideration must be given to
- Effort exerted in performing ex
- Present medications
- Reason for termination of test

Defined by:
- Symptoms produced
- Bong scale (indices of perceived exertion)
- CPx parameters (e.g., Respi exchange ratio)

- *Early HR acceleration:* Ambiguous study reports
- HR recovery
  - Initial steep 30 seconds fa and then gradual fall
  - Abnormal HRR = <12 beats/min after 1 min with post exercise cool down; <18 BPM with 1 min with immediate cessation of movt into either supine position and <42 BPM after 2 mins
- *BP:* SBP increased minimally
- Exaggerated SBP response
  - >210 female and >190 male
  - Indicate future dec of HTN
- Ex induced hypotension
  - Its presence warrants consideration of prompt invasive evaluation
- Other
  - Systolic pr peak is low—associated with severe CAD
  - Recovery systolic pr response—worse or prognosis with abnormal response
  - Double product reserve—better than HR
- ECG response
  - ST depression—flat or down sloping
  - Up sloping ST depression—can be considered abnormal if associated with low workload
  - *aVR:* 1 mm or greater ST elevation—Lm disease
  - ST segment adjustment
    - Complicated method ST/HR slope
    - *Simple method:* ST/HR index
  - ST elevation—poor progno
  - Change in QPSd—CAO if it occurs at lower HR
    - Ex induced RABB—not associated with CAD
  - *T wave alternans:* Strong neg predictive value means its absence indicate who will not benefit from ICD
  - Pseudo normalization of T- non-specific
  - Arrhythmia.

DIAGNOSTIC VALUE OF EX-TEST
- Sensitivity and specificity
  - Cut point of 0.1 MV (1 mm) of horizontal or downslope ST depression in 3 consecutive beats in at least a single lead

  Sensitivity 68%; Specificity 77%
  - Higher sensitivity in patients with TVD rather than SVD
- Ex induced ST depression does not give info about
  - Extent of disease
  - Specific coro vessel involved
  ST elevation can localize transmural infarction
- Pretest probability and post-test probability
  Changes act to age and presentation

  Greatly affects PPV and NPV
- Women
  - Premenopausal women with one or fewer risk factor of CAD with atypical symptoms—Diagnostic value of Ex-test high rate of false positive test

  TMT is limited value in such age group except reassurance
  - Sensitivity 36–76%
  - Specificity 60–86%
  - Non-ST segment variables
    - Peak ex capacity (METS) ⎤
    - Chronotropic response ⎥ More useful
    - HRR for prognosis   ⎥
    - BP response   ⎦
  - TMT is recommended choice for women who are symptomatic, intermediate risk, can exercise and have normal resting ECG.

PROGNOSTIC VALUE

Strongest predictor = Exercise capacity
Weakest predictor = ST depression

Prognostic Score
- Puke treadmill score
  - Ex time (Bruce)
  - mm of ST deviation (except aVR)
  - Anginal score index (1 = non-limiting angina 2 = exercise limiting angina)
Score = Ex time – (5 × ST deviation) – (4 × Angina index)

Prog value independent of
- Coro anatomy
- LV function data

- Sex specific score
  Includes various parameters

Men	Women
Max HR	Max HR
Age	Age
Ex ST dep	Ex ST dep
Angina history	Angina history
Diabetes	Diabetes
Ex test: Induced angina	*Ex test:* Induced angina
Hypercholesterolemia	Smoking
	Estrogen status

  Score given for all variables and prognosis calculated
- Cleveland Clinic score

TMT IN PATIENTS WITH AS

- When peak velocity >5.5 m/sec—TMT should not be done
- Purpose of TMT is As is to induce symptoms or abnormal BP response
- Special emphasis should be given to minute by minute BP response, patients symptoms and heart rhythm
- Terminate of limiting dyspnea, fatigue, angina, dizziness, any decrease in SBP, and complex vent ectopic
- If possible give 2 mins cool down walk and avoid supine position (to prevent acute LVVO).

Appropriate Patient

- Asymptomatic or equivocally symptomatic severe As
- Able to perfusion TMT   ↓
- No CI to AVR   AVA <1 cm²
                                 Mean Gr >40
                                 Peak vel 4–5.5
                                 Normal LV function

Treadmill Specific

- Mod Bruce with less intense early stage
- Min by min BP assessment
- Cool down walk.

Normal Ex Response

- Predict absence of stenosis related symptoms and death for 1 year
  - Valve surgery can be delayed
  Normal BP response
  - NO decreased from baseline
  - Ex associated increase of >20 mm Hg
  - Fall of <10 mm Hg from peak
  No angina/dizziness
  No complex vent ectopy
  Age appropriate ex capacity.

OTHER CONDITIONS WHERE TMT CAN BE PERFORMED

- HCM
  - Define presence of ex-induced LVOTO
  - Identify patient with co existent CAD
  - Detect patients with high risk indicator of abnormal BP response
- Adult CHD
  - Unrepaired adult COA
    To assess for ex induced hypotension
  - Repaired TOF
- Arrhythmia
  Class 1
  - Assess rate adaptive pacemaker
  - Long AHB
  Class 2a
  - Known or suspected ex induced arrhythmias
  - Evaluation of med, surgery and ablative treatment
  - Evaluation of AF
  - Assessment of adequate rate control
  - T wave alternans for diagnosis and risk stratification
  Class 2b
  - Isolated vent ectopy in middle aged
  - 1° HB, Wenkeback, LBBB, RBBB
  - Pre-excitation
  - LQT:
    - LQT1—Ex induced prolongation
    - LQT2—Ex induced shortening (normal)
    - LQT3—Super normal shortening
- Physical activity and exercise prescription
- Disability assessment (e.g., PAD).

PROTOCOLS

- Bruce:
  Adv:
  - Widely used in past
  - Bases of older studies
  - Comparison is easier
  Diasdv:
  - Large increment of change in workload between stages
  - 4th stage can be run or walk—resulting in divergent O_2 cost and workload
- *Modified bruce:*
  Adv:
  - For less fit person
  - Additional stage 0 and ½
  - Lower workload for person with poor CV fitness

- Others
  - Superior to Bruce
  - Gradual increase in workload
  - Can be modified to suite individual
    - Naughton protocol
      - Good for older or debilitated person
    - Balke protocol
      - Good for younger fit person
      - Maintain speed of 3, 3.5, 4 men and increase grade every 2 mins
    - Cornell protocol
      - Good for wide range of fitness level
    - Ramp protocol
      - Advanced computer driven protocols.

STRESS TEST POST MI

Class 1:

- Before (D) for prognostic assessment, activity prescription and evaluation of medical treatment (submaximal test at about 4-6 d)
- Early after (D) for prognostic assessment, cardiac rehabilitation if not performed pre discharge (symptoms limited, about 14-21 d)
- Late after (D) for prognostic assessment, activity prescription, cardiac rehab and evaluation of medical management (symptoms limited; 3-6 weeks).

BASELINE ABNORMALITY THAT MAY OBSCURE ECG CHANGES DURING EX

- LBBB
- LVH with repol abnormality
- Digitalis therapy
- Vent paced rhythm
- WPW synd
- ST abnormality associated with SVT/AF
- ST abnormality with MVP and severe anemia.

Complications

- Cardiac arrest
- *Ischemia:* Angina; MI
- *Arrhythmia:* SVT, AF, VT, VF
- *Bradyarrhythmias:* BBB, AV blocks
- CHF
- HTN/hypotension
- Aneurysm rupture
- Underlying medical condition predisposing to Compli
  - HCM; CAD; Idiopathic LVH
  - Marfan; As; RV dysplasia; CHD; LQTS
  - Myocarditis; pericarditis
  - Amyloidosis; sarcoidosis
  - Sickle cell trait
- Pulm complications
  - Ex induced asthma
  - Bronchospasm
  - Pneumothorax
  - Exacerbation of underlying pulm disease
- GI-vomiting, diarrhea
- *Neurologic:* Dizziness, syncope, CVA
- *Musculoskeletal:* Mechanical injury, back injury, joint pain, muscle cramps/spasm

SECTION 21: ECHO

21.1 INTRACARDIAC FLOW VORTEX IMAGING

INTRODUCTION

- At several points within CV system, blood flow breaks down into nonlaminar spiral flow known as vortices.
  ↓
- It represents important physiological adaptation required to maintain delicate balance between energy conservation, conversion and dissipation

NORMAL BLOODSTREAM

Two types of flow force
1. Pressure head and momentum—driving forward flow
2. Viscosity and shear stress between fluid layers and containing boundaries—try to slow down the blood flow
   ↓
   Fluid in center have highest velocity
   ↓
   As blood enters chamber through valve
   ↓
   Peripheral layer of blood flow loses its contact with the surrounding wall
   ↓
   Outer fluid layer curl or spin away from central core to produce spiral vortices.

VISUALIZATION AND QUANTIFICATION

- *CMR:*
  - Velocity encoded phase—contrast CMR
  - Permits only 20 visualization of blood flow
  - For an assessment, multiple cardiac cycles need to be assessed
  - Can also produce 4D flow CMR

Advantages
- Complete visualization of heart and large vessels
- Good spatial resolution
- High accuracy.

Disadvantages
- Low temporal resolution
- Longer screen time
- Need for breath holding
- Cost
- C—I in patient with device
- Requires gating over several cardiac cycle—not useful for arrhythmia
- *Echo cardiography:*
  - Easy, safer real—time imaging, simultaneous assessment of cardiac function and str
  - Techniques
- Echocardiographic particle imaging velocimetry
  - Most promising
  - Utilize ultrasound contrast
  - Principle similar to speckle tracking
  - Complete 3D flow pattern not possible
- Vector flow mapping or Echo dynamography
  - Color Doppler based
  - Axial and radial velocities combined to calculate flow vector at each site
  - Low temporal resolution
- *Others:*
  - Cross beam ultrasound
  - Combining color flow and speckle tracking

With any of method (MRI/ECHO), quantitative parameters are achieved

- Measure of vortex location
  - Vortex depth
  - Vortex transverse position
- Measure of vortex morphology
  - Vortex length
  - Vortex width
  - Sphericity index
- Measure of vortex pulsatility
  - Vortex relative strength
  - Vortex pulsation correlation.

ABNORMALITY OF VORTEX FLOW IN VARIOUS DISEASE

- LV flow abnormality
  - LV remodeling in patient with global or regional dysfunction
  - LV thrombus in patient with global or regional dysfunction
  - LV remodeling in other cardiomyopathies (LVOTO-HCM)
  - Abnormality of LV diastolic dysfunction
  - LV remodeling in patient with MV disease and following MVR
  - LV mechanical dyssynchrony
- Atrial flow abnormality
  - Risk of atrial arrhythmia
  - Risk of atrial thrombus formation
  - Atrial dysfunction in various CHD
- Abnormality of flow pattern in great vessel
  - Risk of developing aortic dilation, aortic dissection
  - Risk of developing aortic atherosclerosis, carotid art disease, renal artery stenosis
  - Retrograde cerebral embolization from complex plaques in descending thoracic Ao
  - Development of pulm thrombo embolism, pulm HTN, etc.

21.2 SPECKLE TRACKING

INTRODUCTION

- Offline analysis of digitally recorded and ECG triggered come loops
- Use speckle artifacts in echo image
- *Speckles:* Natural acoustic markers for tagging the myocardium motion during cardiac cycle
- Helps in calculation of myocardial velocities
- Speckles are small dots or group of myocardial pixels that are created by the interaction of ultrasonic beam and myocardium
  ↓
  Considered as acoustic fingerprints of that region
  ↓
  It enables to judge the direction of movt, speed of such movement and distance of such movement of any points in myocardium.

METHOD

- Track endocardial and epicardial borders of LV
- Correctly define region of interest in long and short axis
- Post processing software automatically divides ventricle into 6 equally distributed segments
- Mathematical algorithm applied to generate values.

Images Required

- 4 chamber ⎤
- 2 chamber ⎬ To measure LV longitudinal strain
- 3 chamber ⎦
- SAX at basal ⎤ To measure radial and circumferential
- Mid and apical ⎦ strain
- SAX at base and apex ⎤ To measure LV rotation and torsion

Caution

- Utmost imp to quality of image
- Optimize gain setting
- Reduce depth
- On PLAX—avoid foreshortening of LV
- On SAX—LV cavity should be circular
- Grayscale frame rate b/w 30-70 frames/sec
- At lower frame rate, large displacement of speckles between successive from precludes satisfactory tracking of speckles
- At high frame rate, spatial resolution of image gets compromised

Image opened in offline application
↓
Software analyze AV valve movt to determine systole and diastole
↓
Trace endocardial border in end syst frame
↓
Same thing done for all images required
↓
Software perform speckle tracking

STRAIN IMAGING

Basics

- Evaluation of myocardial region with ref to an adjacent myocardial seg
- *Deformation analysis:* Analysis of vent mechanism or shapes during cardiac cycle

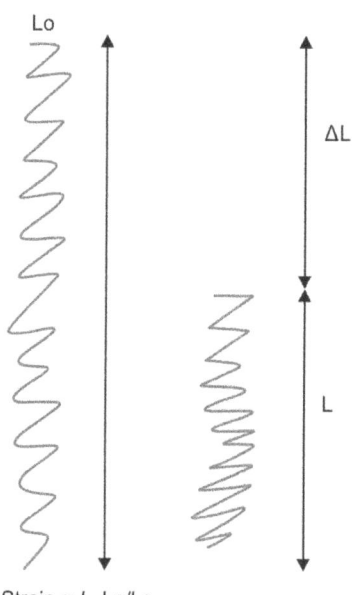

Strain = L–Lo/Lo

- Strain = Percentage thickening or deformation of myocardium during cardiac cycle
- Strain rate = change of strain per unit of time
- Strain calculated in 3 orthogonal planes representing longitudinal, radial and circumferential strain
- Negative strain—shortening of segment
- Positive strain—lengthening of segment

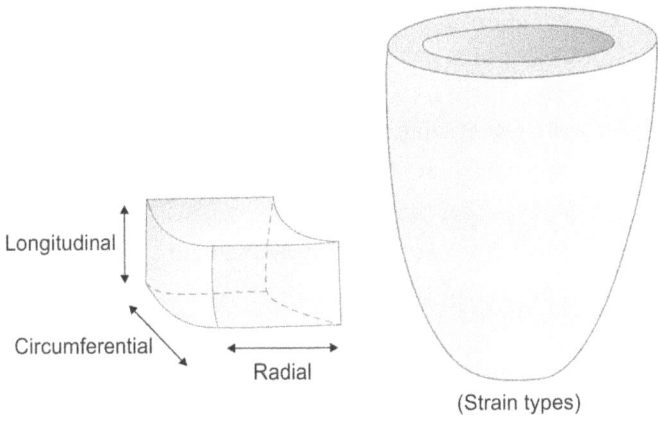

(Strain types)

Methods

- Doppler tissue imaging
  - Two discrete points are compared for change in velocity
  - Strain rate—1° parameter obtained
  - Strain—derived by integrating velocity over time
- Speckle tracking
  - Actual location of discrete myocardial segments calculated
  - Strain is 1° parameter
  - Strain rate derived by calculating change in distance over time

2D speckle tracking	TDI
Deformation analysis in and dimensions	One dimension measurement
Angle independent	Angle dependent
Better spatial resolution	Limited spatial resolution
Less time consuming and Easy data processing	Time consuming
Lower temporal resolution	High temporal resolution
Require high quality image	Not
Lower interobserver variability	High interobserver variability
Optimal frame rate required	

*Strain is not uniform among all myocardium
- *Radial strain:* Magnitude of basal parameters are higher than apical values
- *Longitudinal strain:* Less variability from apex to base
- *Circumferential strain:* Higher in ant and lat wall than in post and septal wall
  Normal longitudinal strain avg −20%
  Normal radial strain about + 40%
- Strain calculated in all segments is represented as bull's eye presentation

PATTERN STRAIN

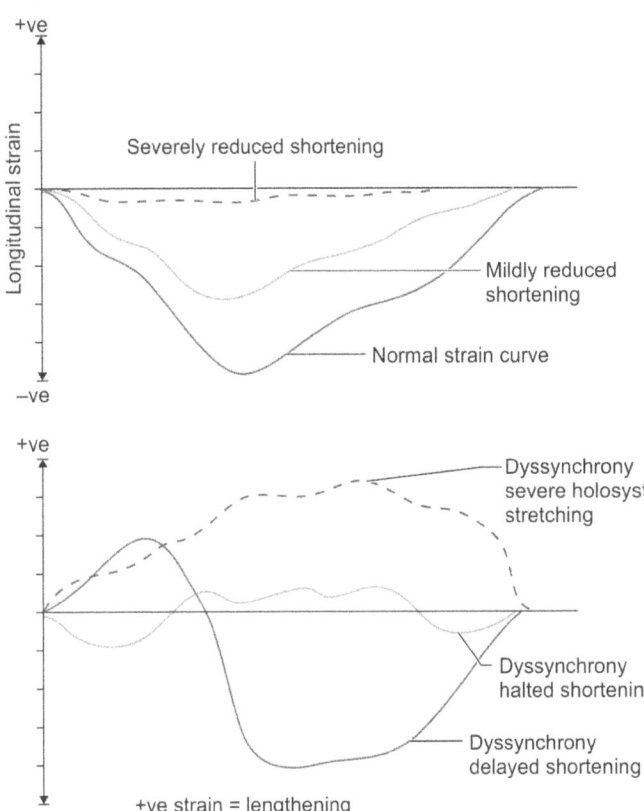

- In normal myocardium strain pattern recorded from all segments moves in equal direction
- In DCMP—It is here

VENT TORSION

- Similar to winding and unwinding of towel
- *IVCT:* The apex and base rotates in counter clockwise
- *Ejection phase:* Apex rotates counterclockwise and base rotates clockwise when reviewed from apex
- *IVRT:* Both apex and base rotate in clockwise
- *Diastole:* Relaxation myocardial fibers—recoiling clockwise apical rotation

  Rotation: Measure of rotational movement of the myocardium in retention to an imaginary line from apex to base

  Twist: Net diff between apical and basal rotation

  Torsion: Twist/ventricle distance between apex and base (degree/cm)

CLINICAL APPLICATIONS

- *CAD:* Myocardial ischemia, infarction, viability
  - Reduction in strain
    - Speckle tracking is more sensitive than traditional visual method of assessing RWMA

- Post systolic thickening by radial strain correlates with severity of ischemia
- Lower circumferential strain in transmural infarct than in subendocardial infarct

■ HFPEF
Reduced and delayed LV untwisting at rest and exercise

■ *Cardiac resynchronize therapy:*
STAR study: (speckle tracking and resync) showed that radial and transverse strains are better than longitudinal and circumferential strain in predicting LVEF response and long term survival post CRT

Lack of dyssynchrony before CRT by speckle tracking strain is associated with poor outcome and high rehospitalization with HF

■ *Other:*
- Stress cardiomyopathy
- Restrictive cardiomyopathy

- Detection of subclinical disease/early myocardial involvement
- Detection of rejection and coronary stenosis in heart transplant patient
- Early detection of chemo induced cardiotoxicity
- Valvular heart disease
- Post chemo cardiotoxicity assessment

■ D/D between athlete's heart and HCM

Athlete	HCM
Normal strain	Decreased long strain
Increased LVEDP (decreased after deconditioning for 3 months)	Decreased LVEDP (no change with deconditioning)
Increased LV Twist	Delayed LV twisting
Increased early LA strain rate	Reduced LA strain and strain rate

21.3 3D-ECHO

Q.1 Compare and contrast 3D-ECHO with TEE (June 14).
Q.2 Discuss characteristics and application of real time 3D-ECHO (Dec 10) (June 13).

TECHNIQUES

- Reconstruction technique
  - External reference system (nonsystematic image acquisition by freehand scanning)
  - Interval reference system (systematic image acquisition by predetermined transducer motion)
- Volumetric real time technique
  - Real time 3D volume acquisition
  - Real time 3D imaging

TECHNICAL ISSUE IN REAL TIME 3D

- Either sacrifice frame rate for image quality (resolution) or resolution for frame rate
- Min frame rate req = 20 Hz (20 frames/sec)

To overcome these limitations
- Increase beam width
- Increase strength of signal
- Parallel receive beam processing—increasing frame rate
- Limit total no of beams by scanning a volume—3D room mode
- Gating—Use ECG signals to acquire smaller subvolumes for each RR interval and then

Stich this subvolumes to produce larger volume.

INNOVATIONS

Phased array transducer
↓
Sparse matrix array transducer
↓
Microbeam former
↓
Dense matrix array transducer

MODE

- Real time mode
  - Narrow angle 60°:30°
  - Real time interventional guidance
  - Higher resolution
  - No stitching artifact
  - Electronic steering of beam
- Zoom mode
  - Focused 30°:30°
  - For valve imaging/masses (thrombi, vegetation)
- Full volume mode
  - Covers wider region 90°:90°
  - Near real image
  - High temporal resolution
  - For spatial relationship of cardiac str
  - For chamber quantification
- Color flow mode
  - Limited angle 60°:60°
  - Limited temporal resolution
  - Used for shape and extension of jets

ARTIFACTS

- Stitch artifacts
- Dropout artifacts
- Blurring and blooming artifacts
- Gain artifacts

PROTOCOLS

- *Aortic valve:*
  - PLAX with and without color (Zeomed mode)
- *Mitral valve:*
  - PLAX with and without color
  - AP 4C with and without color
- *LV/RV:*
  - AP4C—narrow and wide angle
  - Image must be tilted to place RV in center for RV imaging
- *IAS/IVS:* AP4C
- *PV:* Parasternal RVOT view with and without color
- *TV:* AP 4C view with and without color
  Parasternal RV Inflow view with and without color.

APPLICATION

- Left vent function
  - For global and regional function
  - *Adv:* No foresightening
    No geometrical assumptions
  - Can measure
    - End diastolic vol
    - End systolic vol
    - LV mass
    - Color coded regional segmental analysis (volume-time curves)
- Parametric imaging
  - 800 endocardial data points—To: develop a polar map
  - Endocardial motion displayed as shade of
    Blue—inward motion
    Red—outward motion

Black—no motion
↓
Akinetic myocardium—black or red color
Normal or hypokinetic—shades of blue
↓
17 segmental analysis can be achieved from color coded parameter imaging
- LA volume calculation
- RV function
  - Volumetric analysis
  - Systolic and diastolic function
    Adv: No geometric assumption
- Valvular disease
  - MVP-MR
    - Accurate anatomy—which scallop prolapse
    - Vena contracta area-direct measurement
    - Surgeon's view
    Note: TEE is good enough
           TEE view are better than 3D [TEE Better]
  - MS
    - MVA at smallest orifice
    - Better assessment of BMV
    - Planimetry from apical window
    - New GOLD standard [3D ECHO Gold standard]
  - AR
    - Better delineation
    - Vena contracta area [TEE Better]
  - AS
    - AVA measurement
    - Access noncircular LVOT area
- Other application
  - Dyssynchrony
  - Structural heart disease
    - VSD/ASD
  - Stress ECHO
  - Intracardiac mass/thrombus
  - Interventions
    - Real time 3D ECHO
    - ASD closure
    - Septostomy
    - BMV

SUMMARY

	Recommended for clinical practice	Promising clinical studies	Areas of active search	Unstudied
LV function status				
Volume and EF	✓			
Shape			✓	
Dyssynchrony			✓	
Mass		✓		
RV function assess				
Volume		✓		
Shape				✓
EF		✓		
AV - anatomy and Stenosis regurgitation		✓		✓
LA-volume		✓		
RA-volume				✓
MV anatomy	✓			
Stenosis	✓			
Regurgitation			✓	
TV-anatomy				✓
Or PV- stenosis				✓
Regurgitation				✓

3D ECHO

Advantages

- Only one image needed for entire assessment
- Nearly automated analysis
- Display temporal/spatial distribution of timing in bull's eye plot
- Short term improvement in 3D dyssynchrony index s/p CRT

Disadvantages

- Req high end equipment and probe
- Low temporal and spatial resolution
- Highly dependent on image quality
- Incomplete inclusion of apex
- Can't perform in AF or Freq ectopics

21.4 DOBUTAMINE STRESS ECHO

INTRODUCTION
- Stress ECHO is a procedure that allows dynamic evaluation of cardiac str and function during physical exercise or pharmacological stress by increasing HR, cardiac output and myo O_2 demand
- CV stress
  - Exercise
  - Pharmacological agents

BASIC PRINCIPLE

Increased cardiac work load
↓
Increased O_2 demand
↓
If demand supply mismatch
↓
Impair myocardial thickening and endocardial motion

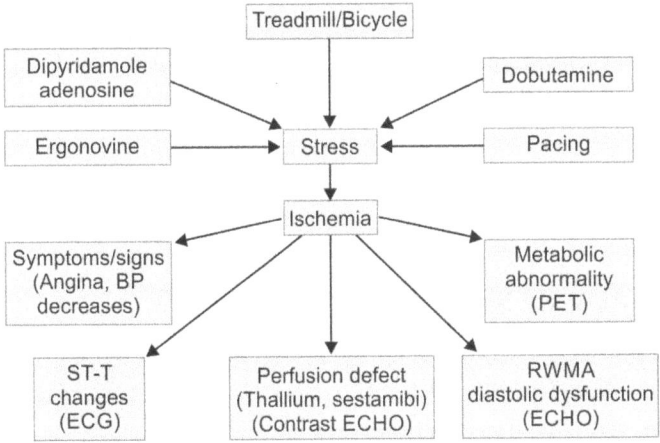

VARIOUS STENOSIS

Exercise	Nonexercise
Treadmill	Dobutamine
Supine bicycle	Dipyridamole
Upright bicycle	Adenosine
Handgrip	Pacing
Stair step	Ergonovine

INFO OBTAINED FROM EXERCISE STRESS BUT NOT FROM PHARMAC TEST
- Exercise duration/tolerance
- Reproducibility of symptoms with activity
- Heart rate response to exercise and BP response
- Detection of stress induced arrhythmias
- Assess control of angina with medical treatment
- Prognosis

INDICATION OF PHARMACOLOGICAL STRESS
- Inability to exercise/inadequate exercise
- LBBB ⎫
- Paced rhythm ⎬ difficult to interpret ECG
- Pre-excitation ⎬
- Other conduction abnormality ⎭
- Evaluation of patient very early post MI (<3 days) or stent (<2 weeks)
- Patient on BB or CCB that interfering with achieving THR

Indication
- *CAD:*
  - Diagnosis and prognosis; location and severity of inducible
  - Ischemia
  - Viability testing
  - Stunned/hibernating myocardium
- *MS:*
  - Severe MS with asymptomatic
  - Symptoms discordant with ECHO findings
  - Assess transvalvular gradient at stress
- *As:* Differentiation of LFLG As
  - Prognosis
- *PHTN:* Assessment of PASP at stress when patient is unable to exercise
- Pre op evaluation in selected patients

- Dobutamine
  - Increased contractility at lower dose
  - Progressive chronotropic response at high dose
  - Recently used in patients with decompensated HF for UA
  - Can be safely used in patients with recent MI, extensive LV dysfunction, AAA, syncope, As, HOCM, H/O VT
- Dobutamine is synthetic catecholamine
  - B1—increased cardiac contractility and HR positive inotropic and positive chronotropic
  - B2—peripheral vasodilatation
  - Alpha1—vasoconstriction
  - Onset of action = 2 mins
  - Half Life = 2 mins (cont IV infusion)
  - For stress ECHO
    - Infusion begun at 5 (or 10) µg/kg/min
    - Increased every 3 min to 10, 20, 30 and 40
  - Low dose images acquired at 5 or 10 µg/kg/min (At first sign of increased contractility)
  - Mid dose images acquired at 20–30 µg/kg/min

- Peak images acquired before termination
- Atropine can be used to augment HR
- Post stress images acquired after return to baseline

ENDPOINTS TO TERMINATE DST
- THR exceeding 85% of predicted
- Dev of significant angina
- Recognition of new WMA
- Decrease in SBP >20 mm Hg from baseline
- Arrhythmias (AF/VT)

CAUTION
- Elderly patients (no guidelines on dose reduction)
- HTN (Dobu can increase or decrease BP—atropine can be used to achieve HR if increased BP is limiting dose
- Migraine can worsen due to vasodilatation
- Schizophrenic patient may not tolerate catecholamine effect of dobutamine.

INTERPRETATION
- Subjective assessment of WMA
  - 17 segment model
  - Wall motion index = Segmental score / No of segments scored

  Give each segment a score
  1 = Normal
  2 = hypokinetic
  3 = akinetic
  4 = dyskinetic
  5 = aneursmal
  WMS ≥2.5—poor progno
- Rest and stress wall motion response

Rest	Stress	Interpretation
Normal	Hyperkinetic	Normal
Normal	Hypo/akinetic	Ischemia
Akinetic	Akinetic	Scar
Hypokinetic	Akinetic/dyskinetic	Ischemia and/or scar
Hypo/akinetic	normal	Viable myo

False +ve	False -ve
Hypertensive response	Suboptimal stress
HCM	Delayed post TMT imaging
Microvasc disease (LVH, synd x, DM, myocarditis)	Single vessel disease – Mod stenosis
Epicardial spasm	Conc LVH
Abnormal IVS motion	Significant MR/AR

- Myocardial viability:
  - Hibernating myocardium refers to viable but underperformed myocardial tissue that regains functionality after revasc
  - >6 mm thickness—viable
  - Increased contractility with dobu—viable
  - Biphasic response—low dose increased contractility and at high dose decreased contractility—viable ← Most sensitive

  ↓

  ASE guidelines recommend that viability assessment induces improvement in at least 2 segments of LV on ECHO
- Other agents
  - Dipyridamole and adenosine
  - Acts by creating maldistribution of blood flow
  - Preventing normal increase in the flow in areas supplied by stenotic coro art (coro steal).

ADV OF STRESS ECHO OVER NUCLEAR STRESS
- Higher specificity
- Visualization of cardiac valves
- Evaluate for presence of pericardial eff
- More accurate assessment of LV and RV syst function
- Low cost
- Lack of radiation
- Doppler interrogation to determine diastolic function.

21.5 TEE

ADVANTAGES

- Transducer 2-3 mm from heart
- Closer to post str, better visualization of LA, LAA, PV, MV, TV, Aorta
- Far from Sx area (intra op monitoring)
- High resolution images

DISADVANTAGES

- Seminvasive procedure
- Chances of injury
- Needs orientation and expertise

INDICATIONS

- Assessment of prosthetic valve/native valve IE
- Prosthetic valve function
- Suspected cardio embolic event
- Cardinal tumor
- Atrial septal abnormality assessment
- Evaluations of AOD
- Evaluation of CHD/CAD
- Critically ill patient
- Intraop imaging
- Nondiagnostic TEE

CONTRAINDICATIONS

- Absolute
  - Esophageal structure/obstruction
  - Suspected or know perforated viscus
  - GI bleeding not evaluated
  - Instability of Cx vertebrae
- Relative
  - Esophageal varices/diverticula
  - Cervical arthritis
  - Esophageal distortion
  - Bleeding diathesis/over—anti coagulation

COMPLICATIONS

Major

- Death
- Esophageal rupture
- Laryngospasm/bronchospasm
- CHF or pulm edema
- Sustained VT/AF/SVT

Minor

- Excessive retching/vomiting
- Hoarseness
- Sore throat
- Minor pharyngeal bleed
- Blood tinged sputum
- NSVT/SVT/AF/Brady/Heart attack
- Transient Hypo/hypertension
- Angina
- Transient hypoxia
- Tracheal intubation

21.6 ICE

Q.1 What is intracardiac ECHO? What are their advantages over TEE? Discuss its use in clinical practice (Dec 1).

- Imaging technique to guide percutaneous interventional procedures
- Principally used during closure of ASA and LAA
- 1st gen introduced in 1980s
  - High resolution image
  - High frequency of transducer (20-40 Hz)—limited tissue penetration
  - Anatomic intracardiac overview not properly obtained
- Newly developed: Steerable phased array ultrasound catheter system with low frequency and Doppler qualities—expanded clinical use of TEE

ADVANTAGES

- G.A/sedation not needed
- Patient discomfort is less
- Communication with patient during procedure is possible as compared to ICE
- Availability of direct online info on the position of catheters and devices
- Possibility of direct monitoring of acute procedure related complications
  E.g.: Thrombus formation
       Pericardial effusion etc.

LIMITATIONS

- Shaft size (10 Fr)
- Lack of additional catheter features
  E.g.: Port for guidewires
        Therapeutic devices and pressure
- Phased array catheter are expensive and for single use only
- Provides only monoplane image
- Difficult for operator to obtain the same views
- No standard views for ICE has been defined

CLINICAL USE

- For interventional procedure
- Evaluation of intracardiac thrombus
- Transseptal puncture
- ASD/PFO closure
- LAA closure
- Interventional EP procedure
  - PV ablation in AF
  - AFL ablation
  - VT ablation
- *Other*
  - Diagnosis/biopsy of intracardiac mass
  - Balloon mitral Transseptal
  - Visualization of CS

TECHNIQUE

- 9 MHz single element transducer incorporated in 8 F catheter
- Piezoelectric crystal is rotated at 1,800 rpm in radial direction (perpendicular to cath shaft)
- Provides cross sectional image in 360° plane
- ICE catheter needs to be filled with 3-5 mL sterile water before it is connected to ultrasound machine

Phased array tipped catheter system uses
- 10 F ultrasound catheter
- 10 F introducer sheath
- Catheter connected to ultrasound system
- Measurement of HD and physiologic variables can be made using Doppler imaging

FUTURE

- Higher resolution
  - More reproducible and more flexible
- Electrophysiology enabled device for imaging and therapy
  - Integration of ultrasound imaging with mapping techniques, fusion, and overlay imaging.

21.7 TISSUE DOPPLER IMAGING

Q. TDI in health and disease (2000, 2010, 2013)

TDI uses principle of Doppler to measure velocity of myocardial motion

DISADV OF 2D IMAGING IN ASSESSING MYOCARDIAL MOTION

- Poor delineation of endocardial borders
- Interobserver variability
- Qualitative analysis (not quantitative)
- Poor regional function assessment
- Diastolic function assessment limited.

ADV OF TDI

- Can obtain data even in suboptimal window
- Less interobserver variation
- Quantitative method
- Important in diastolic function assessment
- Better regional assessment.

PRINCIPLE

- *Doppler effect:* Freq of a reflected ultrasound wave is altered by movement of reflecting surface "away from" or "toward" the source
- Conventional Doppler
  - Based on movement of RBCs
  - RBCs are weak reflector and fast moving
  - So conventional Doppler has to filter the reflected waves
  - *Filters:* Adjusted to exclude highly reflective objects and to maximize less reflective and high velocity objects

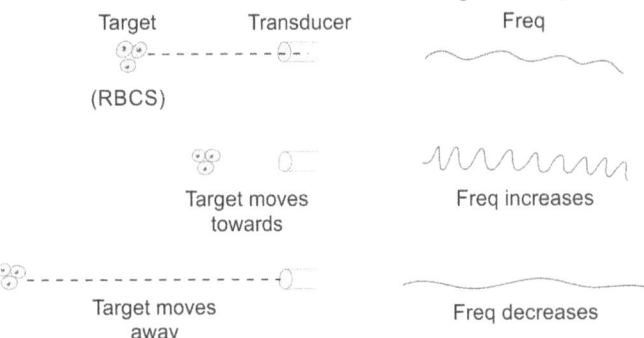

(Principle of Doppler effect or Doppler shift)

- Doppler shift can be calculated as

$$\Delta F = \frac{2f_o V}{C} \times \cos \theta$$

Δf = Doppler shift
f_o = transducer Freq
V = velocity (tissue)
C = velocity (light)
θ = angle of incidence

So velocity alpha ΔF

Velocity Alpha $1/f_o$—high freq transducer can detect low velocity (tissue).

Velocity of alpha $1/\cos \theta$—more angle—velocity underestimated (so angle of transducer and tissue movt has to be parallel).

Routine Doppler imaging	Tissue Doppler imaging
Targets RBC	Targets tissue
↓	↓
Low intensity reflector	High intensity reflector
High velocity	Low velocity

So, sir TDI filter has to be set to exclude high velocity and low intensity signals.

LIMITATION

- TDI measures only the vector of motion that is parallel to the direction of the ultrasound
- Incident angle between the beam and the direction of target motion varies from region to region

↓

Limits ability to provide absolute velocity.

MODES

- Pulse wave TDI
  - Used as measure peak myocardial velocity
  - Suitable for measurement of long axis ventricular motion (apical view)
  - MAPSE/TAPSE
  - Wave forms

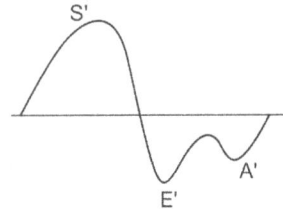

  - Normal annular Doppler pattern
    - Septal S' velocity lower than lateral S' velocity
    - E'/A' >1
    - Peak Tissue velocity is at base and decreases as sampling moves towards apex
    - Age related decreases in peak velocity s' and e'
    - E'/A' reversal after age 50
- Color TDI:
  - Color coded representation of Myocardial velocity superimposed on grayscale 2D and m-mode images
  - Indicate direction and velocity of myocardial motion

- M-mode color Doppler TDI
  - Color coded image of tissue motion along an M-mode interrogation line
  - Combination of color Doppler + M-mode + TDI — High temporal and spatial resolution
  - Can be used for strain rate imaging
  - Can also device epicardial–endocardial gradient (difference between velocity)
    ↓
    Selective decrease in endocardial velocity is a marker of ischemia (very sensitive)
    (*Caution:* It's angle dependent)

CLINICAL APPLICATION

- Assessment of LV systolic function:
  - Systolic Myocardial velocity (S') at lateral mitral annulus measures longitudinal systolic function
  - Well correlated with LVEF
  - Mitral annular displacement velocity decrease in LV dysfunction
  - Regional reduction in S' velocity Suggest RWMA
- Assessment of LV diastolic function
  - Determined by mitral annular plane diastolic motion (e', a', E/e')
  - Mitral valve Inflow (E and A) are preload dependent
  - While TDI diastolic motion is load independent
  - Reduced lateral e' velocity to ≤8 cm/s in older adults indicate impaired LV relaxation
  - Can differentiate between normal and pseudo normal mitral inflow pattern
- Coronary artery disease
  - Reduction in s' velocity within 15 seconds of onset of ischemia
  - <7.5 cm/sec LV wall velocity - RWMA
  - e'/a' reversal
  - Can define endocardial–epicardial gradient
- TDI stress ECHO:
  - Peak S' velocity increases with dobutamine and exercise and decreases with ischemia
    Adv:
    - Better identification of abnormal segments
    - Better reproductivity than standard ECHO
    - Peak s' velocity <5.5 cm/s identify abnormal segment (96% sensitivity and 81% specificity)
- Estimation of LV filling pr: (E/e') (mitral valve)
  - Lateral E/e' ≥10 or ≥ elevated LV filling pr septal E/e' ≥15   (LVEDP)
  - E/e' <=8 => correlated with normal LVEDP
  - E/e' >10 = predicted PCWP >15
- Diff between constriction and restrictive physiology
  - CP and RCMP both have abnormal LV filling
  - In absence of myocardial disease e' velocity typically remain normal

    So, e' < 8 cm/sec—restriction
        e' >8 cm/sec—constriction
- D/D between HCM and athletes heart
  - HCM—Reduced e' velocity
  - Athletes—highly compliant ventricles with brisk e' vel
- Assessment of dyssynchrony
  - TDI can be used to assess relative timing of peak systolic contraction in multiple myocardial regions
  - Deviation of time to peak contraction represents measure of overall vent dyssynchrony
- Assessment of RV function
  - TAPSE

So, overall TDI is
- Complimentary to std ECHO
- Imp for diastolic function assessment
- Can obtain data even in suboptimal window
- Less inter-observer variation
- Better regional assessment

Nuclear Imaging

22.1 RADIONUCLEOTIDE VENTRICULOGRAPHY

INTRODUCTION
- Radionucleotide ventriculography is also known as radionuclide angiography
- Two techniques.

TECHNIQUES
- *Equilibrium technique:*
    - Also known as MUGA (multiple gated acquisition)
    - Data recorded synchronized with R wave
    - Similar to gated SPECT
    - ^{99}Tc labeled RBC or ^{99}Tc labeled albumin used for labeling blood pool
    - Image of heart acquired in 3 std projection anterior, LAD and left lateral
    - Acquisition time 5-10 mins
- *Analysis*
    - Size of heart chamber and great vessels
    - RWMA
    - Global function
    - Vent wall thickness, pericardial effusion, pericardial fat pad or pericardial mass
- *First pass radionuclide angiography or ventriculography:*
    - ^{99}Tc DTPA is recommended
    - Bolus of radioactivity passes through rt side of heart-lung—left side
    - Images acquired rapidly as tracer passes through heart.

ADVANTAGES
- High target to background ratio
- More distinct temporal situation
- Rapidly of imaging.

22.2 VIABILITY, HIBERNATION AND STUNNING

MYOCARDIAL VIABILITY

Definition

Viable myocardium is defined as myocardium that demonstrates abnormal function at rest and improves with revascularization

- Stunning refers to transient myocardial dysfunction, which is often caused by abrupt cessation of flow typical of an acute coronary occlusion
- Hibernation occurs when viable myocardium has altered its metabolism and thus reduced its contractile function as a mechanism to cope with chronically inadequate blood supply (chronic stable angina/or repetitive ischemic injury.

Technique

- Indicated in patient with CAD and resting LV dysfunction
- In patients who are eligible for revascularization
  - SPECT
  - PET with metabolic agents
  - Dobutamine ECHO
  - Contrast ECHO
  - Delayed enhanced MRI.

SPECT

- Thallium 201 and Tc 98 both are perfusion agents taken up by viable myocardium
- Long $t_{1/2}$ of these agents allow for regional distributed which makes them feasible to use in centers without generator or cyclotron
- Stress SPECT can easily diagnose viability

Thallium 201

- Utilize Na^+/K^+ ATPase transport system (present only on viable cells with intact membrane)
- Linear relationship between blood flow and uptake of Thallium at rest and exercise

Rest/redistribution Thallium protocol

- Imaging 30-60 min after Thallium injection
- Reimaging 4 hours later ↓ [Sens - 90% / Spec - 54%]
- Defect in initial image that improves in 4 hours represents area of viable myocardium
- Less sensitive than PET and other Thallium protocols

Stress/redistribution protocol

- Pharmacological/exercise induced stress
- Subsequent Thallium injection
- Imaging immediately and after 4 hours ↓ [Sens-86% / Spec-47%]
- Myocardium not perfused with stress/rest—scar
- Defect on stress but improve on rest—viable ↓ [Less sensitive]
- Imaging 24 hours later to search for late redistribution improves sensitivity but dramatically decrease specificity

Stress/rest/reinjection

- Same as stress-redistribution protocol
- Reinjection of 1 mCi of Thallium with subsequent reimaging
- Increased sensitivity by increasing blood level of Thallium
- Reinjection imaging can be performed immediately after redistribution image (4 hours) or after several hours (sensitivity does not differ significantly between 2 techniques) ↓
- Myocardium with defect that do not improve upon reinjection or redistribution—scar
- Any improvement in uptake with reinjection—viable
- Technetium^{99} depends on mitochondrial function, sarcolemma integrity and intact energy production pathways
- Shorter $t_{1/2}$ (6 hours)—large dose allowed ↓

    Redistribution of ^{99}Tc is significantly less than Thallium—it is less helpful for viability study
- *Fully quantitative analysis* of SPECT image is more accurate to identify high and low risk population
  - Improves sensitivity
- Region showing <60% Thallium uptake on redistribution—very low chance of recovery
- Tc^{99} NEWT has similar redistribution kinetics and may be useful (in future).

PET

- Gold standard for viability testing
- FDG—PET

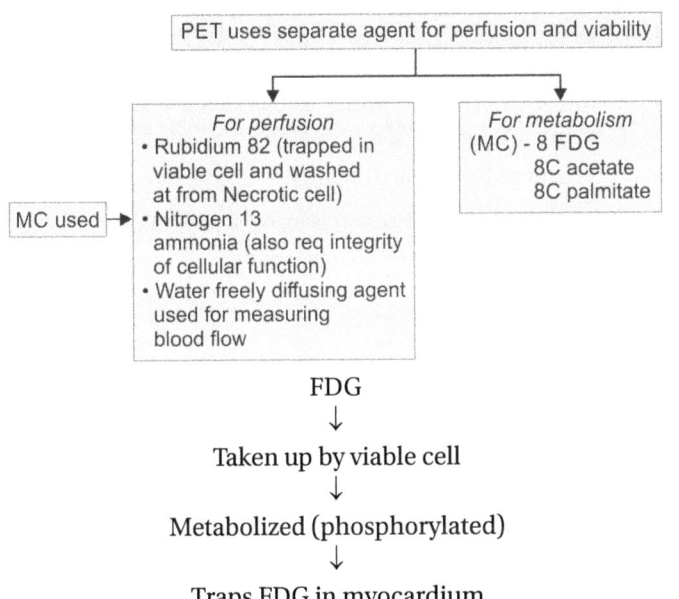

FDG
↓
Taken up by viable cell
↓
Metabolized (phosphorylated)
↓
Traps FDG in myocardium

- During period of ischemia glucose is used as major metabolic to provide energy
- *Limitation:* Diabetes with impaired cellular uptake of glucose.

Combi of Perfusion and Metabolic Tracers

- Normal perfusion indicates viability on its own and does not req specific assessment of metabolism
- Reduced perfusion with intact metabolism (flow-metabolism mismatch)—hibernating, viable myocardium
- Impaired perf and meta both—scar.

Diagnostic Accuracy

- PET and CMRI both are highly accurate
- Image quality better than SPECT
    Sens—71-100%
    Spec—38-91%

Dobutamine ECHO

- In viable myo, with increasing dose of dobutamine, myo O_2 consumption increases and ischemia develops with worsening of WMA
↓
This "Biphasic response" most specific for viable myocardium
- "Uniphasic response" (improve thickening and contractility and does not regression of thickness or contractility at high dose)—much less predictive of improvement after revasc
- Area with reduced thickness and contractility which remains same on Dobu—scar
    Sens = 84%
    Spec = 84%

Cardiac MRI

- No risk of ionizing radiation
- Gadolinium based contrast agents pass quickly through normal areas of myocardium
↓
- In scarred tissue, the interstitial space between collagen fibers is larger than in normal myocardium—causing a delayed within of gadolinium enhancement
↓
So gadolinium remains trapped in scar tissue
↓
Longer washout of gadolinium from infarcted of fibrotic myocardium
↓
So fibrotic or scar area appear as bright (hyperintense) on images taken 10-20 mins after contrast injection
- Transmural extent of hyperenhancement on delayed imaging is used to determine viability
↓
- Segments with 0-25% transmural extent of hyperenhancement—viable tissue
- 75-100% transmural hyperenhancement—scar
- 25-75%—Intermediate viability (Amt of viability in adjacent segment is taken into account)
↓
Amt of hyperenhancement within a region can be correlated with segmental wall function and rest/stress perfusion to determine viability.

Diagnostic accuracy
- Superior than SPECT
- Similar sensitivity and slightly improved specificity than PET
- Main advantage is to delineate transmural extent of infarction.

Choice of Technique

- Dobutamine stress and SPECT are less expensive
- PET and MRI both are robust but costly

ECG

- No clear correlation between Q wave in ECG and presence of viability

- Patients with preserved QT dispersion are likely to have viable myocardium
- Patients with high QT dispersion—predominantly non-viable scar tissue

Approach

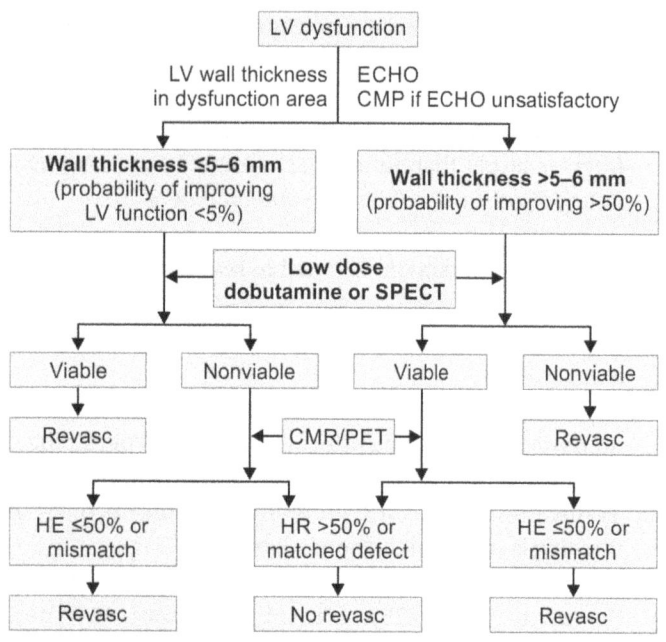

HIBERNATION AND STUNNING

Stunning

Definition

Prolonged and fully reversible dysfunction of the ischemic heart that persists despite normalization of blood flow.

Features

- Normal perfusion
- Depressed myocardial function
- Dissociation of usual relationship between subendocardial flow and function
- Reversible
- Function improves with Inotropic agents.

Various Setting

Stunning occurs in various setting (in viva as well as experimentally)

- Single, completely reversible episode of regional ischemia (<20 min)
- Multiple, completely reversible episode of regional ischemia
- Partly reversible and partly irreversible ischemia in vivo (>20 min and <3 hours)
- After global ischemic (in vitro)
- After global ischemic (in vivo)—cardioplegic arrest
- After exercise—induced ischemia.

Clinical Relevance

In clinical setting stunning can occur

- *Brief period of total coro occlusion:* Patients with angina due to spasm
- Global ischemia after cardio-pulm bypass
- *In combination:* Subendocardium is infarcted overlying subepicardium reversible injured in MI
- Following exercise in flow limiting stenosis
- Ischemic about that is induced by PCI.

Mechanism

- No unified view
- Multiple plausible hypothesis
  - *Oxy radical hypothesis:* Oxidative stress secondary to generation of ROS
  - *Calcium hypothesis:* Results from disturbance of cellular Ca^{++} homeostasis.

Oxy radical hypothesis:

- ROS mediated injury responsible for stunning occurs in initial moments of reperfusion
- Antioxidant therapy alleviates stunning whether begun before ischemia or just prior to reperf. But ineffective when begun after reperf
- None of antioxidant completely prevented myocardial stunning

Ca^{++} hypothesis:

- Transient Ca^{++} overload activates Ca^{++} dependent proteases

↓

Degrades and induce covalent modification of myofilaments

↓

Decreased responsiveness to Ca^{++}

↓

Decreased maximal force of contraction

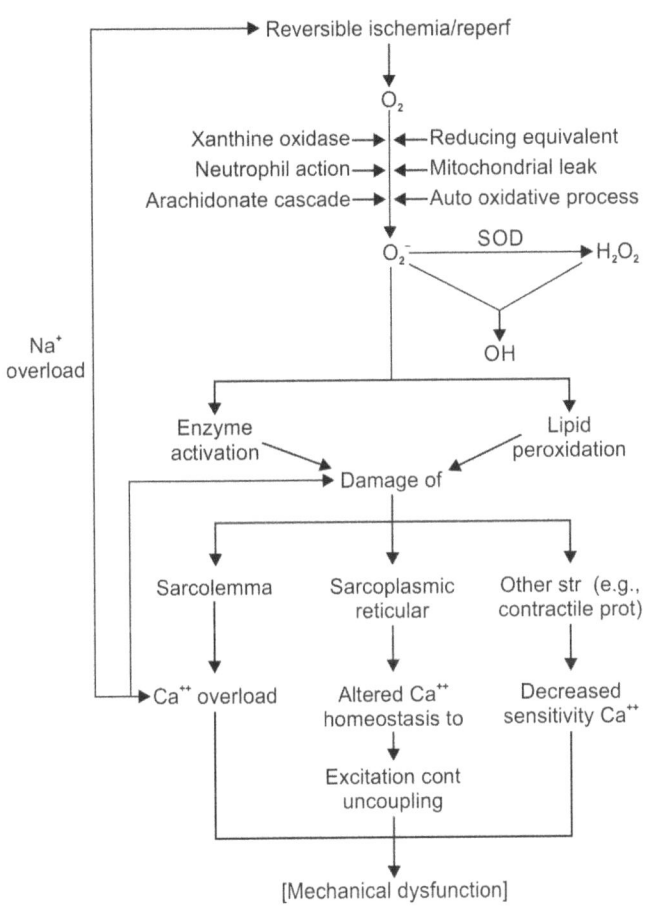

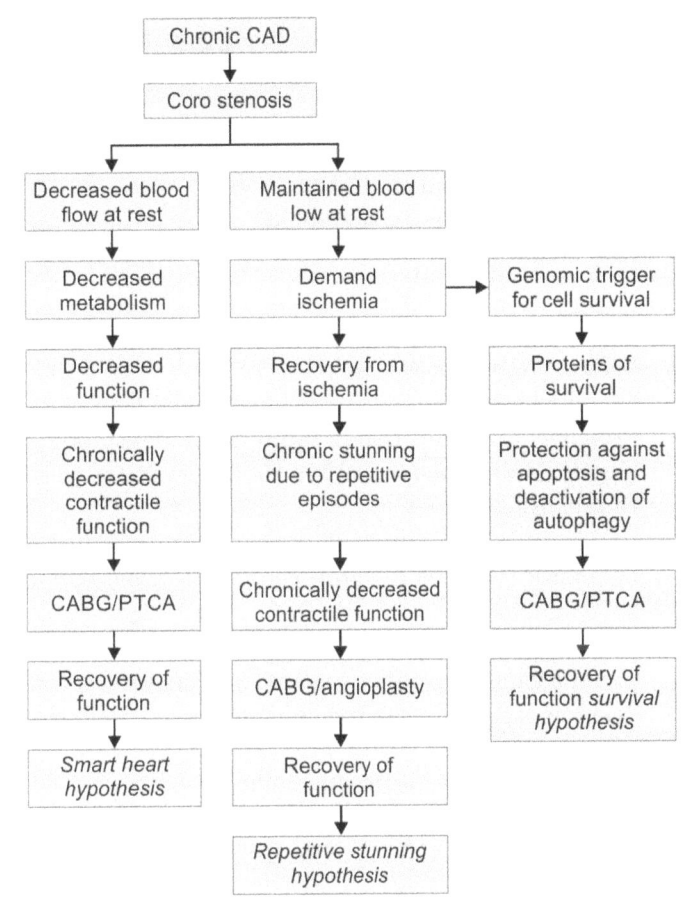

Hibernation

Definition

Hibernation refers to adaptive reduction of myocardial contractile function in response to reduced myo blood flow.

Mechanism

- *Smart heart hypothesis*
  - Myo metabolism and function reduced to match concomitant reduction in CBF which prevents necrosis
- *Repetitive stunning hypothesis*
  - Repetitive epi of ischemia results in sustained depression of contractile function
- *Genomic survival hypothesis*
  - Maintained viability in hibernation suggests possibility of genomic adaptation
  - Major survival gene (anti-apoptotic gene, cytoprotective gene and growth promoting gene) and their corresponding proteins are upregulated in hibernating myo.

Nat History

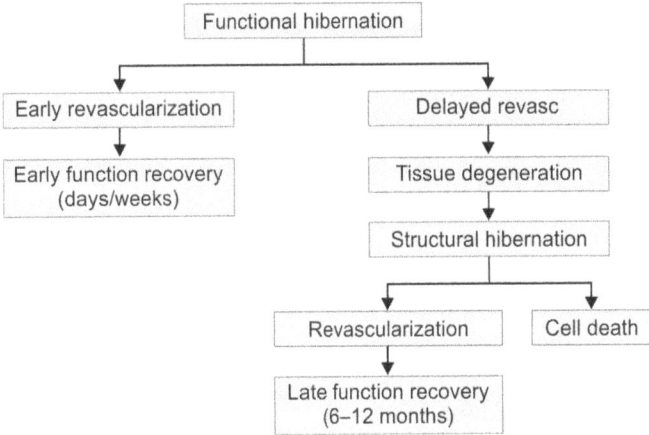

Histology

- Myolysis
- Glycogen accumulation
- Increased interstitial fibrosis.

Clinical Relevance

20–50% patients with chronic ischemic LV dysfunction have significant amt of viable hibernating myocardium—they improve with revasc.

22.3 NUCLEAR CARDIOLOGY

INTRODUCTION
Integral role in
- Noninvasive detection of CAD
- Assessment of myocardial viability
- Risk stratification

SPECT
- Most commonly performed
- SPECT with MI
- *Principle:* After injection of radiotracer, the isotope is extracted from blood by viable myocardium and retained within myocyte
  ↓
  Photons are emitted from myocardium in proportion to tracer uptake
  ↓
  Gamma camera captures this info and converts it into data representing magnitude of uptake and location of emission
  (Collimator used = Parallel hole collimators)

NEW TECHNOLOGY: HIGH SPEED SPECT
- Advanced camera and collimator
- Imaging time greatly reduced
  15 min with conventional
  5-6 min with newer solid-state cameras ⎤
- 2-fold increase in spatial resolution   ⎬ Adv
- Lower dose of tracer requirement   ⎪
- Cost effective.   ⎦

SPECT TRACERS AND PROTOCOL
- *Thallium 201:*
  - Biological property similar to K^+
  - K^+ is major intracellular ion in muscle and is virtually absent in scar tissue
  - ^{201}Tl is suitable to differentiate normal and ischemic myocardium from scar
  - $t_{1/2}$ = 73 hrs
  - First pass excretion fraction = 85%
  - 5% of administered dose is distributed to myocardium
  - Thallium transported to myocyte by Na^+-K^+ ATPase
  - Peak myocardial concentration is achieved within 5 mins
  - After this—a wash at phase, called redistribution begins in 10-15 mins.

  Disadv Energy spectrum is suboptimal for gamma-camera-long $t_{1/2}$ limb reinjection

  - Thallium clearance from normal myocardium is faster than ischemic myocardium called differential washout.

  Protocols
  - After stress, reversal of Thallium defect from the initial peak stress to delayed 3-4 hour or 24 hour redistribution image—a marker of reversibly ischemic, viable myocardium
  - Thallium in resting state, extent of Thallium defect reversibility from initial rest images to delayed redistribution image reflect viable myocardium with hypoperfusion
  - When scarred myocardium present—initial rest or stress Thallium defect persists—termed irreversible or fixed defects
  - In some patients Thallium reinjection is required to identify viable myocardium when there are irreversible defects on stress redistribution image
- *Technetium-99 labeled tracer:*
  - Excellent myocardial extraction and flow kinetic
  - $t_{1/2}$ = 6 hrs
  - *Various Tc^{99} labeled tracers*
    - *Sestamibi:* Available for clinical use
    - *Teboroxime*
    - *Tetrofosmin:* Available for clinical use
  - First pass extraction fraction = 60%
  - Retained within mitochondria
  - Redistribution is minimal
  - Two separate injection required
    1. At peak stress
    2. At rest

Protocols
- *Single day study*
  - Myo blood flow interrogated at rest and peak (or reverse order)
  - First dose is low and 2nd high
- *Two day study*
  - High dose both at rest and stress
- *Dual isotope technique*
  - Ij of Thallium at rest
  - Fl by technitium at peak.

ANALYSIS OF IMAGING
- Key elements to be reported
  - Presence of location of perfusion defect
  - Reversibility of defect on rest imaging
- 17 segmental model used
- Perfusion graded from 0 to 4

- 0 = normal perfusion and 4 is very severe defect
- *Summed stress score* (SSS) represents extent and severity of stress perfusion abnormality
- *Summed rest score*
- *Summed difference score* represents extent and severity of stress induced ischemia

Analysis Method
- Semiquantitative visual analysis ──────┐
- Fully quantitative computer analysis
  ↓   ↓
  Highly reproducible   Depends on experience
                               and training of reader

Other Important Signs in SPECT Imaging beyond MPI
- *Lung uptake*
  - Patients with lung uptake often have severe MVD
  - Exhibit increased PCWP and decreased EF during Ex
    ↓
    Implying extensive MVD
  - Ischemia induced elevation of LAP – increased mean PAP – slows pulm transit of tracer – increased lung uptake
- *Transient ischemic dilatation of LV*
  - LV cavity appears larger on stress imaging
  - Related to extensive ischemia and prolonged post ischemic systolic function
  - In older patients it may also represent diffuse subendocardial ischemia (decreased uptake in subendocardium) - also associated with severe CAD

Normal variation in SPECT imaging falsely interpreted as defect
- Dropout of upper septum 2° to imaging of muscular septum with memb septum
- Apical thinning—mistaken as perfusion defect
- Lateral wall often appears brighter than contrast septum
- *Artifacts (affecting image interpretation)*
  - Breast attenuation
  - Inferior wall attenuation
    - Due to diaphragm overlapping inf call
    - Artifact related to extracardiac tissue uptake
      - When such a str is near to heart, cardiac region appears falsely hotter
      - 2nd possibility is a nearby hot extra cardiac structure causing negative love artifact.

Gated SPECT Imaging
ECG gated SPECT imaging for simultaneous assessment of LV function and perfusion

With MPI, the number of counts recorded during any individual cardiac cycle is insufficient to create an interpretable image to assess vent function
↓
ECG gated SPECT

As peak of R wave detected—Gate opens and a set no of milliseconds of activity recorded in frame-1
↓
Gate closes and opens immediately to record frame –2 similarly
↓
Sequence continues for a prespecified number of frames (e.g., 8 frames each of 125 msec for patients with HR of 60)
↓
Several hundred beats recorded over 10-15 mins
↓
Avg cardiac cycle reconstructed (Req. All beats have homogeneous cardiac cycle length)
↓
- LV function can be calculated
- RWMA can be ascertained.

PET SCAN
Position emitting isotopes (Tracers)

For perfusion imaging	For metabolism imaging
^{15}O - oxygen	^{11}C - carbon
^{13}N - ammonia	^{18}F - fluomdeoxy glucose
^{82}Rb - Rubidium	

*Adv Over SPECT
Measurement of myocardial perfusion and metabolism in absolutely quantitative terms.

*Image Acquisition
Principle: Positron emitting isotope
↓
Positron emitted from nucleus
↓
Travel a few millimeters in tissue
↓
Ultimately collides with electron ⎤ Called
(negatively charged beta particles) ⎦ beta-decay
↓
Complete annihilation of electron and positron
↓
Conversion to energy in form of electromagnetic radiation
↓
Discharged gamma rays travel in opp direction
↓

PET detectors are programmed to detect such photons striking directly opposing detectors

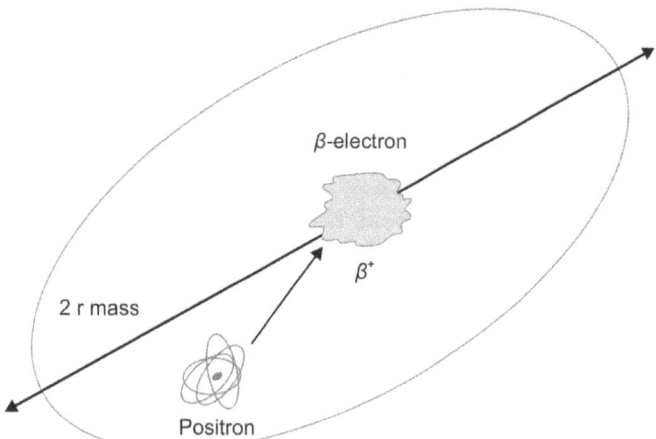

Advantage (Over SPECT)
- Quantitative analysis of perfusion and metabolism
- High spatial resolution
- Improved attenuation and scattered correction
- Potential for quantifying regional blood flow and blood flow reserve

(e.g., patients with MVD–SPECT fails to show balanced ischemic; while PET can detect blood flow and flow reserve- helps early identification of CAD).

Disadv
- On site cyclotron requirement for N-ammonia and other tracer
- High cost of monthly generator replacement for ^{82}Rb
- Relatively short $t_{1/2}$ of ^{82}Rb and N limits the utility of PET perfusion studies to patient undergoing pharmacological stress only.

PET-CT OR SPECT-CT
- Completely anatomical and function imaging
- Decision depends upon: (1) age; (2) underlying heart rhythm; (3) known CAC or metallic implants; (4) lung disease; (5) renal insufficiency
- Hybrid PET-CT should be limited to subset of patients in whom knowledge of both coronary anatomy and physiology would be anticipated to have impact on clinical management (e.g., Anomalies coro anatomy/ myocardial bridge and chest pain).

22.4 USE OF NUCLEAR IMAGING

MYOCARDIAL BLOOD FLOW, MYOCARDIAL METABOLISM, AND VENTRICULAR FUNCTION

Assessment of Myocardial Blood Flow

- *Myocardial blood flow at rest*
  - SPECT tracer require viable myocardium for its uptake and retention
  - Visualization of myocardium suggests presence of working viable cell memb
  - Lack of visualization does not necessarily mean lack of viable cells can indicate 2 things
    1. Lack of functioning intact cell memb in area of infarcted myocardium
    2. Reduced blood flow to hibernating myocardium
       ↓
  - Severe reduction in uptake of tracer signifi infarction
  - But a moderate reduction cannot always differentiate *'hibernating'* from *'partially scarred myocardium'* in patients with LV dysfunction
       ↓

18-FDE PET (metabolic accessor) can be used as adjunct to myocardial blood flow assessment

MI:
- Severely reduced uptake of tracer (due to decreased blood flow as well as non-viable myocardium)
- Infarct size can be assessed by Tc-sestamibi (because of its minimal clearance)
- Two consecutive studies (one pre reperfusion and 2nd later on)—change in defect size represents magnitude of salvaged myocardium by reperfusion.

Assessment of Myocardial Blood Flow/Perfusion at Stress

Determinants of CBF at stress are
- Perfusion pr at head of system (aortic diastolic pr)
- Downstream resistance (predominantly determined by coronary arteriolar bed)
  Major mech responsible

Adenosine
dipyridamole
- Exercise stress = CBF increases 2-3 times above normal
- Pharmacological stress = CBF increases 4-5 times above normal

Magnitude of blood flow increases 2° to any stress relative to flow values at rest is termed coronary blood flow reserve

Ideal tracer to measure CBF reserve should have

- Rapid extraction from blood
- Should be extracted as completely as possible
- Should be retained in myocardium sufficient enough to be imaged
- Should track CBF across entire physiologic range
- Should not interfere with commonly used drugs or ischemia
- In clinical practice

None of tracer have all these qualities

Rb and N ammonia has been validated for detection of CBF and flow reserve
       ↓
Most PET uses pharmacological stress

Detection of Stress-induced Ischemia vs Infarction

Perfusion abnormality

At rest	at stress
Normal perfusion +	Abnormal perfusion—reversible
Abnormal perfusion +	Abnormal perfusion—irreversible

Pharmacological Stress

- *Dipyridamole:* 142 ug/kg/min
  Duration-4 min by injection pump
  Isotope Ij-3 min after completion of infu
- *Adenosine:* 140 ug/kg/min
  Duration-6 min infusion by pump
  Isotope Ij-3 min after completion of infu
- *Regadenoson:* 0.4 mg (5 mL) rapid injection followed by 5 mL saline flush
  Isotope injection—10-20 second after saline

Mech: Dipyridamole metabolized by ADA

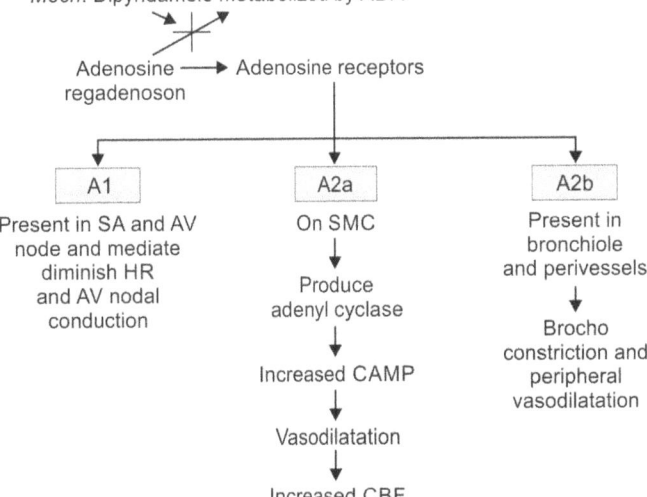

Diff between Pharmacological and Vasodilator
- Higher level of CBF achieved during pharmacological stress—increased sensitivity of detecting CAD
- Vasodilator stress (pharmacological) is less physiological than exercise and symptoms during test cannot be clearly linked to perfusion pattern
- Anti ischemic meals significantly affect the results of MPI during exercise.

Dobutamine Stress
- In some patient vasodilator stress is CI because of reactive brochosporte airways
- Dobutamine has a relative rapid onset of action
- $t_{1/2}$ = 2 mins
- Start at 5 ug/kg/min and increased stepwise by 5 ug/kg/min every 3 mins to mat of 40 ug/kg/min
- Low dose—increased contractility through adrenergic receptors
- Dose >10—HR rises steadily and increase in O_2 demand stimulates increase in myo blood flow
- Increment in myo blood flow during max dose is less than that achieved during vasodilatation

↓

Vasodilator stress is preferred modality for MPI

Assessment of Cellular Metabolism and Physiology
- *Myocardial ischemia and viability*
  - *Programmed cell survival*

    Comprises of Myocardial stunning

    Hibernation

    Ischemic preconditioning
  - If supply demand imbalance is transient—reversible ischemia
  - Prolonged imbalance—phosphate stores depleted and regional function deteriorated progressively
  - Prolonged enough—irreversible injury
  - In stunned and hibernating myocardium
    - Myocardial function is depressed at rest
    - But myocyte remain viable
    - Stunning observed after transient period of ischemia followed by reperfusion
    - Hibernation occurs due to adaptive response of myocardium to repetitive episodes of ischemia resulting in hypoperfusion at rest
  - Cell viability require
    - Sufficient myocardial blood flow
    - Cell memb integrity
    - Preserved metabolic activity
  - So only MBF values done + provide info about stunned and hibernating myocardium

↓

Metabolic parameters need to be assessed

↓

Tracer that reflects cation flux (^{201}Tl), electro-mechanical gradient (^{99}Tc) or metabolic process (^{18}FDC) provide insight into myocardial viability

↓

^{201}Tl = Myocyte uptake represent sarcolemma integrity and cation flux

^{99}Tc = Myocyte uptake represents mitochondrial memb integrity and myocyte memb electro-mechanical gradient

FDG = myocyte uptake provide insight into intact glucose metabolism

- *Myocardial metabolism*
  - ATP generated in
    - Oxidative phosphorylation
    - Glycolysis
  - Major source of energy
    - Fatty acid
    - Glucose
    - Lactate
  - *In fasting state:* Long chain FA are preferred source of energy
  - *In normal oxygen supply:* ATP and tissue citrate formed by breakdown of FA—suppress oxidation of glucose
  - *When O_2 supply decrease:* ATP and citrate level falls—glycolysis accelerated—can maintain ATP supply at cost of generating lactic acid—require adequate blood flow to remove lactate and H^+ ion
  - *Severe hypoperfusion:* End product of glycolytic pathway accumulate—depletion of glycolytic enzyme and depletion of high energy phosphate-cell memb disruption and cell death
- *Imaging of FA mechanisms*
  - Early PET studies
  - C- palmitate
  - I-BMIPP—Investigational
- *Imaging of glucose metabolism*

  Concept: Glucose utilization may be preserved or increased relative to flow in hypoperfused viable (hibernating) myocardium—metabolism perfusion mismatch

Q. PET and hibernating myocardium
- Glucose use absent in scarred and fibrotic tissue
- In hibernating myo—the energy produced by glycolysis may be adequate to maintain myocyte viability and to preserve electromechanical gradient across cell memb. But may not be sufficient to sustain contractile function FDG is useful
- *Imaging of oxidative metabolism and mitochondrial function*
  C acetate—In patients with recent MI and chronic stable angina, clearance rates of C-acetate predicts myocardial viability and function recovery after revasc

Pet Viability

	Contractility	Perfusion	Metabolism
Normal	Normal	Normal	Normal
Stunning	Decreasing	Decreasing-normal	Normal-decreasing
Hibernation	Decreasing	Decreasing	Increasing
Scar	Decreasing	Decreasing	Decreasing

Assessment of Vent Function

- *LV systolic function*
  By radionuclide ventriculography
  Gated SPECT
  Gated PET
  - Can also determine response to stress/exercise
  - In normal healthy subject—EI response to exercise
- *Evaluation of LV volume*
  - Radionuclide ventriculography (RVG)
  - *Adv*: Do not require assumption about vent geometry (if ECHO)
  - Suitable even when geometry is abnormal
  - Can also be calculated with gated SPECT/PET
- *Evaluation of diastolic function*
  Based on analysis of LV time-activity curve, obtained by RVG technique
  Useful in patients with HCM
  HF

DISEASE DETECTION, RISK STRATIFICATION AND CLINICAL DECISION MAKING

Stable Chest Pain Syndrome

Two major goals of testing
1. Ascertain whether CAD present or not
2. To determine long term prognosis
   - To detect patient at hard cardiac events (no fatal MI, cardiac death, all cause death)
   - To detect patient at soft cardiac events (revascularization and hospital admission for ACS/HF)

ACC/AHA
- Low risk = <1% /year risk of hard events
- Intermediate risk = 1–3%/year risk
- High risk = >3%/year risk

Prognosis

- Extent of perfusion abnormality by MPI has an important relationship with subseq likelihood of adv outcome
- In patients with suspected CAD, risk of cardiac death and management increases as no of reversible perfusion defects increases
- Stress MPI has incremental value for prognosis when added to stress ECG preg such as Duke treadmill score
- *Normal MPI associated with low risk outcomes*
  - Even when angiographic CAD is present with stable symptoms complex, normal MPI is associated with low risk outcomes
  - Mech for normal MPI in presence of CAD
    - Not clearly understood
    - May involve normal endothelial function allowing appropriate flow mediated vasodilatation during stress
    - Presence of robust collaterals
- *Dynamic assessment of progno by several studies*
  Extent of ischemia—determine sunseq outcome (specificity of such determination is low)
- *Courage trial* showed benefit of DMT in patients with SIHD
- Whether such Patient would benefit from more aggressive Intervention is concept for future study
- Benefit of serial imaging to assess for presence of residual ischemia is uncertain.

Detecting Presence and Extent of CAD

- CAG is gold standard
- *Many factors* influence sensitivity and specificity of MPI for detecting CAD
  - *Methodological influences*
    - Referral bias
    - Post referral bias
  - *Physiological influences*
    - LBBB
    - HCM
    - LV hypertrophy
    - DCM
    - Endothelial dysfunction
- *Sensitivity and specificity*
  - Sensitivity to detect CAD = 87%
  - Specificity to rule out CAD = 73%
  - ECG gated SPECT enhance specificity

- *Sensitivity affected by*
  - No of vessels involved: single vessel disease has less sensitivity than MVD
- *Cause of false positive*
  - Attenuation defect
  - Technical inadequacy
  - Coro vasospasm
  - Anomalous circulation
  - Cardiomyopathy
  - Conduction defect (LBBB)
- *Cause of false negative*
  - Submaximal ex stress
  - Use of antianginal drugs
  - Collateral circulation
  - Inappropriate interpretation
  - Suboptimal imaging
  - Balance ischemia
  - Delay in stress imaging
- *Influence of tracer*
  - Improved specificity in women with use of ^{99}Tc sestamibi based tracer compared with Tl
  - ^{99}Tc also better in obese person
- *Influence of automated quantitation*
  - Avoid inter and intra observer variations
- *Pharmacological stress test*
  - Better increased in CBF with vasodilators
  - But no reported improved diagnostic or prognostic value of pharmacological stress vs exercise stress
  - Exercised is preferred stressor ⎤
  - For patients who cannot exercise vasodilatation are procedure of choice ⎥ SUMMARY
  - Dobutamine used for patients CI for vasodilators ⎥
  - If person can't reach 85% of exercise capacity—do not give isotope because sensitivity is low for detection of CAD ⎦

Patients with Established CAD

- *Imaging post CABG*
  - Detect graft stenosis
  - SPECT in asymptomatic person is uncertain Indi
  - Extent of SPECT abnormality is important
    - More extensive perfusion abnormality is associated with higher risk of subsequent cardiac death or MI
- *Imaging post PCI*
  - Exercise MPI is superior for detecting presence and location of restenosis after PCI
  - Routine assessment of post PCI is inappropriate

- *LV function during exercise in patients with CAD*
  - EF response to exercise is reflection of impact of regional ischemia
  - Patients with CAD + Abnormal ex response in terms of EF or LV dilatation - high risk.

Detection of Preclinical CAD and Risk Stratification in Asymptomatic Subjects

- Based on Bayesian principle
- Current guidelines do not recommend routine stress MPI in asymptomatic patients
- Appropriate use criteria do not even recommend routine use of MPI in diabetics asymptomatic patients.

SPECT after Abnormal CT CAC

- Stress MPI is appropriate test to determine the need for and potential benefit of catheterization after CT demonstration of CAC (when baseline risk is high and Agatston score is >100)
- Combining CT and SPECT may provide refinement of risk stratification.

Acute Coronary Syndrome

- Diagnostic as well as prognostic
- Typical role in stabilized patient post PCI to determine risk stratification
- *Suspected CAD in ED*
  - Patient with atypical pain can be subjected to ^{99}TC SPECT
  - Improve triage
  - Reversible defect—confirms CAD
  - Absence of any perfusion defect—makes diagnosis of angina unlikely
- *NSTEMI/UA*
  - For patient with Intermediate or low risk. Stress MPI can give risk stratification value
- *STEMI:*
  - Noninvasive risk stratification before (D) is appropriate
- *Assessment of inducible ISCHEMIA Port MI*
  Three major determinants of risk
  1. Residual LV function at rest
  2. Extent of ischemic myocardium
  3. Susceptibility to vent arrhythmias
     ↓
     - Gated SPECT provides these info and is imp test in stable patient after STEMI
     - Pharmacological stress reversible defects are imp marker of residual risk and predictor of cardiac events

Imaging after Heart Failure

- *Is CAD positive causes of heart failure?*

  MPI provide info about subgroup of HF patient also has HF due to reversible ischemia and gets benefited by reperfusion
  - Normal stress MPI in HF is highly predictive of nonischemic HF
  - High sensitivity but moderate specificity
  - More extensive and more severe part defect—CAD
  - Smaller and milder defects—nonischemic cardiomyopathy
  - *Class 2A indi for revascularization:* To improve survival in patients with mild to mod LV system diagnosis function and significant multiversel CAD or prox LAD stenosis when viable myocardium extent

  Imaging protocols for assessing myocardial viability
  - ^{201}Tl
  - ^{99}Tc sestamibi and Tetrofosmin
  - *PET blood flow:* Metabolism mismatch
- Simultaneous assessment of LV function in patients with HF.

Imaging in Inflammatory and Infiltrative Cardiomyopathies

- *Myocarditis*

  "In-labeled Antimyosin scan which specifically target myosin heavy chain is used for detection of necrosis associated with myocarditis and heart transplant rejection
  - Sensitivity 95%
  - NPV 95%
- *Sarcoid heart disease*
  - SPECT MPI or gallium 67 along with CMR/CT ⎤ localize myocardial involvement in sarcoidosis
  - FDG also get accumulated in patients with granulomatous reaction and cannot diffuse out or metabolic further
    - As granuloma matures, number of macrophages and inflammatory cells decrease with subsequent fibrosis
    - FDG in concert with come can detect between acute and chronic involvement by sarcoidosis
- *Cardiac amyloidosis:* Tc pyrophosphate is helpful to identify patient with amyloidosis

Q. Molecular imaging of atherosclerosis (Dec 14)
Q. Role of PET in CV Disease (Dec 1)

Assessment of Cardiac Sympathetic Innervation in HF

- I-MIBG, c-hydrolyephedrive, and F-Fluorobenzyl guanidine
  ↓
  Imaging of sympathetic Innervation in HF
- PET provide higher resolution imaging compared to planner/SPECT imaging

Imaging Prior to Noncardiac Surgery

Normal MPI: Low likelihood of periop or long-term post op cardiac events

Reversible defect: Increase risk of cardiac events

Fixed defects: Lower risk than ischemia

Molecular Imaging of CVS

Imaging of Unstable Atherosclerotic Plague and Platelet Activation

Vulnerable plague = Necrotic lipid core + thin fibrous cap
                  + large amount of macrophage

PET imaging-can characterize coronary and carotid artery plague

- Inflammation and microcalcification by PET—OT
- Macrophage infiltration by 18FDG PET
- Active microcalcification by 18 F—NAF (F Sodium Fluoride)
- ^{18}F galacto RGD can forget Integrin AlphavB3 as well as macrophages ↓
  ↓ Marker of neovascularization

Most of studies using these molecular imaging probs for atherosclerosis are restricted to larger artenol beds such as carotids and aorta rather than coronaries

Coronary lesions that is vulnerable to rupture expresses
- Inflammation
- Intraplaque neovascularization
- Microcalcification
- Apoptosis
- Intraplaque hemorrhage.

Imaging for Apoptosis

- Tc labeled Annexure v. localize apoptotic cells
- Evaluation of patients LV dysfunction after MI to visualize apoptosis.

Imaging of Cell or Gene-based Regenerative Therapy

- Molecular imaging can identify optimal cell type, delivery root, during regimen and timing of cell delivery for understanding and advancing stem cell therapy
- PET, SPECT, PET-CT or optical imaging
- Cardiac micro PET.

Imaging of Interstitial Fibrosis and LV Remodeling

- Radionuclide imaging of RAAS
- ^{18}F-Fluorobenzyl lisinopril
- Increased ACE may be a stimulus for collagen replacement and remodeling
- Recently ATIR is also targeted for imaging human heart.

Imaging of Cardiac Valvular Inflammation and Calcification

FDG and ^{18}NaF techniques.

Imaging of Cardiac Device and Prosthetic Valve Infection

FDG-PET can accurately localize the site and extent of the device infection.

SECTION 23

Cardiac CT MRI and Plaque Rupture

23.1 PLAQUE RUPTURE AND VULNERABLE PLAQUE

LUMINAL THROMBOSIS OCCURS DUE TO VARIOUS PATHOLOGIES

- Plaque rupture (75%)
- Plaque erosion (30–35%)
- Calcified nodule (2–7%)

PLAQUE RUPTURE

Definition

A plaque with deep injury with a real defect or gap in fibrous cap that had separated its lipid rich atheromatous core from flowing blood, thereby exposing thrombogenic core of plaque.

Plaque rupture depends on:
- Its vulnerability (intrinsic property) and
- Rupture trigger (extrinsic forces).

Rupture Triggers

- Blood pressure and pulse pressure
  - Induces circumferential pressure and radial pressure
- Spasm
- Fluid dynamic stress—High blood velocity within stenotic lesions may shear endothelium away.

Vulnerability of Plaque

High risk vulnerable plaque is a nonobstructive, silent coronary lesion that suddenly becomes obstructive and symptomatic.

Histology Features

- Thin-cap fibroatheroma (TCFA) (mc/60–70%)
- Pathologic initial thickening
- Calcific plaque with luminal calcified nodule.

Prospect Trial

- Age, male sex, HTN, DM, HF, and dyslipidemia are predictors of TCFAs
- DM is strongly associated
- *Biomarkers:* hs-CRP, myeloperoxidase, Il - Lr, TNF alpha are postulated to have predictive valve.

Pathophysiology

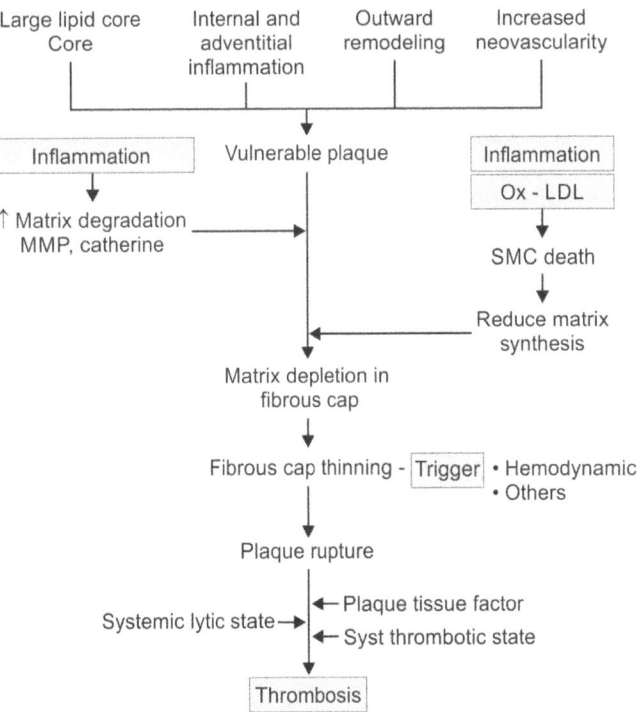

Thin fibrous cap ≤ 64 mm

Imaging Technique

- *CAG:* Any irregular lesion with ulceration, flop or aneurysm on CAG should be labeled as *"suspicious for plaque rupture"*
- *IVUS:* Excellent tool for detecting remodeling. Also detect neo vascularization within plaque. Cannot detect macrophage—poor in detecting inflammation
- *Virtual histology:* Can visualize necrotic core, calcium, collagen and fibrous tissue
  - Better than IVUS alone
- *OCT:* Highest resolution 10-20 mm
  Identify necrotic core, fibrotic cap thickness, and macrophage
  - The only imaging modality that can identify plaque with cap thickness of 65 mm or less
  - Gold standard to quantify plaque neo vascularization
  - However OCT has limited plaque penetration power, which leads to significant limitation in assessing remodeling index
- *Intravascular palpography (elastography):*
  - Determine mechanical property of vascular wall to identify vulnerable plaque
  - Color coding of strain value is performed and superimposed on IVVS image
  - High sensitivity and specificity
- *Intracoronary thermography:*
  - *Basic:* Atherosclerotic lesion with high levels of inflammatory activity produces heat
  - Several coro temperature measuring catheters are under evaluation
  - Can detect temperature of 0.05°C with spatial resolution of 0.5 mm
  - *Disadvantage:* Possible vasc injury due to direct contact with vessel wall
- *Intravascular radiation detector*
  - Very early stage of development
  - If FOG to detect metabolism
  - ^{99}TC Annexin 5 to detect apoptosis
  - ^{99}TC monocyte chemotactic peptide—1 to detect receptor expression
- *Angioscopy*
  - Yellow plagues associated with high concentration of chol—laden crystal and have thin cap
  - White plague usually has thick cap
  - *Limitation:* Does not provide direct information about plague composition
- *MRI:* Intravascular targeting agents that localize to components of atherosclerotic plaque and enhanced by MRI (gado fluorine m)
- *Near infrared spectroscopy:*
  - Used to determine chemical composition
  - *Principle:* Different substances absorb and scatter NIRS light to different degree

  (*Raman spectroscopy* also based on this principle)

Management

- *Plaque stabilization: Systemic*
  - Statin and fibrates
  - ACE-1
  - BB
  - Aspirin
  - Regular exercise
  - Omega-3 F.A.
  - Reverse chol. transport system activator (not approved)
    - App AI milano
  - Vaccination against TIE-2 (the angiopoietic receptor) (Experimental)
- *Plaque stabilization local:*
  - Stenting-neo intimal proliferation-increased thickness of fibrous cap-stabilize vulnerable plaque (theoretically)
- *Plaque stabilization: Regional*
  - Photodynamic therapy
- *Trigger reduction*

23.2 CARDIAC COMPUTED TOMOGRAPHY

INTRODUCTION

Cardiac CT provides info about
- Arterial wall
- LV and RV systolic function
- Cardiac valve function
- Myocardial tissue characterization
- Evaluation of coro physiology with perfusion imaging.

SCAN MODES

- Basic scan modes
  - *Helical scanning*
    - Cont radiation exposure and table movt
  - High pitch helical CT
    - Very rapid table feed
  - *Axial image*
    - Sequential scanner snapshot, in between which x-ray tube is turned off and table is moved to diff position

    ↓

    Reduce radiation exposure

CLINICAL APPLICATION

Seven categories:
1. Detection of CAD in symptomatic patient without known heart disease
2. CAD risk assessment in asymptomatic patient
3. CAD detection in other cardiac disease
4. Use of CT angio after other test results
5. Evaluation after revascularization
6. Evaluation of cardiac str and function
7. Evaluation of intracardiac and extracardiac str.
   CT angio considered most appropriate in which pretest likelihood of CAD is low or intermediate.

Coronary Calcium Scoring—(Noncardiac CT)

- Used is asymptomatic patient to refine their clinically predicted risk of CAD
- CAC alpha extent of atherosclerosis
- Although only approx 20% of plaque contain calcified regions
- Arterial calcification is above process involving deposition of hydroxyapatite, most typically in areas with healed plaque rupture
- Acute pl rupture
  Vulnerable plaque } contain speckled or prog Ca^{++}
- Healed plaque—contain diffuse Ca^{++}
- CT CAC—measurements of areas and density of all foci of calcification, defined using HV

Sum of area and density weighings across the coronary arteries is the unitless CAC score

$$CAC = \frac{\text{Area of each calcified}}{\text{Coronary lesion}} \times \frac{\text{Coefficient of 1 to 4}}{\text{Depending on max CT attenuation}}$$

Indi for CAC Scoring

- *Recommended*
  - Patients with F/H/O pre mat CAD
  - Patient with Intermediate risk of CAD
- *May be considered*
  - Patients with high risk of CAD
- *Not recommended*
  - Patients with loss risk of CAD

> Not all plaques are calcified. Not all healthy calcified plaques are significantly stenotic

CAC score 5 groups
1. 0 = No coronary calcium
2. 100 = mild coro calcification
3. 100 to 399 = mod calcification
4. 400 to 999 = severe calcification
5. >1000 = extensive calcification

- CAC score is age and gender specific
- CAC score has modest reproducibility
  - Interscan variability of 10–20%
  - More reproducible at lower HR and high CAC score
- CAC depends on
  - Age
  - Gender
  - Ethnicity
  - Standard cardiac risk factors
- Detection CAC indicates increased risk of incident CAD
  - CAC > 100 = 2-fold increased risk
  - CAC > 1000 = 11 fold increased risk
- Higher clinical risk associated with
  - Multivessel CAC
  - More no of calcified lesions
  - Diffuse spotty calcification (small foci < 3 mm size)
- CAC score = 0 - very high event free survival
- *"Coronary CAC coverage score"*
  Greater predictive accuracy
- Current guidelines (appropriate use criteria)
  - Intermediate risk patient (on clinical background) CAC can
  - Low risk patients with family H/O premat CD be done
- Once present, CAC tends to progress at a rate of approx 20%/year

- Patients with clinically significant CAC progression (>10%/year)—higher clinical event risk and 3-fold increased risk for all-cause mortality
  ↓
Risk reducing intervention (e.g., statin) do not retard CAC progression—CAC progression is a complex phenomena

Current guidelines do not support performance of serial CAC testing.

Coronary CT Angio (CCTA)

- *For diagnosis of CAD*
  - Accuracy of 64 slice CT
    - Sensitivity 87-99%
    - Specificity 93-96%
  - Most useful in low—intermediate risk patients
  - NPV of CCTA is very high 95-100%
  - CCTA is excellent for ruling out CAD

  Patients who are poor candidate for CCTA
  - Patient likely to have heavily calcified coro art
    - Older than 75 years
    - ESRD
    - Paget's disease
  - AF/APL
  - Freq VPCs
  - Uncontrolled tachy

  Grading: 0 Normal = absence of plaque/no luminal stenosis
  1 minimal = plaque with <25% stenosis
  2 mild = 25-49% stenosis
  3 mod = 50-69% stenosis
  4 severe = 70-99% stenosis
  5 occluded

- *For Prognosis*
  Two approaches
  1. Calculation of segment involvement score
  2. No of involved vessels

  Clinical application of CCTA
  - *In ED*
    - To exclude CAD in patient with atypical/nonspecific chest pain/angina
    - Facilitate triage
  - *Detection of noncalcified plaques*
    - Appealing but unvalidated approach
    - Defined as any coro art wall lesion with an x-ray attenuation detectably below that for iodine contrast medium but higher than for surrounding tissue
    - Difficult to quantify
    - Severity tends to be underestimated
    - 15-50 HU—lipid rich plaque approx 100 HU—fibrous plaque
  - Vulnerable plaque
    - Low attenuation plaque (<30 HU)
    - Outward remodeling
    - Spotty calcification (<3 mm size)
- *Evaluation post CABG*
  - In general patients with known CAD are not good candidate for CCTA because of high pre-test likelihood
  - Evaluation of bypass graft is highly accurate—specification ~ 100% due to its large size and limited mobility
  - Metallic clips and severe CAC limits its use
  - Before redo CABG CCTA is appropriate to delineate relationship of sternal wires to cardiac and graft structures
- *Imaging coro stents*
  - Artifacts from metallic stent limits its use
  - Mod—high accuracy (approaching 90% can be achieved when stent > 3 min or greater in diameter
  - Stent in LMCA may be appropriately imaged
  - Quantitative assessment of contrast density within stent may assist in diagnosis
  - Currently CT is not recommended for suspected Isx.

CT artifacts
- Registration error (seen as horizontal line)
- Respiratory motion
- Poor contrast opacification of coro art
- Coronary duplication artifact (by ectopic)
- Poor signal to noise ratio (grain image)
- Severe coro calcification
- Streak artifact by implanted pacemaker

- *Coronary artery anomalies*
  MDCT with 3D reconstruction.

Ventricular and Valvular Morphology

- Contrast enhanced MDCT provide images of cardiac chamber as well as accurate assessment of RV and LV systolic function
- Myocardial morphology can also be reliably assessed for—previous MI (wall thinning, calcification or fatty replacement)
- Clot in LAA can be identified with high NPV
- High accuracy for LV mural thrombi
- Anatomic evaluation of both native and prosthetic valves
  - *AS:* Valve calcification and orifice area more accurate assessment of annulus
    Detection of potential hazards (Ao root calcification)
  - Imp tool before TAVR
  - AR—malcoaptation of valve

- Prosthetic valve malfunction
  - Size mismatch
  - Tissue ingrowth
  - Valve thrombosis
  - Paravalvular leaks.

Acute Aortic Syndromes and PE

- AK dissection—100% sensitivity and 98% specificity
- Ao intramural hematoma
- Pulm embolism—99% NPV

Pericardial Disease

- Congenital absence of pericat
- Constructive pericarditis
- Pericardial syst
- Neoplasm.

Congenital Heart Disease

Coronary Blood Flow, Physiology and Myocardial Scar

- Myocardial attenuation reflects CBF on 1st pass imaging
  - CECT at rest and during adenosine administration can detect coronary reserve

    ↓

    Limitation: High dose radiation exposure
  - Physiology by CT FFR
  - *Scar*

    Cardiac CT detects regions of myocardial hypo-attenuation + myo thickness <5 mm

    ↓

    Prev MI or nonviable myocardium

23.3 CARDIOVASCULAR MRI

BASIC PRINCIPLE
- Based on imaging of protons within abundant hydrogen atoms in human body
- Hydrogen-proton behave like tiny magnet
  Patient placed inside CMR scanner with a static magnetic field (Bo)
  ↓
  Spin of a proton—hydrogen either align or opposing to spin main direction of Bo
  ↓
  Summation of aligned and opposing spin forms a net magnetization vector that aligns along longitudinal axis (z axis)
  ↓
  3 orthogonal sets of giant cells are placed so that a slight linear alteration in strength of Bo can be created in each of x, y and z direction

CLINICAL APPLICATION OF CMR
Coronary Artery Disease
CMR Protocols
- Cine imaging
- Tz weighed edema imaging
- MPI at rest and stress
- LGE imaging of MI
- *Myocardial ischemia and Infarction*
  - Ischemia
    Cine image: Normal or RWMA
    Edema: Negative
    Perfusion: Reversible subendocardial perfusion defect in a coro distribution
    LGE: Normal
    Other:
    - Subendocardial perfusion defect from significant coro stenosis should persist beyond peak myo enhancement during first pass transit of GBCA bolus
    - Coronary MRA may show luminal stenosis
  - Acute MI
    Cine: RWMA
    Edema: Usually transmural bright region in the segment subtended IRA
    MPI: Subendocardial perfusion defect at rest (post revasc) represent no-reflow
    LGE: Subendocardial or transmural LGE
    Other: Elo myocardial hemorrhage by T2 and T2* imaging intracavitary thrombus.
  - Chronic MI
    Cine: RWMA; Chronic remodeling changes
    Edema: Neg
    MPI: Subendocardial defect at rest matching thinned infarct region
    LGE: Thinned subendocardial or transmural LGE
    Other: Intracavitary thrombus

LGE
- LGE imaging is most accurate noninvasive method for quantifying infarct size and morphology
- Excellent spatial resolution
- LGE provide info of subendocardial infarct beyond SPECT/PET
- Sens 99%; spec 94%
- In acute MI, LGE done within 5 min after contrast injection shows microvascular obst (no flow) seen as hypoenhanced area surround by bright region representing infarct
- In nonacute setting, infarct identified by LGE with history or ECG—strong, predictor of adv event
- Can detect myocardial hemorrhage (2° to reperfusion)
- Can detect acute RV injury—prognostic value
- Infarct tissue heterogenicity on LGE—suggest atherogenic substrate that develop as a result of MI-strong predictor of vent arrhythmia-required ICD
- *Assessment of myocardial viability*
  CMR:
  - Structural assessment
  - Physiology associated with myocardial viability
  - *End diastolic wall thickness*
    - High specificity from low dose dobutamine cine image provide an assessment of mid-myocardium
    - Limited accuracy in predicting recovery of regional function because wall involve irreversibly damaged myocardium and thinned epicardial of viable myocardium
    - EDW thickness ≥5.5 mm ⎤
    - Dobutamine induced systolic ⎬ Predictor of segmental recovery post revasc
      Wall thickness of ≥2 mm ⎦
  - Transmural extent of scar on LGE
    - Predict progressive stepwise decrease in function recovery despite successful coronary revascularization
    - Compared to dobutamine cine CMR, LGE is easy to perform

- 50% transmurality cut off is sensitive in predicting recovery
- Even thin myocardium without LGE increase in thickness post revasc and good choice of regain function
  ↓
- Overall LGE image is sufficient to detect myocardial viability and predict recovery post revasc
- Low dose dobu is complementary in acute post MI period when tissue edema is prominent or when high specificity is required to justify CABG in patients with high risk

	Acute myocardial stunning	*Chronic hibernation*
Cine	RWMA	RWMA regional thinning possible
Edema	Positive	Negative
MPI	Normal at rest	Resting subendocardial perfusion defect in a coro distribution
LGE	Normal	Normal
Other	• Stress perfusion shows perfusion defect during peak vasodilatation • Coro MRA shows Luminal stenosis	• Stress perfusion shows larger extent of perfusion defect than at rest • Intracavitary thrombus may exist

Detecting and quantifying myocardial ischemia
Advantage of CMR- MPI over SPECT
- Not limited by attenuation artifact
- Free from ionizing radiation
- 3-4 fold higher spatial resolution
- Also characterize dynamic range of myo blood flow without being limited by plateau effects at higher flow rate
- Sensitivity 91%
  Specificity 94%
- CMR-MPI can be analyzed quantitatively (fully automated) using signal intensity vs time curves—gives absolute myocardial blood flow and minimize bias
- Dobutamine stress CMR is better than Dobutamine stress ECHO
- Exercise CMR is investigational tool

- *Imaging of atheroscleotic plaque*
  MRI:
  - Most comprehensive noninvasive method to characterize plaque str and activity
  - T1 W image differentiate thin fibrous cap from lipid core ⎤
  - T2 W image can detect intraplaque hemorrhage ⎥ For carotid or aortic plaque
  - Plaque revascularization can also be assessed ⎥
  - Ultrasmall superpara magnetic particles of iron oxide (USP10) may target macrophage activity ⎦
  - Imaging of coronary plaque is challenged by cardiac and respi motion and small vessel size
    ↓
  Future technological improvement with use of exogenous target contrast agents, intravascular coils and high field CMR are promising

- *Assessment of global and regional function*

Cardiomyopathy

- Accurate and highly reproducible
- CMR offer unique ability to detect
  LV dyssynchrony ⎤
  Scar extent   ⎥ Imp for response to CRT
  Coronary venous anatomy

Protocols
- Cine cardiac function/str
- MPI at rest
- Myocardial edema imaging
- LGE imaging

- *Hypertrophic CMP:*
  Cine: Increased vent mass; ASH with/without LVOTO, spade shaped LV chamber in apical HCM
  Edema: Often Abnormal
  MPI: Abnormal in thickened myocardial segment represents
  Abnormal microcirculation

  LGE: LGE at RV insertion into LV or patchy midwall involve in hypertrophied segment
  Other: Outflow Obstruction by phase contrast imaging
         May show reduced intramyocardial motion

- Cine imaging useful in distinguishing physiological from pathological hypertrophy
- EDW thickness to cavity volume ratio <0.15 mm/mL/m² and back of abnormal LGE of myocardium differentiates physiological LVH from pathological LVH
- Superior to ECHO
  - ECHO misses antilat wall hypertrophy in 33%
  - ECHO misses apical aneurysm in 40%

- Markedly elevated LV mass index (>91 gm/m² male and >69 g/m² female) very sensitive for HCM and associated cardiac death
- Max wall thickness >30 mm—highly specific for cardiac death
- Blunted endocardial myocardial blood flow and myocardial fibrosis both related to degree of hypertrophy—possibility that microvascular dysfunction plays a role in dev of hypertrophy
- In patients with HCM, LGE associated with arrhythmias

- ARVC
  Cine: RV dilated/aneurysmal
  Edema: Negative
  Perfusion: Normal
  LGE: RV often full thickness LGE matching location of RV aneurysm
  LV focal LGE
  Other:
  - Fatty infiltration of RV and LV focally seen with T1 W imaging and confirmed by fat suppression technique
  - Nulling of normal myocardial signal in RV and LV require different inversion times (TI)

  CMR better than ECHO
  - Quantitative and volumetric function assessment of RV
  - Characterization of fibrofatty myocardial tissue
  - Also detect LV disease
  - Localized aneurysm
  - Severe global dilatation with Systolic dysfunction } major criterion
  - Severe segmental dilatation of RV
  - CMR sensitivity = 90%; specificity 78%
  - Fat suppression LGE imaging of Rav fibrosis shown high correlation with endomyocardial Bx

- Myocarditis
  Cine: RWMA and/or hypocontractile LV
  Edema: Usually transmural
  Bright regions seen—patchy or diffuse
  MPI: Normal
  LGE: Epicardial and midwall LGE involving IL wall/septum

  CMR target 3 main pathophysiologic components
  1. Myocardial edema by T2 imaging
  2. Regional hyperemia and capillary leak by early gadolinium enhancement
  3. Myocardial necrosis/fibrosis by LGE
     - Combined T2 WI and LGE - Good diagnostic accuracy

- *Cardiac sarcoid*
  Cine: RWMA and/or hypocontractile LV/RV
  MPI: Normal
  Edema: Bright regions
  LGE: Multifocal intense LGE involving septum, IL wall of LV, RA and RV free wall
  Stage of disease edema—noncascading granulomatous infiltration—patchy myocardial fibrosis

- *Amyloidosis*
  Cine: Restrictive morphology
  Edema: Neg
  MPI: Diffuse perfusion defect
  LGE: Diffuse circumferential LGE
  Char: Zebra stripe circumferential pattern of LGE involving LV and even RV subendocardium

- *Idiopathic DCM*
  Cine: Dilated, contractile LV
  Edema: Neg
  MPI: Normal
  LGE: Midwall LGE often in septum
  CMR:
  - Can rule out ischemic cardiomyopathy
  - Pattern of LGE has diagnostic and prognostic implications
  - Monitoring of treatment and disease progression
  - In total absence of LGE-Ischemic case unlikely
  - CMR using combination of LGE and coronary MRA- 96% specific and 100% sensitive

- *Iron overload CM pathy*
  - Global systolic LV dysfunction present
  - CMR T2* image for quantifying myocardial iron

- *Other cardiomyopathy*
  - Chagas disease
  - LV noncompaction
  - Transient LV apical ballooning
  - Endomyocardial fibrosis
  - Loeffler endocarditis

Pericardial Disease

- Protocols
  - Cine imaging
  - T1 W and T2W double inversion black blood FSE sequence
  - LGE imaging and whole heart
- Normal pericardium <2 mm thick and low intensity on T1 and T2W image
- Transverse sinus may be mistaken for AoD
- Oblique sinus may be mistaken for esophageal lesion or bronchogenic cyst

- *Pericardial effusion*
  - Low intensity on T1W
  - High intensity on gradient echo imaging
  - Exception is hemorrhage effusion
- *Constrictive pericarditis*
  - Pericardial thickening ≥4 mm ⎤
  - Tethering of pericardium   ⎬ Char
  - Conical or tubular deformity of vent ⎦
  - 2° changes: Atrial enlargement
    Syst and PV dilatation
    Hepatomegaly, ascites
    Pleural effusion
  - *Cine sequence:* Feature of constrictive physiology (diastolic septal bounce and abrupt limitation of diastolic filling)
    (D/D)(RCMP):
    - Generally delayed diastolic filling pattern
    - Real time cine with free breathing shows vent interdependence with septal bounce
- Congenital absence of pericardium
- Pericardial syst

Disease of Aorta

- *Aortic aneurysm*
  - MRI can detect both as vessel wall and lumen
  - More reliable than CT
- *Aortic dissection*
- *Intramural hematoma and penetrating ulcer*
- *Atherosclerotic disease*
  - Irregular thickening
- Trauma to aorta
- Aortitis
- Aortic stents and grafts

Cong Heart Disease

- *ASD/VSD*
  - Diagnostic purpose
  - Access suitability for transseptal closure
  - Quantify RV function
  - Determine Qp/Qs
  - Coexisting anomaly
  - Residual shunt and proper device deployment
- *Anomalous PV connection*
- *COA*
- *d-TGA*
- *Conotruncal anomalies*
  TOF: Evaluation of planned surgical procedure
       Post op evaluation (RV function)

Valvular Heart Disease

- Provide complementary evaluation that obtained by ECHO
- More sensitive than ECHO in detecting 3D changes in vent size, function and myocardial mass
- *Novel application:* Vortical blood flow in PA
  - Estimate mPAP and differentiate patient with PH
- Clear morphology of valve, planimetry, precise quantification of regurgitant vol, accurate measure of vent vol and function, associated abnormality.

Cardiac Thrombus and Mass

- LGE image detect thrombus with high specificity
- Good sensitivity and specificity for tumors

Novel cardiac MRI techniques

- *T1 and T2 mapping*
  - T1 mapping—demonstrate good correlation with collagen content of interstitial space
  - T2 mapping detect myocardial edema
- *MR spectroscopy*
  - Provides info regarding cellular metabolism
- *CMR imaging at 3 Tesla*
  - High signal to noise ratio—higher quality speed and spatial resolution
  - Pulse sequence such as MPI and LGE are improved from higher signal to noise ratio at 3T
  - Fat suppression imaging can be more precise
- *Molecular cardiac MRI*
- *CMR for testing novel CV therapies*
  Experimental use for stem cell tracking and their survival

CONTRAINDICATION

- Cerebral aneurysm clips
- Metallic foreign bodies
- Cardiac pacemaker and ICD—relative
- Cardiac catheters (PA catheters)—relative
- Intravasc coils/stents/filter (upto 6-8 weeks)
- Heart valve prosthesis
- Metallic cardiac devices (ASD/VSD/PDA closure) (6-8 wks)
- Retained epicardial pacing wire

HYPER ENHANCEMENT WITH MRI IN CV DISEASE

Ischemic

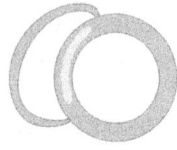 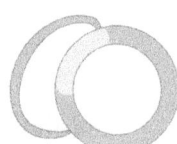

Subendocardial infarct   Transmural infarct

Non-ischemic

(A) *Mid wall HE*

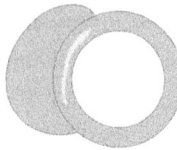 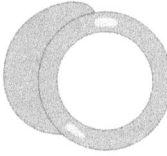 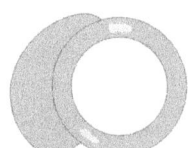

Idiopathic DCM myocarditis   HCM RV pr overload (CHD, PHTN)   Sarcoidosis Anderson-Fabry disease myocarditis chagas disease

(B) *Epicardial HE*

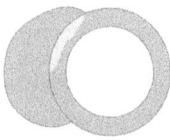 

Sarcoidosis, Myocarditis, Anderson-Fabry disease, Chagas disease

(C) *Global endocardial HE*

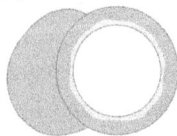

- Amyloidosis
- Systemic sclerosis
- Post-cardiac transplant

SECTION 24

Trials

24.1 AMULET STUDY

INTRODUCTION

Amulet: Percutaneous transcatheter left atrial appendage occluder device
- To prevent thromboembolism from LA appendage among patients with nonvalvular AF
- By St. Jude medical AMPLATZER

Type of study:
- Randomized prospective study
- Competitive study
  (Amulet vs. watchman device)

INCLUSION CRITERIA

- Age ≥18 years
- Nonvalvular AF
- High risk of stroke/systemic embolism
    CHADS2 >2 or CHA2DS2 vasc >3
- Patient with suitable LAA closure
- Patient suitable for short-term oral anticoagulation but not suitable for long-term oral anticoagulation
- Written consent.

EXCLUSION CRITERIA

- Patient has valvular heart disease
- Patient undergone ASD/PFO device closure in past
- Patient with mechanical valve prosthesis
- Stroke/TIA within 90 days
- NYHA class 4 heart failure
- LVEF <30%
- Reversible cause of AF
- Any contraindication to postprocedural dual antiplatelet therapy or OACs
- Active endocarditis
- Known malignancy or other illness where life expectancy is <2 years
- Thrombocytopenia (<70,000 platelets) or anemia (Hb <10 mg/dL).

PRIMARY OUTCOME MEASURES

- Procedure related complications, major bleeding events, all-cause mortality (within 12 months)
- Ischemic stroke/TIA/systemic emboli
    (Within 18 months)
- Device closure (defined on TEE).

SECONDARY OUTCOME MEASURES

- All stroke, systemic emboli or cardiovascular/unexplained death
- Major bleeding post device (18 months).

RESULT: (INTRIM) (EXPECTED COMPLETION: 2020–23)

- Implant success >98% cases
- Implant success, LAA closure rate and device or procedure related complications are comparable to watchman device
- Early mortality (within 7 days) is less (0.3%) compared to watchman device (0.7%)

24.2 BEST (2015)

BACKGROUND
- In patients with MVCAD: IG PCI with 2nd gen stents (DES) non-inferior to CABG with regards to death, MI or target vessel revasc
- CABG is class 1 recommendation for MVD (based on older RCT and data with 1st gen stents).

DESIGN
- Prospective
- Randomized
- N = 880
- Median follow-up 4–6 years
- *Analysis:* Intention to treat
- 1° outcome: (Death, nonfatal MI, TVR) composite.

INCLUSION
- Age ≥18 years
- Angiographically confirmed MVCAD (>70% stenosis in at least 2 major epicardial vessel in 2 separate coro art territories)
- Indication for revasc based on symptoms of angina/objective elo myo ischemia.

EXCLUSION
- Known hypersensitivity to heparin, ASA, clopidogrel, everolimus, or contrast media
- NYHA 3 or more CHF symptoms
- Prev CABG
- Planned simultaneous surgery with CABG (e.g., valve replace)
- Prior PCI with PES within 1 year
- 2 or more CTO in major arteries
- Acute STEMI within 72 hours
- Abnormal CPK, CPKMB or troponin levels
- Previous stroke within 6 months or stroke of >6 months with significant residual
- Life expectancy <2 years
- LM CAD ≥50% stenosis.

INTERVENTION
- Randomization in to PCI and CABG gr 1:1
- Use of IVUS, adjunctive device or Gp2b/3a inhibitors at operator choice
- All patients undergoing received aspirin and clopidogrel before or during PCI
- After PCI all patients received
  Aspirin (100 mg)
  Clopidogrel (75) × 12 months
- Secondary prev medications used as per guidelines
- Follow-up at 1 month, 6, 9, and 12 months and annually.

RESULT
- Non-significant increase in composite of death, non-fatal MI or TVR in PCI group (15.3% vs. 10.6%) — 1° endpoint
- NS increase in all cause death; MI; spont MI; and TVR in PCI group
- Stroke decreased in PCI group (again NS) — 2° endpoint
- TIMI major bleeding was significantly reduced in patients undergoing PCI

CONCLUSION
In patient with MV-CAD, PCI with 2nd gen (everolimus eluting stents) are inferior to CABG and associated with absolute 4–7% increase in death, MI and TVR at 4–6 years
↓
This was due to 3.3% absolute increase in TVR.

CRITICS
- 40% of patients were diabetics—result may have driven by patients with DM—no subgroup analysis of non-diabetics patients had been done
- Open labeled study—*assessment bias*
- Study terminated early due to slow enrollment
- Patient in PCI group were more likely to receive certain medications like DAPT, BB, ACE/ARB, CCB, etc.,—limiting the benefit of CABG over PCI.

24.3 CANTOS TRIAL

CANAKINUMAB ANTI-INFLAMMATORY THROMBOSIS OUTCOMES STUDY

It tests the "Inflammatory hypothesis of atherosclerosis".

Background

Experimental and clinical data suggest that reducing inflammation without affecting lipid levels may reduce risk of cardiovascular disease.

Population

- History of MI
- Blood level of CRP >2 mg/dL

Exclusion

History of chronic or recurrent infection
- Previous cancer other than Basal cell Ca
- Suspected or known immunocompromised
- History or high risk of TB
- HIV
- Ongoing anti-inflammatory treatment.

Randomization

Initially randomly assigned
1:1:1
Placebo Canakinumab or 300 mg
150 mg
↓
After 741 patient
50 mg dose added on request
↓
Final randomization
1.5:1:1:1
(Placebo)

All doses: SC once every 3 months
For 300 mg—every 2 weeks
For 1st 2 doses
And then once every 3 months
↓
Randomization

Endpoint

Primary efficacy endpoint:
- First occurrence of non-fatal MI
- Any non-fatal stroke
  - Cardiovascular death

Secondary efficacy endpoints:
- Incidence of new onset type 2 DM among patients with pre-diabetes at randomization

2 other prespecified secondary endpoints = Death from any cause
Composite of non-fatal MI/any non-fatal stroke or death of any cause.

Result

Canakinumab significantly reduced high sensitivity C-reactive protein from baseline as compared with placebo without reducing LDL cholesterol level and 150 mg dose resulted in significantly lower incidence of recurrent cardiovascular event.

24.4 AIDA

BACKGROUND
In patients with stable or unstable CAD undergoing PCI, are bioresorbable scaffolds superior to DES with regards to target vessel failure?

DESIGN
- Prospective
- Multi-center
- Single-blind
- Duration of follow-up 2 yrs
- *Analysis:* Intention to treat.

1° OUTCOME
Target vessel failure (death, target vessel MI, target vessel revasc).

INCLUSION
Patient is a candidate for DES based on consensus guidelines.

EXCLUSION
- Age <18 years
- Bifurcation lesion with planned 2 stent strategy
- Planned treatment of ISR
- Unsuccessful predilatation of one of the lesion
- One or more lesions treated with scaffold/stent length >70 mm and/or overlapping of 4 or more stents
- Pregnancy
- Life expectancy <1 yr
- Unable to meet clinical follow-up

INTERVENTION
- 1:1 randomization to scaffold and DES
- Patients were blinded/but not providers/operations
- Postdilatation was not required during 1st year of study while during 2nd yr, postdilatation was recommended by manufacturer
- DAPT and other medications as per ESC guidelines
- Follow-up 1 month, 6 months, 1-2-3-4-5 years.

RESULT
- Target vessel failure (death, non-fatal MI or target vessel revasc) was NS diff between 2 groups
- All cause death, MI or any revasc was also NS.

CONCLUSION
- BRS associated with similar rate of target vessel failure as DES at 2 years
- Scaffold were associated with absolute 2-6% increase in probable or definite device thrombosis compared to DES.

CRITICS
- Nonbinding of operator/providers
- Limited follow-up of 2 years.

24.5 CASTLE AF

INTRODUCTION

CASTLE AF = NOVEL [1st time primary endpoint = mortality (Catheter ablation vs. conventional therapy for hospitalized) patients with A fib and LV dysfunction]

397 patients
Symptomatic paroxysmal or persistent AF
left VEF of ≤35%
Randomized

All had implantable/ (CRT-1) cardioverter defibrillator with home capability
- Radiofrequency cardiac ablation
- Conventional drug treatment

Primary endpoint: Composite of all-cause mortality unplanned hospitalization for worsening heart failure

Secondary endpoint: All-cause mortality
Hospitalization
Worsening heart failure
CV mortality
Cerebrovascular accident
Quality of life

INCLUSION

Criteria

- ICD (CRT-1) home monitoring capabilities with 1° or 2° prevention
- LVEF ≤35%
- NYHA class 2 or higher
- Symptomatic paroxysmal or persistent AF
- Failed or intolerant to 1 or more anti arrhythmic medication.

At 5 years
- Catheter ablation led to significant improvement in primary composite endpoint of all-cause mortality and worsening heart failure with relative risk reduction of 38%
- 8% increase in EF vs none in conventional group.

24.6 CAPTAF

INTRODUCTION

CAPTAF is catheter ablation compared with optimized pharmacological therapy for atrial fibrillation.

It showed improvement in quality of life with catheter ablation for atrial fibrillation.

GOAL

Evaluate catheter ablation compared with pharmacological therapy among patients with paroxysmal or persistent atrial fibrillation.

Study design: Randomized parallel
Inclusion Criteria: 155 patients

Paroxysmal or persistent atrial fibrillation
Who failed at least once antiarrhythmic drug
↓ Randomized ↓
Catheter ablation   Pharmacological therapy
Primary outcome, general health score at 12 months.

PRINCIPAL FINDINGS

Primary outcome, general health score at 12 months improved significantly more in ablation group than in drug group.

24.7 CAMERA-MRI TRIAL

CATHETER ABLATION vs MEDICAL RATE CONTROL IN HEART FAILURE

Multicenter randomized control study (open study)
Eligibility: Inclusion criteria
- Paroxysmal or persistent AF
- LVEF <0.45
- DCMP
  Min age = 18, Max age = 85
  Gender = Both males and females.

KEY EXCLUSION CRITERIA
- Non-MRI safe pacemaker, ICD
- Biventricular device
- Renal impairment (Cr >2)
- Left atrial thrombus.

PRIMARY OUTCOME
- Recovery of LV assessed by improvement in EF determined by cardiac MRI and echocardiography (assessed at 6 months)
- Restoration of sinus rhythm assessed by loop recorder interrogation (catheter ablation arr), (Holter monitoring) and ECG (rate control arr)

Loop recorder = 6 weeks, 3 and 6 months
Holter monitoring assessed at 3 and 6 months

Arm 1	Arm 2 pharmacological
Catheter ablation	rate control
(3D mapping)	(Beta-blocker/digoxin)

MRI help to identify those patients with AF/HF following catheter ablation, HF will reverse or completely reverse

Pt with HF display a unique pattern of scarring in heart muscle capable of being detected by MRI.

CONCLUSION
- AF = underappreciated cause of LV dysfunction in patient with an otherwise unexplained
  Cardiomyopathy with rate controlled persistent AF
- Catheter ablation is effective in restoring SR and LV
- Absence of delayed enhancement identified patient likely to recover LV function with catheter ablation.

24.8 VIVA TRIAL

INTRODUCTION
"Vascular endothelial growth factor in ischemia for vascular angiogenesis"

    Double-blind

    Placebo controlled trial

    Designed to evaluate safety and efficacy of intracoronary and IV infusion of rh VEGF.

METHOD
178 patients

    Stable exertional angina

    Unsuitable for revascularization

        ↓Randomized to receive placebo

Low dose rh VEGF   High dose rh VEGF   20 min
17 mg/kg/min   50 mg/kg/min   Intracoronary

By intracoronary infusion

    |On day 0

IV infusion on day 3,6 and 9 (4-hour infusion)

- Exercise treadmill tests   Day 60
- Angina class   Day 120
- Quality of life assessments

   Myocardial perfusion imagine baseline |60

Primary endpoint: Change in ETT time from baseline to day 60 between group

Secondary endpoint: Change in ETT time from baseline to day 120, rest and exercise myocardial perfusion imaging on day 60, angina class and quality of life measurements at day 60/120.

CONCLUSION
rh VEGF
- Safe
- Well tolerated
- No improvement beyond placebo in all measurements by day 60
- By day 120
  High dose rh VEGF
  Significant improvement in angina
  And favorable trends in ETT time and angina frequency.

24.9 COMPASS TRIAL

BACKGROUND

Whether rivaroxaban alone or in combination with aspirin would be more effective than aspirin alone for secondary cardiovascular prevention:
- 602 Caths
- 33 countries
- Double-blind
- Randomized

INCLUSION CRITERIA

- Written concept
- CAD younger than 65 years of age involving at least 2 vascular beds or to have at least additional risk factors
  - Current smoking
  - DM
  - eGFR <60 m/min
  - Heart failure
  - Nonlacunar ischemic stroke ≥1 month.

EXCLUSION CRITERIA

- High bleeding risk
- Recent stroke or previous hemorrhagic or lacunar stroke
- Severe heart failure
- Advance stable kidney disease eGFR <15 mL/m
- Use of dual antiplatelet therapy
  - Anticoagulation or other
  - Antithrombotic therapy

27,395

↓

Stable atherosclerotic vascular disease

Rivaroxaban

- 5 mg 1-0-1
- 2.5 mg 1-0-1 + aspirin 100 mg 1-00
- Aspirin 100 mg 1-00

Primary efficacy outcome: Composite of cardiovascular death, stroke or MI

3 secondary efficacy outcome:
- Composite of ischemic stroke
  MI
  Acute limb ischemia
  Or death from CAD
- Composite of ischemic stroke, MI, acute limb ischemia or cardiovascular death
- Death from any cause.

RESULT

Primary outcome occurred in fewer patients in Rivaroxaban + aspirin group.

CONCLUSION

Patients with stable atherosclerotic disease, those assigned to rivaroxaban 2.5 mg 1-0-1 daily
+ Aspirin
had better cardiovascular outcomes and more major bleeding events than those assigned to Aspirin alone.

Rivaroxaban 5 mg BD alone did not result in better cardiovascular outcomes and resulting in more major bleeding.

24.10 CLARIFY STUDY

■ SUGGEST

Caution in use of blood pressure (BP) lowering treatment in patient with coronary artery disease

22,672 patient 45 counts
↓
Clarify registry

treated for HTN from November 2009 to June 2010
Systolic/diastolic BP before each event averaged and categorized into 10 mm Hg increment

Primary outcome	Secondary outcome
CV death	Each component of primary
MI	Endpoint
or	All cause death and
Stroke	Hospital admission for heart failure

Median follow-up of 5 years

Increased SBP >140 mm Hg or more ⎤ Increased risk of
Increased DBP >80 mm Hg ⎦ cardiovascular events

SBP <120 mm Hg also increases the risk for primary outcome as well as Increased risk for all secondary outcome except stroke.

Study support existence of J curve phenomenon
Low BP goals from randomized study
When translated in routine practice
  Higher adverse effects ⟶
  especially in old

24.11 CULPRIT SHOCK—2017

QUESTION

In patient with AMI and cardiogenic shock, who found to have MVD on CAG—Is mc—PCI superior to culprit-only PCI?

DESIGN

- Multicenter
- Open—labeled
- Randomized
- N = 706
- F/up = 30 days
- Analysis = intention to treat
- 1° outcome = Death from any cause or severe renal failure leading to renal replacement therapy.

INCLUSION

- Planned early revasc by PCI
- MV—CAD with identifiable culprit lesion
- Shock defined as (either of)
  - SBP <90 for >30 minutes
  - Catecholamine required to maintain SBP >90 during systole
- Signs of pulm congestion
- Signs of impaired perfusion (any 1)
  - Altered mentation
  - Cold, clammy skin and extremities
  - Oliguria with U-O <30 mL/h
  - Lactate >2-0 mmol/L.

EXCLUSION

- Resuscitation >30 min
- No intrinsic heart action
- Cerebral deficit with fixed dilated pupils
- Need for 1° urgent CABG
- Single vessel disease
- Mechanical cause of cardiogenic shock
- Onset of shock >12 hrs
- Massive lung emboli
- Age >90 years
- Shock of other cause (hypovolemia, sepsis)
- Limited life expectancy <6 mths.

INTERVENTION

- 1:1 Randomization immediately after CAG
- In patient randomized to MV—PCI,
  - PCI of all lesions with ≥70% stenosis was mandated (including CTO)
- In patient randomized to culprit only—PCI,
  - Revasc of other lesion was staged based on residual ischemic lesion (non-invasive testing or FFR), symptoms and clinical—neurological states.

CONCLUSION

- Culprit only PCI is associated with 95% absolute reduction in rate of death or renal replacement therapy at 30 days
- This was driven primarily by 7-3% absolute risk reduction in all cause mortality.

24.12 CHAMPION PHOENIX—2013

QUESTION
Is congrelor better than clopidogrel in patient undergoing urgent or elective PCI.

DESIGN
- Multicenter
- Double-blind
- Randomized trial
- 11, 142 pts
- Follow-up–48 hrs
- Analysis: modified intention-to-treat
- *1° outcome:* All cause mortality; MI; ischemia—driven revise or stent thrombosis within 48 hrs post randomization.

INCLUSION
- >18 years
- PCI indicated (one of those)
  - Stable angina with diagnostic CAG within 90 days prior to randomization
  - NSTEMI with diagnostic CAG <72 hrs prior to randomization
  - STEMI

EXCLUSION
- Treatment with P2Y12 antagonist, or abciximab within 7 days prior
- Treatment with eptifibatide, tirofiban or fibrinolytic within 12 hrs prior
- HTN (SBP > 180 or DBP > 110)—inadequately controlled
- Impaired hemostasis, coagulopathy or thrombocytopenia
- Planned adm for <12 hrs post PCI
- Allergy or contraindication to cangrelor/clopidogrel
- Preg/lactation.

INTERVENTION
- Randomization in double-blind manner
  - *Congrelor:* 30 mg/kg bolus–4 mg/kg/min for ≥2 hrs or duration of procedure (whichever is longer) + placebo capsules
  - *Clopidogrel:* Placebo infusion and then clopidogrel loading dose of 600 mg or 300 mg
- Both group received
  - Aspirin 75–325 mg + clopidogrel 75mg}- during 48 hours

RESULT
- Cangrelor reduced risk of Ischemic events as compared to clopidogrel
- Cangrelor is iv, fast acting (+ ½ 2.9–5.5 mins) antiplatelet medication with reversible inhibition of P2 Y12
- Cangrelor significantly reduce risk of 1° outcomes
- There was no significant increase in risk of bleeding
- However, congrelor was associated with higher risk of dyspnea

CHAMPION-PHOENIX
CHAMPION-PCI
CHAMPION-PLATFORM
} No difference in risk of 1° outcome between patient treated with cangrelor or clopidogrel

24.13 COURAGE TRIAL

"OPTIMAL MEDICAL THERAPY WITH OR WITHOUT PCI FOR STABLE CORONARY DISEASE"

[Clinical outcomes utilizing revascularization and aggressive drug evaluation]

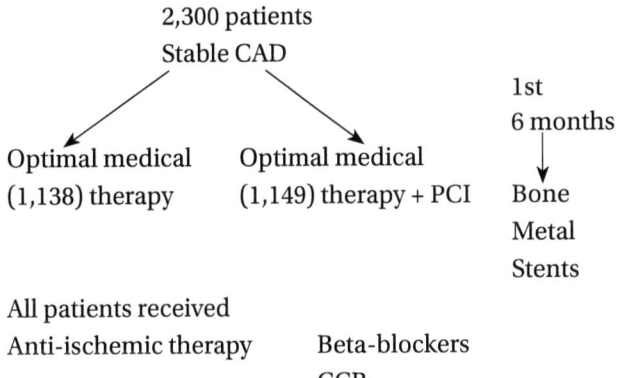

2,300 patients
Stable CAD

Optimal medical (1,138) therapy
Optimal medical (1,149) therapy + PCI

1st 6 months
Bone Metal Stents

All patients received
Anti-ischemic therapy — Beta-blockers, CCB, Nitrates
Lipid lowering therapy
Antiplatelet aspirin or/and clopidogrel
Multi-center
Open-label
RCT
Median follow-up: 4–6 years

Primary outcome: Composite of death from any cause and non-fatal MI.

Inclusion criteria
- Stable CAD
- CCS class 1, 3, 2 or 4 angina (stabilized)
- >70% stenosis in at least 1 coronary artery
- Objective Myocardial ischemia
- Substantial change in ST decreases
- T wave inversion on resting ECG
- Inducible ischemia with exercise or pharmacologic stress test 80% stenosis classic angina without provocative testing

Exclusion criteria
- Persist CCS class 2 angina
- Marked positive treadmill H
- LVEF <30%
- Refractory CHF
- Cardiogenic shock
- >50% main left disease
- Revascularization within previous 6 months
- Coronary lesions deemed unsuitable for PCI

RESULT
- No significant difference in rates of ACS hospitalization between groups
- No significant difference between two treatment strategies for primary outcome of death from any case and non-fatal MI
- Follow-up of cohorts demonstrated trial significantly more patients in PCI arr were free of angina and had high overall quality of life by 6 months, but benefit disappeared by 36 months, reflecting progression of underlying CAD.

24.14 CROSS BOSS FIRST TRIAL

TRIAL

Randomized comparison of a cross boss first vs standard wire escalation strategy for crossing coronary chronic total occlusion.

- Single-blind trial
- *Goal:* Help advance the field of CTO PCI by examining whether upfront use of cross boss catheter for antegrade CTO intervention can help improve outcomes and procedural efficiency as compared to standard guide wire techniques.

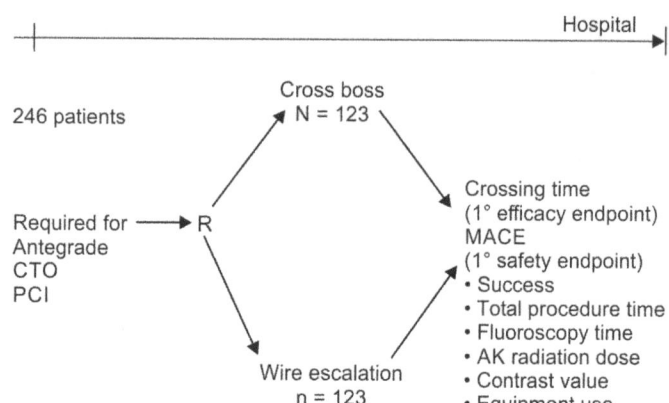

24.15 DECISION-CTO

INTRODUCTION

OMT with or without stenting for CTO

Goal: To assess safety and efficacy of CTO—PCI compared with OMT among patients with at least one CTO.

Study design: Randomized prospective trial

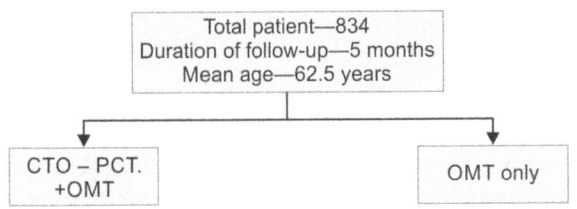

- Revascularization of all
  Significant non-LTO lesions
  Within a vessel diameter
  ≥2.5 mm
- PCI to be completed in 30 days of revascularization.

INCLUSION CRITERIA

- Silent ischemia, stable angina or ACS
- De novo CTO located in a proximal to mid epicardial coronary artery within a reference diameter of ≥2.5 mm
- CTO was defined as a coronary artery obstruction with TIMI flow grade 0 of at least 3 months duration based on patient history.

EXCLUSION CRITERIA

- CTO located in distal coronary
- Three different vessels COTs in any location
- Two proximal CTOs in separate coronary arteries
- Left main lesions/ISR/graft vessel disease
- LVEF <20%
- Severe comorbidities.

PRIMARY ENDPOINTS

Composite outcome of all cause death, MI, stroke and any revascularization for 3 years after randomization.

SECONDARY ENDPOINTS

- All death
- Angina class; quality of life; clinical outcome at 5 years
- MI; stroke; Any revascularization; CTO vessel related revascularization; hospitalization due to ACS/LVEF compromisation.

RESULT

CTO - PCT + OMT is not superior to OMT alone in reducing cardiovascular outcomes among patients with at least one CTO.

24.16 FAVOR 2 STUDIES

INTRODUCTION

Evaluated diagnostic accuracy of quantitative flow ratio, (GFR) novel angiography-based method for delivering fractional flow reserve (FFR) without pressure wire O_2 including hyperemia in diagnosing hemodynamically—significant coronary stenosis as defined by FFR

    308 patients enrolled
    Observational study
    Cohort/prospective

PRIMARY OUTCOME

Diagnostic accuracy of online QFR to determine presence or absence of hemodynamically—significant coronary artery stenosis at vessel level using binary outcomes when compared to FFR.

SECONDARY OUTCOME

In comparison to online 2D QCA, sensitivity and specificity of online QFR to determine presence or absence of hemodynamically significant coronary artery stenosis at vessel level using binary outcomes compared to FFR

Eligibility: 18 years and older
Sexes: All

    Patients—high risk
    ↓
    One or more stenosis
    ↓
    Invasive CAG

Lesions quantified by—QCA

FFR—access functional significance of identified stenosis

QFR = *Novel method* = Functional significance of coronary stenosis by calculation of pressure drop in vessel based on 2 angiographic projections

Inclusion criteria	Exclusion criteria	Angiographic exclusion criteria
• Stable and unstable angina Age > 18 years • Signed informed concert Angiographic • At least 1 stenosis discrete 30–90% by used	• MI within 72 hours • NYHA 3 • GFR < 45 mL/min • Allergy to adenosine/contrast agent • AF/AP bed	• Myocardial bridge • Ostial lesion <3 mm to aortic • Side branches of bifurcation lesions • Poor angiographic image quality • Severe overlap at stenotic segment • Severe overlap at target vesse

RESULT

- *QFR:* Sensitivity 88% US 46% P<0.01
  Specificity 88 vs 77% P<0.01
  Comparison to 2D quantitative CAG
- *QFR:* Superior sensitivity and specificity for detection of functional significant leisure in comparison with 2D quantitative CAC using FFR.

24.17 FAME 1, 2 AND 3 TRIAL

FAME-1 TRIAL

Introduction
F - FFR vs
A - Angiography for
M - Multivessel
E - Evaluation

Background
- Stenting of non-ischemic stenting has no benefit compared to medical treatment only
- Stenting of ischemic related stenting improves symptoms and outcome
- In MVD, it is difficult to identify which stenosis causes ischemia
- FFR is most accurate and selective index to indicate whether a particular stenosis is responsible for inducible ischemia
- FFR is guided PCI in patient with MVD improves outcome.

Hypothesis
FFR guided PCI in MVD is superior to current angiography guided PCI.

Design
- Randomized multicenter study
- 1000 patients
- Stenosis of >50% in at least 2 of 3 major coronary arteries.

Inclusion
- All patients with MVD
- At least 2 stenosis ≥50% in 2 or 3 major epicardial coronary artery disease, amenable for stenting.

Exclusion
- LM disease or prev CABG
- STEMI with ck >1000 U/L within last 5 days
- Extremely tortuous or calcified coronary arteries (Patients with prev PCI were not excluded).

Design

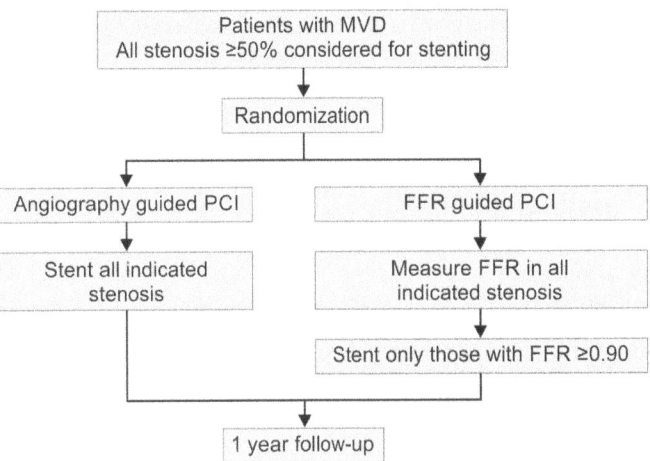

1° Endpoint
Composite of death, myocardial infarction, or repeat revascularization (MACE) at 1 year.

2° Endpoint
- Individual components of MACE @ 1 year
- Functional class
- Use of anti-anginal drugs
- Health related QOL (Euro QOL-50)
- Procedure time
- Amt of contrast agents used
- Cost of procedure.

Procedure
- Only DES were used
- FFR measured by pressure wire
- Hyperemia Induced by adenosine (140 ug/kg/min)
- Ekg, ck, ckMB, etc., during hospital stay
- Follow-up 1 month, 6 months and 1 year.

Conclusion
- Routine measurement of FFR during PCI with DES in patients with MVD (compared to angio guided PCI)
  - Reduce the rate of the composite endpoints of death, MI, re-PCI, and CABG at 1 year by ~30%
  - Reduce mortality and MI at 1 year by ~35%
  - Cost saving
  - Does not prolong procedure
  - Reduce no of stents used
  - Decreased amt of contrast agent used
  - Results in a similar, if not better, function status

- Routine measurement of FFR during DES-stenting in patients with MVD is superior to current angio-guided treatment
- It supports evolving paradigm of "functionally complete revascularization", i.e., stenting of ischemic lesions and medical treatment of nonischemic ones.

5-year Follow-up

- Confirmed long-term safety of FFR-guided PCI in patients with MVD
- Significant decrease in MACE for up to 2 years post index procedure
- From 2 to 5 years risk of both groups developed similarly (31% - CAG vs 28% FFR)
- Lower no of stented arteries in FFR guided group.

FAME-2 TRIAL

Introduction

Compare FFR guided PCI to OMT alone.

Design

- Randomized, prospective, control trial
- Non-blinded
- 888 patients
  - 441 OMT alone
  - 447 FFR guided PCI + OMT
- Mean follow-up—7 months.

1° Endpoints

Composite of all-cause mortality, non-fatal MI and unplanned hospitalization with urgent revasc.

2° Endpoints

- All-cause mortality
- Non-fatal MI
- Urgent revasc
- CV death
- Non-urgent revasc
- Function class
- Stroke
- Stent thrombosis (definite/probable).

Inclusion

- Stable CAD with at least one of the following
  - CCS angina class 1–3
  - CCS class 4 with medical stabilization for 7 days
  - ≥1 stenosis of ≥50% stenosis in ≥1 coro art with an artery diameter ≥2.5 mm with viable myocardium
- PCI candidate

Exclusion

- Age <21 years
- CABG indicated
- LM disease
- STEMI or NSTEMI in <7 days
- DAPT contraindicated
- LVEF <30%
- Severe LVH
- Extremely tortuous/calcified arteries (not amenable to FFR)
- Life expectancy <2 years
- Inability to consent.

Note: Patients with restenosis or previous stent were included.

Those with 100% could be included if recanalization was likely and if there were another significant lesion based on FFR.

Interventions

- Patients with FFR >0.8 were related with OMT alone
- OMT included
  - Aspirin
  - Selective Beta-blocker (metoprolol) +or- CCB
  - ACEI/ARB
  - Statin + Ezetimibe
  - Smoking cessation
  - Good DM control
- PCI group additionally receive
  - Clopidogrel (600 mg loading) + aspirin
  - Clopidogrel (75 mg daily) ≥1 year
- Follow-up 1 month, 6 months and annually up to 5 years
  - EuroQOL-5D tool.

Results

1° Outcomes

All-cause mortality, nonfatal MI or unplanned hospitalization with urgent revasc significantly decreased in FFR guided treatment group (12.7% vs 4.3%).

2° Outcomes

- Urgent revasc and all cause revasc significantly less in FFR group
- No significant change in all-cause mortality, non-fatal MI, CV death or angina function class.

Conclusion

- In patients with SCAD, and at least one stenosis with an FFR ≤0.8, OMT alone was associated with more than 4 fold larger MACE than FFR guided PCI + OMT

- In patients with HD non-significant FFR (>0.80), OMT alone was associated with superior clinical outcome.

Criticism
- Enrollment was prematurely closed—limiting the length of follow-up
- Non-blinded
- OMT did not included lifestyle changes (like COURAGE Trial)
- DAPT used only in FFR-PCI group.

FAME-3 TRIAL
(FFR guided PCI vs CABG)

Background
In SYNTAX trial (at 1 year follow-up)
- Cardiac deaths, MI and repeat revasc was higher in PCI arm compared to CABG
- Similar results obtained at 3 year follow-up.

Hypothesis
FFR-guided PCI using 2nd gen DES (resolute) in patients with result in similar outcomes to CABG.

Design
- Multicenter
- Prospective
- Randomized
- Non-inferiority design
- 1,500 patients from 10 sites
- 2 year enrollment and up to 5 year follow-up.

Inclusion
- Age ≥21 years
- Willing and able to provide informed, written consent
- MVD, defined as ≥50% diameter stenosis in each of 3 major epicardial vessels but not involving LMCA, and amenable to revasc by both PCI and CABG as determined by the heart team.

Exclusion
- LMCA requiring revasc
- Previous CABG
- Reg for other cardiac or non-cardiac surgery (e.g., Valve replacement)
- Cardiogenic shock and/or need for mechanical pharmacological HD support
- Recent STEMI (<5 d)
- Ongoing NSTEMI with increasing biomarkers
- Known LVEF <30%.

1° Endpoint
One year rate of death, MI, stroke and revascularization

2° Endpoint
- 3-year rate of death, MI and stroke and 5 years
- Stent thrombosis and graft occlusion
- Bleeding Compli
- Significant Arrhythmias
- Development of ARF
- Length of hospitalization
- Rehospitalization
- QOL
- Utility of function SYNTAX score.

Conclusion
FAME 3 intended to prove FFR guided PCI non inferiority to CABG.

24.18 FORMA TRIAL

INTRODUCTION

Early feasibility study of Edwards FORMA tricuspid transcatheter repair
- Multicentric, prospective
- Interventional
- Open label

PRIMARY OUTCOME MEASURE

Procedural success (Time Frame: 30 days)
  Device success and freedom from device or procedure related SAE'S at 30 days.

SECONDARY OUTCOME MEASURES

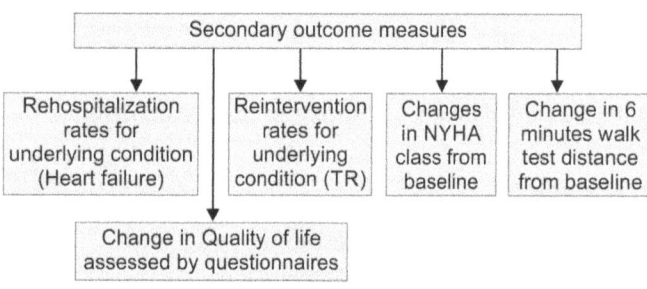

INCLUSION CRITERIA

- Clinically significant, symptomatic (NYHA 2 or greater)
- Functional class 2 or greater
- Functional or secondary tricuspid regurgitation
  - NYHA class 2 or greater or signs of persistent Rt heart failure despite optimal medial therapy
  - Determined by 1 heart team
  - Moderate to severe TR—1.6 million
  - Severe TR = under recognized/under treated condition
  - Severe functional TR—high risk
  - No death, no major complications reported
  - FORMA system is designed to value TR by occupying the regurgitant orifice area and providing a surface for the coaptation at values native leaflets
  - Device consist of foam filled polymer balloon spacer and rail that is anchored at the right ventricular apex
  - Implantation with left axillary vein access.

24.19 FOURIER

BACKGROUND

In patient with atherosclerotic disease and LDL >70 despite high or mod statin treatment, dose addition of PCSK of inhibitor evolocumab reduce major CV events compared to placebo.

DESIGN

- Multicenter
- Randomized
- Double-blinded
- Evolocumab versus placebo
- *Analysis:* Intention to treat.

INCLUSION

- Age ≥40 and ≤85
- Clinical e/o ath disease (any 1)
  - MI/non-hemorrhagic stroke/symptomatic PAO
- Major risk factor for CV events (any 1)
  - DM/age ≥65/MI or non-hemorrhagic stroke within 6 months/additional MI or non-hemorrhagic stroke/current daily smoker/H/O PAD
- Minor risk factors for CV events (any 2 if no major risk factors present)
  - H/O non-MI related coro revasc/residual CAD with stenosis ≥40% in ≥2 large vessels/most recent HDL <40 ♂ or <50 ♀/most resent hs-CRP > 2/most recent LDL ≥130 or ≥70 after 2 weeks of lipid lowering Rp/presence of metabolic cynd/most recent fasting TG ≤400.

EXCLUSION

- MI or stroke within 4 weeks
- NYHA 3 or 4 HF or LVEF <30%
- Hemorrhagic stroke
- Uncontrolled or recurrent VT
- SBP > 180 or PBP > 150
- Use of CETP inhibitor/mipomersen/lomitapide within 12 months
- Prior use of G inhibitor other than evolocumab
- Uncontrolled or inadequately treated hypo/hyperthyroid
- Sever renal or liver dysfunction
- Active malignancy
- Active infection
- Life expectancy <3 years.

INTERVENTION

Evolocumab s/c 140 mg every 2 weeks or 420 mg every month

RESULT

1°outcome—Evolocumab significantly decrease composite endpoint of CV death, MI, Stroke, hospitalization for UA and coro decade

2° outcome—It also reduced CV death; MI; stroke; and Coro revasc

- Injection site reaction was noted with use of evolocumab.

CONCLUSION

- Evolocumab reduced MACE in patient with clinical ATH disease and LDL >70 mg/dL by 15% (absolute risk reduction) at medicine follow-up of 26 months
- These was no overall or CV specific mortality benefit with evolocumab
- Other than injection—site reaction (2%) no major adverse effects noted with evolocumab (including neurocognitive effects)
- Evolocumab resulted in modest reduction in CV events without reduction in overall CV mortality.

LIMITATION

- Median follow-up of 26 months limits study its effects on CV mortality
- Very low CV mortality (≤2%) in both groups may results in under powering to detect mortality benefit.

24.20 HOPE 3 TRIAL: IMPLICATION IN INDIA

INTRODUCTION

HOPE-3: (Heart outcome prevention evaluation-3)
- Initiated in 2007
- To evaluate effect of low dose potent statin to lower LDL-C, low dose fixed combi of ARD + D and their combination to prevent major CV events in patients who are not at intermediate risk and no previous CAD
- 12,705 participants.

INCLUSION CRITERIA

- Elevated WHR
- HDL chol <39 male; <50 female
- Current or recent smoking
- Prediabetes/diet-controlled DM
- Premat CAD in 1st degree relative
- Early renal dysfunction

at least 1 of this as inclusion criteria

- Randomly assigned to 4 groups
    1. Rosuvas 10 mg + combi pill (candesartan 16 mg and HCTZ 12.5 mg)
    2. Rosuvas 10 + placebo
    3. Placebo + combi pill
    4. 2 placebo pill
- Median follow-up 5–6 years

FINDINGS

- Compared with placebo, Rosuvastatin decrease mean LDL-C level by 35 mg/dL and antihypertensive drugs lower mean SBP/DBP by 6/3 mm Hg
- 1st co-primary outcome (CV death, non-fatal stroke or non-fatal MI) occurred significantly less frequently with rosuvas than with placebo
  Absolute reductions were 0.3% - CV related death
  0.4% - MI
  0.5% - stroke
- Overall candesartan + HCTZ did not significantly lower incidence of 1st co primary endpoint. However, it lowered incidence in subgroup with highest baseline SBP (>143)
- Overall outcome with rosuvas + candesartan + HCTZ was not better than outcome with rosuvas alone
- All-cause mortality was not lowered by active Tx compared with placebo
  Neither treatment increased risk of DM
- Significantly differ from JUPITER trial.

24.21 ILUMIEN 3 TRIAL: OPTIMIZE PCI

INTRODUCTION

Optical coherence tomography (OCT) compared to Intravascular ultrasound (IVUS) and angiography to guide coronary stent implantation a multicenter randomized trial in PCI.

AIM

To demonstrate safety and efficacy of an OCT guided strategy for stent implantation

OCT sizing algorithm:

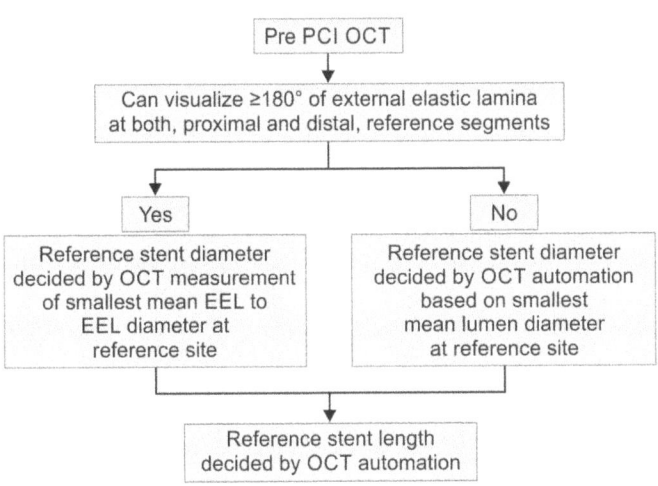

OCT stent optimization algorithm:

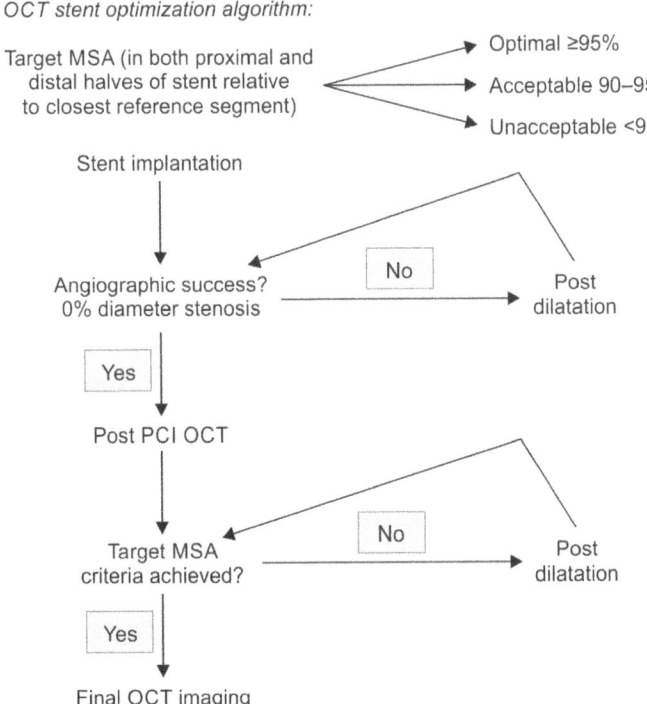

INCLUSION CRITERIA

- Age ≥18 years
- Indication for PCI (angina, stent ischemia, NSTEMI, STEMI >24 hours)
- Single vessel disease
- Reference vessel diameter ≥2–2.5 mm – ≤3.5 mm
- Target lesion length <40 mm

EXCLUSION CRITERIA

- Planned use of BMS/BVS
- Multivessel disease
- LM dimension stenosis ≥30% or LM PCI planned
- Ostial RCA/CTO/Bifurcation/ISR lesions
- CrCl <30

STUDY DESIGN

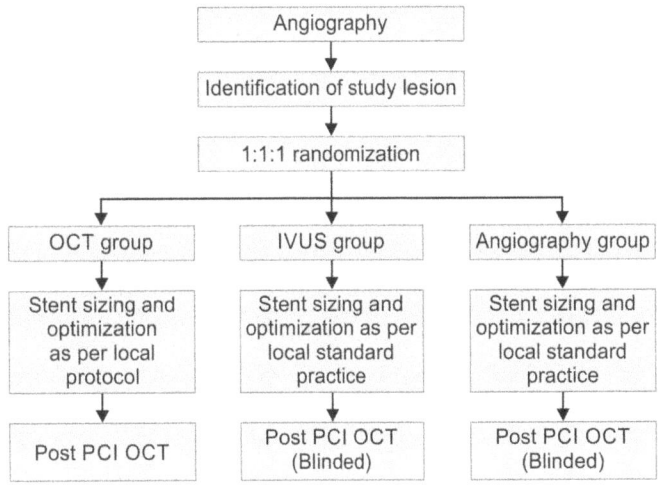

PRIMARY ENDPOINTS

Efficacy Endpoints

- Non-inferiority of OCT guided stenting to IVUS guided stenting
- Superiority of OCT guided stenting to angiography guided stenting
- Superiorly of OCT guided stenting to IVUS guided stenting.

Safety Endpoints

Procedural MACE (procedural complications—perforates dissection; thrombus, acute closure; requiring active interventions—prolonged balloon inflation, additional stent, pericardiocentesis).

SECONDARY ENDPOINTS

- Acute procedural success
- Post PCI stent expansion
- Mean stent expansion
- Intra-stent expansion
- Edge dissections
- Stent malapposition
- Intra-stent lumen area.

RESULT

- OCT guided PCI using EEL based stent optimization was non-inferior to IVUS guided PCI for achieving MSA
- OCT guided PCI resulted in superior stent expansion and procedural success compared to angiography guided PCI
- OCT guided PCI resulted in fewest untreated major dissections and areas of major stent malapposition.

LIMITATIONS

- BVS not included
- Trial was not powered for clinical outcomes.

24.22 IMPACT AF

INTRODUCTION

Multifactored intervention to improve treatment with oral anticoagulants in AF: An International cluster randomized trial

- 2 arm
- Prospective
- Internatum
- Randomized
- Controlled trial

INCLUSION PT—AF

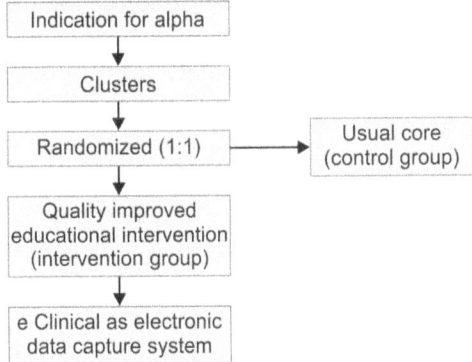

Results significant increase in proportion of patients treated with oral anticoagulants.

PROTECT AF

Left atrial appendage closure (LAAC) with watchman device was equivalent to warfarin for prevailing stroke in AF but has high rate of complication

- Randomized clinical trial
- 2:1 to LAAC or warfarin

PROJECT AF (WATCHMAN LEFT ATRIAL APPENDAGE SYSTEM FOR EMBOLIC PROTECTION IN PATIENTS WITH AF)

Patient population
Non-valvular AF at least
18 years of age
CHADS2 score of at least

- Randomized
- Parallel
- Mean EF = 57%
- F = 30%

Exclusion

- C/I to long-term warfarin therapy
- NYHA 4 HF
- Presence of repair of an ASD
- Planned ablation procedure of atrial fibrillation
- Symptomatic carotid disease
- EF <30%
- LAA thrombus

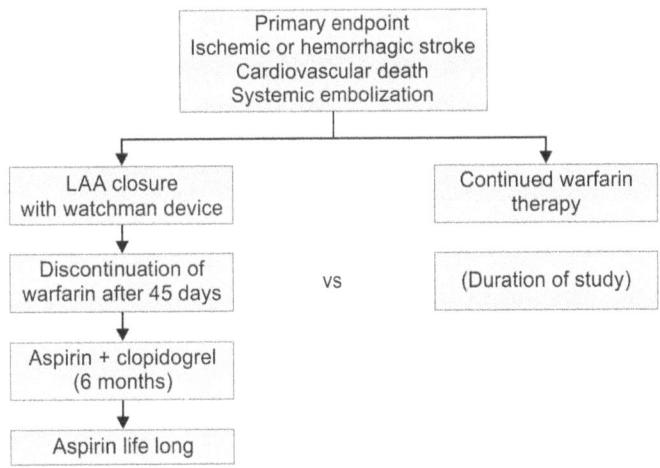

Results/Interpretation

707 patients randomized

	Device group	Control group
Primary efficacy outcome	3/100 patients	4.9/100 patients
Strokes	2.3/100 patients	3.2/100 patients

1 hemorrhagic vs 6 hemorrhagic stroke

Patients of nonvalvular AF, use of watchman device for left atrial appendage ligation in fibrillation

- Noninferior rate of cardiovascular death, stroke or systemic embolism compared to warfarin dose which was sustained to 5 years of follow-up.

Procedural (and long-term) safety of this device will need to be balanced against seductive in hemorrhagic stroke afforded from discontinuation of warfarin

- This device reduces Ischemic stroke
- Long-term follow-up needed.

24.23 FOURIER TRIAL

INTRODUCTION

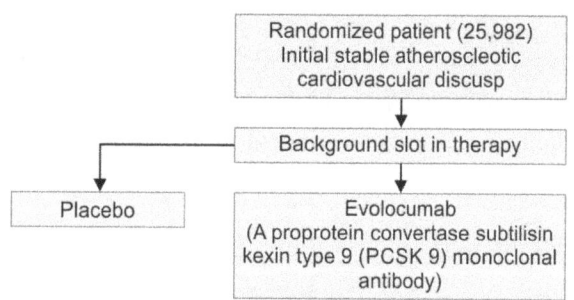

Primary efficacy endpoint
Composite of CV death
MI
Stroke
Coronary revascularization
Hospitalization for unstable angina

Key secondary endpoint
2659 subjects
in lowest LDL-C category
(<0.5 mmol/L) at 4 weeks
experiencing lowest rate for
cardiovascular death or MI

Evolocumab reduce LDL-C levels to a medium of 0.8 mmol/L and significantly reduced risk of cardiovascular event at a median follow-up of 2.2 years

1,154 patients underset formed cognitive testing prior to or on 1st day of study treatment as a part of Ebbinghaus study
No adverse effect on memory
    Executive function
    memory or
    reaction time associated
    with lower LDL-C

CONCLUSION

Very aggressive reduction of LDL-Cholesterol to ultra-low levels associated with progressively fewer cardiovascular event or appears to pose no safety concern in patient in stable atherosclerotic cardiovascular divert over 2.2 years of follow-up

24.24 SYMPLICITY HTN-3 TRIAL

INTRODUCTION

- Due to aging of population and greater trends towards, HTN is growing in prevalence
- Approx 10% of patients have renal hypertension
- Sympathetic nervous system play an important role in resistant HTN
- Catheter based renal denervation can play a role in reducing BP.

TYPE OF STUDY

Multicenter, Randomized, Prospective, single-blinded trial

Goal: To study safety and effectiveness of renal denervation in subjects with uncontrolled hypertension

Device used: Simplicity Catheter—used for RF ablation of bilateral renal denervation.

INCLUSION CRITERIA

- ≥18 years and ≤80 years
- Individual receiving stable medication regimen including full tolerated dose of B anti-HTN medication of different classes (one of them must be a diuretic)
  - No change for minimum of 2 weeks prior to screening
  - Expected to maintain without change for 6 months
- Office SBP ≥160 mm Hg based on an average of 3 BP readings.

EXCLUSION CRITERIA

- eGFR <45 mL/mm/m^2
- Ambulatory BP monitoring avg. SBP <135 mm Hg
- Type 1 DM
- Primary Pulm HTN
- Pregnant, nursing or planning to be pregnant
- Requiring chronic O2 support or mechanical ventilation other than nocturnal respi support for sleep apnea
- Main renal artery <4 mm diameter or <20 mm treatable length
- Multiple renal arteries where main renal artery is supplying <75% of kidney
- Renal artery stenosis >50% or aneurysm in either renal artery
- Prior H/O renal artery intervention.

STUDY PROTOCOL

Screening visit 1: Office BP ≥160: Full dose ≥3 anti-HTN; No med change in 2 wks and no planned change for 6 months

(2 wks)

Screening visit 2: Office BP ≥160; 24 hr ABP SBP ≥135

Renal angiogram To look for eligible subjects

1:1 Randomization

Renal denervation | Sham procedure

Follow-up visits at 1 m, 3 m, 6 m, 12–60 months

PRIMARY ENDPOINTS

- *Safety endpoints:*
  - Rate of MAE (Major Adverse Event)
    All-cause mortality, ESRD, embolic event resulting in end organ damage, renal artery or other vascular complications, hypertensive crisis through 30 days
- *Efficacy endpoints:* Comparison of office SBP change from baseline to 6 months in renal denervation arm compared with change from baseline to 6 months in control arm.

SECONDARY ENDPOINT

Change in 24 h ABPM-SBP.

RESULT

Renal denervation was safe but not associated with significant additional reduction in office or ambulatory BP.

LIMITATIONS

- Drug adherence not measured by blood level
- Biological confirmation of denervation did not occur, as there is no accepted measure.

24.25 PARTNER 1 AND 2 SURTAVI

PARTNER 1

(Placement of aortic transcatheter trial)
- Randomized prospective study
- 2 arms

PARTNER A
- High-risk Sx patients
- Society of thoracic score >10%
- Surgeon assessed risk of mortality >15%

PARTNER B
Inoperable patients (by assessment of 2 surgeons)

Aim

To determine the safety and effectiveness of the device and delivery system (transfemoral and transapical) in high-risk symptomatic patients with severe As.

Inclusion Criteria

- Aortic valve stenosis with
- AVA < 0.8 cm^2
- Gradient >40 mm Hg (mean)
  >64 mm Hg (peak)
- Survival >1 year
- NYHA class ≥2

Exclusion Criteria

- Bicuspid or non-calcific valve
- Coronary artery disease
- Aortic annulus diameter <18 or >25
- Severe MR/AR
- LVEF < 20%
- Severe renal insufficiency.

Device Used

Edwards sapien heart valve system.

Study Design

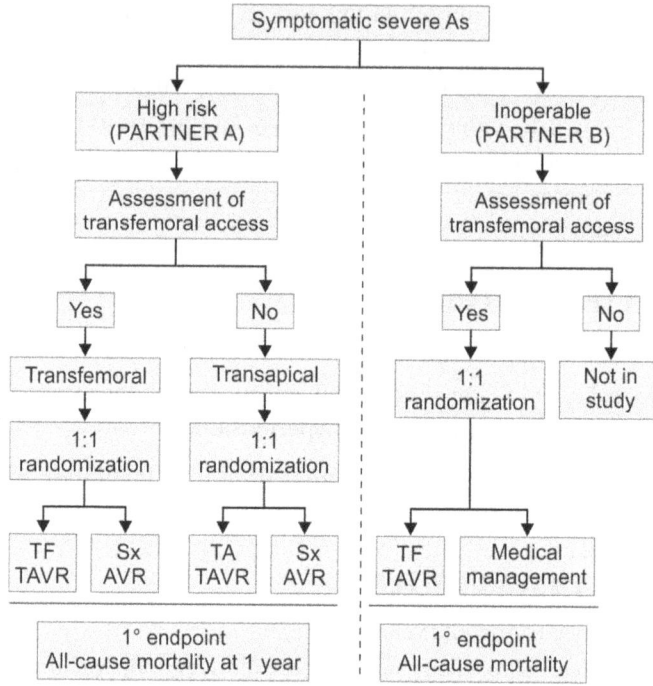

2° endpoints

- Death from cardiovascular cause
- Repeat hospitalization because of valve or procedure related deterioration
- MI/stroke/AKI
- 6 min walk distance
- Valve performance.

Results

- TAVR is non-inferior to AVR in terms of all-cause mortality at 2 year
- 2 fold higher neurologic events and major stroke after TAVR, compared to AVR both at 30 days and 1 year
  However composite endpoint of death and major stroke was similar

- 2 fold increase in major bleeding and AF post AVR (compared to TAVR)
- NYHA functional class and 6 min walk distance improvement at 30 days was more in TAVR, but at 1 year TAVR and AVR are equally effective
- Perivalvular leak post TAVR contribute to significant mortality even at 2 years.

Conclusion

Survival has been reasonably good but stroke and perivalvular leakage require further device development.

PARTNER 2 TRIAL

Aim

- To evaluate 1 year clinical and ECHO outcomes of SAPIEN-3 TAVR in *intermediate risk patients*
- To compare these intermediate risk patient outcomes using SAPIEN-3 TAVR with surgical AVR using pre-specified propensity score analysis.

Inclusion Criteria

- Severe As: AVA ≤0.8 cm² (iAVA <0.5 cm²/m²)
  - Mean AV gradient >40
  - Peak jet velocity >4 m/s
- NYHA ≥2 functional class
- Intermediate risk
  - Determined by heart team
  - STS between 4–8%
  - Adjudicated by case review committee.

Exclusion Criteria

- Bicuspid AV or predominant AR (>3+)
- Aortic annulus diameter <18 or >28
- Severe LV dysfunction (EF <20%)
- Untreated CAD/Unprotected LM disease/SYNTEX score >32
- AMI within 1 month
- CVA or TIA within 6 months
- Sr. Creat >3 mg/dL or dialysis dependent
- Hemodynamic instability
- Life expectancy <24 months.

Device Used

SAPIEN 3 heart valve

Study Design

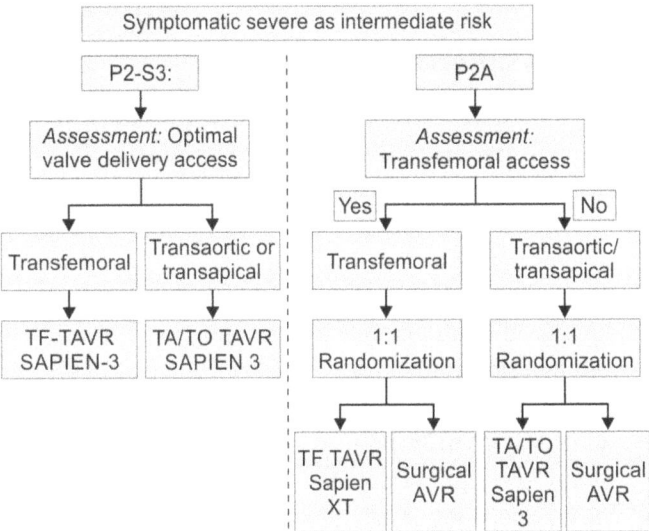

Primary Endpoint

- Composite of all-cause mortality, all stroke, ≥ moderate AR at 2 year
- Propensity score analysis.

Result

- In intermediate risk patients, SAPIEN-3 TAVR resulted in low 1 year rates of all-cause mortality (7.4%), all stroke (4.6%) and moderate or severe AR (1.5%)
- Propensity score analysis (Sapien 3 TAVR vs Sx AVR)
  - Non-inferiority for primary endpoints
  - Superiority of Sapien 3 TAVR for 1° endpoints
  - Superiority of Sx AVR for AR ≥ moderate.

SURTAVI TRIAL

Safety and efficacy study of the medtronic core valve system in the treatment of severe, symptomatic aortic stenosis in intermediate risk subjects who need AVR.

Study Design

Randomized prospective trial.

Inclusion Criteria

- Patients with severe As
  AVA ≤1 cm² or i AVA <0.6 cm²/m² and mean gradient >40 or Vmax >4 m/sec
- *Symptomatic As:* NYHA 2 or more

- Predicted risk of operative mortality ≥3% and <15% at 30 days (intermediate risk).

Exclusion Criteria

- Contraindications for placement of bioprosthetic valve
- Known hypersensitivity or contraindications to anticoagulants/antiplatelets
- Any PCI or peripheral intervention within 30 days of randomization
- Symptomatic carotid or vertebral artery disease or successful treatment of carotid stenosis within 6 weeks of randomization
- Recent CVA/TIA
- Acute MI within 30 days
- Multivessel CAD with syntax score >22
- Severe liver/lung/renal disease
- Unsuitable anatomy (annulus <18 or >29 mm)
- Severe MR or TR
- Congenital bicuspid or unicuspid valve.

Study Protocol

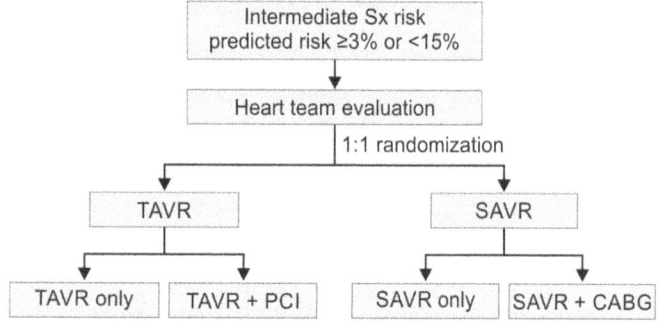

Primary Endpoint Measures

All-cause mortality or disabling stroke at 24 months.

Secondary Endpoint Measures

- *Safety*
  - All-cause mortality
  - All stroke
  - Aortic valve re-intervention
  - Major vascular complications
  - Life threatening or major bleeding
  - Pacemaker implantation
  - MACCE
- *Efficacy*
  - Effective orifice area
  - Mean gradient
  - Moderate/severe As
- Quality of life

Result

- TAVR with self-expanding core valve is noninferior to SAVR for all-cause mortality or disabling stroke at 24 months
- TAVR has significantly less 30 day stoke, AkI, AF and transfusion use
- TAVR related with superior quality of life at 30 days
- TAVR significantly improved AV hemodynamics with lower mean gradients and larger aortic valve areas than SAVR
- SAVR has less residual AR, major vascular complications, and fewer new pacemakers
- Need for new pacemaker after TAVR was not associated with increased mortality.

24.26 SENTINEL TRIAL

INTRODUCTION
Cerebral protection in transcatheter aortic valve replacement.

BACKGROUND
- Neurologic events remain a feared complication after TAVR
- Prior studies with dual filter system during TAVR showed reduction in new cerebral lesion volume.

PURPOSE
To evaluate safety and efficacy of embolic protection in reducing cerebral embolization and associated with neurological consequences during TAVR.

DEVICE USED
- Claret medical sentinel system (from RRA 6F)
- Edwards SAPIEN heart valve
- SAPIEN XT

INCLUSION CRITERIA
- Severe symptomatic AS (without AR & EF >20%)
- Compatible left common carotid artery (6.5-10 mm) and brachiocephalic artery (9-15 mm) without significant stenosis (70%) as determined by CT
- Informed consent.

EXCLUSION CRITERIA
- Right extremity vasculature not suitable
- Brachiocephalic, left carotid or aortic arch not suitable
- CVA or TIA within 6 months
- Neurological disease with persistent defects
- Carotid disease requiring treatment within 6 weeks
- Contraindications to MRI
- Renal insufficiency (CR Cl <30) or RRT
- Severe LV dysfunction (EF <20%)
- Balloon valvuloplasty (BAV) within 30 days.

STUDY DESIGN

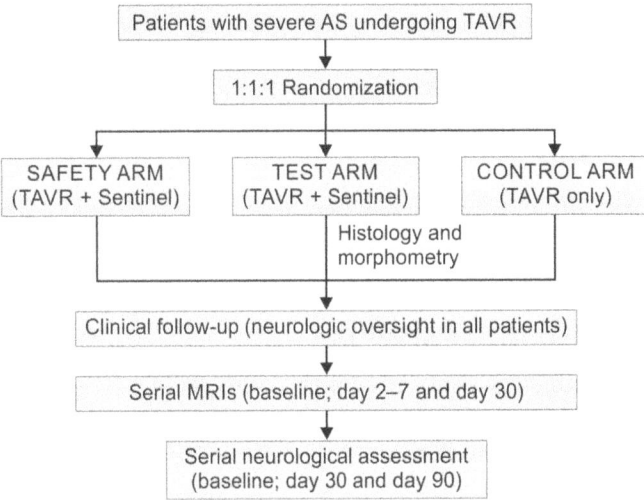

PRIMARY ENDPOINTS
- Safety (non-inferiority)
  - MACCE at 30 days
  - All-cause mortality, stroke, AKI stage 3
- Efficacy (superiority)
  - Reduction in median total new lesion volume in protected territory assessed by DW—MRI at day 2-7 post procedure

CONCLUSION
In high-risk patients undergoing TAVR, the sentinel dual filter embolic protection device was associated with
- A favorable safety profile
  - MACCE 7.3%, which was significantly below historical performance safety goal
  - Low major vascular complication (0.4%)
- Captured embolic debris in almost all patients
- Reduction in 30 days stroke from 9.1 to 5.6% (not statistically significant)
- Reduction in DW—MRI new lesion volume with embolic protection (statistically insignificant)
  - However after adjusting potential confounders, significant reduction in new lesion volume in protected territories.

24.27 PREVAIL TRIAL

INTRODUCTION
Prospective randomized evaluation of the WATCHMAN left atrial appendage closure device in patients with AF versus long-term warfarin therapy.

GOAL
To assess the safety and efficacy of LAA occlusion for stroke prevention in patients with NVAF compared with long-term warfarin therapy.

INCLUSION CRITERIA
- Paroxysmal, persistent or permanent NVAF
- Eligibility for long-term warfarin therapy
- CHAD 2 score of ≥2.

EXCLUSION CRITERIA
- Contraindication or allergy to aspirin
- H/O ASD repair or has ASD/PFO device
- Implanted mechanical valve prosthesis
- NYHA 4 class CHF
- Resting heart rate >110 bpm
- ECHO criteria for exclusion
  - LVEF <30%
  - Existing pericardial diffusion >2 mm
  - High-risk PFO
- Significant MS
- Cardiac tumor
- Complex atheroma with mobile plaque of descending aorta/arch of aorta.

PRIMARY ENDPOINTS
- 7 days procedure rate of death; ischemic stroke; systolic embolism and complication requiring major cardiovascular intervention
- Comparison of composite of stroke, systemic embolism and CV/unexplained death
- Comparison of ischemic stroke and systemic embolism occurring >7 days post randomization.

PRIMARY SAFETY ENDPOINTS
- Device embolization requiring retrieval
- Pericardial effusion requiring intervention
- Cranial bleeds and GI bleeds
- Any bleed that requires ≥2 units PRBC.

RESULTS
- Hemorrhagic stroke risk is significantly lower with the device
- All-cause stroke and all-cause mortality risk are noninferior to warfarin.

24.28 ORBITA TRIAL

[Investigational with optimal medical therapy of angioplasty in stable angina]

INTRODUCTION

- *Study type:* Interventional
- *Study design:* Randomized intervention double-blinded
- *Primary purpose:* Treatment
- *Official title:* Defining a gold standard for ischemic: Effects of interventional revascularization versus Optimum medical therapy on exercise capacity in patients with stable coronary artery disease
- *Primary outcome measures:* Exercise time on treadmill
  Time frame: 6 weeks

Enrollment: 230
Duration of follow-up: 6 weeks

Arms:
- Coronary angioplasty
- Optimum medical therapy

Placebo: Sham procedure and optimum medical therapy

6 weeks of medical optimization

All patients, invasive physiological assessment of FFR and iFR was done

Inclusion criteria	Exclusion criteria
Stable angina and at least 1 lesion with angiographic stenosis ≥70% in single vessel suitable for stent implantation	• ACS • Previous CABG • Left main stem disease • C/I to PCI

Contd...

Inclusion criteria	Exclusion criteria
	• Heavily calcified lesion (tortuous) • CTO in target vessel • Life expectancy <2 year • Pregnancy • Age <18 or >85 years • Angiographic stenosis >50% in non-target vessel • Inability to correct

PRIMARY OUTCOME

Change in exercise time from baseline for PCI vs sham was 28.4 vs 11.8 seconds.

SECONDARY OUTCOME

- Change in Seattle Angina questionnaire (SAQ)—Physical limitation from baseline
- Change in SAQ—angina frequency from baseline
- Change in Duke treadmill score from baseline

INTERPRETATION

- In patients with medically treated angina and severe coronary stenosis. PCI did not increase exercise time by more than the effect of a placebo procedure
- The efficacy of invasive procedure can be assessed with placebo control = standard for pharmacotherapy.

24.29 NOBLE TRIAL

INTRODUCTION
"Prospective randomized trial comparing biolimus-eluting stent and bypass graft surgery in selected patients with left main coronary artery disease".

AIM
PCI with drug eluting stent produce non-inferior clinical results compared with CABG in revascularization of patients with unprotected left main coronary artery stenosis.

INCLUSION CRITERIA
- Stable angina unstable angina or ACS
- Left main lesion
  - Visually assessed stenosis diameter ≥50% or FFR ≤0.80
  - Located in the ostium, mid shaft or bifurcation
- No more than three additional non-complex lesion
- Heart team determines that equivalent revascularization could be achieved with CABG or PCI.

EXCLUSION CRITERIA
- Additional non-LM lesions (complex lesions) [CTO; Bifurcation lesion requiring 2 stent techniques; calcified or tortuous vessels]
- STEMI within 24 hrs
- Being considered too high risk for CABG or PCI
- Expected survival of <1 year

PRIMARY ENDPOINT
- Composite of MACCE
  - Death from any cause
  - Non-procedural MI
  - Repeat revascularization
  - Stroke

SECONDARY ENDPOINTS
- Individual components of primary endpoints
- Definite stent thrombosis
- Symptomatic graft occlusion
- Procedural MI
- Repeat revascularization
  - Target lesion
  - Left main coronary artery target lesion
  - De novo lesion.

CONCLUSION
- PCI did not meet non-inferiority for primary endpoints of 5 year MACCE compared to CABG
- CABG was superior to PCI
- PCI resulted in higher rates of nonprocedural MI
- Repeat revascularization was higher after PCI, primarily due to de novo lesions and non LMCA target lesion revascularization
- All cause mortality was similar for PCI and CABG.

24.30 VAMPIRE 3 TRIAL

INTRODUCTION

It is randomized trial of distal filter protection during PCI of high-risk plaque:
- Randomized
- Open label
- Multi-center study.

OBJECTIVE

Selective use of distal filter protection might decrease the incidence of no-reflow phenomenon after PCI in ACS patients with attenuated plaque ≥5 mm

Inclusion criteria	Exclusion criteria
• Patients with STEMI • Non-STEMI within 2 months from symptom onset or with unstable angina for which PCI was indicated • Vessel diameter = 2.5 and 5 mm	• Cardiogenic shock/cardiac anat • HD or renal insufficiency • Left main trunk or saphenous vein graft lesion • In stent restenosis lesions • Balloon dilation necessary before IVUS innervation

IVUS Eligibility Criteria

- Attenuated plaque with a longitudinal length ≥5 mm by 40 mHz IVUS before PCI
- Attenuated plaque = defined as IVUS images with backward signal attenuation ≥180° behind plaque without dense calculation.

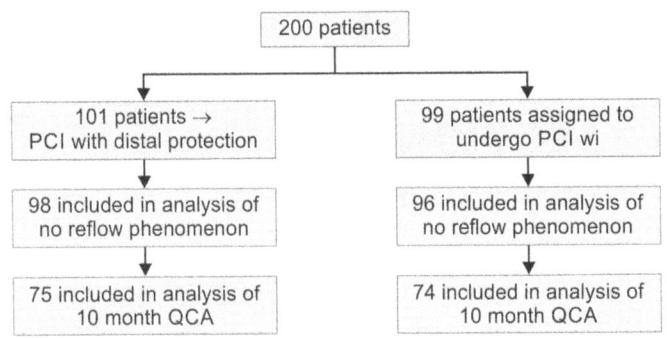

STUDY ENDPOINT

Primary—Incidence of NO reflow phenomenon during PCI.

SECONDARY ENDPOINT

- Post procedural Timi flow
- Corrected Timi frame count
- Ck or CkMB elevation 6 to 24 hours after PCI
- Rate of major adverse cardiac events occurring before discharge.

CONCLUSION

Use of distal embolic protection applied with filter device decreases incidence of NO reflow phenomenon. Fewer serious adverse cardiac events after revascularization than conventional PCI in ACS patients with attenuated plaque ≥5 mm in length.

SECTION 25: RCT versus Registries

RANDOMIZED CONTROLLED TRIAL

- Randomized controlled trials (RCTs) is defined as a study in which the participants are divided by chance into separate groups that compare the effects of a treatment or intervent.
- By random allocation of participants, it is assumed that groups will be similar and comparison is fair.

Advantages

- In all probability, RCTs make the group comparable for known and unknown prognostic factors
  - Genetic factors
  - Age
  - Sex
  - Comorbidities
  - Race
- It is to use for statistical purpose and these statistics are readily interpretable by general public.

Disadvantages

- Only selected population taken
- Artificial conditions tested, less real-life situation
- Generally investigates bard primary points like mortality, however, patients are more concerned about quality of life, rate of hospitalization
- Adverse, effects are not well studied as most RCTs are underpowered for them
- Studied for limited period, so long-term adverse effects are not studied
- Generally, more mules and a particular race is represented more, so generalization may be difficult
- Expensive.

REGISTRIES

It is an organized system that uses observational methods to collect uniform data, to evaluate specified outcomes for a population which has a particular disease, exposure or characteristic.

Advantages

- Large number of varied characteristics patients are included, so more generalizability
- Real life situation is studied and hence effect outside the experimental design is studied
- It identifies risk factors for adverse events and prognostic factors for outcome
- Particularly useful for rare diseases
- Long term effects can be studied
- Inexpensive.

Disadvantages

- Statistical significance cannot be determined
- Because of heterogeneous population, effect of confounding factors cannot be eliminated
- Disease effect changes over long term and also due to environment and lifestyle changes, so a very long-term registry will not give meaningful observations for present scenarios
- Definition and classification of disease change with time, so criteria in initial years may be different from later years
- Patients with worse outcomes may not be registered or under-repeated
- Meta-analysis of registries is difficult.

CONCLUSION

RCTs and registries, both are needed, and are complementary to each other.

Index

A

Abacavir 540
Abdominal aortic aneurysm 4
Aberrant LPA 152
Aberrant RSCA 150
AC
    chest pain, causes of 340, 441
    radiation, symptoms of 416
Academic research consortium 423
ACC/AHA 354, 429, 639
    guidelines 435
        management and lipids 505
Accelerated aging syndrome 120
ACHF, pathophysiology of 308
Acquired immunity, role of 131
ACS, emerging biomarkers of 461
Acute aortic syndromes 11, 647
Acute coronary syndrome 640
Acute perfusion contraction matching 458
Adenosine 58
Adenosine-A1 receptor antagonist 265
Adequate collaterals develop 169
Adipokines 269
Adrenal causes 360
Adrenal gland cortex 244
Adrenergic signaling system 306
Aerobic exercise training 552
Aerobic Gm neg bacilli 366
AF
    nonpharmacological management of 87
    protect 677
    vagotonic 84
AFL
    ablation of 68
    type of 62
AHA guidelines cut-off 99
AHF
    management of 311
    signs of 310
    symptoms of 310
    ultrafiltration for 313
AIDA 656
AKI 532
AL amyloidosis 140
Alagille syndrome 229
ALCAPA 169
Alcohol 121
    consumption, moderate 114
    septal ablation 126
Alport syndrome 1
Alteplase 327
AmBP, indications for 338
Ambrisentan 393
Ambulatory hypertensive patients 337

AMI 99
Amiodarone 32, 54, 126, 246
Amiodarone-iodine risk antiarrhythmic 246
Amulet study 653
Amyloidosis 122, 139
Analysis method 635
Andersen-Tawil
    former LQT 7 60
    syndrome 94
Anemia 440
Aneurysm osteoarthritis syndrome 8
Aneurysmal disease 1, 98
Aneurysm-osteoarthritis syndrome 7
Angelini classification 168
Angina
    develop with exertion 483
    pectoris, stable 483
Angiotensin receptors 267
Anistreplase 326
Ankyrin B syndrome 59
Annular ventricular tachycardia 29
Anomalies 168
Anomalous systemic venous connection 153
Anrep effect 285
ANS, role of 84
Anterograde, technique 379
Antiatherogenic action 488
Anticoagulants 86, 322, 465, 539
Anticoagulants post-MI 481
Anticoagulation 466
    activity 328
    optimal duration of 588
Antihypertensive drugs 347
Anti-inflammatory modulators 100
Antimicrobial treatment 371
Antiplatelet 463, 478
    drugs 320
    newer 322
    periop 543
Antisense oligonucleotide 511
Ao arch
    double 151
    interrupted 207
Ao PR, central 341
Aorta
    coarctation of 159
    disease of 1, 651
Aortex flow in disease, abnormality of 617
Aortic aneurysm 1
Aortic arch anomalies 150
Aortic dissection 7
Aortic intramural hematoma 11
Aortic plaque 649
Aortic pulmonary window 164
Aortic sac 166

Aortic syndrome 12
Aortic-LV tunnel 180
Aortoarteritis 12
    nonspecific 419
Aortopathy 544
AP, ablation of 66
Apixaban factor alpha A inhibitor 334
APLA syndrome 368
Apolipoprotein 515
Apoptosis, imaging for 641
AR
    cause of congenital 180
    causes of severe 180
    congenital 180
Arborization abnormally 214
Arch, left sided 150
Arrhythmia 14, 39, 94, 288, 304, 599
    ablation for 66
    autonomic modulation for 41
    detection 424
    specific 62
    susceptibility, reduced 288
    type of 33
Arrhythmogenesis, mechanism of 71
Arrhythmogenic cardiomyopathy 116
Arterial embolism 571
Arterial stenosis, clinical implication 96
Arterial system position 47
Arterio venous difference 391
Artifacts 412, 621
ARV 188
AS
    congenital 176
    natural history of 426
    supravalvular 179
    valvular 176
ASD 597
ASH/ISH HTN guidelines 354
Aspirin 320, 463
    resistance 320
Asplenia syndrome 225
Assess functional capacity 542
Asteroid 498
Asystolic arrest 18
AT, ablation of 68
Atenolol 479
Atherectomy, rotational 421
Atherogenesis, rupture and inflammation in 97
Atheroma, evolution of 105
Atherosclerosis 96, 98, 103, 104, 515
    accelerated 98, 539
    complication of 96
    molecular imaging of 641
    special cases of 98

Athletes 125
   heart 552
Atrial fibrillation 84, 126
Atrial flutter 62
Atrial tachy 62
Atrial tachyarrhythmias 68
Atrioventricular connections 243
Atrioventricular re-entrant tachycardia 34
Autonomic disorders, CV manifestation of 519
Autonomic dysregulation 521
Autonomic failure
   primary disorder of 24
   secondary 522
Autonomic modulation, device based 275
Autonomic testing 520
Autopsy cases 539
Autosomal dominant syndrome 167
Autosomal recessive syndrome 116, 117
AV
   connection 223
   junction 154
   node 38
      dysfunction 48
AV block
   features 40
   third degree 41
AV O_2 difference calculation 392
AV valve 155
   tensile apparatus of 187
AVNRT 34
   ablation for 67
AVP antagonist 292
AVRT 34
AVSD
   complete 154
   unbalanced 155
Axxess 381
Azygos vein continuation 205

B

BACT pericarditis 568
Balloon
   angioplasty, after 98
   atrial septostomy 193, 241, 594
   PTCA 422
BAMI trial 289
Baroreceptor 519
   reflex testing 47
BB, choice of 479
Behavioral determinants 350
Behcet's syndrome 2
Beraprost 193
Beta-agonist 453
Beta-blocker 10, 54, 462, 475, 478, 487
   agents, characteristics of 487
   periop 543
Beta-hemolytic streptococci 372
Beta-receptor
   action of 487
   desensitization of 255
Bicuspid aortic valve 544
Bifurcation stent system 381

Bile acid binding resins 497
Bilirubin 573
Biochemical tests 484
Biologic death, progression to 19
Biomarker 319
   newer 102
Biphasic technique 65
Bisoprolol 479
BIV repair 211
Bivalirudin 466
Bleeding risk 467
Bleeding, steps to reduce chances of 467
Blood
   pressure, determinants 350
   tests 192
Bloodstream, normal 616
Blunt injury 547
BMS vs. DES-ISR 399
Body surface mapping 47
Bonnet classification 159
Bosentan 193, 393
Bowditch 271
   effect 286
BP
   in acute CVA 339
   management of 349
   measurement of 343
   systolic intervention trial 354
Bradbury-Eggleston syndrome 24
Bradyarrhythmia 18, 30, 40, 440
Breathing 520
Bridge to recovery 258
Bridge to transplant 258
Bronchial art 213
Brugada 31
   syndrome 15, 42, 93-95
Bulboventricular foramen 223
Bundle branch 39
   re-entrant 30
Burr 421
Bypassing bottle neck 195

C

CABG
   first 395
   patch trial 274
Cachexia syndrome 262
CAD
   detection of preclinical 640
   metabolic
      alteration in 456
      management in 456
CAG 119
   guidelines for 492
   restenosis 422
Calcium
   and sodium, sarcolemma control of 270
   channel blockers 93, 347
Calmodulin
   activates 305
   stabilizing 304
Calmodulin-dependent protein kinase 270
CAMERA-MRI trial 659

Canakinumab anti-inflammatory thrombosis 655
Cancer 569
Cangrelor 322
CANTOS trial 655
CAPTAF 658
Carbonic anhydrase inhibitor 293
Carcinoid heart disease 135
Carcinoid syndrome 135
Cardiac allograft vasculopathy 317
Cardiac amyloidosis 139
Cardiac arrest 14, 19
   clinical features of 18
   management of 20
   survivors of 19
Cardiac arrhythmia 202
   diagnosis of 45
   genetics of 38, 59
   therapy of 50, 65
Cardiac biopsy 119
Cardiac cath 157, 162, 165, 170, 172, 175, 178, 179, 183, 193, 200, 208, 211, 215, 218, 221, 224, 228, 237, 241, 558
Cardiac cells 92
Cardiac chamber 221
Cardiac computed tomography 645
Cardiac CT MRI and plaque rupture 643
Cardiac cycle 431
   length, change 602
Cardiac death, prevention of 21
Cardiac destabilization syndrome 418
Cardiac device 642
Cardiac disturbance syndrome 419
Cardiac donor-exclusion criteria 315
Cardiac electrical stimulation 76
Cardiac fibrillation 75
Cardiac fibrosis 256
Cardiac glycoside 296
Cardiac hypertrophy 456
Cardiac imaging 123, 132
Cardiac mapping, direct 49, 101
Cardiac MRI 631
Cardiac myocyte 288
Cardiac myosin activator 264
Cardiac output
   in Fontan 194
   measurement of 392
   normally 391
Cardiac position and orientation 242
Cardiac remodeling 131
Cardiac sympathetic innervation, assessment of 641
Cardiac thrombus and mass 651
Cardiac transplant 275, 314
Cardiac type 227
Cardiac valvular inflammation and calcification, imaging of 642
Cardinal ion channels 89
Cardinal symptoms 272, 574
Cardiogenic shock 311, 442
Cardiomegaly 221
Cardiomyopathy 134, 116, 144, 649
   reversible 136
Cardiopulmonary dynamics 583

Cardiopulmonary exercise test 276
Cardiorenal syndrome 294, 527
    acute 527
    chronic 528
    secondary 527
Cardiotoxins 130
Cardiovascular abnormalities 539
Cardiovascular complications 525
Cardiovascular death 661
Cardiovascular disease 288
    primary prevention of 108
    risk markers of 108
Cardiovascular function and structure 301
Cardiovascular implantable device INF 362
Cardiovascular MRI 648
Cardiovascular regeneration 287
Cardiovascular therapeutics, cells used for 289
Carditis 534
Carotid artery stenting 375
Carotid plaque 649
Carotid stenting, hemodynamic effect of 376
Carpenter classification 188
Carvedilol 479
Castle AF 657
Cat's eye syndrome 225
Catecholaminergic polymorphic ventricular tachycardia 44
Catheter 412
    simplicity 679
CBA 422
CBC 555
CCB 488, 593, 462
CCFA 119
Cell 642
    therapy 287
Cellular metabolism and physiology, assessment of 638
Central sleep apnea 582
Cerebrovasc disease 344
Cervical AO arch 151
Champion phoenix 664
Chaperone heat shock protein 120
CHARGE syndrome 147
CHD
    in preg 597
    markers of 202
Chemoreflex 520
Chest pain
    approach to 340, 441
    D/D of 483
    syndrome of 250
        stable 639
Cheyne stokes respi 582
CHF 210
Chimaric natriuretic peptide 264
Cholesterol
    absorption inhibition 498, 513
    ester transfer protein inhibitor 499
Cholinergic and nitric oxide signaling 307
Chronic autonomic failure, primary 521
Circulatory regulation 470
CKD 344
Clopidogrel 321, 463, 464

CMR 119
    clinical application of 648
CoA
    asymptomatic 162
    collaterals in 161
Coagulation 259, 330
Coarctation, types of 159
Cocaethylene 526
Cocaine 525
    related MI 525
Collateral resistance, regulation of 447
Coma 23
Combined disorders 71
Compartment syndrome 427
Complex clinical syndrome 272
Conduction, ablation and modification of 68
Congestion 309
Congestive heart failure, chronic 16
Conn's syndrome 245
Connective tissue disease 569
Conotruncal anomalies 166
Constrictive pericarditis 557, 560
    mild 559
Constrictive vs restrictive 560
Contractile cell 279
Contractility, contractility of 93
Conus 166
    and truncus, septation of 166
Conventional balloon 422
Conventional risk factors 108
Core valve system (medtronic) 428
Coro art
    anomalies, congenital 168
    spasm 440
    stenosis, physiological assessment of 460
Coro AV fistula, congenital 171
Coro circ, effect on 489
Coro embolism 440
Coro endothelial dysfunction 440
Coronary aneurysm 171
Coronary artery
    disease 15, 17, 648
    in rheumatic rise 548
    revascularization 274
Coronary blood flow 444
    auto regulation 444
    control of 444
    physiology 647
Coronary calcium scoring 645
    indication for 645
Coronary collateral circulation 447
Coronary CT angio 646
Coronary CTO refractor 379
Coronary disease, stable 665
Coronary flow reserve 445, 448
Coronary lesion, types of 431
Coronary microcirculation
    regulation of 493
    structure and function of 455
Coronary perforation 378
Coronary sinus, anomalies of 153, 206
Coronary vascular resistance, determinants of 455
Coronary vasospasm 469

Courage trial 665
CPVT 32
Crocortin-2 264
Cross Boss first trial 666
CRP 99
CRS, secondary 529
CRT 282
    indication 283
Crusade bleeding risk score 467
Cryothermal ablation 66
CSA and CV disease 582
CT
    and MRI 208, 228, 559
    angio 485
    artifacts 646
CTEPH 594
CTO intervention 379
Culprit shock 663
Cushing syndrome 111, 244, 361
Cutting balloon 422
CV
    compilations 548, 549
    effect 244, 252
    manifestation 247
    metabolic disease 501
    radiation, clinical presentation of 416
    response to exercise 552
    risk 550
        stratification 343
    system 548
CV disease 247, 515, 541, 596
    adrenal and 244
    associations and risk 581
    growth hormone in 247
    hyper enhancement with MRI in 652
    mechanism 580
CVE examination 172
CVS, molecular imaging of 641
Cyanosis 210, 230
Cyanotic CHD, associated with 151
Cyanotic congenital heart disease 234
Cytoskeleton 119

D

Dabigatran 334
Dacron syndrome 158
DAD 72
DASH diet 114
DC cardioversion 65
DCMP 539
Death
    mode of 298
    short-term risk for 441
Deep vein thrombosis 583
    classification of 584
Deferred stenting 383
Delayed rectifier 94
Depression 112
Destination therapy 262
Determine visceral situs 242
Device used 679
DFT, minimum shock strength 76
Diabetic cardiomyopathy 121

Diagnostic scoring system 586
Diastolic driving pressure, concept of 455
Dietary chol, higher 501
Dietary interventions 346
Dietary supplements 114
DiGeorge syndrome 147, 149, 213
Dilated cardiomyopathy 119
    genetics of 119
Diltiazem 57, 488
Direct renin inhibitor 347
Discrepancy, reason for 322
Disease detection
    clinical decision making 639
    risk stratification 639
Dissection, type B 11
Distal coronary bed 431
    antegrade flow into 431
Distal platelet emboli 439
Distal protection devices 384
Diuretic resistance 293, 312
Dobutamine 313
    echo 623, 631
    stress 623, 638
Dofetilide 57
Dopamine 313
Doppler effect, principle of 627
DORV 181
Down syndrome 150, 154, 156, 204, 232
DPVR, determinants of 299
Dronedarone 55
Drug therapy, complication of 540
Drug-eluting balloons 380
Drug-induced torsades 28, 60
DT, criteria for 259
Duct dependent circulation 185
    diagnosis of 185
Ductus venosus, anomalies of 153
Dynamic auscultation 601
Dynamic LVOT obstruction after AMI 443
Dysautonomia 521
Dyslipidemia 515
    treatment, emerging therapies for 513
Dyslipoproteinemia 515
Dysplasia, triangle of 116
Dyspnea 230, 368
Dyssynchrony and dyssynergy, role of 299

E

Early repolarization syndrome 42
Ebstein's anomaly 187
    left sided 190
ECG 45, 116, 119, 124, 132, 134, 139, 148, 157, 161, 165, 170, 172, 174, 177, 179, 183, 192, 200, 204, 205, 208, 210, 214, 218, 221, 223, 227, 231, 240, 244, 247, 251, 555, 558, 569, 609, 631
    atrial rate 62
    gated SPECT imaging 635
    hospital recording 46
    in EO, indication and contraindication for exercise 340, 441
    parameters 64
    resting 484
    twelve lead 189
Echo 119, 134, 145, 148, 157, 162, 165, 170, 172, 174, 177, 179, 180, 183, 189, 193, 200, 204, 205, 206, 208, 210, 215, 218, 221, 224, 227, 232, 237, 240, 251, 370, 537, 555, 558, 578, 616
    for LVAD 263
    imaging, approach to 370
    limitation of 237
Echocardiographic criteria 128
Echo-Doppler assessment 263
ECMO 139
Edoxaban-engage-AF traial 335
EDS, indications for 48
Edward's classification 150
Effusive-constrictive pericarditis 559
Eisenmenger syndrome 157, 191
    chest pain 148
Elastography 415
Electrical instability, assessment of 482
EMB, condition identifiable with 385
Embolic protection devices 376
Embryogenesis 234
Endarterectomy 375
Endocardial cushion, maldevelopment of 209
Endocarditis 369
Endocardium 89
Endocrine
    disorder 247
    system 244
Endomyocardial biopsy 132, 139, 385
Endomyocardial fibrosis 136
Endothelin
    antagonist 539
    receptor antagonist 594
Endothelium in coronary tone regulation, role of 446
Enterococci 366, 372
Enterococcus 539
Enzyme
    processing 515
    receptor 515
    and processing 515
Epicardial dilatation 386
Epicardial ventricular tachycardia 64
Epicardium 89
Epoprostenol 193, 393
EPS, complication of 49
Erosion, superficial 97
Erythema marginatum 535
Esmolol, short acting iv beta-blocker 475
Estrogen's cardioprotective effect 115
Ethanol 545
    and heart 545
Exercise
    capacity, decrease 553
    physiology, basic principle of 552
    primarily stressing skeletal muscular system 552
    testing 46, 611, 612
        physiology of 611
        requirement for performing 340, 441
Exertion, greater level of 483
Exertional leg pain, D/D of 574
Extracellular matrix 300
Ezetimibe 513

F

Fabry disease 134
Familial and senile systemic amyloidosis 141
Familial thoracic Ao aneurysm syndrome 1
Fascicular ventricular tachycardia 29
Fastidious gram-negative bacilli 366
Fatal echo 597
Fats and CV disorder 501
FCI, closed 203
Fetal aortic valvuloplasty 203
Fetal echo 202
Fetal life 169
Fetal pacing 203
Fetal pulm valvuloplasty 203
Fetal-atrial septostomy 203
Fetus 210
Fever, persistence of 368
FFR 386
    noninvasive 387
    role of 386
    strategy 490
FFRCT, limitation of 389
Fibrates 498
Fibrinolysis 326, 328
    contraindication to 475
    regulation of 331
Fibrinolytic activity 329
Fibrinolytic system 331
Fibrinolytic therapy on mortality, effect of 476
Fick's oxygen method 392
Fick's principle 391
Fish oils 499
Flecainide 32
Flexstome 422
FMD 419, 578
Fondaparinux 324, 466
Fontan
    and exercise 195
    circulation 194
    complication of 197
    failing 195, 197
    successful 195
    types of 194
Forgotten HD criteria 176
FOURIER 673
    trial 678
Fractional flow reserve 448
Frailty 277, 429
Frank starling relationship 285
    role of 281
Free wall rupture 443
Fungi 366

G

Gamma, secretase activity 120
GAS pharyngitis 533
Gaucher and glycogen storage disease 134
Gemfibrozil 499

Gene
  delivery system 287
  therapy 287
Gene-based regenerative therapy, imaging of 642
Genetic lipoprotein disorder 506
  classification of 506
Genetic syndrome 199
  evaluation of 202
Genotype-phenotype 42, 60
Giant cell arthritis 548
Glycerophospholipid 515
Goldenhar's syndrome 229
Gorlin's formula 433, 435
Gp 2b/3a inhibitors 321, 465
Gram-negative bacilli and fungi 372
Great arteries 166, 223
Great vessel 375
  situs 243

H

HACEK organism 366, 372
Hand grip 602
HAS-BLED score 86
HCM
  and athlete's heart, distinguish 125
  phenotype 123
HCS syndrome, mech of 40
HD 164, 176, 205–207, 217
  consequences, determinants of 561
  related to pacing 76
  theory 159
HDL
  cholesterol 110
  non-cholesterol 510
  receptors for 515
Heart
  muscle 451
  parts of 89
  rate and force frequency relationship 286
  rate modulation 520
  sound, second 605
Heart disease 249, 550, 579, 596
  care of end stage 277
  congenital 16, 147, 647, 651
  management of 277
Heart failure 124, 253, 266, 272, 288, 355, 451
  acute 308
    and subacute 16
    decomposition in 300
  advanced 277
  apoptosis role in 255
  categorization of 272, 319
  catheter ablation 659
  diagnosis 296
  hospitalization for worsening 657
  imaging after 641
  medical rate control in 659
  pathogenesis of 266
  prime symptom of 276
  with preserved ejection fraction 298, 299
    management 290
    pathophysiology of 298

Helminths 130
Hemochromatosis 134
Hemodialysis 359
Hemodynamic 160, 169, 171, 192, 200, 210, 220, 223, 226, 230, 234, 396, 590
  assessment 480
  changes 596
  classification 480
  role of 299
  subtypes 350
Hemostasis 328
Hemostatic system 320, 328
Heparin 322, 477
  reversal 466
Hepatic function 259
Heritable arrhythmia syndrome 42, 44
Heterogeneous clinical syndrome 308
Heterotaxy syndrome 156
HF 290
  assessment of 641
  device for monitoring 318
    and managing 282
  diuretic for 293
  mechanical causes of 442
  medical management of 126
  potential new therapies for 264
  refractory 275
  stages of 272
HFPEF
  causes of 300
  clinical features of 300
Hibernating myocardium 495
  chronic 495
Hibernation 633
  and stunning 632
  short-term 495
His bundle 39
HIV 539
  disease 568
  infection, CV complications of 539
Holter monitoring 46
Homocysteine 101
HOPE 3 trial, implication in India 518, 674
Hormonal mechanism 353
HP, surgical management of 274
HTN 573
  add-on drugs for difficult 348
  and erectile dysfunction 356
  and sprint trial, management of 354
  causes of true resistant 356
  device based treatment for 342
  evidence based approach to 349
  in pregnancy 345
  resistant 356
  secondary 359
  systemic management 346
HTN-3 trial, symplicity 679
Hybrid revascularization 395
Hydration 531
Hyper perf synd 376
Hypercoagulable states 332
  classification of 332
Hyperemia 386

Hyperlipidemia
  secondary causes of 504
  type 2 506
Hyperoxia test 185
Hyperparathyroidism 249
Hypersensitive carotid sinus 30, 40
Hypertension 109, 337
  mechanism and diagnosis 350
  systolic 299
  uncontrolled 679
Hypertensive crisis 162
  management of 356, 357
Hypertensive heart disease 344
  pathogenesis of 355
Hyperthyroidism 250
  increased risk of MACE 246
Hypertonic saline 313
Hypertrophic cardiomyopathy 16, 122
Hypertrophy 254
  early stage of 254
Hypocalcemia 249
Hypoperfusion, predominant related to 310
Hypoplastic left heart syndrome 197, 199
Hypoplastic rt heart syndrome 209
Hypotension 440
Hypothesis 7, 669, 671
Hypothyroidism 251
Hypothyroid-related Hoffmann syndrome 251
Hypoxemia 453
Hypoxic spells 230

I

IA agents, class 51
IABP 396
IAS 155
IB agents, class 52
Ibutilide 50, 56, 63
ICD 76
  and HF, current role of 283
  dilemmas with 437
  troubleshooting 81
Idiopathic RCM, c/f of 139
Idiopathic ventricular tachycardia 29
Idiopathic VF 29
IE agents, class 53
iFR 389
  advantage of 389
IMH, fate of 12
Impaired coronary vasodilatation reserve 355
Implantable cardioverter-defibrillator 437
  indications for 22
  subcutaneous 424
Implantable device 275
Implantable loop recorder 46
Implantation procedure 406
Impulse conduction, disorder of 71, 73
Increased parasymp tone, disorder of 524
Increased sympathetic outflow, disorders of 524
Indicator dilution method 393
Infarct expansion 471
Infarct size, limitation of 475
Infection 98

Infective endocarditis 362, 365, 539
    factors influencing risk of 365
    prophylaxis 364
Infiltrative cardiomyopathy 139
Inflammation, biomarkers of 100
Inflammatory and infiltrative cardiomyopathies, imaging in 641
Inhibit PCSK9, strategies to 513
Injury, mode of 530
Innate immunity, role of 131
Innominate art arise 375
Inotropic agents, positive 454
Inotropic and vasodilating agent 454
Insulin 512
    resistance and DM 111
Intensive statin therapy, categories of 505
Interstitial fibrosis, imaging of 642
Intracardiac flow vortex imaging 616
Intracardiac site records 47
Intracellular LDL
    conc 515
    receptor 515
Intracoronary thermography 415
Intraluminal pressure force 493
Intravascular imaging, modalities of 415
Intravascular paleography 415
Intravascular radiation detector 415
Intravascular ultrasound 401
Intrinsic coro art anatomy, anomalies of 168
Ion channels 90, 91, 120
Ip3 receptor 72
Irreversible injury and death 458
Ischemia
    acute 255
    consequences of 459
    management of 444
    metabolic and functional consequences of 458
    vs. infarction, stress-induced 637
Ischemic cardiomyopathy 274
Ischemic heart disease 439
    stable 483
Ischemic pain 453
Ischemic postconditioning 459
Ischemic preconditioning 459, 483
Isolated atrial amyloidosis 141
Isometric exercise 602
Istaroxime 265
Ivabradine 58, 490
IVC
    anomalies of 153
    mask syndrome 242
    to LA, anomalous 206
IVS 155
IVUS
    eligibility criteria 687
    limitation of 403

J

J wave syndrome 29
Jaccoud arthritis 534
Jacobsen syndrome 176
Jones criteria 535, 536
JUPITER trial 100

K

Kawasaki disease 549
Kearns–sayre syndrome 17
Kidney damage, progression of 532
Kindwall 31
Klebsiella 539
Kugel's artery 172
Kutsche and VCM merop, morphological classification 164

L

LA appendage and closure 404
LA(A) and SGLT2 511
LAA, device therapy for 405
Lamivudine 540
Laplace's law 285
LDL
    cholesterol 110
    lipoprotein 506
LDL-C, reduction of 513
Left ventricular
    noncompaction 128
    reconstruction 274
    remodelling 253
LGE imaging 648
Lidocaine 32
Life care, end of 278
Life threatening syndrome 33
Lifestyle modification 346
Limb ischemia, acute 571
Lipid 515
    biochemistry of 515
    disorders 497
    metabolism 510
Lipid-lowering therapy 467
Lipodystrophy syndrome 120
Lipoprot(A) 101, 511
Lipoprotein 515
    disorders 506
    metabolism and transport 516
    transport system 515
Liraglutide (leader trial) 512
LMWH 323, 466
Loeffler endocarditis 135
Loeys-Dietz syndrome 1
Lone AF 84
Loop diuretics 292
Low birth weight 352
Low LDL level 498
Lown–Ganong–Levine syndrome 36
LQTS syndrome, acquired 270
Lung receive blood 214
LV
    diastolic dysfunction 539
    diastolic stiffness 299
    dysfunction, valve surgery in 274
    function, assessment of 482
    hypertrophy 123
    pacing, leadless 406, 407
    relaxation 298
    remodeling 266
        imaging of 642
    remodelling, reversibility of 257
    systolic dysfunction 539
LVAD
    adverse events with 262
    implantation, after 263
LVF in STEMI 453
LVH criteria 609
LVOT 155
    obstruction 123
Lymphoma 540

M

Macitentan 393
Macrophage express receptor 515
MADIT-CRT 283
Mahaim fibers 34, 36
Malformation syndrome 122
Malignancy 540
Malperfusion syndrome 7
Maneuvers 601
MAPCA 229
Mapping technologies 70
Marfan syndrome 1, 8
Mechanical circulation support device 258
    temporary 260
Mehran system 398
Menal function, neurohormonal alteration of 268
Menopause hormone therapy 115
Mental stress 112
Metabolic syndrome 23, 102, 109, 111, 113, 510
Metabolism, inborn error of 122
Metoprolol 479
Mexiletine 32
MI
    and healing, cellular events during 451
    criteria for 439
    pericarditis and dressler 569
    related to
        CABG 440
        stent thrombosis 440
    short term risk for 340
    without coronary atherosclerosis, causes of 468
Microvascular dilatation 386
Microvascular dysfunction 124
Miller 31
Milrinone 313, 454
Mineralocorticoid antagonist 293
Mineralocorticoid excess, syndromes of 360
Minimally invasive CABG 491
Mipomersen 511
Miracal-EF 283
Mitochondria 279
Mitochondrial disease 122
MitraClip 408, 410
    procedure 408
Mitral valve apparatus 123
MOA 51, 320, 323, 325, 326, 334, 422, 480, 487, 499
Monophasic technique 65
Morphine 462

Morris classification 164
    modified 164
MRI techniques, novel cardiac 651
MUFA 501
Müller maneuver 601
Multipolar electrodes in venous 47
Murmur
    diastolic 602
    presystolic 603
MV incompetence 169
MVA calculation 433 637
Mycobacterium 539
Myectomy, surgical 126
Myo ischemia
    assessment of 482
    evidence of 482
Myocardial blood flow 439, 440, 637
    assessment of 637
Myocardial consumption, determinants
    of 444
Myocardial injury, causes of 451, 452
Myocardial ischemia, infant develop 169
Myocardial metabolism 637
Myocardial motion, disadv of 2D imaging in
    assessing 627
Myocardial necrosis, patterns of 451
Myocardial neurosis 439
Myocardial perfusion imaging 660
Myocardial salvage index 476
Myocardial scar 647
Myocardial viability 630
Myocarditis 129
Myocardium 17
    changes 255
Myocyte
    damage, markers of 461
    structure of 279
Myocytolysis 254
Myosin, role of 280

N

Natiuretic peptide 264, 268, 319
Natriuretic peptides 319
Naxos syndrome 146
Neonatal PVR falls 169
Nephrotic syndrome 332
Neprilysin 269
Neural circulatory control 519
Neural control 493
Neural mechanism 350
Neurocardiogenic syncope, variants of 524
Neurohormonal antagonist 264
Neurohormonal mechanism 266
Neurohumoral and CNS influence, electrical
    instability related to 17
Neuromuscular disease 122
NHANES criteria 291
Nicotine acid 499
Nielsen syndrome 94
Nifedipine 488
Nile stent 382
Nitrate 462, 480, 488
    administration of 480
    tolerance 489

Nitroprusside 435
NOACs 334
    pros of 335
    reversal 335
Nodule, subcutaneous 535
Nonbacterial thrombotic endocarditis 539
Noncardiac surgery 541, 542
    imaging prior to 641
Noncatecholamine 454
Nonglycoside 454
Noninvasive testing, based on 485
Noonan syndrome 1, 159
Normal arteries, layers of 104
Norwood surgery 201
Novel agents 499
Novel risk markers 99
NSTE-ACS 461, 466
NSVT 32
Nuclear cardiology 634
Nuclear envelope 120
Nuclear imaging 629
    use of 637
Nuclear MPI 170
Nuclear testing 484
Nutrition 260, 501
Nutritionally variant streptococci 372

O

Obesity 113, 346
    induced CM-pathy 136
Obstructive sleep apnea 579
OCT, clinical application of 413
Omecamtiv mecarbil 264
Optical coherence tomography 412
Optical engine 412
Orbita trial 685
Orbital atherectomy system 421
Organs, pathophysiology of 471
Origin and course, anomalies of 168
Orthostatic hypotension 23
OSA CV disease 580
OSA, pathophysiologic consequence of 580
OT obstruction 124
Otamixaban 466
Oxacillin-resistant 372
Oxidation 304
Oxidative stress 268
Oxidatively modified LDL 515

P

PA
    absence of 152
    arising from asc Ao 152
    with intact vent septum 209
Pacemaker 76
    leadless 406
    syndrome 80, 406
        cause of 76
Paclitaxel 380
PAD
    risk factors for 573
    testing for 575

PAH approved drugs, initiate treatment
    with 593
Palliative shunts 232
Palliative surgical treatment 158, 170
Palpitation 49
    distressing syndrome of 63
Papillary muscle rupture 443
Paracrine vasoactive mediators 494
Parasympathetic activity, withdrawal of 267
Parathyroid disease 249
Paroxysmal AV block 41
Passive cardiac support device 275
PCI
    antiplatelet therapy for 478
    selection for 491
    vs. OMT 490
PCM, therapy for 121
PCSK9 inhibitors 513
PCWP error 434
PDE-5 inhibitor 539, 594
PE with hypotension, massive 586
Pediatric cardiology 436
Pediatric RAS 419
Penetrating atherosclerotic ulcer 12
Penicillin resistance 371
Percutaneous coronary angioscopy 415
Percutaneous mitral valve 408
Percutaneous therapy 275
Pericardial disease 539, 554, 565, 568, 569,
    647, 650
    specific causes of 568
Pericardial effusion 539, 561
Pericarditis 539
    acute 554
    recurrent 567
Pericardium
    cardiomyopathy 137
    in heart disease, passive role of 566
Peripheral artery disease 571, 573
Peripheral vasculature, neurohormonal
    alteration of 269
Permeability 90
Persistent ductus venosus 206
Persistent LSVC 205
PET
    and hibernating myocardium 639
    scan 630, 635
    viability 639
PET-CT 636
PGE1 185
    monitoring 185
Pharmacological stress, indication of 623
Pheochromocytoma 252
Phosphodiesterase inhibitor 454
Phospholamban inhibits SERCA 304
Physical activity 113, 346
Phytosterols 499
PJRT 34, 36
Plaque
    rupture 96, 643
    susceptibility 97
    vulnerability of 643
Platelet 329
    activation, imaging of 641
    inhibition 328

Poiseuille's law 436
Poland's syndrome 229
Polypill 112
Polysomnography 581
Polysplenia syndrome 156, 225
Postcardiac arrest care 20
Postmenopausal hormone therapy 115
Postshock arrhythmia 66
Post-STEMI, risk stratification 482
Potassium
  channel 93
  sparing 292, 293
PPI, troubleshooting 80
Prasugrel 464
Pre-excitation syndrome 35, 74
Pregnancy 596
PreHTN, pathophysio of 338
Premature atrial contractions 62
Premature ventricular complexes 31
Pressure overload hypertrophy 355
Pressure wire 386
Primitive vent 166
Prinzmetal angina 473
Procainamide 32
Proinflammatory cytokines 246
Prophylactic antiarrhythmics 480
Prophylaxis 362
Prostacyclin 539
Prostanoids 593
Prosthetic valve 599
  infection 642
Protease-activated receptor-1 antagonist 465
Protein 279
Prothrombin 330
Protozoa 130
Provocative test 473
Prox tubule 292, 511
Pseudoaneurysm 443
PUFA 501
Pulm art
  anomalies of 152
  distribution, multiple source 214
  HTN, signs and symptoms of 591
Pulm AV fistula, congenital 217
Pulm HTN, primary 539
Pulmonary arterial HTN 591
Pulmonary atresia 213
Pulmonary diseases 579
Pulmonary embolism 583
  classification of 584
  severity index criteria 586
Pulmonary function 259
Pulmonary hypertension 589, 598
Pulmonary vasculature in Fontan 195
Pulselessness 578
Pumps 270
Pure autonomic failure 24
PV disease, pathogenesis of 204

Q

Q waves, D/D of 610
QRS tachy in AP, wide 36
QT syndrome
  long 59
  short 59, 60

R

RA abnormality 609
RAAS, activation of 267
Radiation
  effect of 416
  exposure, assessment of 416
  hazards 416
Radical hypothesis 632
Radionucleotide ventriculography 629
Raghib's complex 205
Ranolazine 58, 462, 489
RAPS inhibitors 479
RAS, causes of 418
Rastelli classification 156
Rayment model 280
RCM, approach to 139
RCTs of ICD 283
Refractory period, prolongs 288
Regional dysfunction 117
Relapsing 567
Relative penicillin resistance 371
Relax cycle 304
Renal angioplasty 418
Renal artery stenosis 418
  clinical clues for 418
Renal denervation 419
  effectiveness of 679
  used for RF ablation of bilateral 679
Renal disease 568
  acute 359
  and CV illness 530
  chronic 359
Renal dysfunction 466
Renal insufficiency 290
Renal mechanism 352
Renal parenchymal disease 359
Renal stenting and denervation 418
Renal transplant 359
Renal vein sampling 361
Rendu-Osler-Weber syndrome 217
Renin secreting tumor 360
Renocardiac syndrome
  acute 527
  chronic 527, 528
Renocardial CRS, acute 528
Renoprotective agents 265
Renovascular HTN 359
  causes of 359
Reperfusion arrhythmias 476
Reperfusion injury 474, 476
  increase 474
  mediators of 474
  protection against 476
Repetitive ischemia, consequences of 459
Repolarization abnormality 117
Resistance exercise 552
Respiration
  failure 440
  normal 601

Restenosis after PCI 98
Restenosis cutting balloon trial 422
Restless leg syndrome 456
Restrictive cardiomegaly 560
Restrictive cardiomyopathy 139
Reteplase 327
Retrograde, technique 379
Revascularization 490
  guidelines for 492
Reversible posterior leukoencephalopathy syndrome 357
RF ablation 64
  for VT 69
Rheumatic disease 548
Rheumatic factor 533
Right aortic arch 151
Rivaroxaban 334
RNA binding 120
Rolofylline 265
Rubella syndrome 176, 179
Rupture 3
  of IVS 443
  triggers 643
RV
  function 259
  inlet portion of 187
RVH criteria 610
RVMI 442

S

S2
  abnormal splitting of 605
  characteristics of 605
SA
  nodal arrhythmias, ablation of 68
  node 38
SACT 48
Salt leading suppression test 361
Salt wasting syndrome 350
SAPIEN-3 428
Sarcoid cardiomyopathy 142
Sarcoidosis 139
Sarcomere 119
Sarcopenia 277
Sarcoplasmic reticula 120
Saturated fatty acid 501
Saturn 498
Scavenger lipoprotein receptor 515
Segmental artery pulm circ 213
Semaglutide 512
Semi lunar valves 166
Senile syst amyloidosis 141
Sentinel trial 683
Serelaxin 264
SGLT 2 inhibitor 511
Shock trial 274
S-ICD, implementation of 424
Sick sinus syndrome 40, 42, 150
Sildenafil 193, 393
Single ventricle 222
Sinus
  node, dysfunction 48
  tachy 62
  venosus, anomalies of valves of 153

Sinus of Valsalva 219
    aneurysm of 219
SLE like syndrome 52
Sleep apnea 579
SLV, formation of 166
Smoking 108
SNRT 48
Sodium channel 92
Solid state system 401
Soluble guanylyl cyclase stimulator 594
Sotalol 56
Speckle tracking 618
SPECT
    high speed 634
    imaging falsely interpreted as defect 635
    tracers and protocol 634
SPECT-CT 636
Spinal cord stimulation 490
Spironolactone 296
Split, abnormal 605
Staircase
    negative 93
    positive 93
Staphylococcal species 366
Staphylococci 372
Statin 497
    controversy with 108
    in particular population, use of 498
    intolerance 502
        increasing risk of 502
        management of 502
Stavudine 540
Stem cell
    classification of 288
    delivery 289
    therapy 288
STEMI
    anticoagulant therapy 477
    clinical features 439
    management 475
    pathology 439
    pathophysiology of 439, 470
Stenosis 623
    pressure flow relationship 460
    severity 460
Stent 98, 375, 376
    bifurcation 381
    drawbacks of cover 378
    restenosis 398
    thrombosis 328, 423
        prevention of 423
    used 381
Stimulate cardiac electrical activity 47
Stimuli repetitive stimuli 93
Stokes-Adams syndrome 41
Strain imaging 618
Streptococcal
    pharyngitis 533
    skin infection 534
    species 365
Streptococci 371
Streptococcus gallolyticus 371
Streptokinase 326

Stress
    cardiomyopathy 145
    copin 264
    echo over nuclear stress 624
    perfusion 637
    pharmacological 637
    under 445
Stress test 609
    contraindications to 612
    noninvasive 484
    post MI 615
Stroke 373, 661, 673
Stunned myocardium 495
Stunning 632
Subclavian steal syndrome 160
Subendocardial ischemia 458
    onset of 445
Subendocardium 445
Subepicardium 445
Sudden cardiac death 14, 21
    causes of 15
    prevention of 126
Sudden death 125
    syndrome 93
Sudden infant death syndrome 14, 17, 92, 93
Supravalvular aortic stenosis 178
Surgical palliative procedure,
        second stage 224
SURTAVI 429, 681
SVC
    abnormality of 153
    syndrome 8
Sydenham chorea 533, 535
Sympathetic nervous system,
        activation of 266
Syncope
    and hypotension 23
    causes of 23
    management of 26
    unexplained 48
Systolic wall stress 285

T

Tachyarrhythmias, pathophysiologic
        mechanisms of 18
Tachy-Brady syndrome 40
Tachycardia 48, 144, 440
Tacrolimus 122
Tadalafil 193, 393
Takayasu's arteritis 548
Takotsubo cardiomyopathy 145
Tamponade 10, 561, 563
    signs of 563
Taussig-Bing 182
TAVI, valve-in-valve 430
TAVR for AR 430
Tenecteplase 327
Terminal purkinje fibers 39
Terminating TMT, indication for 612
Termination, anomalies of 168
Tetralogy of Fallot 229
TG, reduction of 514
Thiazide diuretic 292, 293

Thienopyridines 321
Thin cap fibro atheroma 413
Thin filament 280
Three-D
    CT 426
    echo 621, 622
    MR 426
    TEE 426
Thrombin inhibitor, direct 466
Thromboangiitis obliterans 578
Thromboembolism 87
Thrombolysis, cath based 572
Thrombosis 97, 328
    complications 96
    threshold 332
Thrombus in situs 571
Thyroid 249
    function 246
Thyroiditis mediated 246
Ticagrelor 321, 464
Tilt table test 47
TIMI
    grading 431
    myocardial blush grade 431
Timothy syndrome 59, 60, 93
Tissue
    characterization of wall 117
    Doppler imaging 627
    engineered valve 428
Titin in contraction, role of 280
TMT in AS 614
Torsades de pointer 28
Transcatheter therapy
    addressing
        chordae 410
        leaflet 409
        MV annulus 409
        papillary muscle and LV 410
    for MR 408, 409
Transcutaneous MV replacement 410
Transfatty acid 501
Transient arterial occlusion 602
Transient CP 559
Transmural penetrating arteries 493
Transmural variability, concept of 455
Transplanted heart, physiology of 314
Traumatic heart disease 547
Treadmill specific 614
Treppe effect 286
Treppe phenomena 271
Treprostinil 193, 393
Tricuspid atresia 234
Triggered activity 71
Triglyceride 111
Troponin release, mechanism of 461
Truncus 166
    arteriosus 147
        hemodynamics 148
Tryton SV stent 381
Tuberculosis 568
Turner syndrome 159, 176
TV leaflet 187
Two-D echo 597

U

Ularitide 264
Unstable atherosclerotic plague, imaging of 641
Urocortin-2 264
Urodilatin 264
Urokinase 327

V

Vaccines 538
VAD, monitoring of 262
Valsalva 601
Valve
    area calculation 433
    right-sided 373
    second generation 428
Valvular heart disease 16, 598, 651
Valvular morphology 646
Vampire 3 trial 687
Vascular biology 103
Vascular causes 574
Vascular endothelium 328
Vascular heart disease 544
Vascular mechanism 352
Vascular resistance 436
Vascular ring 150
Vascular steal syndrome 23
Vascular stiffness 299
Vasoconstrictors 269
Vasodilating agents 264
Vasodilation, pharmacological 469

Vasodilators 269
Vasopressin antagonists 293
Vaughan Williams classification 50
Velocardiofacial syndrome 167, 229
Vent dilatation 471
Vent function, assessment of 639
Vent hypertrophy 17
Vent recovery, measure of 609
Vent remodeling 470
Vent torsion 619
Ventricle 169
    in fontan 195
Ventricular dyssynchrony 282
Ventricular function 637
Ventricular hypertrophy 16
Ventricular looping 243
Ventricular morphology 646
Ventricular pattern 222
Ventricular premature contraction 31
Ventricular tachycardia 29, 31
    bidirectional 29
    outflow tract 29
    storm 33
Ventriculoarterial connection 243
Ventriculoarterial impedance 551
Verapamil 57
Viability, hibernation and stunning 630
Viable dysfunctional myocardium 496
Viral infection 130
Viral pericarditis 568
Viridans group 371
Virus 129
Vitamin D 249, 550
    deficiency, risk factors for 550

Vorapaxar 322, 465
VSD 213
    doubly committed 182
    subaortic 182
    subpulmonic 182
    to arterial relationship 181
    type of 181
VT
    caused by nonreentrant mech 75
    drugs for 32
    storm 33
    treatment of 32
    with decreased EI 32
    with normal EF 32
VT/VF
    electrical therapy for 79
    in ICD, detection of 78
Vulnerable plaque 643

W

Wall stress 285
    measurement of 285
Warfarin 325
Wavelengths, function of 415
Weight loss 113
William syndrome 179
William-Beuren syndrome 159
Wound healing 97

Z

Zidovudine 540

EU GSPR Authorised Reprsentative
Logos Europe, 9 rue Nicolas Poussin
1700, La Rochelle, France
Phone: +33 (0) 6 67 93 73 78
E-mail: contact@logoseurope.eu